NURSE'S REFERENCE LIBRARY®

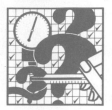

Signs & Symptoms

Nursing86 Books™
Springhouse Corporation
Springhouse, Pennsylvania

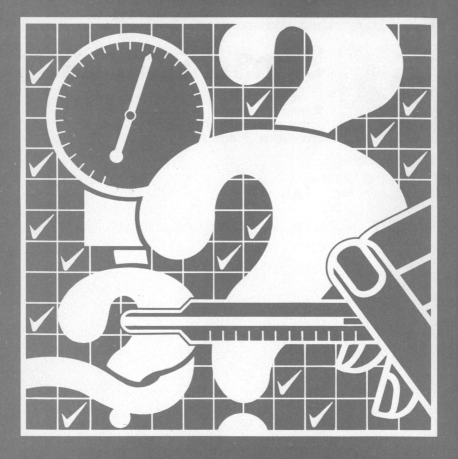

NURSE'S REFERENCE LIBRARY®

Signs & Symptoms

Nursing86 Books™
Springhouse Corporation
Springhouse, Pennsylvania

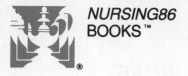

NURSING86
BOOKS ™

Springhouse Corporation Book Division

CHAIRMAN
Eugene W. Jackson

PRESIDENT
Daniel L. Cheney

VICE-PRESIDENT AND DIRECTOR
Timothy B. King

VICE-PRESIDENT, BOOK OPERATIONS
Thomas A. Temple

VICE-PRESIDENT, PRODUCTION AND PURCHASING
Bacil Guiley

PROGRAM DIRECTOR, REFERENCE BOOKS
Stanley E. Loeb

© 1986 by Springhouse Corporation, 1111 Bethlehem Pike, Springhouse, Pa. 19477

Printed in the United States of America.

NRL9-011285

Library of Congress Cataloging in Publication Data
Main entry under title:

Signs & Symptoms.

   (Nurse's reference library)
   "Nursing86 books."
   Bibliography: p.
   Includes index.
   1. Diagnosis.   2. Nursing.   3. Symptomatology.
   I. Springhouse Corporation.   II. Series.
[DNLM: 1. Diagnosis—nurses' instruction.
2. Nursing Process—methods.   WB 143 S5784]
RT48.S555   1986   616.07'5   85-17353
ISBN 0-916730-96-4

NURSE'S REFERENCE LIBRARY®

Staff for this volume

EXECUTIVE EDITOR
Matthew Cahill

CLINICAL DIRECTOR
Minnie Bowen Rose, RN, BSN, MEd

ART DIRECTOR
Sonja E. Douglas

Editorial Manager: Jill Lasker

Clinical Editors: Joanne Patzek DaCunha, RN; Donna L. Hilton, RN, CCRN, CEN

Contributing Clinical Editors: Margaret L. Belcher, RN, BSN; Marren Cummings Berthold, RN; Mary Chapman Gyetvan, RN, BSEd; Sandra Ludwig-Nettina, RN, BSN: Maryann Mackell, RN, BSN; Paulette Schank, RN, CCRN, CEN; Nina Poorman Welsh, RN

Text Editors: H. Nancy Holmes, Patricia Minard Shinehouse

Associate Editors: Kevin J. Law, Elizabeth L. Mauro, June Norris

Contributing Editors: Andrea F. Barrett, June Gomez, Barbara Hodgson, Roberta Kangilaski, Diana Odell Potter, Nancy J. Priff, Rebecca S. Van Dine

Drug Information Manager: Larry Neil Gever, PharmD

Copy Supervisor: David R. Moreau

Copy Editors: Traci A. Deraco, Diane M. Labus, Doris Weinstock

Contributing Copy Editors: Andrew Goodwin, JoAnn Learman, Amy S. Norwitz, Donna Lynne Rondolone

Production Coordinator: Sally Johnson

Senior Designer: Matie Anne Patterson

Designers: Jacalyn Bove, Maryanne Buschini, Carol Cameron-Sears, Lynn Foulk, Linda Franklin, Christopher Laird

Illustrators: Michael Adams, Dimitrios Bastos, David Christiana, John Cymerman, Design Management, Marie Garafano, Jean Gardner, Peter Gerritsen, Ira Alan Grunther, Robert Jackson, Mark Mancini, Robert Phillips, Kathleen Pierson, George Retsick, Melodye Rosales, Dennis Schofield

Art Production Manager: Robert Perry

Art Assistants: Suzanne Centola, Donald Knauss, Sandra Sanders, Louise Stamper, Joan Walsh, Bob Wieder

Typography Manager: David C. Kosten

Typography Assistants: Elizabeth DiCicco, Amanda C. Erb, Ethel Halle, Diane Paluba, Nancy Wirs

Senior Production Manager: Deborah C. Meiris

Production Manager: Wilbur D. Davidson

Production Assistant: Tim A. Landis

Assistants: Maree E. DeRosa, Marlene C. Rosensweig

Special thanks to Susan Hatch Brunt; Bernadette M. Glenn; Loralee Choman Moclock; Diane Schweisguth, RN, BSN; and Caroline M. Swider; who assisted in the preparation of this volume.

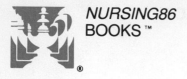

NURSING86
BOOKS ™

NURSE'S REFERENCE LIBRARY®

This volume is part of a series conceived by the publishers of *Nursing86®* magazine and written by hundreds of nursing and medical specialists. This series, the NURSE'S REFERENCE LIBRARY, is the most comprehensive reference set ever created exclusively for the nursing profession. Each volume brings together the most up-to-date clinical information and related nursing practice. Each volume informs, explains, alerts, guides, educates. Taken together, the NURSE'S REFERENCE LIBRARY provides today's nurse with the knowledge and the skills that she needs to be effective in her daily practice and to advance in her career.

Other volumes in the series:

Diseases	Drugs	Procedures	Practices
Diagnostics	Assessment	Definitions	Emergencies

Other publications:

NEW NURSING SKILLBOOK™ SERIES
Giving Emergency Care Competently
Monitoring Fluid and Electrolytes Precisely
Assessing Vital Functions Accurately
Coping with Neurologic Problems Proficiently
Reading EKGs Correctly

Combatting Cardiovascular Diseases Skillfully
Nursing Critically Ill Patients Confidently
Dealing with Death and Dying
Managing Diabetes Properly
Giving Cardiovascular Drugs Safely

NURSING PHOTOBOOK™ SERIES
Providing Respiratory Care
Managing I.V. Therapy
Dealing with Emergencies
Giving Medications
Assessing Your Patients
Using Monitors
Providing Early Mobility
Giving Cardiac Care
Performing GI Procedures
Implementing Urologic Procedures

Controlling Infection
Ensuring Intensive Care
Coping with Neurologic Disorders
Caring for Surgical Patients
Working with Orthopedic Patients
Nursing Pediatric Patients
Helping Geriatric Patients
Attending Ob/Gyn Patients
Aiding Ambulatory Patients
Carrying Out Special Procedures

NURSING NOW™ SERIES
Shock
Hypertension
Drug Interactions

Cardiac Crises
Respiratory Emergencies
Pain

NURSE'S CLINICAL LIBRARY™
Cardiovascular Disorders
Respiratory Disorders
Endocrine Disorders
Neurologic Disorders

Renal and Urologic Disorders
Gastrointestinal Disorders
Neoplastic Disorders
Immune Disorders

Nursing86 DRUG HANDBOOK™

MediQuik Cards™

CLINICAL POCKET MANUAL™ SERIES
Diagnostic Tests
Emergency Care
Fluids and Electrolytes
Signs and Symptoms

Cardiovascular Care
Respiratory Care
Critical Care
Neurologic Care

NURSE REVIEW™ SERIES
Cardiac Problems

Respiratory Problems

Contents

Appendices and Index

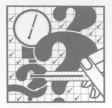

Advisory Board

At the time of publication, the advisors, clinical consultants, and contributors held the following positions.

Clinical Consultants

Jeannette E. Anders, RN, Nurse Clinician, Department of Dermatology, Columbia–Presbyterian Medical Center, New York

John M. Bertoni, MD, PhD, Associate Professor of Neurology, Thomas Jefferson University, Philadelphia

Laura P. Borden, RN, BSN, Child Life Coordinator, East Tennessee Children's Hospital, Knoxville

Heather Boyd-Monk, RN, SRN, BSN, Assistant Director of Nursing for Education Programs, Wills Eye Hospital, Philadelphia

Barbara Gross Braverman, RN, MSN, CS, Psychiatric Clinical Nurse Specialist, Medical College of Pennsylvania, Philadelphia

George J. Brodmerkel, Jr., MD, Head, Division of Gastroenterology, Allegheny General Hospital, Pittsburgh

Mimi Callanan, RN, MSN, CNRN, Epilepsy Clinical Specialist, Graduate Hospital, Philadelphia

James M. Cerletty, MD, Associate Professor of Medicine, Medical College of Wisconsin, Milwaukee

Joanne K. Condi, RN, MN, CNRN, Assistant Administrator, Neuroscience Division, Shadyside Hospital, Pittsburgh; President, Neurolore, Inc., Pittsburgh

Jean A. Cross, RN, BSN, CCRN, Head Nurse, Coronary Intensive Care, Cleveland Clinic Foundation

Elise C. Deutsch, MD, Instructor, Department of Otolaryngology–Head and Neck Surgery, University of Illinois, Chicago

Brian B. Doyle, MD, Clinical Professor of Psychiatry and Family and Community Medicine, Georgetown University School of Medicine, Washington, D.C.

Thaddeus P. Dryja, MD, Assistant Professor of Ophthalmology, Harvard Medical School–Massachusetts Eye and Ear Infirmary, Boston

Laura Johnson Farling, RN, CNRN, CCRN, Clinical Instructor, Neurosurgical ICU, Cleveland Clinic Foundation

Mary T. Folkerth, RN, MSN, Assistant Professor, Pediatrics, Department of Nursing, College of Allied Health Professions, Temple University, Philadelphia

Cindy Frisbie, RN, BA, Pediatric Neurosurgery Clinician, Children's Memorial Hospital, Chicago

William J. Fulkerson, MD, Assistant Professor of Medicine, Duke University School of Medicine, Durham, N.C.

Susan Gauthier, RN, MSN, Assistant Professor, Department of Nursing, College of Allied Health Professions, Temple University, Philadelphia

Leon I. Gilner, MD, Assistant Professor of Neurosurgery, Medical College of Pennsylvania, Philadelphia

Sandra K. Crabtree Goodnough, RN, MSN, Pulmonary Clinical Nurse Specialist, Hermann Hospital, Houston; Assistant Professor, School of Nursing, University of Texas Health Science Center at Houston

Donna H. Groh, RN, MSN, Assistant Director of Nursing, Children's Hospital of Los Angeles

A. Hadi Hakki, MD, FRCS, Assistant Professor of Surgery, Hahnemann University Hospital, Philadelphia; Associate Attending Surgeon, Bryn Mawr (Pa.) Hospital

Barbara S. Henzel, RN, BSN, Nurse, Gastrointestinal Department, Hospital of the University of Pennsylvania, Philadelphia

Denise A. Hess, RN, BS, Supervisor, Cardiac and Nuclear Exercise Labs, Hospital of the University of Pennsylvania, Philadelphia

Mark P. Jacobson, DO, Assistant Professor, Department of Pediatrics, University of Medicine and Dentistry of New Jersey, Camden

Sheila Scannell Jenkins, RN, MSN, Milford, Conn.

Joan P. Jones, RN, MS, Coordinator, Maternal/Newborn Services, St. Luke's Episcopal Hospital, Houston

Lynn Joseph, RN, Head Nurse, Neurology Unit, Ottawa Civic Hospital

Kathy Keuch, RN, MSN, Educational Coordinator, Parent Child Health, Alexandria (Va.) Hospital

Robert L. Klaus, MD, Acting Chief, Urology Division, Department of Surgery, Albert Einstein Medical Center, Philadelphia

Peter G. Lavine, MD, Director, Coronary Care Unit, Crozer-Chester Medical Center, Chester, Pa.

Gary Lees, RN, BSN, Nurse Clinician, Philadelphia Child Guidance Clinic

June Levine, RN, MSN, Assistant Director of Nursing, Children's Hospital of Los Angeles

Herbert A. Luscombe, MD, Professor and Chairman, Department of Dermatology, Jefferson Medical College, Thomas Jefferson University, Philadelphia

Neil R. MacIntyre, MD, Assistant Professor of Medicine, Duke University Medical Center, Durham, N.C.

Thomas E. Mackell, MD, FAAOS, Active Staff, Department of Orthopedic Surgery, Doylestown (Pa.) Hospital

Margaret E. Miller, RN, MSN, Head and Neck Nurse Coordinator, Illinois Masonic Medical Center, Chicago

Roger M. Morrell, MD, PhD, FACP, Diplomate, American Board of Psychiatry and Neurology; Professor, Neurology and Immunology, Wayne State University School of Medicine, Detroit; Chief, Neurology Service, Veteran's Administration Medical Center, Allen Park, Mich.

Dennis G. Ross, RN, MSN, MAE, CNOR, Associate Professor of Nursing, Castleton (Vt.) State College

Gizell Maria Rossetti, MD, Staff Neurologist, Nicolet Clinic, Neenah, Wis.

Grannum R. Sant, MD, Assistant Professor of Urology, Tufts University School of Medicine, Boston

Edith W. Schmidt, MEd, CCC, Director, Speech/Language Pathology, Magee Rehabilitation Hospital, Philadelphia

Harrison J. Schull, Jr., MD, FACP, Assistant Clinical Professor of Medicine (GI), Vanderbilt University, Nashville, Tenn.

Eric Zachary Silfen, MD, Staff Physician, Montgomery General Hospital, Olney, Md.; Attending Physician, Departments of Internal Medicine and Emergency Medicine, Georgetown University Hospital, Washington, D.C.

Barbara Lee Barrat Solomon, RN, MS, CCNS, Clinical Nurse Specialist, National Institutes of Health, Bethesda, Md.

Michael I. Sorkin, MD, Associate Professor of Medicine, University of Pittsburgh

Arlene B. Strong, RN, MN, ANP, Cardiac Clinical Specialist and Adult Nurse Practitioner, Anticoagulation Clinic, Veterans Administration Medical Center, Portland, Ore.

Lawrence L. Tretbar, MD, Professor, Clinical Surgery, University of Missouri–Kansas City School of Medicine

Richard W. Tureck, MD, Assistant Professor of Obstetrics and Gynecology, Hospital of the University of Pennsylvania, Philadelphia

Susan A. VanDeVelde-Coke, RN, MA, MBA, Director of Nursing, General Hospital, Health Sciences Centre, Winnipeg, Manitoba

D. Vidyasagar, MBBS, Professor of Pediatrics and Director of Neonatology, University of Illinois College of Medicine, Chicago

Connie A. Walleck, RN, MS, CNRN, Clinical Nurse Supervisor/Clinical Nurse Specialist, Neurotrauma Center, Maryland Institute of Emergency Medical Services Systems, Baltimore

Bertha Warren, MSN, Pulmonary Nurse Specialist, Veterans Administration Medical Center, Sepulveda, Calif.

John K. Wiley, MD, FACS, Associate Clinical Professor, Neurosurgery, Wright State University School of Medicine, Dayton, Ohio

Sandi Wind, RN, ET, Enterostomal Therapist, Hahnemann University Hospital, Philadelphia

Joseph H. Zeccardi, MD, Director, Emergency Department, Thomas Jefferson University, Philadelphia

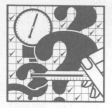 # Contributors

Deborah G. Althoff, RN, BSN, CNOR, Operating Room Staff Nurse, Rutland (Vt.) Regional Medical Center

Sherry L. Altschuler, PhD, Chief, Audiology/Speech Pathology, Veterans Administration Hospital, Philadelphia

Linda M. Appenheimer, RN, MS, Unit Leader/Assistant Professor, College of Nursing, Rush–Presbyterian–St. Luke's Medical Center, Chicago

Charold L. Baer, RN, PhD, Professor, Oregon Health Sciences University, Portland

Roxanne Aubol Batterden, RN, CCRN, Primary Nurse II, Surgical ICU, University of Maryland Medical Systems, Baltimore

Barbara Gross Braverman, RN, MSN, CS, Psychiatric Clinical Nurse Specialist, Medical College of Pennsylvania, Philadelphia

Sally A. Brozenec, RN, MS, Practitioner–Teacher, Rush University of Chicago

June M. Buckle, RN, MSN, Assistant Director of Nursing, Department of Medicine, The Johns Hopkins Hospital, Baltimore

Laura J. Burke, RN, MSN, Cardiovascular Clinical Nurse Specialist, St. Luke's Hospital, Milwaukee

Dorothea Caldwell, MPH, NP, Nurse Practitioner, Rockefeller University, New York

Mimi Callanan, RN, MSN, Epilepsy Clinical Specialist, Mid-Atlantic Regional Epilepsy Center, Medical College of Pennsylvania, Philadelphia

Jeanette K. Chambers, RN, MS, CS, Renal Clinical Nurse Specialist, Riverside Methodist Hospital, Columbus, Ohio

Mary Katherine Crathern, RN, BSN, Assistant Professor, New Hampshire Vocational Technical Institute, Berlin

Betty Dale, RN, BSN, Head Nurse, Urology, University of Minnesota Hospitals and Clinics, Minneapolis

Nancy B. Davis, RN, BSN, FNP, Nurse Practitioner and RN First Assistant, Cardiovascular and Chest Surgical Associates, Boise, Idaho

Linda J. Dec, RN, ADN, Staff Nurse, Medical City Dallas Hospital

Gloria Ferraro Donnelly, RN, PhD, FAAN, Chairman, Department of Nursing, La Salle University, Philadelphia

Linda M. Duffy, RN, MS, CURN, CANP, Clinical Specialist for Urology, Veterans Administration Medical Center, Minneapolis

Elizabeth A. Ely, RN, MS, Assistant Professor of Nursing, University of New Hampshire, Durham

Susan Hann Eshleman, RN, MS, MSN, Neurosensory Nursing Instructor, Chester County Hospital School of Nursing, West Chester, Pa.

Roslyn M. Gleeson, RNC, MSN, Clinical Specialist/Nursing of Children, Alfred I. Du Pont Institute, Wilmington, Del.

Susan Gauthier, RN, MSN, Assistant Professor, Department of Nursing, College of Allied Health Professions, Temple University, Philadelphia

Sandra K. Crabtree Goodnough, RN, MSN, Pulmonary Clinical Nurse Specialist, Hermann Hospital, Houston; Assistant Professor, School of Nursing, University of Texas Health Science Center at Houston

Diana W. Guthrie, RN, C, PhD, FAAN, Associate Professor/Diabetes Nurse Specialist, University of Kansas School of Medicine, Wichita

Mary Chapman Gyetvan, RN, BSEd, Clinical Consultant, Springhouse Corporation, Springhouse, Pa.

Marcia J. Hill, RN, MS, Clinical Practitioner/Teacher, Methodist Hospital, Houston; Clinical Assistant Professor, Baylor College of Medicine, Houston

Esther Holzbauer, OSB, MSN, Assistant Professor, Nursing, Mount Marty College, Yankton, S. D.

Kathryn M. Kater, RN, MSN, Neuro-Cardiothoracic Clinical Specialist, Barnes Hospital, St. Louis

Lee Ann Kelly, RN, MS, PNP, Head Nurse, Antepartum/Postpartum, Hermann Hospital, Houston

Mary Ann Myrick King, RN, BSN, Staff Nurse, Outpatient Dermatology Clinic, Veterans Administration Medical Center, Washington, D.C.

JoAnne Konick-McMahan, RNC, BSN, Level 4 Staff Nurse, Hospital of the University of Pennsylvania, Philadelphia

Susan L. W. Krupnick, RN, MSN, CCRN, CEN, CS, Administrator, Education Division, and Independent Clinical Nurse Specialist (Psychiatry), Skilled Nursing, Inc., Springhouse, Pa.

Karen A. Landis, RN, MS, CCRN, Pulmonary Clinical Nurse Specialist, Lehigh Valley Hospital Center, Allentown, Pa.

Melvina J. Lohmann, RNC, MEd, ANP, Assistant Professor of Nursing, Cedar Crest College, Allentown, Pa.

Chris Platt Moldovanyi, RN, MSN, Clinical Nurse Specialist, Endocrinology, Cleveland Clinic Foundation

Mary Lou Moore, RNC, PhD, ACCE, FAAN, Nurse Researcher/Educator, Bowman Gray School of Medicine, Winston-Salem, N.C.

Janice Overdorff, RN, BSN, Administrative Nurse III, University of Illinois, Chicago

Amy Perrin-Ross, RN, MSN, CNRN, Clinical Nurse Specialist, Neuroscience, Loyola University Medical Center, Maywood, Ill.

Frances W. Quinless, RN, PhD, Assistant Professor, Rutgers University College of Nursing, Newark, N.J.

Patricia L. Radzewicz, RN, BSN, Head Nurse, University of Illinois Eye and Ear Infirmary, Chicago

Dennis G. Ross, RN, MSN, MAE, CNOR, Associate Professor of Nursing, Castleton (Vt.) State College

Linda C. Rothfield, RN, MSN, CANP, Specialty Instructor II, The Johns Hopkins Hospital, Baltimore

Susan Rumsey, RN, BSN, MPH, Perinatal Outreach Education Coordinator, Wake Area Health Education Center, Raleigh, N.C.

Mary Jo Sagaties, RN, MSN, FNP-C, Nurse Practitioner/Ophthalmic Photographer, Leahey Eye Clinic, Lowell, Mass.; PhD Candidate, Boston University School of Medicine

Sheron L. Salyer, RNC, BSN, Perinatal Research Nurse, Vanderbilt Medical Center, Vanderbilt University School of Medicine, Nashville, Tenn.

Kay Freeman Sauers, RN, BSN, MS, Clinical Nurse Specialist in Orthopedics, Trauma Rehabilitation Center/Montebello Hospital Center, Baltimore

Kristine Ann Scordo, RN, BSN, MS, Clinical Nurse Specialist, Cardiology, Bethesda Hospital, Cincinnati

Karen N. Shine, RN, BSN, Quality Assurance–Risk Management Coordinator, Dana-Farber Cancer Institute, Boston

Katherine Small, RN, MS, Nurse Supervisor, University of Maryland Hospital, Baltimore

Carol E. Smith, RN, PhD, Associate Professor, University of Kansas School of Nursing, Kansas City

June L. Stark, RN, BSN, CCRN, Critical Care Instructor/Renal Nurse Consultant, New England Medical Center, Boston

Clare M. Stearns, RN, MS, CNOR, ARNP, Orthopedic Nurse Practitioner, St. Luke Medical Center, Berlin, N.H.; Adjunct Faculty, Department of Nursing, University of New Hampshire, Durham

Christina M. Stewart, RN, MSN, CNRN, CCRN, Clinical Nurse Specialist, Loyola University of Chicago, Maywood, Ill.

Frances J. Storlie, RN, PhD, CANP, Director, Personal Health Services, Southwest Washington Health District, Vancouver

Arlene B. Strong, RN, MN, ANP, Cardiac Clinical Specialist, Adult Nurse Practitioner—Anticoagulation Clinic, Veterans Administration Medical Center, Portland, Ore.

Alicia Alphin Tollison, RNCS, BSN, MN, Educational Coordinator, Alexandria (Va.) Hospital

Naomi Walpert, RN, MS, Clinical Nurse Specialist for Endocrinology and Metabolism, Sinai Hospital, Baltimore

Maryann Banko Wee, RN, BSN, Risk Management Consultant, Virginia Professional Underwriters, Inc., Jackson, Miss.

Bunny Weiss, RN, BSN, Urology Nurse Specialist, Albert Einstein Medical Center–Northern Division, Philadelphia

Janette R. Yanko, RN, MN, CNRN, Neurological/Neurosurgical Clinical Specialist, Youngstown (Ohio) Hospital Association

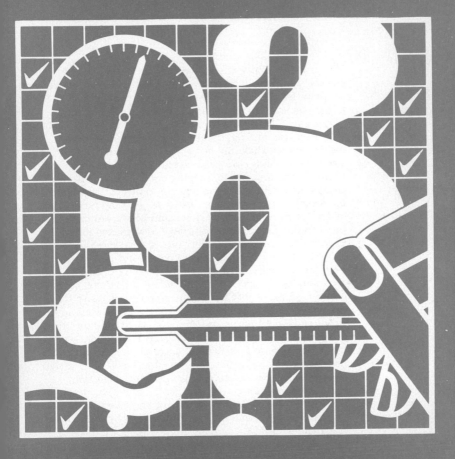

Foreword

You probably know nurses who can recognize a new sign or symptom in virtually any patient and can quickly pinpoint its probable cause. These nurses always seem to know just what to assess and just what their findings may mean. This skill and understanding, once uncommon as a prerequisite of nursing practice, is today becoming increasingly important for maintaining your status as a health care professional. Why? One important reason is the impact of sweeping changes in our health care system. With cost-containment policies, ever-increasing demands on your time, and growing numbers of gravely ill patients, you're constantly pressed to expand the scope of your duties. And that means improving your present skills and acquiring new ones.

To meet these challenges confidently and provide the best possible patient care, you obviously need more than a passing familiarity with only the most common signs and symptoms of disease. You need comprehensive information on how to recognize and interpret even the most subtle indicators of disease. You also need to know what to assess after you've identified a sign or symptom—and, if necessary, how to intervene to prevent or contain complications. And, of course, you need to know what a sign or symptom forecasts about your patient's condition.

Signs & Symptoms, the latest volume in the Nurse's Reference Library, puts this body of knowledge at your fingertips. This handy reference thoroughly covers 300 signs and symptoms, ranging from common indicators of disease, such as fever and vomiting, to less common but still significant indicators, such as nystagmus and tracheal deviation. What's more, the volume's alphabetical arrangement helps you quickly locate any sign or symptom.

Each sign or symptom is covered in a standard format, beginning with an introduction that defines and describes the sign or symptom, discusses its significance and incidence, and summarizes its possible causes. For an elicited sign, such as Kernig's sign, the introduction also describes the technique for evoking a response.

From here on, the arrangement of each entry reflects your probable thinking when faced with the patient's problem. *Assessment* discusses what to do immediately after you've identified a sign or the patient has reported a symptom. If the sign or symptom can signal a life-, limb-, or organ-threatening disorder, you'll find emergency assessment and intervention steps highlighted first. Or, if it doesn't signal a crisis, you'll find assessment steps that explore the patient's complaint and direct the history and physical examination.

The next section, *Medical causes,* covers disorders that can produce the sign or symptom. When appropriate, this section first characterizes the sign or symptom in each disorder according to its severity, onset, location, duration, or aggravating and alleviating factors. Then, it describes other signs and symptoms that a patient with the disorder is likely to have. Additional causes of the sign or symptom—such as drugs, diagnostic tests, and surgery—appear next, under *Other causes.*

The following section, *Special considerations,* discusses pertinent nursing care measures—monitoring the patient for signs of complications, promoting comfort, administering drugs, and carrying out patient teaching. This section also reviews diagnostic tests the patient may undergo.

The final section, *Pediatric pointers,* lists disorders that cause the sign or symptom primarily in children. It also alerts you to key differences between adult and pediatric patients in a sign's significance or severity and in your assessment and intervention techniques.

Throughout the book, you'll find numerous charts, graphs, and illustrations that provide important background information or clarify difficult points. For example, graphically highlighted charts help you quickly match assessment findings with possible causes for abdominal pain, dyspnea, hematuria, and many more signs and symptoms. A special graphic symbol—*Emergency*—calls your attention to signs and symptoms that require emergency assessment and intervention. Another graphic symbol, *Assessment tip,* highlights a special assessment technique or information that can help you pinpoint or further characterize a particular sign or symptom. And *Patient-teaching aids* provide instructions that you can photocopy and give to your patients to promote participation in their own care.

A special appendix provides summaries of an additional 250 signs and symptoms, including infrequently elicited signs, psychiatric signs and symptoms, and nail and tongue signs.

Signs & Symptoms is an organized and comprehensive reference. I heartily recommend it to nurses and other health professionals who wish to confirm, update, and expand their knowledge of this clinically significant subject. The times demand this knowledge—and *Signs & Symptoms* delivers it.

Gloria Ferraro Donnelly, RN, PhD, FAAN

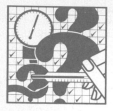

Overview

Never before has there been so great a need for nurses to correctly identify and thoroughly assess signs and symptoms. Obviously, this ability will improve the quality of patient care—and perhaps even save a life. After all, as the patient's chief monitor, we're usually the first to notice any change in his condition.

But there are other reasons. First, our role as nurses has expanded. We've assumed new duties and taken on greater responsibility in diagnostic testing, patient teaching, administration and, perhaps most importantly, patient assessment. Modern nursing practice requires us to make independent judgments about a patient's condition. We're expected not only to follow the doctor's orders, but also to recognize significant signs and symptoms—and to do something about them. And we're expected to keep up-to-date with new drugs and procedures, which means more side effects and complications to watch for and guard against.

Over the last 20 years, nurses by the thousands have accepted the challenge of coronary, burn, shock, respiratory, and other intensive care specialties. These nurses have led the way in developing the skills necessary to recognize and assess signs and symptoms on a moment-by-moment basis. Today, *all* of us must become equally informed, equally skilled. To protect our gains and continue to grow professionally, we must be ever more confident in our analytical skills, more certain in our knowledge and expertise.

There are yet other reasons for correctly identifying and thoroughly assessing signs and symptoms. For example, along with our expanded role has come increased liability for our nursing judgments, decisions, and actions—and for those of others. The trend toward licensing health care assistants (HCAs) in many states further magnifies the need for us to expand our knowledge of the mechanisms and indicators of disease. Why? An HCA doesn't have the in-depth training that you have and must rely on your expertise. If you're his certifying professional, legal responsibility for the safety of his practice rests with *you*.

Moreover, in this country, we're experiencing a health care revolution that's shifting the emphasis from treating illness to promoting wellness. As a result, the demand for hospital care is shrinking while clinics and community health centers are being called upon increasingly to provide direct patient care. Combined with this shift away from hospital care is a new cost consciousness in health care, brought on by the federal government's implementation of diagnosis-related groups (DRGs) to control Medicare costs. Hospitals, forced to operate more like businesses in order to survive, are discharging patients earlier to avoid exceeding the costs allowable under the DRG system. This trend is making hospitals the province of the very ill, who need the most proficient nursing care available. It also means that more patients are discharged still needing acute care and sophisticated equipment. And that home care, hospices, and extended care facilities are becoming increasingly common alternatives to a prolonged hospital stay. The result? A growing demand for highly skilled nurses in out-of-hospital settings—and mounting pressure on these nurses to personally provide the expert level of care traditionally found in a hospital.

In a nutshell, increased professional responsibility and liability, supervision of other health care workers, profound changes in hospital care, new emphasis on alternative health care settings, the appearance of more and more new drugs and procedures—all of these developments are radically changing the art and science of nursing. We nurses have always responded to changing demands—and now our evolving professional status demands that we increase our knowledge and skill in all areas of nursing. Obviously, there's much to learn—and too much to remember.

For all of us, *Signs & Symptoms* is a necessary resource for providing a safe and effective nursing practice. I believe that every nurse—from practitioner to intensive care, from medical/surgical unit to home care—would do well to invest in a copy of this book. We've done without it too long already.

Frances J. Storlie, RN, PhD, CANP

abdominal distention • abdominal mass • abdominal pain • abdominal rigidi
use • agitation • alopecia • amenorrhea • amnesia • analgesia • anhidrosis • a
anuria • anxiety • aphasia • apnea • apneustic respirations • apraxia • arm p
athetosis • aura • Babinski's reflex • back pain • barrel chest • Battle's sign • I
bladder distention • blood pressure decrease • blood pressure increase • bowe
bowel sounds—hyperactive • bowel sounds—hypoactive • bradycardia • brad
dimpling • breast nodule • breast pain • breast ulcer • breath with ammonia
odor • breath with fruity odor • Brudzinski's sign • bruits • buffalo hump • b
lait spots • capillary refill time—prolonged • carpopedal spasm • cat cry • che
asymmetrical • chest pain • Cheyne-Stokes respirations • chills • chorea • Chv
cogwheel rigidity • cold intolerance • confusion • conjunctival injection • cons
reflex—absent • costovertebral angle tenderness • cough—barking • cough—n
productive • crackles • crepitation—bony • crepitation—subcutaneous • cry—
cyanosis • decerebrate posture • decorticate posture • deep tendon reflexes—h
reflexes—hypoactive • depression • diaphoresis • diarrhea • diplopia • dizzin
absent • drooling • dysarthria • dysmenorrhea • dyspareunia • dyspepsia • dy
dystonia • dysuria • earache • edema—generalized • edema of the arms • ede
of the legs • enophthalmos • enuresis • epistaxis • eructation • erythema • exc
discharge • eye pain • facial pain • fasciculations • fatigue • fecal incontinenc
fever • flank pain • flatulence • fontanelle bulging • fontanelle depression • foo
abnormalities • gait—bizarre • gait—propulsive • gait—scissors • gait—spast
gait—waddling • gallop—atrial • gallop—ventricular • genital lesions in the r
respirations • gum bleeding • gum swelling • gynecomastia • halitosis • halo
hearing loss • heat intolerance • Heberden's nodes • hematemesis • hematoche
hemianopia • hemoptysis • hepatomegaly • hiccups • hirsutism • hoarseness
hyperpigmentation • hyperpnea • hypopigmentation • impotence • insomnia •
claudication • Janeway's spots • jaundice • jaw pain • jugular vein distention
sign • leg pain • level of consciousness—decreased • lid lag • light flashes • lc
lymphadenopathy • masklike facies • McBurney's sign • McMurray's sign • m
metrorrhagia • miosis • moon face • mouth lesions • murmurs • muscle atrop
muscle spasms • muscle spasticity • muscle weakness • mydriasis • myocloni
nausea • neck pain • night blindness • nipple discharge • nipple retraction •
rigidity • nystagmus • ocular deviation • oligomenorrhea • oliguria • opisthot
dyskinesia • orthopnea • orthostatic hypotension • Ortolani's sign • Osler's no
palpitations • papular rash • paralysis • paresthesias • paroxysmal nocturnal
d'orange • pericardial friction rub • peristaltic waves—visible • photophobia
rub • polydipsia • polyphagia • polyuria • postnasal drip • priapism • prurit
psychotic behavior • ptosis • pulse—absent or weak • pulse—bounding • pul
pulse pressure—widened • pulse rhythm abnormality • pulsus alternans • pu
paradoxus • pupils—nonreactive • pupils—sluggish • purple striae • purpur
pyrosis • raccoon's eyes • rebound tenderness • rectal pain • retractions—cos
rhinorrhea • rhonchi • Romberg's sign • salivation—decreased • salivation—i
scotoma • scrotal swelling • seizure—absence • seizure—focal • seizure—ger
seizure—psychomotor • setting-sun sign • shallow respirations • skin—bronz
skin—mottled • skin—scaly • skin turgor—decreased • spider angioma • sple
respirations • stool—clay-colored • stridor • syncope • tachycardia • tachypne
tearing—increased • throat pain • tic • tinnitus • tracheal deviation • trachea
trismus • tunnel vision • uremic frost • urethral discharge • urinary frequenc
urinary incontinence • urinary urgency • urine cloudiness • urticaria • vagin
postmenopausal • vaginal discharge • venous hum • vertigo • vesicular rash

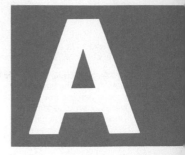

Abdominal Distention

Abdominal distention refers to increased abdominal girth—the result of increased intraabdominal pressure forcing the abdominal wall outward. Distention may be mild or severe, depending on the amount of pressure. It may be localized or diffuse and may occur gradually or suddenly. Acute abdominal distention may signal life-threatening peritonitis or acute bowel obstruction.

Abdominal distention results from accumulation of fluid or gas (or both) within the lumen of the gastrointestinal (GI) tract or peritoneal cavity. Both fluid and gas are normally present in the GI tract, but not in the peritoneal cavity. However, if fluid and gas are unable to pass freely through the GI tract, abdominal distention occurs. In the peritoneal cavity, distention may reflect acute bleeding, accumulation of ascitic fluid, or air from perforation of an abdominal organ.

Abdominal distention doesn't always signal pathology. For example, in anxious patients or those with digestive distress, localized distention in the left upper quadrant can result from aerophagia—the unconscious swallowing of air. Generalized distention can result from ingestion of fruits or vegetables with large amounts of unabsorbable carbohydrates, such as legumes, or from abnormal food fermentation by microbes.

Assessment

If the patient displays abdominal distention, quickly check for signs of hypovolemia, such as pallor, diaphoresis, hypotension, and a rapid, thready pulse. Ask the patient if he's experiencing severe abdominal pain or difficulty breathing. Find out about any recent accidents and observe the patient for signs of trauma and of peritoneal bleeding, such as a bluish tinge around the umbilicus (Cullen's sign). Then auscultate all abdominal quadrants, noting rapid and high-pitched, diminished, or absent bowel sounds. (If you don't hear bowel sounds immediately, listen for at least 5 minutes.) *Gently* palpate the abdomen for rigidity. Remember that deep or extensive palpation may increase pain and aggravate hemorrhage or perforation.

If you detect abdominal distention, pain, and rigidity along with abnormal bowel sounds, have another nurse notify the doctor immediately, and begin emergency interventions. Place the patient in a supine position, administer oxygen, and insert an I.V. line for fluid

DETECTING ASCITES

To differentiate ascites from other causes of distention, check for shifting dullness, fluid wave, or puddle sign, as described here:

Shifting dullness
Step 1. With the patient supine, percuss from the umbilicus outward to the flank. Draw a line on the patient's skin to mark the change from tympany to dullness.

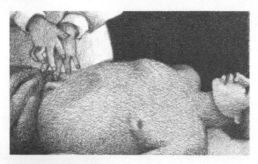

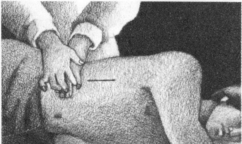

Step 2. Turn the patient onto his side, which causes ascitic fluid to shift. Percuss again and mark the change from tympany to dullness. Any difference between these lines can indicate ascites.

Fluid wave
Have another nurse press deeply into the patient's midline to prevent vibration from traveling along the abdominal wall. Place one of your palms on one of the patient's flanks. Strike the opposite flank with your other hand. If you feel the blow in the opposite palm, ascitic fluid is present.

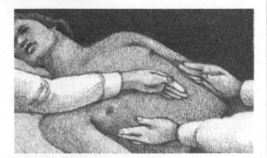

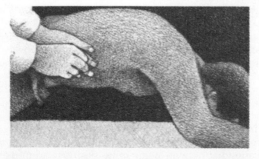

Puddle sign
Position the patient on his elbows and knees, which causes ascitic fluid to pool in the most dependent part of the abdomen. Percuss the abdomen from the flank to the midline. The percussion note becomes louder at the edge of the puddle, or ascitic pool.

replacement, as ordered. Prepare to insert, or assist with insertion of, a GI tube to relieve acute intraluminal distention. Reassure the patient and prepare him for surgery, as ordered.

If the patient's abdominal distention isn't acute, ask about the onset and duration of distention and its associated signs. The patient with localized distention may report a sensation of pressure, fullness, or tenderness in the affected area. The patient with generalized distention may report a bloated feeling, a pounding heart, and difficulty breathing deeply or when lying flat. He may also feel unable to bend at his waist. Be sure to ask about abdominal pain, fever, nausea, vomiting, anorexia, altered bowel habits, and weight gain or loss.

Obtain a medical history, noting GI or biliary disorders that may cause peritonitis or ascites, such as cirrhosis, hepatitis, or inflammatory bowel disease. Also note chronic constipation. Has the patient recently had abdominal surgery, which might lead to abdominal distention? Also ask about recent accidents, even minor ones, like falling off a stepladder.

Next, perform a physical examination. Stand at the foot of the bed and observe the recumbent patient for abdominal asymmetry to determine if distention is localized or generalized. Then assess abdominal contour by stooping at his side. Inspect for tense, glistening skin and bulging flanks, which may indicate ascites. Note the umbilicus. An everted umbilicus may indicate ascites or umbilical hernia. An inverted umbilicus may indicate gas distention; it's also common in obesity. Inspect the abdomen for signs of inguinal or femoral hernia and for incisions that may point to adhesions. Both may lead to intestinal obstruction. Then auscultate for bowel sounds, abdominal friction rubs (indicating peritoneal inflammation), and bruits (indicating an aneurysm). Listen for succussion splash—a splashing sound normally heard in the stomach when the patient moves or when palpation disturbs the viscera. However, an abnormally loud splash indicates fluid accumulation, suggesting gastric dilatation or obstruction.

Next, percuss and palpate the abdomen to determine if distention results from air, fluid, or both. A tympanic note in the left lower quadrant suggests an air-filled descending or sigmoid colon. A tympanic note throughout a generally distended abdomen suggests an air-filled peritoneal cavity. A dull percussion note throughout a generally distended abdomen suggests a fluid-filled peritoneal cavity. Remember that obesity also causes a dull note throughout the abdomen.

Palpate the abdomen for tenderness, noting if it's localized or generalized. Finally, measure abdominal girth for a baseline. Mark the flanks with a felt-tipped pen as a reference for subsequent measurements.

Medical causes

• **Abdominal cancer.** Generalized abdominal distention may occur when the cancer—most often, an ovarian or pancreatic tumor—produces ascites. Shifting dullness and a fluid wave accompany distention. Associated signs and symptoms may include severe abdominal pain, an abdominal mass, anorexia, jaundice, GI hemorrhage (hematemesis or melena), dyspepsia, and weight loss that progresses to muscle weakness and atrophy.

• **Abdominal trauma.** When brisk internal bleeding accompanies trauma, abdominal distention may be acute and dramatic. Associated signs of this life-threatening disorder include abdominal rigidity with guarding, decreased or absent bowel sounds, vomiting, tenderness, and abdominal bruising. Pain may occur over the trauma site, or over the scapula if abdominal bleeding irritates the phrenic nerve. Signs of hypovolemic shock, such as hypotension and rapid, thready pulse, will appear with significant blood loss.

• **Bladder distention.** Various disorders

ABDOMINAL DISTENTION: CAUSES AND ASSOCIATED FINDINGS

CAUSES	Abdominal mass	Abdominal pain	Abdominal rigidity	Anorexia	Bowel sounds—absent	Bowel sounds—hyperactive	Bowel sounds—hypoactive	Constipation	Diarrhea
Abdominal cancer	●	●		●					
Abdominal trauma		●	●		●		●		
Bladder distention	●								
Cirrhosis		●		●				●	●
Congestive heart failure		●							
Gastric dilatation (acute)		●			●		●		
Irritable bowel syndrome		●						●	●
Large-bowel obstruction		●				●		●	
Mesenteric artery occlusion (acute)		●	●	●	●			●	●
Nephrotic syndrome				●					
Ovarian cysts	●	●							
Paralytic ileus		●			●		●	●	
Peritonitis		●	●		●		●		
Small-bowel obstruction		●				●		●	
Toxic megacolon (acute)		●			●		●		

Edema	Fever	Hepatomegaly	Hypotension	Jaundice	Jugular vein distention	Nausea	Oliguria	Rebound tenderness	Succussion splash	Tachycardia	Tachypnea	Urinary frequency	Vomiting	Weight change
				•										•
			•										•	
												•		
•	•	•		•		•							•	•
•		•			•	•							•	
									•				•	
						•								
													•	
	•		•							•	•		•	
•							•							
													•	
	•		•			•		•		•			•	
						•		•					•	
	•							•		•				

cause bladder distention, which in turn causes lower abdominal distention. Slight dullness on percussion above the symphysis indicates mild bladder distention. A palpable, smooth, rounded, fluctuant suprapubic mass suggests severe distention; a fluctuant mass extending to the umbilicus indicates extremely severe distention. Urinary dribbling, frequency, or urgency may occur with urinary obstruction. Suprapubic discomfort is also common.

• *Cirrhosis.* In this disorder, ascites causes generalized distention and is confirmed by a fluid wave, shifting dullness, and a puddle sign. Umbilical eversion and caput medusae (dilated veins around the umbilicus) are common. The patient may report a feeling of fullness or weight gain. Associated findings include vague abdominal pain, fever, anorexia, nausea, vomiting, constipation or diarrhea, bleeding tendencies, severe pruritus, palmar erythema, spider angiomas, leg edema, and possibly splenomegaly. Jaundice is usually a late sign. Hepatomegaly occurs initially, but the liver may not be palpable in advanced disease.

• *Congestive heart failure (CHF).* Generalized abdominal distention caused by ascites is confirmed by shifting dullness and a fluid wave. Accompanying the distention are the hallmarks of CHF: peripheral edema, jugular vein distention, dyspnea, and tachycardia. Common associated signs include hepatomegaly, which may cause right upper quadrant pain; nausea; vomiting; productive cough; rales; cool extremities; and cyanotic nail beds.

• *Gastric dilatation (acute).* Left upper quadrant distention is characteristic in acute gastric dilatation. It's accompanied by persistent, copious vomiting and, possibly, epigastric pain. Physical examination reveals tympany, gastric tenderness, and a succussion splash. Initially, visible peristalsis may occur. Later, hypoactive or absent bowel sounds confirm ileus.

• *Irritable bowel syndrome.* This disorder may produce intermittent, local-

ized distention—the result of periodic intestinal spasms. Lower abdominal pain or cramping typically accompanies these spasms. Pain is usually relieved by defecation or passage of gas and aggravated by stress or ingestion of raw fruits and vegetables. Associated signs and symptoms include diarrhea that alternates with constipation or normal bowel function, nausea, mucus-streaked stool, and dyspepsia.

• *Large-bowel obstruction.* Dramatic abdominal distention is characteristic in this life-threatening disorder; in fact, loops of the large bowel may become visible on the abdomen. Constipation precedes the distention and, in fact, may be the only symptom for days. Associated findings may include tympany, high-pitched bowel sounds, and sudden onset of colicky lower abdominal pain that becomes persistent. Fecal vomiting is a late sign.

• *Mesenteric artery occlusion (acute).* In this life-threatening disorder, abdominal distention usually occurs several hours after the sudden onset of severe, colicky periumbilical pain that later becomes constant and diffuse. Related signs include severe abdominal tenderness with guarding and rigidity, absent bowel sounds, and, occasionally, a bruit in the right iliac fossa. There may be vomiting, anorexia, diarrhea, or constipation. Late signs include fever, tachycardia, tachypnea, hypotension, and cool, clammy skin.

• *Nephrotic syndrome.* This may produce massive edema, causing generalized abdominal distention with a fluid wave and shifting dullness. It may also produce elevated blood pressure, possibly hematuria or oliguria, fatigue, anorexia, depression, and pallor.

• *Ovarian cysts.* Typically, large ovarian cysts produce lower abdominal distention accompanied by umbilical eversion. Because they're thin-walled and fluid-filled, these cysts produce a fluid wave and shifting dullness—signs that mimic ascites. Lower abdominal pain and a palpable mass may be present.

• *Paralytic ileus.* This disorder produces generalized distention with a tympanic percussion note. It's accompanied by absent or hypoactive bowel sounds and, occasionally, mild abdominal pain and vomiting. The patient may be severely constipated or may pass flatus and small, liquid stools.

• *Peritonitis.* In this life-threatening disorder, abdominal distention may be localized or generalized, depending on the extent of peritonitis. Fluid accumulates first within the peritoneal cavity and then within the bowel lumen, causing a fluid wave and shifting dullness. Typically, distention is accompanied by sudden and severe abdominal pain that worsens with movement, rebound tenderness, and abdominal rigidity.

The skin over the patient's abdomen may appear taut. Associated signs and symptoms usually include hypoactive or absent bowel sounds, fever, chills, hyperalgesia, nausea, and vomiting. Signs of shock, such as tachycardia and hypotension, will appear with significant fluid loss into the abdomen.

• *Small-bowel obstruction.* Abdominal distention is characteristic in this life-threatening disorder. It's most pronounced in late obstruction, especially in the distal small bowel. Auscultation reveals hyperactive bowel sounds, whereas percussion produces a tympanic note. Accompanying distention are colicky periumbilical pain, constipation, nausea, and vomiting; the higher the obstruction, the earlier and more severe the vomiting. Rebound tenderness reflects intestinal strangulation with ischemia. Associated signs and symptoms may include drowsiness, malaise, and signs of dehydration. Signs of hypovolemic shock will appear with progressive dehydration and plasma loss.

• *Toxic megacolon (acute).* This life-threatening complication of infectious or ulcerative colitis produces dramatic abdominal distention that usually develops gradually. It's accompanied by a tympanic percussion note, diminished or absent bowel sounds, and mild

rebound tenderness. The patient will also have abdominal pain and tenderness, fever, and tachycardia.

Special considerations

Position the patient comfortably, using pillows for support. Place him on his left side to help flatus escape. Or, if he has ascites, elevate the head of the bed to ease his breathing. If the patient's anxiety triggers air swallowing or deep breathing that causes discomfort, advise him to take slow breaths. Administer drugs to relieve pain, as ordered, and offer emotional support. If the patient has an obstruction or ascites, explain food and fluid restrictions. Stress good oral hygiene to prevent dry mouth.

Prepare the patient for diagnostic tests, such as abdominal X-rays, endoscopy, laparoscopy, ultrasonography, computed tomography, or possibly paracentesis.

Pediatric pointers

Because the young child's abdomen is normally rounded, distention may be difficult to observe. Fortunately, though, the abdominal wall is less developed than an adult's, making palpation easier. When percussing the abdomen, remember that children normally swallow air when eating and crying, resulting in louder than normal tympany. Minimal tympany with abdominal distention may result from fluid accumulation or solid masses. To check for abdominal fluid, test for shifting dullness instead of for a fluid wave. (In a child, air swallowing and incomplete abdominal muscle development make the fluid wave hard to interpret.)

In the neonate, ascites usually results from GI or urinary perforation; in an older child, it may result from heart failure, cirrhosis, or nephrosis. Besides ascites, congenital malformations of the GI tract (such as intussusception and volvulus) may cause abdominal distention. A hernia may cause distention if it produces an intestinal obstruction. In addition, overeating and constipation can also cause distention.

Abdominal Mass

Often detected on routine physical examination, an abdominal mass is a localized swelling in one of the abdominal quadrants. Typically, this sign develops insidiously and may represent an enlarged organ, a neoplasm, an abscess, a vascular defect, or a fecal mass.

Distinguishing an abdominal mass from normal structures requires skillful palpation. At times, palpation must be repeated with the patient in a different position or performed by a second examiner to verify initial findings. A palpable abdominal mass is an important clinical sign and usually represents a serious—and perhaps life-threatening—disorder.

Assessment

If the patient has a pulsating midabdominal mass and severe abdominal pain, suspect an aortic aneurysm. Quickly take his vital signs, and have another nurse notify the doctor immediately. Because the patient may require emergency surgery, withhold food or fluids until the doctor can examine him. Prepare to start an I.V. infusion for fluid and blood replacement and to administer oxygen. Obtain routine preoperative tests, and prepare the patient for angiography. Frequently monitor blood pressure, pulse, respirations, and urinary output. Be alert for signs of shock, such as tachycardia, hypotension, and cool, clammy skin, which may indicate significant blood loss.

If the patient's abdominal mass doesn't suggest an aortic aneurysm, continue with a detailed history. Ask the patient if the mass is painful. If so, is the pain constant, or does it occur only on palpation? Is it localized or generalized? Determine if the patient was already aware of the mass. If he was, has he noticed any change in its size or location? Next, review the pa-

tient's medical history, especially noting gastrointestinal (GI) disorders. Ask about GI signs and symptoms, such as constipation, diarrhea, rectal bleeding, abnormally colored stools, and vomiting. Has the patient noticed a change in appetite? If the patient's female, ask about the regularity of her menstrual cycles.

Begin the physical examination by auscultating for bowel sounds in each quadrant. Listen for bruits or friction rubs, and check for enlarged veins. Lightly palpate and then deeply palpate the abdomen, assessing any painful or suspicious areas last. (If your patient has an abdominal mass that's known to be cancerous, do *not* perform deep palpation to avoid spreading tumor cells.) Be sure to note the patient's position when you locate the mass. Some masses can only be detected with the patient supine; others require a side-lying position.

Estimate the size of the mass in centimeters. Is it round or sausage-shaped? Describe its contour as smooth, rough, sharply defined, nodular, or irregular. Does the mass have a doughy, soft, solid, or hard consistency? Percuss the mass: a dull sound indicates a fluid-filled mass; a tympanic sound indicates an air-filled mass.

Next, determine if the mass moves with your hand or in response to respiration. Is the mass free-floating or attached to intraabdominal structures? To determine whether the mass is located in the abdominal wall or the abdominal cavity, ask the patient to lift his head and shoulders off the examination table, thereby contracting his abdominal muscles. While these muscles are contracted, try to palpate the mass. If you can, the mass is in the abdominal wall; if you can't, the mass is within the abdominal cavity.

Medical causes

• *Abdominal aortic aneurysm.* This disorder may persist for years, producing only a pulsating periumbilical mass with a systolic bruit over the aorta.

However, it may become life-threatening if the aneurysm expands and its walls weaken. In such cases, the patient initially reports constant upper abdominal pain or, less often, low back or dull abdominal pain. If the aneurysm ruptures, he'll report severe abdominal and back pain. And after rupture, the aneurysm no longer pulsates.

Associated signs and symptoms may include mottled skin below the waist, absent femoral and pedal pulses, lower blood pressure in the legs than in the arms, mild-to-moderate tenderness with guarding, and abdominal rigidity. Signs of shock—such as tachycardia and cool, clammy skin—will appear with significant blood loss.

● **Bladder distention.** A smooth, rounded, fluctuant suprapubic mass is characteristic. In extreme distention, the mass may extend to the umbilicus. Severe suprapubic pain and urinary frequency and urgency may also occur.

● **Cholecystitis.** Deep palpation below the liver border may detect a smooth, firm, sausage-shaped mass. However, in acute inflammation, the gallbladder is usually too tender to palpate. Cholecystitis can cause severe right upper quadrant pain that may radiate to the right shoulder, chest, or back; abdominal rigidity and tenderness; fever; pallor; diaphoresis; anorexia; nausea; and vomiting.

● **Cholelithiasis.** Usually, a stone-filled gallbladder produces a painless right upper quadrant mass that's smooth and sausage-shaped. However, passage of a stone through the bile or cystic duct may cause severe right upper quadrant pain that radiates to the epigastrium, back, or shoulder blades. Accompanying signs and symptoms include anorexia, nausea, vomiting, chills, diaphoresis, restlessness, and low-grade fever. Jaundice may occur with obstruction of the common bile duct.

● **Colonic cancer.** A right lower quadrant mass may occur in cancer of the right colon, which may also cause black, tarry stools and abdominal aching, pressure, or dull cramps. Associated signs and symptoms include weakness, fatigue, exertional dyspnea, vertigo, and signs of intestinal obstruction, such as obstipation and vomiting.

Occasionally, cancer of the left colon also causes a palpable mass. Most often, though, it produces rectal bleeding, intermittent abdominal fullness or cramping, and rectal pressure. Later, the patient develops obstipation, diarrhea, or pencil-shaped, grossly bloody, or mucus-streaked stools. Typically, defecation relieves pain.

● **Crohn's disease.** In this disorder, tender, sausage-shaped masses are usually palpable in the right lower quadrant and, at times, in the left lower quadrant. Attacks of colicky right lower quadrant pain and diarrhea are common. Associated signs and symptoms include fever, anorexia, weight loss, hyperactive bowel sounds, nausea, and abdominal tenderness with guarding.

● **Diverticulitis.** Most common in the sigmoid colon, this disorder may produce a left lower quadrant mass. It also produces intermittent abdominal pain that's relieved by defecation or passage of flatus. Other findings may include alternating constipation and diarrhea, nausea, and a low-grade fever.

● **Gallbladder carcinoma.** This disorder may produce a moderately tender, irregular mass in the right upper quadrant. Accompanying it is chronic, progressively severe epigastric or right upper quadrant pain that may radiate to the right shoulder. Associated signs and symptoms include nausea, vomiting, anorexia, weight loss, jaundice, and, at times, hepatosplenomegaly.

● **Gastric carcinoma.** Advanced gastric carcinoma may produce an epigastric mass. Early symptoms include chronic dyspepsia and epigastric discomfort, whereas late findings include weight loss, a feeling of fullness after eating, fatigue, and, occasionally, coffee-ground vomitus or melena.

● **Hepatic carcinoma.** This disorder produces a tender, nodular mass in the right upper quadrant or right epigastric area accompanied by severe pain.

ABDOMINAL MASS: LOCATIONS AND CAUSES

The location of an abdominal mass provides an important clue to the causative disorder. Here are the disorders responsible for abdominal masses and the quadrants where the masses occur.

Right upper quadrant
- Aortic aneurysm (epigastric area)
- Cholecystitis/cholelithiasis
- Gallbladder, gastric, hepatic carcinoma
- Hepatomegaly
- Hydronephrosis
- Pancreatic abscess/pseudocysts
- Renal cell carcinoma

Left upper quadrant
- Aortic aneurysm (epigastric area)
- Gastric carcinoma (epigastric area)
- Hydronephrosis
- Pancreatic abscess (epigastric area)
- Pancreatic pseudocysts (epigastric area)
- Renal cell carcinoma
- Splenomegaly

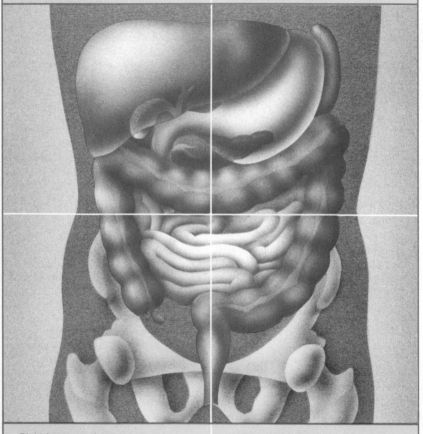

Right lower quadrant
- Bladder distention (suprapubic area)
- Colonic cancer
- Crohn's disease
- Ovarian cyst (suprapubic area)
- Uterine leiomyomas (suprapubic area)

Left lower quadrant
- Bladder distention (suprapubic area)
- Colonic cancer
- Diverticulitis
- Ovarian cyst (suprapubic area)
- Uterine leiomyomas (suprapubic area)
- Volvulus

Its other effects can include weight loss, weakness, anorexia, nausea, fever, dependent edema, and, occasionally, jaundice and ascites. A large tumor can also cause a bruit or hum.

● *Hepatomegaly.* This produces a firm, blunt, irregular mass in the epigastric region or below the right costal margin. Associated signs and symptoms depend on the causative disorder but commonly include ascites, right upper quadrant pain and tenderness, anorexia, nausea, vomiting, leg edema, jaundice, and, possibly, splenomegaly.

● *Hydronephrosis.* Enlarging one or both kidneys, this disorder produces a smooth, boggy mass in one or both flanks. Other findings vary with the degree of hydronephrosis. There may be severe colicky renal pain or dull flank pain that radiates to the groin. There may also be hematuria, pyuria, dysuria, alternating oliguria and polyuria, nausea, and vomiting.

● *Ovarian cyst.* A large ovarian cyst may produce a smooth, rounded, fluctuant mass resembling a distended bladder, in the suprapubic region. Large or multiple cysts may also cause mild pelvic discomfort, low back pain, and menstrual irregularities. A twisted or ruptured cyst may cause abdominal tenderness, distention, and rigidity.

● *Pancreatic abscess.* Occasionally, this disorder may produce a palpable epigastric mass accompanied by epigastric pain and tenderness. The patient's temperature usually rises abruptly but may climb steadily. Nausea, vomiting, diarrhea, tachycardia, and hypotension may also occur.

● *Pancreatic pseudocysts.* After pancreatitis, pseudocysts may form on the pancreas, causing a palpable nodular mass in the epigastric area. Other findings include nausea, vomiting, diarrhea, abdominal pain and tenderness, low-grade fever, and tachycardia.

● *Renal cell carcinoma.* Usually occurring in only one kidney, this disorder produces a smooth, firm, nontender mass near the affected kidney. Accompanying it are dull, constant abdominal or flank pain and hematuria. Other signs and symptoms include elevated blood pressure, fever, and urinary retention. Weight loss, nausea, vomiting, and leg edema occur late.

● *Splenomegaly.* The lymphomas, leukemias, hemolytic anemias, and inflammatory diseases are among the many disorders that may cause splenomegaly. Typically, the smooth edge of the enlarged spleen is palpable in the left upper quadrant. Associated signs and symptoms vary with the causative disorder but often include a feeling of abdominal fullness, left upper quadrant abdominal pain and tenderness, splenic friction rub, splenic bruits, and low-grade fever.

● *Uterine leiomyomas (fibroids).* If large enough, these common, benign uterine tumors produce a round, multinodular mass in the suprapubic region. Most often, the patient's chief complaint is menorrhagia. There may also be a feeling of heaviness in the abdomen; pressure on surrounding organs may cause back pain, constipation, and urinary frequency or urgency.

Special considerations
Discovery of an abdominal mass often causes anxiety. Offer emotional support to the patient and his family as they await the diagnosis. Position the patient comfortably, and administer drugs for pain or anxiety, as ordered.

Carefully explain diagnostic tests, which may include blood and urine studies, abdominal X-rays, barium enema, computed tomography, ultrasonography, radioisotope scans, and gastroscopy or sigmoidoscopy. The doctor may also perform a pelvic or rectal examination.

If an abdominal mass causes bowel obstruction, watch for signs of peritonitis—abdominal pain and rebound tenderness—and for signs of shock, such as tachycardia and hypotension.

Pediatric pointers
Detecting an abdominal mass in an infant can be quite a challenge. However,

these tips will make palpation easier for you: allow an infant to suck on his bottle or pacifier to prevent crying, which causes abdominal rigidity and interferes with palpation. Avoid tickling him, since laughter also causes abdominal rigidity. Also reduce his apprehension by distracting him with cheerful conversation. Rest your hand on his abdomen for a few moments before palpation. If he remains sensitive, place his hand under yours as you palpate.

In newborns, most abdominal masses result from renal disorders, such as polycystic kidney disease or congenital hydronephrosis. In older infants and children, abdominal masses usually result from enlarged organs, such as the liver and spleen.

Other common causes include Wilms' tumor, neuroblastoma, intussusception, volvulus, Hirschsprung's disease (congenital megacolon), pyloric stenosis, and abdominal abscess.

Abdominal Pain

Usually, abdominal pain results from gastrointestinal (GI) disorders, but it can also result from reproductive, genitourinary (GU), musculoskeletal, and vascular disorders; drug use; and the effects of toxins. At times, it signals life-threatening complications.

Abdominal pain arises from the abdominopelvic viscera, the parietal peritoneum, or the capsules of the liver, kidney, or spleen. It may be acute or chronic, diffuse or localized. Visceral pain develops slowly into a dull, aching pain that's poorly localized in the epigastric, periumbilical, or lower midabdominal region. In contrast, somatic pain produces a bright, sharp, more intense, and well-localized discomfort that rapidly follows the insult. Movement or coughing aggravates this pain.

Pain may also be referred to the abdomen from another site with the same

or similar nerve supply. This sharp, well-localized, referred pain is felt in skin or deeper tissues and may coexist with skin hyperesthesia and muscle hyperalgesia.

Mechanisms that produce abdominal pain include stretching or tension of the gut wall, traction on the peritoneum or mesentery, vigorous intestinal contraction, inflammation, ischemia, or sensory nerve irritation.

Assessment

If the patient is experiencing sudden and severe abdominal pain, quickly take his vital signs, palpate pulses below the waist, and have another nurse notify the doctor—especially if the patient has signs of hypovolemic shock, such as tachycardia and hypotension. If the patient also has mottled skin below the waist and a pulsating epigastric mass, or rebound tenderness and rigidity, prepare to administer oxygen and I.V. fluids or volume expanders. As ordered, insert an indwelling (Foley) catheter to monitor urine output, and insert a GI tube if vomiting occurs. Prepare the patient for surgery, if required.

If the patient has no life-threatening signs or symptoms, take his history. Ask if the pain is constant or intermittent and when it began. Typically, abdominal pain lasting more than 6 hours in a previously healthy patient requires surgery to correct its cause. Constant, steady pain suggests organ perforation, ischemia, or inflammation or the presence of blood in the peritoneal cavity. Intermittent, cramping pain suggests obstruction of a hollow organ.

If the pain is intermittent, find out the duration of a typical episode. Then ask where the pain is located and if it radiates to other areas. Find out if movement, coughing, exertion, vomiting, eating, elimination, or walking worsens or relieves the pain. Remember that the patient may report abdominal pain as indigestion or gas pain, so have him describe it in detail.

Ask about drug and alcohol use and

ABDOMINAL PAIN: TYPES AND LOCATION

AFFECTED ORGAN	VISCERAL PAIN	PARIETAL PAIN	REFERRED PAIN
Stomach	Middle epigastrium	Middle epigastrium and left upper quadrant	Shoulders
Small intestine	Periumbilical area	Over affected site	Midback (rare)
Appendix	Periumbilical area	Right lower quadrant	Right lower quadrant
Proximal colon	Periumbilical area and right flank for ascending colon	Over affected site	Right lower quadrant and back (rare)
Distal colon	Hypogastrium and left flank for descending colon	Over affected site	Left lower quadrant and back (rare)
Gallbladder	Middle epigastrium	Right upper quadrant	Right subscapular area
Ureters	Costovertebral angle	Over affected site	Groin; scrotum in men, labia in women (rare)
Pancreas	Middle epigastrium and left upper quadrant	Middle epigastrium and left upper quadrant	Back and left shoulder
Ovaries, fallopian tubes, and uterus	Hypogastrium and groin	Over affected site	Inner thighs

a history of vascular, GI, GU, or reproductive disorders. As appropriate, ask the female patient about the date of her last menses, changes in her menstrual pattern, or dyspareunia.

Ask your patient about appetite changes; the onset and frequency of any nausea or vomiting; and any changes in bowel habits, such as constipation, diarrhea, and changes in stool consistency. When was the last bowel movement? Ask about urinary frequency, urgency, or pain. Is the urine cloudy or pink?

Perform a physical examination. Take vital signs and assess skin turgor and mucous membranes. Inspect the abdomen for distention or visible peristaltic waves and, if indicated, measure abdominal girth. Auscultate for bowel sounds and characterize their motility. Percuss all quadrants, carefully noting the percussion sounds. Palpate the entire abdomen for masses, rigidity, and tenderness. Check specifically for costovertebral angle (CVA) tenderness, abdominal tenderness with guarding, and rebound tenderness.

Medical causes

● *Abdominal aortic aneurysm (dissecting).* Initially, this life-threatening disorder may produce dull abdominal, low back, or severe chest pain. More often, it produces constant upper abdominal pain, which may worsen when the patient lies down and abate when he leans forward or sits up. Palpation may reveal an epigastric mass that pulsates before rupture but not after it.

Other findings may include mottled skin below the waist, absent femoral and pedal pulses, lower blood pressure in the legs than in the arms, mild-to-moderate abdominal tenderness with guarding, and abdominal rigidity. Signs of shock appear, such as tachycardia and tachypnea.

● *Abdominal cancer.* Abdominal pain usually occurs late in this disorder. It may be accompanied by anorexia, weight loss, weakness, depression, and abdominal mass and distention.

● *Abdominal trauma.* Generalized or localized abdominal pain occurs with possible ecchymoses on the abdomen; abdominal tenderness; vomiting; and, with hemorrhage into the peritoneal cavity, abdominal rigidity.

● *Adrenal crisis.* Severe abdominal pain appears early, along with nausea, vomiting, weakness, anorexia, and fever. Later signs are progressive loss of consciousness, hypotension, tachycardia, oliguria, and cool, clammy skin.

● *Appendicitis.* In this life-threatening disorder, dull discomfort in the epigastric or umbilical region typically precedes anorexia, nausea, and vomiting. Pain localizes at McBurney's point in the right lower quadrant, accompanied by abdominal rigidity, increasing tenderness (especially over McBurney's point), rebound tenderness, and retractive respirations. Later signs include constipation (or diarrhea), slight fever, and tachycardia.

● *Cholecystitis.* Severe pain in the right upper quadrant may arise suddenly or increase gradually over several hours and may radiate to the right shoulder, chest, or back. Accompanying it are anorexia, nausea, vomiting, fever, abdominal rigidity, tenderness and a palpable mass in the right upper quadrant, pallor, and diaphoresis.

● *Cholelithiasis.* Sudden, severe, and paroxysmal pain in the right upper quadrant may last several minutes to several hours and may radiate to the epigastrium, back, or shoulder blades. It's accompanied by anorexia, nausea, vomiting (sometimes bilious), low-

grade fever, diaphoresis, restlessness, a palpable abdominal mass, and abdominal tenderness with guarding over the gallbladder or biliary duct.

● *Cirrhosis.* Dull abdominal aching occurs early, usually with anorexia, indigestion, nausea, vomiting, constipation, or diarrhea. Subsequent right upper quadrant pain worsens when the patient sits up or leans forward. Associated signs include fever, ascites, leg edema, weight gain, hepatomegaly, jaundice, severe pruritus, bleeding tendencies, palmar erythema, and spider angiomas.

● *Congestive heart failure.* Right upper quadrant pain commonly accompanies this disorder's hallmarks: neck vein distention, dyspnea, tachycardia, and peripheral edema. Other findings may include nausea, vomiting, ascites, productive cough, rales, cool extremities, and cyanotic nail beds.

● *Crohn's disease.* An *acute* attack causes severe, cramping pain in the lower abdomen, typically preceded by weeks or months of milder, cramping pain. It may also cause diarrhea or constipation, bloody stools, hyperactive bowel sounds, high fever, abdominal tenderness with guarding, and possibly a palpable mass in a lower quadrant.

Milder *chronic* symptoms include right lower quadrant pain with diarrhea, steatorrhea, and weight loss.

● *Cystitis.* Abdominal pain and tenderness are usually suprapubic. Associated signs and symptoms include malaise, flank pain, low back pain, nausea, vomiting, urinary frequency, nocturia, dysuria, fever, and chills.

● *Diabetic ketoacidosis.* Rarely, severe, sharp, shooting, and girdling pain may persist for several days. Fruity breath odor, a weak and rapid pulse, Kussmaul's respirations, and poor skin turgor also appear.

● *Diverticulitis.* Mild diverticulitis usually produces intermittent, diffuse abdominal pain, which is sometimes relieved by defecation or passage of flatus. Other signs and symptoms include nausea, constipation, low-grade fever, and frequently a palpable abdominal mass. Rupture causes left lower quadrant pain, abdominal rigidity, and possible signs of sepsis and shock (high fever, chills, and hypotension).

• *Duodenal ulcer.* Localized abdominal pain—described as steady, gnawing, burning, aching, or hungerlike—may occur high in the midepigastrium or slightly off center, usually on the right. It usually doesn't radiate unless pancreatic penetration occurs. Commonly, pain begins 2 to 4 hours after meals and may cause nocturnal awakening. Ingestion of food or antacids brings relief until the cycle starts again but also may produce weight gain. Other symptoms include changes in bowel habits, and heartburn or retrosternal burning.

• *Ectopic pregnancy.* Lower abdominal pain may be sharp, dull, or cramping, and constant or intermittent in this potentially life-threatening disorder. Vaginal bleeding, nausea, and vomiting may occur, along with urinary frequency, a tender adnexal mass, and a 1- to 2-month history of amenorrhea. Rupture of the fallopian tube produces sharp lower abdominal pain, which may radiate to the shoulders and neck and become extreme with cervical or adnexal palpation. Signs of shock, such as pallor, tachycardia, and hypotension, may also appear.

• *Endometriosis.* Constant, severe pain in the lower abdomen usually begins 5 to 7 days before menstruation begins and may be aggravated by defecation. Depending on the location of the ectopic tissue, the pain may be accompanied by constipation, abdominal tenderness, dysmenorrhea, dyspareunia, and deep sacral pain.

• *Gastric ulcer.* Diffuse, gnawing, burning pain in the left upper quadrant or epigastric area often occurs 1 to 2 hours after meals and may be relieved by food or antacids. Vague bloating and nausea after eating are common. Indigestion, weight change, anorexia, and episodes of GI bleeding also occur.

• *Gastritis.* In *acute gastritis*, abdominal pain can range from mild epigastric discomfort to burning pain in the left upper quadrant. Other typical features include belching, fever, malaise, anorexia, nausea, bloody or coffee-ground vomitus, and melena. In *chronic gastritis*, weight loss may also occur.

• *Gastroenteritis.* Cramping or colicky abdominal pain, which can be diffuse, originates in the left upper quadrant and radiates or migrates to the other quadrants. It's accompanied by diarrhea, hyperactive bowel sounds, headache, myalgia, nausea, and vomiting.

• *Hepatic abscess.* Abdominal pain that is steady, severe, and located in the right upper quadrant or midepigastrium frequently accompanies this rare disorder, although right upper quadrant tenderness is the most important finding. Other signs and symptoms are anorexia, diarrhea, nausea, fever, diaphoresis, and, infrequently, vomiting.

• *Hepatic amebiasis.* This disorder, rare in the United States, causes relatively severe right upper quadrant pain and tenderness over the liver and possibly the right shoulder. Accompanying signs and symptoms include fever, weakness, weight loss, chills, diaphoresis, and jaundiced or brownish skin.

• *Hepatitis.* Liver enlargement from any type of hepatitis will cause discomfort or dull pain and tenderness in the right upper quadrant. Associated signs and symptoms may include dark urine, clay-colored stools, nausea, vomiting, anorexia, jaundice, and pruritus.

• *Herpes zoster.* Herpes zoster of the thoracic, lumbar, or sacral nerves can cause localized abdominal and chest pain in the area these nerves serve. Pain, tenderness, and fever can precede or accompany erythematous papules.

• *Insect toxins.* Generalized, cramping abdominal pain usually occurs with low-grade fever, nausea, vomiting, abdominal rigidity, tremors, and burning sensations in the hands or feet.

• *Intestinal obstruction.* Short episodes of intense, colicky, cramping pain alternate with pain-free intervals in this life-threatening disorder. Accompa-

ABDOMINAL PAIN: CAUSES AND ASSOCIATED FINDINGS

S&S CAUSES	\<MAJOR ASSOCIATED SIGNS AND SYMPTOMS\> Abdominal distention	Abdominal mass	Abdominal rigidity	Abdominal tenderness	Amenorrhea	Anorexia	Bowel sounds—absent	Bowel sounds—hyperactive	Bowel sounds—hypoactive	Breath odor, fruity	
Abdominal aortic aneurysm		●	●	●							
Abdominal cancer	●	●				●					
Adrenal crisis						●					
Appendicitis			●	●		●					
Cholecystitis		●	●	●		●					
Cholelithiasis		●		●		●					
Cirrhosis	●					●					
Congestive heart failure	●										
Crohn's disease		●		●				●			
Cystitis				●							
Diabetic ketoacidosis										●	
Diverticulitis		●	●								
Duodenal ulcer											
Ectopic pregnancy		●			●						
Endometriosis				●							
Gastric ulcer						●					
Gastritis						●					
Gastroenteritis								●			
Hepatic abscess				●		●					
Hepatic amebiasis				●							
Hepatitis				●		●					

Chest pain	Constipation	Cough	CVA tenderness	Diarrhea	Dyspnea	Fever	Kussmaul's respirations	Nausea	Oliguria/anuria	Skin lesions	Skin mottling	Tachycardia	Tachypnea	Urinary frequency	Vomiting	Weakness	Weight change
•											•	•	•				
																•	•
						•		•	•			•			•	•	
	•			•		•		•				•			•		
•						•		•							•		
						•		•							•		
	•			•		•		•							•		•
		•			•			•				•			•		
	•			•		•											•
						•		•						•	•		
							•					•					
	•					•		•									
•	•		•														•
								•						•	•		
	•																
								•									•
						•		•							•		•
				•				•							•		
				•		•		•							•		
						•										•	•
								•							•		

(continued)

ABDOMINAL PAIN: CAUSES AND ASSOCIATED FINDINGS *(continued)*

S&S CAUSES	MAJOR ASSOCIATED SIGNS AND SYMPTOMS										
	Abdominal distention	Abdominal mass	Abdominal rigidity	Abdominal tenderness	Amenorrhea	Anorexia	Bowel sounds—absent	Bowel sounds—hyperactive	Bowel sounds—hypoactive	Breath odor, fruity	
Herpes zoster				•							
Intestinal obstruction	•			•			•	•	•		
Irritable bowel syndrome	•			•							
Mesenteric artery ischemia			•	•		•					
Myocardial infarction											
Ovarian cyst	•	•		•	•						
Pancreatitis			•	•					•		
Pelvic inflammatory disease		•		•							
Perforated ulcer			•	•			•				
Peritonitis	•		•	•			•		•		
Pleurisy											
Pneumonia			•	•							
Pneumothorax											
Prostatitis											
Pyelonephritis				•							
Renal calculi											
Sickle cell crisis											
Ulcerative colitis				•		•			•		
Uremia				•		•					

Chest pain	Constipation	Cough	CVA tenderness	Diarrhea	Dyspnea	Fever	Kussmaul's respirations	Nausea	Oliguria/anuria	Skin lesions	Skin mottling	Tachycardia	Tachypnea	Urinary frequency	Vomiting	Weakness	Weight change
•						•				•							
	•							•				•	•		•		
	•			•				•									
	•			•								•	•		•		
•					•			•							•	•	
						•		•							•		
						•		•				•			•		
						•		•							•		
						•						•					
						•		•				•	•		•		
•													•				
•		•			•	•											
•					•							•	•	•			
						•											
			•			•		•							•	•	
			•			•		•							•		
•					•	•										•	
				•		•		•							•		•
				•				•	•						•		

nying signs and symptoms may include abdominal distention, tenderness, and guarding; visible peristaltic waves; high-pitched, tinkling, or hyperactive sounds proximal to obstruction and hypoactive or absent sounds distally; obstipation; and pain-induced agitation. In jejunal and duodenal obstruction, nausea and bilious vomiting occur early. In distal small-bowel or large-bowel obstruction, nausea and vomiting are often feculent. Complete obstruction produces absent bowel sounds. Late-stage obstruction produces signs of hypovolemic shock, such as hypotension and tachycardia.

• *Irritable bowel syndrome.* Lower abdominal cramping or pain is aggravated by eating coarse or raw foods and may be alleviated by defecation or passage of flatus. Related findings include abdominal tenderness, diurnal diarrhea alternating with constipation or normal bowel function, and small stools with visible mucus. Dyspepsia, nausea, and abdominal distention may also occur. Stress, anxiety, and emotional lability intensify the symptoms.

• *Mesenteric artery ischemia.* Severe, constant, and diffuse abdominal pain is preceded by 2 to 3 days of colicky periumbilical pain and diarrhea. Associated findings include vomiting, anorexia, alternating periods of diarrhea and constipation, and, in late stages, extreme abdominal tenderness with rigidity, tachycardia, tachypnea, and cool, clammy skin.

• *Myocardial infarction.* Substernal chest pain may radiate to the abdomen in this life-threatening disorder. Associated signs and symptoms include weakness, diaphoresis, nausea, vomiting, anxiety, and dyspnea.

• *Ovarian cyst.* Torsion or hemorrhage causes pain and tenderness in the right or left lower abdominal quadrant. Sharp and severe if the patient suddenly stands or stoops, the pain becomes brief and intermittent if the torsion self-corrects, or dull and diffuse after several hours if it doesn't. Pain is accompanied by slight fever, mild nausea and vomiting, abdominal tenderness and a palpable mass, and possibly amenorrhea. Abdominal distention may occur with large cysts. Peritoneal irritation, or rupture and peritonitis, causes high fever and severe nausea and vomiting.

• *Pancreatitis.* Life-threatening *acute pancreatitis* produces fulminating, continuous upper abdominal pain that may radiate to both flanks and to the back. To relieve this flain, the patient may bend forward, draw his knees to his chest, or move restlessly about. Early findings include abdominal tenderness, nausea, vomiting, fever, pallor, tachycardia, and, in some patients, abdominal rigidity, rebound tenderness, and hypoactive bowel sounds. Grey Turner's or Cullen's sign signals hemorrhagic pancreatitis. As inflammation subsides, jaundice may occur.

Chronic pancreatitis produces severe left upper quadrant or epigastric pain that radiates to the back. Abdominal tenderness, a midepigastric mass, jaundice, fever, and splenomegaly may occur. Steatorrhea and weight loss are common.

• *Pelvic inflammatory disease.* Pain in the right or left lower quadrant ranges from vague discomfort worsened by movement to deep, severe, and progressive pain. Sometimes, metrorrhagia precedes or accompanies the onset of pain. Extreme pain accompanies cervical or adnexal palpation. Associated findings may include abdominal tenderness, a palpable abdominal or pelvic mass, fever, occasional chills, nausea, vomiting, and abnormal vaginal bleeding.

• *Perforated ulcer.* In this life-threatening disorder, sudden, severe, and prostrating epigastric pain may radiate through the abdomen to the back. Other signs and symptoms include boardlike abdominal rigidity, tenderness with guarding, generalized rebound tenderness, absent bowel sounds, grunting and shallow respirations, and, often, fever, tachycardia, and hypotension.

• *Peritonitis.* In this life-threatening disorder, sudden and severe pain can be diffuse or localized in the area of the underlying disorder; movement worsens the pain. The degree of abdominal tenderness usually depends on the disease's extent. Typical findings include fever; chills; nausea; vomiting; hypoactive or absent bowel sounds; abdominal tenderness, distention, and rigidity; rebound tenderness and guarding; hyperalgesia; tachycardia; hypotension; and tachypnea.

• *Pleurisy.* This disorder may produce upper abdominal or costal margin pain referred from the chest. Characteristic sharp, stabbing chest pain increases with inspiration and movement. Frequently, a pleural friction rub and rapid, shallow breathing occur.

• *Pneumonia.* Lower lobe pneumonia can cause pleuritic chest pain and referred, severe upper abdominal pain, tenderness, and rigidity that diminish with inspiration. It can also cause fever, shaking chills, achiness, headache, blood-tinged or rusty sputum, a dry, hacking cough, and dyspnea.

• *Pneumothorax.* This potentially life-threatening disorder can cause pain across the upper abdomen and costal margin that's referred from the chest. Characteristic chest pain arises suddenly and worsens with deep inspiration or movement. Accompanying signs and symptoms include anxiety, dyspnea, cyanosis, decreased or absent breath sounds over the affected area, tachypnea, and tachycardia.

• *Prostatitis.* Vague abdominal pain or discomfort in the lower abdomen, groin, perineum, or rectum may develop. Other findings may include dysuria, urinary frequency and urgency, fever, chills, lower back pain, myalgia, and arthralgia.

• *Pyelonephritis (acute).* Progressive lower quadrant pain in one or both sides, flank pain, and CVA tenderness characterize this disorder. Pain may radiate to the lower midabdomen or to the groin. Additional signs and symptoms may include abdominal and back tenderness, high fever, shaking chills, nausea, vomiting, and urinary frequency and urgency.

• *Renal calculi.* Depending on the location of calculi, severe abdominal or back pain may occur. However, the classic symptom is severe, colicky pain that travels from the CVA to the flank, the suprapubic region, and the external genitalia. The pain may be excruciating or dull and constant. Pain-induced agitation, nausea, vomiting, abdominal distention, fever, chills, and urinary urgency may occur.

• *Sickle cell crisis.* Sudden, severe abdominal pain may accompany chest, back, hand, or foot pain. Associated signs and symptoms may include weakness, aching joints, dyspnea, and scleral jaundice.

• *Splenic infarction.* Fulminating pain in the left upper quadrant occurs along with chest pain that may worsen on inspiration. Pain often radiates to the left shoulder with splinting of the left diaphragm, abdominal guarding, and occasionally a splenic friction rub.

• *Systemic lupus erythematosus.* Generalized abdominal pain is unusual but may occur after meals. Butterfly rash, photosensitivity, alopecia, mucous membrane ulcers, and nondeforming arthritis are characteristic. Other common signs and symptoms include anorexia, vomiting, abdominal tenderness with guarding, and abdominal distention after meals.

• *Ulcerative colitis.* This disorder may begin with vague abdominal discomfort that leads to cramping lower abdominal pain. As the disorder progresses, pain can become steady and diffuse, increasing with movement and coughing. The most common symptom—recurrent and possibly severe diarrhea with blood, pus, and mucus—may relieve the pain. The abdomen may feel soft, squashy, and extremely tender. High-pitched, infrequent bowel sounds may accompany nausea, vomiting, anorexia, weight loss, and mild, intermittent fever.

• *Uremia.* Characterized by generalized or periumbilical pain that shifts and varies in intensity, this disorder causes diverse GI symptoms, such as nausea, anorexia, vomiting, and diarrhea. Abdominal tenderness that changes in location and intensity may occur, along with visual disturbances, bleeding, headache, decreased level of consciousness, vertigo, and oliguria or anuria.

Other causes
● *Drugs.* Salicylates and nonsteroidal anti-inflammatory drugs commonly cause burning, gnawing pain in the left upper quadrant or epigastric area, along with nausea and vomiting.

Special considerations
Help the patient find a comfortable position, if possible, to ease his distress. Closely monitor his status because abdominal pain can signal a life-threatening disorder. Notify the doctor immediately if you detect tachycardia, hypotension, clammy skin, abdominal rigidity, rebound tenderness, a change in the pain's location or intensity, or sudden relief from pain.

Before diagnosis, withhold analgesics since they may mask symptoms. Also withhold food and fluids, since surgery may be needed, and prepare for I.V. infusion. If ordered, prepare to insert a nasogastric or other intestinal tube and to assist with peritoneal lavage or abdominal paracentesis.

As ordered, prepare the patient for procedures to help establish diagnosis. These may include pelvic or rectal examination; blood, urine, and stool tests; X-rays; barium studies; ultrasonography; endoscopy; or biopsy.

Pediatric pointers
Because a child often has difficulty describing abdominal pain, pay close attention to nonverbal cues—wincing, lethargy, or unusual positioning (such as a side-lying position with knees flexed to the abdomen).

In children, abdominal pain can signal a disorder with greater severity or different associated signs than in adults. Appendicitis, for example, has a higher rupture rate and mortality in children, and vomiting may be the only

other sign. Acute pyelonephritis may cause abdominal pain, vomiting, and diarrhea, but not the classic urologic signs found in adults. Peptic ulcer, which is becoming increasingly common in teenagers, causes nocturnal pain and colic that, unlike peptic ulcer in adults, may not be relieved by food.

Abdominal pain in children can also result from lactose intolerance, allergic-tension-fatigue syndrome, volvulus, Meckel's diverticulum, intussusception, mesenteric adenitis, diabetes mellitus, juvenile rheumatoid arthritis, and many uncommon disorders, such as heavy metal poisoning. Remember, too, that a child's complaint of abdominal pain may reflect an emotional need, such as a wish to avoid school or to gain adult attention.

Abdominal Rigidity
[Abdominal muscle spasm, involuntary guarding]

Detected by palpation, abdominal rigidity refers to abnormal muscle tension or inflexibility of the abdomen. Rigidity may be voluntary or involuntary. Voluntary rigidity reflects the patient's fear or nervousness upon palpation, while involuntary rigidity reflects potentially life-threatening peritoneal irritation or inflammation.

Involuntary rigidity most commonly results from gastrointestinal disorders, but may also result from pulmonary and vascular disorders and from the effects of insect toxins. Usually, it occurs with nausea, vomiting, and abdominal tenderness, distention, and pain.

Assessment
After palpating abdominal rigidity, quickly take the patient's vital signs and have another nurse notify the doctor. Even

though the patient may not appear gravely ill or have markedly abnormal vital signs, his abdominal rigidity calls for emergency intervention. Prepare to administer oxygen and to insert an I.V. line for fluid and blood replacement. The doctor may also order drugs to support blood pressure. Prepare to catheterize the patient, as ordered, and monitor intake and output. Also be ready to assist with insertion of an intestinal tube to relieve abdominal distention. Because emergency surgery may be necessary, prepare the patient for laboratory tests and X-rays, as ordered.

If the patient's condition allows further assessment, take a brief history. Find out when the abdominal rigidity began. Is it associated with abdominal pain? If so, did the pain begin at the same time? Determine whether abdominal rigidity is localized or generalized. Is it always present? Has its site changed or remained constant? Next ask about aggravating or alleviating factors, such as position changes, coughing, vomiting, elimination, and walking.

Then explore other signs and symptoms. Inspect the abdomen for peristaltic waves, which may be visible in very thin patients. Also check for a visible distended bowel loop. Next, auscultate bowel sounds. Perform light palpation to locate the rigidity and determine its severity. Avoid deep palpation, which may exacerbate abdominal pain. Finally, check for poor skin turgor and dry mucous membranes, indicating dehydration.

Medical causes

● *Dissecting abdominal aortic aneurysm.* Mild-to-moderate abdominal rigidity occurs in this life-threatening disorder. Typically, it's accompanied by constant upper abdominal pain that may radiate to the lower back. The pain may worsen when the patient lies down and may be relieved when he leans forward or sits up. Before rupture, the aneurysm may produce a pulsating mass in the

---

RECOGNIZING VOLUNTARY RIGIDITY

Distinguishing voluntary and involuntary abdominal rigidity is a must for accurate nursing assessment. Review this comparison so that you can quickly tell the two apart.

Voluntary rigidity is:
● usually symmetric
● more rigid on inspiration (expiration causes muscle relaxation)
● eased by relaxation techniques, such as positioning the patient comfortably and talking to him in a calm, soothing manner
● painless when the patient sits up using his abdominal muscles alone.

Involuntary rigidity is:
● usually asymmetric
● equally rigid on inspiration and expiration
● unaffected by relaxation techniques
● painful when the patient sits up using his abdominal muscles alone.

---

epigastrium, accompanied by a systolic bruit over the aorta. However, the mass stops pulsating after rupture. Associated signs and symptoms may include mottled skin below the waist, absent femoral and pedal pulses, lower blood pressure in the legs than in the arms, and mild-to-moderate tenderness with guarding. Significant blood loss causes signs of shock, such as tachycardia, tachypnea, and cool, clammy skin.

● *Insect toxins.* Insect stings and bites, especially black widow spider bites, release toxins that can produce generalized, cramping abdominal pain usually accompanied by rigidity. These toxins may also cause low-grade fever, nausea, vomiting, tremors, and burning sensations in the hands and feet.

● *Mesenteric artery ischemia.* Two to three days of persistent, low-grade abdominal pain and diarrhea precede abdominal rigidity in this life-threatening disorder. Rigidity occurs in the central or periumbilical region and is accompanied by severe abdominal tenderness, fever, and signs of shock such as tachycardia and hypotension. Other findings may include vomiting, anorexia, diarrhea, or constipation.

• **Peritonitis.** Depending on the cause of peritonitis, abdominal rigidity may be localized or generalized. For example, if an inflamed appendix causes local peritonitis, rigidity may be localized in the right lower quadrant. If a perforated ulcer causes widespread peritonitis, rigidity may be generalized and, in severe cases, boardlike.

Peritonitis also causes sudden and severe abdominal pain that can be localized or generalized. It can also produce abdominal tenderness and distention, rebound tenderness, guarding, hyperalgesia, hypoactive or absent bowel sounds, nausea, and vomiting. Usually, the patient also displays fever, chills, tachycardia, tachypnea, and hypotension.

• **Pneumonia.** In lower lobe pneumonia, severe upper abdominal pain and tenderness accompany rigidity that diminishes with inspiration. Associated signs and symptoms include a dry, hacking cough, blood-tinged or rusty sputum, dyspnea, achiness, headache, fever, and sudden onset of chills.

Special considerations

Continue to monitor the patient closely for signs of shock. Position him as comfortably as possible. Until the doctor makes a tentative diagnosis, withhold analgesics since they may mask symptoms. Because emergency surgery may be required, withhold food and fluids and, if ordered, administer I.V. antibiotics. Prepare the patient for diagnostic tests, which may include blood, urine, and stool studies; chest and abdominal X-rays; peritoneal lavage; and gastroscopy or colonoscopy. A pelvic or rectal examination may also be done.

Pediatric pointers

Voluntary rigidity may be difficult to distinguish from involuntary rigidity if associated pain makes the child restless, tense, or apprehensive. However, in any child with suspected involuntary rigidity, your priority is early detection of dehydration and shock, which can rapidly become life-threatening.

Abdominal rigidity in the child can stem from gastric perforation, hypertrophic pyloric stenosis, duodenal obstruction, meconium ileus, intussusception, cystic fibrosis, celiac disease, and appendicitis.

Accessory Muscle Use

The accessory muscles—the sternocleidomastoid, scalene, pectoralis major, trapezius, internal intercostals, and abdominal muscles—help the diaphragm maintain respiration when breathing requires *extra* effort. Some accessory muscle use normally takes place during singing, talking, coughing, defecating, and exercising. However, more pronounced use of these muscles may signal acute respiratory distress. It may also result from chronic respiratory disease or the effects of tests and treatments. Typically, the extent of accessory muscle use reflects the severity of the underlying cause.

Assessment

If the patient displays increased accessory muscle use, quickly observe for signs of acute respiratory distress: decreased level of consciousness, shortness of breath when speaking, tachypnea, intercostal and sternal retractions, cyanosis, external breath sounds like wheezing or stridor, diaphoresis, nasal flaring, and extreme apprehension or agitation. If you detect most of these signs, quickly auscultate for abnormal, diminished, or absent breath sounds and have another nurse notify the doctor immediately. Check for airway obstruction and, if detected, attempt to restore airway patency. Insert an airway or assist with intubation. Then begin suctioning and manual or me-

REVIEWING ACCESSORY MUSCLE LOCATION AND FUNCTION

Physical exertion and pulmonary disease often increase the work of breathing, taxing the diaphragm and external intercostal muscles. When this happens, accessory muscles provide the extra effort needed to maintain respirations. The upper accessory muscles assist with inspiration, while the upper chest, sternum, the internal intercostal and abdominal muscles assist with expiration.

In inspiration, the scalene muscles elevate, fix, and expand the upper chest.

The sternocleidomastoid muscles raise the sternum, expanding the chest's anteroposterior and longitudinal dimensions. The pectoralis majors elevate the chest, increasing its anteroposterior size, and trapezius muscles raise the thoracic cage.

In expiration, the internal intercostals depress the ribs, decreasing the chest size. The abdominal muscles pull the lower chest down, depress the lower ribs, and compress the abdominal contents, which exerts pressure on the chest.

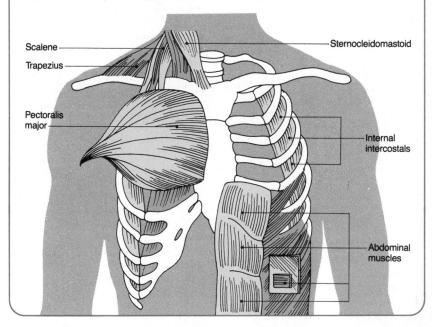

Scalene — Sternocleidomastoid
Trapezius —
Pectoralis major —
Internal intercostals
Abdominal muscles

chanical ventilation. Administer oxygen; if the patient has chronic obstructive pulmonary disease (COPD), use a low flow rate. Insert an I.V. line, if ordered.

When appropriate, assess the patient more fully. Ask him about the onset, duration, and severity of associated symptoms, such as dyspnea, chest pain, cough, or fever. Then explore his medical history, focusing on respiratory disorders, such as infection or COPD. Also ask about cardiac disorders, such as congestive heart failure, which may

lead to pulmonary edema; and about neuromuscular disorders, such as amyotrophic lateral sclerosis, which may affect respiratory muscle function. Note a history of allergies or asthma. Because collagen diseases can cause diffuse infiltrative lung disease, ask about such conditions as rheumatoid arthritis and lupus erythematosus. Next, ask about recent trauma, especially to the spine or chest. Also determine if the patient has recently undergone pulmonary function tests or received respiratory therapy. Ask about smoking, which can aggravate respiratory disorders, and about occupational exposure to chemical fumes or mineral dusts such as asbestos, which can cause diffuse infiltrative lung disease. Explore the family history for such disorders as cystic fibrosis and neurofibromatosis, which can cause diffuse infiltrative lung disease.

Perform a detailed chest examination, noting abnormal respiratory rate, rhythm, or depth. Assess the color, temperature, and turgor of the patient's skin, and check for clubbing.

Medical causes

• *Adult respiratory distress syndrome.* In this life-threatening disorder, accessory muscle use increases in response to hypoxia. It's accompanied by intercostal, supracostal, and sternal retractions on inspiration and by grunting on expiration. Other characteristics include tachypnea, dyspnea, diaphoresis, diffuse crackles, and a cough with pink, frothy sputum. Worsening hypoxia produces anxiety, tachycardia, and mental sluggishness.

• *Airway obstruction.* Acute upper airway obstruction can be life-threatening—fortunately, most obstructions are subacute or chronic. Typically, this disorder increases accessory muscle use. Its most telling sign, however, is inspiratory stridor. Associated signs and symptoms often include dyspnea, tachypnea, gasping, wheezing, coughing, intercostal retractions, cyanosis, and tachycardia.

• *Amyotrophic lateral sclerosis.* Typically, this progressive motor neuron disorder affects the diaphragm, but not the accessory muscles. As a result, increased accessory muscle use is characteristic. It's accompanied by fasciculations, muscle atrophy and weakness, spasticity, bilateral Babinski's reflex, and hyperactive deep tendon reflexes. Incoordination makes carrying out routine activities difficult for the patient. Associated signs and symptoms include impaired speech; difficulty chewing, swallowing, and

breathing; urinary frequency and urgency; and, occasionally, choking and excessive drooling. Although the patient's mental status remains intact, his poor prognosis may cause periodic depression.

• *Asthma.* During acute asthmatic attacks, the patient usually displays increased accessory muscle use. Accompanying it are severe dyspnea, tachypnea, wheezing, productive cough, nasal flaring, and cyanosis. Auscultation reveals faint breath sounds, musical crackles, and rhonchi. Other signs and symptoms include tachycardia, diaphoresis, and apprehension caused by air hunger. Chronic asthma may also cause barrel chest and clubbing.

• *Chronic bronchitis.* In this form of COPD, increased accessory muscle use is preceded by productive cough and exertional dyspnea. It's accompanied by wheezing, basal crackles, tachypnea, neck vein distention, prolonged expiration, barrel chest, and clubbing. Cyanosis and weight gain from edema account for the characteristic label of "blue bloater." Low-grade fever may occur with secondary infection.

• *Diffuse infiltrative (or fibrotic) lung disease.* In this disorder, progressive pulmonary degeneration eventually increases accessory muscle use. Typically, though, the patient reports progressive dyspnea on exertion as his chief complaint. He may also have cough, anorexia, weakness, fatigue, vague chest pain, tachypnea, and crackles at the base of the lungs.

• *Emphysema.* Increased accessory muscle use occurs with progressive dyspnea on exertion and minimally productive cough in this form of COPD. Sometimes called the "pink puffer," the patient will display pursed-lip breathing and tachypnea. Associated signs and symptoms include peripheral cyanosis, anorexia, weight loss, malaise, barrel chest, and clubbing. Auscultation reveals distant heart sounds; percussion detects hyperresonance.

• *Pneumonia.* Bacterial pneumonia

most commonly produces increased accessory muscle use. Initially, this infection produces sudden high fever with chills. Its associated signs and symptoms include chest pain, productive cough, dyspnea, tachypnea, tachycardia, expiratory grunting, cyanosis, diaphoresis, and fine crackles.

● *Pulmonary edema.* In acute pulmonary edema, increased accessory muscle use is accompanied by dyspnea, tachypnea, orthopnea, crepitant crackles, wheezing, and a cough with pink, frothy sputum. Other findings: restlessness, tachycardia, ventricular gallop, and cool, clammy, cyanotic skin.

● *Pulmonary embolism.* Although signs and symptoms vary with the size, num-

ACCESSORY MUSCLE USE: CAUSES AND ASSOCIATED FINDINGS

CAUSES	Barrel chest	Chest pain	Cough	Crackles	Cyanosis	Diaphoresis	Dyspnea	Fever	Muscle weakness	Paralysis	Stridor	Tachycardia	Tachypnea	Wheezing
Adult respiratory distress syndrome			●	●		●	●					●	●	
Airway obstruction			●		●		●				●	●	●	●
Amyotrophic lateral sclerosis							●		●					
Asthma	●		●	●	●	●	●					●	●	●
Chronic bronchitis	●		●	●	●		●	●					●	●
Diffuse infiltrative lung disease		●	●	●			●						●	
Emphysema	●		●		●		●						●	
Pneumonia		●	●	●	●	●	●	●				●	●	
Pulmonary edema			●	●	●		●					●	●	●
Pulmonary embolism		●	●	●	●		●	●				●	●	●
Spinal cord injury									●	●				
Thoracic injury		●			●		●					●		

ber, and location of the emboli, this life-threatening disorder may cause increased accessory muscle use. Commonly, it produces dyspnea and tachypnea that may be accompanied by pleuritic or substernal chest pain. Other signs include restlessness, tachycardia, productive cough, low-grade fever, and, with a large embolus, hemoptysis, cyanosis, syncope, neck vein distention, scattered crackles, or focal wheezing.

• *Spinal cord injury.* Increased accessory muscle use may occur, depending on the location and severity of injury. Injury below L1 typically doesn't affect the diaphragm or accessory muscles, whereas injury between C3 and C5 affects only the upper respiratory muscles and diaphragm, causing increased accessory muscle use.

Associated signs and symptoms of spinal cord injury may include unilateral or bilateral Babinski's reflex; hyperactive deep tendon reflexes; spasticity; and variable or total loss of pain and temperature sensation, proprioception, and motor function. Horner's syndrome (unilateral ptosis, pupillary constriction, facial anhydrosis) may occur with lower cervical cord injury.

• *Thoracic injury.* Increased accessory muscle use may occur, depending on the type and extent of injury. Associated signs and symptoms of this potentially life-threatening injury may include an obvious chest wound or bruising, chest pain, dyspnea, cyanosis, and agitation. Signs of shock, such as tachycardia and hypotension, occur with significant blood loss.

Other causes
• *Diagnostic tests and treatments.* Pulmonary function tests, incentive spirometry, and widely used intermittent positive pressure breathing can increase accessory muscle use.

Special considerations
Because labored breathing can make the patient apprehensive, provide emotional support. If the patient is alert,

elevate the head of the bed to make his breathing as easy as possible. Allow him to get plenty of rest, and encourage fluid intake to liquefy secretions. Administer oxygen, as ordered. Prepare him for such tests as pulmonary function studies, chest X-rays, lung scans, arterial blood gas analysis, complete blood count, and sputum culture.

If appropriate, stress how smoking endangers the patient's health, and refer him to an organized program to stop smoking. Also teach him how to prevent infection. Explain the purpose of prescribed drugs, such as bronchodilators and mucolytics, and make sure he knows their dosage and schedule.

Pediatric pointers
Because an infant or child tires sooner than an adult, respiratory distress can more rapidly precipitate respiratory failure. Upper airway obstruction—caused by edema, bronchospasm, or a foreign object—most commonly produces respiratory distress and increased accessory muscle use. Disorders associated with airway obstruction include acute epiglottitis, croup, pertussis, cystic fibrosis, and asthma.

Agitation

Agitation refers to a state of hyperarousal, increased tension, and irritability that can lead to confusion, hyperactivity, and overt hostility. This common sign can result from various disorders, pain, fever, anxiety, drug use and withdrawal, and hypersensitivity reactions. It can arise gradually or suddenly and last for minutes or months. Whether it's mild or severe, agitation worsens with increased fever, pain, stress, or external stimuli.

By itself, agitation merely signals a change in the patient's condition. But when considered in light of his history, current status, and other signs and symptoms, it becomes a more useful indicator of a developing disorder.

Assessment

Determine the severity of the patient's agitation by assessing the number and quality of agitation-induced behaviors, such as emotional lability, confusion, memory loss, hyperactivity, and hostility. If possible, obtain a history from the patient or a family member, including diet and known allergies. Ask if the patient is currently being treated for any illnesses. Has he had any recent infections, trauma, stress, or changes in sleep patterns? Ask about the use and dosage of any prescribed or over-the-counter drugs. Check for signs of drug abuse, such as needle tracks or dilated pupils. Ask about the patient's usual alcohol intake and the time of his last drink.

To obtain baseline data for future comparison, check and record the patient's vital signs and neurologic status.

Medical causes

● *Alcohol withdrawal syndrome.* Mild-to-severe agitation occurs in this syndrome, which is marked by hyperactivity, tremors, and anxiety. In *delirium tremens*, the potentially life-threatening stage of alcohol withdrawal, severe agitation occurs with visual hallucinations, insomnia, diaphoresis, and depression. Pulse rate and temperature rise as withdrawal progresses, and status epilepticus, cardiac exhaustion, and shock can occur.

● *Anxiety.* This common symptom produces varying degrees of agitation. The patient may be unaware of his anxiety or may complain of it without knowing its cause. Associated findings may include nausea, vomiting, diarrhea, cool and clammy skin, frontal headache, back pain, insomnia, and tremors.

● *Chronic renal failure.* Moderate-to-severe agitation occurs here, marked especially by confusion and memory loss. It's accompanied by diverse signs and symptoms, such as nausea, vomiting, anorexia, mouth ulcers, ammonia

breath odor, GI bleeding, pallor, edema, dry skin, and uremic frost.

● *Dementia.* Mild-to-severe agitation can result from many common syndromes, such as Alzheimer's disease and Huntington's chorea. The patient may display a decrease in memory, attention span, problem-solving ability, and alertness. Hypoactivity, wandering behavior, hallucinations, aphasia, and insomnia may also occur.

● *Drug withdrawal syndrome.* Mild-to-severe agitation occurs in this syndrome. Related findings vary with the specific drug but may include anxiety, abdominal cramps, diaphoresis, and anorexia. In narcotic or barbiturate withdrawal, a decreased level of consciousness can occur as well as seizures and elevated blood pressure, heart, and respiratory rates.

● *Hepatic encephalopathy.* Agitation occurs only with fulminating encephalopathy. Other findings may include drowsiness, stupor, fetor hepaticus, asterixis, and hyperreflexia.

● *Hypersensitivity reaction.* Moderate-to-severe agitation appears, possibly as the first sign of a reaction. Depending on the reaction's severity, agitation may be accompanied by urticaria, pruritus, and facial and dependent edema.

In *anaphylactic shock*, a potentially life-threatening hypersensitivity reaction, agitation occurs rapidly along with apprehension or uneasiness, urticaria or diffuse erythema, warm, moist skin, paresthesias, pruritus, edema, dyspnea, wheezing, stridor, hypotension, and tachycardia. Abdominal cramps, vomiting, and diarrhea can also occur.

● *Hypoxemia.* Beginning as restlessness, agitation rapidly worsens. The patient may be confused and have impaired judgment and motor coordination. He may also have tachycardia, tachypnea, dyspnea, and cyanosis.

● *Increased intracranial pressure (ICP).* No matter what causes increased ICP, agitation usually precedes other symptoms. Other early indicators may include headache, nausea, and vomiting.

Increased ICP produces respiratory changes, such as Cheyne-Stokes, cluster, ataxic, or apneustic breathing. It also produces sluggish, nonreactive, or unequal pupils; widening pulse pressure; tachycardia; decreased level of consciousness; seizures; and motor changes, such as decerebrate or decorticate posture.

• *Organic brain syndrome.* In this syndrome, the patient's agitation is manifested as hyperactivity, emotional lability, confusion, and memory loss. In addition, the patient may display slurred or incoherent speech and paranoid behavior.

• *Post-head-trauma syndrome.* Shortly after or even years after injury, mild-to-severe agitation develops, characterized by disorientation, loss of concentration, angry outbursts, and emotional lability. Other findings include fatigue, wandering behavior, and poor judgment.

• *Vitamin B₆ deficiency.* Agitation can range from mild to severe in this deficiency. Other classic signs and symptoms include seizures, peripheral paresthesias, and dermatitis. Oculogyric crisis may also occur.

Other causes

• *Drugs.* Mild-to-moderate agitation, frequently dose-related, develops as a side effect of central nervous system stimulants—especially appetite suppressants, such as amphetamines and amphetamine-like drugs; sympathomimetic drugs such as ephedrine; caffeine; and theophylline.

• *Radiographic contrast medium.* Reaction to the contrast medium injected during various diagnostic tests produces moderate-to-severe agitation along with other signs of hypersensitivity.

Special considerations

Because agitation can be an early sign of diverse disorders, continue to monitor the patient's vital signs and neurologic status while the cause is being determined. Eliminate stressors, which can increase agitation. Provide adequate lighting, maintain a calm environment, and allow the patient ample time to sleep. Ensure a balanced diet, and provide vitamin supplements as ordered.

Encourage the patient to discuss his feelings, but be sure to remain calm, nonjudgmental, and nonargumentative. Use restraints sparingly, since they tend to increase agitation.

If appropriate, prepare the patient for diagnostic tests, such as computed tomography scanning, skull X-rays, magnetic resonance imaging, and blood studies.

Pediatric pointers

A common sign in children, agitation accompanies the expected childhood diseases as well as the more severe disorders that can lead to brain damage: hyperbilirubinemia, phenylketonuria, vitamin A deficiency, hepatitis, frontal lobe syndrome, increased ICP, and lead poisoning. In neonates, agitation can stem from alcohol or drug withdrawal if the mother abused these substances.

When assessing the agitated child, remember to use words that he can understand and to look for nonverbal cues. For instance, if you suspect that pain is causing agitation, ask him to tell you where it hurts, but be sure to watch for other indicators, such as wincing, crying, or moving away.

Alopecia

[Hair loss]

Occurring most often on the scalp, alopecia usually develops gradually and may be diffuse or patchy. It can be classified as scarring or nonscarring. Scarring alopecia, or permanent hair loss, results from hair follicle destruction, which smooths the skin surface, erasing follicular openings. Nonscarring alopecia, or temporary hair loss, results from hair follicle damage that spares follicular openings, allowing future hair growth.

Probably the most common cause of alopecia is use of antineoplastic drugs. However, alopecia may also result from use of other drugs; radiotherapy; skin, connective tissue, endocrine, nutritional, and psychological disorders; neoplasms; infection; burns; and the effects of toxins.

Normally, everyone loses about 50 hairs a day, and these hairs are replaced by new ones. However, aging, genetic predisposition, and hormonal changes may contribute to gradual recession of the hairline and hair thinning. This alopecia occurs in about 40% of adult men and may also occur in postmenopausal women. In men, hair loss commonly affects the temporal areas, producing an M-shaped hairline. In women, diffuse thinning marks the centrofrontal area. In both sexes, hair loss also occurs on the trunk, pubic area, axillae, arms, and legs. Another normal pattern of alopecia occurs 2 to 4 months postpartum. This temporary, diffuse hair loss on the scalp may be scant or dramatic and possibly accentuated at the frontal areas. Acute anxiety, high fever, and even certain hair styles or grooming methods may also cause alopecia.

Assessment

If the patient isn't receiving antineoplastic drugs or radiation therapy, begin by asking when he first noticed the hair loss or thinning. Does it affect the scalp alone or occur elsewhere on the body? Is it accompanied by itching? Then carefully explore other signs and symptoms to help distinguish between normal and pathologic hair loss. Ask about recent weight change, anorexia, nausea, vomiting, and altered bowel habits. Also ask about any urinary changes, such as hematuria or oliguria. Has the patient been especially tired or irritable? Does he have a cough or difficulty breathing? Ask about joint pain or stiffness and about heat or cold in-

tolerance. Inquire about exposure to insecticides. If the patient's female, find out if she has had menstrual irregularities. Also note her pregnancy history. Ask the male patient about impotence or decreased libido.

Next, ask about hair care. Does the patient frequently use a hot blow dryer or electric curlers? Periodically dye or bleach hair, or receive a permanent? Ask the black patient about hot combing to straighten hair. Also ask about frequent use of a long-toothed comb to achieve an Afro look, or braiding the hair in cornrows. Check for a family history of alopecia, and ask about nervous habits, such as pulling the hair or twirling it around a finger.

Begin the physical examination by assessing the extent and pattern of scalp hair loss. Is it patchy or symmetrical? Is the hair surrounding a bald area brittle or lusterless? Is it a different color than other scalp hair? Does it fall out easily? Inspect the underlying skin for follicular openings, erythema, loss of pigment, scaling, induration, broken hair shafts, and hair regrowth.

Then examine the rest of the skin. Note the size, color, texture, and location of any lesions. Check for jaundice, edema, hyperpigmentation, pallor, or duskiness. Examine nails for vertical or horizontal pitting, thickening, brittleness, or whitening. As you do so, watch for fine tremors in the hands. Observe for muscle weakness and ptosis. Palpate for lymphadenopathy, enlarged thyroid or salivary glands, and masses in the abdomen or chest. Finally, take vital signs.

Medical causes

● *Alopecia areata.* Well-circumscribed patches of nonscarring scalp alopecia usually occur in this disorder, without skin changes. Occasionally, however, the patches also appear on the beard, axillae, pubic area, arms, legs, or the entire body (alopecia universalis). "Exclamation point" hairs—loose hairs with rough, brushlike tips on narrow, less-pigmented shafts—typically border expanding patches of alopecia. Although this disorder is recurrent, hair growth usually returns after several months. In about 20% of patients, alopecia areata also causes horizontal or vertical nail pitting.

• *Alopecia mucinosa.* This uncommon disorder causes hair loss with follicular papules or plaques primarily on the head and neck; keratin and oil commonly plug these follicles.

• *Arsenic poisoning.* Most common in chronic poisoning, alopecia is diffuse and mainly affects the scalp. Related signs may include muscle weakness and wasting, areflexia, partial or total vision loss, bronze skin, and others.

• *Arterial insufficiency.* Patchy alopecia occurs in this disorder, typically on the legs, feet, and toes. It's accompanied by thin, shiny, atrophic skin and thickened nails. The skin turns pale when the patient's legs are elevated and dusky when they're dependent. Associated signs include weak or absent peripheral pulses, cool extremities, paresthesias, and intermittent claudication.

• *Burns.* Full-thickness or third-degree burns completely destroy the dermis and epidermis, leaving translucent, charred, or ulcerated skin. Scarring or keloid formation associated with these burns causes permanent alopecia.

• *Cutaneous T-cell lymphoma.* Common in older patients, this disorder may be associated with alopecia mucinosa in its first, or premycotic, stage. Scattered papules or plaques may occur on clothed areas, such as breasts and buttocks, or a zebra-like pattern of scaly erythema may form on the trunk. Alopecia may persist through the plaque and tumor stages.

• *Dissecting cellulitis of the scalp.* Resulting from infection, this disorder is characterized by small nodules that eventually rupture and drain. Keloid formation during healing causes permanent alopecia.

• *Exfoliative dermatitis.* In this transient disorder, loss of scalp and body hair is preceded by several weeks of generalized scaling and erythema. Nail loss commonly occurs, along with pruritus, malaise, fever, weight loss, lymphadenopathy, and gynecomastia.

• *Folliculitis decalvans.* This rare disorder eventually causes scarring alopecia, especially on the scalp, axillae, groin, and beard. It's characterized by inflamed hair follicles with small pustules, erythema, and scaling that leave smooth, shiny, depressed scars.

• *Fungal infections.* Tinea capitis (ringworm), the most common fungal infection, produces irregular balding areas, scaling, and erythematous lesions. As these lesions enlarge, their centers heal, causing the classic ring-shaped appearance. Surrounding the balding areas are lusterless and broken scalp hairs. When they break off at the scalp surface, hairs resemble black dots. Other findings may include pruritus and thick, whitish nails.

• *Hodgkin's lymphoma.* Permanent alopecia may occur if the lymphoma infiltrates the scalp. It's accompanied by edema, pruritus, and hyperpigmentation. Associated signs vary with the degree and location of lymphadenopathy.

• *Hypopituitarism.* In adults, this disorder typically varies greatly, depending on its severity and the number of deficient hormones. Gonadotropin deficiency in the female causes sparse or absent pubic and axillary hair accompanied by infertility, amenorrhea, and breast atrophy. A similar deficiency in the male decreases facial and body hair and causes infertility, decreased libido, poor muscle development, and undersized testes, penis, and prostate gland. A human growth hormone deficiency at an early age may cause short stature. Deficiency of thyroid-stimulating hormone produces signs of hypothyroidism; deficiency of adrenocorticotropic hormone produces signs of adrenocortical insufficiency.

• *Hypothyroidism.* In this disorder, the hair on the face, scalp, and genitals thins and becomes dull, coarse, and brittle. Most characteristic, though, is loss of the outer third of the eyebrows. Typically, it's preceded by fatigue, con-

RECOGNIZING PATTERNS OF ALOPECIA

Distinctive patterns of alopecia result from different causes. These illustrations show four of the most common patterns.

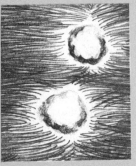

Tinea capitis, a fungal infection, produces irregular bald patches with scaly, red lesions.

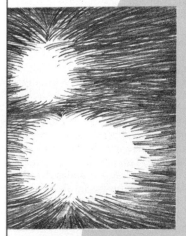

Alopecia areata causes patchy, nonscarring hair loss. "Exclamation point" hairs border expanding patches of alopecia.

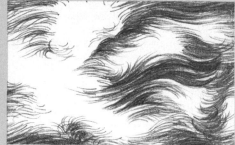

Trauma from habitual hair pulling or injudicious grooming habits may cause permanent peripheral alopecia.

Antineoplastic drugs produce diffuse, yet temporary, hair loss.

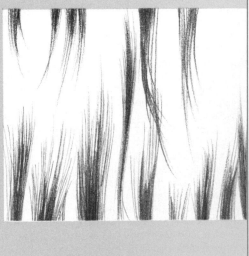

stipation, cold intolerance, and weight gain. Other signs and symptoms include dry, flaky, inelastic skin; puffy face, hands, and feet; hoarseness; thick, brittle nails; impaired mental function; bradycardia; menorrhagia; and myalgias.

• *Lichen planus.* Occasionally, this skin disorder produces patchy hair loss on the scalp with skin inflammation. Angular, flat, purple papules typically develop on the lower back, genitalia, ankles, and lower legs. Related findings include pruritus and nail changes, ranging from grooves to nail loss.

• *Lupus erythematosus.* In both discoid and systemic lupus, hair tends to become brittle and may fall out in patches. Short, broken hairs ("lupus hairs") commonly appear above the forehead. Both types of lupus are characterized by raised, red, scaling plaques with follicular plugging, telangiectasia, and central atrophy. Facial plaques often assume a distinctive butterfly pattern.

In systemic lupus, however, this rash may vary in severity from malar erythema to discoid lesions. Unlike discoid lupus, systemic lupus affects multiple body systems. It may produce photosensitivity, weight loss, fatigue, lymphadenopathy, emotional lability, and others.

• *Myotonic dystrophy.* Premature baldness characterizes the adult form of this muscular dystrophy. However, myotonia—the inability to normally relax a muscle after its contraction—is its primary sign. Associated signs include muscle wasting and cataracts.

• *Progressive systemic sclerosis.* A late sign in this disease, permanent alopecia is accompanied by thickening of the skin, especially on the arms and hands. The skin appears taut and shiny and loses its pigment. Other findings include dysphagia, dyspepsia, abdominal pain, altered bowel habits, cough, dyspnea, and signs of renal failure.

• *Protein deficiency.* This disorder produces brittle, fine, dry, and thinning hair and, occasionally, changes in its pigment. Characteristic muscle wast-

ing may be accompanied by edema, hepatomegaly, apathy, irritability, anorexia, diarrhea, and dry, flaky skin.

• *Sarcoidosis.* This disorder may produce scarring alopecia if it infiltrates the scalp. Accompanied by various lesions on the face and the oral and nasal mucosa, it may also produce fever, weight loss, fatigue, lymphadenopathy, substernal pain, visual muscle weakness, arthralgias, myalgias, and cranial nerve palsies.

• *Seborrheic dermatitis.* Erupting in areas with many sebaceous glands and in skin folds, this disorder most commonly produces hair loss on the scalp. Alopecia begins at the vertex and frontal areas and may spread to other scalp areas. The patient's skin is reddened and dry with branlike scales that flake off easily. Pruritus is common.

• *Secondary syphilis.* This infection produces temporary, patchy hair loss that gives the scalp and beard a "motheaten" appearance. It also produces loss of eyelashes and eyebrows. Accompanying alopecia is a pruritic rash that may be macular, papular, pustular, or nodular. Associated signs and symptoms may include slight fever, weight loss, sore throat, malaise, anorexia, nausea, vomiting, and headache.

• *Skin metastases.* Occasionally, cancer from an internal site, such as the lung, metastasizes to the skin, causing scarring alopecia that may develop slowly along with scalp induration and atrophy. Related findings include weight loss, fever, altered bowel habits, abdominal pain, and lymphadenopathy.

• *Thallium poisoning.* This type of poisoning produces diffuse, but temporary, hair loss on the scalp. Nausea and vomiting are also common. In acute poisoning, there may be arm and leg pain, bilateral ptosis, ataxia, fever, nasal congestion, conjunctival injection, and abdominal pain. In chronic poisoning, the skin appears translucent, thin, and shiny; signs of renal damage, such as oliguria, commonly occur.

• *Thyrotoxicosis.* Diffuse hair loss, possibly accentuated at the temples, occurs with this disorder. Hair becomes fine, soft, and friable. Uniform flushing and thickening of the skin occurs, marked by red, raised, pruritic patches. Characteristically, this disorder produces fine tremors, nervousness, an enlarged thyroid, sweating, heat intolerance, menstrual changes, palpitations, weight loss despite increased appetite, diarrhea, and possibly exophthalmos.

Other causes

• *Drugs.* Chemotherapy especially can cause alopecia. For example, bleomycin, cyclophosphamide, dactinomycin, daunorubicin, doxorubicin, fluorouracil, and methotrexate may cause patchy, reversible alopecia a few weeks after administration. Usually, hair loss is limited to the scalp, but with long-term chemotherapy, the axillae, arms, legs, face, and pubic area may also shed hair. New hair, which may differ in thickness, texture, and color from the patient's normal hair, may begin to grow after discontinuing the drug or between successive treatments.

Other common drugs may cause diffuse hair loss on the scalp a few weeks after administration. These include oral contraceptives, colchicine, heparin, warfarin, excessive doses of vitamin A, trimethadione, indomethacin, methysergide, valproic acid, carbamazepine, gentamicin, allopurinol, lithium, beta-adrenergic blockers, and antithyroid drugs. Hair growth usually returns when these drugs are discontinued.

• *Radiotherapy.* Like certain drugs, radiotherapy produces temporary, reversible hair loss a few weeks after exposure. Because X-rays damage hair follicles at the site of therapy, head or scalp X-rays cause the most obvious hair loss.

Special considerations

Alopecia can have a devastating impact on the patient's self-image, especially if it's extensive and sudden, as with antineoplastic drugs. So clearly explain to the patient what to expect and re-assure him that his hair will grow back. Occasionally, scalp hypothermia methods, such as a cryogen or ice-filled cap or a scalp tourniquet, may be used before, during, and after drug administration to cause scalp vasoconstriction and to decrease drug delivery to the hair follicles. However, these methods are contraindicated in cancers with circulating malignant cells, such as lymphoma, or with scalp metastases.

Encourage gentle hair care to avoid further hair loss. Also suggest a wig, cap, or scarf, if appropriate. Remind the patient to cover his head in cold weather to prevent loss of body heat.

The doctor may order a skin biopsy to determine the cause of the alopecia, especially if skin changes are evident. Microscopic examination of a plucked hair may also aid diagnosis.

In patients with partial baldness or alopecia areata, topical application of minoxidil (a common antihypertensive drug) for several months stimulates localized hair growth. However, hair loss may recur if the drug is discontinued.

Pediatric pointers

Alopecia normally occurs in the first six months of life. It may involve sudden, diffuse hair loss or gradual thinning that's hardly noticeable. Reassure the infant's parents that this hair loss is normal and temporary. If bald areas result from leaving the infant in one position for too long, advise the parents to change his position regularly.

Common causes of alopecia include use of antineoplastics and radiotherapy, seborrheic dermatitis (known as cradle cap in infancy), alopecia mucinosa, tinea capitis, and hypopituitarism. In children, tinea capitis may produce a kerion lesion—a boggy, raised, tender, and hairless lesion. Trichotillomania, a psychological disorder more common in children than adults, may produce patchy baldness with stubby hair growth due to habitual hair pulling. Other causes include progeria and congenital hair shaft defects, such as trichorrhexis nodosa.

Amenorrhea

Amenorrhea—the absence of menstrual flow—can be classified as primary or secondary. In *primary amenorrhea,* menstruation fails to begin before the age of 18. In *secondary amenorrhea,* it begins at an appropriate age but later ceases for 3 or more months in the absence of normal physiologic causes, such as pregnancy, lactation, and menopause.

Pathologic amenorrhea results from anovulation or physical obstruction to menstrual outflow, such as from an imperforate hymen, cervical stenosis, or intrauterine adhesions. Anovulation itself may result from hormonal imbalance, debilitating disease, stress or emotional disturbances, demanding and continuous exercise, malnutrition, obesity, and anatomic abnormalities, such as genetic absence of the ovaries

HOW AMENORRHEA DEVELOPS

A disruption at any point in the menstrual cycle can produce amenorrhea, as illustrated in the flowchart below.

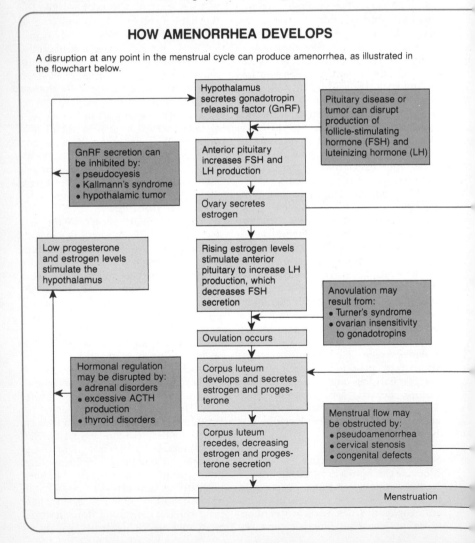

or uterus. Amenorrhea may also result from certain treatments.

Assessment

Begin your assessment by determining if the amenorrhea is primary or secondary. If it's primary, ask the patient at what age her mother first menstruated, since age of menarche is fairly consistent in families. Form an overall impression of the patient's physical, mental, and emotional development, since these factors as well as heredity and climate may delay menarche until after the age of 18.

If menstruation began at an appropriate age but has since ceased, determine the frequency and duration of the patient's previous menstrual cycles. Ask her about the onset and nature of any changes in her normal menstrual pattern, and determine the date of her last menstruation. Find out if she has noticed any related signs, such as breast swelling or weight changes.

Determine when the patient last had a physical examination. Review her health history, noting especially any long-term illnesses, such as anemia, or use of oral contraceptives. Ask about exercise habits, especially running, and stress on the job or at home. Probe the patient's eating habits, including the number and size of daily meals and snacks.

Carefully observe the patient's appearance. Are secondary sex characteristics evident? Are signs of virilization present?

If you're responsible for performing a pelvic examination, check for anatomic aberrations of the outflow tract, such as cervical adhesions or an imperforate hymen.

Medical causes

• **Adrenal tumor.** Amenorrhea may be accompanied by acne, thinning scalp hair, hirsutism, increased blood pressure, and truncal obesity.

• **Adrenocortical hyperplasia.** Amenorrhea precedes characteristic cushingoid signs, such as truncal obesity, moon face, buffalo hump, bruises, purple striae, and widened pulse pressure. Acne, thinning scalp hair, and hirsutism typically appear.

• **Adrenocortical hypofunction.** Besides amenorrhea, this disorder may cause fatigue, irritability, weight loss, nausea, vomiting, and orthostatic hypotension.

• **Amenorrhea-lactation disorders.** These disorders, such as Forbes-Albright and Chiari-Frommel syndromes, produce secondary amenorrhea accompanied

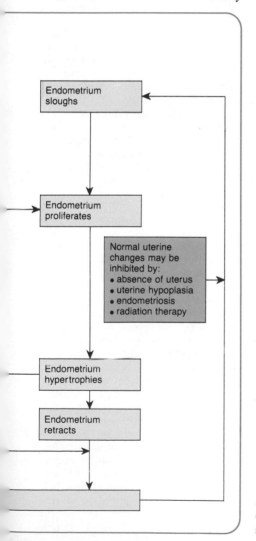

Endometrium sloughs

Endometrium proliferates

Normal uterine changes may be inhibited by:
• absence of uterus
• uterine hypoplasia
• endometriosis
• radiation therapy

Endometrium hypertrophies

Endometrium retracts

by lactation in the absence of breast-feeding. Associated features include large, engorged breasts and vaginal atrophy.

• *Anorexia nervosa.* This psychological disorder can cause either primary or secondary amenorrhea. Related findings often include significant weight loss, a thin or emaciated appearance, compulsive behavior patterns, blotchy or sallow complexion, constipation, reduced libido, decreased pleasure in once-enjoyable activities, dry skin, loss of scalp hair, skeletal muscle atrophy, and sleep disturbances.

• *Asherman's syndrome.* This relatively rare sequela of vigorous curettage produces secondary amenorrhea. Pelvic examination may reveal cervical adhesions and occlusion.

• *Cervical stenosis.* An uncommon disorder, cervical stenosis obstructs menstrual flow, producing amenorrhea. Examination may reveal a scarred cervix without an external os.

• *Congenital absence of the ovaries.* This anomaly results in primary amenorrhea and absence of secondary sex characteristics.

• *Congenital absence of the uterus.* Primary amenorrhea occurs with this disorder.

• *Corpus luteum cysts.* Often causing sudden amenorrhea, these cysts may also produce acute abdominal pain and breast swelling. Examination may reveal a tender adnexal mass as well as vaginal and cervical hyperemia.

• *Hypothalamic tumor.* In addition to amenorrhea, a hypothalamic tumor can cause endocrine and visual field defects, gonadal underdevelopment or dysfunction, and short stature.

• *Hypothyroidism.* Deficient thyroid hormone levels can cause primary or secondary amenorrhea. Typically vague early findings include fatigue, forgetfulness, cold intolerance, unexplained weight gain, and constipation. Subsequent signs include bradycardia; decreased mental acuity; dry, flaky, inelastic skin; puffy face, hands, and feet; hoarseness; periorbital edema; ptosis;

dry, sparse hair; and thick, brittle nails. Other common findings include anorexia, abdominal distention, decreased libido, ataxia, intention tremor, nystagmus, and delayed reflex relaxation time, especially in the Achilles tendon.

• *Kallmann's syndrome.* This rare familial form of hypothalamic dysfunction causes primary amenorrhea and infantile sexual development. Associated findings include mental retardation, anosmia, and midline facial defects, such as cleft lip and palate.

• *Mosaicism.* This genetic disorder results in primary amenorrhea and absence of secondary sex characteristics.

• *Ovarian insensitivity to gonadotropins.* This hormonal disturbance leads to amenorrhea and an absence of secondary sex characteristics.

• *Pelvic inflammatory disease (PID).* Rarely, PID destroys the ovaries and produces secondary amenorrhea. In acute PID, the patient may also display high fever, chills, severe lower abdominal pain and tenderness, nausea, and vomiting.

• *Pituitary infarction.* This disorder usually causes postpartum failure to lactate and to resume menses. Associated signs and symptoms depend on the infarction's severity but may include headaches, visual field defects, oculomotor palsies, and an altered level of consciousness.

• *Pituitary tumor.* Amenorrhea may be the first sign of several types of pituitary tumor. Associated findings may include headache; visual disturbances, such as bitemporal hemianopia; and acromegaly. Cushingoid signs include moon face, buffalo hump, hirsutism, truncal obesity, bruises, purple striae, and widened pulse pressure.

• *Polycystic ovary syndrome.* Typically, menarche occurs at a normal age, followed by irregular menstrual cycles, oligomenorrhea, and secondary amenorrhea. Or periods of profuse bleeding may alternate with periods of amenorrhea. Obesity, hirsutism, slight deepening of the voice, and enlarged, "oysterlike" ovaries may also accompany this disorder.

● **Pseudoamenorrhea.** An anatomic anomaly, such as imperforate hymen, obstructs menstrual flow, causing primary amenorrhea and possibly abdominal cramps. Examination may reveal a pink or blue bulging hymen.

● **Pseudocyesis.** Amenorrhea may be accompanied by lordosis, abdominal distention, nausea, and breast enlargement in this disorder.

● **Sertoli-Leydig cell tumor.** This ovarian tumor may produce amenorrhea along with acne, hirsutism, deepening of the voice, and clitoral enlargement.

● **Testicular feminization.** Primary amenorrhea may signal this form of male pseudohermaphroditism. The patient, outwardly female but genetically male, shows breast and external genital development, but scant or absent pubic hair.

● **Thyrotoxicosis.** Thyroid hormone overproduction may result in amenorrhea. Classic signs and symptoms include an enlarged thyroid (goiter), nervousness, heat intolerance, sweating, tremors, palpitations, tachycardia, dyspnea, weakness, and weight loss despite increased appetite.

● **Turner's syndrome.** Primary amenorrhea and failure to develop secondary sex characteristics may signal this syndrome of genetic ovarian dysgenesis. Typical features include short stature, webbing of the neck, low nuchal hairline, a broad chest with widely spaced nipples and poor breast development, underdeveloped genitalia, and edema of the legs and feet.

● **Uterine hypoplasia.** Primary amenorrhea results from underdevelopment of the uterus, which is detectable on physical examination.

● **Vaginal agenesis.** A rare cause of primary amenorrhea, this anomaly may also produce cyclic moliminal symptoms but without abdominal pain.

Other causes

● **Drugs.** Cyclophosphamide, busulfan, chlorambucil, and phenothiazines may cause amenorrhea. Oral contraceptives may cause anovulation and amenorrhea after discontinuation.

● **Radiation therapy.** Irradiation of the abdomen may destroy the endometrium or ovaries, causing amenorrhea.

● **Surgery.** Surgical removal of both ovaries or the uterus produces amenorrhea.

Special considerations

In patients with secondary amenorrhea, physical and pelvic examinations must rule out pregnancy before diagnostic testing begins. Typical tests include progestin withdrawal, serum hormone and thyroid function studies, and endometrial biopsy.

After diagnosis, answer the patient's questions about the type of treatment that will be provided and its expected outcome. Because amenorrhea can cause severe emotional distress, provide emotional support. Be sure to encourage the patient to discuss her fears, and, if necessary, refer her for psychological counseling.

Pediatric pointers

Adolescent girls are especially prone to amenorrhea caused by emotional upsets, typically stemming from school, social, or family problems.

Amnesia

Amnesia—a disturbance in or loss of memory—may be partial or complete, and anterograde or retrograde. Anterograde amnesia denotes memory loss for events that occurred *after* onset of the causative trauma or disease; retrograde amnesia denotes memory loss for events that occurred *before* onset. Depending on the cause, amnesia may arise suddenly or slowly and may be temporary or permanent.

Organic, or *true*, amnesia results from temporal lobe dysfunction and characteristically spares patches of memory. A common symptom in patients with seizures and head trauma, organic amnesia can also be an early indicator of Alzheimer's disease. *Hysterical amnesia* has a psychogenic origin and characteristically causes complete memory loss. *Treatment-induced amnesia* is usually transient.

Assessment

Because the patient often isn't aware of his amnesia, you'll usually need help in gathering information from his family or friends. Throughout your assessment, notice the patient's general appearance, behavior, mood, and train of thought. Ask when the amnesia first appeared and what types of things the patient's unable to remember. Can he learn new information? How long does he remember it? Does the amnesia encompass a recent or a remote time period?

Test the patient's recent memory with such questions as "How did you get here?" "What was the day before yesterday?" Test his intermediate memory by asking, "Who was the president before this one?" "What was the last type of car you bought?" Test remote memory with such questions as "How old are you?" "Where were you born?"

Take the patient's vital signs and assess his level of consciousness (LOC). Check his pupils: they should be equal in size and should constrict quickly when exposed to direct light. Also assess his extraocular movements. Test motor function by having the patient move his arms and legs through their range of motion. Evaluate sensory function with pinpricks on the patient's skin (see *Testing for Analgesia*, pages 44 and 45).

Medical causes

• *Alzheimer's disease.* This disease usually begins with retrograde amnesia, which progresses slowly over many months or years to include anterograde amnesia, producing severe and permanent memory loss. Associated findings include agitation, inability to concentrate, disregard for personal hygiene, confusion, irritability, and emotional lability. Later signs include aphasia, dementia, incontinence, and muscle rigidity.

• *Cerebral hypoxia.* After recovery from hypoxia (brought on by such conditions as carbon monoxide poisoning or acute respiratory failure), the patient may experience total amnesia for the event, along with sensory disturbances, such as numbness and tingling.

• *Head trauma.* Depending on the trauma's severity, amnesia may last for minutes, hours, or longer. Usually, amnesia for the event persists, as well as brief retrograde and longer anterograde amnesia. Severe head trauma can cause permanent amnesia or difficulty in retaining recent memories. Related findings may include altered respirations and LOC; headache; dizziness; confusion; visual disturbances, such as blurred or double vision; and motor and sensory disturbances, such as hemiparesis and paresthesias, on the side of the body opposite the injury.

• *Herpes simplex encephalitis.* Recovery from this disease often leaves the patient with severe and possibly permanent amnesia. Associated findings include signs and symptoms of meningeal irritation, such as headache, fever, and altered LOC, along with seizures and motor and sensory disturbances (such as paresis, paralysis, numbness, and tingling).

• *Hysteria.* Hysterical amnesia, a complete and long-lasting memory loss, begins and ends abruptly. It's typically accompanied by confusion.

• *Seizure.* In temporal lobe seizures, amnesia occurs suddenly and lasts for several seconds to minutes. The patient may recall an aura or nothing at all.

An irritable focus on the left side of the brain primarily causes amnesia for verbal memories; an irritable focus on the right side of the brain, graphic *and* verbal amnesia. Associated signs may include decreased LOC during the seizure; confusion; motor and sensory

AMNESIA: CAUSES AND ASSOCIATED FINDINGS

S&S CAUSES	MAJOR ASSOCIATED SIGNS AND SYMPTOMS												
	Agitation	Ataxia	Confusion	Decreased LOC	Diplopia	Dizziness	Emotional lability	Headache	Nausea	Paresthesias	Vertigo	Visual blurring	Vomiting
Alzheimer's disease	•		•				•						
Cerebral hypoxia				•						•			
Head trauma			•	•	•	•		•		•		•	
Herpes simplex encephalitis				•				•	•				
Hysteria			•										
Vertebrobasilar circulatory disorders		•		•	•	•			•		•	•	•
Wernicke-Korsakoff syndrome		•	•	•	•			•		•			

disturbances, such as hemiparesis, unusual tastes, and paresthesias; and blurred vision.

• *Vertebrobasilar circulatory disorders.* Vertebrobasilar ischemia, infarction, embolus, or hemorrhage typically causes complete amnesia that begins abruptly, lasts for several hours, and ends abruptly. Associated findings include dizziness, decreased LOC, ataxia, blurred or double vision, vertigo, nausea, and vomiting.

• *Wernicke-Korsakoff syndrome.* Retrograde and anterograde amnesia can become permanent without treatment in this syndrome. Accompanying clinical findings include apathy, an inability to concentrate or to put events into sequence, and confabulation to fill memory gaps. The syndrome may also cause diplopia, decreased LOC, headache, ataxia, and symptoms of periph-

eral neuropathy, such as numbness and tingling.

Other causes

• *Drugs.* Anterograde amnesia can be precipitated by general anesthetics, especially fentanyl, halothane, and isoflurane; barbiturates, most commonly thiopental and pentobarbital; and certain benzodiazepines, especially triazolam.

• *Electroconvulsive therapy.* Sudden onset of retrograde or anterograde amnesia occurs with electroconvulsive therapy. Typically, the amnesia lasts for several minutes to several hours, but severe, prolonged amnesia occurs with treatments given frequently over a prolonged period.

• *Temporal lobe surgery.* Usually performed on only one lobe, this surgery causes brief, slight amnesia. However, removal of both lobes leaves permanent amnesia.

Special considerations

As ordered, prepare the patient for diagnostic tests, such as computed tomography scan, electroencephalography, or cerebral angiography.

Provide reality orientation for the patient with retrograde amnesia, and encourage his family members to help by supplying familiar photos, objects, or music.

Adjust your patient-teaching techniques for the patient with anterograde amnesia, since he can't acquire new information. Include his family in teaching sessions. In addition, write down all instructions—particularly medication dosages and schedules—so the patient won't have to rely on his memory.

Consider basic needs, such as safety, elimination, and nutrition, for the patient with severe amnesia. If necessary, arrange for placement in an extended-care facility.

Pediatric pointers

A child who suffers amnesia during seizures may be mistakenly labeled as "learning disabled." To prevent this mislabeling, stress the importance of adhering to the prescribed medication schedule, and discuss ways that the child, his parents, and his teachers can cope with amnesia.

Analgesia

Analgesia, the absence of sensitivity to pain, is an important sign of central nervous system disease, often indicating a specific type and location of spinal cord lesion. It always occurs with loss of temperature sensation (thermanesthesia), since these sensory nerve impulses travel together in the spinal cord. It can also occur with other sensory deficits, such as paresthesia, loss of proprioception and vibratory sense, and tactile anesthesia in various disorders involving the peripheral nerves, spinal cord, and brain. However, when accompanied only by thermanesthesia, analgesia points to an incomplete lesion of the spinal cord.

Analgesia can be partial or total below the level of the lesion, and unilateral or bilateral, depending on the cause and level of the lesion. Its onset may be slow and progressive with a tumor, or abrupt with trauma. Often transient, analgesia may resolve spontaneously.

Assessment

If the patient complains of unilateral or bilateral analgesia over a large body area, accompanied by paralysis, suspect spinal cord injury. Have another nurse notify the doctor immediately, while you immobilize the patient's spine in proper alignment, using a cervical collar and a long backboard if possible. If a collar or backboard isn't available, position the patient supine on a flat surface, and place sandbags around his head, neck, and torso. Use correct technique and extreme caution when moving him, to prevent exacerbating spinal injury. Continuously monitor respiratory rate and rhythm, and observe for accessory muscle use, since a complete lesion above the T6 level may cause diaphragmatic and intercostal muscle paralysis. Have an artificial airway and Ambu bag on hand, and be prepared to initiate emergency resuscitation measures in the event of respiratory failure.

Once you're satisfied that the patient's spine and respiratory status are stabilized—or if the analgesia is less severe and isn't accompanied by signs of spinal cord injury—perform a physical examination and baseline neurologic assessment. Begin by taking the patient's vital signs and assessing his level of consciousness. Then test pupillary, corneal, cough, and gag reflexes to rule out brain stem and cranial nerve involvement. If the patient is conscious, assess his speech and ability to swallow.

If possible, observe the patient's gait and posture, and assess his balance and coordination. Evaluate muscle tone and strength in all extremities. Test for other sensory deficits over all dermatomes (individual skin segments innervated by a specific spinal nerve) by applying light tactile stimulation with a tongue depressor or cotton swab. Repeat a more thorough check of pain sensitivity, if necessary, using a pin (see *Testing for Analgesia*, pages 44 and 45). Also test temperature sensation over all dermatomes, using two test tubes—one filled with hot water, the other with cold water. In each arm and leg, test vibration sense (using a tuning fork), proprioception, and both superficial and deep tendon reflexes. If the patient is paralyzed, palpate his muscles to determine whether paralysis is spastic or flaccid.

Focus your history taking on the onset of analgesia—sudden or gradual—and on any recent trauma—a fall, sports injury, or automobile accident. Obtain a complete medical history, noting especially any incidence of cancer in the patient or his family.

Medical causes

• *Anterior cord syndrome.* In this syndrome, analgesia and thermanesthesia occur bilaterally below the level of the lesion, along with flaccid paralysis and hypoactive DTRs.

• *Central cord syndrome.* Typically, analgesia and thermanesthesia occur bilaterally in several dermatomes, frequently extending in a capelike fashion over the arms, back, and shoulders. Early weakness in the hands progresses to weakness and muscle spasms in the arms and shoulder girdle. Hyperactive DTRs and spastic weakness of the legs may develop. However, if the lesion affects the lumbar spine, hypoactive DTRs and flaccid weakness may occur.

With brain stem involvement, additional findings may include facial analgesia and thermanesthesia, vertigo, nystagmus, atrophy of the tongue, and dysarthria. The patient may also have dysphagia, urinary retention, anhidrosis, decreased intestinal motility, and hyperkeratosis.

• *Spinal cord hemisection.* Contralateral analgesia and thermanesthesia occur below the level of the lesion. In addition, loss of proprioception, spastic paralysis, and hyperactive DTRs develop ipsilaterally. The patient may experience urinary retention with overflow incontinence.

Other causes

• *Drugs.* Analgesia may occur with use of topical and local anesthetics, although numbness and tingling are more common.

Special considerations

Prepare the patient for spinal X-rays, and maintain spinal alignment and stability during transport to the laboratory.

Focus your nursing care on preventing further injury to the patient, since analgesia can mask injury or developing complications. Prevent formation of decubiti through meticulous skin care, massage, use of lamb's wool pads, and frequent repositioning, especially when significant motor deficits hamper the patient's movement. Guard against scalding by testing the patient's bathwater temperature before he bathes; advise him to test it at home using a thermometer or a body part with intact sensation.

Pediatric pointers

Since a child may have difficulty describing analgesia, observe him carefully during the assessment for nonverbal clues to pain—facial expressions, crying, retraction from stimulus. Remember that pain thresholds are high in infants, so your assessment findings may not be reliable. Also remember to test bathwater carefully for a child who's too young to test it himself.

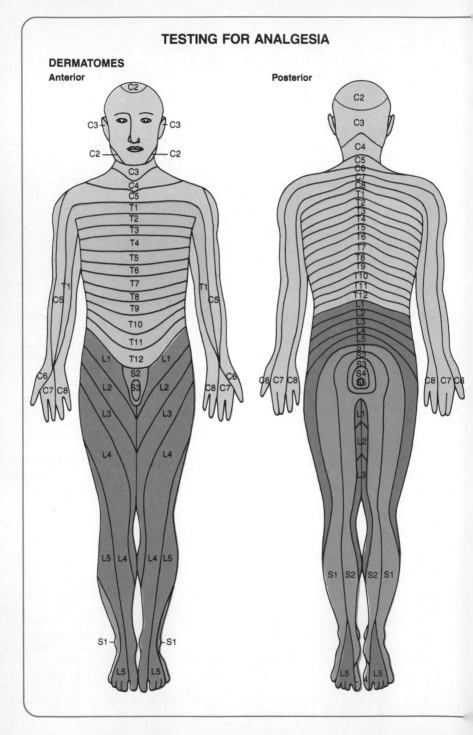

By carefully and systematically testing your patient's sensitivity to pain, you can determine whether his nerve damage has a segmental or peripheral distribution and help locate the causative lesion.

Tell the patient to relax, and explain that you're going to lightly touch areas of his skin with a small pin. Have him close his eyes. Apply the pin firmly enough to produce pain without breaking the skin. (Practice on yourself first to learn how to apply the correct pressure.)

Starting with the patient's head and face, move down his body, pricking his skin on alternating sides. Have the patient report when he feels pain. Occasionally use the blunt end of the pin, and vary your test pattern to gauge the accuracy of his response.

Document your findings thoroughly, clearly demarcating any areas of lost pain sensation on either a dermatome chart (shown at left) or on appropriate peripheral nerve diagrams (shown below).

PERIPHERAL NERVES

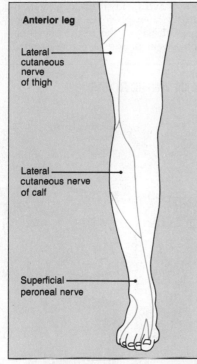

Anterior leg

Lateral cutaneous nerve of thigh

Lateral cutaneous nerve of calf

Superficial peroneal nerve

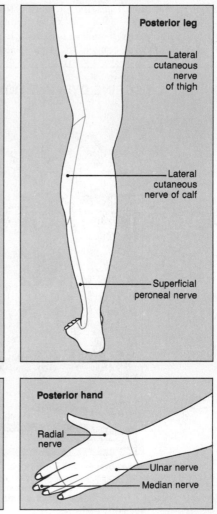

Posterior leg

Lateral cutaneous nerve of thigh

Lateral cutaneous nerve of calf

Superficial peroneal nerve

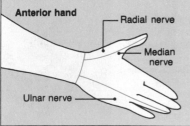

Anterior hand

Radial nerve

Median nerve

Ulnar nerve

Posterior hand

Radial nerve

Ulnar nerve

Median nerve

Anhidrosis

Anhidrosis—an abnormal deficiency of sweat in response to heat—can be generalized (complete) or localized (partial). Generalized anhidrosis can lead to life-threatening impairment of thermoregulation. Localized anhidrosis rarely interferes with thermoregulation, since it affects only a small percentage of the body's eccrine (sweat) glands.

Anhidrosis results from neurologic and skin disorders; congenital, atrophic, or traumatic changes to sweat glands; and use of certain drugs. Neurologic disorders disturb central or peripheral nervous pathways that normally activate sweating, causing retention of excess body heat and perspiration. The absence, obstruction, atrophy, or degeneration of sweat glands can produce anhidrosis at the skin surface, even if neurologic stimulation is normal.

Anhidrosis may go unrecognized until significant heat or exertion fails to raise sweat. However, localized anhidrosis often provokes compensatory hyperhidrosis in the remaining functional sweat glands. Often the patient's

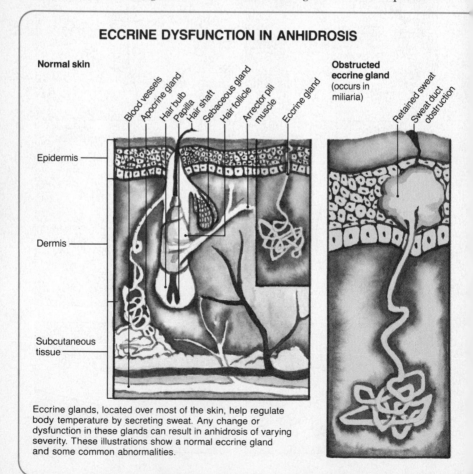

ECCRINE DYSFUNCTION IN ANHIDROSIS

Normal skin

Blood vessels
Apocrine gland
Hair bulb
Papilla
Hair shaft
Sebaceous gland
Hair follicle
Arrector pili muscle
Eccrine gland

Obstructed eccrine gland (occurs in miliaria)

Retained sweat
Sweat duct obstruction

Epidermis

Dermis

Subcutaneous tissue

Eccrine glands, located over most of the skin, help regulate body temperature by secreting sweat. Any change or dysfunction in these glands can result in anhidrosis of varying severity. These illustrations show a normal eccrine gland and some common abnormalities.

chief complaint, this hyperhidrosis can flood the skin surface, masking areas of sweat gland deficiency.

Assessment

If you detect anhidrosis in a patient whose skin feels hot and flushed, ask if the patient's also experiencing nausea, dizziness, palpitations, and substernal tightness. If so, quickly take rectal temperature and other vital signs, and assess the patient's level of consciousness. If rectal temperature exceeding 102.2° F. (39° C.) occurs with tachycardia, tachypnea, altered blood pressure, and decreased level of consciousness, suspect life-threatening anhidrotic asthenia (heatstroke). Have another nurse immediately notify the doctor, while you start rapid cooling measures, such as immersing the patient in ice or very cold water and giving I.V. fluid replacements. Continue these measures, and frequently check vital signs and neurologic status until the patient's temperature drops below 102° F. Then place him in an air-conditioned room.

If anhidrosis is localized or the patient reports local hyperhidrosis or unexplained fever, take a brief history. Ask the patient to characterize his sweating during heat spells or strenuous activity. Does he usually sweat

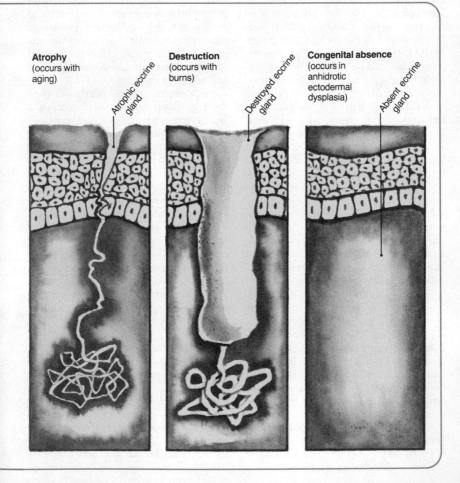

Atrophy
(occurs with aging)

Atrophic eccrine gland

Destruction
(occurs with burns)

Destroyed eccrine gland

Congenital absence
(occurs in anhidrotic ectodermal dysplasia)

Absent eccrine gland

slightly? Profusely? Ask about recent prolonged or extreme exposure to heat and about the onset of anhidrosis or hyperhidrosis. Obtain a complete medical history, focusing on neurologic disorders; skin disorders, such as psoriasis and scleroderma; systemic diseases that can cause peripheral neuropathies, such as diabetes mellitus; and drug use.

Inspect skin color, texture, and turgor. If you detect any skin lesions, document their location, size, color, texture, and pattern.

Medical causes

● *Anhidrotic asthenia.* This life-threatening disorder causes acute, generalized anhidrosis. In early stages, sweating may still occur and the patient may be rational, but his rectal temperature may already exceed 102.2° F. Associated signs and symptoms include severe headache and muscle cramps, which later disappear; fatigue; nausea and vomiting; dizziness; palpitations; substernal tightness; and elevated blood pressure followed by hypotension. Within minutes, anhidrosis and hot, flushed skin develop, accompanied by tachycardia, tachypnea, and confusion progressing to loss of consciousness.

● *Burns.* Depending on their severity, burns may cause permanent anhidrosis in affected areas. Other possible signs include blistering, edema, and increased pain or loss of sensation.

● *Cerebral lesions.* Cerebral cortex and brain stem lesions may cause anhidrotic palms and soles, along with various motor and sensory disturbances specific to the site of the lesions.

● *Horner's syndrome.* A supraclavicular spinal cord lesion produces unilateral facial anhidrosis with compensatory contralateral hyperhidrosis. Other findings include ipsilateral pupillary constriction and ptosis.

● *Miliaria crystallina.* This usually innocuous form of miliaria causes anhidrosis and tiny, clear, fragile blisters, usually under the arms and breasts.

● *Miliaria profunda.* If severe and extensive, this form of miliaria can progress to life-threatening anhidrotic asthenia. Typically, though, it produces localized anhidrosis with compensatory facial hyperhydrosis. Whitish papules appear mostly on the trunk, but also on the extremities. Associated signs include inguinal and axillary lymphadenopathy, weakness, shortness of breath, palpitations, and fever.

● *Miliaria rubra (prickly heat).* Like miliaria profunda, this common form of miliaria can progress to life-threatening anhidrotic asthenia if it's severe and extensive. Typically, though, it produces localized anhidrosis. Small, erythematous papules with centrally placed blisters appear on the trunk and neck and rarely on the face, palms, or soles. Pustules may also appear in extensive and chronic miliaria. Related symptoms include paroxysmal itching and paresthesias.

● *Peripheral neuritis.* Anhidrosis over the legs often appears with compensatory hyperhidrosis over the head and neck. Associated findings mainly involve the extremities and may include glossy red skin; paresthesias, hyperesthesia or anesthesia in the hands and feet; diminished or absent deep tendon reflexes; flaccid paralysis and muscle wasting; footdrop; and burning pain.

● *Shy-Drager syndrome.* This degenerative neurologic syndrome causes ascending anhidrosis in the legs. Other signs and symptoms include severe orthostatic hypotension, loss of leg hair, impotence, constipation, urinary retention or urgency, decreased salivation and tearing, mydriasis, and impaired visual accommodation. Eventually, focal neurologic signs may appear, such as leg tremors, incoordination, and muscle wasting and fasciculation.

● *Spinal cord lesions.* Anhidrosis may occur symmetrically below the level of the lesion, with compensatory hyperhidrosis in adjacent areas. Other findings depend on the site and extent of the lesion but may include partial or total loss of motor and sensory function below the lesion. The patient's cardiovascular and respiratory function may also be impaired.

Other causes
• *Drugs.* Anticholinergics, such as atropine and scopolamine, can cause generalized anhidrosis.

Special considerations
Because even a careful assessment can be inconclusive, you may need specific tests to evaluate anhidrosis. These include wrapping the patient in an electric blanket or placing him in a heated box to observe the skin for sweat patterns, applying topical agents that detect sweat on the skin, or administering systemic cholinergic drugs, which stimulate sweating.

Advise the patient with anhidrosis to remain in cool environments, to move slowly during warm weather, and to avoid strenuous exercise and hot foods. Warn him about the anhidrotic effects of any drugs he's receiving.

Pediatric pointers
In both infants and children, miliaria rubra and congenital skin disorders, such as ichthyosis and anhidrotic ectodermal dysplasia, are the most common causes of anhidrosis.

Since delayed development of the thermoregulatory center renders an infant—especially a premature one—anhidrotic for several weeks after birth, caution parents against overdressing their infant.

Anorexia

Anorexia, a lack of appetite in the presence of a physiologic need for food, is a common symptom of gastrointestinal (GI) and endocrine disorders. It's also characteristic of certain severe psychological disturbances. This symptom can also result from such factors as anxiety, chronic pain, poor oral hygiene, increased blood temperature due to hot weather or fever, and alterations in taste or smell that normally accompany aging. Anorexia can result from drug therapy or abuse, too. Short-term anorexia rarely jeopardizes the patient's health. However, chronic anorexia can lead to life-threatening malnutrition.

Assessment
Begin your assessment by taking the patient's vital signs and weight. Ask him to provide his previous minimum and maximum weights. Explore his dietary habits by asking such questions as, "Do you eat regular meals or mainly snacks?" "What do you usually eat for breakfast?" "For dinner?" Ask about favorite and disliked foods, and the reasons for such preferences; he may identify certain tastes and smells that nauseate him and cause loss of appetite. Also ask about any dental problems that interfere with chewing, including poor-fitting dentures. Find out if he has difficulty or pain when he swallows or if he vomits or has diarrhea after meals. Also ask about the frequency and intensity of physical exercise.

Check for a history of stomach or bowel disorders, which can interfere with the ability to digest, absorb, or metabolize nutrients. Find out if the patient has experienced any change in bowel habits. Ask about drug use and dosage and about alcohol use.

If the medical history doesn't reveal an organic basis for anorexia, consider psychological factors. Ask the patient if he knows what's causing his decreased appetite. Situational factors, such as a death in the family or problems at school or on the job, can lead to depression and subsequent loss of appetite. Check for signs of malnutrition (see *Is Your Patient Malnourished?*, page 50). If the patient has any of these signs, consistently refuses food, and has lost 7% to 10% of his body weight within the last month, notify the doctor.

IS YOUR PATIENT MALNOURISHED?

When assessing a patient with anorexia, be sure to check for these common signs of malnutrition.

Hair. Dull, dry, thin, fine, straight, and easily plucked; areas of lighter or darker spots and hair loss

Face. Generalized swelling; dark areas on cheeks and under eyes; lumpy or flaky skin around the nose and mouth; enlarged parotid glands

Eyes. Dull appearance; dry and either pale or red membranes; triangular, shiny gray spots on conjunctivae; red and fissured eyelid corners; bloodshot ring around cornea

Lips. Red and swollen, especially at corners

Tongue. Swollen, purple, and raw-looking, with sores or abnormal papillae

Teeth. Missing, or emerging abnormally; visible cavities or dark spots; spongy, often bleeding gums

Neck. Swollen thyroid gland

Skin. Dry, flaky, swollen, and dark, with lighter or darker spots, some resembling bruises; tight and drawn, with poor skin turgor

Nails. Spoon-shaped, brittle, and ridged

Musculoskeletal system. Muscle wasting, knock-knee or bowlegs, bumps on ribs, swollen joints, musculoskeletal hemorrhages

Cardiovascular system. Heart rate above 100 beats/minute; dysrhythmias; elevated blood pressure

Abdomen. Enlarged liver and spleen

Reproductive system. Decreased libido; amenorrhea

Nervous system. Irritability; confusion; paresthesias in hands and feet; loss of proprioception; decreased ankle and knee reflexes

Medical causes

• *Adrenocortical hypofunction.* In this disorder, anorexia may begin slowly and subtly, causing gradual weight loss. Other common signs and symptoms include nausea and vomiting, abdominal pain, diarrhea, weakness, fatigue, malaise, vitiligo, bronze-colored skin, and purple striae on the breasts, abdomen, shoulders, and hips.

• *Alcoholism.* Chronic anorexia commonly accompanies alcoholism, eventually leading to malnutrition. Other findings: signs of liver damage (jaundice, spider angiomas, ascites, edema), paresthesias, tremors, increased blood pressure, bruising, GI bleeding, and abdominal pain.

• *Anorexia nervosa.* Chronic anorexia begins insidiously and eventually leads to life-threatening malnutrition, evidenced by skeletal muscle atrophy, loss of fatty tissue, constipation, amenorrhea, dry and blotchy or sallow skin, alopecia, sleep disturbances, distorted self-image, anhedonia, and decreased libido. Paradoxically, the patient often exhibits extreme restlessness and vigor and may exercise avidly.

• *Appendicitis.* Anorexia closely follows the abrupt onset of generalized or localized epigastric pain, nausea, and vomiting. It can continue as pain localizes in the right lower quadrant (McBurney's point) and other signs appear: abdominal rigidity, rebound tenderness, constipation (or diarrhea), slight fever, and tachycardia.

• *Cancer.* Chronic anorexia occurs, with possible weight loss, weakness, apathy, and cachexia.

• *Chronic renal failure.* Chronic anorexia is common and insidious. It's accompanied by changes in all body systems, such as nausea, vomiting, mouth ulcers, ammonia breath odor, GI bleeding, constipation or diarrhea, drowsiness, confusion, tremors, pallor, dry and scaly skin, pruritus, alopecia, purpuric lesions, and edema.

• *Cirrhosis.* Anorexia occurs early and may be accompanied by weakness, nausea, vomiting, constipation or diarrhea, and dull abdominal pain. It continues after these early signs subside and is accompanied by lethargy, slurred speech, bleeding tendencies, ascites, severe pruritus, dry skin, poor skin turgor, hepatomegaly, fetor hepaticus, jaundice, edema of the legs, and right upper quadrant pain.

• *Crohn's disease.* Chronic anorexia causes marked weight loss. Associated signs vary according to the site and extent of the lesion and may include diarrhea, abdominal pain, fever, abdominal mass, weakness, and, rarely, clubbing of the fingers. Acute inflammatory symptoms—right lower quadrant pain, cramping, tenderness, flatulence, fever, nausea, diarrhea, and bloody stools—mimic appendicitis.

• *Depressive syndrome.* Anorexia reflects anhedonia in this syndrome. Accompanying symptoms may include poor concentration, indecisiveness, delusions, menstrual irregularities, decreased libido, insomnia or hypersomnia, fatigue, mood swings, and gradual social withdrawal.

• *Gastritis.* In *acute gastritis,* the onset of anorexia may be sudden; in *chronic gastritis,* it's insidious. In both types, postprandial epigastric distress may occur with nausea, vomiting (often with hematemesis), fever, belching, and malaise.

• *Hepatitis.* In *viral hepatitis,* anorexia begins in the preicteric phase, accompanied by fatigue, malaise, headache, arthralgia, myalgia, photophobia, cough, sore throat, rhinitis, nausea and vomiting, mild fever, hepatomegaly, and lymphadenopathy. It may continue throughout the icteric phase, along with mild weight loss, dark urine, claycolored stools, jaundice, right upper quadrant pain, and, possibly, irritability and severe pruritus.

In *nonviral hepatitis,* anorexia and its accompanying signs usually resemble those of viral hepatitis but may vary depending on the causative agent and the extent of liver damage.

• *Hypopituitarism.* Anorexia usually develops slowly in this disorder. Its accompanying signs vary with the disorder's severity and the number and type of deficient hormones. These signs may include amenorrhea; decreased libido; lethargy; cold intolerance; pale, thin, and dry skin; dry, brittle hair; and decreased temperature, blood pressure, and pulse rate.

• *Hypothyroidism.* Anorexia is common and usually insidious in thyroid hormone deficiency. Typically vague early findings include fatigue, forgetfulness, cold intolerance, unexplained weight gain, and constipation. Subsequent findings include decreased mental stability; dry, flaky, and inelastic skin; edema of the face, hands, and feet; ptosis; hoarseness; thick, brittle nails; coarse, broken hair; and signs of decreased cardiac output, such as bradycardia. Other common findings include abdominal distention, menstrual irregularities, decreased libido, ataxia, intention tremor, nystagmus, and slow reflex relaxation time.

• *Ketoacidosis.* Anorexia usually arises gradually and is accompanied by dry, flushed skin; fruity breath odor; polydipsia; hypotension; weak, rapid pulse; dry mouth; abdominal pain; and vomiting.

• *Pernicious anemia.* In this disorder, insidious anorexia may cause considerable weight loss. Related findings include the classic triad of burning tongue, general weakness, and numbness and tingling in the extremities; alternating constipation and diarrhea; abdominal pain; nausea and vomiting; bleeding gums; ataxia; positive Babinski's and Romberg's signs; diplopia and blurred vision; irritability, headache, malaise, and fatigue.

Other causes

• *Drugs.* Anorexia results from use of amphetamines, chemotherapeutic agents, sympathomimetics such as ephedrine, and some antibiotics. It also signals digitalis toxicity.

• *Radiation therapy.* Radiation treatments can cause anorexia, possibly due to metabolic disturbances.

• *Total parenteral nutrition.* Maintenance of blood glucose levels by I.V. therapy may cause anorexia.

Special considerations

Because the causes of anorexia are diverse, diagnostic procedures may include thyroid function studies, esophagography, upper GI series, gallbladder series, barium enema, liver and kidney function tests, hormone assays, computed tomography scans, ultrasonography, and blood studies to assess nutritional status.

When caring for the anorexic patient, promote protein and caloric intake by providing high-calorie snacks or frequent, small meals. Encourage the patient's family to supply his favorite foods to help stimulate his appetite. Take a 24-hour diet history daily. If the patient consistently exaggerates his food intake (a common occurrence in anorexia nervosa), ask the dietitian to maintain strict calorie and nutrient counts for the patient's meals. In severe malnutrition, provide supplemental nutritional support, such as total parenteral nutrition.

Because anorexia and poor nutrition increase susceptibility to infection, monitor the patient's vital signs and white blood cell count and closely observe any wounds.

Pediatric pointers

In children, anorexia commonly accompanies many illnesses, but usually resolves promptly. However, in preadolescent and adolescent girls, be alert for the often subtle signs of anorexia nervosa.

Anosmia

Although usually an insignificant consequence of nasal congestion or obstruction, anosmia—absence of the sense of smell—occasionally heralds a serious neural defect. Temporary anosmia can result from any condition that causes irritation and swelling of the nasal mucosa and obstructs the olfactory area in the nose, such as heavy smoking, rhinitis, or sinusitis. Permanent anosmia, on the other hand, usually indicates a lesion in the olfactory nerve pathway. Permanent or temporary anosmia can also result from inhalation of irritants, such as cocaine or acid fumes, that paralyze the nasal cilia. Anosmia may also be reported—without an identifiable organic cause—by patients suffering from hysteria, depression, or schizophrenia.

Anosmia is invariably perceived as bilateral; unilateral anosmia can occur but can't be recognized by the patient. Because combined stimulation of taste buds and olfactory cells produces the sense of taste, anosmia is usually accompanied by ageusia, loss of the sense of taste.

Assessment

Begin the patient history by asking about the onset and duration of anosmia and any related symptoms—stuffy nose, nasal discharge or bleeding, postnasal drip, sneezing, dry or sore mouth and throat, loss of sense of taste or appetite, excessive tearing, and facial or eye pain. Pinpoint any history of nasal disease, allergies, or head trauma. Ask about heavy smoking and the use of prescribed or over-the-counter nasal drops or sprays. Be sure to rule out cocaine use.

Inspect and palpate nasal structures for obvious injury, inflammation, deformities, and septal deviation or perforation. Observe the contour and color of the nasal mucosa and the size and color of the turbinates. Check for polyps, which appear as translucent, white masses around the middle meatus. Note the source and character of any nasal discharge. Palpate the sinus areas for tenderness and contour.

Assess for nasal obstruction by occluding one nostril at a time with your thumb as the patient breathes quietly; listen for breath sounds and for sounds

THE SENSE OF SMELL

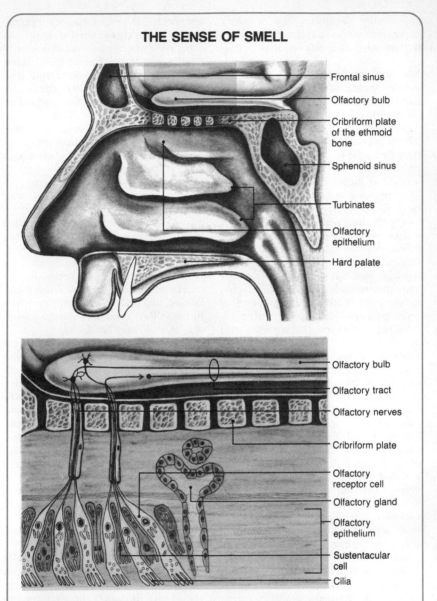

- Frontal sinus
- Olfactory bulb
- Cribriform plate of the ethmoid bone
- Sphenoid sinus
- Turbinates
- Olfactory epithelium
- Hard palate

- Olfactory bulb
- Olfactory tract
- Olfactory nerves
- Cribriform plate
- Olfactory receptor cell
- Olfactory gland
- Olfactory epithelium
- Sustentacular cell
- Cilia

Our noses can distinguish the odors of thousands of chemicals, but researchers haven't yet discovered why. They do know, however, that the olfactory epithelium contains olfactory receptor cells, along with olfactory glands and sustentacular cells, both of which secrete mucus to keep the epithelial surface moist. The mucus covering the olfactory cells probably traps airborne odorous molecules, which then fit into the appropriate receptors on the cell surface. In response to this stimulus, the receptor cell then transmits an impulse along the olfactory nerve (cranial nerve I) to the olfactory area of the cortex, where it's interpreted. Any disruption along this transmission pathway, or any obstruction of the epithelial surface due to dryness or congestion, can cause anosmia.

of moisture or mucus. Test olfactory nerve (cranial nerve I) function by having the patient identify common odors.

Medical causes

• *Anterior cerebral artery occlusion.* Permanent anosmia may follow vascular damage involving the olfactory nerve. Associated symptoms include contralateral weakness and numbness (especially in the leg), confusion, and impaired motor and sensory functions.

• *Diabetes mellitus.* Insidious, permanent anosmia may occur, along with fatigue, polyuria, polydipsia, weight loss, polyphagia, and weakness.

• *Head trauma.* Permanent anosmia may follow damage to the olfactory nerve. Depending on the type and severity of trauma, associated signs and symptoms may include epistaxis, headache, nausea and vomiting, altered level of consciousness, blurred or double vision, raccoon's eyes, Battle's sign, and otorrhea.

• *Lead poisoning.* Anosmia may be permanent or temporary, depending on the extent of damage to the nasal mucosa. Associated findings include abdominal pain, weakness, headache, nausea, vomiting, constipation, wristdrop or footdrop, lead line on the gums, metallic taste, convulsions, delirium, and possibly coma.

• *Lethal midline granuloma.* Permanent anosmia accompanies this slowly progressive disease. Examination reveals ulcerative granulation tissue in the nose, sinuses, and palate; often widespread crust formation and tissue necrosis; septal cartilage destruction; and possible purulent rhinorrhea, serous otitis media, and inflammation of the eyelids and lacrimal apparatus.

• *Nasal or sinus neoplasms.* Anosmia may be permanent if the neoplasm destroys or displaces the olfactory nerve. Associated signs and symptoms may include unilateral or bilateral epistaxis, swelling and tenderness in the affected area, proptosis, diplopia, and decreased tearing.

• *Pernicious anemia.* Anosmia may be temporary or permanent. It's accompanied by the classic triad of weakness; sore, pale tongue; and numbness and tingling in the extremities. Related findings include distortion of taste, pallor, headache, irritability, dizziness, nausea, vomiting, diarrhea, and shortness of breath.

• *Polyps.* Temporary anosmia occurs when multiple polyps obstruct nasal cavities. Examination reveals the smooth, pale, grapelike polyp clusters.

• *Rhinitis.* In common *acute viral rhinitis,* temporary anosmia occurs with nasal congestion; sneezing; watery or purulent nasal discharge; red, swollen nasal mucosa; dryness or a tickling sensation in the nasopharynx; headache; low-grade fever; and chills.

In *allergic rhinitis,* temporary anosmia accompanies nasal congestion; itching mucosa; pale, edematous turbinates; thin nasal discharge; sneezing; tearing; and headache.

In *atrophic rhinitis,* anosmia resolves with successful treatment of the disorder. Purulent, yellow-green, foul-smelling crusts on sclerotic mucous membranes are characteristic, with paradoxical complaints of nasal congestion in an airway that's more open than normal. Turbinates are thin and atrophic. The nasopharynx and pharynx appear smooth, dry, and shiny rather than pink and moist.

In *vasomotor rhinitis,* temporary anosmia is accompanied by chronic nasal congestion, watery nasal discharge, postnasal drip, sneezing, and pale nasal mucosa.

• *Septal fracture.* Anosmia is usually temporary; sense of smell returns with septal repositioning. Examination reveals septal deviation and swelling, epistaxis, hematoma, nasal congestion, and ecchymoses.

• *Septal hematoma.* Anosmia is temporary, resolving with repair of the nasal mucosa or absorption of the hematoma. Associated signs include epistaxis; dusky-red, inflamed nasal mucosa; headache; and mouth breathing.

• *Sinusitis.* Temporary anosmia may be

associated with nasal congestion; sinus pain, tenderness, and swelling; severe headache; watery or purulent nasal discharge; postnasal drip; inflamed throat and nasal mucosa; enlarged, purulent turbinates; malaise; low-grade fever; and chills.

Other causes

• *Drugs.* Anosmia can result from prolonged use of nasal decongestants, which produces rebound nasal congestion. Occasionally, it results from naphazoline, a local decongestant that may cause paralysis of nasal cilia. It can also result from reserpine and, less commonly, amphetamines, phenothiazines, and estrogen, which cause nasal congestion.

• *Radiation therapy.* Permanent anosmia may follow radiation damage to the nasal mucosa or olfactory nerve.

• *Surgery.* Temporary anosmia may result from damage to the olfactory nerve or nasal mucosa during nasal or sinus surgery. Permanent anosmia accompanies a permanent tracheostomy, which disrupts nasal breathing.

Special considerations

If the patient's anosmia results from nasal congestion, administer local decongestants or antihistamines, and provide a vaporizer or humidifier to prevent mucosal drying and to help thin purulent nasal discharge. Advise the patient to avoid excessive use of local decongestants, which can lead to rebound nasal congestion.

If anosmia doesn't result from simple nasal congestion, prepare the patient for diagnostic tests, such as sinus transillumination, skull X-ray, or computed tomography scan, as ordered.

Although permanent anosmia usually doesn't respond to treatment, vitamin A given orally or by injection occasionally provides improvement.

Pediatric pointers

Anosmia in children most commonly results from nasal obstruction by a foreign body or enlarged adenoids.

Anuria

Clinically defined as urine output of less than 75 ml daily, anuria indicates either urinary tract obstruction or acute renal failure due to various mechanisms (see *Major Causes of Acute Renal Failure,* page 56). Fortunately, anuria rarely occurs—even in renal failure, the kidneys usually produce at least 75 ml of urine daily.

Because urine output is easily measured, anuria rarely goes undetected. However, without immediate treatment, anuria can rapidly cause uremia and other complications of urinary retention.

Assessment

After detecting anuria, your priorities are to determine if urine formation is occurring and to intervene appropriately. First, notify the doctor and prepare to catheterize the patient to relieve any lower urinary tract obstruction and to check for residual urine. You may find that an obstruction hinders catheter insertion and that urine return is cloudy and foul-smelling. If you collect more than 75 ml of urine, suspect lower urinary tract obstruction; less than 75 ml, renal dysfunction or obstruction higher in the urinary tract.

Next, take the patient's vital signs and obtain a complete patient history. Start by asking about any changes in the patient's usual voiding pattern. Determine the amount of fluid normally ingested each day, the amount of fluid ingested in the last 24 to 48 hours, and the time and amount of his last urination. Review the patient's medical history, noting especially previous kidney disease, urinary tract obstruction or infection, prostate enlargement, renal calculi, neurogenic bladder, or congenital abnormalities. Ask about recent abdominal, renal, or urinary tract surgery. Also ask about drug use.

MAJOR CAUSES OF ACUTE RENAL FAILURE

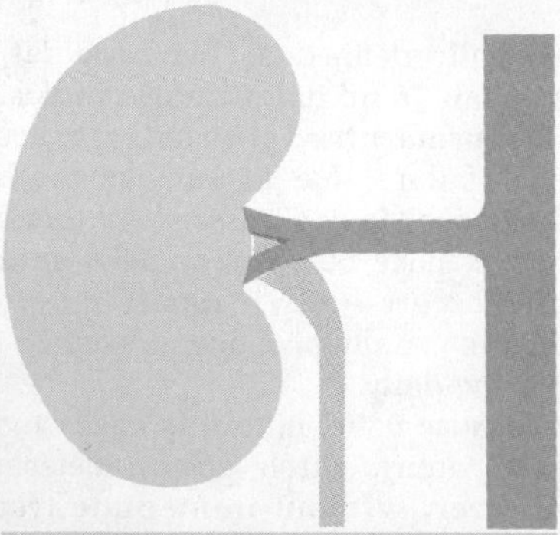

Intrarenal causes
Acute tubular necrosis
Cortical necrosis
Glomerulonephritis
Papillary necrosis
Renal vascular occlusion
Vasculitis

Postrenal causes
Bladder obstruction
Ureteral obstruction
Urethral obstruction

Prerenal causes
Decreased cardiac output
Hypovolemia
Peripheral vasodilation
Renovascular obstruction
Severe vasoconstriction

Inspect and palpate the abdomen for asymmetry, distention, or bulging. Inspect the flank area for edema or erythema, and percuss and palpate the bladder. Palpate the kidneys both anteriorly and posteriorly, and percuss them at the costovertebral angle. Auscultate over the renal arteries, listening for bruits.

Medical causes

• *Acute tubular necrosis.* Prolonged (up to 2 weeks) anuria or, more commonly,

oliguria is a common finding in this disorder. It precedes the onset of diuresis, which is heralded by polyuria. Associated findings reflect the underlying cause and may include signs of hyperkalemia (muscle weakness, cardiac dysrhythmias), uremia (anorexia, nausea, vomiting, confusion, lethargy, twitching, convulsions, pruritus, uremic frost, and Kussmaul's respirations), and congestive heart failure (edema, jugular vein distention, rales, and dyspnea).

• *Cortical necrosis (bilateral).* This disorder is characterized by a sudden change from oliguria to anuria, along with gross hematuria, flank pain, and fever.

• *Glomerulonephritis (acute).* This disorder produces anuria or oliguria. Related effects include mild fever, malaise, flank pain, hematuria, facial and generalized edema, elevated blood pressure, headache, nausea, vomiting, abdominal pain, and signs of pulmonary congestion (rales, dyspnea).

• *Hemolytic-uremic syndrome.* Anuria often occurs in the initial stages of this disorder and may last from 1 to 10 days. The patient may have vomiting, diarrhea, abdominal pain, hematemesis, melena, purpura, fever, elevated blood pressure, hepatomegaly, ecchymoses, edema, hematuria, and pallor. He may also show signs of upper respiratory tract infection.

• *Papillary necrosis (acute).* Bilateral papillary necrosis produces anuria or oliguria. It also produces flank pain, costovertebral angle tenderness, renal colic, abdominal pain and rigidity, fever, vomiting, decreased bowel sounds, hematuria, and pyuria.

• *Renal artery occlusion (bilateral).* This disorder produces anuria or severe oliguria, often accompanied by severe, continuous upper abdominal and flank pain; nausea and vomiting; decreased bowel sounds; and fever up to 102° F. (39° C.).

• *Renal vein occlusion (bilateral).* This disorder occasionally causes anuria; more typical signs and symptoms include acute low back pain, fever, flank tenderness, and hematuria. Development of pulmonary emboli, a common complication, produces sudden dyspnea, pleuritic pain, tachypnea, tachycardia, rales, pleural friction rub, and possibly hemoptysis.

• *Urinary tract obstruction.* Severe obstruction can produce acute and sometimes total anuria, alternating with or preceded by burning and pain on urination, overflow incontinence or dribbling, increased urinary frequency and nocturia, voiding of small amounts, or altered urinary stream. Associated findings may include bladder distention, pain and a sensation of fullness in the lower abdomen and groin, upper abdominal and flank pain, nausea and vomiting, and signs of secondary infection, such as fever, chills, malaise, and cloudy, foul-smelling urine.

• *Vasculitis.* This disorder occasionally produces anuria. More typical findings include malaise, myalgia, polyarthralgia, fever, elevated blood pressure, hematuria, dysrhythmias, pallor, and possibly skin lesions, urticaria, and purpura.

Other causes

• *Diagnostic tests.* Contrast media used in radiographic studies can cause nephrotoxicity, producing oliguria and, rarely, anuria.

• *Drugs.* Many classes of drugs can cause anuria or, more commonly, oliguria through their nephrotoxic effects. Antibiotics, especially the aminoglycosides, are the most commonly nephrotoxic. Adrenergic and anticholinergic drugs can cause anuria by affecting the nerves and muscles of micturition to produce urinary retention.

Special considerations

If catheterization fails to initiate urine flow, prepare the patient for diagnostic studies, such as ultrasonography, cystoscopy, retrograde pyelography, and renal scan, to detect possible obstruction higher in the urinary tract. If these tests reveal an obstruction, prepare the

patient for immediate surgery to remove the obstruction, and insert a nephrostomy or ureterostomy tube, as ordered, to drain the urine. However, if these tests fail to reveal an obstruction, prepare the patient for further kidney function studies.

While the diagnostic workup is being completed, carefully monitor the patient's vital signs and intake and output. Restrict the patient's daily fluid allowance to 600 ml more than the previous day's total urine output. Restrict foods and juices high in potassium and sodium, and make sure the patient maintains a balanced diet with controlled protein levels. Provide low-sodium hard candy to help decrease his thirst. Record fluid intake and output, and weigh the patient daily.

Pediatric pointers

Anuria in neonates is clinically defined as the absence of urinary output for 24 hours. It can be classified as primary or secondary. Primary anuria results from bilateral renal agenesis, aplasia, or multicystic dysplasia. Secondary anuria, associated with edema or dehydration, results from renal ischemia, renal vein thrombosis, or congenital anomalies of the genitourinary tract.

Anxiety

Anxiety, a subjective reaction to a real or imagined threat, can best be described as a nonspecific feeling of uneasiness or dread. It may be mild, moderate, or severe. Mild anxiety may cause slight physical or psychological discomfort, whereas severe anxiety may be incapacitating or even life-threatening.

Everyone experiences anxiety from time to time—it's a normal response to actual danger, prompting the body (through stimulation of the sympathetic and parasympathetic nervous systems) to purposeful action. It's also a normal response to physical and emotional stress, which can be produced by virtually any illness. In addition, anxiety can be precipitated or exacerbated by many nonpathologic factors, including lack of sleep, poor diet, and excessive intake of caffeine or other stimulants. However, excessive, unwarranted anxiety may indicate an underlying psychological problem.

Assessment
If the patient displays acute, severe anxiety, quickly take his vital signs and determine his chief complaint. Because anxiety is a notoriously nonspecific symptom, you'll need this information to guide your subsequent assessment and interventions. For example, if the patient's severe anxiety were accompanied by chest pain and shortness of breath, you might suspect myocardial infarction and act accordingly.

During your assessment, try to calm the patient as much as possible. Suggest relaxation techniques, and talk to him in a reassuring, soothing voice. Remember that uncontrolled anxiety can alter vital signs and often exacerbate the causative disorder.

If the patient displays mild or moderate anxiety, ask about its duration. Is his anxiety constant or sporadic? Did he notice any precipitating factors? Find out if his anxiety is exacerbated by stress, lack of sleep, or excessive caffeine intake and alleviated by rest, tranquilizers, or exercise.

Obtain a complete medical history, especially noting drug use. Then perform a physical examination, focusing on any complaints that may trigger or be aggravated by anxiety.

If the patient's anxiety isn't accompanied by significant physical signs, suspect a psychological basis. Assess the patient's level of consciousness and observe his behavior. If appropriate, refer him for psychiatric evaluation.

Medical causes
● *Adult respiratory distress syndrome.* Acute anxiety occurs along with tachy-cardia, mental sluggishness, and, in severe cases, hypotension. Associated respiratory signs include dyspnea, tachypnea, intercostal and suprasternal retractions, rales, and rhonchi.

● *Affective disorder.* In the depressive form of this disorder, chronic anxiety occurs with varying severity. The hallmark sign, though, is depression upon awakening, which abates over the course of the day. Associated signs and symptoms vary but may include dysphoria, anger, insomnia or hypersomnia, decreased libido, and multiple somatic complaints.

● *Anaphylactic shock.* Acute anxiety usually signals the onset of this shock state. It's accompanied by urticaria, angioedema, pruritus, and shortness of breath. Shortly thereafter, other signs and symptoms develop: light-headedness, hypotension, tachycardia, nasal congestion, sneezing, wheezing, dyspnea, barking cough, abdominal cramps, vomiting, diarrhea, and urinary urgency and incontinence.

● *Angina pectoris.* Acute anxiety may either precede or follow an attack of angina pectoris. An attack produces sharp and crushing substernal or anterior chest pain that may radiate to the back, neck, arms, or jaw. The pain is often relieved by nitroglycerin or rest, which eases anxiety.

● *Asthma.* In allergic asthma attacks, acute anxiety occurs with dyspnea, wheezing, productive cough, accessory muscle use, hyperresonant lung fields, diminished breath sounds, coarse rales, cyanosis, tachycardia, and diaphoresis.

● *Autonomic hyperreflexia (AHR).* The earliest sign of AHR may be acute anxiety accompanied by severe headache and dramatic hypertension. Pallor and motor and sensory deficits occur below the level of the lesion, while flushing occurs above it.

● *Cardiogenic shock.* Acute anxiety occurs along with cool, pale, clammy skin, tachycardia, weak and thready pulse, tachypnea, ventricular gallop, rales, neck vein distention, decreased urine output, hypotension, narrowing pulse pressure, and peripheral edema.

• *Chronic obstructive pulmonary disease.* Acute anxiety, dyspnea on exertion, cough, wheezing, rales, hyperresonant lung fields, tachypnea, and accessory muscle use characterize this disorder.

• *Congestive heart failure.* In this disorder, acute anxiety is frequently the first symptom of inadequate oxygenation. Associated signs and symptoms include restlessness, shortness of breath, tachypnea, decreased level of consciousness, edema, rales, ventricular gallop, hypotension, diaphoresis, and cyanosis.

• *Conversion disorder.* Chronic anxiety is characteristic along with one or two specific somatic complaints that have no physiologic basis. Common complaints are dizziness, chest pain, palpitations, a lump in the throat, and choking.

• *Hyperthyroidism.* Acute anxiety may be an early sign of this disorder. Classic signs include heat intolerance, weight loss despite increased appetite, nervousness, tremor, palpitations, sweating, an enlarged thyroid, and diarrhea. Exophthalmos may occur.

• *Hyperventilation syndrome.* This disorder produces acute anxiety, pallor, circumoral and peripheral paresthesia, and, occasionally, carpopedal spasms.

• *Hypochondriacal neurosis.* Mild-to-moderate chronic anxiety occurs in this disorder. Typically, the patient has vague or detailed physical complaints and is convinced they result from a fatal disease. Difficulty swallowing and back pain are but two of the common complaints. The patient tends to "physician hop" and isn't reassured by any number of favorable physical examinations and laboratory test results.

• *Hypoglycemia.* Anxiety resulting from hypoglycemia is usually mild to moderate and associated with hunger, mild headache, palpitations, blurred vision, weakness, and diaphoresis.

• *Myocardial infarction.* In this life-threatening disorder, acute anxiety commonly occurs with persistent, crushing substernal pain that may radiate to the left arm, jaw, neck, or shoulder blades. It can be accompanied by shortness of breath, nausea, vomiting, diaphoresis, and cool, pale skin.

• *Obsessive-compulsive disorders.* Chronic anxiety occurs in these psychiatric disorders, which are characterized by recurrent, unshakable thoughts or impulses to perform ritualistic acts that the patient recognizes as irrational but cannot control. The patient's anxiety builds if he can't perform these acts and diminishes after he does so.

• *Pheochromocytoma.* Acute, severe anxiety accompanies this disorder's cardinal sign—persistent or paroxysmal hypertension. Common associated signs and symptoms include tachycardia, diaphoresis, postural hypotension, tachypnea, flushing, severe headache, palpitations, nausea, vomiting, epigastric pain, and paresthesias.

• *Phobic disorder.* In this disorder, chronic anxiety occurs with persistent fear of an object, activity, or situation that results in a compelling desire to avoid it. The patient recognizes the fear as irrational but can't suppress it.

• *Pneumonia.* Acute anxiety may occur in pneumonia associated with hypoxemia. Related signs and symptoms include productive cough, pleuritic chest pain, fever, chills, rales, diminished breath sounds, and hyperresonant lung fields.

• *Pneumothorax.* Acute anxiety occurs in moderate-to-severe pneumothorax associated with profound respiratory distress. It's accompanied by sharp pleuritic pain, coughing, shortness of breath, cyanosis, asymmetrical chest expansion, weak and rapid pulse, pallor, and neck vein distention.

• *Postconcussion syndrome.* This syndrome may produce chronic anxiety or periodic attacks of acute anxiety. Associated symptoms include irritability, insomnia, dizziness, and mild headache. Usually, the anxiety is most pronounced in situations demanding attention, judgment, or comprehension.

• *Posttraumatic stress disorder.* This disorder produces chronic anxiety of varying severity. It's accompanied by intrusive, vivid memories and thoughts of the traumatic event. The patient also relives the event in dreams and nightmares. Insomnia, depression, and feelings of numbness and detachment are common.

• *Pulmonary edema.* In this disorder, acute anxiety occurs with dyspnea, orthopnea, cough with frothy sputum, tachycardia, tachypnea, rales, ventricular gallop, hypotension, and thready pulse. The patient's skin may be cool, clammy, and cyanotic.

• *Pulmonary embolism.* Acute anxiety is usually accompanied by dyspnea, tachypnea, chest pain, tachycardia, blood-tinged sputum, and low-grade fever.

• *Rabies.* Anxiety signals the beginning of the acute phase of this rare disorder. It's commonly accompanied by painful laryngeal spasms associated with difficulty swallowing and, as a result, hydrophobia.

• *Somatization disorder.* Most common in adolescents and young adults, this disorder is characterized by chronic anxiety and various somatic complaints that have no physiologic basis. Anxiety and depression may be prominent or hidden by dramatic, flamboyant, or seductive behavior.

Other causes

• *Drugs.* Many drugs cause anxiety, especially sympathomimetics and central nervous system stimulants. Tricyclic antidepressants may cause paradoxical anxiety.

Special considerations

Often your supportive nursing care can do much to help relieve the patient's anxiety. First, provide a calm, quiet atmosphere and make the patient comfortable. Encourage him to freely express his feelings and concerns. Take a short walk with him while you're talking, if this helps him. Or try anxiety-reducing measures, such as distraction, relaxation techniques, or biofeedback.

Pediatric pointers

Anxiety in children usually results from painful physical illness or inadequate oxygenation. Its autonomic signs tend to be more common and dramatic than in adults.

Aphasia

[Dysphasia]

Aphasia, impaired expression or comprehension of written or spoken language, reflects disease or injury of the brain's language centers (see *Where Language Originates*). Depending on its severity, aphasia may slightly impede communication or may make it impossible. It can be classified as Broca's, Wernicke's, anomic, or global aphasia (see *Identifying Types of Aphasia,* page 62). Anomic aphasia eventually resolves in more than 50% of patients, but global aphasia is irreversible.

Assessment

If the patient *suddenly* develops aphasia, have another nurse notify the doctor immediately. Quickly assess the patient for signs of increased intracranial pressure (ICP), such as pupillary changes, decreased level of consciousness, vomiting, seizures, bradycardia, widening pulse pressure, and irregular respirations. If you detect signs of increased ICP, administer mannitol I.V., as ordered, to decrease cerebral edema. Also, make sure that emergency resuscitation equipment is readily available to support respiratory and cardiac function, if necessary. If ordered, prepare the patient for emergency surgery.

If the patient doesn't display signs of increased ICP, or if his aphasia has developed gradually, perform a thorough neurologic assessment, starting with the patient history. You'll probably need to obtain this history from the patient's

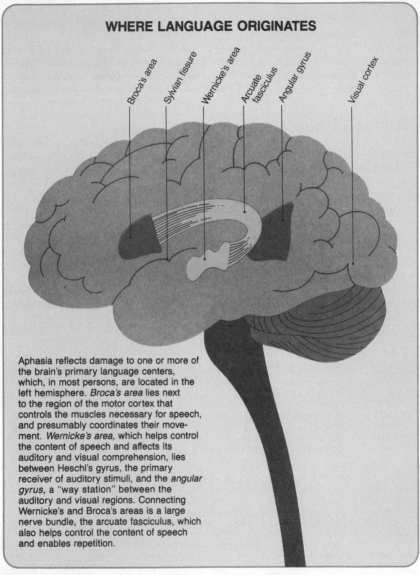

WHERE LANGUAGE ORIGINATES

Broca's area

Sylvian fissure

Wernicke's area

Arcuate fasciculus

Angular gyrus

Visual cortex

Aphasia reflects damage to one or more of the brain's primary language centers, which, in most persons, are located in the left hemisphere. *Broca's area* lies next to the region of the motor cortex that controls the muscles necessary for speech, and presumably coordinates their movement. *Wernicke's area,* which helps control the content of speech and affects its auditory and visual comprehension, lies between Heschl's gyrus, the primary receiver of auditory stimuli, and the *angular gyrus,* a "way station" between the auditory and visual regions. Connecting Wernicke's and Broca's areas is a large nerve bundle, the arcuate fasciculus, which also helps control the content of speech and enables repetition.

family or companion because of the patient's impairment. Ask about a history of headaches, hypertension, or seizure disorders and about drug use. Also ask about the patient's ability to communicate and to perform routine activities before aphasia began.

Check for obvious signs of neurologic deficit—such as ptosis or fluid leakage from the nose and ears. Take the pa-

tient's vital signs and assess his level of consciousness. Recognize, though, that assessing level of consciousness is often difficult because the patient's verbal responses may be unreliable. Also recognize that dysarthria (impaired articulation due to weakness or paralysis of the muscles necessary for speech) or speech apraxia (inability to voluntarily control the muscles of speech) may accompany aphasia; speak slowly and distinctly, and allow the patient ample time to respond. Assess pupillary response, eye movements, and motor function, especially mouth and tongue movement and swallowing. To best assess motor function, first demonstrate and then have the patient imitate responses, rather than merely providing verbal directions.

Medical causes

● *Alzheimer's disease.* In this degenerative disease, anomic aphasia may begin insidiously and then progress to Wernicke's and, finally, global aphasia. Associated signs include behavioral changes, memory loss, poor judgment, restlessness, myoclonus, and muscle rigidity. Incontinence is a late sign.

● *Brain abscess.* Any type of aphasia may occur in brain abscess. Usually, aphasia develops insidiously and may be accompanied by hemiparesis, ataxia, facial weakness, and signs of increased ICP.

● *Brain tumor.* Anomic aphasia may be an early sign of this disorder. As the tumor enlarges, other aphasias may occur along with behavioral changes, memory loss, motor weakness, seizures, auditory hallucinations, and visual field deficits.

● *Cerebrovascular accident.* The most common cause of aphasia, this disorder may produce Wernicke's, Broca's, or global aphasia. Associated findings usually include decreased level of consciousness, right-sided hemiparesis, homonymous hemianopia, and paresthesia and loss of sensation. (These symptoms may appear on the left side, if the right hemisphere contains the language centers.)

● *Encephalitis.* This disorder usually produces transient aphasia. Its earlier

IDENTIFYING TYPES OF APHASIA

TYPE	LOCATION OF LESION	CLINICAL FINDINGS
Broca's aphasia (expressive aphasia)	Broca's area; usually in third frontal convolution of the left hemisphere	Patient's understanding of written and spoken language is slightly impaired, but his motor impairment causes nonfluent speech. His speech also displays word-finding difficulty, jargon, paraphasias (inaccurate, sometimes unintelligible sound/word substitutions or neologisms), limited vocabulary, and simple sentence construction. Also, the patient can't repeat words or phrases.
Wernicke's aphasia (receptive aphasia)	Wernicke's area; usually in posterior/superior temporal lobe	Patient has difficulty understanding written and spoken language. He can't repeat words or phrases or follow directions. His speech is fluent, but it contains paraphasias and tends to be rapid and rambling. Also, the patient has difficulty naming objects (anomia).
Anomic aphasia	Temporal-parietal area; may extend to angular gyrus, but sometimes poorly localized	Patient's understanding of written and spoken language is relatively unimpaired. His speech, though fluent, lacks meaningful content. Word-finding difficulty and circumlocution (roundabout sentence construction) are characteristic. Rarely, the patient also displays paraphasias.
Global aphasia	Broca's and Wernicke's areas	Patient has profoundly impaired receptive and expressive ability. He can't repeat words or phrases and can't follow directions. His occasional speech is marked by paraphasias or jargon.

signs include fever, headache, and vomiting. Accompanying aphasia may be convulsions, confusion, stupor or coma, hemiparesis, asymmetrical deep tendon reflexes, positive Babinski's reflex, ataxia, myoclonus, nystagmus, ocular palsies, and facial weakness.

• *Head trauma.* Any type of aphasia may accompany severe head trauma; typically, it occurs suddenly and may be transient or permanent, depending on the extent of brain damage. Associated signs and symptoms may include blurred or double vision, headache, pallor, diaphoresis, numbness and paresis, cerebrospinal otorrhea or rhinorrhea, altered respirations, tachycardia, disorientation, behavioral changes, and signs of increased ICP.

• *Transient ischemic attack (TIA).* This disorder can produce any type of aphasia. Usually, the aphasia occurs suddenly and resolves within 24 hours of the TIA. Associated symptoms include transient hemiparesis, hemianopia, and paresthesia (all usually right-sided), dizziness, and confusion.

Other causes
• *Drug abuse.* Heroin overdose can cause any type of aphasia.

Special considerations
Immediately after aphasia develops, the patient may become confused or disoriented. Help to restore a sense of reality by frequently telling him what has happened, where he is and why, and the date. Carefully explain diagnostic tests, such as skull X-rays, computed tomography scan, angiography, and electroencephalography. Later, expect periods of depression as the patient recognizes his handicap. Help him to communicate by providing a relaxed, accepting environment with a minimum of distracting stimuli.

Be alert for sudden outbursts of profanity by the patient. This common behavior usually reflects intense frustration with his impairment. Deal with such outbursts as gently as possible to ease embarrassment.

When you speak to the patient, don't assume that he understands you. He may simply be interpreting subtle clues to meaning, such as social context, facial expressions, and gestures. To help avoid misunderstanding, speak to him in simple phrases, and use demonstration to clarify your verbal directions, when appropriate.

Remember that aphasia is a *language* disorder, not an emotional or auditory one, so speak to the patient in a normal tone of voice. Make sure he has necessary aids, such as eyeglasses or dentures, to facilitate communication.

Refer the patient to a speech pathologist early to help him cope with his aphasia. Support from social services may be necessary later, if the patient is unable to return to work.

Pediatric pointers
Recognize that the term *childhood aphasia* is sometimes mistakenly applied to children who fail to develop normal language skills but who aren't considered mentally retarded or developmentally delayed. Aphasia refers solely to loss of previously developed communication skills.

Brain damage associated with aphasia in children most commonly follows anoxia—the result of near-drowning or airway obstruction.

Apnea

Apnea is the cessation of spontaneous respiration. Occasionally, it's temporary and self-limiting, as occurs during Cheyne-Stokes and Biot's respirations. More often, though, it's a life-threatening emergency that requires immediate intervention to prevent death.

Apnea usually results from one or more of six pathophysiologic mechanisms, each of which has numerous causes (see *Causes of Apnea,* page 65). Its most common causes include trauma, cardiac arrest, neurologic disease, aspiration of foreign objects, bronchospasm, and drug overdose.

Assessment

If you detect apnea, your first priority is to establish and maintain a patent airway. Position the patient supine and open his airway using the head-tilt or chin-lift technique. (*Caution:* Use the jaw-thrust technique on a patient with an obvious or suspected head or neck injury, to prevent hyperextending the neck.) Next, quickly look, listen, and feel for spontaneous respiration; if it's absent, begin artificial ventilation until it occurs or until mechanical ventilation can be initiated.

Because apnea may result from cardiac arrest (or may cause it), be sure to assess the patient's carotid pulse immediately after you've established a patent airway. Or, if the patient's an infant or small child, assess the brachial pulse instead. If you can't palpate a pulse, begin cardiac compression.

Once you're satisfied that the patient's respiratory and cardiac status is stable, begin to investigate the underlying cause of apnea. Ask the patient (or, if he's unable to answer, anyone who witnessed the episode) about the onset of apnea and the events immediately preceding it. The cause may become readily apparent, as in trauma.

Take a patient history, noting especially any reports of headache, chest pain, muscle weakness, sore throat, or dyspnea. Ask about any history of respiratory, cardiac, or neurologic disease and about allergies and drug use.

Inspect the head, face, neck, and trunk for soft-tissue injury, hemorrhage, or skeletal deformity. Don't overlook obvious clues, such as oral and nasal secretions reflecting fluid-filled airways and alveoli or facial soot and singed nasal hair suggesting thermal injury to the tracheobronchial tree.

Auscultate over all lung lobes for adventitious breath sounds, particularly rales and rhonchi, and percuss the lung fields for increased dullness or hyper-resonance. Move on to the heart, auscultating for murmurs, pericardial friction rub, and dysrhythmias. Check for cyanosis, pallor, jugular vein distention, and edema. If appropriate, perform a neurologic assessment. Evaluate level of consciousness, orientation, and mental status; test cranial nerve function and motor function, sensation, and reflexes in all extremities.

Medical causes

• *Airway obstruction.* Occlusion or compression of the trachea, central airways, or smaller airways can cause sudden apnea by blocking airflow and producing acute respiratory failure.

• *Alveolar gas diffusion impairment.* An occlusion at the alveolar-capillary membrane level or an accumulation of fluid within the alveoli themselves produces apnea by interfering with pulmonary gas exchange and producing acute respiratory failure. Apnea may arise suddenly, as in near-drowning and acute pulmonary edema, or more gradually, as in emphysema. It may be preceded by rales and labored respirations with accessory muscle use.

• *Brain stem dysfunction.* Primary or secondary brain stem dysfunction can cause apnea by destroying the brain stem's ability to initiate respirations. Apnea may arise suddenly (as in trauma, hemorrhage, or infarction) or gradually (as in degenerative disease or tumor). It may be preceded by decreased level of consciousness and various motor and sensory deficits.

• *Pleural pressure gradient disruption.* Conversion of normal negative pleural air pressure to positive pressure by chest wall injuries (such as flail chest) causes lung collapse, producing respiratory distress and, if untreated, apnea. Associated signs include an asymmetrical chest wall and asymmetrical or paradoxical respirations.

• *Pulmonary capillary perfusion decrease.* Apnea can stem from obstructed pulmonary circulation, most commonly due to heart failure or lack of circulatory patency. It occurs suddenly in cardiac arrest, massive pulmonary embolism, and most cases of severe shock. In contrast, it occurs progressively in septic shock and pulmonary hypertension. Related findings include hypotension, tachycardia, and edema.

• *Respiratory muscle failure.* Trauma or disease can disrupt the mechanics of respiration, causing sudden or gradual apnea. Associated findings may include diaphragmatic or intercostal muscle paralysis from injury, or respiratory weakness or paralysis from acute or degenerative disease.

Other causes
• *Drugs.* Central nervous system (CNS) depressants—such as narcotic analgesics, barbiturates, anesthetics, and alcohol—may cause hypoventilation and apnea. Intravenous infusion of benzodiazepines, such as diazepam, may cause respiratory depression and apnea when given with other CNS depressants, especially in elderly or acutely ill patients. Neuromuscular blocking agents—such as curariform drugs (especially when given concomitantly with aminoglycosides) and anticholinesterase inhibitors—may produce sudden apnea due to respiratory muscle paralysis.

Special considerations
Closely monitor the apneic patient's cardiac and respiratory status to prevent further apneic episodes.

Pediatric pointers
Premature infants are especially susceptible to periodic apneic episodes due to CNS immaturity. Other common causes of apnea in infants include sepsis, intraventricular and subarachnoid hemorrhage, seizures, bronchiolitis, and sudden infant death syndrome.

In toddlers and older children, the primary cause of apnea is acute airway obstruction from aspiration of foreign objects. Other causes include acute epiglottitis, croup, asthma, and systemic disorders such as muscular dystrophy and cystic fibrosis.

CAUSES OF APNEA

Airway obstruction
• Airway edema
• Airway occlusion by tongue
• Airway occlusion by tumor
• Asthma
• Bronchospasm
• Chronic bronchitis
• Diffuse atelectasis
• Foreign body aspiration
• Hemothorax or pneumothorax
• Mucous plugging
• Obstructive sleep apnea
• Secretion retention
• Tracheal/bronchial rupture

Alveolar gas diffusion impairment
• Adult respiratory distress syndrome
• Diffuse pneumonia
• Emphysema
• Near-drowning
• Pulmonary edema
• Pulmonary fibrosis
• Secretion retention

Brain stem dysfunction
• Brain abscess
• Brain stem injury
• Brain tumor
• Cerebral hemorrhage
• Cerebral infarction
• Encephalitis
• Head trauma
• Hypoventilatory sleep apnea
• Increased intracranial pressure
• Meningitis
• Pontine/medullary hemorrhage or infarction
• Transtentorial herniation

Pleural pressure gradient disruption
• Flail chest
• Open chest wounds

Pulmonary capillary perfusion decrease
• Cardiac arrest
• Dysrhythmias
• Myocardial infarction
• Pulmonary embolism
• Pulmonary hypertension
• Shock

Respiratory muscle failure
• Amyotrophic lateral sclerosis
• Botulism
• Diphtheria
• Guillain-Barré syndrome
• Myasthenia gravis
• Phrenic nerve paralysis
• Rupture of the diaphragm
• Spinal cord injury

Apneustic Respirations

This irregular breathing pattern is characterized by prolonged, gasping inspiration and brief, inefficient expiration. It's an important localizing sign of severe brain stem damage.

Involuntary breathing is primarily regulated by groups of neurons, or respiratory centers, in the medulla oblongata and the pons. In the medulla, neurons react to impulses from the pons and other areas to regulate respiratory rate and depth. In the pons, two respiratory centers regulate respiratory rhythm by interacting with the medullary respiratory center to smooth the transition from inspiration to expiration and back. The apneustic center in the pons stimulates inspiratory neurons in the medulla to precipitate inspiration. These inspiratory neurons, in turn, stimulate the pneumotaxic center in the pons to precipitate expiration. Destruction of neural pathways by pontine lesions disrupts regulation of respiratory rhythm, causing apneustic respirations.

Apneustic respirations must be differentiated from bradypnea and hyperpnea (disturbances in rate and depth, but not in rhythm), Cheyne-Stokes respirations (rhythmic alterations in rate and depth, followed by periods of apnea), and Biot's respirations (irregularly alternating periods of hyperpnea and apnea).

Assessment

Your first priority for the patient with apneustic respirations is to ensure adequate ventilation. Have another nurse notify the doctor while you prepare to insert an artificial airway and administer oxygen until mechanical ventilation can begin. Next, thoroughly assess the patient's neurologic status, using a standardized tool such as the Glasgow Coma Scale. Obtain a brief patient history from a family member or companion, if possible.

Medical cause
● **Pontine lesions.** Apneustic respirations invariably result from extensive damage to the upper or lower pons, whether due to infarction, hemorrhage, herniation, severe infection, tumor, or trauma. Typically, they're accompanied by profound stupor or coma; pinpoint midline pupils; ocular bobbing (a spontaneous downward jerk, followed by a slow drift up to midline); quadriplegia or, less commonly, hemiplegia with pupils pointing toward the affected side; a positive Babinski's reflex; negative oculocephalic and oculovestibular reflexes; and, possibly, decorticate posture.

Special considerations
Constantly monitor the patient's neurologic and respiratory status. Notify the doctor immediately of prolonged apneic periods or signs of neurologic deterioration. Monitor the patient's arterial blood gas levels. If appropriate, prepare him for neurologic tests, such as electroencephalography and computed tomography.

Pediatric pointers
In young children, avoid using the Glasgow Coma Scale since it requires verbal responses and assumes a certain level of language development.

Apraxia

Apraxia is the inability to perform purposeful movements in the absence of significant weakness, sensory loss, poor coordination, or lack of comprehension or motivation. This uncommon neurologic sign usually indicates a lesion in the cerebral cortex. Its onset, severity, and duration vary, depending on the location and extent of the lesion.

Apraxia is classified as *ideational,*

HOW APRAXIA INTERFERES WITH PURPOSEFUL MOVEMENT

TYPE OF APRAXIA	DESCRIPTION	ASSESSMENT TECHNIQUE
Ideational apraxia	The patient can physically perform the steps required to complete a task but fails to remember the sequence in which they're performed.	Ask the patient to tie his shoelace. Typically, he'll be able to grasp the shoelace, loop it, and pull on it. However, he'll fail to remember the sequence of steps needed to tie a knot.
Ideomotor apraxia	The patient understands and can physically perform the steps required to complete a task but can't formulate a plan to carry them out.	Ask the patient to wave or cross his arms. Typically, he won't respond. Later, he'll be able to perform the gesture spontaneously.
Kinetic apraxia	The patient understands the task and formulates a plan but fails to set the proper muscles in motion.	Ask the patient to comb his hair. Typically, he'll fail to move his arm and hand correctly to do so. However, he'll be able to state that he needs to pick up the comb and draw it through his hair.

ideomotor, or *kinetic,* depending on the stage at which voluntary movement is impaired (see *How Apraxia Interferes with Purposeful Movement*). It can also be classified by type of motor or skill impairment. For example, *facial* and *gait* apraxia involve specific motor groups and are easily perceived. *Constructional* apraxia refers to the inability to copy simple drawings or patterns. *Dressing* apraxia refers to the inability to dress oneself correctly. *Callosal* apraxia refers to normal motor function on one side of the body accompanied by the inability to reproduce movements on the other side.

Assessment

If you detect apraxia, ask about previous neurologic disease. If the patient fails to report such disease, notify the doctor and begin a neurologic assessment. First, take the patient's vital signs and assess his level of consciousness (LOC). Be alert for any evidence of aphasia or dysarthria. Ask the patient if he has recently experienced headache or dizziness. Then test motor function, observing for weakness and tremors. Next, use a small pin or other pointed object to test sensory function. Check deep tendon reflexes for quality and symmetry. Finally, test the patient for visual field deficits.

During your assessment, be alert for signs of increased intracranial pressure, such as headache and vomiting. If you detect these, elevate the head of the bed 30° and monitor the patient closely for altered pupil size and reactivity, bradycardia, widened pulse pressure, and irregular respirations. Have emergency resuscitation equipment nearby, and be prepared to give mannitol I.V. to decrease cerebral edema.

If you detect seizures, stay with the patient and have another nurse notify the doctor immediately. Avoid restraining the patient. Help him to a lying position, loosen any tight clothing, and place a pillow or other soft object beneath his head. If the patient's teeth are clenched, don't force anything into his mouth. If his mouth is open, protect the tongue by placing a soft object, such as a washcloth, between his teeth. Turn the patient's head to provide an open airway.

After completing the examination and ensuring the patient's safety, take a history. Ask about previous cerebrovascular disease, atherosclerosis, neoplastic disease, infection, or hepatic disease. Then assess the apraxia further to help determine its type.

Medical causes

• *Alzheimer's disease.* This disorder sometimes causes gradual and irreversible ideomotor apraxia. It can also cause amnesia, anomia, decreased attention span, apathy, aphasia, restlessness, agitation, paranoid delusions, incontinence, social withdrawal, ataxia, and tremors.

• *Brain abscess.* Apraxia occasionally results from a large brain abscess but usually resolves spontaneously after the infection subsides. Typically, its type depends on the location of the abscess. The apraxia is accompanied by headache, fever, drowsiness, decreased mental acuity, aphasia, dysarthria, hemiparesis, focal or generalized seizures, and ocular disturbances such as nystagmus, decreased visual acuity, and unequal pupils.

• *Brain tumor.* In this disorder, progressive apraxia may be preceded by decreased mental acuity, headache, dizziness, and seizures. It may occur with or directly after early signs of increased intracranial pressure, such as pupil changes. It may also occur with other localizing signs of the tumor, such as aphasia, visual field deficits, weakness, stiffness, and hyperreflexia in the extremities.

• *Cerebrovascular accident (CVA).* This disorder commonly causes sudden onset of apraxia. Although apraxia often resolves spontaneously, it may persist after massive CVA. Associated signs and symptoms vary according to the affected artery but can include confusion, stupor or coma, hemiplegia, unilateral or bilateral visual field deficits, aphasia, agnosia, dysarthria, and urinary incontinence.

• *Hepatic encephalopathy.* This disorder may cause gradual onset of constructional apraxia, which may be reversible with treatment. Early associated signs and symptoms include disorientation, amnesia, slurred speech, asterixis, and lethargy. Later signs include hyperreflexia, positive Babinski's reflex, agitation, seizures, fetor hepaticus, stupor, and coma.

Other cause

• *Hemodialysis.* Long-term hemodialysis occasionally causes a syndrome known as dialysis dementia or dialysis encephalopathy. In this syndrome, speech apraxia accompanies other speech deficits, seizures, and behavioral changes.

Special considerations

Prepare the patient for diagnostic studies, such as computed tomography and radionuclide brain scans.

Because weakness, sensory deficits, confusion, and seizures may accompany apraxia, take measures to ensure safety. For example, assist the patient with gait apraxia in walking.

Explain the patient's apraxia to him, and encourage his participation in normal activities. Help him to overcome his frustrations at being unable to perform routine tasks. Demonstrate each step in these tasks, and give the patient sufficient time to imitate each step. Avoid giving complex directions, and enlist the help of family members in rehabilitation. Also refer the patient to a physical or occupational therapist.

Pediatric pointers

Detecting apraxia in children is often difficult. However, any sudden inability to perform a previously accomplished movement warrants prompt neurologic evaluation, since brain tumor—the most common cause of

APRAXIA: CAUSES AND ASSOCIATED FINDINGS

CAUSES	Amnesia	Aphasia	Decreased LOC	Decreased mental acuity	Dysarthria	Fetor hepaticus	Headache	Hyperreflexia	Incontinence	Seizures	Tremors	Visual field deficits
Alzheimer's disease	•	•							•		•	
Brain abscess		•		•	•		•			•		
Brain tumor		•		•			•	•	•	•		•
Cerebrovascular accident		•	•		•				•			•
Hepatic encephalopathy	•			•		•		•		•	•	

apraxia in children—can be treated effectively if detected early.

Brain damage in a young child may cause developmental apraxia, which interferes with the ability to learn activities that require sequential movement, such as hopping, jumping, hitting or kicking a ball, or dancing. When caring for a child with apraxia, be aware of his limitations, yet provide an environment that's conducive to rehabilitation. Provide emotional support since playmates will often tease a child who's unable to perform normal physical activities.

Arm Pain

Usually, arm pain results from musculoskeletal disorders, but it can also result from neurovascular or cardiovascular disorders. Its location, onset, and character provide clues to its cause. The pain may affect the entire arm or only the upper arm or forearm. It may arise suddenly or gradually and be constant or intermittent. Arm pain can be described as sharp or dull, burning or numbing, shooting or penetrating. Diffuse arm pain, though, may be difficult to describe, especially if it isn't associated with injury.

Assessment
If the patient reports arm pain after an injury, take a brief history of the injury from the patient or his companion. Then quickly assess for severe injuries requiring immediate treatment. If you've ruled out severe injuries, check pulses, capillary refill time, sensation, and movement distal to the affected area, since circulatory impairment or nerve injury may require immediate surgery. Inspect the arm for deformity, assess the level of pain, and immobilize the arm to prevent further injury.

CAUSES OF LOCAL PAIN

Various disorders cause hand, wrist, elbow, or shoulder pain. In some disorders, pain may radiate from the injury site to other areas.

Hand pain
Arthritis
Buerger's disease
Carpal tunnel syndrome
Dupuytren's contracture
Elbow tunnel syndrome
Fracture
Ganglion
Infection
Occlusive vascular disease
Radiculopathy
Raynaud's disease
Shoulder-hand syndrome (reflex
   sympathetic dystrophy)
Sprain or strain
Thoracic outlet syndromes
Trigger finger

Wrist pain
Arthritis
Carpal tunnel syndrome
Fracture
Ganglion
Sprain or strain
Tenosynovitis (de Quervain's disease)

Elbow pain
Arthritis
Bursitis
Dislocation
Fracture
Lateral epicondylitis (tennis elbow)
Tendonitis

Shoulder pain
Acromioclavicular separation
Acute pancreatitis
Adhesive capsulitis (frozen shoulder)
Angina pectoris
Arthritis
Bursitis
Cholecystitis/cholelithiasis
Clavicle fracture
Diaphragmatic pleurisy
Dislocation
Dissecting aortic aneurysm
Gastritis
Humeral neck fracture
Infection
Pancoast's syndrome
Perforated ulcer
Pneumothorax
Ruptured spleen (left shoulder)
Shoulder-hand syndrome
Subphrenic abscess
Tendonitis

If the patient reports generalized or intermittent arm pain, ask him to describe the pain and relate when it began. Is pain associated with repetitive or specific movements or positions? Ask him to point out other painful areas, since arm pain may be referred. For example, arm pain may accompany the characteristic chest pain of myocardial infarction. Ask him if the pain worsens in the morning or in the evening, if it prevents him from performing his job, or if it restricts any movements. Also ask if heat, rest, or drugs relieve it. Finally, ask about any preexisting illnesses, a family history of gout or arthritis, and current drug therapy.

Next, perform a focused examination. Observe the way the patient walks, sits, and holds his arm. Inspect the entire arm, comparing it to the opposite arm for symmetry, movement, and muscle atrophy. Palpate the entire arm for swelling, nodules, and tender areas. In both arms, compare active range of motion, muscle strength, and reflexes.

If the patient reports numbness or tingling, check his sensation to vibration and pinprick. Compare bilateral hand grasps and shoulder strength to detect weakness.

If a patient has a cast, splint, or restrictive dressing, check for circulation, sensation, and mobility distal to the dressing. Ask the patient about edema and if the pain has worsened within the last 24 hours. Also ask what activities he has been performing.

Medical causes

• **Angina.** This disorder may cause inner arm pain, as well as chest and jaw pain. Typically, the pain follows exertion and persists for a few minutes. Accompanied by dyspnea, diaphoresis, and apprehension, the pain is relieved by rest or vasodilators, such as nitroglycerin.

• **Biceps rupture.** Rupture of the biceps after excessive weight lifting or osteoarthritic degeneration of bicipital tendon insertion at the shoulder can cause pain in the upper arm. Forearm

ARM PAIN: CAUSES AND ASSOCIATED FINDINGS

CAUSES	MAJOR ASSOCIATED SIGNS AND SYMPTOMS											
	Chest pain	Crepitus	Decreased motion	Decreased reflex response	Deformity	Ecchymosis	Edema	Impaired circulation	Muscle weakness	Nausea	Paresthesia	Vomiting
Angina	●											
Biceps rupture					●		●		●			
Cellulitis							●					
Cervical nerve root compression				●					●		●	
Compartment syndrome				●			●	●	●		●	
Fractures		●	●		●	●	●	●			●	
Muscle contusion						●	●					
Muscle strain			●						●			
Myocardial infarction	●									●		●
Neoplasms of the arm							●	●			●	
Osteomyelitis			●				●					

flexion and supination aggravate the pain. Other signs include muscle weakness, deformity, and edema.

• **Cellulitis.** Typically, this disorder affects the legs, but it can also affect the arms. It produces pain as well as redness, tenderness, edema, and, at times, fever, chills, tachycardia, headache, and hypotension.

• **Cervical nerve root compression.** Compression of the cervical nerves supplying the upper arm produces chronic arm and neck pain, which may worsen with movement or prolonged sitting.

The patient may also experience muscle weakness, paresthesia, and decreased reflex response.

• **Compartment syndrome.** Severe pain with passive muscle stretching is the cardinal sign of this syndrome. It may also impair distal circulation and cause muscle weakness, decreased reflex response, paresthesia, and edema. Ominous signs include paralysis and absent pulse.

• **Fractures.** In fractures of the cervical vertebrae, humerus, scapula, clavicle, radius, or ulna, pain can occur at the injury site and radiate throughout the entire arm. Pain at a fresh fracture site is intense and worsens with movement. Associated signs and symptoms include crepitus, felt and heard from bone ends rubbing together (do not attempt to elicit this sign); deformity, if bones are unaligned; local ecchymosis and edema; impaired distal circulation; paresthesia; and decreased sensation distal to the injury site.

● **Muscle contusion.** This disorder may cause generalized pain in the area of injury. It may also cause local swelling and ecchymosis.

● **Muscle strain.** Acute or chronic muscle strain causes mild-to-severe pain with movement. The resultant reduction in arm movement may cause muscle weakness and atrophy.

● **Myocardial infarction.** In this life-threatening disorder, the patient may complain of left arm pain as well as the characteristic deep and crushing chest pain. He may display weakness, pallor, nausea, vomiting, diaphoresis, altered blood pressure, tachycardia, dyspnea, and feelings of apprehension or impending doom.

● **Neoplasms of the arm.** This disorder produces continuous, deep, and penetrating arm pain that worsens at night. Occasionally, redness and swelling accompany arm pain; later, skin breakdown, impaired circulation, and paresthesia may occur.

● **Osteomyelitis.** This disorder typically begins with the sudden onset of localized arm pain and fever. It's accompanied by local tenderness, painful and restricted movement, and later, swelling. Associated findings include malaise and tachycardia.

Special considerations

If you suspect a fracture, apply a sling or a splint to immobilize the arm, and monitor for worsening pain, numbness, or decreased circulation distal to the injury site. Also monitor vital signs, and be alert for tachycardia, hypotension, and diaphoresis. Withhold food, fluids, and analgesics until the doctor evaluates potential fractures. Promote the patient's comfort by elevating his arm and applying ice. Cleanse abrasions and lacerations and apply dry, sterile dressings, if necessary.

Also prepare the patient for X-rays or other diagnostic tests.

Pediatric pointers

In children, arm pain commonly results from fractures, muscle sprain, muscular dystrophy, or rheumatoid arthritis. In young children especially, the exact location of the pain may be difficult to establish. Watch for nonverbal clues, such as wincing or guarding.

If the child has a fracture or sprain, obtain a complete account of the injury. Closely observe interactions between the child and his family, and don't rule out the possibility of child abuse.

Asterixis

[Liver flap, flapping tremor]

A bilateral, coarse tremor, asterixis is characterized by rapid, nonrhythmic extensions and flexions. This elicited sign is most commonly observed in the wrists and fingers but also appears in the ankles, the corners of the mouth, the eyelids, and the tongue. Typically, it signals the onset of coma in end-stage hepatic, renal, and pulmonary disease.

To elicit asterixis, have the patient extend his arms, dorsiflex his wrists, and spread his fingers (or do this for him, if necessary). Briefly observe for asterixis. Alternately, if the patient has a decreased level of consciousness but can follow verbal commands, ask him to squeeze two of your fingers. Consider rapid clutching and unclutching positive for asterixis. Or elevate the patient's leg off the bed and dorsiflex the foot. Briefly observe for asterixis in the ankle. If the patient can tightly close his eyes and mouth, observe for irregular tremulous movements of the eyelids and corners of the mouth. If he can stick out his tongue, observe for continuous quivering.

Assessment

Because asterixis usually signals impending coma, quickly assess neurologic status and vital signs. Compare this data to the patient's baseline, and report acute changes to the doctor immediately. Continue to closely monitor neurologic status, vital signs, and urine output. Watch for signs of respiratory insufficiency, and be prepared to assist with endotracheal intubation and ventilatory support. Also be alert for complications of end-stage hepatic, renal, or pulmonary disease.

If the patient has hepatic disease, assess for early signs of hemorrhage, including restlessness, tachypnea, and cool, moist, pale skin. (If the patient is jaundiced, check for pallor in the conjunctiva and mucous membranes of the mouth.) Recognize that hypotension, oliguria, hematemesis, and melena are late signs of hemorrhage. If any of these signs develop, notify the doctor immediately. Prepare to insert a large-bore I.V. for fluid and blood replacement. Position the patient flat in bed with his legs elevated 20°. Begin or continue to administer oxygen.

If the patient has renal disease, briefly review what type of therapy he's received. If he's on dialysis, ask about the frequency of treatments to help gauge the severity of disease. Question a family member if the patient's level of consciousness is significantly decreased. Then assess for hyperkalemia and metabolic acidosis. Look for tachycardia, nausea, diarrhea, abdominal cramps, muscle weakness, hyperreflexia, and Kussmaul's respirations. If you detect any of these signs, notify the doctor immediately. Prepare to administer sodium bicarbonate, calcium gluconate, dextrose, insulin, or Kayexalate, as ordered.

If the patient has pulmonary disease, assess for labored respirations, tachypnea, accessory muscle use, and cya-

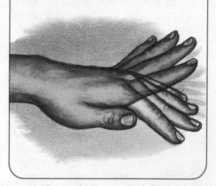

ASTERIXIS: A CHARACTERISTIC FLAPPING TREMOR

In asterixis, the wrists and fingers "flap" in rapid, nonrhythmic extension and flexion when the arms are extended, wrists dorsiflexed, and fingers spread.

nosis. If you detect any of these signs, notify the doctor immediately. Prepare to assist with ventilatory support via nasal cannula, mask, or intubation and mechanical ventilation.

Medical causes

• *Hepatic encephalopathy.* This life-threatening disorder initially causes slight personality changes (disorientation, forgetfulness, slurred speech) and a slight tremor. This tremor progresses into asterixis—the hallmark of hepatic encephalopathy—and is accompanied by lethargy, aberrant behavior, and apraxia. Eventually, the patient becomes stuporous and displays hyperventilation. When he slips into coma, hyperactive reflexes, a positive Babinski's reflex, and fetor hepaticus are characteristic. There may also be bradycardia, decreased respirations, and seizures.

• *Severe respiratory insufficiency.* Characterized by life-threatening respiratory acidosis, this disorder initially produces headache, restlessness, confusion, apprehension, and decreased reflexes. Eventually, the patient becomes somnolent and may demonstrate asterixis before slipping into coma. Associated signs and symptoms of respiratory insufficiency include difficulty breathing and rapid, shallow respirations. The patient may be hypertensive in early disease but may develop hypotension later.

• *Uremic syndrome.* This life-threatening disorder initially causes lethargy, somnolence, confusion, disorientation, behavior changes, and irritability. Eventually, though, signs and symptoms appear in diverse body systems. Asterixis is accompanied by stupor, paresthesias, muscle twitching, fasciculations, and foot drop. Other signs and symptoms include polyuria and nocturia followed by oliguria and, then, anuria; elevated blood pressure; signs of congestive heart failure and pericarditis; Kussmaul's respirations; anorexia; nausea; vomiting; diarrhea; GI bleeding; weight loss; ammonia breath odor; and metallic taste. Uremic syndrome also produces pallor, bleeding tendency, uremic frost, pruritus, brittle and thin nails, hair loss, muscle wasting, and pathologic fractures. Impotence may occur in the male, amenorrhea in the female.

Special considerations
Provide simple patient comfort measures, such as frequent rest periods to minimize fatigue. Elevate the head of the bed to relieve dyspnea and orthopnea. Administer oil baths and avoid soap to relieve itching caused by jaundice and uremia. Provide emotional support to the patient and his family.

Provide enteral or parenteral nutrition if the patient is intubated or has a decreased level of consciousness. Closely monitor serum and urine glucose levels to evaluate hyperalimentation. Since the patient will probably be on bed rest, reposition him at least once every 2 hours to prevent skin breakdown. Also, recognize that his debilitated state makes him prone to infection. Observe strict hand washing and aseptic technique when changing dressings and caring for invasive lines.

Pediatric pointers
End-stage hepatic, renal, and pulmonary disease may also cause asterixis in children.

Ataxia

Classified as cerebellar or sensory, ataxia refers to incoordination and irregularity of voluntary, purposeful movements. *Cerebellar* ataxia results from disease of the cerebellum and its pathways to and from the cerebral cortex, brain stem, and spinal cord. It causes gait, trunk, limb, and possibly speech disorders. *Sensory* ataxia results from impaired position sense (proprioception) caused by interruption of afferent nerve fibers in the peripheral nerves, posterior roots, posterior columns of the spinal cord, or medial lemnisci, or occasionally by a lesion in both parietal lobes. It causes gait disorders.

Ataxia occurs in acute and chronic forms. *Acute* ataxia, usually cerebellar, may result from hemorrhage or a large tumor in the posterior fossa. In this life-threatening condition, the cerebellum may herniate downward through the foramen magnum behind the cervical spinal cord or upward through the tentorium upon the cerebral hemispheres. Herniation may also compress the brain stem. Acute ataxia may also result from drug toxicity or poisoning. *Chronic* ataxia can be progressive and, at times, can result from acute disease. It can also occur in metabolic and chronic degenerative neurologic disease.

Assessment
If you observe ataxic movements, assess the patient for signs of increased intracranial pressure and impending herniation. Assess his level of consciousness and be alert for pupillary abnormalities, motor weakness or paralysis, neck stiffness or pain, and vomiting. Check

the patient's vital signs, especially respirations; abnormal respiratory patterns may quickly lead to respiratory arrest. Report any untoward signs at once, and elevate the head of the bed. Have emergency resuscitation equipment readily available and, if ordered, prepare the patient for computed tomography scanning or surgery.

If the patient isn't in distress, review his history. Ask about previous cerebrovascular accident, multiple sclerosis, diabetes, central nervous system infection, neoplastic disease, and a family history of ataxia. Also ask about chronic alcohol abuse or prolonged exposure to industrial toxins, such as mercury. Determine if the patient's ataxia arose suddenly or gradually.

If necessary, perform the Romberg test to distinguish between cerebellar and sensory ataxia. Instruct the patient to stand with his feet together and his arms at his side. Note his posture and balance, first with his eyes open, then closed. Test results may indicate normal posture and balance (minimal swaying), cerebellar ataxia (swaying and inability to maintain balance with eyes open or closed), or sensory ataxia (increased swaying and inability to maintain balance with eyes closed). Stand close to the patient during this test to prevent his falling.

If you test for gait and limb ataxia, be aware that motor weakness may mimic ataxic movements, so check motor strength, too. In gait ataxia, ask the patient if he tends to fall to one side or if falling occurs more often at night. In truncal ataxia, remember that the patient's inability to walk or stand, combined with the absence of other signs while he's lying down, may give the impression of hysteria or drug or alcohol intoxication.

Medical causes
● *Behçet's disease.* This rare, chronic meningitis causes cerebellar ataxia. It's accompanied by focal neurologic signs, such as cranial nerve palsy, mental disturbances, aphasia, and hemiparesis.

● *Cerebellar abscess.* This disorder commonly causes limb ataxia on the side opposite the lesion, as well as gait and truncal ataxia. Typically, the initial symptom is headache behind the ear or in the occipital region, followed by ocular motor palsy, fever, vomiting, altered level of consciousness, and coma.

● *Cerebellar hemorrhage.* In this life-threatening disorder, ataxia usually occurs acutely but is transient. Unilateral or bilateral ataxia affects the trunk, gait, or limbs.

The patient initially experiences repeated vomiting, occipital headache, vertigo, ocular motor palsy, dysphagia, and dysarthria. Later signs, such as decreased level of consciousness or coma, signal impending herniation.

● *Cerebrovascular accident (CVA).* In this life-threatening disorder, occlusions in the vertebrobasilar arteries cause infarction in the medulla, pons, or cerebellum that may lead to ataxia. The ataxia may occur at the onset of CVA and remain as a residual deficit. Worsening ataxia during the acute phase may indicate extension of the CVA. The ataxia may be accompanied by unilateral or bilateral motor weakness, possible altered level of consciousness, sensory loss, vertigo, nausea, vomiting, ocular motor palsy, and dysphagia.

● *Cranial trauma.* This disorder rarely produces ataxia. Usually, it's unilateral; bilateral ataxia suggests traumatic hemorrhage. Associated features include vomiting, headache, decreased level of consciousness, irritability, and focal neurologic defects. If the cerebral hemispheres are also affected, focal or generalized seizures may occur.

● *Diabetic neuropathy.* Peripheral nerve damage caused by diabetes mellitus may cause sensory ataxia as well as extremity pain, slight leg weakness, skin changes, and bowel and bladder dysfunction.

● *Diphtheria.* Within 4 to 8 weeks of the onset of symptoms, a life-threatening neuropathy can produce sensory ataxia. Diphtheria can be accompanied by fever, paresthesia, and paral-

IDENTIFYING ATAXIA

Ataxia may be observed in the patient's speech, in the movements of his trunk and limbs, or in his gait.

In **speech ataxia,** a form of dysarthria, the patient typically speaks slowly and stresses usually unstressed words and syllables. Speech content is not affected.

In **truncal ataxia,** a disturbance in equilibrium, the patient cannot sit or stand without falling. Also, his head and trunk may bob and sway (titubation). If he's able to walk, his gait is reeling.

In **limb ataxia,** the patient loses the ability to gauge distance, speed, and power of movement, resulting in poorly controlled, variable, and inaccurate voluntary movements. He may move too quickly or too slowly, or his movements may break down into component parts, giving him the appearance of a puppet or a robot. Other effects include a coarse, irregular tremor in purposeful movement (but not at rest) and weak, flaccid muscles.

In **gait ataxia,** the patient's gait is wide-based, unsteady, and irregular. In cerebellar ataxia, the patient may stagger or lurch in zigzag fashion, turn with extreme difficulty, and lose his balance when his feet are together. In sensory ataxia, the patient moves abruptly and stomps or taps his feet. This occurs because he throws his feet forward and outward, then brings them down first on the heels, then on the toes. The patient also fixes his eyes on the ground, watching his steps. However, if he's unable to watch them, staggering worsens. When he stands with his feet together and eyes closed, he sways.

ysis of the limbs and, sometimes, the respiratory muscles.

• *Encephalomyelitis.* This complication of measles, smallpox, chicken pox, or rubella, or of rabies or smallpox vaccination may damage cerebrospinal white matter. Rarely, it's accompanied by cerebellar ataxia. Other signs include headache, fever, vomiting, altered level of consciousness, paralysis, seizures, ocular motor palsy, and pupillary changes.

• *Friedreich's ataxia.* This progressive familial disorder affects the spinal cord and cerebellum. It causes gait ataxia, followed by truncal, limb, and speech ataxia. Other features include pes cavus, kyphoscoliosis, cranial nerve palsy, and motor and sensory deficits. A positive Babinski's reflex may appear.

• *Guillain-Barré syndrome.* Peripheral nerve involvement usually follows mild viral infection, rarely leading to sensory ataxia. This syndrome can also cause ascending paralysis and possible respiratory distress.

• *Hepatocerebral degeneration.* Patients who survive hepatic coma are occasionally left with residual neurologic defects, including a mild cerebellar ataxia with a wide-based, unsteady gait. The ataxia may be accompanied by altered level of consciousness, dysarthria, rhythmic arm tremors, and choreoathetosis of the face, neck, and shoulders.

• **Hyperthermia.** In this disorder, cerebellar ataxia occurs if the patient survives the coma and convulsions characteristic of the acute phase. Subsequent findings include slowly resolving confusion, dementia, and spastic paralysis.

• **Hypothyroidism.** Rarely, cerebellar ataxia may occur as the chief sign in this disorder. It's accompanied by lethargy, constipation, cold intolerance, dry skin, menorrhagia, and other signs.

• **Metastatic carcinoma.** Carcinoma that metastasizes to the cerebellum may cause gait ataxia accompanied by headache, dizziness, nystagmus, decreased level of consciousness, nausea, and vomiting.

• **Multiple sclerosis.** Nystagmus and cerebellar ataxia often occur in this disorder, but they aren't always accompanied by limb weakness and spasticity. Speech ataxia (especially scanning) may occur, as well as sensory ataxia from spinal cord involvement. During remissions, ataxia may subside or even disappear. During exacerbations, it may worsen or even become permanent.

Multiple sclerosis also causes optic neuritis, optic atrophy, numbness and weakness, diplopia, dizziness, and bladder dysfunction.

• **Olivopontocerebellar atrophy.** This disease produces gait ataxia and, later, limb and speech ataxia. Rarely, it produces intention tremor. It's accompanied by choreiform movements, dysphagia, and loss of sphincter tone.

• **Pellagra.** This rare disorder associated with niacin deficiency may cause sensory ataxia, photosensitive dermatitis, dementia, and diarrhea.

• **Poisoning.** Chronic *arsenic* poisoning may cause sensory ataxia, along with headache, seizures, altered level of consciousness, motor deficits, and muscle aching. Chronic *mercury* poisoning causes gait ataxia and limb ataxia, principally of the arms. It also causes tremors of the extremities, tongue, and lips; mental confusion; mood changes; and dysarthria.

• **Polyarteritis nodosa.** Acute or subacute polyarteritis may cause sensory ataxia, abdominal and limb pain, hematuria, fever, and elevated blood pressure.

• **Polyneuropathy.** Carcinomatous and myelomatous polyneuropathy may occur before detection of the primary tumor in carcinoma, multiple myeloma, or Hodgkin's disease. Signs and symptoms include ataxia, severe motor weakness, muscle atrophy, and sensory loss in the limbs. Pain and skin changes may also occur.

• **Porphyria.** This disorder affects the sensory and, more frequently, the motor nerves, possibly leading to ataxia. It also causes abdominal pain, mental disturbances, vomiting, headache, focal neurologic defects, altered level of consciousness, generalized seizures, abdominal pain, and skin lesions.

• **Posterior fossa tumor.** Gait, truncal, or limb ataxia is an early sign of this tumor and may worsen as the tumor enlarges. It's accompanied by vomiting (the most common sign), headache, papilledema, vertigo, ocular motor palsy, decreased level of consciousness, and motor and sensory impairments.

• **Spinocerebellar ataxia.** In this disorder, the patient may initially experience fatigue, followed by stiff-legged gait ataxia. Eventually, limb ataxia, dysarthria, static tremor, nystagmus, cramps, paresthesias, and sensory deficits occur.

• **Syringomyelia.** This chronic, degenerative disorder may cause a mixed spastic-ataxic gait. It's associated with loss of pain and temperature sensation (but preservation of touch sensation), skin changes, amyotrophy, and thoracic scoliosis.

• **Tabes dorsalis.** This rare syndrome appears 25 to 30 years after syphilitic infection. Sensory ataxia, a major sign, is accompanied by paresthesia, sensory deficits, incontinence, impotence, trophic joint degeneration, optic atrophy, pupillary changes, and sharp, stabbing, and brief pain.

• **Wernicke's disease.** The result of thiamine deficiency, this disease produces gait ataxia and, rarely, intention tremor or speech ataxia. In severe ataxia, the patient may be unable to stand or walk. Ataxia decreases with thiamine therapy. Associated signs include nystagmus, diplopia, ocular palsies, confusion, tachycardia, exertional dyspnea, and postural hypotension.

Other causes

• **Drugs.** Toxic levels of anticonvulsants, especially phenytoin, may result in gait ataxia. Toxic levels of anticholinergics and tricyclic antidepressants may also result in ataxia. Aminoglutethimide causes ataxia in about 10% of patients; however, this effect usually disappears 4 to 6 weeks after cessation of drug therapy.

Special considerations

As ordered, prepare the patient for laboratory studies, such as blood tests for toxic drug levels and radiologic tests. Then, focus your care on helping the patient adapt to his condition. Promote goals of rehabilitation and help ensure the patient's safety. For example, instruct the patient with sensory ataxia to move slowly, especially when turning or getting up from a chair. Provide a cane or walker for extra support. Ask the patient's family to check his home for hazards, such as uneven surfaces or absence of handrails on stairs. If appropriate, refer the patient with progressive disease for counseling.

Pediatric pointers

In children, ataxia occurs in acute and chronic forms, resulting from congenital or acquired disease. Acute ataxia may stem from febrile infection, brain tumors, mumps, and other disorders. Chronic ataxia may stem from Gau-

cher's disease, Refsum's disease, and other inborn errors of metabolism.

When assessing a child for ataxia, consider his level of motor skills and emotional state. Your examination may be limited to observing the child in spontaneous activity and carefully questioning his parents about changes in his motor activity, such as increased unsteadiness or falling. If you suspect ataxia, refer the child for neurologic evaluation to rule out brain tumor.

Athetosis

Athetosis, an extrapyramidal sign, is characterized by slow, continuous, and twisting involuntary movements. Typically, these movements involve the face, neck, and distal extremities, such as the forearm, wrist, and hand. Facial grimaces, jaw and tongue movements, and occasional phonation are associated with neck movements. Athetosis worsens during stress and voluntary activity, may subside during relaxation, and may even disappear during sleep. Commonly a lifelong affliction, athetosis is sometimes difficult to distinguish from chorea (hence the term *choreoathetosis*). Typically, though, athetoid movements are slower than choreiform movements.

Athetosis most often begins during childhood, resulting from hypoxia at birth, kernicterus, or genetic disorders. In adults, athetosis most commonly results from vascular or neoplastic lesions, degenerative disease, or drug toxicity.

Assessment

Begin your neurologic evaluation by taking a comprehensive prenatal and postnatal history, covering maternal and child health, labor and delivery, and possible trauma. Obtain a family health history because many genetic disorders can cause athetosis. Also ask about current drug therapy.

DISTINGUISHING ATHETOSIS FROM CHOREA

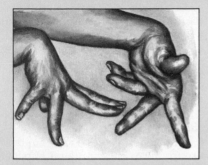

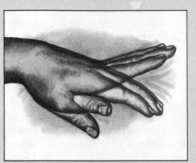

In *athetosis*, movements are typically slow, twisting, and writhing. They're associated with spasticity and most commonly involve the face, neck, and distal extremities.

In *chorea*, movements are brief, rapid, jerky, and unpredictable. They can occur at rest or during normal movement. Typically, they involve the hands, lower arm, face, and head.

Ask about the decline in the patient's functional abilities: When was he last able to roll over, sit up, or carry out daily activities? Find out what problems—uncontrollable movements, mental deterioration, or speech impediment—prompted him to seek medical help. Ask about the effects of rest, stress, and routine activity on symptoms.

Test the patient's muscle strength and tone, range of motion, fine muscle movements, and ability to perform rapidly alternating movements. Observe the limb muscles during voluntary movements, noting the rhythm and duration of contraction and relaxation.

Medical causes

• *Brain tumor.* This disorder affects the basal ganglia, causing contralateral choreoathetosis and dystonia. Associated signs vary markedly with the type of tumor and its degree of invasion.

• *Calcification of the basal ganglia.* This unilateral or bilateral disorder is characterized by choreoathetosis and rigidity. Usually, it arises in adolescence or early adult life.

• *Cerebral infarction.* In this disorder, contralateral athetosis is accompanied by altered level of consciousness. The patient may also display contralateral paralysis of the face or limbs.

• *Hepatic encephalopathy.* Episodic or persistent choreoathetosis occurs in the chronic stage of this encephalopathy. It's accompanied by cerebellar ataxia, myoclonus of the face and limbs, asterixis, dysarthria, and dementia.

• *Huntington's disease.* In this hereditary degenerative disease, athetosis and chorea progressively develop in early or middle adult life. Accompanying signs and symptoms include dystonia, dysarthria, facial apraxia, rigidity, depression, and progressive mental deterioration leading to dementia.

• *Pick's disease.* This rare degenerative disease occasionally causes mild athetosis accompanied by dementia (its chief sign) and dysphagia.

• *Wilson's disease.* In this inherited metabolic disorder, choreoathetoid movements initially involve the fingers and hands and then spread to the arms, head, trunk, and legs. Associated signs and symptoms include Kayser-Fleischer rings (rusty brown rings around the corneas), arm and hand tremors, facial and muscular rigidity, dysarthria, dysphagia, drooling, and progressive dementia. Hepatomegaly, splenomegaly, jaundice, hematemesis, and spider angiomas may also occur.

Other causes

• *Levodopa and phenytoin.* Toxic levels of these drugs may cause athetoid or choreoathetoid movements.

• *Phenothiazines and other antipsychotics.* The piperazine derivatives, such as acetophenazine and prochlorperazine, frequently cause athetosis. The aliphatic phenothiazines, such as chlorpromazine and triflupromazine, occasionally cause it. A third derivative, the piperidine phenothiazines, such as thioridazine and piperacetazine, rarely cause it. Other antipsychotics—such as haloperidol, thiothixene, and loxapine—frequently cause athetosis.

Special considerations

As ordered, prepare the patient for diagnostic tests, such as urine and blood studies, lumbar puncture, electroencephalography, and computed tomography scan.

Occasionally, athetosis can be prevented or treated (by decreasing body copper stores in Wilson's disease or by adjusting drug dosages). Typically, though, it has a lifelong impact on the patient's ability to carry out even routine activities. As a result, you'll need to help the patient adapt to his condition. For example, supply him with assistive devices, such as a long-handled shoehorn, to help him carry out fine-motor tasks. When appropriate, assist in rehabilitation; some patients can be taught to control erratic movements or convert them into purposeful ones. Also, encourage swimming, stretching, and balance and gait exercises to help maintain coordination, slow deterioration, and minimize antisocial behavior.

Encourage the patient and his family to discuss their feelings about athetosis and its cause. Refer the patient to a self-help group and appropriate support services, such as physical therapy.

Pediatric pointers

Childhood athetosis may be acquired or inherited. It can result from hypoxia at birth, which causes an athetoid cerebral palsy; kernicterus; Sydenham's chorea (in school-age children); and paroxysmal choreoathetosis. Inherited causes of athetosis include Lesch-Nyhan syndrome, Tay-Sachs disease, and phenylketonuria.

Focus your nursing care on helping the child develop self-esteem and a positive self-image. Encourage the child and his family to set realistic goals, tailoring educational plans to the child's level of intelligence. Refer the child to special education services, rehabilitation centers, and support groups. Provide emotional support during the frequent medical evaluations required for athetosis.

Aura

An aura is a sensory or motor phenomenon that marks the initial stage of a seizure or the approach of a classic migraine headache. It may be classified as cognitive, affective, psychosensory, or psychomotor (see *Recognizing Types of Aura*).

When associated with a seizure, an aura stems from an irritable focus in the brain that spreads throughout the cortex. Although an aura was once considered a sign of impending seizure, it's now considered an actual stage of a seizure. Typically, it occurs seconds to minutes before the ictal phase. Its intensity, duration, and type depend on the origin of the irritable focus. For example, an aura of bitter taste often accompanies a frontal lobe lesion. Unfortunately, an aura is difficult to describe because the postictal phase of a seizure temporarily alters the patient's level of consciousness, impairing his memory of the event.

The aura associated with classic migraine headache results from cranial vasoconstriction. Diagnostically important, it helps distinguish classic migraine from other types of headache.

Typically, the aura develops over 10 to 30 minutes and varies in intensity and duration. If the patient recognizes the aura as a warning sign, he may be able to prevent the headache by taking appropriate drugs.

Assessment

When an aura rapidly progresses to the ictal phase of a seizure, quickly evaluate the seizure and be alert for life-threatening complications, such as apnea (see "Seizure").

When an aura heralds a classic migraine, make the patient as comfortable as possible. Place him in a dark, quiet room and administer drugs to prevent headache, as ordered. Later, obtain a thorough history of the patient's headaches. Ask him to describe any sensory or motor phenomena that precede each headache. Find out how long each headache typically lasts. Does anything make it worse, such as bright lights, noise, or caffeine? Does anything make it better? Ask the patient about drugs for pain relief.

Medical cause

• *Classic migraine headache.* This disorder is preceded by a vague premonition and then, usually, a visual aura involving flashes of light. The aura develops over 10 to 30 minutes and may intensify until it completely obscures the patient's vision. A classic migraine may also cause numbness or tingling of the lips, face, or hands, slight confusion, and dizziness before the characteristic unilateral, throbbing headache appears. This headache slowly intensifies and, when it peaks, may cause photophobia, nausea, and vomiting.

Special considerations

Advise the patient to keep a diary of factors that precipitate each headache as well as associated symptoms to evaluate the effectiveness of drug therapy and recommended life-style changes. Measures to reduce stress frequently play a role here.

RECOGNIZING TYPES OF AURA

Determining whether an aura marks the patient's thought processes, emotions, or sensory or motor function frequently requires keen nursing assessment. An aura is typically difficult to describe and is only dimly remembered when associated with seizure activity. Among the types of aura the patient may experience are:

COGNITIVE AURAS

Déjà vu (familiarity with unfamiliar events or environments)
Jamais vu (unfamiliarity with a known event)
Time standing still
Flashback of past events

AFFECTIVE AURAS

Fear
Paranoia
Other emotions

PSYCHOSENSORY AURAS

Visual: flashes of light, or scintillations
Olfactory: foul odors
Gustatory: acidic, metallic, or bitter tastes
Auditory: buzzing or ringing in the ears
Tactile: numbness or tingling
Vertigo

PSYCHOMOTOR AURAS

Automatisms (inappropriate, repetitive movements): lip smacking, chewing, swallowing, grimacing, picking at clothes, climbing stairs

Pediatric pointers

Auras in children rarely result from classic migraine headache. Most commonly, they herald seizure activity. Watch for nonverbal clues possibly associated with aura, such as rubbing the eyes, coughing, and spitting.

When taking the seizure history, recognize that children—like adults—tend to forget the aura. Ask simple, direct questions: Do you see anything funny before the seizure? Do you get a bad taste in your mouth? Give the child ample time to respond, since he may have difficulty describing the aura.

Babinski's reflex • back pain • barrel chest • Battle's sign • Biot's respirations
blood pressure decrease • blood pressure increase • bowel sounds—absent •
hyperactive • bowel sounds—hypoactive • bradycardia • bradypnea • breast
nodule • breast pain • breast ulcer • breath with ammonia odor • breath wit
with fruity odor • Brudzinski's sign • bruits • buffalo hump • butterfly rash •
capillary refill time—prolonged • carpopedal spasm • cat cry • chest expansi
pain • Cheyne-Stokes respirations • chills • chorea • Chvostek's sign • clubbin
cold intolerance • confusion • conjunctival injection • constipation • corneal
costovertebral angle tenderness • cough—barking • cough—nonproductive • c
crackles • crepitation—bony • crepitation—subcutaneous • cry—high-pitched
posture • decorticate posture • deep tendon reflexes—hyperactive • deep tend
depression • diaphoresis • diarrhea • diplopia • dizziness • doll's eye sign—a
dysarthria • dysmenorrhea • dyspareunia • dyspepsia • dysphagia • dyspnea
earache • edema—generalized • edema of the arms • edema of the face • ede
enophthalmos • enuresis • epistaxis • eructation • erythema • exophthalmos
pain • facial pain • fasciculations • fatigue • fecal incontinence • fetor hepati
flatulence • fontanelle bulging • fontanelle depression • footdrop • gag reflex
bizarre • gait—propulsive • gait—scissors • gait—spastic • gait—steppage •
gallop—atrial • gallop—ventricular • genital lesions in the male • grunting r
bleeding • gum swelling • gynecomastia • halitosis • halo vision • headache
intolerance • Heberden's nodes • hematemesis • hematochezia • hematuria •
hemoptysis • hepatomegaly • hiccups • hirsutism • hoarseness • Homans' sig
hyperpnea • hypopigmentation • impotence • insomnia • intermittent claudic
jaundice • jaw pain • jugular vein distention • Kehr's sign • Kernig's sign • l
consciousness—decreased • lid lag • light flashes • low birth weight • lymph
facies • McBurney's sign • McMurray's sign • melena • menorrhagia • metro
face • mouth lesions • murmurs • muscle atrophy • muscle flaccidity • muscl
spasticity • muscle weakness • mydriasis • myoclonus • nasal flaring • nause
blindness • nipple discharge • nipple retraction • nocturia • nuchal rigidity
deviation • oligomenorrhea • oliguria • opisthotonos • orofacial dyskinesia •
hypotension • Ortolani's sign • Osler's nodes • otorrhea • pallor • palpitation
paralysis • paresthesias • paroxysmal nocturnal dyspnea • peau d'orange • p
peristaltic waves—visible • photophobia • pica • pleural friction rub • polyd
polyuria • postnasal drip • priapism • pruritus • psoas sign • psychotic beh
absent or weak • pulse—bounding • pulse pressure—narrowed • pulse press
rhythm abnormality • pulsus alternans • pulsus bisferiens • pulsus paradox
pupils—sluggish • purple striae • purpura • pustular rash • pyrosis • racco
tenderness • rectal pain • retractions—costal and sternal • rhinorrhea • rhor
salivation—decreased • salivation—increased • salt craving • scotoma • scro
absence • seizure—focal • seizure—generalized tonic-clonic • seizure—psyc
sign • shallow respirations • skin—bronze • skin—clammy • skin—mottled
turgor—decreased • spider angioma • splenomegaly • stertorous respirations
stridor • syncope • tachycardia • tachypnea • taste abnormalities • tearing—
tic • tinnitus • tracheal deviation • tracheal tugging • tremors • trismus • tu
frost • urethral discharge • urinary frequency • urinary hesitancy • urinary
urgency • urine cloudiness • urticaria • vaginal bleeding—postmenopausal •
venous hum • vertigo • vesicular rash • violent behavior • vision loss • visua
floaters • vomiting • vulvar lesions • weight gain—excessive • weight loss—
wristdrop• abdominal distention • abdominal mass • abdominal pain • abd
accessory muscle use • agitation • alopecia • amenorrhea • amnesia • analg

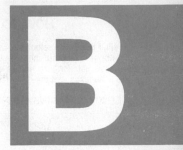

Babinski's Reflex

[Extensor plantor reflex]

Babinski's reflex—dorsiflexion of the great toe with extension and fanning of the other toes—is an abnormal reflex elicited by firmly stroking the sole of the foot. In some patients, this reflex can be triggered by noxious stimuli, such as pain, noise, or even bumping of the bed. It indicates corticospinal damage and helps differentiate neurologic and metabolic coma. Because the corticospinal tract is right- and left-sided, Babinski's reflex may occur unilaterally or bilaterally. It may also be temporary or permanent. A temporary Babinski's reflex commonly occurs during the postictal phase of a seizure, whereas a permanent Babinski's reflex occurs with irreparable corticospinal damage.

Assessment

After eliciting a positive Babinski's reflex, assess the patient for other neurologic signs. Evaluate muscle strength in each extremity by having the patient push or pull against your resistance. Passively flex and extend the extremity to assess muscle tone. Intermittent resistance to flexion and extension indicates spasticity; lack of resistance indicates flaccidity, which allows greater-than-normal range of motion. Next, check for incoordination by asking the patient to perform a repetitive activity. Test deep tendon reflexes in the elbow, antecubital area, wrist, knee, and ankle by striking the tendon with a reflex hammer. An exaggerated muscle response indicates hyperactive deep tendon reflexes; little or no muscle response indicates hypoactivity. Then assess pain sensation and proprioception in the feet. As you move the patient's toes up and down, ask him to identify the direction without looking at his feet. Notify the doctor immediately of any changes in his neurologic status.

Medical causes

• *Amyotrophic lateral sclerosis (ALS).* In this progressive motor neuron disorder, bilateral Babinski's reflex may occur with hyperactive deep tendon reflexes and spasticity. Typically, ALS produces fasciculations accompanied by muscle atrophy and weakness. Incoordination makes carrying out activities of daily living difficult for the patient. Associated signs and symptoms include impaired speech; difficulty chewing, swallowing, and breathing; urinary frequency and urgency; and occasionally, choking and excessive drooling. Although his mental status remains intact, the patient's poor prognosis may cause periodic de-

HOW TO ELICIT BABINSKI'S REFLEX

To elicit Babinski's reflex, stroke the lateral aspect of the sole of the patient's foot with your thumbnail or another moderately sharp object. Normally, this elicits flexion of all toes (a negative Babinski's reflex), as shown at left. In a positive Babinski's reflex, the great toe dorsiflexes and the other toes fan out, as shown at right.

NEGATIVE BABINSKI'S REFLEX

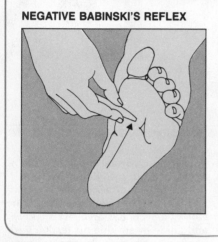

POSITIVE BABINSKI'S REFLEX

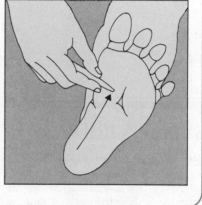

pression. Progressive bulbar palsy may cause crying spells or inappropriate laughter.

• *Brain tumor.* When it involves the corticospinal tract or the cerebellum, a brain tumor may produce Babinski's reflex unilaterally or bilaterally. Accompanying it are hyperactive deep tendon reflexes (unilateral or bilateral), spasticity, seizures, cranial nerve dysfunction, hemiparesis or hemiplegia, decreased pain sensation, unsteady gait, incoordination, headache, emotional lability, and decreased level of consciousness.

• *Cerebrovascular accident (CVA).* Babinski's reflex varies with the site of the CVA. If the CVA involves the cerebrum, it produces unilateral Babinski's reflex accompanied by hemiplegia or hemiparesis, unilateral hyperactive deep tendon reflexes, hemianopia, and aphasia. If it involves the brain stem, it produces bilateral Babinski's reflex accompanied by bilateral weakness or paralysis, bilateral hyperactive deep tendon reflexes, cranial nerve dysfunction, incoordination, and unsteady

gait. Generalized signs and symptoms of CVA may include headache, vomiting, fever, disorientation, nuchal rigidity, convulsions, and coma.

• *Familial spastic paralysis.* This disorder may produce bilateral Babinski's reflex accompanied by hyperactive deep tendon reflexes and progressive spasticity with ataxia and weakness.

• *Friedreich's ataxia.* This disorder may produce bilateral Babinski's reflex. Accompanying it are hypoactive deep tendon reflexes, hypotonia, ataxia, head tremor, weakness, and paresthesias.

• *Head trauma.* Unilateral or bilateral Babinski's reflex may occur here—the result of primary corticospinal damage or secondary injury associated with increased intracranial pressure. Hyperactive deep tendon reflexes and spasticity commonly occur with Babinski's reflex. Occasionally, the patient also has weakness and incoordination. Other signs and symptoms vary with the type of head trauma. There may be headache, vomiting, behavior changes, altered vital signs, and decreased level of consciousness with abnormal pupillary size and response to light.

• *Hepatic encephalopathy.* Babinski's reflex occurs late in this disorder when the patient slips into a coma. It's accompanied by hyperactive reflexes and fetor hepaticus.

• *Meningitis.* Bilateral Babinski's reflex commonly occurs in this infection. It's preceded by fever, chills, and malaise and accompanied by nausea and vomiting. As meningitis progresses, it also causes decreased level of consciousness, nuchal rigidity, positive Brudzinski's and Kernig's signs, hyperactive deep tendon reflexes, and opisthotonos. Associated signs and symptoms include irritability, photophobia, diplopia, delirium, and deep stupor that may progress to coma.

• *Multiple sclerosis (MS).* In most patients with this demyelinating disorder, Babinski's reflex occurs bilaterally. It follows initial signs and symptoms of MS—most commonly, paresthesias, nystagmus, and blurred or double vision. Associated signs and symptoms include scanning speech, dysphagia, intention tremor, weakness, incoordination, spasticity, gait ataxia, seizures, paraparesis or paraplegia, bladder incontinence, and, occasionally, loss of pain and temperature sensation and proprioception. Emotional lability is also characteristic.

• *Pernicious anemia.* Bilateral Babinski's reflex occurs late in this disorder when vitamin B_{12} deficiency affects the central nervous system. Typically, this anemia begins insidiously but eventually causes widespread GI, neurologic, and cardiovascular effects. Characteristic GI signs and symptoms include nausea, vomiting, anorexia, weight loss, flatulence, diarrhea, and constipation. Gingival bleeding and a sore, inflamed tongue may make eating painful and intensify anorexia. The lips, gums, and tongue also appear markedly pale. There may be jaundice, ranging from pale to bright yellow skin. Characteristic neurologic signs and symptoms include neuritis; weakness; peripheral paresthesias; disturbed position sense; incoordination; ataxia; positive Romberg's sign; light-headedness; altered vision (diplopia, blurred vision), taste, and hearing (tinnitus); and bowel and bladder incontinence. The disorder may also produce irritability, poor memory, headache, depression, impotence, and delirium. Characteristic cardiovascular signs include palpitations, wide pulse pressure, dyspnea, orthopnea, and tachycardia.

• *Rabies.* Bilateral Babinski's reflex—possibly elicited by nonspecific noxious stimuli alone—appears in the excitation phase of rabies. This phase occurs 2 to 10 days after the onset of prodromal symptoms, such as fever, malaise, and irritability. (These symptoms occur 30 to 40 days after an animal bite.) It's characterized by marked restlessness and extremely painful pharyngeal muscle spasms. Difficulty swallowing causes excessive drooling and hydrophobia in about 50% of affected patients. Seizures and hyperactive deep tendon reflexes may also occur.

• *Spinal cord injury.* In acute injury, spinal shock temporarily erases all reflexes. As shock resolves, Babinski's reflex occurs—unilaterally when injury affects only one side of the spinal cord (Brown-Séquard syndrome), bilaterally when injury affects both sides. Rather than signaling the return of neurologic function, this reflex confirms corticospinal damage. It's accompanied by hyperactive deep tendon reflexes; spasticity; and variable or total loss of pain and temperature sensation, proprioception, and motor function. Horner's syndrome, characterized by unilateral ptosis, pupillary constriction, and facial anhidrosis, may occur with lower cervical cord injury.

• *Spinal cord tumor.* In this disorder, bilateral Babinski's reflex occurs with variable loss of pain and temperature sensation, proprioception, and motor function. Spasticity, hyperactive deep tendon reflexes, absent abdominal reflexes, and incontinence are also characteristic. Diffuse pain may occur at the level of the tumor.

• **Spinal paralytic poliomyelitis.** Unilateral or bilateral Babinski's reflex occurs 5 to 7 days after the onset of fever in this disorder. It's accompanied by progressive weakness, paresthesias, muscle tenderness, spasticity, irritability, and, later, atrophy. Resistance to neck flexion is characteristic, as are Hoyne's, Kernig's, and Brudzinski's signs.

• **Spinal tuberculosis.** This disorder may produce bilateral Babinski's reflex accompanied by variable loss of pain and temperature sensation, proprioception, and motor function. It also causes spasticity, hyperactive deep tendon reflexes, bladder incontinence, and absent abdominal reflexes.

• **Syringomyelia.** In this disorder, bilateral Babinski's reflex occurs with muscle atrophy and weakness that may progress to paralysis. It's accompanied by spasticity, ataxia, and, occasionally, deep pain. Deep tendon reflexes may be hypoactive or hyperactive. Cranial nerve dysfunction, such as dysphagia and dysarthria, commonly appears late in the disorder.

Special considerations

Typically, Babinski's reflex is accompanied by incoordination, weakness, and spasticity, all of which increase the patient's risk of injury. To prevent injury, assist the patient with activity, especially ambulation. Also, keep his environment tidy and clutter-free.

The doctor may order a computed tomography scan of the brain or spine, an angiogram or myelogram, or possibly a lumbar puncture to clarify or confirm the cause of Babinski's reflex; prepare the patient, as necessary.

Pediatric pointers

Babinski's reflex occurs normally in children under age 2 and reflects immaturity of the corticospinal tract. After age 2, Babinski's reflex is pathologic and may result from hydrocephalus or any of the causes more commonly seen in adults.

Back Pain

Back pain affects an estimated 80% of the population; in fact, it's second only to the common cold for lost time from work. Although this symptom may herald a spondylogenic disorder, it may also result from genitourinary, gastrointestinal, cardiovascular, or neoplastic disorders. Postural imbalance associated with pregnancy may also cause back pain.

The onset, location, and distribution of pain and its response to activity and rest provide important clues about the causative disorder. Pain may be acute or chronic, constant or intermittent. It may remain localized in the back or radiate along the spine or down one or both legs. Pain may be exacerbated by activity—most commonly, bending, stooping, or lifting—and alleviated by rest, or it may be unaffected by both.

Intrinsic back pain results from muscle spasm, nerve root irritation, fracture, or a combination of these mechanisms. It most commonly occurs in the lower back, or lumbosacral area. Back pain may also be referred from the abdomen or flank, possibly signaling life-threatening perforated ulcer, acute pancreatitis, or dissecting abdominal aortic aneurysm.

Assessment

If the patient reports *acute, severe back pain,* quickly take his vital signs and have another nurse notify the doctor immediately. Then perform a rapid, well-directed assessment to rule out life-threatening causes. Ask the patient when the pain began. Can he relate it to any causative factors? For example, did pain occur after eating? After lifting 20 lb? After falling on the ice? Have the patient describe the pain. Is it burning, stabbing, shooting, throbbing, or aching? Is it constant or intermittent? Does pain radiate to the buttocks or legs? Or does it seem to originate in the abdomen and radiate to the back? What makes the pain better or worse? Is it affected by activity or rest? Is it worse in the morning or the evening? Typically, visceral referred back pain is unaffected by activity and rest. In contrast, pain of spondylogenic origin worsens with activity and improves with rest. Pain of neoplastic origin is frequently relieved by walking and worsens at night.

If the patient describes *deep lumbar pain unaffected by activity*, palpate for a pulsating epigastric mass. If this sign is present, suspect dissecting abdominal aortic aneurysm. Withhold food and fluid in anticipation of emergency surgery. Prepare for I.V. fluid replacement and oxygen administration.

If the patient describes *severe epigastric pain that radiates through the abdomen to the back,* assess for absent bowel sounds and for abdominal rigidity and tenderness. If these signs occur, suspect perforated ulcer or acute pancreatitis. Prepare to start an I.V. for fluids and drugs, to administer oxygen, and to insert a nasogastric tube.

However, if life-threatening causes of back pain are ruled out, continue with a more complete history and physical examination. Be aware of the patient's expressions of pain as you do so. Obtain a medical history, including past injuries and illnesses, and a family history. Ask about diet and alcohol intake. Also take a drug history, including past and present prescriptions and over-the-counter drugs. Next, perform a thorough physical examination. Observe skin color, especially in the patient's legs, and palpate skin temperature. Palpate femoral, popliteal, posterior tibial, and pedal pulses. Ask about unusual sensations in the legs, such as numbness and tingling. Observe the patient's posture if pain doesn't prohibit standing. Does he stand erect or tend to lean toward one side? Observe the level of the shoulders and pelvis and the curvature of the back. Ask the patient to bend forward, backward, and from side to side while you palpate for

paravertebral spasms. Note rotation of the spine on the trunk. Palpate the back for tenderness. Then ask the patient to walk first on his heels, then on his toes. Protect him from falling as he does so. Weakness may reflect a muscular disorder or spinal nerve root irritation. Place the patient in a sitting position to evaluate and compare patellar tendon (knee), Achilles tendon, and Babinski's reflexes. Evaluate the strength of the extensor hallucis longus by asking the patient to hold up his big toe against resistance. Measure leg length and hamstring and quadriceps muscles bilaterally. Note a difference of more than 1 cm in muscle size, especially in the calf.

To reproduce leg and back pain, position the patient supine on the examining table. Grasp his heel and slowly lift his leg. If he feels pain, note its exact location and the angle between the table and his leg when it occurs. Repeat this maneuver with the opposite leg. Pain along the sciatic nerve may indicate disk herniation or sciatica. Also note range of motion of the hip and knee.

Medical causes

● *Abdominal aortic aneurysm (dissecting).* Life-threatening dissection of this aneurysm may initially cause low back pain or dull abdominal pain. More often, it produces constant upper abdominal pain. A pulsating abdominal mass may be palpated in the epigastrium; after rupture, though, it no longer pulses. Aneurysmal dissection can also cause mottled skin below the waist, absent femoral and pedal pulses, lower blood pressure in the legs than in the arms, mild-to-moderate tenderness with guarding, and abdominal rigidity. Signs of shock, such as cool, clammy skin, will appear if blood loss is significant.

● *Ankylosing spondylitis.* This chronic, progressive disorder causes sacroiliac pain, which radiates up the spine and is aggravated by lateral pressure on the pelvis. The pain is usually most severe in the morning or after a period of inactivity and isn't relieved by rest. Abnormal rigidity of the lumbar spine with forward flexion is also characteristic. This disorder can also cause local tenderness, fatigue, fever, anorexia, weight loss, and occasional iritis.

• *Appendicitis.* In this life-threatening disorder, a vague and dull discomfort in the epigastric or umbilical region migrates to McBurney's point in the right lower quadrant. In retrocecal appendicitis, pain may also radiate to the back. The shift in pain is preceded by anorexia and nausea. It's accompanied by fever, occasional vomiting, abdominal tenderness (especially over McBurney's point), and rebound tenderness. Some patients also have painful, urgent urination.

• *Cholecystitis.* This disorder produces severe pain in the right upper quadrant that may radiate to the right shoulder, chest, or back. The pain may arise suddenly or may increase gradually over several hours. Accompanying signs and symptoms include anorexia, fever, nausea, vomiting, right upper quadrant tenderness, abdominal rigidity, pallor, and diaphoresis.

• *Chordoma.* A slow-developing malignant tumor, chordoma causes persistent pain in the lower back, sacrum, and coccyx. As the tumor expands, pain may be accompanied by constipation and bowel and bladder incontinence.

• *Endometriosis.* This disorder causes deep sacral pain and severe, cramping pain in the lower abdomen. The pain worsens just before or during menstruation and may be aggravated by defecation. It's accompanied by constipation, abdominal tenderness, dysmenorrhea, and dyspareunia.

• *Intervertebral disk rupture.* This disorder produces gradual or sudden low back pain with or without leg pain (sciatica). Rarely, it produces leg pain alone. More often, pain begins in the back and radiates to the buttocks and leg. The pain is exacerbated by activity, coughing, and sneezing and is eased by rest. It's accompanied by paresthesia (most commonly, numbness or tingling in the lower leg and foot), paravertebral muscle spasm, and decreased reflexes on the affected side. This disorder also affects posture and gait. The patient's spine is slightly flexed and he leans toward the painful side. He walks slowly and rises from a sitting to standing position with extreme difficulty.

• *Lumbosacral sprain.* This disorder causes aching, localized pain and tenderness associated with muscle spasm on lateral motion. The recumbent patient will typically flex his knees and hips to help ease pain. Flexion of the spine intensifies pain, whereas rest helps relieve it.

• *Metastatic tumors.* These tumors commonly spread to the spine, causing low back pain in at least 25% of patients. Typically, the pain begins abruptly, is accompanied by cramping muscular pain, and isn't relieved by rest.

• *Myeloma.* Back pain caused by this primary malignant tumor frequently begins abruptly and worsens with exercise. It may be accompanied by arthritic symptoms, such as achiness, joint swelling, and tenderness. Other clinical effects include fever, malaise, peripheral paresthesias, and weight loss.

• *Pancreatitis (acute).* This life-threatening disorder usually produces fulminating, continuous upper abdominal pain that may radiate to both flanks and to the back. To relieve this pain, the patient may bend forward, draw his knees to his chest, or move restlessly about.

Early associated signs and symptoms include abdominal tenderness, nausea, vomiting, fever, pallor, tachycardia and, in some patients, abdominal guarding, rigidity, rebound tenderness, and hypoactive bowel sounds. A late sign may be jaundice. Occurring as inflammation subsides, Grey Turner's sign or Cullen's sign signals hemorrhagic pancreatitis.

• *Perforated ulcer.* In some patients, perforation of a duodenal or gastric ulcer causes sudden, prostrating epigastric pain that may radiate throughout the abdomen and to the back. This life-threatening disorder also causes boardlike abdominal rigidity, tenderness with guarding, generalized rebound tenderness, the absence of bowel sounds, and grunting, shallow respi-

EXERCISES FOR CHRONIC LOW BACK PAIN

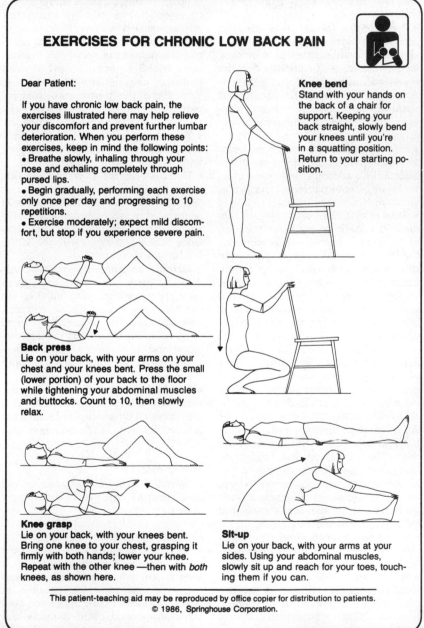

Dear Patient:

If you have chronic low back pain, the exercises illustrated here may help relieve your discomfort and prevent further lumbar deterioration. When you perform these exercises, keep in mind the following points:
• Breathe slowly, inhaling through your nose and exhaling completely through pursed lips.
• Begin gradually, performing each exercise only once per day and progressing to 10 repetitions.
• Exercise moderately; expect mild discomfort, but stop if you experience severe pain.

Back press
Lie on your back, with your arms on your chest and your knees bent. Press the small (lower portion) of your back to the floor while tightening your abdominal muscles and buttocks. Count to 10, then slowly relax.

Knee grasp
Lie on your back, with your knees bent. Bring one knee to your chest, grasping it firmly with both hands; lower your knee. Repeat with the other knee —then with *both* knees, as shown here.

Knee bend
Stand with your hands on the back of a chair for support. Keeping your back straight, slowly bend your knees until you're in a squatting position. Return to your starting position.

Sit-up
Lie on your back, with your arms at your sides. Using your abdominal muscles, slowly sit up and reach for your toes, touching them if you can.

ration. Associated signs often include fever, tachycardia, and hypotension.

● *Prostatic carcinoma.* Chronic, aching back pain may be the only symptom of prostatic carcinoma. Or this disorder may also produce cloudy urine or hematuria.

● *Pyelonephritis (acute).* This disorder produces progressive flank and lower abdominal pain accompanied by back pain or tenderness (especially over the costovertebral angle). It may also produce high fever and chills, nausea and vomiting, flank and abdominal tenderness, and urinary frequency and urgency.

● *Reiter's syndrome.* In some patients, sacroiliac pain is the first sign of this disorder. It's accompanied by the classic triad of conjunctivitis, urethritis, and arthritis.

● *Renal calculi.* The colicky pain of this disorder usually results from irritation of the ureteral lining, which increases the frequency and force of peristaltic contractions. This pain travels from the costovertebral angle to the flank, the suprapubic region, and the external genitalia. Its intensity varies but may become excruciating if calculi travel down a ureter. If calculi are in the renal pelvis and calyces, dull and constant flank pain may occur. Renal calculi also cause nausea, vomiting, urinary urgency (if a calculus lodges near the bladder), and agitation due to pain.

● *Sacroiliac strain.* This disorder causes sacroiliac pain that may radiate to the buttock, hip, and lateral aspect of the thigh. The pain is aggravated by weight bearing on the affected extremity and by abduction with resistance of the leg. Associated signs and symptoms include tenderness of the symphysis pubis and a limp or Trendelenburg lurch.

● *Spinal neoplasm (benign).* Typically, this disorder causes severe, localized back pain and scoliosis.

● *Spinal stenosis.* Resembling a ruptured intervertebral disk, this disorder produces back pain with or without sciatica. Frequently, sciatica affects both legs and is accompanied by clau-dication. The pain may progress to numbness or weakness unless the patient rests for relief.

● *Spondylolisthesis.* A major structural disorder characterized by forward slippage of one vertebra onto another, spondylolisthesis may be asymptomatic or cause low back pain with or without nerve root involvement. Associated symptoms of nerve root involvement include paresthesias, buttock pain, and pain radiating down the leg. Palpation of the lumbar spine may reveal a "step-off" of the spinous process. Flexion of the spine may be limited.

● *Transverse process fracture.* This fracture causes severe localized back pain with muscle spasm and hematoma.

● *Vertebral compression fracture.* Initially, this fracture may be painless. Several weeks later, it causes back pain aggravated by weight bearing and local tenderness. Fracture of a thoracic vertebra may cause referred pain in the lumbar area.

● *Vertebral osteomyelitis.* Initially, this disorder causes insidious back pain. As it progresses, the pain may become constant, more pronounced at night, and aggravated by spinal movement. Accompanying symptoms include vertebral and hamstring spasms, tenderness of the spinous processes, fever, and malaise.

● *Vertebral osteoporosis.* This disorder causes chronic, aching back pain that is aggravated by activity and somewhat relieved by rest. Tenderness may also occur.

Other causes

● *Neurologic tests.* Lumbar puncture and myelography can produce transient back pain.

Special considerations

If back pain suggests a life-threatening cause, monitor the patient closely. Be alert for increasing pain, altered neurovascular status in the legs, loss of bowel or bladder control, altered vital signs, diaphoresis, and cyanosis. Report changes to the doctor immediately.

Until the doctor makes a tentative diagnosis, withhold analgesics, which may mask symptoms. Also withhold food and fluids in case surgery is necessary. Make the patient as comfortable as possible by elevating the head of the bed and placing a pillow under his knees. Encourage relaxation techniques, such as deep breathing. Prepare the patient for a rectal or pelvic exam, if ordered. The doctor may also order routine blood tests; urinalysis; X-rays of the chest, abdomen, and spine; computed tomography scan; and appropriate biopsies.

If the patient has chronic back pain, reinforce instructions regarding bed rest, analgesics, anti-inflammatory drugs, and exercise (see *Exercises for Chronic Low Back Pain*, page 89). Also suggest daily warm baths to help relieve pain. Help the patient to recognize and make necessary life-style changes; for example, advise him to lose weight or correct poor posture.

Fit the patient for a corset or lumbosacral support, if ordered. Instruct him not to wear this in bed. The doctor may also order heat or cold therapy, a backboard, an egg-crate mattress, or pelvic traction; explain these pain-relief measures to the patient. Teach him about alternatives to analgesic drugs, such as biofeedback and transcutaneous electrical nerve stimulation.

Be aware that back pain is notoriously associated with malingering. Refer the patient to other professionals, such as a physical therapist, occupational therapist, or psychologist, when indicated.

Pediatric pointers

Because a child may have difficulty describing back pain, be alert for nonverbal clues, such as wincing or refusal to walk. Closely observe family dynamics during history taking for clues suggesting child abuse.

Back pain in the child may stem from intervertebral disk inflammation (diskitis), neoplasms, idiopathic juvenile osteoporosis, and spondylolisthesis.

Disk herniation typically doesn't cause back pain. Scoliosis, a common disorder in adolescents, also rarely causes back pain.

Barrel Chest

In barrel chest, the normal elliptical configuration of the chest is replaced by a rounded one in which the anteroposterior diameter enlarges to approximate the transverse diameter. The diaphragm is depressed and the sternum pushed forward with the ribs attached in a horizontal, not angular, fashion. As a result, the chest appears continuously in the inspiratory position.

Typically a late sign of chronic obstructive pulmonary disease (COPD), barrel chest results from augmented lung volumes due to chronic airflow obstruction. It may go unnoticed by the patient because of its gradual development. In the elderly, senile kyphosis of the thoracic spine may be mistaken for barrel chest. However, unlike barrel chest, senile kyphosis lacks signs of pulmonary disease.

Assessment

Begin by asking about a history of pulmonary disease. Note chronic exposure to environmental irritants, such as asbestos. Also ask about the patient's smoking habits. Then explore other symptoms of pulmonary disease. Does the patient have a cough? Is it productive or nonproductive? If it's productive, have him describe sputum color and consistency. Does the patient experience shortness of breath? Is it related to activity? Although dyspnea is common in COPD, many patients fail to associate it with the disease. Instead, they'll blame "old age" or "getting out of shape" for causing dyspnea.

Auscultate for abnormal breath sounds, such as crackles and wheezes. Then percuss the chest; hyperresonant sounds indicate trapped air, whereas

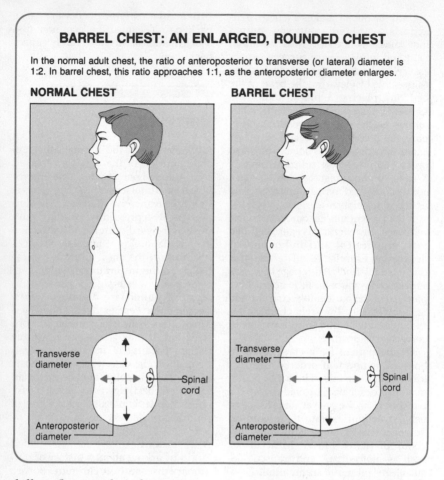

BARREL CHEST: AN ENLARGED, ROUNDED CHEST

In the normal adult chest, the ratio of anteroposterior to transverse (or lateral) diameter is 1:2. In barrel chest, this ratio approaches 1:1, as the anteroposterior diameter enlarges.

NORMAL CHEST

BARREL CHEST

Transverse diameter

Spinal cord

Anteroposterior diameter

Transverse diameter

Spinal cord

Anteroposterior diameter

dull or flat sounds indicate mucus buildup. Be alert for accessory muscle use, intercostal retractions, and tachypnea, which may signal respiratory distress. If these signs develop, notify the doctor immediately.

Finally, assess the patient's general appearance. Look for central cyanosis in the cheeks, the nose, and the mucosa inside the lips. Look for peripheral cyanosis in the nail beds. If cyanosis develops, notify the doctor immediately. Also note clubbing, a late sign of COPD.

Medical causes

● *Asthma.* Typically, barrel chest develops only in chronic asthma. An acute asthmatic attack causes severe dys-

pnea, wheezing, and productive cough. It can also cause prolonged expiratory time, accessory muscle use, tachycardia, tachypnea, perspiration, and flushing.

● *Chronic bronchitis.* A late sign in chronic bronchitis, barrel chest is characteristically preceded by productive cough and exertional dyspnea. This form of COPD may also cause cyanosis, tachypnea, wheezing, prolonged expiratory time, and accessory muscle use.

● *Emphysema.* In this form of COPD, barrel chest is also a late sign. Typically, the disorder begins insidiously, with dyspnea the predominant symptom. Eventually, emphysema may also cause chronic cough, anorexia, weight loss, malaise, accessory muscle use, pursed-lip breathing, tachypnea, peripheral cyanosis, and clubbing.

Special considerations

Advise the patient to avoid bronchial irritants—especially smoking—which may exacerbate COPD. Have him notify the doctor of purulent sputum production, which may indicate upper respiratory infection. Instruct him to space his activities to help minimize exertional dyspnea. To ease breathing, have the patient sit and lean forward, resting his hands on his knees to support the upper torso (tripod position). This position allows maximum diaphragmatic excursion, facilitating chest expansion.

Pediatric pointers

In infants, the ratio of anteroposterior to transverse diameter normally approximates 1:1. As the child grows, this ratio gradually changes to 1:2 by age 5 or 6. Cystic fibrosis and chronic asthma may cause barrel chest in the child.

Battle's Sign

Battle's sign—ecchymosis over the mastoid process of the temporal bone—is often the only outward sign of basilar skull fracture. In fact, this type of fracture may go undetected by skull X-rays. If left untreated, it can be fatal because of associated injury to the nearby cranial nerves and brain stem as well as to blood vessels and the meninges.

Appearing behind one or both ears, Battle's sign is easily overlooked or even hidden by the patient's hair. Also, during emergency care of the trauma victim, it may be overshadowed by imminently life-threatening or more apparent injuries.

Force exerted on the head great enough to fracture the base of the skull causes Battle's sign by damaging supporting tissues of the mastoid area. Or

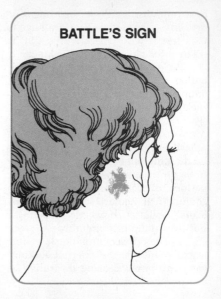

BATTLE'S SIGN

the sign may result from seepage of blood from the fracture site to the mastoid. Battle's sign usually develops 24 to 36 hours after the fracture and may persist for several days to weeks.

Assessment

Report Battle's sign immediately to the doctor. Then perform a complete neurologic examination. Begin with the history. Ask about recent trauma to the head. Did the patient sustain a severe blow to the head? Was he involved in a motor vehicle accident? Note level of consciousness as the patient responds. Does he respond quickly or slowly? Are his answers appropriate or does he appear confused? Check the patient's vital signs; be alert for widening pulse pressure and bradycardia, signs of increased intracranial pressure. Assess cranial nerve function, focusing on nerves III, IV, VI, VII, and VIII. Evaluate pupillary size and response to light as well as motor and verbal responses. Relate this data to the Glasgow Coma Scale. Note cerebrospinal fluid (CSF) leakage from the nose or ears. Ask about postnasal drip, which may reflect CSF drainage down the throat. Also look for the halo sign—blood encircled by a yellowish ring—on bed linens or dressings. To confirm that drainage is CSF, test it with a Dextrostix; CSF is positive for glucose, whereas mucus is not. Follow up the neurologic examination with a complete physical examination to detect other injuries associated with basilar skull fracture.

Medical cause

• *Basilar skull fracture.* Battle's sign may be the only outward sign of this fracture. Or it may be accompanied by periorbital ecchymosis (raccoon eyes), conjunctival hemorrhage, nystagmus, ocular deviation, epistaxis, anosmia, a bulging tympanic membrane (from CSF or blood accumulation), visible fracture lines on the external auditory canal, tinnitus, hearing difficulty, facial paralysis, and vertigo.

Special considerations

Expect the patient with basilar skull fracture to be on bed rest for several days to weeks. Keep him flat to decrease pressure on dural tears and minimize CSF leakage. Monitor neurologic status closely. Avoid nasogastric intubation and nasopharyngeal suction, which may cause cerebral infection. Also caution the patient against blowing his nose, which may worsen a dural tear.

The doctor may order skull X-rays and a computed tomography scan to help confirm basilar skull fracture and to evaluate the severity of head injury. Typically, basilar skull fracture and any associated dural tears heal spontaneously within several days to weeks. However, if the patient has a large dural tear, a craniotomy may be necessary to repair the tear with a graft patch.

Pediatric pointers

Children who are victims of abuse frequently sustain basilar skull fractures from severe blows to the head. As in adults, Battle's sign may be the only outward sign of fracture and, perhaps, the only clue to child abuse. If you suspect child abuse, follow hospital protocol for reporting the incident.

Biot's Respirations

A late and ominous sign of neurologic deterioration, Biot's respirations are characterized by breaths of equal volume interrupted by irregular periods of apnea. This rare breathing pattern may appear abruptly and reflects increased pressure on the medulla coinciding with brain stem herniation.

Assessment

Because Biot's respirations signal life-threatening neurologic deterioration, notify the doctor immediately when you recognize them. (Be sure you've observed the patient's breathing pattern for several minutes to avoid confusing Biot's with Cheyne-Stokes respirations.) Prepare to assist with intubation and mechanical ventilation. Next, take vital signs, noting especially increased systolic pressure.

Medical cause

• *Brain stem herniation.* Biot's respirations are characteristic in this neurologic emergency. Associated signs include pupillary changes, such as inequality and unresponsiveness to light; decorticate or decerebrate posture; bradycardia; and increased systolic pressure.

Special considerations

Monitor vital signs frequently. Elevate the head of the patient's bed 30° to help reduce ICP.

If ordered, prepare the patient for emergency surgery to relieve pressure on the brain stem. A computed tomography scan may be ordered to confirm the cause of brain stem herniation.

Because Biot's respirations typically reflect a grave prognosis, give the patient's family emotional support.

Pediatric pointers

Biot's respirations are rarely seen in children.

DISTINGUISHING BIOT'S AND CHEYNE-STOKES RESPIRATIONS

To avoid confusing Biot's and Cheyne-Stokes respirations, remember this telling characteristic: whether deep or shallow, the volume of each breath in Biot's respirations is equal. Conversely, Cheyne-Stokes respirations wax and wane, with breaths fluctuating from shallow to deep to shallow.

BIOT'S   **CHEYNE-STOKES**

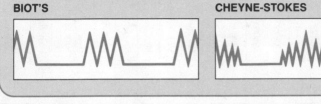

Bladder Distention

Bladder distention—the abnormal enlargement of the bladder—results from an inability to excrete urine, causing its accumulation. Distention can result from mechanical and anatomic obstructions, neuromuscular disorders, and drugs. Relatively common in all ages and both sexes, it occurs most frequently in older men with prostate disorders, leading to urine retention.

Typically, bladder distention occurs gradually, but occasionally its onset may be sudden. Gradual distention usually remains asymptomatic until stretching of the bladder produces discomfort. Acute distention produces perineal fullness, pressure, and pain. If severe distention isn't corrected promptly by catheterization or massage, the bladder rises within the abdomen, its walls become thin, and the risk of rupture increases.

Bladder distention is aggravated by intake of caffeine, alcohol, large quantities of fluid, and diuretics.

Assessment

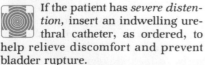 If the patient has *severe distention,* insert an indwelling urethral catheter, as ordered, to help relieve discomfort and prevent bladder rupture.

If distention isn't severe, begin your assessment by reviewing the patient's voiding patterns. Find out the time and amount of his last voiding and the amount of fluid consumed since then. Ask if the patient has difficulty initiating urination. Does he ever use Valsalva's or Credé's maneuver to initiate it? Also ask if urination occurs with urgency or without warning and if it causes pain or irritation. Remember to ask about the force and continuity of the patient's urinary stream and if he feels that his bladder is empty after voiding.

Explore the patient's history for urinary tract obstruction or infections; venereal disease; neurologic, intestinal, or pelvic surgery; lower abdominal or urinary tract trauma; and systemic or neurologic disorders. Note his drug history as well, including use of over-the-counter preparations.

Take the patient's vital signs, and percuss and palpate the bladder. (Remember that an empty bladder can't be palpated through the abdominal wall.) Inspect the urethral meatus and measure its diameter. Describe the appearance and amount of any discharge. Test for perineal sensation and anal sphincter tone, and in the male patient examine the prostate.

Medical causes
• *Benign prostatic hypertrophy.* In this disorder, bladder distention gradually

BLADDER DISTENTION: CAUSES AND ASSOCIATED FINDINGS

CAUSES (S&S)	MAJOR ASSOCIATED SIGNS AND SYMPTOMS												
	Ataxia	Constipation	Dysuria	Fatigue	Fever	Hematuria	Muscle weakness	Myalgia	Nausea	Nocturia	Pain, buttock and sacral	Pain, flank	Pain, lower back
Benign prostatic hypertrophy		•				•				•			
Bladder calculi			•			•							
Bladder neoplasms			•			•				•	•	•	•
Diabetes mellitus				•									
Multiple sclerosis	•						•						
Prostatic neoplasms		•	•	•						•			
Prostatitis (acute)			•	•	•	•		•	•				
Prostatitis (chronic)			•			•						•	•
Spinal neoplasms		•	•			•	•			•			
Urethral calculi												•	
Urethral strictures			•										

develops as the prostate enlarges. Occasionally, its onset is acute. Initially, the patient experiences urinary hesitancy, straining, frequency, reduced force of his urinary stream, nocturia, and post-voiding dribbling. As the disorder progresses, it produces prostatic enlargement, sensations of perineal fullness and incomplete bladder emptying, perineal pain, constipation, and hematuria.

• *Bladder calculi.* This disorder may produce bladder distention, but more often it produces pain as its only symptom. The pain is usually referred to the tip of the penis or the vulvar area. It worsens during walking or exercise and abates when the patient lies down. It can be accompanied by urinary frequency and urgency, hematuria, and dysuria.

• *Bladder neoplasms.* By blocking the urethral orifice, neoplasms can cause bladder distention. Associated signs and symptoms include hematuria (most common one); urinary frequency and urgency; nocturia; dysuria; pyuria; pain in the bladder, rectum, pelvis, flank, back, or legs; vomiting; diarrhea; and sleeplessness.

• *Diabetes mellitus.* If this disorder affects the autonomic nervous system, it may cause neurogenic bladder, leading to urinary retention and bladder distention. Other findings include fatigue, dry mucous membranes, poor skin turgor, incomplete bladder emptying, polydipsia, and polyphagia.

	Pain, pelvic	Pain, penile	Pain, perineal	Pain, vulvar	Perineal fullness	Polydipsia	Polyphagia	Prostatic enlargement	Prostatic rigidity	Pyuria	Urethral discharge	Urinary frequency	Urinary stream changes	Urinary urgency	Vomiting
			•	•				•				•	•		
		•		•								•		•	
	•									•		•		•	•
						•	•								
		•							•			•			
		•		•				•				•	•	•	•
	•	•		•				•		•	•	•	•	•	
												•		•	
		•	•	•							•				
										•	•	•	•	•	

- **Multiple sclerosis.** In this neuromuscular disorder, urinary retention and bladder distention result from interruption of upper motor neuron control of the bladder. Associated signs and symptoms include optic neuritis, paresthesias, impaired position and vibratory senses, diplopia, nystagmus, dizziness, abnormal reflexes, dysarthria, muscle weakness, emotional lability, Lhermitte's sign (transient, electric-like shocks that spread down the body when the head is flexed), and ataxia.
- **Prostatic neoplasms.** This disorder eventually causes bladder distention in up to 25% of patients. Its clinical features include dysuria (most common symptom), urinary frequency, nocturia, weight loss, fatigue, perineal pain, constipation, and a rigid, irregular prostate. Some patients exhibit urinary retention and bladder distention as their only signs.
- **Prostatitis.** In *acute prostatitis*, bladder distention occurs rapidly along with perineal discomfort and fullness. Accompanying signs and symptoms include perineal pain, prostatic enlargement, decreased libido, decreased volume and force of the urinary stream, dysuria, hematuria, and urinary frequency and urgency. Other findings include fatigue, malaise, myalgia, fever, chills, nausea, and vomiting.

In *chronic prostatitis*, bladder distention usually occurs gradually. It's accompanied by sensations of perineal discomfort and fullness, prostatic tenderness, decreased libido, urinary frequency and urgency, dysuria, pyuria, hematuria, persistent urethral discharge, and dull pain radiating to the lower back, buttocks, penis, or perineum.

• **Spinal neoplasms.** Disrupting upper neuron control of the bladder, spinal neoplasms cause neurogenic bladder and resultant distention. Associated symptoms include a sense of pelvic fullness; back pain, often mimicking sciatica-like pain; constipation; tender vertebral processes; sensory deficits; and muscle weakness, flaccidity, and atrophy. Signs of urinary tract infection (dysuria, urinary frequency and urgency, nocturia, tenesmus, hematuria, and weakness) may also occur.

• **Urethral calculi.** In this disorder, urethral obstruction leads to bladder distention. This obstruction causes pain radiating to the penis or vulva and referred to the perineum or rectum. It may also produce a palpable stone and urethral discharge.

• **Urethral stricture.** This disorder results in urinary retention and bladder distention with chronic urethral discharge (most common symptom), urinary frequency (also common), dysuria, urgency, decreased force and diameter of the urinary stream, and pyuria.

Other causes

• **Drugs.** Parasympatholytics, ganglionic blockers, sedatives, anesthetics, and opiates can produce urinary retention and bladder distention.

• **Catheterization.** Use of an indwelling urethral catheter can result in urinary retention and bladder distention. While the catheter is in place, inadequate drainage due to kinked tubing or an occluded lumen may lead to urinary retention. After removal of the catheter, irritation may cause edema, blocking urine outflow.

Special considerations

Monitor the patient's vital signs and the extent of bladder distention. Encourage the patient to change positions to alleviate discomfort, and give analgesics if ordered.

If the patient doesn't require immediate urethral catheterization, provide privacy and suggest that he assume the normal voiding position. Teach the patient to perform Valsalva's maneuver, or gently perform Credé's maneuver. You can also stroke or intermittently apply ice to the inner thigh or help the patient relax in a warm tub or sitz bath. Use the power of suggestion to stimulate voiding. For example, run water in the sink, pour warm water over the patient's perineum, place his hands in warm water, or play tapes of aquatic sounds.

Prepare the patient for diagnostic tests (such as endoscopy and radiologic studies) to determine the cause of bladder distention. Or prepare him for surgery if nursing interventions fail to relieve bladder distention and obstruction prevents catheterization.

Pediatric pointers

Assess for urinary retention and bladder distention in any infant who fails to void normal amounts. (Within the first 48 hours of life, an infant excretes about 60 ml of urine; during the next week, he excretes about 300 ml of urine daily.) In male infants, posterior urethral valves, meatal stenosis, phimosis, and other congenital defects may cause urinary obstruction and resultant bladder distention.

Blood Pressure Decrease

[Hypotension]

Low blood pressure refers to inadequate blood pressure to perfuse or oxygenate the body's tissues. Although commonly linked to shock, this sign may also result from cardiovascular, respiratory, neurologic, and metabolic disorders. Low blood pressure may be drug-induced or may accompany diagnostic tests—most often, those using contrast media. It may stem from stress or change of position—specifically, rising abruptly from a supine or sitting position to a standing position (postural hypotension).

Normal blood pressure varies considerably; what may qualify as low blood pressure for one person may be perfectly normal for another. Consequently, every blood pressure reading must be compared against the patient's baseline. Typically, a reading below 90/60 mm Hg or a drop of 30 mm Hg from the baseline is considered low blood pressure.

Low blood pressure can reflect an expanded intravascular space (as in vasodilatation), a reduced intravascular volume (as in dehydration and hemorrhage), or a decreased cardiac output (as in impaired cardiac muscle contractility). Because the body's pressure-regulating mechanisms are complex and interrelated, a combination of these factors usually contributes to low blood pressure.

Assessment

If the patient's systolic pressure is less than 80 mm Hg or 30 mm Hg below his baseline, suspect shock immediately. To confirm shock, quickly assess for a decreased level of consciousness. Check apical pulse for tachycardia and respirations for tachypnea. Also inspect for cool, clammy skin. If these signs are present, have another nurse notify the doctor immediately. Elevate the patient's legs above the level of his heart. Then start an I.V. line to replace fluids and blood or to administer drugs. Prepare to administer oxygen with mechanical ventilation, if necessary. Monitor the patient's intake and output; insert an indwelling (Foley) catheter for most accurate measurement of urine output. Also prepare to assist with insertion of a central venous line or a Swan-Ganz catheter to evaluate fluid status. Prepare for cardiac monitoring to evaluate cardiac rhythm. Be ready to insert a nasogastric tube to prevent aspiration in the comatose patient. During emergency assessment and care, keep the patient's spinal column immobile until spinal cord trauma is ruled out.

If the patient is conscious, ask him about associated symptoms. For example, does he feel unusually weak or fatigued? Is his vision blurred? Gait unsteady? Does he have chest or abdominal pain or difficulty breathing? Has he had episodes of dizziness or fainting? Do these episodes occur when he stands up suddenly? If so, take blood pressure with the patient lying down, sitting, and then standing; compare readings. A drop in systolic or diastolic pressure of 10 to 20 mm Hg or more between position changes suggests postural hypotension.

Next, continue with a physical examination. Inspect the skin for pallor, diaphoresis, and clamminess. Palpate peripheral pulses. Note paradoxical pulse—an accentuated fall in systolic pressure during inspiration—which suggests pericardial tamponade. Then auscultate for abnormal heart sounds (gallops, murmurs), rates (bradycardia, tachycardia), or rhythms. Auscultate the lungs for abnormal breath sounds (diminished sounds, crackles, wheezing), rates (bradypnea, tachypnea), or rhythms (agonal respirations, Cheyne-Stokes respirations). Look for signs of hemorrhage, including visible bleeding and palpable masses, bruising, and tenderness. Assess for abdominal rigidity and rebound tenderness; auscultate for abnormal bowel sounds.

Medical causes

• *Acute adrenal insufficiency.* Postural hypotension is characteristic in this disorder. Accompanying it are fatigue, weakness, nausea, vomiting, abdominal discomfort, weight loss, fever, and tachycardia. There may also be hyper-

ENSURING ACCURATE BLOOD PRESSURE MEASUREMENT

When taking the patient's blood pressure, begin by applying the cuff properly, as shown here.

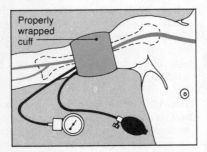

Properly wrapped cuff

Then, be alert for these common pitfalls to avoid recording an inaccurate blood pressure measurement.

• *Wrong-sized cuff.* Select the appropriate size cuff for the patient. This ensures that adequate pressure is applied to compress the brachial artery during cuff inflation. If the cuff bladder is too narrow, the reading will be falsely high. If it's too wide, the reading will be falsely low. The cuff bladder width should be about 40% of the circumference of the midpoint of the limb; bladder length should be twice the width. If the arm circumference is less than 33 cm, select a regular-sized cuff; if it's between 33 and 41 cm, a large-sized cuff; if it's more than 41 cm, a thigh cuff. Pediatric cuffs are also available.

• *Slow cuff deflation, causing venous congestion in the extremity.* Don't deflate the cuff more slowly than 2 mm Hg/heartbeat or you'll get a spuriously high reading.

• *Cuff wrapped too loosely, reducing its*

effective width. Tighten the cuff to avoid a falsely elevated reading.

• *Mercury column not read at eye level.* Read the mercury column at eye level. If the column is below eye level, you may record a falsely low reading; if it's above eye level, a falsely high reading.

• *Tilted mercury column.* Keep the mercury column vertical to avoid a spuriously high reading.

• *Poorly timed measurement.* Don't take blood pressure if the patient appears anxious or has just eaten or ambulated; you'll get a falsely high reading.

• *Incorrect position of the arm.* Keep the patient's arm level with his heart to avoid a falsely low reading.

• *Cuff overinflation, causing venospasm or pain.* Don't overinflate the cuff or you'll get a falsely high reading.

• *Failure to notice an auscultatory gap* (sound fades out for 10 to 15 mm Hg, then returns). To avoid missing the top Korotkoff sound, estimate systolic pressure by palpation first. Then inflate the cuff rapidly—at a rate of 2 to 3 mm Hg/second—to about 30 mm Hg above the palpable systolic pressure.

• *Inaudibility of feeble sounds.* Before reinflating the cuff, have the patient raise his arm to reduce venous pressure and amplify low-volume sounds. After inflating the cuff, lower the patient's arm. Then deflate the cuff and listen. Or, with the patient's arm positioned at heart level, inflate the cuff and have the patient make a fist. Have him rapidly open and close his hand 10 times before you begin to deflate the cuff. Then listen. Be sure to document that the blood pressure reading was augmented.

---

pigmentation of fingers, nails, nipples, scars, and body folds; pale, cool, clammy skin; restlessness; decreased urinary output; tachypnea; and coma.

• *Alcohol toxicity.* Low blood pressure occurs infrequently here. More often, alcohol toxicity produces distinct alcohol breath odor, tachycardia, bradypnea, hypothermia, decreased level of consciousness, seizures, staggering gait, nausea, vomiting, diuresis, and slow, stertorous breathing.

• *Anaphylactic shock.* Following exposure to an allergen, such as penicillin or insect venom, a dramatic fall in blood pressure and narrowed pulse pressure signal this severe allergic reaction. Initially, anaphylactic shock causes anxiety, restlessness, a feeling of doom, intense itching (especially of the hands and feet), and pounding headache. Later, it may also produce coughing, difficulty breathing, nausea, abdominal cramps, involuntary defecation, seizures, flushing, change or loss of voice due to laryngeal edema, urinary incontinence, and tachycardia.

• *Cardiac contusion.* In this disorder, low blood pressure occurs along with tachycardia and, at times, anginal pain and dyspnea.

• *Cardiac dysrhythmias.* In dysrhythmias, blood pressure may fluctuate between normal and low readings. Dizziness, light-headedness, weakness, fatigue, and palpitations may also occur. Auscultation typically reveals a pulse rate greater than 100 beats/minute or less than 60 beats/minute, or an irregular rhythm.

• *Cardiac tamponade.* An accentuated fall in systolic pressure (greater than 10 mm Hg) during inspiration, known as pulsus paradoxus, is characteristic in cardiac tamponade. This disorder also causes cyanosis, tachycardia, neck vein distention, muffled heart sounds, dyspnea, and Kussmaul's respirations.

• *Cardiogenic shock.* In this disorder, systolic pressure falls to less than 80 mm Hg, or 30 mm Hg less than the patient's baseline. Accompanying low blood pressure are narrowed pulse pressure, diminished Korotkoff sounds, peripheral cyanosis, and pale, cool, clammy skin. Cardiogenic shock also causes restlessness and anxiety, which may progress to disorientation and confusion. Associated signs and symptoms include anginal pain, dyspnea, neck vein distention, oliguria, ventricular gallop, tachypnea, and weak, rapid pulse.

• *Congestive heart failure (CHF).* In this disorder, blood pressure may fluctuate between normal and low readings. However, a precipitous drop in blood pressure may signal cardiogenic shock. Other features of CHF include dyspnea of abrupt or gradual onset, fatigue, weight gain, pallor or cyanosis, diaphoresis, and anxiety. Auscultation reveals ventricular gallop, tachycardia, bilateral crackles, and tachypnea. Dependent edema, neck vein distention, prolonged capillary refill time, and hepatomegaly may also occur.

• *Diabetic ketoacidosis.* Hypovolemia triggered by osmotic diuresis in hyperglycemia is responsible for low blood pressure in this disorder. It also commonly produces polydipsia, polyuria, polyphagia, dehydration, weight loss, abdominal pain, nausea, vomiting, Kussmaul's respirations, tachycardia, seizures, and stupor that may progress to coma.

• *Hyperosmolar hyperglycemic nonketotic coma.* This disorder decreases blood pressure—at times dramatically, if the patient loses significant fluid from diuresis. It also produces dry mouth, poor skin turgor, tachycardia, confusion progressing to coma, and, occasionally, focal grand mal seizures.

• *Hypovolemic shock.* In this disorder, systolic pressure falls to less than 80 mm Hg, or 30 mm Hg less than the patient's baseline. Accompanying it are diminished Korotkoff sounds, narrowed pulse pressure, and rapid, weak, and occasionally irregular pulse. Peripheral vasoconstriction causes cyanosis of the extremities and pale, cool, clammy skin. Other signs and symptoms include oliguria, confusion, disorientation, restlessness, and anxiety.

• *Hypoxemia.* In this condition, blood pressure may be alternately low and normal. There may be cyanosis, unsteady gait, and Cheyne-Stokes respirations. Tachycardia may progress to ventricular fibrillation or asystole; restlessness, confusion, and disorientation may progress to coma.

• *Myocardial infarction (MI).* In this life-threatening disorder, blood pressure may be low or high. However, a precipitous drop in blood pressure may signal cardiogenic shock. Associated signs and symptoms of MI include chest pain that may radiate to the jaw, shoulder, arm, or epigastrium; dyspnea; anxiety; nausea or vomiting; diaphoresis; and cool, pale, or cyanotic skin. Auscultation reveals an atrial gallop, murmur, and, occasionally, irregular pulse.

• *Neurogenic shock.* The result of sympathetic denervation due to cervical injury or anesthesia, neurogenic shock produces low blood pressure and bradycardia. However, the patient's skin remains warm and dry because of cutaneous vasodilation and sweat gland denervation. Depending on the cause of shock, there may also be motor weakness of the limbs and diaphragm.

• **Pulmonary embolism.** This disorder causes sudden chest pain and dyspnea accompanied by cyanosis and, occasionally, fever. Low blood pressure occurs with narrowed pulse pressure and diminished Korotkoff sounds. Associated signs include tachycardia, tachypnea, neck vein distention, and hemoptysis.

• **Septic shock.** Initially, this disorder produces fever, chills, and rash. Low blood pressure, tachycardia, and tachypnea may also develop early, but the patient's skin remains warm. Later, low blood pressure becomes increasingly severe—less than 80 mm Hg, or 30 mm Hg less than the patient's baseline—and is accompanied by narrowed pulse pressure. Other late signs include pale skin, cyanotic extremities, oliguria, and coma.

• **Vasovagal syncope.** This transient attack is characterized by low blood pressure, pallor, cold sweats, nausea, and weakness.

Other causes

• **Diagnostic tests.** These include the gastric acid stimulation test using histamine, and X-ray studies using contrast media. The latter may trigger an allergic reaction, which causes low blood pressure.

• **Drugs.** Calcium channel blockers, diuretics, vasodilators, antihypertensives, general anesthetics, narcotic analgesics, monoamine oxidase inhibitors, antianxiety agents (such as benzodiazepines), tranquilizers, and most I.V. antiarrhythmics (especially bretylium tosylate) can cause low blood pressure.

Special considerations

Check the patient's vital signs frequently to determine if low blood pressure is constant or intermittent. If blood pressure is extremely low, assist with insertion of an arterial catheter, or use a Doppler flow meter, to allow close monitoring of pressures.

Place the patient on bed rest, if ordered. Keep the side rails of the bed up. If the patient is ambulatory, assist him, as necessary. To avoid falls, don't leave a dizzy patient unattended when he's sitting or walking. If the patient has postural hypotension, instruct him to stand up slowly. Evaluate his need for a cane or walker.

Prepare the patient for laboratory tests, which may include urinalysis, routine blood studies, EKG, and chest, cervical, and abdominal X-rays.

Pediatric pointers

Normal blood pressure in children is lower than in adults (see *Guide to Pe-*

GUIDE TO PEDIATRIC BLOOD PRESSURE

AGE	NORMAL SYSTOLIC PRESSURE	NORMAL DIASTOLIC PRESSURE
Birth to 3 months	40 to 80 mm Hg	Not detectable
3 months to 1 year	80 to 100 mm Hg	Not detectable
1 to 4 years	100 to 108 mm Hg	60 mm Hg
4 to 12 years	Add 2 mm Hg for every year to 100 mm Hg	60 to 70 mm Hg

diatric Blood Pressure).

Because accidents occur frequently in children, suspect trauma or shock first as a possible cause of low blood pressure. Remember that low blood pressure typically doesn't accompany head injury in adults because intracranial hemorrhage is insufficient to cause hypovolemia. However, it does accompany head injury in infants and young children; their expandable cranial vaults allow significant blood loss into the cranial space, resulting in hypovolemia.

Another common cause of low blood pressure in children is dehydration—the result of failure to thrive or of persistent diarrhea and vomiting for as little as 24 hours.

Blood Pressure Increase

Elevated blood pressure—an intermittent or sustained increase in blood pressure exceeding 140/86 mm Hg—strikes men more often than women and blacks twice as often as whites. By itself, this common sign is easily ignored by the patient; after all, he can't see or feel it. However, its causes can be life-threatening.

Elevated blood pressure may develop suddenly or gradually. A sudden, severe rise in blood pressure (exceeding 200/120 mm Hg) indicates life-threatening hypertensive crisis. However, even a less dramatic rise may be equally significant if it heralds dissecting aortic aneurysm, increased intracranial pressure, eclampsia, or thyrotoxicosis.

Most commonly associated with essential hypertension, elevated blood pressure may also result from renal and endocrine disorders; treatments that affect fluid status, such as dialysis; and drug side effects. Ingestion of large amounts of certain foods, such as black licorice and cheddar cheese, may temporarily elevate blood pressure.

Unfortunately, elevated blood pressure may simply reflect inaccurate blood pressure measurement (see *Ensuring Accurate Blood Pressure Measurement,* page 100). However, careful measurement alone doesn't ensure a clinically useful reading. To be useful, each blood pressure reading must be compared to the patient's baseline. Also, serial readings may be necessary to establish elevated blood pressure.

Assessment

If you detect sharply elevated blood pressure, you'll need to perform a rapid assessment to rule out life-threatening causes. (See *Managing Elevated Blood Pressure,* page 106.)

After ruling out life-threatening causes of elevated blood pressure, complete a more leisurely history and physical examination. Ask about a family history of elevated blood pressure, a likely finding in essential hypertension, pheochromocytoma, and polycystic kidney disease. Then ask about its onset. Did elevated blood pressure appear abruptly? Also find out the patient's age. Sudden onset of elevated blood pressure in middle-aged or elderly patients suggests renovascular stenosis. Although essential hypertension may begin in childhood, it typically isn't diagnosed until near age 35. Pheochromocytoma and primary aldosteronism most frequently occur between ages 40 and 60. If you suspect either of these two, check for postural hypotension. Take blood pressures with the patient in a supine position, then sitting and standing. Normally, systolic pressure falls and diastolic pressure rises on standing. In postural hypotension, both pressures fall.

Also, note headache, palpitations, and sweating. Ask about urinary burning or frequency, which suggests pyelonephritis, and about wine-colored urine and decreased urine output, which suggest glomerulonephritis.

Obtain a drug history, including past and present prescriptions and over-the-

PATHOPHYSIOLOGY OF ELEVATED BLOOD PRESSURE

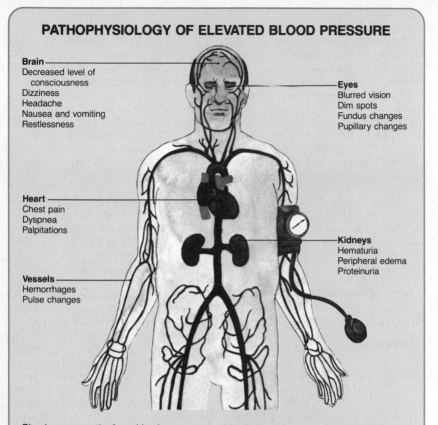

Brain
Decreased level of
 consciousness
Dizziness
Headache
Nausea and vomiting
Restlessness

Eyes
Blurred vision
Dim spots
Fundus changes
Pupillary changes

Heart
Chest pain
Dyspnea
Palpitations

Kidneys
Hematuria
Peripheral edema
Proteinuria

Vessels
Hemorrhages
Pulse changes

Blood pressure—the force blood exerts on vessels as it flows through them—depends on cardiac output, peripheral resistance, and blood volume. A brief review of its regulating mechanisms—nervous system control, capillary fluid shifts, kidney excretion, and hormonal changes—will help you understand how elevated blood pressure develops.

• *Nervous system control* involves the sympathetic division, chiefly baroreceptors and chemoreceptors, which promotes moderate vasoconstriction to maintain normal blood pressure. When this system responds inappropriately, increased vasoconstriction enhances peripheral resistance, resulting in elevated blood pressure.

• *Capillary fluid shifts* regulate blood volume by responding to arterial pressure. Increased pressure forces fluid into the interstitial space; decreased pressure allows it to be drawn back into the arteries by osmosis. However, this fluid shift may take several hours to adjust blood pressure.

• *Kidney excretion* also helps regulate

blood volume by increasing or decreasing urine formation. Normally, an arterial pressure of about 60 mm Hg maintains urine output. When pressure drops below this reading, urine formation ceases, thereby increasing blood volume. Conversely, when arterial pressure exceeds this reading, urine formation increases, thereby reducing blood volume. Like capillary fluid shifts, this mechanism may take several hours to adjust blood pressure.

• *Hormonal changes* reflect stimulation of the kidney's renin-angiotensin system in response to low arterial pressure. This system effects vasoconstriction, which increases arterial pressure, and stimulates aldosterone release, which regulates sodium retention—a key determinant of blood volume.

Elevated blood pressure signals the breakdown or inappropriate response of these pressure-regulating mechanisms. Its associated signs and symptoms concentrate in the target organs and tissues illustrated here.

counter drugs. If the patient is already taking antihypertensive drugs, determine how well he complies with the regimen. Determine the patient's perception of elevated blood pressure. How serious does he believe it is? Does he expect drug therapy to help?

Follow up the history with a well-directed physical examination. Using a funduscope, check for intraocular hemorrhage, exudate, and papilledema, which characterize severe hypertension. Perform a thorough cardiovascular assessment. Check for carotid bruits and neck vein distention. Assess skin color, temperature, and turgor. Palpate peripheral pulses. Auscultate for abnormal heart sounds (gallops, murmurs), rates (bradycardia, tachycardia), or rhythms. Then auscultate for abnormal breath sounds (crackles, wheezing), rates (bradypnea, tachypnea), or rhythms.

Palpate the abdomen for tenderness, masses, or liver enlargement. Auscultate for abdominal bruits. Renal artery stenosis produces bruits over the upper abdomen or in the costovertebral angles. Easily palpable, enlarged kidneys and a large, tender liver suggest polycystic kidney disease.

Medical causes
● *Aldosteronism (primary).* This disorder causes elevated diastolic pressure, which may be accompanied by postural hypotension. Associated signs and symptoms include constipation, muscle weakness, polyuria, polydipsia, and personality changes.
● *Anemia.* Accompanying elevated systolic pressure in this disorder are pulsations in the capillary beds, bounding pulse, tachycardia, systolic ejection murmur, pale mucous membranes, and, in sickle cell anemia, ventricular gallop and crackles.
● *Aortic aneurysm (dissecting).* Initially, this life-threatening disorder causes a sudden rise in systolic pressure, but no change in diastolic pressure. However, this increase is short-lived; the body's ability to compensate fails, resulting in

hypotension. Associated signs vary between abdominal and thoracic aortic aneurysms. In an abdominal aneurysm, there may be persistent abdominal and back pain, weakness, sweating, tachycardia, dyspnea, a pulsating abdominal mass, restlessness, confusion, and cool, clammy skin. In a thoracic aneurysm, there may be a ripping or tearing sensation in the chest, which may radiate to the neck, shoulders, lower back, or abdomen; pallor; syncope; sweating; dyspnea; tachycardia; cyanosis; leg weakness; murmur; and absent radial and femoral pulses.
● *Atherosclerosis.* Here, systolic pressure rises while diastolic pressure remains normal. The patient may show no other signs or he may have weak pulse, flushed skin, tachycardia, anginal pain, and claudication.
● *Cushing's syndrome.* Twice as common in females as in males, this disorder causes elevated blood pressure and widened pulse pressure. There may also be truncal obesity, moon face, and other cushingoid signs.
● *Hypertension. Essential hypertension* develops insidiously and is characterized by a gradual increase in blood pressure from decade to decade. Except for this elevated blood pressure, the patient may be asymptomatic or he may complain of suboccipital headache, light-headedness, tinnitus, and fatigue. In *malignant hypertension,* diastolic pressure abruptly rises above 120 mm Hg, and systolic pressure may exceed 200 mm Hg. Typically, there is pulmonary edema marked by neck vein distention, dyspnea, tachypnea, tachycardia, and coughing of pink, frothy sputum. Other characteristic signs include severe headache, confusion, tinnitus, epistaxis, muscle twitching, nausea, and vomiting.
● *Increased intracranial pressure (ICP).* Initially, this condition causes increased respirations. Then, systolic pressure rises and pulse pressure widens. Increased ICP affects heart rate last, causing bradycardia. Associated signs include headache, projectile

MANAGING ELEVATED BLOOD PRESSURE

Elevated blood pressure can signal various life-threatening disorders. However, if blood pressure exceeds 200/120 mm Hg, the patient is experiencing hypertensive crisis and requires prompt treatment. First, have another nurse notify the doctor immediately. Maintain a patent airway in case the patient vomits. Also, institute seizure precautions. Prepare to administer I.V. antihypertensive drugs and diuretics. Insert an indwelling (Foley) catheter to accurately monitor urine output.

If blood pressure is less severely elevated, continue to rule out other life-threatening causes. If the patient is pregnant, suspect preeclampsia or eclampsia. Place her on bed rest and insert an I.V. line. Administer magnesium sulfate to decrease neuromuscular irritability and antihypertensive drugs, as ordered. Monitor vital signs closely for the next 24 hours. If diastolic blood pressure continues to exceed 100 mm Hg despite drug therapy, prepare the patient for induced labor and delivery or for cesarean section. Offer emotional support if the patient must face delivery of a premature infant.

If the patient isn't pregnant, quickly observe for equally obvious clues. Assess for exophthalmos and an enlarged thyroid gland. If these signs are present, ask about a history of hyperthyroidism. Then assess for other associated signs, including tachycardia, widened pulse pressure, palpitations, severe weakness, diarrhea, fever exceeding 100° F., and nervousness. Report these signs immediately to the doctor. Prepare to administer antithyroid drugs orally or by nasogastric tube, if necessary. Also evaluate fluid status; look for signs of dehydration, such as poor skin turgor. Prepare for I.V. fluid replacement and temperature control by cooling blanket, if necessary.

If the patient shows signs of increased intracranial pressure (such as decreased level of consciousness and fixed or dilated pupils), ask him or his companion about recent head trauma. Then check for increased respirations and bradycardia. Report these signs immediately to the doctor. Maintain a patent airway in case the patient vomits. Also institute seizure precautions. Prepare to give I.V. diuretics. Insert a Foley catheter and monitor intake and output. Check vital signs every 15 minutes until stable.

If the patient has absent or weak peripheral pulses, ask about chest pressure or pain, which suggests dissecting aortic aneurysm. Enforce bed rest until the doctor establishes this diagnosis. If ordered, give I.V. antihypertensive drugs or prepare the patient for surgery.

---

vomiting, decreased level of consciousness, and fixed or dilated pupils.

• *Myocardial infarction.* This life-threatening disorder may cause high or low blood pressure. Common findings include crushing chest pain that may radiate to the jaw, shoulder, arm, or epigastrium. Other findings: dyspnea, anxiety, nausea, vomiting, weakness, diaphoresis, atrial gallop, and murmurs.

• *Pheochromocytoma.* Paroxysmal or sustained elevated blood pressure characterizes pheochromocytoma and may be accompanied by postural hypotension. Associated signs and symptoms include anxiety, diaphoresis, palpitations, tremors, pallor, nausea, weight loss, and headache.

• *Polycystic kidney disease.* Elevated blood pressure is typically preceded by flank pain. Other signs include enlarged kidneys; enlarged, tender liver; and intermittent gross hematuria.

• *Preeclampsia/eclampsia.* Potentially life-threatening to both mother and fetus, this disorder characteristically increases blood pressure. It's defined as a reading of 140/90 mm Hg or more in the first trimester, a reading of 130/80 mm Hg or more in the second or third trimester, an increase of 30 mm Hg above the patient's baseline systolic pressure, or an increase of 15 mm Hg above the patient's baseline diastolic pressure. Accompanying elevated blood pressure are generalized edema, sudden weight gain of 3 lb or more per week during the second or third trimester, severe frontal headache, blurred or double vision, decreased urinary output or oliguria, midabdominal pain, neuromuscular irritability, nausea, and possibly convulsions (eclampsia).

• *Pyelonephritis (chronic).* In some patients, this disorder produces no overt signs until severely elevated systolic and diastolic pressures develop. In others, it may produce recurrent, abrupt episodes of malaise, backache, chills, fever, and pain in one or both loins. Within 24 hours of such episodes, the patient experiences urinary frequency, burning, and occasionally, hematuria.

• *Renovascular stenosis.* This disorder produces abruptly elevated systolic and diastolic pressure. Other characteristic signs and symptoms include bruits over the upper abdomen or in the costovertebral angles, hematuria, and acute flank pain.

• *Thyrotoxicosis.* Accompanying elevated systolic pressure in this potentially life-threatening disorder are widened pulse pressure, tachycardia, bounding pulse, pulsations in the capillary nail beds, palpitations, weight loss, exophthalmos, an enlarged thyroid gland, weakness, diarrhea, fever (over 100° F.), and warm, moist skin. The patient may appear nervous and emotionally unstable, displaying occasional outbursts or even psychotic behavior. There may also be heat intolerance, exertional dyspnea, and, in females, decreased or absent menses.

Other causes

• *Drugs.* Central nervous system stimulants (such as amphetamines), sympathomimetics, corticosteroids, oral contraceptives, monoamine oxidase inhibitors, and cocaine abuse can increase blood pressure.

• *Treatments.* Kidney dialysis and transplantation cause transient elevation of blood pressure.

Special considerations

If routine screening detects elevated blood pressure, stress the need for follow-up diagnostic tests. Prepare the patient for routine blood tests and urinalysis. Depending on the suspected cause of elevated blood pressure, the doctor may also order radiographic studies, especially of the kidneys.

If the patient has essential hypertension, explain the importance of long-term control of elevated blood pressure. Make sure he understands the purpose, dosage, schedule, route, and side effects of prescribed antihypertensive drugs. Reassure him that several drugs are available to treat this disorder in case the one he's taking isn't effective or causes intolerable side effects. Encourage him to report side effects; drug dosage or schedule may simply need adjustment. Also encourage him to lose weight, if necessary, and to restrict dietary sodium. Suggest participation in an exercise or stress management program, too. Teach the patient how to monitor his blood pressure to evaluate the effectiveness of drug therapy and life-style changes. Have him record blood pressure readings as well as symptoms. Advise him to share this information with his doctor during regular follow-up visits.

Pediatric pointers

Normally, blood pressure in children is lower than in adults, an essential point to recognize when assessing for elevated blood pressure (see *Guide to Pediatric Blood Pressure,* page 102).

Elevated blood pressure in children may result from lead or mercury poisoning, essential hypertension, renovascular stenosis, chronic pyelonephritis, coarctation of the aorta, patent ductus arteriosus, glomerulonephritis, adrenogenital syndrome, and neuroblastoma. Treatment typically begins with drug therapy. Surgery may then follow in patent ductus arteriosus, coarctation of the aorta, neuroblastoma, and some cases of renovascular stenosis. Diuretics and antibiotics are used to treat glomerulonephritis and chronic pyelonephritis; hormonal therapy, to treat adrenogenital syndrome.

Bowel Sounds—Absent

[Silent abdomen]

Absent bowel sounds refers to the inability to hear any bowel sounds through a stethoscope after listening for at least 5 minutes in each abdominal quadrant.

Bowel sounds cease when mechanical or vascular obstruction or neurogenic inhibition halts peristalsis. When peristalsis halts, gas from bowel contents and fluid secreted from the intestinal walls accumulate and distend the lumen, leading to life-threatening complications such as perforation, peritonitis and sepsis, or hypovolemic shock.

Simple mechanical obstruction, resulting from adhesions, hernia, or tumor, causes loss of fluids and electrolytes and induces dehydration. Vascular obstruction cuts off circulation to the intestinal walls, leading to ischemia, necrosis, and shock. Neurogenic inhibition, affecting innervation of the intestinal wall, may result from infection, bowel distention, or trauma. It may also follow mechanical or vascular obstruction or metabolic derangement, such as hypokalemia.

Abrupt cessation of bowel sounds, when accompanied by abdominal pain, rigidity, and distention, signals a life-threatening crisis requiring immediate intervention. Absent bowel sounds following a period of hyperactivity are equally ominous and may indicate strangulation of a mechanically obstructed bowel.

Assessment

If you fail to detect bowel sounds and the patient reports sudden, severe abdominal pain and cramping or exhibits severe abdominal distention, call the doctor immediately. Prepare to assist with insertion of a nasogastric or intestinal tube to suction lumen contents and decompress the bowel. Administer I.V. fluids and electrolytes, as ordered, to offset any dehydration and imbalances caused by the dysfunctioning bowel. Because the patient may require surgery to relieve an obstruction, withhold oral intake, as ordered. Take the patient's vital signs, and be alert for signs of shock, such as hypotension, tachycardia, and cool, clammy skin. Measure abdominal girth as a baseline for gauging subsequent changes.

If the patient's condition permits, proceed with a brief history. Ask first about abdominal pain: When did it begin? Has it gotten worse? Where do you feel it? Also ask about a sensation of bloating and about flatulence. Find out if the patient has had diarrhea or passed pencil-thin stools—possible signs of a developing luminal obstruction. Or the patient may have had no bowel movements at all—a possible sign of complete obstruction and paralytic ileus.

Ask about conditions that commonly lead to mechanical obstruction, such as abdominal tumors, hernias, and adhesions from past surgery. Determine if the patient was involved in an accident—even a seemingly minor one, such as falling off a stepladder—that may have caused vascular clots. Check for a history of acute pancreatitis, diverticulitis, or gynecologic infection, which may have led to intraabdominal infection and bowel dysfunction. Be sure to ask about previous toxic conditions, such as uremia, and about spinal cord injury, which can lead to paralytic ileus.

If the patient's pain isn't severe or accompanied by other life-threatening signs, obtain a detailed medical and surgical history and perform an abdominal assessment.

Start your assessment by inspecting abdominal contour. Stoop at the recumbent patient's side and then at the foot of his bed to detect localized or generalized distention. Percuss and palpate the abdomen gently. Listen for dullness over fluid-filled areas and tympany over pockets of gas. Palpate for abdominal rigidity and guarding, suggesting peritoneal irritation that can lead to paralytic ileus.

Medical causes

• *Complete mechanical intestinal obstruction.* Absent bowel sounds follow a period of hyperactive bowel sounds in this potentially life-threatening disorder. This silence accompanies acute, colicky abdominal pain that arises in the quadrant of obstruction and may radiate to the flank or lumbar regions. Associated signs and symptoms include abdominal distention and bloating, constipation, and nausea and vomiting (the higher the blockage, the earlier and more severe the vomiting). In late stages, signs of shock may occur with fever, rebound tenderness, and abdominal rigidity.

• *Mesenteric artery occlusion.* In this life-threatening disorder, bowel sounds disappear after a brief period of hyperactive sounds. Sudden, severe midepigastric or periumbilical pain occurs next, followed by abdominal distention and possible bruits, vomiting, constipation, and signs of shock. Fever is common. Abdominal rigidity may appear late.

• *Paralytic (adynamic) ileus.* The cardinal sign of this potentially life-threatening disorder is absent bowel sounds. Associated signs and symptoms include abdominal distention, generalized discomfort, and constipation or passage of flatus and small, liquid stools. If the disorder follows acute abdominal infection, fever and abdominal pain may also occur.

Other cause

• *Abdominal surgery.* Bowel sounds are normally absent after abdominal surgery—the result of anesthetics and surgical manipulation.

Special considerations

After you've inserted a nasogastric or intestinal tube, elevate the head of the patient's bed at least 30°, and turn the

ARE BOWEL SOUNDS REALLY ABSENT?

Before concluding that your patient has absent bowel sounds, ask yourself these three questions:

Did you use the diaphragm of your stethoscope to auscultate for the bowel sounds?
The diaphragm detects high-frequency sounds, such as bowel sounds, whereas the bell detects low-frequency sounds, such as a vascular bruit or a venous hum.

Did you listen in the same spot for at least 5 minutes for the presence of bowel sounds?
Normally, bowel sounds occur every 5 to 15 seconds, but the duration of a single sound may be less than 1 second.

Did you listen for bowel sounds in all quadrants?
Bowel sounds may be absent in one quadrant, but present in another.

patient as ordered to facilitate passage of the tube through the GI tract. Remember not to tape an intestinal tube to the patient's face. Assure tube patency by checking for drainage and for properly functioning suction devices, and irrigate as ordered. Closely monitor GI drainage losses.

Continue to give I.V. fluids and electrolytes, as ordered, and send a serum specimen to the laboratory for electrolyte analysis at least once a day. Recognize that the patient may need X-ray studies and further blood work to determine the cause of absent bowel sounds.

Once mechanical obstruction and intraabdominal sepsis have been ruled out as causes of absent bowel sounds, give drugs, as ordered, to control pain and stimulate peristalsis.

Pediatric pointers

Absent bowel sounds in children may result from Hirschsprung's disease or intussusception, both of which can lead to life-threatening obstruction.

Bowel Sounds— Hyperactive

Sometimes audible without a stethoscope, hyperactive bowel sounds reflect increased intestinal motility (peristalsis). They're commonly characterized as rapid, rushing, gurgling waves of sounds. They may stem from life-threatening bowel obstruction or gastrointestinal (GI) hemorrhage. However, hyperactive sounds may also stem from GI infection, inflammatory bowel disease (which usually follows a chronic course), food allergies, and stress.

Assessment

After detecting hyperactive bowel sounds, quickly check vital signs and ask the patient about associated symptoms, such as abdominal pain, vomiting, and diarrhea. If the patient reports cramping abdominal pain or vomiting, continue to auscultate for bowel sounds and have another nurse notify the doctor. If bowel sounds stop abruptly, suspect complete bowel obstruction and prepare to assist with GI suction and decompression, as ordered, and to give I.V. fluids and electrolytes. If ordered, prepare the patient for surgery.

If the patient has diarrhea, record its frequency, amount, color, and consistency. If you detect excessive watery diarrhea or bleeding, prepare to ad-

HYPERACTIVE BOWEL SOUNDS: CAUSES AND ASSOCIATED FINDINGS

S&S CAUSES	MAJOR ASSOCIATED SIGNS AND SYMPTOMS											
	Abdominal distention	Abdominal pain	Anorexia	Constipation	Diarrhea	Fever	Nausea	Perianal lesions	Rectal bleeding	Tenesmus	Vomiting	Weight loss
Crohn's disease	●	●	●		●	●		●				●
Food hypersensitivity					●		●				●	
Gastroenteritis		●			●	●	●				●	
Gastrointestinal hemorrhage	●	●			●				●			
Mechanical intestinal obstruction	●	●		●			●				●	
Ulcerative colitis (acute)			●		●	●				●		●

minister antidiarrheal drugs, I.V. fluids and electrolytes, and possibly blood transfusions, as ordered.

If you've ruled out life-threatening conditions, obtain a detailed medical and surgical history. Ask the patient about hernia and abdominal surgery, since these may cause mechanical intestinal obstruction. Does the patient have a history of inflammatory bowel disease? Ask about recent eruptions of gastroenteritis among family members, friends, or co-workers. If the patient has traveled recently, even within the United States, was he aware of any endemic illnesses?

Determine if stress may have contributed to the patient's problem. Ask about food allergies and recent ingestion of unusual foods or fluids. Check for fever, which suggests infection. Having already auscultated, now gently inspect, percuss, and palpate the abdomen.

Medical causes

• **Crohn's disease.** Hyperactive bowel sounds usually arise insidiously. Associated signs and symptoms include diarrhea, cramping abdominal pain, anorexia, low-grade fever, abdominal distention and tenderness, and often a fixed mass in the right lower quadrant. Perianal lesions are common. With progression of the disorder, muscle wasting, weight loss, and signs of dehydration may occur.

• **Food hypersensitivity.** Hyperactive bowel sounds follow ingestion of allergenic foods. Associated findings include diarrhea and, possibly, nausea and vomiting.

• **Gastroenteritis.** Hyperactive bowel sounds follow sudden nausea and vomiting and accompany "explosive" diarrhea. Abdominal cramping or pain is common. Fever may occur, depending on the causative organism.

• **Gastrointestinal hemorrhage.** Hyperactive bowel sounds provide the most immediate indication of persistent bleeding. Associated signs and symptoms may include abdominal disten-

> ## CHARACTERISTICS OF BOWEL SOUNDS
>
> The sounds of swallowed air and fluid moving through the gastrointestinal tract are known as bowel sounds. These sounds usually occur every 5 to 15 seconds, but their frequency may be irregular. For example, bowel sounds are normally more active just before and after a meal. Bowel sounds may last less than 1 second or up to several seconds.
>
> *Normal bowel sounds* can be characterized as murmuring, gurgling, or tinkling. *Hyperactive bowel sounds* can be characterized as loud, gurgling, splashing, and rushing; they're higher pitched and occur more frequently than normal sounds. *Hypoactive bowel sounds* can be characterized as soft or lower in tone and less frequent than normal sounds.

tion, bloody diarrhea, rectal passage of bright red blood clots and jellylike material, and pain during bleeding. Decreased urinary output, tachycardia, and hypotension accompany blood loss.

• **Mechanical intestinal obstruction.** Hyperactive bowel sounds occur simultaneously with cramping abdominal pain every few minutes in this potentially life-threatening disorder; bowel sounds may later become hypoactive and then disappear. In small-bowel obstruction, nausea and vomiting occur earlier and with greater severity than in large-bowel obstruction. In complete bowel obstruction, hyperactive sounds are also accompanied by abdominal distention and constipation, although the bowel distal to the obstruction may continue to empty for up to 3 days.

• **Ulcerative colitis (acute).** Hyperactive bowel sounds arise abruptly in this disorder. They're accompanied by bloody diarrhea, anorexia, abdominal pain, nausea, vomiting, fever, and tenesmus. Weight loss may occur.

Special considerations

If ordered, prepare the patient for diagnostic tests. These may include endoscopy to view a suspected lesion, barium X-rays, or stool analysis.

Explain prescribed dietary changes to the patient. These may vary from complete food and fluid restrictions to a liquid or bland diet. Because stress often precipitates or aggravates bowel hyperactivity, teach the patient relaxation techniques, such as deep breathing. Encourage rest and restrict the patient's physical activity, as ordered.

Pediatric pointers
Hyperactive bowel sounds in children usually result from gastroenteritis, erratic eating habits, excessive ingestion of certain foods (such as unripened fruit), or food allergy.

Bowel Sounds— Hypoactive

Hypoactive bowel sounds, detected by auscultation, are diminished in regularity, tone, or loudness from normal bowel sounds. In themselves, hypoactive bowel sounds don't herald an emergency; in fact, they're considered normal during sleep. However, they may portend the absence of bowel sounds, which can indicate a life-threatening disorder.

Hypoactive bowel sounds result from decreased peristalsis, which, in turn, can result from a developing bowel obstruction. Such obstruction may be mechanical (as from hernia, tumor, or twisting), vascular (as from an embolism or thrombosis), or neurogenic (as from mechanical, ischemic, or toxic impairment of bowel innervation).

Hypoactive bowel sounds can also result from certain drugs and from abdominal surgery and irradiation.

Assessment
After detecting hypoactive bowel sounds, assess for related symptoms. Ask the patient about the location, on-

set, duration, frequency, and severity of any pain. Cramping or colicky abdominal pain usually indicates a mechanical bowel obstruction, whereas diffuse abdominal pain usually indicates intestinal distention in paralytic ileus.

Ask the patient about recent vomiting: When did it begin? How often does it occur? Does the vomitus look bloody? Also ask about any changes in bowel habits: Does he have a history of constipation? When was the last time he had a bowel movement or expelled gas?

Obtain a detailed medical and surgical history of any conditions, such as an abdominal tumor or hernia, that may cause mechanical bowel obstruction. Does the patient have a history of conditions that can cause paralytic ileus, such as pancreatitis; bowel inflammation or gynecologic infection, which may produce peritonitis; toxic conditions, such as uremia; severe pain; or trauma? Has the patient recently had radiation therapy or abdominal surgery, or ingested drugs such as codeine, which can decrease peristalsis and cause hypoactive bowel sounds?

Once the history is complete, perform a careful physical examination. Inspect the abdomen for distention, noting surgical incisions and obvious masses. Gently percuss and palpate the abdomen for masses, gas, fluid, tenderness, and rigidity. Measure abdominal girth to detect any subsequent increase in distention. Also check for poor skin turgor, hypotension, narrowed pulse pressure, and other signs of dehydration and electrolyte imbalance, which may result from paralytic ileus.

Medical causes
• *Mechanical intestinal obstruction.* Bowel sounds may become hypoactive after a period of hyperactivity. The patient may also have acute colicky abdominal pain in the quadrant of obstruction, possibly radiating to the flank or lumbar regions; nausea and vomiting (the higher the obstruction, the earlier and more severe the vom-

iting); constipation; and abdominal distention and bloating. If the obstruction becomes complete, signs of shock may occur.

● **Mesenteric artery occlusion.** After a brief period of hyperactivity, bowel sounds become hypoactive and then quickly disappear, signifying a life-threatening crisis. Associated signs and symptoms include fever, sudden and severe midepigastric or periumbilical pain followed by abdominal distention and possible bruits, vomiting, constipation, and signs of shock. Abdominal rigidity may appear late.

● **Paralytic (adynamic) ileus.** Bowel sounds are hypoactive and may become absent. Associated signs and symptoms include abdominal distention, generalized discomfort, and constipation or passage of flatus and small, liquid stools. If the disorder follows acute abdominal infection, fever and abdominal pain may occur.

Other causes

● **Drugs.** Certain classes of drugs reduce intestinal motility and thus produce hypoactive bowel sounds. These include opiates, such as codeine; anticholinergics, such as propantheline bromide; phenothiazines, such as chlorpromazine; and vinca alkaloids, such as vincristine. General or spinal anesthetics produce transient hypoactive sounds.

● **Radiation therapy.** Hypoactive bowel sounds and abdominal tenderness may occur following irradiation of the abdomen.

● **Surgery.** Hypoactive bowel sounds may occur after manipulation of the bowel. Motility and bowel sounds in the small intestine usually resume in 24 hours; colonic bowel sounds in 3 to 5 days.

Special considerations

Frequently assess the patient with hypoactive bowel sounds for indications of shock (thirst; anxiety; restlessness; cool clammy skin; tachycardia; weak, thready pulse), which can develop if

peristalsis continues to diminish and fluid is lost from the circulation. Be alert for sudden absence of bowel sounds, especially in postoperative and hypokalemic patients, since they're at increased risk for paralytic ileus. Monitor vital signs and auscultate for bowel sounds every 2 to 4 hours. Immediately report sudden absence of bowel sounds, particularly when accompanied by severe pain, abdominal rigidity, guarding, and fever, since this may indicate paralytic ileus from peritonitis. Then prepare for emergency interventions (see "Bowel Sounds—Absent").

The patient with hypoactive bowel sounds may require gastrointestinal suction and decompression, using a nasogastric or intestinal tube. If so, restrict the patient's oral intake and assist with tube insertion, as ordered. Then elevate the head of the bed at least 30°, and turn the patient, as ordered, to facilitate passage of the tube through the GI tract. Remember not to tape an intestinal tube to the patient's face. Assure tube patency by assessing for drainage and for properly functioning suction devices. Irrigate the tube, as ordered, and closely monitor drainage.

Continue to give I.V. fluids and electrolytes, as ordered, and send a serum specimen to the laboratory for electrolyte analysis at least once a day. Recognize that the patient may need X-ray studies, endoscopic procedures, and further blood work to determine the cause of hypoactive bowel sounds.

Provide comfort measures, as needed. Semi-Fowler's position offers the best relief for the patient with paralytic ileus. Sometimes, ambulating the patient can reactivate the sluggish bowel. However, if the patient can't tolerate ambulation, range-of-motion exercises or turning from side to side may stimulate peristalsis.

If unexpelled flatus makes the patient uncomfortable, insert a rectal tube and leave it in place for 1 to 2 hours. During that time, turn the patient from side to side to help move gas through the intestines and out the tube.

Pediatric pointers

Hypoactive bowel sounds in a child may simply be due to bowel distention from excessive swallowing of air while eating or crying. However, be sure to observe the child for further signs of illness. As with an adult, sluggish bowel sounds may signal the onset of paralytic ileus or peritonitis.

Bradycardia

Bradycardia refers to a heart rate of fewer than 60 beats/minute. It occurs normally in young adults, trained athletes, the elderly, and during sleep. It's also a normal response to vagal stimulation caused by coughing, vomiting, or straining during defecation. When bradycardia results from these causes, the heart rate rarely drops below 40 beats/minute. However, when it results from pathologic causes (such as cardiovascular disorders), the heart rate may be as slow as 1 beat/minute.

By itself, bradycardia is a nonspecific sign. However, in conjunction with such symptoms as chest pain, dizziness, and shortness of breath, it can signal a life-threatening disorder.

Assessment

After detecting bradycardia, check for related signs of life-threatening disorders. (See *Managing Severe Bradycardia*.) If the patient's bradycardia *isn't* accompanied by untoward signs, take a brief history. Ask the patient if he or a family member has a history of slow pulse rate, since this sign may be inherited. Find out if the patient has an underlying metabolic disorder, such as hypothyroidism, which can precipitate bradycardia. Ask what medications he's taking and if he's complying with prescribed schedule and dosage.

Medical causes

● *Cardiac dysrhythmia.* Depending on the type and the patient's tolerance of dysrhythmia, bradycardia may be transient or sustained, and benign or life-threatening. Related findings vary but may include hypotension, palpitations, dizziness, weakness, and fatigue.

● *Cardiomyopathy.* This potentially life-threatening disorder causes transient or sustained bradycardia. Associated signs and symptoms include dizziness, syncope, edema, fatigue, jugular vein distention, orthopnea, dyspnea, and peripheral cyanosis.

● *Cervical spinal injury.* Bradycardia may be transient or sustained, depending on the severity of injury. Its onset coincides with sympathetic denervation. Associated signs and symptoms may include hypotension, decreased body temperature, slowed peristalsis, leg paralysis, and partial arm and respiratory muscle paralysis.

● *Hypothermia.* Bradycardia usually appears when core temperature drops below 89.6° F. (32° C.). It's accompanied by shivering, peripheral cyanosis, confusion leading to stupor, muscle rigidity, and bradypnea.

● *Hypothyroidism.* This disorder causes severe bradycardia along with fatigue, constipation, unexplained weight gain, and sensitivity to cold. Related signs include confusion leading to stupor; cool, dry, thick skin; sparse, dry hair; facial swelling; periorbital edema; and thick, brittle nails.

● *Increased intracranial pressure.* Bradycardia occurs as a late sign of this condition along with rapid respirations, elevated systolic pressure, decreased diastolic pressure, and widened pulse pressure. Associated signs and symptoms include persistent headache, projectile vomiting, decreased level of consciousness, and fixed, unequal, possibly dilated pupils.

● *Myocardial infarction.* Mild or severe bradycardia occurs in about 65% of patients with an inferior MI. Accompanying signs and symptoms of MI include an aching, burning, or viselike pressure in the chest that may radiate to the jaw, shoulder, arm, back, or epi-

MANAGING SEVERE BRADYCARDIA

Bradycardia can signal a life-threatening disorder when accompanied by pain, shortness of breath, and other symptoms; prolonged exposure to cold; or head or neck trauma. In such patients, quickly take vital signs and have another nurse immediately notify the doctor. Connect the patient to a cardiac monitor, and insert an I.V. line. Depending on the cause of bradycardia, you'll need to administer fluids, atropine, steroids, or thyroid medication. If indicated, insert an indwelling (Foley) catheter. Assist with intubation and mechanical ventilation if the patient's respiratory rate falls.

If appropriate, perform a focused assessment to help pinpoint the cause of bradycardia. Ask, for example, about pain. Viselike, crushing, or burning chest pain that radiates to the arms, back, or jaw may indicate acute myocardial infarction (MI), whereas severe headache may signal increased intracranial pressure. Also ask about nausea, vomiting, or shortness of breath—symptoms associated with acute MI and cardiomyopathy. Observe the patient for peripheral cyanosis, edema, or neck vein distention, which may indicate cardiomyopathy. Look for a thyroidectomy scar because severe bradycardia may result from hypothyroidism caused by failure to take thyroid hormone replacements.

If the cause of bradycardia is evident, you'll need to provide supportive care. For example, keep the hypothermic patient warm by applying blankets, and monitor his core temperature until it reaches 99° F. (37.2° C.). Or, in the trauma patient, stabilize the head and neck until cervical spinal injury is ruled out.

---

gastric area; nausea and/or vomiting; cool, clammy, and either pale or cyanotic skin; anxiety; and dyspnea. Blood pressure may be elevated or depressed. Auscultation may reveal abnormal heart sounds.

Other causes

• *Diagnostic tests.* Cardiac catheterization and electrophysiologic studies can induce temporary bradycardia.

• *Drugs.* Beta-adrenergic and calcium channel blockers, cardiac glycosides, topical miotics (such as pilocarpine), I.V. nitroglycerin, protamine sulfate, quinidine, and sympatholytics may cause transient bradycardia. Failure to take thyroid hormone replacements may cause bradycardia.

• *Invasive treatments.* Suctioning can induce hypoxia and vagal stimulation, causing bradycardia. Cardiac surgery can cause edema or damage to conduction tissues, causing bradycardia.

Special considerations

Continue to monitor vital signs frequently. Be especially alert for changes in cardiac rhythm, respiratory rate, and level of consciousness.

Prepare the patient for laboratory tests, which can include CBC; cardiac enzyme, serum electrolyte, blood glucose, and thyroid function tests; ABG and BUN levels; and a 12-lead EKG. If appropriate, prepare the patient for 24-hour Holter monitoring.

Pediatric pointers

Heart rates are normally higher in children than in adults. Fetal bradycardia—a heart rate of fewer than 120 beats/minute—may occur during prolonged labor or complications of delivery, such as compression of the umbilicus, partial abruptio placentae, and placenta previa. Intermittent bradycardia, sometimes accompanied by apnea, commonly occurs in premature infants. Bradycardia rarely occurs in full-term infants or children. However, it can result from congenital heart defects, acute glomerulonephritis, and transient or complete heart block associated with cardiac catheterization or cardiac surgery.

Bradypnea

Often preceding life-threatening apnea or respiratory arrest, bradypnea is a pattern of regular respirations with a rate of fewer than 12 breaths/minute. This sign results from neurologic and metabolic disorders and drug overdose, which depress the brain's respiratory control centers.

Assessment

Depending on the degree of central nervous system (CNS) depression, the patient with severe bradypnea may require constant stimulation to breathe. If the patient seems excessively sleepy, try to arouse him by shaking him and instructing him to breathe. Have another nurse immediately notify the doctor, and quickly take the patient's vital signs. Assess his neurologic status by checking pupil size and reactions and by evaluating

NEUROLOGIC CONTROL OF BREATHING

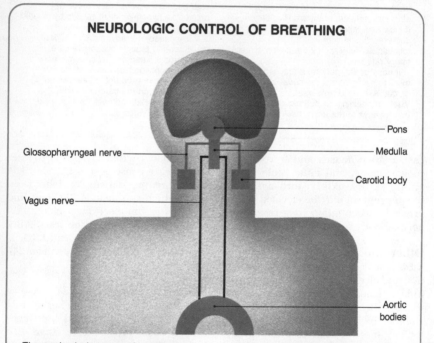

Glossopharyngeal nerve

Vagus nerve

Pons

Medulla

Carotid body

Aortic bodies

The mechanical aspects of breathing are regulated by *respiratory centers*, groups of discrete neurons in the medulla and pons that function as a unit. In the *medullary respiratory center*, neurons associated with inspiration and neurons associated with expiration interact to control respiratory rate and depth. In the pons, two additional centers interact with the medullary center to regulate rhythm: the *apneustic center* stimulates inspiratory neurons in the medulla to precipitate inspiration; these, in turn, stimulate the *pneumotaxic center* to inhibit inspiration, allowing passive expiration to occur.

Normally, the breathing mechanism is stimulated by increased carbon dioxide levels and decreased oxygen levels in the blood. Chemoreceptors in the medulla and in the carotid and aortic bodies respond to changes in $PaCO_2$, pH, and PaO_2, signaling respiratory centers to adjust respiratory rate and depth. Respiratory depression occurs when decreased cerebral perfusion inactivates respiratory center neurons, when changes in $PaCO_2$ and arterial blood pH affect chemoreceptor responsiveness, or when neuron responsiveness to $PaCO_2$ changes is reduced—for example, due to narcotic overdose.

his level of consciousness and his ability to move extremities. Place him on an apnea monitor, keep emergency airway equipment available, and be prepared to assist with intubation and mechanical ventilation if spontaneous respirations cease. To prevent aspiration, position the patient on his side and clear his airway with suction or finger sweeps, if necessary.

Obtain a brief history from the patient, if possible, or whoever accompanied him to the hospital. Ask if there's a possibility of drug overdose, and, if so, try to determine what drug(s) the patient took, how much, when, and by what route. Check the patient's arms for needle marks, indicating possible drug abuse. You may need to administer I.V. naloxone, a narcotic antagonist.

If you rule out drug overdose, ask about chronic illnesses, such as diabetes and renal failure. Check for Medic Alert jewelry or an I.D. card that identifies an underlying condition. Also ask whether the patient has a history of head trauma, brain tumor, neurologic infection, or stroke.

Medical causes
• *Diabetic ketoacidosis.* Bradypnea occurs late in severe, uncontrolled diabetes. Associated signs and symptoms include decreased level of consciousness, fatigue, weakness, fruity breath odor, and oliguria.
• *Hepatic failure.* Occurring in end-stage hepatic failure, bradypnea may be accompanied by coma, hyperactive reflexes, a positive Babinski's sign, fetor hepaticus, and other signs.
• *Increased intracranial pressure.* A late sign of this life-threatening condition, bradypnea is preceded by decreased level of consciousness, deteriorated motor function, and fixed, dilated pupils. The triad of bradypnea, bradycardia, and hypertension is a classic sign of late medullary strangulation.
• *Renal failure.* Occurring in end-stage renal failure, bradypnea may be accompanied by convulsions, decreased

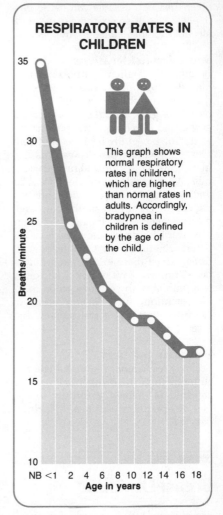

RESPIRATORY RATES IN CHILDREN

This graph shows normal respiratory rates in children, which are higher than normal rates in adults. Accordingly, bradypnea in children is defined by the age of the child.

Breaths/minute vs. Age in years (NB <1 2 4 6 8 10 12 14 16 18)

level of consciousness, gastrointestinal bleeding, hypo- or hypertension, uremic frost, and diverse other signs.
• *Respiratory failure.* Bradypnea occurs in end-stage respiratory failure. Its accompanying signs include cyanosis, diminished breath sounds, tachycardia, mildly increased blood pressure, and decreased level of consciousness.

Other causes
• *Drugs.* An overdose of narcotic analgesics and, less commonly, sedatives, barbiturates, phenothiazines, and

other CNS depressants can cause bradypnea. Use of any of these drugs with alcohol can also cause bradypnea.

Special considerations

Because the patient with bradypnea may develop apnea, check his respiratory status frequently and be prepared to give ventilatory support, if necessary. Don't leave the patient unattended, especially if his level of consciousness is decreased. Keep his bed in the lowest position and raise the side rails. As ordered, obtain blood for ABG and electrolyte studies, and ready the patient for chest and skull X-rays and, maybe, a computed tomography scan.

Administer drugs and oxygen, as ordered. Avoid giving CNS-depressant drugs, since these exacerbate bradypnea. Similarly, give oxygen judiciously to a patient with chronic carbon dioxide retention, such as may occur in chronic obstructive pulmonary disease.

Pediatric pointers

Because respiratory rates are higher in children than in adults, bradypnea in children is defined according to age (see *Respiratory Rates in Children,* page 117).

Breast Dimpling

Breast dimpling—the puckering or retraction of skin on the breast—results from the abnormal attachment of the skin to underlying tissue. It suggests an inflammatory or malignant mass beneath the surface of the skin and most often represents a late sign of breast cancer; benign lesions usually don't produce this effect. Dimpling most commonly affects women over age 40 but also occasionally occurs in males.

Because breast dimpling occurs over a mass or induration, the patient usually discovers other signs before becoming aware of dimpling. However, a thorough breast examination may reveal dimpling and may alert the patient and nurse to a breast problem.

Assessment

Obtain a medical, reproductive, and family history, noting factors that place the patient at a high risk for breast cancer. Ask about her pregnancy history, since women who don't experience a full-term pregnancy until after age 30 are at a higher risk for developing breast cancer. How old was the patient when she began menstruation? How old was she at menopause? More than 30 years of menstrual activity increases the risk of breast cancer. Has her mother or a sister had breast cancer? Has she herself had a previous malignancy, especially cancer in the other breast? Ask about the patient's dietary habits, since a high-fat diet predisposes the patient to breast cancer.

Ask your patient if she's noticed any changes in the shape of her breast. Is any area painful or tender, and is the pain cyclical? If she's lactating, has she recently experienced high fever, chills, malaise, muscle aches, fatigue, or other flulike symptoms? Can she remember sustaining any trauma to the breast?

Carefully inspect the dimpled area. Is it swollen, red, or warm to the touch? Are there bruises or contusions present? Ask your patient to tense her pectoral muscles by pressing her hips with both hands or by raising her hands over her head. Does puckering increase? Gently pull the skin upward toward the clavicle. Is dimpling exaggerated?

Observe the breast for nipple retraction. Do both nipples point in the same direction? Are the nipples flattened or inverted? Does the patient report nipple discharge? If so, ask her to describe the color and character of the discharge. Observe the contour of both breasts. Are they symmetrical?

Examine both breasts with your patient supine, sitting, and leaning forward. Does the skin move freely over both breasts? If you can palpate a lump, describe its size, location, consistency, mobility, and delineation. What relation does the lump have to breast dimpling? Gently mold the breast skin around the lump. Is dimpling exaggerated? Also examine breast and axillary lymph nodes, noting any enlargement.

Medical causes

• *Breast abscess.* Breast dimpling sometimes accompanies chronic breast abscess. Associated findings include a firm, irregular, nontender lump and signs of nipple retraction, such as deviation, inversion, or flattening. Axillary lymph nodes may be enlarged.

• *Breast cancer.* Breast dimpling is an important but somewhat *late* sign of malignancy. A neoplasm that causes dimpling is usually close to the skin and at least 1 cm in diameter; it feels irregularly shaped and fixed to underlying tissue. Other signs of breast cancer may include peau d'orange; changes in breast symmetry or size; or retraction; and a unilateral, spontaneous, nonmilky nipple discharge that is serous or bloody. (*Bloody nipple discharge in the presence of a lump is a classic sign of breast cancer.*) Axillary lymph nodes may be enlarged. Pain may be present but isn't a reliable symptom of breast cancer. A breast ulcer may appear as a late sign.

• *Fat necrosis.* Breast dimpling from fat necrosis follows inflammation and trauma to fatty tissue of the breast. Tenderness, erythema, bruising, and contusions may occur, although the patient often can't remember an incident of breast injury or trauma. Findings include a hard, indurated, poorly delineated lump, which is fibrotic and fixed to underlying tissue or overlying skin, as well as signs of nipple retraction.

• *Mastitis.* Breast dimpling may signal bacterial mastitis, which most often results from duct obstruction and milk stasis during lactation. Heat, erythema, swelling, induration, pain, and tenderness usually accompany mastitis. Dimpling more likely occurs with diffuse induration than with a single hard mass. The skin on the breast may

BREAST DIMPLING

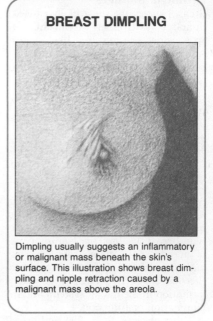

Dimpling usually suggests an inflammatory or malignant mass beneath the skin's surface. This illustration shows breast dimpling and nipple retraction caused by a malignant mass above the areola.

feel fixed to underlying tissue. Other possible findings include nipple retraction, nipple cracks, a puslike discharge, and enlarged axillary lymph nodes. Flulike signs and symptoms, such as fever, malaise, fatigue, and aching, often occur.

Special considerations

Remember that any breast problem can arouse fears of mutilation, loss of sexuality, and death. Allow the patient to express her feelings.

Provide a clear explanation of diagnostic tests that may be ordered, such as mammography, thermography, ultrasound, cytology of nipple discharge, and biopsy.

Discuss breast self-examination, and provide follow-up teaching when the patient expresses a readiness to learn. (See *How to Examine Your Breasts*, pages 122 and 123.) Advise the lactating mother with mastitis to pump her breasts to prevent further milk stasis, to discard the milk, and to substitute formula until the breast infection responds adequately to antibiotics.

Pediatric pointers

Breast cancer, the most likely cause of dimpling, is extremely rare in children. So consider trauma as a likely cause. As in the adult, breast dimpling may occur in the adolescent as a result of fatty tissue necrosis due to trauma.

Breast Nodule

[Breast lump]

A frequently reported gynecologic sign, a breast nodule has two chief causes: benign breast disease and cancer. Benign breast disease, the leading cause of nodules, can stem from cyst formation in obstructed and dilated lactiferous ducts, hypertrophy or tumor formation in the ductal system, and inflammation or infection.

Although less than 20% of breast nodules are malignant, the clinical signs of breast cancer aren't easily distinguished from those of benign breast disease. Breast cancer is a leading cause of death among women but can occur occasionally in men, with signs and symptoms mimicking those found in women. Thus, breast nodules in both sexes should always be evaluated.

A woman who's familiar with the feel of her breasts and performs monthly breast self-examination can detect a nodule 5 mm or less in size, considerably smaller than the 1-cm nodule that's readily detectable by an experienced examiner. However, a woman may not report a nodule because of fear of breast cancer.

Assessment

If your patient reports a lump, ask her how and when she discovered it. Does the size and tenderness of the lump vary with her menstrual cycle? Has the lump changed since she first noticed it? Is she aware of any other breast signs, such as discharge or nipple changes?

Find out if the patient has noticed a change in breast shape, size, or contour. Is she lactating? Does she have fever, chills, fatigue, or other flulike symptoms? Ask her to describe any pain or tenderness associated with the lumps. Is the pain in one breast only? Has she sustained recent trauma to the breast?

Explore the patient's medical and family history for factors that increase her risk of breast cancer. These include a high-fat diet, having a mother or sister with breast cancer, or having a history of malignancies, especially cancer in the other breast. Other risk factors include nulliparity, a first pregnancy after age 30, and early menarche or late menopause.

Next, perform a thorough breast examination. Pay special attention to the upper outer quadrant of each breast, where half the ductal tissue is located. This is the most common site of breast malignancies.

Carefully palpate a suspected breast nodule, noting its location, shape, size, consistency, mobility, and delineation. Does the nodule feel soft, rubbery, and elastic, or hard? Is it mobile, slipping away from your fingers as you palpate it, or is it firmly fixed to adjacent tissue? Does the nodule seem to limit the mobility of the entire breast? Note the nodule's delineation. Are the borders clearly defined or indefinite? Or does the area feel more like a hardness or diffuse induration than a nodule with definite borders?

Do you feel one nodule or several small ones? Is the shape round, oval, lobular, or irregular? Inspect and palpate the skin over the nodule for warmth, redness, and edema. Palpate the lymph nodes of the breast and axilla for enlargement.

Observe the contour of your patient's breasts, looking for asymmetry and irregularities. Be alert for signs of retraction, such as skin dimpling and nipple deviation, retraction, or flattening. (To exaggerate dimpling, have your patient raise her arms over her head or press her hands against her hips.)

Gently pull the breast skin toward the clavicle. Is dimpling evident? Mold the breast skin and again observe for dimpling.

Be alert for nipple discharge that's spontaneous, unilateral, and nonmilky (serous, bloody, or purulent). Be careful not to confuse it with the grayish discharge that can often be elicited from the nipples of a woman who has been pregnant.

Medical causes

• *Adenofibroma.* The extremely mobile or "slippery" feel of this benign neoplasm helps distinguish it from other breast nodules. The nodule usually occurs singly and characteristically feels firm, elastic, and round or lobular, with well-defined margins. It doesn't cause pain or tenderness, can vary from pinhead size to very large, often grows rapidly, and usually lies around the nipple or on the lateral side of the upper outer quadrant.

• *Areolar gland abscess.* Tender, palpable abscesses on the periphery of the areola follow inflammation of the se-

BREAST NODULE: CAUSES AND ASSOCIATED FINDINGS

CAUSES	MAJOR ASSOCIATED SIGNS AND SYMPTOMS							
	Breast dimpling	Breast pain/ tenderness	Erythema	Fever	Lymph-adenopathy	Nipple discharge	Nipple retraction signs	Peau d'orange
Areolar gland abscess		•		•				
Breast abscess (acute)		•	•	•				•
Breast abscess (chronic)	•					•	•	•
Breast cancer	•	•	•		•	•	•	•
Fat necrosis	•	•	•				•	
Intraductal papilloma		•				•		
Mammary duct ectasia		•	•		•	•	•	•
Mastitis	•	•	•	•			•	•
Proliferative breast disease		•				•		

HOW TO EXAMINE YOUR BREASTS

Dear Patient:

Examining your breasts at least once a month will help detect any abnormalities early. Perform this examination on the 4th to 7th day after your menstrual period ends, since your breasts are least congested at that time. If you're past menopause, choose the same date each month. Follow the steps below, and call your doctor if you notice any abnormalities.

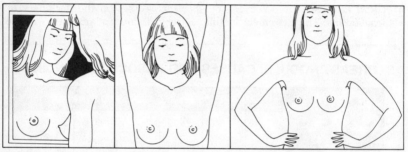

Undress to the waist, then stand in front of a mirror with your arms at your sides. Carefully look for the following: changes in breast shape, size, or symmetry; skin puckering or dimpling; ulceration; lumps; nipple secretions; or retraction of the skin, nipple, or areola. Repeat the inspection with your arms over your head, and with your hands on your hips and elbows out to the sides.

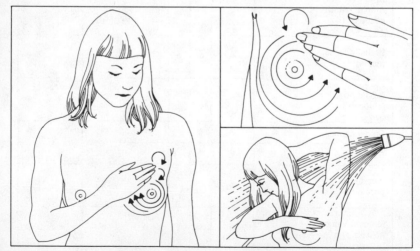

Now, examine your left breast with your right hand. Using the pads of your fingers, move clockwise around your breast to feel for lumps; don't be afraid to press firmly. Start at the outer area of your breast and work inward toward the nipple. You may feel a ridge of firm tissue along the lower part of your breast; this is normal. Repeat the procedure, examining your right breast with your left hand. You may prefer to examine your breasts while standing in the shower, with one hand placed behind your head.

Also using the pads of your fingers, feel the opposite armpit. Repeat the examination on the other armpit. Don't be alarmed if you feel a small lump that moves freely; this area contains the lymph glands. But do check the size of the lump daily. If it doesn't go away or if it gets larger, notify your doctor.

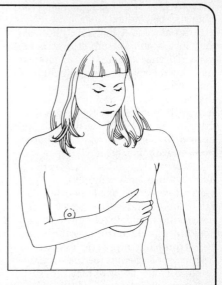

Next, check your nipples for secretions by gently squeezing one nipple between your thumb and forefinger. Check the other nipple the same way. Notify your doctor if you see any secretions, and describe the color and amount.

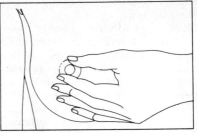

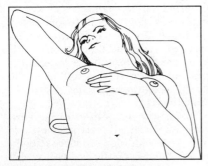

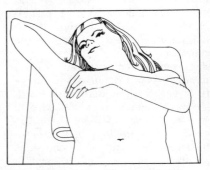

Now, lie down with a rolled-up towel or a small pillow under your right shoulder and your arm behind your head. Using your left hand, examine your right breast and armpit as you did while standing. Repeat the procedure with your left breast.

If you do feel a lump while examining your breasts, note if you can easily lift the skin covering it, if the lump moves under the skin, and if it's soft or hard. Be sure to give your doctor this information when you call him.

baceous glands of Montgomery. Fever may also be present.

● **Breast abscess.** A localized, hot, tender, fluctuant mass with erythema and peau d'orange typifies *acute abscess.* Associated symptoms often include fever, chills, malaise, and generalized discomfort. In *chronic abscess,* the nodule is nontender, irregular, and firm and may feel like a thick wall of fibrous tissue. It's often accompanied by skin dimpling, peau d'orange, and nipple retraction and sometimes by axillary lymphadenopathy.

● **Breast cancer.** A hard, poorly delineated nodule that is fixed to the skin or underlying tissue suggests breast cancer. Malignant nodules often cause breast dimpling, nipple deviation or retraction, or flattening of the nipple or breast contour. Forty to fifty percent of malignant nodules occur in the upper outer quadrant.

Nodules usually occur singly, although satellite nodules may surround the main one. Nipple discharge may be serous or bloody. (*Bloody nipple discharge in the presence of a nodule is a classic sign of breast cancer.*) Additional findings may include edema (peau d'orange) of the skin overlying the mass, erythema, tenderness, and axillary lymphadenopathy. A breast ulcer may occur as a late sign. Breast pain, an unreliable symptom, may be present.

● **Fat necrosis.** This rare, benign mass mimics the poorly delineated nodule of breast cancer. The hard, indurated, and fibrotic nodule is usually fixed to overlying skin or underlying tissue. Erythema, skin dimpling, nipple retraction signs, bruising, and contusions may appear, but local tenderness may never develop, and the patient often can't remember breast injury or trauma.

● **Intraductal papilloma.** The tiny nodules of this benign lesion usually resist palpation. Nodules large enough to be palpated usually occur singly, but they may be multiple and diffuse. Soft and poorly delineated, the nodules usually

lie in the subareolar margin. The primary sign of this disorder is serous or bloody nipple discharge. Breast pain and tenderness may occur.

● **Mammary duct ectasia.** The rubbery breast nodule in this menopausal or postmenopausal disorder usually lies under the areola. It's often accompanied by pain, itching, tenderness, and erythema of the areola; thick, sticky, multicolored nipple discharge; and nipple retraction. The skin overlying the mass may show bluish-green discoloration or edema (peau d'orange). Axillary lymphadenopathy is possible.

● **Mastitis.** In this disorder, breast nodules feel firm and indurated or tender, flocculent, and discrete. Gentle palpation defines the area of maximum purulent accumulation. Skin dimpling and nipple deviation, retraction, or flattening may be present, and the nipple may show a crack or abrasion. Accompanying signs and symptoms include breast warmth, erythema, tenderness, and edema (peau d'orange), plus high fever, chills, malaise, and fatigue.

● **Nipple adenoma.** Although similar in symptoms to Paget's disease, adenomas rarely produce a deep-seated mass.

● **Paget's disease.** This slow-growing intraductal carcinoma begins as a scaling, eczematoid nipple lesion. Later, the nipple becomes reddened and excoriated; complete destruction of the structure may result. The process extends along the skin as well as in the ducts, usually progressing to a deep-seated mass.

● **Proliferative breast disease.** The most common cause of breast nodules, this fibrocystic condition produces smooth, round, slightly elastic nodules, which increase in size and tenderness just before menstruation. The nodules may occur in fine, granular clusters in both breasts or as widespread, well-defined lumps of varying sizes. A thickening of adjacent tissue may be palpable. Cystic nodules are mobile, which helps differentiate them from malignant ones. Because cystic nodules aren't fixed to underlying breast tissue, they don't produce retraction signs, such as nipple deviation or dimpling. A clear, watery (serous), or sticky nipple discharge may appear in one or both breasts. Symptoms of premenstrual syndrome, including headache, irritability, bloating, nausea, vomiting, and abdominal cramping, may also be present.

Special considerations
To many women, a breast nodule immediately signals breast cancer, when, in fact, nodules are usually benign. As a result, try to avoid alarming your patient further. Provide a simple explanation of your examination, and encourage the patient to express her feelings.

Prepare the patient for diagnostic tests, which may include transillumination, mammography, thermography, needle aspiration or open biopsy of the nodule for tissue examination, and cytologic examination of nipple discharge.

Postpone teaching the patient how to perform breast self-examination until she overcomes her initial anxiety at discovering a nodule. Regular breast self-examination is especially important for women who've had a previous malignancy, who have a family history of breast cancer, who are nulliparous or had their first child after age 30, and who had an early menarche or late menopause. (See *How to Examine Your Breasts,* pages 122 and 123.)

Although most nodules occurring during lactation result from mastitis, the possibility of cancer demands careful evaluation. Advise the lactating mother with mastitis to pump her breasts to prevent further milk stasis, to discard the milk, and to substitute formula until the infection responds to antibiotics.

Pediatric pointers
Most nodules in children and adolescents reflect the normal response of breast tissue to hormonal fluctuations. For instance, the breasts of young teenage girls may normally contain cordlike nodules that become tender just before menstruation.

A transient breast nodule in young boys (as well as women between ages 20 and 30) may result from juvenile mastitis. Signs of inflammation are present in a firm mass beneath the nipple. Usually, one breast is affected.

Breast Pain

[Mastalgia]

An unreliable indicator of malignancy, this symptom commonly results from benign breast disease. It may occur during rest or movement and may be aggravated by manipulation or palpation. (Breast *tenderness* refers to pain *elicited* by physical contact.) Breast pain may be unilateral or bilateral; cyclic, intermittent, or constant; and dull or sharp. It may result from surface cuts, furuncles, contusions, and similar lesions (superficial pain); nipple fissures and inflammation in the papillary ducts and areolae (severe, localized pain); stromal distention in the breast parenchyma; a tumor that affects nerve endings (severe, constant pain); or inflammatory lesions that not only distend the stroma but also irritate sensory nerve endings (severe pain). Breast pain may radiate to the back, the arms, and sometimes the neck.

Breast tenderness in women may occur before menstruation and during pregnancy. Before menstruation, breast pain or tenderness stems from increased mammary blood flow resulting from hormonal changes. During pregnancy, breast tenderness and throbbing, tingling, or pricking sensations may occur, also influenced by hormonal changes.

In men, breast pain may stem from gynecomastia (especially during puberty and senescence), reproductive tract anomalies, and organic disease of the pituitary, adrenal cortex, and thyroid glands.

Assessment

Begin by asking the patient if breast pain is constant or intermittent. For either type, ask about onset and character. If it's intermittent, determine the relationship of pain to the phase of the menstrual cycle. Determine if the patient is a nursing mother. If not, ask about any nipple discharge and have her describe it. Is she pregnant? Has she reached menopause? Has she recently experienced any flulike symptoms or sustained any injury to the breast? Has she noticed any change in breast shape or contour?

Ask your patient to describe the pain. She may describe it as sticking, stinging, shooting, stabbing, throbbing, or burning. Determine if the pain affects one breast or both, and ask the patient to point to the painful area.

Instruct the patient to place her arms at her sides, and inspect the breasts. Note their size, symmetry, and contour, and the appearance of the skin. Remember that breast shape and size vary widely and that breasts normally change during the menstrual cycle, pregnancy, and lactation and with aging. Are the breasts red or edematous? Are the veins prominent?

Note the size, shape, and symmetry of the nipples and areolae. Is ecchymosis, rash, ulceration, or discharge present? Do the nipples point in the same direction? Do you see signs of retraction, such as skin dimpling or nipple inversion or flattening?

Repeat your inspection, first with the patient's arms raised above her head and then with her hands pressed against her hips.

Palpate the breasts, first with the patient seated and then with her lying down and a pillow placed under her shoulder on the side being examined. Use the pads of your fingers to compress breast tissue against the chest wall. Proceed systematically from the ster-

num to the midline and from the axilla to the midline, noting any warmth, tenderness, nodules, masses, or irregularities. Palpate the nipple, noting tenderness and nodules, and check for discharge. Palpate axillary lymph nodes, noting any enlargement.

Medical causes

● *Areolar gland abscess.* Tender, palpable abscesses on the periphery of the areola follow inflammation of the sebaceous glands of Montgomery. Fever may also occur.

● *Breast abscess (acute).* In the affected breast, local pain, tenderness, erythema, peau d'orange, and warmth are associated with a nodule. Malaise, fever, and chills may also occur.

● *Breast cancer.* Breast pain is an infrequent symptom. However, when reported, the pain may be described as momentary and snatching, a pricking sensation, or infrequent but bothersome twinges. Notable signs may include a palpable mass, nipple discharge, nipple retraction, breast dimpling, peau d'orange, erythema, change in breast contour, and axillary lymphadenopathy.

● *Breast cyst.* A breast cyst that enlarges rapidly may cause acute, localized, and usually unilateral pain. A palpable breast nodule may be present.

● *Fat necrosis.* Local pain and tenderness may develop in this benign disorder. A history of trauma may be present. Associated findings include ecchymosis, erythema of the overlying skin, a firm, irregular, fixed mass, and skin retraction signs, such as skin dimpling and nipple retraction.

● *Intraductal papilloma.* Unilateral breast pain or tenderness may accompany this condition, although the primary sign is a serous or bloody nipple discharge. Associated signs include a small (usually 2- to 3-mm), soft, poorly delineated mass in the ducts beneath the areola.

● *Mammary duct ectasia.* Burning pain and itching around the areola may occur, although ectasia is frequently

BREAST PAIN: CAUSES AND ASSOCIATED FINDINGS

S&S CAUSES	MAJOR ASSOCIATED SIGNS AND SYMPTOMS							
	Breast nodule	Erythema	Fever	Itching	Lymph-adenopathy	Nipple discharge	Nipple retraction signs	Peau d'orange
Areolar gland abscess	●		●					
Breast abscess (acute)	●	●	●					●
Breast cancer	●	●			●	●	●	●
Breast cyst	●							
Fat necrosis	●	●					●	
Intraductal papilloma	●					●		
Mammary duct ectasia	●	●		●	●		●	●
Mastitis	●	●	●				●	●
Proliferative breast disease	●					●		
Sebaceous cyst (infected)	●	●						

asymptomatic at first. The history may include one or more episodes of inflammation with pain, tenderness, erythema, and acute fever, or with pain and tenderness alone, which develop and then subside spontaneously within 7 to 10 days. Other findings may include a rubbery, subareolar breast nodule; swelling and erythema around the nipple; nipple retraction; a bluish-green discoloration or edema (peau d'orange) of the skin overlying the nodule; a thick, sticky, multicolored nipple discharge; and possible axillary lymphadenopathy. Breast ulcer may occur in late stages.

● *Mastitis.* Unilateral pain may be severe, particularly when the inflammation occurs near the skin surface. Breast skin is frequently red and warm at the inflammation site, and may have an orange-peel appearance. Palpation reveals a firm area of induration. Skin retraction signs, such as breast dimpling and nipple deviation, inversion, or flattening, may be present. Systemic signs and symptoms, such as high fever, chills, malaise, and fatigue, may also be present.

• *Proliferative (fibrocystic) breast disease.* In this common cause of breast pain, cysts develop and may cause pain before menstruation and be asymptomatic after it. Later in the disease's course, pain and tenderness may persist throughout the cycle. The cysts feel firm, mobile, and well defined; they are frequently bilateral and found in the upper outer quadrant of the breast but may also be unilateral and generalized. A clear, watery (serous) nipple discharge may be present in one or both breasts. Symptoms of premenstrual syndrome, including headache, irritability, bloating, nausea, vomiting, and abdominal cramping, may also be present.

• *Sebaceous cyst (infected).* Breast pain may be reported with this cutaneous cyst. Associated symptoms include a small, well-delineated nodule, localized erythema, and induration.

Special considerations

Administer pain medication, as ordered. Suggest that the patient wear a well-fitting brassiere for support, especially if her breasts are large or pendulous.

Provide emotional support for the patient and, when appropriate, emphasize the importance of monthly breast self-examination (see *How to Examine Your Breasts,* pages 122 and 123). Teach the patient how to perform this examination, and instruct her to call the doctor immediately if she detects any breast changes.

If ordered, prepare the patient for diagnostic tests, such as mammography, thermography, cytology of nipple discharge, biopsy, or culture of any aspirate.

Pediatric pointers

Transient gynecomastia can cause breast pain in males during puberty.

Breast Ulcer

Appearing on the nipple, areola, or the breast itself, an ulcer indicates destruction of the skin and subcutaneous tissue. Usually, a breast ulcer is a late sign of cancer, appearing well after confirming diagnosis. However, it may be the presenting sign of breast cancer in men, who are more apt to dismiss earlier breast changes. Breast ulcer can also result from trauma, infection, or radiation.

Assessment

Begin the history by asking when the patient first noticed the ulcer and if it was preceded by other breast changes, such as nodules, edema, or nipple discharge, deviation, or retraction. Has she noticed any change in breast shape? Does the ulcer seem to be getting better or worse? Does it cause pain or produce drainage? Has the patient noticed a skin rash? If she has been treating the ulcer at home, find out how.

Review the patient's personal and family history for factors that increase the risk of breast cancer. Ask, for example, about previous malignancy, especially of the breast, and mastectomy. Determine if the patient's mother or sister has had breast cancer. Ask the patient's age at menarche and menopause, since more than 30 years of menstrual activity increases the risk of breast cancer. Also ask about pregnancy, since nulliparity or birth of a first child after age 30 also increases the risk of breast cancer.

If the patient recently gave birth, ask if she breast-feeds her infant or has recently weaned him. Ask if she's currently taking any oral antibiotics and if she's diabetic. All these factors predispose *Candida* infections.

Inspect the patient's breast, noting any asymmetry or flattening. Look for a rash, scaling, cracking, or red excoriation on the nipples, areola, and inframammary fold. Check especially for skin changes, such as warmth, erythema, or edema (peau d'orange). Palpate the breast for masses, noting any induration beneath the ulcer. Then carefully palpate for tenderness or nodules around the areola and the axillary lymph nodes.

Medical causes

• *Breast cancer.* A breast ulcer that doesn't heal within a month usually indicates cancer. Ulceration along a mastectomy scar may indicate metastatic cancer; a nodule beneath the ulcer may be a late sign of a fulminating tumor. Other signs include a palpable breast nodule, skin dimpling, nipple retraction, bloody or serous nipple discharge, erythema, peau d'orange, and enlarged axillary lymph nodes.

• *Breast trauma.* Tissue destruction with inadequate healing may produce breast ulcers. Associated signs depend on the type of trauma but may include ecchymosis, lacerations, abrasions, swelling, and hematoma.

• **Candida albicans** *infection.* Severe *Candida* infection can cause maceration of breast tissue followed by ulceration. Well-defined, bright red papular patches—usually with scaly borders—characterize the infection, which can develop in the breast folds. In breast-feeding women, cracked nipples predispose to infection.

• *Paget's disease.* Bright red nipple excoriation can extend to the areola and ulcerate. Serous or bloody nipple discharge and extreme nipple itching may accompany ulceration.

Other cause

• *Radiation therapy.* After treatment, the breasts appear "sunburned." Subsequently, the skin ulcerates and the surrounding area becomes red and tender.

Special considerations

Because breast ulcers become easily infected, teach the patient how to apply topical antifungal ointment or cream, as ordered. Instruct her to keep the ul-

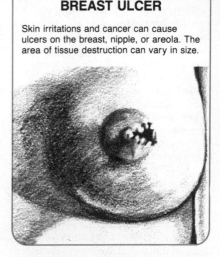

BREAST ULCER

Skin irritations and cancer can cause ulcers on the breast, nipple, or areola. The area of tissue destruction can vary in size.

cer dry to reduce chafing and to wear loose-fitting undergarments.

If breast cancer is suspected, provide emotional support and encourage the patient to express her feelings. Prepare her for diagnostic tests, such as ultrasonography, thermography, mammography, nipple discharge cytology, and breast biopsy. If a *Candida* infection is suspected, prepare her for skin or blood cultures.

Pediatric pointers
None.

Breath with Ammonia Odor

[Uremic fetor]

The odor of ammonia on the breath—described as urinous or "fishy" breath—typically occurs in end-stage chronic renal failure. This sign improves slightly after hemodialysis and persists throughout the disorder's course, but isn't of great concern.

Ammonia breath odor reflects the

long-term metabolic disturbances and biochemical abnormalities associated with uremia and end-stage chronic renal failure. Metabolic end products, blown off by the lungs, produce the ammonia odor, but a specific uremic toxin has not yet been identified. In animals, breath odor analysis has revealed toxic metabolites, such as dimethylamine and trimethylamine, which contribute to the "fishy" odor. The source of these amines, although still unclear, may be intestinal bacteria acting on dietary chlorine.

Assessment
When you detect ammonia breath odor, the diagnosis of chronic renal failure is well established. However, you'll need to assess for associated GI symptoms so that palliative care and support can be individualized.

Inspect the patient's oral cavity for bleeding, swollen gums or tongue, and for ulceration with drainage. Ask the patient if he has experienced a metallic taste, loss of smell, increased thirst, heartburn, difficulty swallowing, or loss of appetite at the sight of food. Ask about early morning vomiting. Since GI bleeding is common in chronic renal failure, ask about bowel habits, noting especially melenous stools or constipation.

Take the patient's vital signs. Inform the doctor of any *abnormal* hypertension (the patient with end-stage chronic renal failure is usually somewhat hypertensive) or significant hypotension. Assess for other signs of shock (such as tachycardia, tachypnea, and cool, clammy skin) and altered mental status. Any significant changes can indicate complications, such as massive GI bleeding or pericarditis with tamponade.

Medical cause
• *End-stage chronic renal failure.* Ammonia breath odor is a late finding. Accompanying signs and symptoms include anuria, skin pigmentation changes and excoriation, brown arcs under the nail margins, tissue wasting, Kussmaul's respirations, neuropathy, lethargy, somnolence, confusion, disorientation, behavior changes with irritability, and mood lability. Later neurologic signs that signal impending uremic coma include muscle twitching and fasciculation, asterixis, paresthesias, and footdrop. Cardiovascular findings may include hypertension and signs of congestive heart failure and pericarditis. GI findings include anorexia, nausea, heartburn, vomiting, constipation, hiccups, and a metallic taste, with oral manifestations such as stomatitis, gum ulceration and bleeding, and a coated tongue. Weight loss is common and uremic frost, pruritus, and signs of hormonal changes, such as impotence or amenorrhea, also appear.

Special considerations
Ammonia breath odor is offensive to others, but the patient may become accustomed to it. As a result, remind him to perform frequent mouth care, particularly before meals, since reducing foul mouth taste and odor may stimulate his appetite. A half-strength hydrogen peroxide mixture or lemon juice gargle helps neutralize the ammonia; the patient may also want to use commercial lozenges or breath sprays or to suck on hard candy. Advise him to use a soft toothbrush or sponge to prevent trauma. If the patient is unable to perform mouth care, do it for him and teach his family members how to assist him.

Maximize dietary intake by offering the patient frequent small meals of his favorite foods, within dietary limitations. Encourage him to take the ordered antacids.

Pediatric pointers
Ammonia breath odor occurs in the child with end-stage chronic renal failure. Provide hard candies to relieve bad mouth taste and odor. If the child is able to gargle, try mixing hydrogen peroxide with flavored mouthwashes.

Breath with Fecal Odor

Fecal breath odor may follow an episode of prolonged vomiting associated with long-standing intestinal obstruction or gastrojejunocolic fistula. It represents an important late diagnostic clue to a potentially life-threatening gastrointestinal (GI) disorder, since complete obstruction of any part of the bowel, if untreated, can cause death within hours from vascular collapse and shock.

Fecal breath odor accompanies fecal vomiting, which results when the obstructed or adynamic intestine attempts self-decompression by regurgitating its contents; vigorous peristaltic waves propel bowel contents backward into the stomach. When the stomach fills with intestinal fluid, further reverse peristalsis results in vomiting. The odor of feculent vomitus lingers in the mouth.

Fecal breath odor may also occur in the patient with a nasogastric or intestinal tube. It's detected only while the underlying disorder persists and abates soon after its resolution.

Assessment

Because fecal breath odor signals a potentially life-threatening intestinal obstruction, you'll need to quickly assess your patient's condition. Monitor vital signs and be alert for signs of shock, such as hypotension, tachycardia, narrowed pulse pressure, and cool, clammy skin.

Ask the patient if he's experiencing nausea and if he has vomited. Ask about the frequency of vomiting and have him describe the color, odor, amount, and consistency of the vomitus. Have an emesis basin nearby to collect and accurately measure any vomitus. Immediately inform the doctor of the patient's vital signs and vomiting history.

Anticipating possible surgery to relieve an obstruction or repair a fistula, withhold all food and fluids. Be prepared to insert a gastric tube or to assist with insertion of an intestinal tube for GI tract decompression. Insert a peripheral I.V. line for vascular access, or assist with central line insertion for large-bore access and central venous pressure monitoring. Obtain a blood sample and send it to the laboratory for complete blood count and electrolyte analysis, since large fluid losses and shifts can produce electrolyte imbalances. Maintain adequate hydration and support circulatory status with additional fluids. Give a physiologic solution with a potassium supplement, such as Ringer's lactate or Plasmanate, as ordered, to prevent metabolic acidosis from gastric losses and metabolic alkalosis from intestinal fluid losses.

If the patient's condition permits continued assessment, ask about previous abdominal surgery, since adhesions can cause an obstruction. Also ask about loss of appetite. Determine if he's experiencing abdominal pain and have him describe its onset, duration, and location. Ask if the pain is intense, persistent, or spasmodic.

Have the patient describe his normal bowel habits, noting especially constipation, diarrhea, or leakage of stool. Ask when his last bowel movement occurred and have him describe its color and consistency.

Auscultate for bowel sounds—hyperactive, high-pitched sounds may indicate *impending* bowel obstruction, whereas hypoactive or absent sounds occur *late* in obstruction and paralytic ileus. Inspect the abdomen, noting contour and any surgical scars. Measure abdominal girth to provide baseline data for subsequent assessment of distention. Palpate for tenderness, distention, and rigidity. Percuss for tympany, indicating a gas-filled bowel, and dullness, indicating fluid.

Medical causes

• **Distal small-bowel obstruction.** In late obstruction, nausea is present although vomiting may be delayed. Initially,

FECAL BREATH ODOR: CAUSES AND ASSOCIATED FINDINGS

S&S CAUSES	MAJOR ASSOCIATED SIGNS AND SYMPTOMS									
	Abdominal distention	Abdominal pain	Anorexia	Constipation	Diarrhea	Hyperactive bowel sounds	Hypoactive/absent bowel sounds	Nausea	Vomiting	Weight loss
Distal small-bowel obstruction	•	•		•	•	•		•	•	
Gastrojejunocolic fistula	•	•	•	•					•	•
Large-bowel obstruction	•	•		•				•	•	

vomitus is gastric contents, changing to bilious and then to fecal contents with resultant fecal breath odor. Accompanying symptoms may include achiness, malaise, drowsiness, and polydipsia. Bowel changes range from diarrhea to constipation and occur with abdominal distention, persistent epigastric or periumbilical colicky pain, and hyperactive bowel sounds and borborygmi, changing to hypoactive or absent sounds in later stages as the obstruction becomes complete. Fever, hypotension, tachycardia, and rebound tenderness may indicate strangulation or perforation.

• *Gastrojejunocolic fistula.* In this disorder, symptoms may be variable and intermittent because of temporary plugging of the fistula. Fecal vomiting with resulting fecal breath odor may occur. Diarrhea is the most frequent presenting sign, and abdominal pain commonly occurs. Related GI findings include anorexia, weight loss, and abdominal distention.

• *Large-bowel obstruction.* Vomiting is usually absent at first, but fecal vomiting with resultant fecal breath odor occurs as a late sign. Typically, symptoms develop more slowly than in small-bowel obstruction. Colicky abdominal pain appears suddenly, followed by continuous hypogastric pain. Marked abdominal distention and tenderness occur, and loops of large bowel may be visible through the abdominal wall. Although constipation develops, defecation may continue for up to 3 days after complete obstruction because of stool remaining in the bowel below the obstruction. Leakage of stool is common with partial obstruction.

Special considerations
After you insert a gastric or intestinal tube, keep the head of the bed elevated at least 30°, and turn the patient as ordered to facilitate gravity passage of the intestinal tube through the GI tract. Remember not to tape the intestinal tube to the patient's face. Ensure tube patency by assessing for drainage and for properly functioning suction devices, and irrigate as ordered. Closely monitor GI drainage losses, and send

serum specimens to the laboratory for electrolyte analysis at least once a day and as ordered. Prepare the patient for diagnostic tests, such as abdominal X-rays, barium enema, and proctoscopy.

Encourage the patient to brush his teeth and gargle with a flavored mouthwash or half-strength hydrogen peroxide mixture to minimize offensive breath odor. Assure him that the fecal odor is temporary and will abate after treatment of the underlying cause.

Pediatric pointers
Carefully monitor the child's fluid and electrolyte status, since dehydration can occur rapidly from persistent vomiting.

Breath with Fruity Odor

Fruity breath odor results from respiratory elimination of excess acetone. This sign characteristically occurs in ketoacidosis—a potentially life-threatening condition that requires immediate treatment to prevent severe dehydration, irreversible coma, and death.

Ketoacidosis results from the excessive catabolism of fats for cellular energy in the absence of usable carbohydrates. This occurs when insulin levels are insufficient to transport glucose into the cells, as in diabetes mellitus, or when glucose is unavailable and hepatic glycogen stores are depleted, as in low-carbohydrate diets and malnutrition. Lacking glucose, the cells burn fat faster than enzymes can handle the ketones, the acidic end products. As a result, the ketones (acetone, beta-hydroxybutyric acid, and acetoacetic acid) accumulate in the blood and urine. To compensate for increased acidity, Kussmaul's respirations expel carbon dioxide with enough acetone to flavor the breath. Eventually, this compensatory mechanism fails, producing ketoacidosis.

Assessment
When you detect fruity breath odor, quickly check for Kussmaul's respirations, and assess the patient's level of consciousness. Take vital signs and check skin turgor. If rapid, deep respirations, stupor, and poor skin turgor accompany fruity breath odor, immediately call the doctor.

Try to obtain a brief history, noting especially diabetes mellitus, nutritional problems such as anorexia nervosa, and fad diets with little or no carbohydrate. Obtain venous and arterial blood samples for glucose, electrolyte, acetone, complete blood count, and arterial blood gas (ABG) studies. Also obtain a urine sample, and test for glucose and acetone. As ordered, administer I.V. fluids and electrolytes to maintain hydration and electrolyte balance and, in diabetic ketoacidosis, regular insulin to reduce blood glucose levels.

If the patient is obtunded, assist with insertion of endotracheal and nasogastric tubes. Suction, as needed. If ordered, insert an indwelling (Foley) catheter and carefully monitor intake and output. Assist with insertion of central venous pressure and arterial lines to monitor the patient's fluid status and blood pressure. Place the patient on a cardiac monitor, monitor vital signs and neurologic status, and draw blood hourly for glucose, acetone, electrolyte, and ABG studies.

If the patient isn't in severe distress, obtain a thorough history. Ask the patient and his family about the onset and duration of fruity breath odor. Find out if and when they've noticed a change in the patient's breathing pattern—for example, to deep, rapid respirations. Ask about increased thirst, frequent urination, weight loss, weakness, fatigue, and abdominal pain. Ask the female patient if she has had monilial vaginitis and if she currently has vaginal secretions with itching. If the patient has a history of diabetes mellitus, ask about stress, past and current infections, and noncompliance with therapy—the most common causes of ketoacidosis in the known diabetic. For the patient with suspected severe weight loss, obtain a dietary and weight history.

Medical causes

• *Diabetic ketoacidosis.* Fruity breath odor often occurs as the ketoacidosis develops over 1 or 2 days. Associated signs and symptoms include polydipsia, polyuria, weak and rapid pulse, hunger, weight loss, weakness, fatigue, nausea, vomiting, and abdominal pain. As the disorder progresses, Kussmaul's respirations, orthostatic hypotension, dehydration, tachycardia, confusion, and stupor occur. Symptoms progressively worsen and may lead to coma.

• *Starvation ketoacidosis.* Fruity breath odor often appears in this potentially life-threatening disorder. Associated signs and symptoms include Kussmaul's respirations; anorexia; weight loss; orthostatic hypotension; bradycardia; dry, scaling skin; sore tongue; muscle and tissue wasting; weakness; fatigue; abdominal pain and distention; poor wound healing; nausea; and possible disorientation, which may progress to stupor and coma.

Special considerations

Provide emotional support for the patient and his family because of the disorder's uncertain outcome. Give them clear explanations of tests and treatments, and allow them to express their concerns.

When the patient becomes more alert and his condition stabilizes, remove any nasogastric tube and start him on an appropriate diet, as ordered. The doctor will then switch the diabetic patient's insulin from I.V. to the subcutaneous route.

Provide appropriate patient teaching or referral. For example, teach the patient with uncontrolled diabetes mellitus to recognize signs of hyperglycemia. Refer the patient with starvation ketoacidosis to a psychologist or support group, and recognize the need for possible long-term follow-up.

Pediatric pointers

Fruity breath odor in an infant or child usually stems from uncontrolled diabetes mellitus. Ketoacidosis, however, develops rapidly in this age group because of low glycogen reserves. As a result, prompt administration of insulin and correction of fluid and electrolyte imbalance is necessary to prevent shock and death.

Brudzinski's Sign

A positive Brudzinski's sign (flexion of the hips and knees in response to passive flexion of the neck) signals meningeal irritation from the pressure of blood or exudate collecting around the spinal nerve roots. Passive flexion of the neck stretches the nerve roots, causing pain and involuntary flexion of the knees and hips. This sign is a common and important early indicator of life-threatening meningitis and subarachnoid hemorrhage. It can be elicited in children as well as in adults, although more reliable indicators of meningeal irritation exist for infants.

Normally, testing for Brudzinski's sign isn't part of a routine examination, unless meningeal irritation is suspected. (See *Testing for Brudzinski's Sign.*)

Assessment

Immediately report a positive Brudzinski's sign. Then, if the patient's alert, ask him about headache, neck pain, nausea, and visual disturbances (blurred or double vision and photophobia)—all symptoms of increased intracranial pressure (ICP). Next, observe for signs of increased ICP, such as altered level of consciousness (restlessness, irritability, confusion, lethargy, personality changes, and coma), pupillary

TESTING FOR BRUDZINSKI'S SIGN

Here's how to test for Brudzinski's sign when you suspect meningeal irritation:

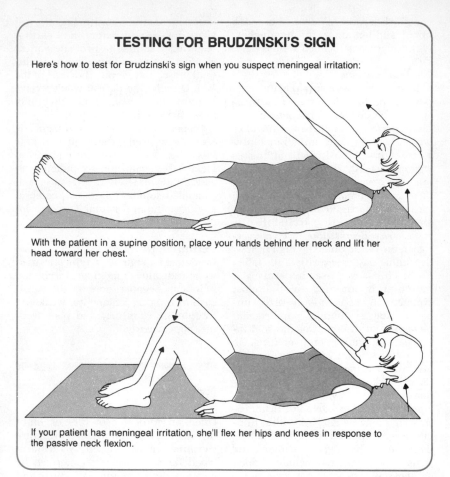

With the patient in a supine position, place your hands behind her neck and lift her head toward her chest.

If your patient has meningeal irritation, she'll flex her hips and knees in response to the passive neck flexion.

changes, bradycardia, widened pulse pressure, irregular respiratory patterns (Cheyne-Stokes or Kussmaul's respirations), vomiting, and moderate fever. Report any of these signs and symptoms to the doctor.

Keep artificial airways, intubation equipment, an Ambu bag, and suction equipment on hand, since your patient's condition may deteriorate suddenly. Elevate the head of the patient's bed 30° to 60° to promote venous drainage. If ordered, administer an osmotic diuretic, such as mannitol, to reduce cerebral edema. Assist with ICP monitoring and, if ICP continues to rise, notify the doctor. You may have to provide mechanical ventilation, to admin-

ister barbiturates and additional doses of diuretics, and to assist with cerebrospinal fluid (CSF) drainage.

Continue your neurologic assessment by evaluating cranial nerve function and noting any motor or sensory deficits. Also assess for Kernig's sign (resistance to leg extension after flexion of the hip and knee), a further indication of meningeal irritation. Look for signs of central nervous system infection, such as fever and nuchal rigidity.

Ask the patient or his family, if necessary, about a history of hypertension, spinal arthritis, or recent head trauma. Ask about dental work and any abscessed teeth (a common cause of meningitis) and about open head injury, endocarditis, and I.V. drug abuse. Ask about sudden onset of headaches, which may be associated with SAH.

Medical causes

• **Arthritis.** In severe spinal arthritis, a positive Brudzinski's sign can occasionally be elicited. The patient may also report back pain (especially after weight bearing) and limited mobility.

• **Meningitis.** A positive Brudzinski's sign can usually be elicited 24 hours after the onset of this life-threatening disorder. Accompanying findings may include headache; a positive Kernig's sign; nuchal rigidity; irritability or restlessness; deep stupor or coma; vertigo; fever (which may be high or low, depending on the severity of the infection); chills; malaise; hyperalgesia; muscular hypotonia; opisthotonos; symmetrical deep tendon reflexes; unequal, sluggish pupils; papilledema; photophobia; diplopia; ocular and facial palsies; nausea; and vomiting. As ICP rises, arterial hypertension, bradycardia, widened pulse pressure, and Cheyne-Stokes or Kussmaul's respirations may appear.

• **Subarachnoid hemorrhage.** Brudzinski's sign may be elicited within minutes after initial bleeding in this life-threatening disorder. Accompanying signs and symptoms include sudden onset of severe headache, nuchal rigidity, altered level of consciousness, dizziness, photophobia, cranial nerve palsies (as evidenced by ptosis, pupil dilation, and limited extraocular muscle movement), nausea and vomiting, fever, and a positive Kernig's sign. Focal signs, such as hemiparesis, visual disturbances, or aphasia, may also occur. As ICP rises, arterial hypertension, bradycardia, widened pulse pressure, and Cheyne-Stokes or Kussmaul's respirations may appear.

Special considerations

The patient with a positive Brudzinski's sign is often critically ill and requires constant ICP monitoring, frequent neurologic checks, and intensive assessment and monitoring of vital signs, intake and output, and cardiorespiratory status. To promote patient comfort, maintain low lights and minimal noise, and elevate the head of the bed. Usually, the patient won't receive narcotic analgesics, since they may mask signs of increased ICP.

Prepare the patient for diagnostic tests, if ordered. These may include blood, urine, and sputum cultures to identify bacteria; lumbar puncture to assess CSF and relieve pressure; and computed tomography scan, cerebral angiography, and spinal X-rays to locate a hemorrhage.

Pediatric pointers

Brudzinski's sign isn't typically used as an indicator of meningeal irritation in infants, because more reliable signs, such as bulging fontanelles, weak cry, fretfulness, vomiting, and poor feeding, appear early.

Bruits

Often an indicator of life- or limb-threatening vascular disease, bruits are swishing sounds caused by turbulent blood flow. They're characterized by location, duration, intensity, pitch, and time of onset in the cardiac cycle. Loud bruits produce intense vibration and a palpable *thrill*. A thrill, however, doesn't provide any further clue to the causative disorder or to its severity.

Bruits are most significant when heard over the abdominal aorta; the renal, carotid, femoral, popliteal, and subclavian arteries; and the thyroid gland. They're also significant when heard consistently despite changes in patient position and when heard during diastole.

Assessment

 If you detect bruits over the abdominal aorta, check for a pulsating mass or a bluish discol-

PREVENTING FALSE BRUITS

Auscultating bruits accurately requires practice and skill. Typically, bruits result from arterial luminal narrowing or arterial dilation. But bruits can also result from excessive pressure applied to the stethoscope's bell during auscultation. This compresses the artery, creating turbulent blood flow and a *false bruit.*

To prevent this, place the bell lightly on the patient's skin. Also, if you're auscultating for a popliteal bruit, you'll need to position the patient supinely, place your hand behind his ankle, and lift his leg slightly before placing the bell behind the knee.

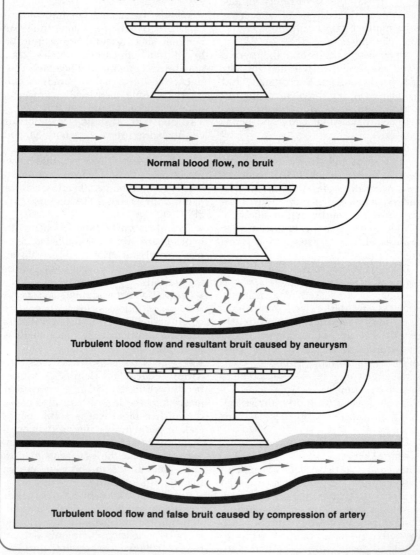

Normal blood flow, no bruit

Turbulent blood flow and resultant bruit caused by aneurysm

Turbulent blood flow and false bruit caused by compression of artery

oration around the umbilicus (Cullen's sign). Either sign—or severe, tearing pain in the abdomen, flank, or lower back—may signal life-threatening dissection of an aortic aneurysm. If you suspect dissection, notify the doctor immediately; emergency surgery may be necessary. Monitor the patient's vital signs constantly, and withhold food and fluids. Watch for signs of hypovolemic shock, such as thirst; hypotension; tachycardia; weak, thready pulse; tachypnea; altered level of consciousness; mottled knees and elbows; and cool, clammy skin.

If you detect bruits over the thyroid gland, ask the patient if he has a history of hyperthyroidism. Report signs and symptoms of life-threatening thyroid storm, such as tremor, restlessness, diarrhea, abdominal pain, and hepatomegaly.

If you detect carotid artery bruits, be alert for signs and symptoms of a transient ischemic attack (TIA), such as dizziness, diplopia, slurred speech, and syncope, which may indicate an impending cerebrovascular accident (CVA). Assess the patient frequently for changes in level of consciousness and muscle function.

If you detect bruits over the femoral, popliteal, or subclavian arteries, watch for signs of decreased or absent peripheral circulation—edema, weakness, and paresthesias. Frequently check distal pulses and skin color and temperature. Immediately report sudden absence of pulse, pallor, or coolness, which may indicate a threat to the affected limb.

If you detect a bruit over any vessel, be sure to check for further vascular damage.

Medical causes

● *Abdominal aortic aneurysm.* A pulsating periumbilical mass accompanied by a systolic bruit over the aorta characterizes this disorder. Associated findings may include abdominal rigidity and tenderness, mottled skin, diminished peripheral pulses, and clau-

dication. Sharp, tearing pain in the abdomen, flank, or lower back signals imminent dissection.

● *Abdominal aortic atherosclerosis.* Loud systolic bruits in the epigastric and midabdominal areas are common. They may be accompanied by leg weakness, numbness, paresthesias, or paralysis; leg pain; and decreased or absent femoral, popliteal, and pedal pulses. Abdominal pain is rarely present.

● *Anemia.* Increased cardiac output causes increased blood flow. In severe anemia, short systolic bruits may be heard over both carotid arteries. They may be accompanied by headache, fatigue, dizziness, pallor, jaundice, palpitations, mild tachycardia, dyspnea, nausea, anorexia, and glossitis.

● *Carotid artery stenosis.* Systolic bruits can be heard over one or both carotid arteries. Other signs and symptoms may be absent. However, dizziness, vertigo, headache, syncope, aphasia, dysarthria, vision loss, hemiparesis, or hemiparalysis signal TIA and may herald CVA.

● *Carotid cavernous fistula.* Continuous bruits heard over the eyeballs and temples are characteristic, as are visual disturbances and protruding, pulsating eyeballs.

● *Peripheral arteriovenous fistula.* A rough, continuous bruit with systolic accentuation may be heard over the fistula; in addition, a palpable thrill is often present.

● *Peripheral vascular disease.* This condition characteristically produces bruits over the femoral artery and other arteries in the legs. It can also cause diminished or absent femoral, popliteal, or pedal pulses; intermittent claudication; numbness, weakness, pain, and cramping in the legs, feet, and hips; and cool, shiny skin and hair loss on the affected extremity.

● *Renal artery stenosis.* Systolic bruits commonly are heard over the abdominal midline and flank on the affected side. Hypertension commonly accompanies stenosis; headache, palpitations, tachycardia, anxiety, dizziness, retinopathy, and mental sluggishness may also appear.

• *Subclavian steal syndrome.* In this syndrome, systolic bruits may be heard over one or both subclavian arteries as a result of narrowing of the arterial lumen. They may be accompanied by decreased blood pressure and claudication in the affected arm, hemiparesis, visual disturbances, vertigo, and dysarthria.

• *Thyrotoxicosis.* A systolic bruit is often heard over the thyroid gland. Accompanying signs and symptoms appear in all body systems, but the most characteristic ones include thyroid enlargement, fatigue, nervousness, tachycardia, heat intolerance, sweating, tremor, diarrhea, and weight loss despite increased appetite. Exophthalmos may also be present.

Special considerations

Because bruits can signal a life-threatening vascular disorder, frequently check the patient's vital signs and auscultate over the affected arteries. Be especially alert for bruits that become louder or develop a diastolic component.

Administer medications, such as vasodilators, anticoagulants, antiplatelets, or antihypertensives, as ordered.

Prepare the patient for diagnostic tests, such as blood studies, radiographs, an EKG, cardiac catheterization, and ultrasonography.

Instruct the patient to inform the doctor if he develops dizziness or pain, since this may indicate a worsening of his condition.

Pediatric pointers

Bruits are common in young children but are usually of little significance; for example, cranial bruits are normal until age 4. However, certain bruits may be significant. Since birthmarks often accompany congenital arteriovenous fistulas, carefully auscultate for bruits in a child with port-wine spots or cavernous or diffuse hemangiomas.

Buffalo Hump

An accumulation of cervicodorsal fat, buffalo hump usually indicates hypercortisolism, or Cushing's syndrome. Hypercortisolism itself may result from adrenal carcinoma, adrenal adenoma, ectopic adrenocorticotropic hormone (ACTH) production, excessive pituitary secretion of ACTH (Cushing's disease), or long-term glucocorticoid therapy.

Buffalo hump doesn't help distinguish between the underlying causes of hypercortisolism, but it may help direct diagnostic testing.

Assessment

Ask the patient about recent weight gain and when he first noticed the buffalo hump. Typically, a history of moderate-to-extreme obesity, with accumulation of adipose tissue in the nape of the neck, face, and trunk and thinning of the arms and legs, indicates hypercortisolism. If the patient has an old photograph, use it to compare his current and former weight and the distribution of adipose tissue. Ask if the patient or any family member has a history of endocrine disorders, malignant disease, or obesity. If the patient's a female of childbearing age, ask the date of her last menses and about any changes in her normal menstrual pattern. Next, ask about any changes in diet or drug use. If the patient's receiving glucocorticoid therapy, ask about the dosage, schedule, route of administration, and any recent changes in therapy.

Take the patient's vital signs, height, and weight. Form an impression of his appearance, noting obvious signs such as hirsutism, diaphoresis, and moon face. Inspect the arms, legs, and trunk for striae, and note skin turgor. Assess muscle function by asking the patient to rise from a squatting position; note any difficulty since this may indicate

RECOGNIZING HYPERCORTISOLISM

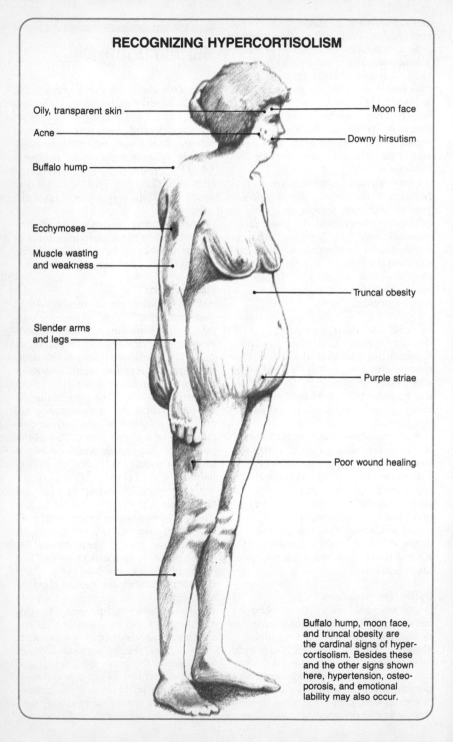

Oily, transparent skin

Acne

Buffalo hump

Ecchymoses

Muscle wasting and weakness

Slender arms and legs

Moon face

Downy hirsutism

Truncal obesity

Purple striae

Poor wound healing

Buffalo hump, moon face, and truncal obesity are the cardinal signs of hypercortisolism. Besides these and the other signs shown here, hypertension, osteoporosis, and emotional lability may also occur.

quadriceps muscle weakness.

During your assessment, observe the patient's behavior. Extreme emotional lability along with depression, irritability, or confusion may signal hypercortisolism.

Medical causes
• *Hypercortisolism.* Buffalo hump varies in size depending on the severity of the disorder and the amount of weight gain. It's often accompanied by hirsutism, moon face, and truncal obesity with slender arms and legs. The skin may appear transparent, with purple striae and ecchymoses. Other findings may include acne, muscle weakness and wasting, fatigue, poor wound healing, elevated blood pressure, personality changes, and amenorrhea or oligomenorrhea in women or impotence in men.

• *Morbid obesity.* The size of the buffalo hump depends on the amount of weight gain and the distribution of adipose tissue. Associated signs and symptoms may include generalized adiposity, silver striae, elevated blood pressure, and hypogonadism.

Other causes
• *Drugs.* Buffalo hump may result from excessive dosages of glucocorticoids, such as cortisone, hydrocortisone, and prednisone.

Special considerations
Prepare the patient for diagnostic tests, if ordered. Blood and urine tests can confirm hypercortisolism. Ultrasonography, computed tomography (CT) scan, or arteriography can localize adrenal tumors. Chest X-rays, bronchography, and an abdominal CT scan can determine ectopic involvement. Visual field testing and a skull CT scan can identify pituitary tumors.

Pediatric pointers
Although rare in children, buffalo hump may occur at any age. In children over age 7, this sign usually results from pituitary oversecretion of ACTH in bilateral adrenal hyperplasia. In younger children, it often results from glucocorticoid therapy—for example, overuse of glucocorticoid eyedrops.

Butterfly Rash

When present, butterfly rash is a cardinal sign of systemic lupus erythematosus. However, it can also signal dermatologic disorders.

Typically, butterfly rash appears in a malar distribution across the nose and cheeks. Similar rashes may appear on the neck, scalp, and other areas. Butterfly rash is sometimes mistaken for sunburn, since it can be provoked or aggravated by ultraviolet rays.

Assessment
Ask the patient when he first noticed the butterfly rash and if he has been recently exposed to sun. Next, ask about recent weight or hair loss and about the presence of rashes elsewhere on his body. Does he have a family history of lupus erythematosus? Is he taking hydralazine or procainamide (common causes of drug-induced lupus erythematosus)?

Inspect the rash, noting any macules, papules, pustules, and scaling. Is the rash edematous? Are areas of hypopigmentation or hyperpigmentation present? Look for blisters or ulcers in the mouth, and note any inflamed lesions. Check for rashes elsewhere on the body.

Medical causes
• *Discoid lupus erythematosus.* This benign form of lupus erythematosus may present with a unilateral or butterfly rash that consists of mildly scaling, erythematous, raised, sharply demarcated plaques with follicular plugging and central atrophy. The rash may also involve the scalp, ears, chest, or any part of the body exposed to sun. Telangiectases, scarring alopecia, and

BUTTERFLY RASH

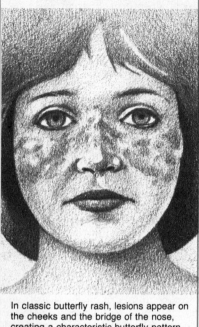

In classic butterfly rash, lesions appear on the cheeks and the bridge of the nose, creating a characteristic butterfly pattern. The rash may vary in severity from malar erythema to discoid lesions (plaques).

hypopigmentation or hyperpigmentation may occur later. A destructive distortion of the nose ("parrot beak") and ears may develop. Other accompanying signs include conjunctival redness, dilated capillaries of the nail fold, bilateral parotid gland enlargement, oral lesions, and mottled, reddish-blue skin on the legs.

● **Erysipelas.** In this streptococcal infection, butterfly rash appears as warm, indurated, tender, pruritic, edematous, and erythematous plaques, enlarging peripherally with sharply elevated margins; vesicles and bullae may form. Commonly, the rash appears abruptly and covers the bridge of the nose and one or both cheeks, halting at the hairline of the scalp or beard. However, the rash may also appear on the hands and genitals. Associated

signs and symptoms include fever, malaise, headache, vomiting, sore throat, and cervical lymphadenopathy.

● **Polymorphous light eruption.** Butterfly rash appears as erythema, vesicles, plaques, and multiple small papules that may later become eczematized, lichenified, and excoriated. Provoked by ultraviolet rays, the rash appears on the cheeks and bridge of the nose, the hands and arms, and other areas, beginning a few hours to several days after exposure. The rash may be accompanied by pruritus.

● **Rosacea.** Initially, the butterfly rash may appear as a prominent, nonscaling, intermittent erythema limited to the lower half of the nose or including the chin, cheeks, and central forehead. As rosacea develops, the duration of the rash increases; instead of disappearing after each episode, the rash varies in intensity and is often accompanied by telangiectasia. In advanced rosacea, the skin is oily, with papules, pustules, nodules, and telangiectases restricted to the central third of the face. In men with severe rosacea, butterfly rash may be accompanied by rhinophyma—a thickened, lobulated overgrowth of sebaceous glands and epithelial connective tissue on the lower half of the nose and, possibly, the adjacent cheeks.

● **Seborrheic dermatitis.** The butterfly rash appears as greasy, scaling, slightly yellow macules and papules of varying size; the scalp, beard, eyebrows, portions of the forehead above the bridge of the nose, nasolabial fold, or trunk may also be involved. Associated signs and symptoms may include crusts and fissures (particularly when the external ear and scalp are involved), pruritus, redness, blepharitis, styes, severe acne, and oily skin.

● **Systemic lupus erythematosus (SLE).** Occurring in about 40% of patients with this connective tissue disorder, butterfly rash appears as a red, scaly, sharply demarcated macular eruption. The rash may be transient in acute SLE or may progress slowly to include the forehead, chin, the area around the

BUTTERFLY RASH: CAUSES AND ASSOCIATED FINDINGS

CAUSES	Acne	Alopecia	Erythema	Fever	Maculopapular lesions	Malaise	Mucous membrane lesions	Photosensitivity	Plaques	Pruritus	Scaling	Telangiectases
Discoid lupus erythematosus		•	•				•	•	•		•	•
Erysipelas			•	•		•				•		
Polymorphous light eruption			•		•			•	•	•		
Rosacea			•		•							•
Seborrheic dermatitis	•				•					•		
Systemic lupus erythematosus		•	•	•	•	•	•	•			•	•

ears, and other exposed areas. Common associated skin findings include photosensitivity; scaling; patchy alopecia; mucous membrane lesions; mottled erythema of the palms and fingers; periungual erythema with edema; macular, reddish-purple lesions on the volar surfaces of the fingers; telangiectasia of the base of the nails or eyelids; purpura; petechiae; or ecchymoses.

Butterfly rash may also be accompanied by joint pain, stiffness, and deformities—particularly ulnar deviation of the fingers and subluxation of the proximal interphalangeal joints. Related findings include periorbital and facial edema, dyspnea, low-grade fever, malaise, weakness, fatigue, weight loss, anorexia, nausea, vomiting, lymphadenopathy, and hepatosplenomegaly.

Other causes
• *Drugs.* Hydralazine and procainamide can cause an SLE-like syndrome.

Special considerations
Prepare the patient for immunologic studies, complete blood count, and possibly liver studies. If ordered, obtain a urine specimen.

Withhold photosensitizing drugs, such as phenothiazines, sulfonamides, sulfonylureas, and thiazide diuretics. Instruct the patient to avoid exposure to the sun or to use a sunscreen. Suggest that he use hypoallergenic makeup to help conceal facial lesions.

Pediatric pointers
Butterfly rash occurs rarely in pediatric patients and may consist only of an erythematous blush or scaly, erythematous papules.

café-au-lait spots • capillary refill time—prolonged • carpopedal spasm • cat
asymmetrical • chest pain • Cheyne-Stokes respirations • chills • chorea • Ch
cogwheel rigidity • cold intolerance • confusion • conjunctival injection • cor
reflex—absent • costovertebral angle tenderness • cough—barking • cough—r
productive • crackles • crepitation—bony • crepitation—subcutaneous • cry—
cyanosis • decerebrate posture • decorticate posture • deep tendon reflexes—
reflexes—hypoactive • depression • diaphoresis • diarrhea • diplopia • dizzir
absent • drooling • dysarthria • dysmenorrhea • dyspareunia • dyspepsia • d
dystonia • dysuria • earache • edema—generalized • edema of the arms • ed
of the legs • enophthalmos • enuresis • epistaxis • eructation • erythema • ex
discharge • eye pain • facial pain • fasciculations • fatigue • fecal incontinen
fever • flank pain • flatulence • fontanelle bulging • fontanelle depression • fo
abnormalities • gait—bizarre • gait—propulsive • gait—scissors • gait—spas
gait—waddling • gallop—atrial • gallop—ventricular • genital lesions in the
respirations • gum bleeding • gum swelling • gynecomastia • halitosis • halo
hearing loss • heat intolerance • Heberden's nodes • hematemesis • hematoch
hemianopia • hemoptysis • hepatomegaly • hiccups • hirsutism • hoarseness
hyperpigmentation • hyperpnea • hypopigmentation • impotence • insomnia
claudication • Janeway's spots • jaundice • jaw pain • jugular vein distentior
sign • leg pain • level of consciousness—decreased • lid lag • light flashes •
lymphadenopathy • masklike facies • McBurney's sign • McMurray's sign • n
metrorrhagia • miosis • moon face • mouth lesions • murmurs • muscle atro
muscle spasms • muscle spasticity • muscle weakness • mydriasis • myoclor
nausea • neck pain • night blindness • nipple discharge • nipple retraction •
rigidity • nystagmus • ocular deviation • oligomenorrhea • oliguria • opisthc
dyskinesia • orthopnea • orthostatic hypotension • Ortolani's sign • Osler's n
palpitations • papular rash • paralysis • paresthesias • paroxysmal nocturna
d'orange • pericardial friction rub • peristaltic waves—visible • photophobia
rub • polydipsia • polyphagia • polyuria • postnasal drip • priapism • pruri
psychotic behavior • ptosis • pulse—absent or weak • pulse—bounding • pu
pulse pressure—widened • pulse rhythm abnormality • pulsus alternans • p
paradoxus • pupils—nonreactive • pupils—sluggish • purple striae • purpu
pyrosis • raccoon's eyes • rebound tenderness • rectal pain • retractions—co
rhinorrhea • rhonchi • Romberg's sign • salivation—decreased • salivation—
scotoma • scrotal swelling • seizure—absence • seizure—focal • seizure—ge
seizure—psychomotor • setting-sun sign • shallow respirations • skin—bror
skin—mottled • skin—scaly • skin turgor—decreased • spider angioma • sp
respirations • stool—clay-colored • stridor • syncope • tachycardia • tachypr
tearing—increased • throat pain • tic • tinnitus • tracheal deviation • trach
trismus • tunnel vision • uremic frost • urethral discharge • urinary frequer
urinary incontinence • urinary urgency • urine cloudiness • urticaria • vagi
postmenopausal • vaginal discharge • venous hum • vertigo • vesicular rash
loss • visual blurring • visual floaters • vomiting • vulvar lesions • weight ga
loss—excessive • wheezing • wristdrop• abdominal distention • abdominal
abdominal rigidity • accessory muscle use • agitation • alopecia • amenorrl
analgesia • anhidrosis • anorexia • anosmia • anuria • anxiety • aphasia •
respirations • apraxia • arm pain • asterixis • ataxia • athetosis • aura • Ba
pain • barrel chest • Battle's sign • Biot's respirations • bladder distention •
blood pressure increase • bowel sounds—absent • bowel sounds—hyperact
hypoactive • bradycardia • bradypnea • breast dimpling • breast nodule • l

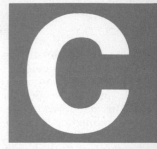

Café-au-Lait Spots

An important indicator of neurofibromatosis and other congenital melanotic disorders, café-au-lait spots appear as flat, light brown, uniformly hyperpigmented macules on the skin surface. They usually appear in childhood (most often before age 10) and can be differentiated from freckles and other benign birthmarks by their larger size (ranging from a few millimeters to 1.5 cm or larger) and more irregular shape. Although one to three spots may be a normal finding, the presence of café-au-lait spots usually indicates an underlying disorder.

Assessment

Ask the patient or his parents when the café-au-lait spots first appeared. Also ask about a family history of these spots and of neurofibromatosis. Review the patient's history for seizures, frequent fractures, or mental retardation.

Inspect the skin, noting the location and pattern of the spots. Observe for distinctive skin lesions, such as axillary freckling, mottling, small spherical patches, and areas of depigmentation. Check for subcutaneous neurofibromas along major nerve branches, especially on the trunk. Also check for bony abnormalities, such as scoliosis or kyphosis.

Medical causes

● *Albright's syndrome.* In this syndrome, café-au-lait spots are smaller (about 1 cm) and more irregularly shaped than those in neurofibromatosis. They may stop abruptly at the midline and seem to follow a dermatomal distribution. Usually, fewer than six spots appear, often unilaterally on the forehead, neck, and lower back. When they occur on the scalp, the hair overlying them may be more deeply pigmented. Associated signs may include skeletal deformities, frequent fractures, and, in females, sexual precocity.

● *Neurofibromatosis.* The most common cause of café-au-lait spots, this disorder is characterized by six or more large, smooth-bordered spots. Associated signs include axillary freckling; irregular, hyperpigmented, and mottled skin; and, most significantly, multiple skin-colored pedunculated nodules clustered along nerve sheaths. These nodules develop during childhood and proliferate throughout life, affecting all body tissues and causing marked deformity. Mental impairment, seizures, hearing loss, exophthalmos, decreased visual acuity, and GI bleeding can eventually occur.

● *Tuberous sclerosis.* Mental retardation and seizures characteristically appear first, followed several years later by cutaneous facial lesions—multiple café-au-lait spots, spherical areas of rough skin, and areas of yellow-red or depigmented nevi.

Special considerations

Although café-au-lait spots require no treatment, you'll obviously need to provide emotional support for the patient and his family. Also, refer them for genetic counseling. If ordered, prepare the patient for diagnostic tests, such as tissue biopsy and radiographic studies.

Capillary Refill Time— Prolonged

Capillary refill time is the duration required for color to return to the nail bed of a finger or toe after application of slight pressure, which causes blanching. This duration reflects the quality of peripheral vasomotor function. Normal capillary refill time is less than 3 seconds.

Prolonged refill time isn't diagnostic of any disorder but must be evaluated along with other signs and symptoms. However, this sign usually signals obstructive peripheral arterial disease or decreased cardiac output.

Capillary refill time is typically tested during a routine cardiovascular assessment. It isn't tested in suspected life-threatening disorders, because other, more characteristic signs and symptoms appear earlier.

Assessment

If you detect prolonged capillary refill time, take the patient's vital signs and check pulses in the affected limb. Does the limb feel cold or look cyanotic? Does the patient report pain or any unusual sensations in his fingers or toes, especially after exposure to cold?

Take a brief medical history, noting especially previous peripheral vascular disease. Find out what medications the patient is taking.

Medical causes

● *Aortic aneurysm (dissecting).* Capillary refill time is prolonged in the fingers and toes with a dissecting aneurysm in the thoracic aorta, and is prolonged in just the toes with a dissecting aneurysm in the abdominal aorta. Common accompanying signs and symptoms include a pulsating abdominal mass, systolic bruit, and substernal or abdominal pain.

● *Aortic arch syndrome.* Prolonged capillary refill time in the fingers occurs early in this syndrome. The patient displays absent carotid pulses and possibly unequal radial pulses. Other signs and symptoms usually precede loss of pulses and include fever, night sweats, arthralgia, weight loss, anorexia, nausea, malaise, skin rash, splenomegaly, and pallor.

● *Aortic bifurcation occlusion (acute).* Prolonged capillary refill time in the toes is a late sign in this rare but usually fatal disorder. All lower extremity pulses are absent, and the patient complains of sudden, moderate-to-severe pain in the legs and, less often, in the abdomen, lumbosacral area, or perineum. Both legs are cold, pale, totally numb, and flaccid.

● *Arterial occlusion (acute).* Prolonged capillary refill time occurs early in the affected limb. Arterial pulses are usually absent distal to the obstruction; the affected limb appears cool and pale or cyanotic. Intermittent claudication, moderate-to-severe pain, numbness, and paresthesias or paralysis of the affected limb may occur.

● *Buerger's disease.* Capillary refill time is prolonged in the toes. Exposure to low temperatures turns the feet cold, cyanotic, and numb; later they redden, become hot, and tingle. Other findings include intermittent claudication of the instep, weak peripheral pulses, and, in later stages, ulceration, muscle atrophy, and gangrene.

If the disease affects the hands, prolonged capillary refill may accompany painful fingertip ulcerations.

● *Cardiac tamponade.* Prolonged capillary refill time represents a late sign of decreased cardiac output. Associated signs include tachycardia, cyanosis, dyspnea, neck vein distention, and hypotension.

• **Hypothermia.** Prolonged capillary refill time may appear early as a compensatory response. Associated signs and symptoms depend on the degree of hypothermia and may include some combination of shivering, fatigue, weakness, decreased level of consciousness, slurred speech, ataxia, muscle stiffness or rigidity, tachycardia or bradycardia, hyporeflexia or areflexia, diuresis, oliguria, bradypnea, decreased blood pressure, and cold, pale skin.

• **Peripheral arterial trauma.** Any trauma to a peripheral artery that reduces distal blood flow also prolongs capillary refill time in the affected extremity. Related findings in that extremity include bruising or pulsating bleeding; weakened pulse; cool, pale skin; cyanosis; paresthesias; and sensory loss.

• **Peripheral vascular disease.** Prolonged capillary refill time in the affected extremities is a late sign. Peripheral pulses gradually weaken and then disappear. Intermittent claudication, coolness, pallor, and decreased hair growth are associated signs. Impotence may accompany arterial occlusion in the descending aorta or femoral areas.

• **Raynaud's disease.** Capillary refill time is prolonged in the fingers, the usual site of this disease's characteristic episodic arterial vasospasm. Exposure to cold or stress produces blanching in the fingers, then cyanosis, and then erythema before fingers return to normal temperature. Warmth relieves symptoms, which may include paresthesias. Chronic disease may produce trophic changes, such as sclerodactyly, ulcerations, or chronic paronychia.

• **Shock.** Prolonged capillary refill time appears late in almost all types of shock. Accompanying signs include hypotension, tachycardia, tachypnea, and cool, clammy skin.

• **Volkmann's contracture.** Prolonged capillary refill time results from this contracture's characteristic vasospasm. Associated signs include loss of mobility and loss of strength in the affected extremity.

Other causes

• **Diagnostic tests.** Cardiac catheterization can cause arterial hematoma or clot formation and prolonged capillary refill time.

• **Drugs.** Drugs that cause vasoconstriction (particularly alpha-adrenergics) prolong capillary refill time.

• **Treatments.** Prolonged capillary refill time can result from an arterial line or umbilical line, which can cause arterial hematoma and obstructed distal blood flow; or an improperly fitting cast, which constricts circulation.

Special considerations

Frequently assess the patient's vital signs, level of consciousness, and affected extremity, and report any changes, such as progressive cyanosis or loss of an existing pulse.

Prepare the patient for diagnostic tests, which may include arteriography or Doppler ultrasonography, to help confirm or rule out arterial occlusion.

Pediatric pointers

Capillary refill time may be prolonged in newborns with acrocyanosis, but this is a normal finding. Typically, prolonged capillary refill time is associated with the same disorders in children as in adults. However, its most common pediatric cause is cardiac surgery, such as repair of congenital heart defects.

Carpopedal Spasm

Carpopedal spasm is the violent, painful contraction of the muscles in the hands and feet. It's an important sign of tetany, a potentially life-threatening condition characterized by increased neuromuscular excitation and sus-

CARPOPEDAL SPASM

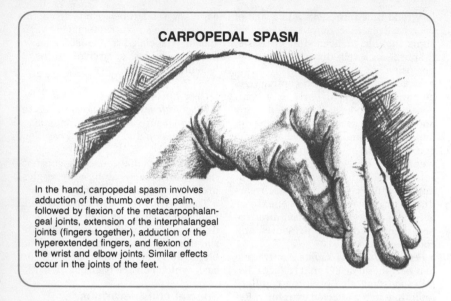

In the hand, carpopedal spasm involves adduction of the thumb over the palm, followed by flexion of the metacarpophalangeal joints, extension of the interphalangeal joints (fingers together), adduction of the hyperextended fingers, and flexion of the wrist and elbow joints. Similar effects occur in the joints of the feet.

tained muscle contraction and commonly associated with hypocalcemia.

Carpopedal spasm requires prompt evaluation and intervention; untreated, it can cause laryngospasm, seizures, cardiac dysrhythmias, and cardiac and respiratory arrest.

Assessment

If you detect carpopedal spasm, quickly assess the patient for signs of respiratory distress (laryngospasm, stridor, loud crowing noises, cyanosis) or cardiac dysrhythmias, which indicate hypocalcemia. If you detect these signs, call a doctor immediately, administer an I.V. calcium preparation as ordered, and give emergency respiratory and cardiac support as needed. If calcium infusion doesn't control seizures, administer a sedative, such as chloral hydrate or phenobarbital, as ordered.

If the patient isn't in distress, obtain a detailed history. Ask about the onset and duration of the spasms and the degree of pain they produce. Also ask about related signs of hypocalcemia, such as numbness and tingling of the fingertips and feet; other muscle cramps or spasms; and nausea, vom-

iting, and abdominal pain. Check for previous neck surgery, calcium or magnesium deficiency, and hypoparathyroidism.

During the history, form a general impression of the patient's mental status and behavior. If possible, ask the patient's family members or friends if they've noticed changes in the patient's behavior. Mental confusion or even personality changes may occur with hypocalcemia.

Inspect the patient's skin and fingernails, noting any dryness or scaling and the presence of ridged, brittle nails.

Medical cause

• *Hypocalcemia.* Carpopedal spasm is an early sign of hypocalcemia. It's usually accompanied by paresthesias of the fingers, toes, and perioral area; muscle weakness, twitching, and cramping; hyperreflexia; chorea; fatigue; and palpitations. Positive Chvostek's and Trousseau's signs can be elicited. Laryngospasm, stridor, and seizures may appear in severe hypocalcemia.

Chronic hypocalcemia may be accompanied by mental status changes; cramps; dry, scaly skin; brittle nails; and thin, patchy hair and eyebrows.

Other causes
• *Treatments.* Multiple blood transfusions and parathyroidectomy may cause hypocalcemia, resulting in carpopedal spasm. Surgical procedures that impair calcium absorption, such as ileostomy formation and gastric resection with gastrojejunostomy, may also cause hypocalcemia.

Special considerations
Carpopedal spasm can cause severe pain and anxiety, leading to hyperventilation. If this occurs, help the patient slow his breathing through your relaxing touch, reassuring attitude, and clear directions for what he should do. Provide a quiet, dark environment to reduce the patient's anxiety.

As ordered, prepare the patient for laboratory tests, such as complete blood count and serum calcium, phosphorus, and parathyroid hormone studies.

Pediatric pointers
Idiopathic hypoparathyroidism is a common cause of hypocalcemia in children. You'll need to carefully monitor children with this condition, since carpopedal spasm may herald the onset of epileptiform seizures or generalized tetany followed by prolonged tonic spasms.

Cat Cry

Occurring during infancy, this mewing, kittenlike sound is the primary indicator of cri du chat, or cat cry, syndrome. This syndrome affects 1 in 20,000 newborns, occurs more commonly in females, and causes profound mental retardation and, frequently, death before age 1. The chromosomal defect responsible (deletion of the short arm of chromosome 5) usually appears spontaneously, but may be inherited from a carrier parent. The characteristic cry is thought to result from abnormal laryngeal development.

Assessment
If you detect cat cry in a newborn, suspect cri du chat and immediately inform the doctor. Be alert for signs of respiratory distress, such as nasal flaring; irregular, shallow respirations; cyanosis; and a respiratory rate over 60 breaths/minute. Prepare to suction the infant and to administer warmed oxygen. Keep emergency resuscitation equipment nearby since bradycardia may develop. Perform a physical examination and note any abnormalities.

If you detect cat cry in an older infant, ask the parents when it developed. Sudden onset of an abnormal cry in an infant with a previously normal, vigorous cry suggests other disorders, not cri du chat. (See "Cry—High-pitched.")

Medical cause
• *Cri du chat syndrome.* A kittenlike cry appears at birth or shortly thereafter. It's accompanied by profound mental retardation, microcephaly, low birth weight, hypotonia, failure to thrive, and feeding difficulties. Typically, the infant displays a round face with wide-set eyes; strabismus; a broad-based nose with oblique or downward-sloping epicanthal folds; abnormally shaped, low-set ears; and an unusually small jaw. He may also have a short neck, webbed fingers, and a simian crease.

Special considerations
Connect the infant to an apnea monitor, and check for signs of respiratory distress. Keep suction equipment and warmed oxygen available. Watch for signs of increased intracranial pressure. As ordered, obtain a blood sample for chromosomal analysis. Prepare the infant for a computed tomography scan to rule out other causes of microcephaly, and an ear, nose, and throat examination to evaluate vocal cords.

Because the infant with cri du chat is usually a poor eater, monitor intake, output, and weight. Instruct the parents to offer small, frequent feedings.

Chest Expansion— Asymmetrical

Asymmetrical chest expansion is the uneven extension of portions of the chest wall during inspiration. During normal respiration, the thorax uniformly expands upward and outward, then contracts downward and inward. When this process is disrupted, breathing becomes uncoordinated, causing asymmetrical chest expansion.

Asymmetrical expansion may develop suddenly or gradually and may affect one or both sides of the chest wall. It may occur as *delayed expiration* (chest lag); as *abnormal movement during inspiration* (for example, intercostal retractions, paradoxical movement, or chest-abdomen asynchrony); or as *unilateral absence of movement.* It most commonly results from pleural disorders, such as life-threatening hemothorax or tension pneumothorax. However, this sign can also result from musculoskeletal or neurologic disorders, airway obstruction, or trauma. Regardless of its underlying cause, asymmetrical chest expansion produces rapid and shallow or deep respirations that increase the work of breathing.

Assessment

If you detect asymmetrical chest expansion, first consider traumatic injury to the patient's ribs or sternum, which can cause flail chest—a life-threatening emergency characterized by paradoxical chest movement. Quickly take the patient's vital signs and assess for signs of acute respiratory distress—rapid and shallow respirations, tachycardia, and cyanosis. If you detect these signs, have another nurse immediately notify the doctor. Then, use tape or sandbags to temporarily splint the unstable flail segment. Depending on the severity of respiratory distress, administer oxygen by nasal cannula, mask, or mechanical ventilator. Insert an I.V. line to allow fluid replacement and administration of pain medication, which helps prevent splinting. If ordered, draw a blood sample for arterial blood gas analysis and connect the patient to a cardiac monitor.

Remember that asymmetrical chest expansion may also result from hemothorax, tension pneumothorax, bronchial obstruction, and other life-threatening causes—although it's not a cardinal sign of these disorders. Because *any* form of asymmetrical chest expansion can compromise the patient's respiratory status, don't leave him unattended. Be alert for signs of respiratory distress, and notify the doctor immediately if they occur.

If you don't suspect flail chest, and if the patient isn't experiencing acute respiratory distress, obtain a brief history. Asymmetrical chest expansion often results from mechanical airflow obstruction, so find out if the patient's experiencing dyspnea or pain during breathing. If so, does he feel constantly short of breath or have intermittent attacks of breathlessness? Does the pain worsen his feeling of breathlessness? Does repositioning, coughing, or any other activity relieve or worsen the dyspnea or pain? Is the pain more noticeable during inspiration or expiration? Can he inhale deeply?

Ask if the patient has a history of pulmonary or systemic illness—frequent upper respiratory infections, asthma, tuberculosis, pneumonia, or cancer. Has he had thoracic surgery? (This typically produces asymmetrical chest expansion on the affected side.) Also ask about blunt or penetrating chest trauma, which may have caused pulmonary injury. And obtain an occupational history to find out if the patient may have inhaled toxic fumes or aspirated a toxic substance.

Now perform a physical examination. Begin by gently palpating the trachea for midline positioning. Then ex-

RECOGNIZING LIFE-THREATENING CAUSES OF ASYMMETRICAL CHEST EXPANSION

As you know, asymmetrical chest expansion can result from several life-threatening disorders. Two common causes—bronchial obstruction and flail chest—produce distinctive chest wall movements that provide important clues about the underlying disorder.

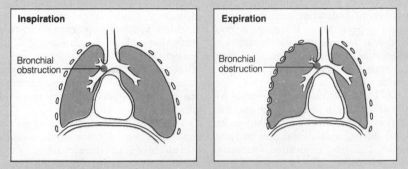

In *bronchial obstruction*, only the unaffected portion of the chest wall expands during inspiration. Intercostal bulging during expiration may indicate that air is trapped in the chest.

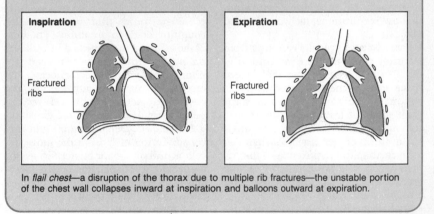

In *flail chest*—a disruption of the thorax due to multiple rib fractures—the unstable portion of the chest wall collapses inward at inspiration and balloons outward at expiration.

amine the posterior chest wall for areas of tenderness or deformity. To evaluate the extent of asymmetrical chest expansion, place your hands—fingers together and thumbs abducted toward the spine—flat on both sections of the lower posterior chest wall. Position your thumbs at the 10th rib, and grasp the lateral rib cage with your hands. As the patient inhales, note the uneven separation of your thumbs and gauge the distance between them. Then repeat this technique on the upper posterior chest wall. Next, use the ulnar surface of your hand to palpate for vocal or tactile fremitus on both sides of the chest. To check for vocal fremitus, ask the patient to repeat "99" as you proceed. Note any asymmetrical vibrations and areas of enhanced, diminished, or absent fremitus. Then percuss and auscultate to detect air and fluid in the lungs and pleural spaces. Finally, auscultate all lung fields for normal and adventitious breath sounds.

Now examine the patient's anterior chest wall, using the same assessment techniques.

Medical causes

● *Bronchial obstruction.* Life-threatening loss of airway patency may occur gradually or suddenly. Typically, lack of chest movement indicates complete obstruction; chest lag signals partial obstruction. If air is trapped in the chest, you may detect intercostal bulging during expiration and hyperresonance on percussion. You may also note dyspnea; accessory muscle use; suprasternal, substernal, or intercostal retractions; or decreased or absent breath sounds.

● *Flail chest.* In this life-threatening injury to the ribs or sternum, the unstable portion of the chest wall collapses inward during inspiration and balloons outward during expiration (paradoxical movement). The patient will have ecchymoses, severe localized pain, and other signs of traumatic injury to the chest wall. He may also have rapid, shallow respirations, tachycardia, and cyanosis.

● *Hemothorax.* Typically resulting from trauma, this fulminating and life-threatening bleeding into the pleural space causes chest lag during inspiration. Associated findings may include signs of traumatic chest injury, stabbing pain at the injury site, anxiety, dullness on percussion, tachypnea, tachycardia, and hypoxemia. If the patient becomes hypovolemic, you'll note signs of shock, such as hypotension and a rapid, weak pulse.

● *Kyphoscoliosis.* Abnormal curvature of both the anteroposterior thoracic spine (kyphosis) and the lateral spine (scoliosis) gradually compresses one lung and distends the other. This produces decreased chest wall movement on the compressed-lung side and ballooning of the intercostal muscles during inspiration on the opposite side. It can also produce ineffective coughing, dyspnea, back pain, and fatigue.

● *Myasthenia gravis.* Progressive loss of ventilatory muscle function produces chest-abdominal asynchrony that can lead to acute respiratory distress. Typically, the patient's shallow respirations and increased muscle weakness cause severe dyspnea, tachypnea, and possible apnea.

● *Phrenic nerve dysfunction.* In this disorder, the paralyzed hemidiaphragm fails to contract downward, causing asynchrony of the thorax and upper abdomen on the affected side during inspiration. Onset from trauma may be sudden; gradual onset may result from infection or spinal cord disease. If the patient has underlying pulmonary dysfunction that contributes to hyperventilation, his inability to breathe deeply or to cough effectively may cause atelectasis of the affected lung.

● *Pleural effusion.* Chest lag at end-inspiration occurs gradually in this life-threatening accumulation of fluid, blood, or pus in the pleural space. Usually, some combination of dyspnea, tachypnea, and tachycardia precedes chest lag; the patient may also have pleuritic pain that worsens with coughing or deep breathing. The area of the effusion is delineated by dullness on percussion and by egobronchophony, whispered pectoriloquy, decreased or absent breath sounds, and decreased tactile fremitus. Fever appears if infection causes the effusion.

● *Pneumonia.* Depending on whether consolidation of fluid in the lungs develops unilaterally or bilaterally, asymmetrical chest expansion occurs as inspiratory chest lag or as chest-abdomen asynchrony. The patient will typically have fever, chills, tachycardia, tachypnea, and dyspnea along with rales, rhonchi, and chest pain that worsens during deep breathing. The patient may also be fatigued and anorexic and have a productive cough with rust-colored sputum.

● *Pneumothorax.* Entrapment of air in the pleural space can cause chest lag at end-inspiration. This life-threatening condition also causes sudden, stabbing chest pain that may radiate to the arms, face, back, or abdomen and dyspnea unrelated to the chest pain's severity. Other findings may include tachypnea, decreased tactile fremitus, tympany on percussion, decreased or absent breath sounds over the trapped air, tachycardia, restlessness, and anxiety.

In *tension pneumothorax,* the same signs and symptoms occur as in pneumothorax, but they're much more severe. A tension pneumothorax rapidly compresses the heart and great vessels, causing cyanosis, hypotension, tachycardia, restlessness, and anxiety. The patient may also have subcutaneous crepitation of the upper trunk, neck, and face and mediastinal and tracheal deviation away from the affected side. You may auscultate a crunching sound over the precordium with each heartbeat; this indicates pneumomediastinum.

• *Poliomyelitis.* In this rare disorder, paralysis of the chest wall muscles and the diaphragm produces chest-abdomen asynchrony, fever, muscle pain, and weakness. The patient most commonly experiences decreased reflex response in the affected muscles and difficulty in swallowing and speaking.

• *Pulmonary embolism.* This acute, life-threatening disorder causes chest lag, sudden, stabbing chest pain, and tachycardia. The patient usually has severe dyspnea, blood-tinged sputum, pleural friction rub, and acute anxiety.

Other causes

• *Treatments.* Asymmetrical chest expansion can result from pneumonectomy and surgical removal of several ribs. Chest lag or absence of chest movement may also result from intubation of a mainstem bronchus—a serious complication typically due to incorrect insertion of an endotracheal tube or movement of the tube while it's in the trachea.

Special considerations

If you're caring for an intubated patient, regularly auscultate breath sounds in the lung peripheries to help detect a misplaced tube. If this occurs, prepare the patient for a chest X-ray to allow rapid repositioning of the tube.

Pediatric pointers

Children have a greater risk than adults of mainstem bronchus (especially left bronchus) intubation. However, because a child's breath sounds are frequently referred from one lung to the other due to the small size of the thoracic cage, use chest wall expansion as an indicator of correct tube position.

Congenital abnormalities, such as cerebral palsy and diaphragmatic hernia, can cause asymmetrical chest expansion. In *cerebral palsy,* asymmetrical facial muscles usually accompany chest-abdomen asynchrony. In life-threatening *diaphragmatic hernia,* asymmetrical expansion usually occurs on the left side of the chest.

Chest Pain

This symptom most often results from disorders that affect thoracic or abdominal organs—the heart, pleurae, lungs, gallbladder, pancreas, or stomach. It's an important indicator of several acute and life-threatening cardiopulmonary and GI disorders. However, it can also result from musculoskeletal and hematologic disorders, anxiety, and drug therapy.

The cause of chest pain may be difficult to distinguish initially. Chest pain can arise suddenly or gradually. It can radiate to the arms, neck, jaw, or back. It can be steady or intermittent, mild or acute. And it can range in character from a sharp shooting sensation to a feeling of heaviness, fullness, or even indigestion. It can be provoked or aggravated by stress, anxiety, exertion, deep breathing, or eating certain foods.

Assessment

Ask the patient when his chest pain began. Did it arise suddenly or gradually? Is it more severe or frequent now than when it first started? Sudden, severe chest pain requires prompt evaluation and treatment since it may her-

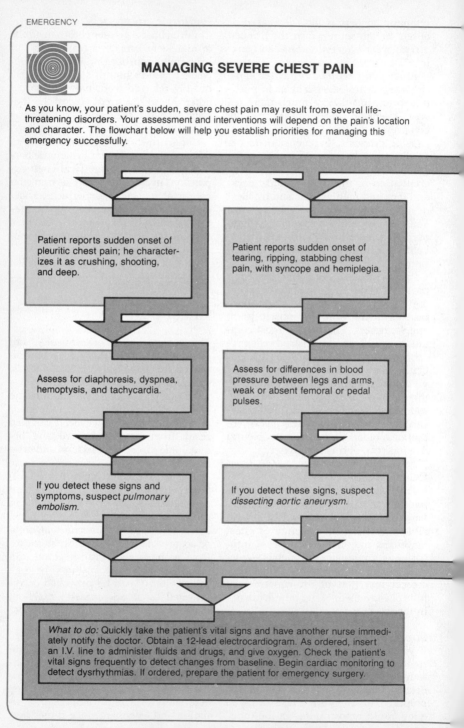

MANAGING SEVERE CHEST PAIN

As you know, your patient's sudden, severe chest pain may result from several life-threatening disorders. Your assessment and interventions will depend on the pain's location and character. The flowchart below will help you establish priorities for managing this emergency successfully.

Patient reports sudden onset of pleuritic chest pain; he characterizes it as crushing, shooting, and deep.

Patient reports sudden onset of tearing, ripping, stabbing chest pain, with syncope and hemiplegia.

Assess for diaphoresis, dyspnea, hemoptysis, and tachycardia.

Assess for differences in blood pressure between legs and arms, weak or absent femoral or pedal pulses.

If you detect these signs and symptoms, suspect *pulmonary embolism*.

If you detect these signs, suspect *dissecting aortic aneurysm*.

What to do: Quickly take the patient's vital signs and have another nurse immediately notify the doctor. Obtain a 12-lead electrocardiogram. As ordered, insert an I.V. line to administer fluids and drugs, and give oxygen. Check the patient's vital signs frequently to detect changes from baseline. Begin cardiac monitoring to detect dysrhythmias. If ordered, prepare the patient for emergency surgery.

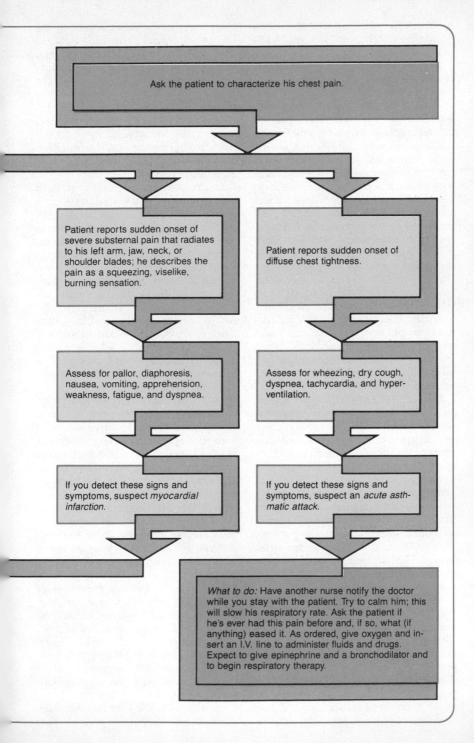

Ask the patient to characterize his chest pain.

Patient reports sudden onset of severe substernal pain that radiates to his left arm, jaw, neck, or shoulder blades; he describes the pain as a squeezing, viselike, burning sensation.

Patient reports sudden onset of diffuse chest tightness.

Assess for pallor, diaphoresis, nausea, vomiting, apprehension, weakness, fatigue, and dyspnea.

Assess for wheezing, dry cough, dyspnea, tachycardia, and hyperventilation.

If you detect these signs and symptoms, suspect *myocardial infarction.*

If you detect these signs and symptoms, suspect an *acute asthmatic attack.*

What to do: Have another nurse notify the doctor while you stay with the patient. Try to calm him; this will slow his respiratory rate. Ask the patient if he's ever had this pain before and, if so, what (if anything) eased it. As ordered, give oxygen and insert an I.V. line to administer fluids and drugs. Expect to give epinephrine and a bronchodilator and to begin respiratory therapy.

ald a life-threatening disorder. (See *Managing Severe Chest Pain*, pages 154 and 155.)

If the patient's chest pain isn't severe, proceed with the history. Ask the patient if he can point to the painful area or if he feels diffuse pain. Sometimes a patient won't perceive the sensation he's feeling as pain, so ask whether he has any discomfort radiating to his neck, jaw, arms, or back. If he does, ask him to describe it: Is it a dull, aching, pressurelike sensation? A sharp, stabbing, knifelike pain? Does he feel it on the surface or deep inside? Find out whether it's constant or intermittent. If it's intermittent, how long does it last? Also ask the patient if movement, exertion, breathing, position changes, or eating certain foods worsens or helps relieve the pain. Does anything in particular seem to bring it on?

Review the patient's history for cardiac or pulmonary disease, chest trauma, intestinal disease, or sickle cell anemia. Find out what medications he's taking, if any, and ask about recent dosage or schedule changes.

Take the patient's vital signs, noting especially fever, tachycardia, hypertension, or hypotension. Assess for jugular vein distention and peripheral edema, observe his breathing pattern, and inspect his chest for asymmetrical expansion. Auscultate the lungs for pleural friction rub, crackles, rhonchi, wheezes, or diminished or absent breath sounds. Next, auscultate for murmurs, clicks, gallops, or pericardial friction rub. Palpate for lifts, heaves, thrills, gallops, tactile fremitus, an abdominal mass, and tenderness.

Medical causes

● *Angina.* In *angina pectoris*, the patient may experience a feeling of tightness or pressure in the chest that he describes as pain or a sensation of indigestion or expansion. Usually, the pain occurs in the retrosternal region over a palm-sized or larger area. It may radiate to the neck, jaw, and arms—classically, to the inner aspect of the left arm. Anginal pain tends to begin gradually, build to its maximum, then slowly subside. Provoked by exertion, emotional stress, or a heavy meal, the pain typically last 2 to 10 minutes. Associated signs and symptoms may include dyspnea, nausea, vomiting, tachycardia, dizziness, diaphoresis, belching, or palpitations. You may hear an atrial gallop (S_4) or murmur during an anginal episode.

In *Prinzmetal's angina*, chest pain occurs when the patient's at rest—or it may awaken him. It may be accompanied by shortness of breath, nausea, vomiting, dizziness, and palpitations. During an attack, you may hear an atrial gallop.

● *Anxiety.* Acute anxiety can produce intermittent, sharp, stabbing pain, often located in the left breast. This pain isn't related to exertion and lasts only a few seconds, but the patient may experience a precordial ache or a sensation of heaviness that lasts for hours or days. Associated signs and symptoms may include precordial tenderness, palpitations, fatigue, headache, insomnia, breathlessness, nausea, vomiting, diarrhea, and tremors.

● *Aortic aneurysm (dissecting).* The chest pain associated with this disorder usually begins suddenly and is most severe at its onset. The patient describes an excruciating tearing, ripping, stabbing pain in his chest and neck that radiates to his upper back, abdomen, and lower back. He may also have abdominal tenderness; a palpable abdominal mass; tachycardia; murmurs; syncope; weakness or transient paralysis of the legs; a systolic bruit; systemic hypotension; lower blood pressure in the legs than in the arms; and weak or absent femoral or pedal pulses. His skin is pale, cool, diaphoretic, and mottled below the waist. Capillary refill time is prolonged in the toes, and palpation reveals decreased pulsation of one or both carotid arteries.

● *Asthma.* In a life-threatening asthmatic attack, diffuse and painful chest tightness arises suddenly along with a dry cough and mild wheezing, which progress to a productive cough, audible wheezing, and severe dyspnea. Related respiratory findings include rhonchi, crackles, prolonged expirations, intercostal and supraclavicular retractions on inspiration, accessory muscle use, flaring nostrils, and tachypnea. Other clinical features: anxiety, tachycardia, diaphoresis, flushing, and cyanosis.

• *Blastomycosis.* Besides pleuritic chest pain, this disorder initially produces signs and symptoms that mimic those of viral upper respiratory infection: a dry, hacking, or productive cough (and sometimes hemoptysis), fever, chills, anorexia, weight loss, fatigue, night sweats, and malaise.

• *Bronchitis.* In its acute form, this disorder produces a burning chest pain or a sensation of substernal tightness. It also produces a cough, initially dry but later productive, that worsens the chest pain. Other findings: a low-grade fever, chills, sore throat, tachycardia, muscle and back pain, rhonchi, crackles, and wheezes. Severe bronchitis causes fever of 101° F. to 102° F. and possible bronchospasm with worsening wheezing and increased coughing.

• *Cardiomyopathy.* In hypertrophic cardiomyopathy, angina-like chest pain may be accompanied by dyspnea, a cough, dizziness, syncope, gallops, and murmurs.

• *Cholecystitis.* This disorder typically produces abrupt epigastric or right upper quadrant pain, which may be sharp or intensely aching. The pain, either steady or intermittent, may radiate to the back. Commonly associated signs and symptoms include nausea, vomiting, fever, diaphoresis, and chills. Palpation of the right upper quadrant may detect an abdominal mass, rigidity, distention, and tenderness.

• *Coccidioidomycosis.* In this disorder, pleuritic chest pain occurs with a dry or slightly productive cough. Other effects include fever, rhonchi, wheezing, occasional chills, sore throat, backache, headache, malaise, marked weakness, anorexia, and macular rash.

• *Costochondritis.* Pain and tenderness occur at the costochondral junctions, especially at the second costocartilage.

• *Distention of the colon's splenic flexure.* Central chest pain may radiate to the left arm in this disorder. The pain may be relieved by defecation or passage of flatus.

• *Esophageal spasm.* In this disorder, substernal chest pain may last up to an hour and can radiate to the neck, jaw, arms, or back. It often mimics anginal pain—a squeezing or dull sensation. Associated signs and symptoms include dysphagia for solids, bradycardia, and nodal rhythm.

• *Herpes zoster (shingles).* The pain of pre-eruptive herpes zoster may mimic that of myocardial infarction. Initially, the pain—characteristically unilateral—is sharp and shooting. About 4 or 5 days after its onset, small, red, nodular lesions erupt on the painful areas—usually the thorax, arms, and legs—and the chest pain becomes burning. Associated findings may include fever, malaise, pruritus, or paresthesia or hyperesthesia of the affected areas.

• *Hiatal hernia.* Typically, this disorder produces an angina-like sternal burning, ache, or pressure that may radiate to the left shoulder and arm. The discomfort often occurs after a meal when the patient bends over or lies down. Other findings: a bitter taste and pain while eating or drinking, especially hot drinks and spicy foods.

• *Interstitial lung disease.* As this disease advances, the patient may have pleuritic chest pain along with progressive dypsnea, cellophane-type crackles, nonproductive cough, fatigue, weight loss, clubbing, or cyanosis.

• *Legionnaire's disease.* This disorder produces pleuritic chest pain along with malaise, headache, and possibly diarrhea, anorexia, diffuse myalgias, and general weakness. Within 12 to 24 hours, sudden high fever and chills develop as a nonproductive cough progresses to mucoid and then to muco-

CHEST PAIN: CAUSES AND ASSOCIATED FINDINGS

CHIEF CAUSES	Abdominal mass	Abdominal tenderness	Atrial gallop	Breath sounds—decreased	Cough	Crackles	Cyanosis	Diaphoresis	Dizziness	Dyspnea	Fever	Hemoptysis	Murmur
Angina pectoris			●					●	●	●			●
Aortic aneurysm (dissecting)	●	●						●					●
Asthma (acute)					●	●	●	●		●			
Bronchitis (acute)					●	●					●		
Cardiomyopathy			●		●					●	●		●
Cholecystitis	●	●						●			●		
Interstitial lung disease					●	●	●			●			
Lung abscess				●	●	●		●		●	●	●	
Lung cancer					●					●	●	●	
Mitral prolapse									●	●			●
Myocardial infarction			●			●		●		●	●		●
Pancreatitis		●				●					●		
Peptic ulcer		●											
Pericarditis										●	●		
Pleurisy				●		●	●			●	●		
Pneumonia				●	●	●	●	●		●	●		
Pneumothorax				●	●		●			●			
Pulmonary embolism					●	●	●	●		●	●	●	
Pulmonary hypertension					●					●		●	

Nausea/vomiting	Pericardial friction rub	Pleural friction rub	Skin mottling	Syncope	Tachycardia	Tachypnea	Wheezes
●					●		
			●	●	●		
					●	●	●
					●		●
				●			
●							
		●					
							●
					●		
●							
●				●	●		
●							
	●				●		
		●				●	
					●	●	
					●	●	
		●			●	●	●
			●				

purulent sputum, with possibile hemoptysis. Many patients are flushed, mildly diaphoretic, and prostrated and have nausea, vomiting, mild temporary amnesia, confusion, dyspnea, crackles, tachypnea, or tachycardia.

● *Lung abscess.* Pleuritic chest pain develops insidiously in this disorder along with a pleural friction rub and a cough that raises copious amounts of purulent, foul-smelling, blood-tinged sputum. The affected side is dull to percussion, and decreased breath sounds and crackles may be heard. The patient will also display diaphoresis, anorexia, weight loss, fever, chills, fatigue, weakness, dyspnea, and clubbing.

● *Lung cancer.* The chest pain associated with lung cancer is often described as an intermittent aching felt deep within the chest. If the tumor metastasizes to the ribs or vertebrae, the pain becomes localized, continuous, and gnawing. Associated findings may include cough (sometimes bloody), wheezing, dyspnea, fatigue, anorexia, weight loss, or fever.

● *Mediastinitis.* This disorder produces severe retrosternal chest pain that radiates to the epigastrium, back, or shoulder and may worsen with breathing, coughing, or sneezing. Its accompanying signs and symptoms include chills, fever, and dysphagia.

● *Mitral prolapse.* Typically, the patient with a prolapsed mitral valve will experience sharp, stabbing precordial chest pain or precordial ache. The pain can last for seconds or for hours; it occasionally mimics the pain of ischemic heart disease. However, the characteristic sign of mitral prolapse is a midsystolic click followed by a systolic murmur at the apex. The patient may experience migraine headache, dizziness, episodic severe fatigue, dyspnea, tachycardia, mood swings, or palpitations.

● *Muscle strain.* Strained chest, arm, or shoulder muscles may cause a superficial and continuous ache or "pulling" sensation in the chest. Lifting, pulling, or pushing heavy objects may aggravate this discomfort. In acute muscle strain, the patient may experience fatigue, weakness, and rapid swelling of the affected area.

• *Myocardial infarction (MI).* The chest pain in MI lasts from 15 minutes to hours. Typically a crushing substernal pain, unrelieved by rest or nitroglycerin, it may radiate to the patient's left arm, jaw, neck, or shoulder blades. The patient may have pallor, clammy skin, dyspnea, diaphoresis, nausea, vomiting, anxiety, restlessness, and a feeling of impending doom. He may develop hypotension or hypertension, an atrial gallop, murmurs, and crackles. A low-grade fever may arise within 4 days.

• *Nocardiosis.* This disorder causes pleuritic chest pain with a cough that produces thick, tenacious, purulent or mucopurulent, and possibly blood-tinged sputum. Nocardiosis also may cause fever, night sweats, anorexia, malaise, weight loss, and diminished or absent breath sounds.

• *Pancreatitis.* In its acute form, this disorder usually causes intense pain in the epigastric area that radiates to the back and worsens when the patient is supine. Nausea, vomiting, fever, abdominal tenderness and rigidity, diminished bowel sounds, and crackles at lung bases may also occur. A patient with severe pancreatitis may be extremely restless and have mottled skin, tachycardia, and cold, sweaty extremities. Fulminant pancreatitis causes massive hemorrhage resulting in shock and coma.

• *Peptic ulcer.* In this disorder, sharp and burning pain usually arises in the epigastric region. This pain characteristically arises hours after food intake, often occurring during the night. It lasts longer than angina-like pain and is relieved by food or antacids. Other findings may include nausea, vomiting, and epigastric tenderness.

• *Pericarditis.* This disorder produces precordial or retrosternal pain aggravated by deep breathing, coughing, position changes, and occasionally by swallowing. Frequently, the pain is sharp or cutting and radiates to the shoulder and neck. Associated signs and symptoms may include pericardial friction rub, fever, tachycardia, and dyspnea.

• *Pleurisy.* The chest pain of pleurisy arises abruptly and reaches maximum intensity within a few hours. It's sharp, even knifelike, usually unilateral, and located in the lower and lateral aspects of the chest. Deep breathing, coughing, or thoracic movement characteristically aggravates it. Auscultation over the painful area may reveal decreased breath sounds, inspiratory crackles, and a pleural friction rub. Other effects may be dyspnea, rapid, shallow breathing, cyanosis, fever, or fatigue.

• *Pneumonia.* This disorder produces pleuritic chest pain that increases with deep inspiration and is accompanied by shaking chills and fever. The patient has a dry cough that later becomes productive. Other signs and symptoms may include crackles, rhonchi, tachycardia, tachypnea, myalgias, fatigue, headache, dyspnea, abdominal pain, anorexia, cyanosis, decreased breath sounds, and diaphoresis.

• *Pneumothorax.* Spontaneous pneumothorax, a life-threatening disorder, causes sudden sharp chest pain that's severe, often unilateral, and rarely localized; it increases with chest movement. When it's located centrally and radiates to the neck, it may mimic an MI. After the pain's onset, dyspnea and cyanosis progressively worsen. Breath sounds are decreased or absent on the affected side with hyperresonance or tympany, subcutaneous crepitation, and decreased vocal fremitus. Asymmetrical chest expansion, accessory muscle use, a nonproductive cough, tachypnea, tachycardia, anxiety, and restlessness also occur.

• *Psittacosis.* This disorder may produce pleuritic chest pain on rare occasions. It typically begins abruptly with chills, fever, headache, myalgias, epistaxis, and prostration.

• *Pulmonary actinomycosis.* This disorder causes pleuritic chest pain with a cough that's initially dry but later produces purulent sputum. The patient may also display hemoptysis, fever, weight loss, fatigue, weakness, dyspnea, and night sweats.

● *Pulmonary embolism.* This disorder produces a substernal pain or choking sensation. Typically, the patient first experiences sudden dyspnea with intense angina-like or pleuritic pain aggravated by deep breathing and thoracic movement. Other findings may include tachycardia, tachypnea, cough (which may be nonproductive or productive of blood-tinged sputum), a low-grade fever, restlessness, diaphoresis, crackles, a pleural friction rub, diffuse wheezing, dullness to percussion, signs of circulatory collapse (weak, rapid pulse; hypotension), signs of cerebral ischemia (transient unconsciousness, coma, convulsions), signs of hypoxia (restlessness), and—particularly in the elderly—hemiplegia and other focal neurologic deficits. Less common signs include massive hemoptysis, chest splinting, and leg edema. A patient with a large embolus may have cyanosis and distended neck veins.

● *Pulmonary hypertension (primary).* Angina-like pain develops late in this disorder, usually on exertion. The precordial pain may radiate to the neck but doesn't characteristically radiate to the arms. Typical accompanying signs and symptoms include exertional dyspnea, fatigue, syncope, weakness, cough, and hemoptysis.

● *Rib fracture.* The chest pain due to fractured ribs is usually sharp, severe, and aggravated by inspiration, coughing, or pressure on the affected area. Besides shallow, splinted respirations, dyspnea, and cough, the patient experiences tenderness and slight edema at the fracture site.

● *Sickle cell crisis.* Chest pain associated with sickle cell crisis typically has a bizarre distribution. It may start as a vague pain, often located in the back, hands, or feet. As the pain worsens, it becomes generalized or localized to the abdomen or chest, causing severe pleuritic pain. The patient may also have abdominal distention and rigidity, dyspnea, fever, and jaundice.

● *Thoracic outlet syndrome.* Often causing paresthesias along the ulnar distribution of the arm, this syndrome can be confused with angina. The patient usually experiences angina-like pain after lifting his arms above his head, working with his hands above his shoulders, or lifting a weight. The pain disappears immediately when he lowers his arms. Other signs and symptoms may include a difference in blood pressure between arms and cool, pale skin.

● *Tuberculosis.* In a patient with this disorder, pleuritic chest pain and fine crackles occur after coughing. Associated signs and symptoms may include night sweats, anorexia, weight loss, fever, malaise, dyspnea, easy fatigability, mild-to-severe productive cough, occasional hemoptysis, dullness to percussion, increased tactile fremitus, and amphoric breath sounds.

Other causes

● *Chinese restaurant syndrome.* This benign condition—a reaction to excessive ingestion of monosodium glutamate (a common additive in Chinese foods)—mimics the signs of acute MI. The patient may complain of retrosternal burning, ache, or pressure and a burning sensation over his arms, legs, and face; a sensation of facial pressure; shortness of breath; or tachycardia.

● *Drugs.* Abrupt withdrawal of beta blockers can cause rebound angina in patients with coronary heart disease—especially those who've received high doses for a prolonged period.

Special considerations

As needed, prepare the patient for cardiopulmonary studies, such as an EKG and lung scan. Perform venipuncture to collect a serum sample for cardiac enzyme and other studies.

Explain the purpose and procedure of each diagnostic test to the patient, to help alleviate his anxiety. Also explain the purpose of any prescribed medications, and make sure the patient understands the dosage, schedule, and possible side effects.

Keep in mind that a patient with chest pain may deny his discomfort, so stress the importance of reporting symptoms to allow adjustment of his treatment.

Pediatric pointers

Even children old enough to talk may have difficulty describing chest pain, so be alert for nonverbal clues such as restlessness, facial grimaces, or holding the painful area. Ask the child to point to the painful area and then (to find out if it's radiating) to where the pain goes. Determine the pain's severity by asking his parents if the pain interferes with the child's normal activities and behavior. Remember, a child may complain of chest pain in an attempt to get attention or to avoid attending school.

Cheyne-Stokes Respirations

The most common pattern of periodic breathing, Cheyne-Stokes is characterized by a waxing and waning period of hyperpnea that alternates with a shorter period of apnea. This pattern can occur normally in people who live at high altitudes and in the elderly during sleep. Most often, though, it indicates increased intracranial pressure from a deep cerebral or brainstem lesion (usually bilateral), or a metabolic disturbance in the brain.

Cheyne-Stokes respirations always indicate a major change in the patient's condition—usually for the worse. For example, in a patient who's had head trauma or brain surgery, Cheyne-Stokes respirations may signal increasing intracranial pressure.

Assessment

If you detect Cheyne-Stokes respirations in a patient with a history of head trauma, recent brain surgery, or other brain insult, quickly take his vital signs. Immediately notify the doctor. Keep the patient's head elevated 30°, and perform a rapid neurologic assessment to obtain baseline data. Reassess his neurologic status often. If intracranial pressure continues to rise, you'll detect changes in his level of consciousness, pupillary reactions, and ability to move his extremities. Be prepared to assist with intracranial pressure monitoring, as ordered.

Time the periods of hyperpnea and apnea for 3 or 4 minutes to evaluate respirations and to obtain baseline data. Be alert for prolonged periods of apnea. Frequently check blood pressure; also check skin color to detect signs of hypoxemia. Maintain airway patency and administer oxygen as needed. If the patient's condition worsens, assist with endotracheal intubation.

When the patient's condition permits, obtain a brief history. Ask especially about drug use—large doses of narcotics, hypnotics, or barbiturates can precipitate Cheyne-Stokes respirations.

Medical causes

● *Heart failure.* In left ventricular failure, Cheyne-Stokes respirations may occur with exertional dyspnea and orthopnea. Related findings include fatigue, weakness, tachycardia, tachypnea, and crackles. Cough, generally nonproductive but occasionally producing clear or blood-tinged sputum, may also occur.

● *Hypertensive encephalopathy.* In this life-threatening disorder, severe hypertension precedes Cheyne-Stokes respirations. The patient's level of consciousness will be decreased, and he may experience vomiting or seizures, severe headaches, visual disturbances (including transient blindness), and transient paralysis.

• **Increased intracranial pressure (ICP).**
As ICP rises, Cheyne-Stokes is the first
irregular respiratory pattern to occur.
It's preceded by decreased level of consciousness and accompanied by hypertension, headache, vomiting, impaired or unequal motor movement,
and visual disturbances (blurring,
diplopia, photophobia, and pupillary
changes). In late stages of increased
ICP, bradycardia and widened pulse
pressure occur.

• **Renal failure.** In end-stage chronic
renal failure, Cheyne-Stokes respirations may occur along with bleeding
gums, oral lesions, ammonia breath
odor, and marked changes in every
body system.

• **Stokes-Adams attacks.** Cheyne-Stokes
respirations may follow a Stokes-
Adams attack—a syncopal episode associated with atrioventricular block.
The patient is hypotensive, with a heart
rate between 20 and 50. He may also
appear pale, shaking, and confused.

Other causes

• **Drugs.** Large doses of hypnotics, narcotics, or barbiturates can precipitate
Cheyne-Stokes respirations.

Special considerations

When evaluating Cheyne-Stokes respirations, be careful not to mistake periods of hypoventilation or decreased
tidal volume for apnea.

Pediatric pointers

Cheyne-Stokes respirations rarely occur in children, except in late heart
failure.

Chills

[Rigors]

Chills are extreme, involuntary muscle
contractions with characteristic paroxysms of violent shivering and teeth-
chattering. Commonly accompanied by
fever, chills tend to arise suddenly, most
often heralding the onset of infection.
Certain diseases, such as pneumococcal pneumonia, produce only a single,
shaking chill. Other diseases, such as
malaria, produce intermittent chills
with recurring high fever. Still others
produce continuous chills for up to 1
hour, precipitating a high fever.

Chills can also result from lymphomas, transfusion reactions, and certain
drugs. Of course, chills without fever
occur as a normal response to exposure
to cold.

Assessment

Ask the patient when the chills began
and if they're continuous or intermittent. Because fever often accompanies
chills, take the patient's rectal temperature to obtain a baseline reading.
Then, check his temperature often to
monitor fluctuations and to determine
his temperature curve. Typically, a localized infection produces sudden onset of shaking chills, sweats, and high
fever. A systemic infection, in contrast,
produces intermittent chills with recurring episodes of high fever or continuous chills that may last up to 1 hour
and precipitate a high fever.

Ask the patient about related signs
and symptoms, such as headache, confusion, abdominal pain, nausea, or
muscle disturbances. Does he have any
known allergies, an infection, or a history of an infectious disorder? Find out
what medications he's taking and if any
drug has improved or worsened his
symptoms. Ask about recent exposure
to farm animals, guinea pigs, ham-
sters, dogs, and birds such as pigeons,
parrots, and parakeets. Also ask about
recent insect or animal bites and travel
to foreign countries.

Medical causes

• **Cholangitis.** Charcot's triad—chills
with spiking fever, abdominal pain,
and jaundice—characterizes sudden
obstruction of the common bile duct.
The patient may have associated pru-

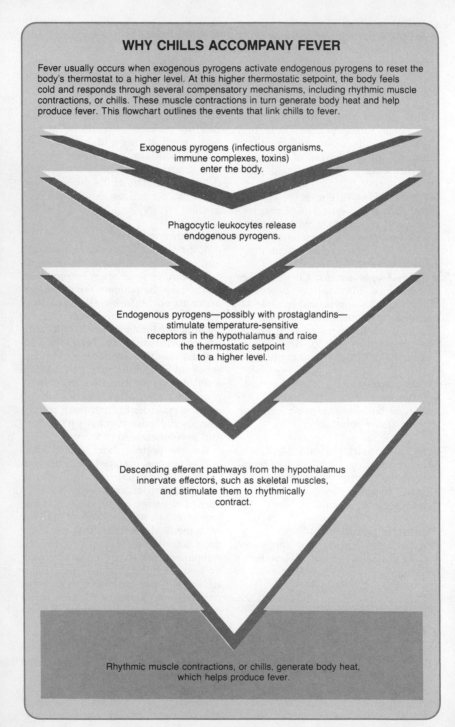

WHY CHILLS ACCOMPANY FEVER

Fever usually occurs when exogenous pyrogens activate endogenous pyrogens to reset the body's thermostat to a higher level. At this higher thermostatic setpoint, the body feels cold and responds through several compensatory mechanisms, including rhythmic muscle contractions, or chills. These muscle contractions in turn generate body heat and help produce fever. This flowchart outlines the events that link chills to fever.

Exogenous pyrogens (infectious organisms, immune complexes, toxins) enter the body.

Phagocytic leukocytes release endogenous pyrogens.

Endogenous pyrogens—possibly with prostaglandins—stimulate temperature-sensitive receptors in the hypothalamus and raise the thermostatic setpoint to a higher level.

Descending efferent pathways from the hypothalamus innervate effectors, such as skeletal muscles, and stimulate them to rhythmically contract.

Rhythmic muscle contractions, or chills, generate body heat, which helps produce fever.

ritus, weakness, and fatigue.

• *Gram-negative bacteremia.* This infection causes sudden chills and fever. It also causes nausea, vomiting, diarrhea, and prostration.

• *Hemolytic anemia.* In acute hemolytic anemia, fulminating chills occur with fever and abdominal pain. The patient has rapidly developing jaundice, hepatomegaly, and possibly splenomegaly.

• *Hepatic abscess.* Although this infection can occur insidiously, it most commonly arises abruptly, with chills, fever, nausea, vomiting, diarrhea, anorexia, and severe upper abdominal tenderness and pain that may radiate to the right shoulder.

• *Hodgkin's lymphoma.* In some patients, this lymphoma produces a cyclical fever with intermittent chills. The patient characteristically experiences several days or weeks of fever and chills alternating with periods of no fever and no chills. This disorder commonly produces regional lymphadenopathy that may progress to hepatosplenomegaly. Other findings: diaphoresis, fatigue, and pruritus.

• *Infective endocarditis.* This infection produces abrupt onset of intermittent, shaking chills with fever. Petechiae commonly develop, and the patient may also have Janeway lesions on his hands and feet and Osler's nodes on his palms and soles. Associated findings include hematuria, eye hemorrhage, Roth's spots, and signs of cardiac failure (dyspnea, peripheral edema).

• *Influenza.* Initially, this disorder causes abrupt onset of chills, high fever, malaise, headache, myalgias, and nonproductive cough. Some patients may also suddenly develop rhinitis, rhinorrhea, laryngitis, conjunctivitis, hoarseness, and sore throat. Chills generally subside after the first few days, but intermittent fever, weakness, and cough may persist up to 1 week.

• *Legionnaire's disease.* Within 12 to 48 hours after onset of this disease, the patient suddenly develops chills and a high fever. Prodromal signs and symptoms characteristically include malaise, headache, and possibly diarrhea, anorexia, diffuse myalgias, and general weakness. An initially nonproductive cough progresses to a productive cough with mucoid or mucopurulent sputum and possibly hemoptysis. Usually, the patient also has nausea, vomiting, confusion, mild, temporary amnesia, pleuritic chest pain, dyspnea, tachypnea, crackles, tachycardia, and flushed and mildly diaphoretic skin.

• *Lung abscess.* Besides chills, this disorder causes sweating, pleuritic chest pain, dyspnea, clubbing, weakness, headache, malaise, anorexia, weight loss, and a cough that produces large amounts of purulent, foul-smelling, often bloody sputum.

• *Lymphangitis.* Acute lymphangitis produces chills and other systemic symptoms, such as fever, malaise, and headache. Its characteristic signs: red streaks radiating from a wound or cellulitis draining toward tender, regional lymph nodes.

• *Lymphogranuloma venereum.* Along with chills and lymphadenopathy, this disorder produces fever, headache, anorexia, myalgias, arthralgias, and weight loss. The primary genital lesion is a papule or small erosion, which precedes lymphatic involvement and heals spontaneously within a few days.

• *Malaria.* The malarial paroxysm begins with a period of chills that lasts 1 to 2 hours. A high fever lasting 3 to 4 hours follows, and 2 to 4 hours of profuse diaphoresis complete the paroxysmal cycle. In benign malaria, the paroxysm may be interspersed with periods of well-being. The patient also has headache, muscle pain, and possibly hepatosplenomegaly.

• *Miliary tuberculosis.* In its acute form, this illness presents with intermittent chills, high fever, and night sweats. The patient may also have epididymal or testicular nodules and splenomegaly.

• *Otitis media.* Acute suppurative otitis media produces chills accompanied by fever and severe, deep, and throbbing ear pain. The patient usually displays a mild conductive hearing loss and a bulging, hyperemic tympanic membrane. He may also have dizziness, nausea, and vomiting.

• *Pelvic inflammatory disease.* This infection causes chills and fever with, typically, lower abdominal pain and tenderness; profuse, purulent vaginal discharge; or abnormal menstrual bleeding. The patient may also have nausea, vomiting, an abdominal mass, and dysuria.

• *Pneumonia.* A single shaking chill usually heralds the sudden onset of pneumococcal pneumonia; other pneumonias characteristically cause intermittent chills. In any type of pneumonia, related findings may include fever, productive cough with bloody sputum, pleuritic chest pain, dyspnea, tachypnea, and tachycardia. The patient may be cyanotic and diaphoretic, with bronchial breath sounds and crackles, rhonchi, increased tactile fremitus, and grunting respirations. He may also experience achiness, anorexia, fatigue, and headache.

• *Psittacosis.* This disease typically begins with abrupt onset of chills, fever, headache, myalgias, epistaxis, and prostration. Initial dry, hacking cough progresses to pneumonia with a cough that produces small amounts of mucoid, blood-streaked sputum. The patient also has tachypnea, fine crackles, photophobia, abdominal distention and tenderness, nausea, vomiting, a faint macular rash and, rarely, chest pain.

• *Puerperal or postabortal sepsis.* Chills and high fever occur as early as 6 hours or as late as 10 days postpartum or postabortion. The patient may also have purulent vaginal discharge, an enlarged and tender uterus, abdominal pain, backache, and possibly nausea, vomiting, and diarrhea.

• *Pyelonephritis.* In acute pyelonephritis, the patient develops chills, high fever, and possibly nausea and vomiting over several hours to days. He generally also has anorexia, fatigue, myalgia, flank pain, marked costovertebral angle tenderness, hematuria or cloudy urine, and urinary frequency, urgency, and burning.

• *Renal abscess.* This disorder initially produces sudden chills and fever. Its later effects include flank pain, costovertebral angle tenderness, abdominal muscle spasm, and transient hematuria.

• *Rocky Mountain spotted fever.* This disorder begins with sudden onset of chills, fever, malaise, excruciating headache, and muscle, bone, and joint pain. Typically, the patient's tongue is covered with a thick white coating that gradually turns brown. After 2 to 6 days of fever and occasional chills, a macular or maculopapular rash appears on the hands and feet and then becomes generalized; after a few days, the rash becomes petechial.

• *Septic arthritis.* Chills and fever accompany the characteristic red, swollen, and painful joints this disorder causes.

• *Septic shock.* Initially, septic shock produces chills, fever, and possibly nausea, vomiting, and diarrhea. The patient's skin is typically flushed, warm, and dry; his blood pressure is normal or slightly low; and he has tachycardia and tachypnea. As septic shock progresses, the patient's arms and legs become cool and cyanotic, and

---

RARE CAUSES OF CHILLS

Chills can result from disorders that rarely occur in the United States but may be fairly common worldwide. So remember to ask about recent foreign travel when you obtain a patient's history. And keep in mind this partial list of rare disorders that produce chills:
• Brucellosis (undulant fever)
• Dengue (breakbone fever)
• Epidemic typhus (louse-borne typhus)
• Leptospirosis
• Lymphocytic choriomeningitis
• Plague
• Pulmonary tularemia
• Rat bite fever
• Relapsing fever

he develops oliguria, thirst, anxiety, restlessness, confusion, and hypotension. Later, his skin becomes cold and clammy; his pulse becomes rapid and thready; and he develops severe hypotension, persistent oliguria or anuria, signs of respiratory failure, and coma.

• *Sinusitis.* In acute sinusitis, chills occur along with fever, headache, and pain, tenderness, and swelling over the affected sinuses. Maxillary sinusitis produces pain over the cheeks and upper teeth; ethmoid sinusitis, pain over the eyes; frontal sinusitis, pain over the eyebrows; and sphenoid sinusitis, pain behind the eyes. The primary indicator of sinusitis is nasal discharge, which is often bloody for 24 to 48 hours before gradually becoming purulent.

• *Snake bite.* Most pit viper bites that result in envenomation cause chills, typically with fever. Other systemic signs and symptoms may include sweating, weakness, dizziness, fainting, hypotension, nausea, vomiting, diarrhea, and thirst. The area around the snake bite may be marked by immediate swelling and tenderness, pain, ecchymoses, petechiae, blebs, bloody discharge, and local necrosis. The patient may have difficulty speaking, blurred vision, and paralysis. He may also show bleeding tendencies and signs of respiratory distress and shock.

• *Typhoid fever.* This disorder may initially cause sudden chills and a sharply rising fever. More often, though, the patient's body temperature gradually increases for 5 to 7 days with accompanying chilliness or frank chills. Headache, abdominal discomfort, constipation, and demonstrable splenomegaly appear by the end of the first week. A characteristic rash called "rose spots" develops on the upper abdomen and anterior thorax during the second week but lasts only 2 or 3 days. Later, the patient may have a dry cough, epistaxis, mental dullness or delirium, marked abdominal distention, significant weight loss, profound fatigue, and diarrhea.

• *Violin spider bite.* The bite of this spider produces chills, fever, malaise, weakness, nausea, vomiting, and joint pain within 24 to 48 hours. The patient may also develop skin rash and delirium.

Other causes

• *Drugs.* Amphotericin B heads the list of common drugs associated with chills. However, I.V. bleomycin and intermittent administration of oral antipyretics can also cause chills.

• *I.V. therapy.* Infection at the I.V. insertion site can cause chills, high fever, and local redness, warmth, induration, and tenderness.

• *Transfusion reaction.* Hemolytic reaction may cause chills during the transfusion or immediately afterward. A nonhemolytic febrile reaction may also cause chills.

Special considerations

Check the patient's vital signs often— especially if his chills result from a known or suspected infection. Be alert for such signs of progressive septic shock as hypotension, tachycardia, and tachypnea. If appropriate, obtain samples of blood, sputum, or wound drainage for culture to determine the causative organism. Give antibiotics, as ordered. You may also be asked to prepare the patient for radiographic studies and to obtain serum and urine samples.

Because chills are an involuntary response to an increased body temperature set by the hypothalamic thermostat, providing the patient with blankets won't stop his chills or shivering. However, do keep the temperature of the patient's room as even as possible. Provide adequate hydration and nutrients, and give antipyretics to help control fever; remember, however, that irregular use of antipyretics can trigger compensatory chills.

Pediatric pointers

Infants don't get chills because they have poorly developed shivering mechanisms. What's more, most classic febrile childhood infections—such as measles and mumps—don't typically produce chills. However, older children and teenagers do experience chills in mycoplasma pneumonia and acute pyogenic osteomyelitis.

Chorea

[Choreiform movements]

Chorea—brief, unpredictable bursts of rapid, jerky motion that interrupt normal coordinated movement—indicates dysfunction of the extrapyramidal system. Unlike tics, choreiform movements are seldom repetitive, but tend to appear purposeful despite their involuntary nature. Although any muscle can be affected, chorea most often involves the face, head, lower arms, and hands. It can affect both sides of the body or only one, but when it affects the face, both sides are always involved. Chorea may be aggravated by excitement or fatigue and may disappear during sleep. In some patients, it may be difficult to distinguish from athetosis (snakelike, writhing movements), although choreiform movements are generally more rapid than athetoid ones. (See *Distinguishing Athetosis from Chorea*, page 79.)

Assessment
Ask the patient and his family when they first noticed the choreiform movements. Do the movements disappear when the patient's asleep? Find out if anyone in the patient's family has the same type of movements, and ask about a family history of such diseases as Huntington's chorea. Also ask what medications the patient's taking. Obtain an occupational history, noting especially prolonged exposure to manganese dioxide or lead. As you obtain history information, observe the patient for excessive restlessness and periodic facial grimaces that may interrupt his speech.

Perform a physical examination to evaluate the severity of the patient's chorea. Ask him to stick out his tongue and keep it out. Typically, he'll be unable to do this; instead, his tongue will dart in and out of his mouth. Observe the patient's arms and legs separately for involuntary jerky movements. Ask him to extend and flex his hand as if halting traffic, and note the choreiform movements—they'll be extremely evident in this position. Also check for such related signs as athetosis, rigidity, or tremor.

To assess for choreoathetotic gait, ask the patient to walk. He may change the positions of his trunk and upper body parts with each step and jerk and tilt his head to one side. And because of superimposed involuntary movements and postures, the patient's legs may move only slowly and awkwardly. (An involuntary movement suspending his leg momentarily with each step may give a dancing quality to his gait.)

Medical causes
• *Carbon monoxide poisoning.* A patient who survives severe carbon monoxide poisoning may have neurologic sequela, such as chorea, rigidity, dementia, impaired sensory function, masklike face, generalized seizures, and myoclonus.
• *Cerebral infarction.* An infarction that involves the thalamic area produces unilateral or bilateral chorea. The patient may also experience dysarthria, tremors, rigidity, weakness, and sensory disturbances, such as paresthesias.
• *Encephalitis.* Chorea occurs in the recovery phase of this disorder. Low-grade fever and athetotis may also be present, along with such focal neurologic signs as hemiparesis, hemiplegia, and facial droop.
• *Huntington's chorea.* In this inherited disorder, chorea may be the first sign or may occur with intellectual decline that leads to emotional disturbances

and dementia. The patient's movements tend to be choreoathetotic and may be accompanied by dysarthria, dystonia, prancing gait, dysphagia, and facial grimacing.

• *Lead poisoning.* In the later stages of lead poisoning, chorea occurs along with seizures, headache, memory lapses, and severe mental impairment. The patient may also have a masklike face, footdrop, wristdrop, dizziness, ataxia, weakness, lethargy, abdominal pain, anorexia, nausea, vomiting, constipation, lead line on the gums, and a metallic taste in his mouth.

• *Manganese poisoning.* In miners who've been exposed to manganese dioxide for prolonged periods, chorea characteristically occurs with propulsive gait, dystonia, and rigidity. Initially, the patient may have a masklike face, resting tremor, and personality changes; later, extreme muscle weakness and lethargy occur.

• *Wilson's disease.* Chorea is an early indicator of this disorder along with dystonia affecting the arms and legs. The patient typically experiences dysarthria, tremors, hoarseness, dysphagia, and slowed body movements; he may also have emotional and behavioral disturbances, drooling, rigidity, and mental deterioration. The pathognomonic Kayser-Fleischer ring in the cornea appears as the disease progresses.

Other causes

• *Drugs.* Phenothiazines (especially the piperazine derivatives), haloperidol, thiothixene, and loxapine frequently produce chorea. Metoclopramide, metyrosine, oral contraceptives, levodopa, and phenytoin may also cause this sign.

Special considerations

Because the patient's movements are involuntary and increase his risk of severe injury, pad the side rails of his bed and keep sharp objects out of his environment. Help him minimize physical activity and emotional upset, to avoid aggravating the chorea, and provide adequate periods of rest and sleep.

Pediatric pointers

Sydenham's chorea occurs in childhood as a delayed manifestation of rheumatic fever. In Hallervorden-Spatz disease—a rare and inherited degenerative disorder—choreoathetotic movements occur in late childhood or early adolescence. Chorea can also occur in children with athetoid cerebral palsy.

Chvostek's Sign

Chvostek's sign is an abnormal spasm of the facial muscles that's elicited by lightly tapping the patient's facial nerve near his lower jaw. This sign usually suggests hypocalcemia but can occur normally in about 25% of patients. Typically, it precedes other signs of hy-

ELICITING CHVOSTEK'S SIGN

Begin by telling the patient to relax his facial muscles. Then stand directly in front of him and tap the facial nerve either just anterior to the earlobe and below the zygomatic arch or between the zygomatic arch and the corner of his mouth. A positive response varies from twitching of the lip at the corner of the mouth to spasm of all facial muscles, depending on the severity of hypocalcemia.

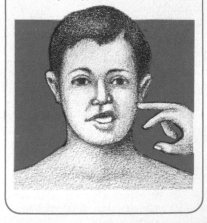

pocalcemia and persists until the onset of tetany. It can't be elicited during tetany because of strong muscle contractions.

Normally, eliciting Chvostek's sign is attempted only in patients with suspected hypocalcemic disorders. But because the parathyroid gland regulates calcium balance, Chvostek's sign may also be tested in patients before neck surgery, to provide a baseline.

Assessment
If you elicit Chvostek's sign, notify the doctor. Then, test for Trousseau's sign, a more reliable indicator of hypocalcemia. Closely monitor the patient for signs of tetany, such as carpopedal spasms or circumoral and extremity paresthesias.

Obtain a brief history. Find out if the patient has had surgical removal of the parathyroid glands or has a history of hypoparathyroidism, hypomagnesemia, or malabsorption disorder. Ask the patient or his family if he's experienced any mental changes, such as depression or slowed responses, which can accompany chronic hypocalcemia.

Medical cause
• *Hypocalcemia.* The degree of Chvostek's sign response reflects the patient's serum calcium level. Initially, hypocalcemia produces paresthesias in the fingers, toes, and circumoral area that progress to muscle tension and carpopedal spasms. The patient may also complain of muscle weakness, fatigue, and palpitations. Muscle twitching, hyperactive deep tendon reflexes, choreiform movements, and muscle cramps may also occur. The patient with chronic hypocalcemia may have mental status changes; diplopia; difficulty swallowing; abdominal cramps; dry, scaly skin; brittle nails; and thin, patchy scalp and eyebrow hair.

Other cause
• *Blood transfusion.* Massive transfusion can lower serum calcium levels and allow Chvostek's sign to be elicited.

Special considerations
As ordered, collect serum samples for serial calcium studies to evaluate the severity of hypocalcemia and the effectiveness of therapy. Such therapy involves oral or I.V. calcium supplements.

Pediatric pointers
Because Chvostek's sign may be present in healthy infants, it isn't elicited to detect neonatal tetany.

Clubbing

A nonspecific sign of pulmonary and cyanotic cardiovascular disorders, clubbing is the painless, usually bilateral increase in soft tissue around the terminal phalanges of the fingers or toes. It doesn't involve changes in the underlying bone. In early clubbing, the normal 160° angle between the nail and the nail base approximates 180°. As clubbing progresses, this angle widens and the base of the nail becomes visibly swollen. In late clubbing, the angle where the nail meets the now-convex nail base extends more than halfway up the nail.

Assessment
You'll probably detect clubbing while assessing other signs of known pulmonary or cardiovascular disease. Therefore, review the patient's current plan of treatment, since clubbing may resolve with correction of the underlying disorder. Also evaluate the extent of clubbing in both the fingers and toes.

Medical causes
• *Bronchiectasis.* Clubbing occurs commonly in the late stage of this disorder. You may also see this classic sign: a cough producing copious, foul-smelling, and mucopurulent sputum. Hemoptysis and coarse crackles over the affected area, heard during inspiration, are also characteristic. The patient may complain of weight loss, fa-

tigue, weakness, and dyspnea on exertion. He may also have rhonchi, fever, malaise, and halitosis.

• **Bronchitis.** In chronic bronchitis, clubbing may occur as a late sign and is unrelated to the severity of the disease. The patient has a chronic productive cough. He may display barrel chest, dyspnea, wheezing, increased use of accessory muscles, cyanosis, tachypnea, crackles, scattered rhonchi, and prolonged expiration.

• **Congestive heart failure.** Clubbing occurs as a late sign along with wheezing, dyspnea, and fatigue. Other findings may include neck vein distention, hepatomegaly, tachypnea, palpitations, dependent edema, unexplained weight gain, nausea, anorexia, chest tightness, slowed mental response, hypotension, diaphoresis, narrow pulse pressure, pallor, oliguria, a gallop rhythm (S_3), and crackles on inspiration.

• **Emphysema.** Clubbing occurs late in this disease. The patient may have anorexia, malaise, dyspnea, tachypnea, diminished breath sounds, peripheral cyanosis, and pursed lip breathing. He may also display accessory muscle use, barrel chest, and productive cough.

• **Endocarditis.** In subacute infective endocarditis, clubbing may be accompanied by fever, anorexia, pallor, weakness, night sweats, fatigue, tachycardia, and weight loss. The patient may also have arthralgia, petechiae, Osler's nodes, splinter hemorrhages, Janeway lesions, splenomegaly, and Roth's spots. Cardiac murmurs are usually present.

• **Interstitial fibrosis.** Clubbing occurs in almost all patients with advanced interstitial fibrosis. Typically, the patient will also have intermittent chest pain, dyspnea, crackles, fatigue, weight loss, and possible cyanosis.

• **Lung abscess.** Initially, this disorder produces clubbing, which may reverse with resolution of the abscess. It can also produce pleuritic chest pain; dyspnea; crackles; productive cough with a large amount of purulent, foul-smell-

ing, often bloody sputum; and halitosis. The patient may also experience weakness, fatigue, anorexia, headache, malaise, weight loss, and fever with chills. You may hear decreased breath sounds.

• **Lung and pleural cancer.** Clubbing occurs commonly here. Associated findings may include hemoptysis, dyspnea,

EVALUATING CLUBBED FINGERS

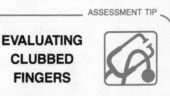

To quickly assess a patient's fingers for early clubbing, gently palpate the bases of his nails. Normally, they'll feel firm—but in early clubbing, nail bases will feel springy when palpated. To evaluate late clubbing, have the patient place the first phalanges of the forefingers together, as shown. Normal nail bases are concave and create a small, diamond-shaped space when the first phalanges are opposed (top). In late clubbing, however, the now-convex nail bases can touch without leaving a space (bottom).

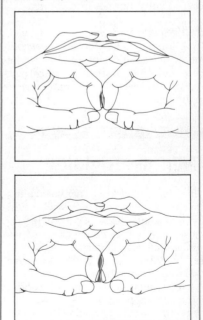

wheezing, chest pain, weight loss, anorexia, fatigue, and fever.

Special considerations
Don't mistake curved nails—a normal variation—for clubbing. How? Always remember that the angle between the nail and its base remains normal in curved nails, but not in clubbing.

Pediatric pointers
In children, clubbing occurs most commonly in cyanotic congenital heart disease and cystic fibrosis. Surgical correction of heart defects may reverse clubbing.

Cogwheel Rigidity

This cardinal sign of Parkinson's disease is characterized by muscle rigidity that abates in a series of jerking movements when the muscle is passively stretched. This sign can be elicited by stabilizing the patient's forearm and then moving his hand through the range of motion. (Cogwheel rigidity most often appears in the arms, but it can sometimes be elicited in the ankle.) Both the patient and the examiner can see and feel these characteristic move-

ments, thought to be a combination of rigidity and tremor.

Assessment
After you've elicited cogwheel rigidity, take the patient's history to determine when he first noticed associated signs of Parkinson's disease. For example, how long has he experienced tremors? Did he notice tremors of his hands first? Does he have "pill-rolling" hand movements? When did he first notice that his movements were becoming slower? How long has he experienced stiffness in his arms and legs? While taking the history, observe for signs of pronounced Parkinsonism, such as drooling, a masklike face, dysphagia, speaking in a monotone, and altered gait.

Find out what medications the patient is taking, and ask if they've helped relieve some of his symptoms. If he's taking levodopa and his symptoms have worsened, find out if he's exceeded the prescribed dosage. If you suspect an overdosage, inform the doctor and withhold the drug, as ordered.

If the patient's taking a phenothiazine or other antipsychotic and has no history of Parkinson's disease, he may be having an adverse reaction to his medication. Inform the doctor and withhold the drug, as ordered.

Medical cause
• *Parkinson's disease.* In this disorder, cogwheel rigidity occurs together with an insidious tremor, which usually begins in the fingers (unilateral pill-roll tremor), increases during stress or anxiety, and decreases with purposeful movement and sleep.

Bradykinesia (slowness of voluntary movements and speech) also occurs. The patient walks with difficulty; his gait lacks normal parallel motion and may be retropulsive or propulsive. He has a high-pitched monotonal way of speaking and a masklike facial expression, and he may experience drooling; loss of posture control, so that he walks with his body bent forward; dysphagia; or dysarthria. An oculogyric crisis (eyes fixed upward and involutary tonic movements) or blepharospasm (complete eyelid closure) may also occur.

Other causes
• **Drugs.** Phenothiazines and other antipsychotics—such as haloperidol, thiothixene, and loxapine—can cause cogwheel rigidity. Metoclopramide and metyrosine infrequently cause it.

Special considerations
If the patient has associated muscular dysfunction, assist him with ambulation, feeding, and other activities of daily living, as needed. Provide symptomatic care, as appropriate. For example, administer stool softeners if the patient has constipation; or, if he has dysphagia, offer a soft diet with small, frequent feedings. Refer the patient to the National Parkinson Foundation or the American Parkinson Disease Association, which provide educational materials and support.

Pediatric pointers
Cogwheel rigidity doesn't occur in children.

Cold Intolerance

Usually developing gradually, this increased sensitivity to cold temperatures reflects damage to the body's temperature-regulating mechanism (located in the hypothalamus) or a decreased basal metabolic rate (BMR). Typically, this symptom results from tumors or hormonal deficiency. In the elderly, though, it reflects normal age-related decreases in BMR and muscle mass.

Assessment
Find out when the patient first noticed cold intolerance: When did he begin using more blankets? Wearing heavier clothing? Ask about associated signs and symptoms, such as changes in vision or in the texture or amount of body hair. If the patient is female, ask about changes in her normal menstrual pattern.

Before proceeding with the physical examination, obtain a brief history. Does the patient have a history of hypothyroidism or hypothalamic disease? Is he currently taking any medications? If so, is he complying with the prescribed schedule and dosage? Has the regimen been changed recently?

Now perform a physical examination. Begin by taking the patient's vital signs and checking for dry skin and hair loss. Then ask the patient to straighten and extend his arms. Are his hands shaking? During the examination, note if the patient shivers or complains of chills. Provide a blanket, if necessary.

Medical causes
• **Hypopituitarism.** Clinical features usually develop slowly in this disorder and vary with its severity. Cold intolerance and shivering typically accompany cold, dry, and thin skin with a waxy pallor, and fine wrinkles around the mouth. Other findings may include fatigue, lethargy, menstrual disturbances, impotence, decreased libido, nervousness, irritability, headache, and hunger. If hypopituitarism results from a pituitary tumor, expect neurologic signs and symptoms, such as headache, bilateral temporal hemianopia, loss of visual acuity, and possibly blindness.

• **Hypothalamic lesion.** A patient with hypothalamic damage may show unexplained fluctuations from cold intolerance to heat intolerance. Cold intolerance develops suddenly; the patient typically complains of feeling chilled, shivering, and wearing extra clothes to keep warm. Related findings may include amenorrhea, sleep-pattern disturbances, increased thirst and urination, vigorous appetite with weight gain, decreased vision, headache, and such personality changes as attacks of rage, laughing, and crying.

• *Hypothyroidism.* Cold intolerance develops early in this disorder and progressively worsens. Other early findings include fatigue, anorexia with weight gain, constipation, and menorrhagia. As hypothyroidism progresses, the patient has loss of libido and slowed intellectual and motor activity. The hair becomes dry and sparse, the nails thick and brittle, the skin dry, pale, cool, and doughy. Eventually, the patient displays a characteristic dull expression with periorbital and facial edema and puffy hands and feet. Deep tendon reflexes are delayed. Bradycardia, abdominal distention, and ataxia may also occur.

Special considerations
Help increase the patient's comfort by regulating his room temperature and by providing extra clothing and blankets. Allow the patient to openly express his concerns about body image changes related to his cold intolerance. Instruct him and his family to adapt the patient's environment to meet his needs.

Prepare the patient for diagnostic tests, as ordered, to determine the cause of cold intolerance. Once the cause is known, explain the disease process to the patient and his family to help alleviate their anxiety. Also explain that, with proper treatment, he can expect relief from his symptoms.

Pediatric pointers
In an infant, some degree of cold intolerance is normal, because fat distribution is decreased and the temperature-regulating mechanism is immature at birth. Make sure the parents understand that their infant will quickly lose body heat if he's exposed to cold temperatures. Instruct them to dress the infant warmly for sleep and before going outdoors, and to avoid chilling him during his bath.

An infant with cold intolerance due to hypothyroidism may have subtle, nonspecific signs of the underlying disorder—or none at all. Typically, the infant shivers and has a subnormal temperature (below 86° F., or 30° C.); cold, mottled skin, especially on the extremities; and blue lips.

Confusion

An umbrella term for puzzling or inappropriate behavior or responses, *confusion* reflects the inability to think quickly and coherently. Depending on its cause, confusion may arise suddenly or gradually and may be temporary or irreversible. Aggravated by stress and sensory deprivation, confusion often occurs in hospitalized patients—especially the elderly, in whom it may be mistaken for senility.

When severe confusion arises suddenly and the patient also has hallucinations and psychomotor hyperactivity, his condition is classifed as *delirium.* Long-term, progressive confusion with deterioration of all cognitive functions is classified as *dementia.*

Confusion can result from hypoxemia due to pulmonary disorders. However, it can also have a metabolic, neurologic, cardiovascular, cerebrovascular, or nutritional origin or can result from a severe systemic infection or the effects of toxins, drugs, or alcohol. Confusion may signal worsening of an underlying and perhaps irreversible disease. It's often an early sign of fluid and electrolyte imbalance.

Assessment
When you take his history, ask the patient to describe what's bothering him. He probably won't report confusion as his chief complaint—instead, he may complain of memory loss, a nagging sense of apprehension, or an inability to concentrate. Ask when this feeling began and if he feels this way all the time or just occasionally. Find out, too, if the patient has a history of head trauma or a cardiopulmonary, meta-

bolic, cerebrovascular, or neurologic disorder. What medication is he taking, if any? Ask about any changes in eating or sleeping habits and in drug or alcohol use.

Now, perform a neurologic assessment to establish the patient's level of consciousness. (See *Glasgow Coma Scale: Grading Level of Consciousness*, page 454.)

Medical causes

• *Brain tumor.* In the early stages of brain tumor, confusion is usually mild and difficult to detect. As the tumor impinges on cerebral structures, however, the patient's confusion worsens, and he may display personality changes, bizarre behavior, or sensory and motor deficits. He may also have visual field deficits and aphasia.

• *Cerebrovascular disorders.* These disorders produce confusion due to tissue hypoxia and ischemia. Confusion may be insidious and fleeting, as in a transient ischemic attack, or acute and permanent, as in cerebrovascular accident.

• *Dementia.* This group of progressive brain diseases—such as Alzheimer's disease—eventually produces severe and irreversible confusion along with memory loss and intellectual deterioration. Disorientation, tremors, and gait disturbances may also occur.

• *Fluid and electrolyte imbalance.* The extent of imbalance determines the severity of the patient's confusion. Typically, he'll show signs of dehydration, such as lassitude, poor skin turgor, dry skin and mucous membranes, and oliguria. He may also have hypotension and a low-grade fever.

• *Head trauma.* Concussion, contusion, and brain hemorrhage may produce confusion at the time of injury, shortly afterward, or months or even years afterward. The patient may be delirious, with periodic loss of consciousness. Vomiting, severe headache, pupillary changes, and sensory and motor deficits are also common.

• *Heat stroke.* This disorder causes pronounced confusion that gradually worsens as body temperature rises. Initially, the patient may be irritable and dizzy; later, he may become delirious, have seizures, and lose consciousness.

• *Heavy metal poisoning.* Chronic ingestion or inhalation of heavy metals (such as lead, arsenic, mercury, and manganese) eventually produces confusion and, typically, weakness and drowsiness. The patient may also experience headache, vomiting, seizures, tremors, gait disturbances, and mental deterioration.

• *Hypothermia.* Confusion may be an early sign of this disorder. Typically, the patient displays slurred speech, cold and pale skin, hyperactive deep tendon reflexes, rapid pulse, and decreased blood pressure and respirations. As his body temperature continues to drop, his confusion progresses to stupor and coma, his muscles develop rigidity, and his respirations become depressed further.

• *Hypoxemia.* Acute pulmonary disorders that result in hypoxemia produce confusion that can range from mild disorientation to delirium. Chronic pulmonary disorders produce persistent confusion.

• *Infection.* Severe generalized infection, such as sepsis, often produces delirium. Central nervous system (CNS) infections, such as meningitis, cause varying degrees of confusion along with headache and nuchal rigidity.

• *Low perfusion states.* Mild confusion is an early sign of decreased cerebral perfusion. Associated findings usually include hypotension, tachycardia or bradycardia, irregular pulse, ventricular gallop, edema, and cyanosis.

• *Metabolic encephalopathy.* Both hyperglycemia and hypoglycemia can produce sudden onset of confusion. A patient with hypoglycemia may also experience transient delirium and seizures. Uremic and hepatic encephalopathies produce gradual confusion that may progress to seizures and coma. Usually, the patient also experiences tremors and restlessness.

● *Nutritional deficiencies.* Inadequate dietary intake of thiamine, niacin, or vitamin B_{12} produces insidious, progressive confusion and possible mental deterioration.

● *Seizure disorders.* Mild-to-moderate confusion may immediately follow any type of seizure. The confusion usually disappears within several hours.

● *Thyroid hormone disorders.* Hyperthyroidism produces mild-to-moderate confusion along with nervousness, inability to concentrate, weight loss, flushed skin, and tachycardia. Hypothyroidism produces mild, insidious confusion and memory loss; weight gain; bradycardia; and fatigue.

Other causes

● *Alcohol.* Intoxication causes confusion and stupor, and alcohol withdrawal may cause delirium and seizures.

● *Drugs.* Large doses of CNS depressants produce confusion that can persist for several days after the drug is discontinued. Narcotic and barbiturate withdrawal also causes acute confusion, possibly with delirium. Other drugs that commonly cause confusion include lidocaine, digitalis, indomethacin, cycloserine, chlorequine, atropine, and cimetidine.

Special considerations

Never leave a confused patient unattended, to prevent injury to himself and others. (Apply restraints, however, only if necessary to ensure his safety.) Keep the patient calm and quiet, and plan uninterrupted rest periods. To help him stay oriented, keep a large calendar and a clock visible, and make a list of his activities with specific dates and times. Always reintroduce yourself to the patient each time you enter his room.

Pediatric pointers

Confusion can't be determined in infants and very young children. However, older children with acute febrile illnesses commonly experience transient delirium or acute confusion.

Conjunctival Injection

A common ocular sign associated with inflammation, conjunctival injection is nonuniform redness of the conjunctiva from hyperemia. This redness can be diffuse, localized, or peripheral—or it may encircle a clear cornea.

Most often, conjunctival injection results from bacterial or viral conjunctivitis. But it can also signal a severe ocular disorder that, if untreated, may lead to permanent blindness. In particular, conjunctival injection is an early sign of trachoma—a leading cause of blindness in Third World countries and in American Indians living in the southwestern United States.

Of course, conjunctival injection can also result from minor eye irritation due to inadequate sleep, overuse of contact lenses, environmental irritants, and excessive eye rubbing.

Assessment

If the patient with conjunctival injection reports a chemical splash to the eye, immediately irrigate the eye with copious amounts of normal saline solution. (Be sure to first remove contact lenses, if present.) Remember to evert the lids and wipe the fornices with a cotton-tipped applicator to remove any foreign body particles and as much of the chemical solution as possible.

Whatever the cause of your patient's conjunctival injection, when you take his history, ask if he has any associated pain. If so, when did the pain begin, and where is it located? Is it constant or intermittent? Also ask about itching, burning, or a foreign body sensation in his eye. Find out if the patient has photophobia, halo vision, or excessive tearing. Does he have a history of eye disease or trauma?

If the patient has suffered ocular

trauma, avoid touching the affected eye. Test his visual acuity and intraocular pressure (IOP) only if his eyelids can be opened without applying pressure. Place a metal shield over the affected eye to protect it, if necessary.

If the patient's condition permits, examine the affected eye. First, determine the location and severity of conjunctival injection. Is it circumcorneal or localized? Peripheral or diffuse? Note any conjunctival or lid edema, ocular deviation, conjunctival follicles, ptosis, or exophthalmos. Also note the type and amount of any discharge.

Test the patient's visual acuity to establish a baseline. Note if the patient has had vision changes: Is his vision blurred or his visual acuity markedly decreased? Next, test pupillary reaction to light.

Assist the doctor with IOP measurements. To assess for increased IOP without a tonometer, gently place your index finger over the closed eyelid—if the globe feels rock-hard, intraocular pressure is elevated.

Medical causes

- *Astigmatism.* An uncorrected or poorly corrected astigmatism can produce diffuse conjunctival injection. The patient complains of headache, eye pain, and eye fatigue.
- *Blepharitis.* This disorder produces diffuse conjunctival injection. Ulcerations appear on the eyelids, which burn, itch, and have no lashes.
- *Chemical burns.* In this ocular emergency, diffuse conjunctival injection occurs, but severe pain is the most prominent symptom. The patient also has photophobia, blepharospasm, and decreased visual acuity in the affected eye; the cornea may appear gray, and the pupil may be unilaterally smaller.
- *Conjunctival foreign bodies and abrasions.* These conditions feature localized conjunctival injection with sudden, severe eye pain. The patient may have increased tearing and photophobia, but usually his visual acuity isn't impaired.

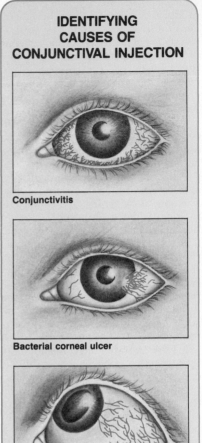

IDENTIFYING CAUSES OF CONJUNCTIVAL INJECTION

Conjunctivitis

Bacterial corneal ulcer

Episcleritis

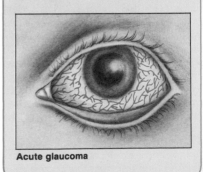

Acute glaucoma

● *Conjunctivitis.* *Allergic conjunctivitis* produces a milky, diffuse, peripheral conjunctival injection. The patient complains of photophobia and a feeling of fullness around the eyes. He'll have watery, stringy eye discharge, increased tearing, itching, palpebral conjunctival follicles, and (in hay fever) conjunctival edema.

Bacterial conjunctivitis causes diffuse peripheral conjunctival injection along with thick, purulent eye discharge that contains mucous threads. The patient's lids and lashes stick together, and he has excessive tearing, photophobia, burning, and itching. He may experience pain and a foreign body sensation if the cornea is involved.

Besides diffuse peripheral conjunctival injection, the patient with *fungal conjunctivitis* complains of photophobia and increased tearing, itching, and burning. The discharge is thick and purulent, making his eyelids crusted, sticky, and swollen. Corneal involvement causes pain.

In *viral conjunctivitis,* the conjunctival injection is brilliant red, diffuse, and peripheral. The patient may also have conjunctival edema, follicles on the palpebral conjunctiva, and lid edema. The patient complains of itching, increased tearing, and possibly a foreign body sensation. He may also have a local viral skin rash or signs of upper respiratory infection.

● *Corneal abrasion.* In this disorder, diffuse conjunctival injection is extremely painful—especially when the eyelids move over the abrasion. The patient may also experience photophobia, excessive tearing, blurred vision, and a foreign body sensation.

● *Corneal erosion.* Recurrent corneal erosion produces diffuse conjunctival injection. The patient has severe, continuous pain from rubbing of the eyelid over the eroded area of the cornea. He also complains of photophobia.

● *Corneal ulcer.* Bacterial, viral, and fungal corneal ulcers produce diffuse conjunctival injection that increases in the circumcorneal area. Accompany-ing findings include severe photophobia, severe pain in and around the eye, markedly decreased visual acuity, and copious and purulent eye discharge and crusting. If the patient has associated iritis, physical examination will also reveal corneal opacities and abnormal pupil response to light.

● *Dacryoadenitis.* In this disorder, the patient has large, diffuse conjunctival injection and complains of pain over the temporal part of the eye. He also has considerable lid swelling and, possibly, purulent eye discharge.

● *Episcleritis.* Conjunctival injection is localized and raised and may be violet or purplish-pink in this disorder. The sclera is also inflamed. Associated signs and symptoms include deep pain, photophobia, increased tearing, and conjunctival edema.

● *Glaucoma.* In acute closed-angle glaucoma, conjunctival injection is typically circumcorneal. The patient has severe eye pain along with nausea and vomiting. His intraocular pressure is severely elevated and his vision is blurred. He also sees rainbow-colored halos around lights, and his corneas appear steamy because of corneal edema. The pupil of the affected eye will be moderately dilated and completely unresponsive to light.

● *Hyphema.* Depending on the type and extent of traumatic injury, a hyphema produces diffuse conjunctival injection, possibly with lid and orbital edema. The patient may complain of pain in and around the eye. The extent of visual impairment depends on the hyphema's size and location.

● *Iritis.* In acute iritis, marked conjunctival injection is located mainly around the cornea. The patient has moderate-to-severe pain and photophobia. His vision is blurred, his pupils are constricted, and his pupillary response to light is poor.

● *Keratoconjunctivitis sicca.* This disorder produces severe diffuse conjunctival injection. The patient has generalized eye pain along with burning, itching, a foreign body sensation, excessive mucous secretion from the eye, absence of tears, and photophobia.

• *Ocular lacerations and intraocular foreign bodies.* Diffuse conjunctival injection may be increased in the area of injury. The patient will experience impaired visual acuity and moderate-to-severe pain, depending on the type and extent of injury. He may also have lid edema, photophobia, excessive tearing, and abnormal pupillary response.

• *Ocular tumors.* If a tumor is located in the orbit behind the globe, conjunctival injection may occur together with exophthalmos. With muscle involvement, conjunctival edema, ocular deviation, and diplopia usually occur.

• *Scleritis.* In this relatively rare disorder, conjunctival injection can be diffuse or localized over the area of the scleritis nodule. The patient has severe pain on moving the eye, photophobia, tenderness, and tearing.

• *Stevens-Johnson syndrome.* This disorder produces diffuse conjunctival injection, purulent eye discharge, severe eye pain, photophobia, decreased tearing, entropion, and trichiasis.

• *Uveitis.* Diffuse conjunctival injection, which may be increased in the circumcorneal area, characterizes this disorder. It's accompanied by constricted, irregularly shaped pupils; blurred vision; tenderness; and photophobia. It may cause sudden, severe ocular pain.

Special considerations

As indicated, prepare the patient for such diagnostic tests as eye and orbit X-rays, ocular ultrasonography, and fluorescein staining. If the patient complains of photophobia, darken the room, or suggest that he wear sunglasses. Obtain cultures of any eye discharge, and record its appearance, consistency, and amount. If the patient's visual acuity is markedly decreased, orient him to his environment to ensure his comfort and safety.

Because most forms of conjunctivitis are contagious, the infection can easily spread to the other eye or to other family members. Stress the importance of hand washing and of not touching the affected eye to prevent contagion.

Pediatric pointers

An infant can develop self-limiting chemical conjunctivitis at birth from ocular instillation of silver nitrate. Or, 2 to 5 days after birth, he may develop bacterial conjunctivitis due to contamination in the birth canal. An infant with congenital syphilis has prominent conjunctival injection and grayish pink corneas.

Constipation

Constipation is defined as small, infrequent, and difficult bowel movements. Because normal bowel movements can vary in frequency from twice a day to once every 3 days, constipation must be determined in relation to the patient's normal elimination pattern. Constipation may be a minor annoyance or, uncommonly, a sign of a life-threatening disorder, such as acute intestinal obstruction. Untreated, constipation can lead to headache, anorexia, and abdominal discomfort, and can adversely affect the patient's lifestyle and well-being.

Most often, constipation occurs when the urge to defecate is suppressed and the muscles associated with bowel movements remain contracted. Because the autonomic nervous system controls bowel movements—by sensing rectal distention from fecal contents and by stimulating the external sphincter—any factor that influences this system may cause bowel dysfunction. (See *How Habits and Stress Cause Constipation,* page 181.)

Assessment

Ask the patient to describe the size, consistency, and frequency of his bowel movements. How long has he experienced constipation? Acute constipation usually has an organic cause, such as an anal or rectal disorder. In a patient over age 45, recent onset of constipation may be an early sign of colorectal cancer. Conversely, chronic constipation typically has a functional cause and may be related to stress.

Does the patient have pain related to constipation? If so, when did he first notice the pain, and where is it located? Cramping abdominal pain and distention suggest obstipation—extreme, persistent constipation due to intestinal tract obstruction. Ask the patient if elimination worsens or helps relieve the pain. Elimination usually worsens pain, but, in such disorders as irritable bowel syndrome, it may relieve it.

Ask the patient to describe a typical day's menu. Then estimate his daily fiber and fluid intake. Ask him, too, about any changes in eating habits, in medication or alcohol use, or in physical activity. Has he experienced recent emotional distress? Has constipation affected his family life or social contacts? Also ask about the patient's job. A sedentary or stressful job can contribute to constipation.

Find out whether the patient has a history of gastrointestinal, rectoanal, neurologic, or metabolic disorders; abdominal surgery; or radiation therapy. Then ask about the medications he's taking, including over-the-counter preparations such as laxatives, mineral oil, stool softeners, and enemas.

Inspect the abdomen for distention or scars from previous surgery. Then auscultate for bowel sounds, and characterize their motility. Percuss all four quadrants, and gently palpate for abdominal tenderness, a palpable mass, and hepatomegaly. Next, examine the patient's rectum. Spread his buttocks to expose the anus, and inspect for inflammation, lesions, scars, fissures, and external hemorrhoids. Use a disposable glove and lubricant to palpate the anal sphincter for laxity or stricture. Also palpate for rectal masses and fecal impaction. Finally, obtain a stool sample and test it for occult blood.

As you assess the patient, remember that constipation can also result from several life-threatening disorders, such as acute intestinal obstruction and mesenteric artery ischemia—but it doesn't herald these conditions.

Medical causes

● *Anal fissure.* A crack or laceration in the lining of the anal wall can cause acute constipation—usually due to the patient's fear of the severe tearing or burning pain associated with bowel movements. He may notice a few drops of blood streaking toilet tissue or his underclothes.

● *Anorectal abscess.* In this disorder, constipation occurs together with severe, throbbing, localized pain and tenderness at the abscess site. The patient may also have localized inflammation, swelling, and purulent drainage and complain of fever and malaise.

● *Cirrhosis.* In the early stages of cirrhosis, the patient has constipation along with nausea, vomiting, and a dull pain in the right upper quadrant. Other early findings include indigestion, anorexia, flatulence, hepatomegaly, and possibly splenomegaly and diarrhea.

● *Crohn's disease.* Although most patients with this disorder experience diarrhea, some develop chronic constipation due to strictures. Other findings include cramping abdominal pain, anorexia, weight loss, a palpable mass in the right or left lower quadrant, perianal lesions, and (rarely) clubbing. Acute inflammatory signs may include nausea, fever, tachycardia, abdominal tenderness and guarding, hyperactive bowel sounds, and abdominal distention along with the abdominal pain and diarrhea.

● *Diabetic neuropathy.* This neuropathy produces episodic constipation or diarrhea. Other signs and symptoms may include dysphagia, postural hypotension, syncope, and painless bladder distention with overflow incontinence. A male patient may also experience impotence and retrograde ejaculation.

• *Diverticulitis.* In this disorder, constipation occurs together with left lower quadrant pain and tenderness and possibly a palpable abdominal mass. The patient may have mild nausea, flatulence, or a low-grade fever.

• *Hemorrhoids.* Thrombosed hemorrhoids cause constipation as the patient tries to avoid the severe pain of defecation.The hemorrhoids may bleed during defecation.

• *Hepatic porphyria.* Abdominal pain—which may be severe, colicky, local-ized, or generalized—precedes constipation in hepatic porphyria. The patient may also have fever, sinus tachycardia, labile hypertension, excessive diaphoresis, severe vomiting, photophobia, urinary retention, nervousness or restlessness, disorientation, and possibly visual hallucinations. His deep tendon reflexes may be diminished or absent. Some patients have skin lesions causing itching, burning, erythema, altered pigmentation, and edema in areas exposed to

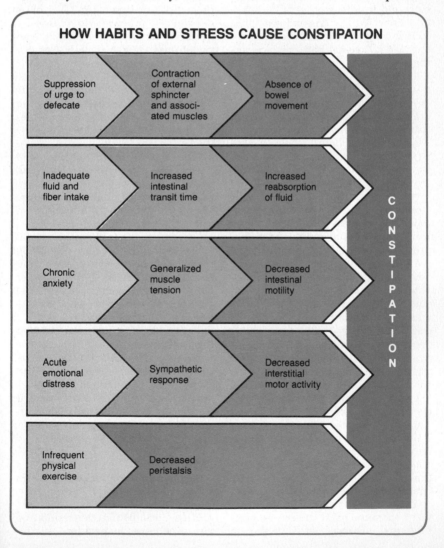

HOW HABITS AND STRESS CAUSE CONSTIPATION

			C O N S T I P A T I O N
Suppression of urge to defecate	Contraction of external sphincter and associated muscles	Absence of bowel movement	
Inadequate fluid and fiber intake	Increased intestinal transit time	Increased reabsorption of fluid	
Chronic anxiety	Generalized muscle tension	Decreased intestinal motility	
Acute emotional distress	Sympathetic response	Decreased interstitial motor activity	
Infrequent physical exercise	Decreased peristalsis		

light. Severe hepatic porphyria can produce delirium, coma, seizures, paraplegia, or complete flaccid quadriplegia.

● *Hypercalcemia.* In this disorder, constipation usually occurs along with anorexia, nausea, vomiting, and polyuria. The patient may also have dysrhythmias, bone pain, muscle weakness and atrophy, hypoactive deep tendon reflexes, and personality changes.

● *Hypothyroidism.* This disorder causes early and insidious onset of constipation. Other early signs and symptoms include fatigue, sensitivity to cold, anorexia with weight gain, and menorrhagia.

● *Intestinal obstruction.* Constipation associated with this disorder varies in severity and onset with the location and extent of the obstruction. In partial obstruction, constipation may alternate with leakage of liquid stool. In complete obstruction, obstipation may occur. Constipation can be the earliest sign of partial colon obstruction, but it usually occurs later if the level of the obstruction is more proximal. Associated findings may include episodes of colicky abdominal pain, abdominal distention, nausea, or vomiting. The patient may also have hyperactive bowel sounds, visible peristaltic waves, a palpable abdominal mass, and abdominal tenderness.

● *Irritable bowel syndrome.* Usually, this common syndrome produces chronic constipation, although some patients may have intermittent, watery diarrhea and others may complain of alternating constipation and diarrhea. Stress may trigger nausea and abdominal distention and tenderness, but defecation usually relieves these symptoms. Typically, the stools are scybalous and contain visible mucus.

● *Mesenteric artery ischemia.* This life-threatening disorder produces sudden constipation with failure to expel stool or flatus. Initially, it also produces severe abdominal pain, tenderness, vomiting, and anorexia. Later, the patient

may develop abdominal guarding, rigidity, and distention; tachycardia; tachypnea; fever; and signs of shock, such as cool, clammy skin and hypotension. A bruit may be heard.

● *Multiple sclerosis.* This disorder can produce constipation along with ocular disturbances, such as nystagmus, blurred vision, and diplopia; vertigo; and sensory disturbances. The patient may also have motor weakness, seizures, paralysis, muscle spasticity, gait ataxia, intention tremor, hyperreflexia, dysarthria, or dysphagia. This disorder can also produce urinary urgency, frequency, and incontinence and emotional instability. A male patient may experience impotence.

● *Spinal cord lesion.* Constipation may occur in this disorder along with urinary retention, sexual dysfunction, pain, and possibly motor weakness, paralysis, or sensory impairment below the level of the lesion.

● *Tabes dorsalis.* In this disorder, constipation occurs with an ataxic gait; paresthesias; loss of sensation of body position, deep pain, and temperature; Charcot's joints; Argyll Robertson pupil; and possibly impotence.

● *Ulcerative colitis.* In chronic ulcerative colitis, constipation may occur—but bloody diarrhea with pus and/or mucus is the hallmark of this disorder. Other signs and symptoms may include cramping lower abdominal pain, tenesmus, anorexia, low-grade fever, and, occasionally, nausea and vomiting. Bowel sounds may be hyperactive. Later, weight loss and weakness occur.

● *Ulcerative proctitis.* This disorder produces acute constipation with tenesmus. The patient feels an intense urge to defecate but is unable to do so. Instead, he may eliminate mucus, pus, or blood.

Other causes

● *Diagnostic tests.* Constipation can result from retention of barium given during certain GI studies.

● *Drugs.* Constipation often results from use of codeine, meperidine, methadone, and morphine. Less frequently, it may be due to hydrocodone, hydromorphone, levorphanol, oxycodone, oxymorphone, or pentazocine.

Constipation may result from drugs other than narcotic analgesics. These include vinca alkaloids, polystyrene sodium sulfonate, antacids containing aluminum or calcium, anticholinergics, and drugs with anticholinergic effects (such as tricyclic antidepressants). Constipation may also result from excessive use of laxatives or enemas.

• *Surgery and radiotherapy.* Constipation can result from rectoanal surgery, which may traumatize nerves, and abdominal irradiation, which may cause intestinal stricture.

Special considerations
As indicated, prepare the patient for diagnostic tests, such as proctosigmoidoscopy, barium enema, plain abdominal films, and upper GI series.

Stress the importance of a high-fiber diet, and encourage the patient to drink sufficient fluids. (Explain that he may experience temporary bloating or flatulence after adding fiber to his diet.) Also encourage him to exercise at least 1½ hours each week, if possible. If the patient's on bedrest, reposition him frequently, and help him perform active or passive exercises, as indicated. Teach abdominal toning exercises, if his abdominal muscles are weak, and relaxation techniques to help reduce stress related to constipation.

Caution the patient not to strain during defecation, to prevent injuring rectoanal tissue. Instruct him to avoid using laxatives or enemas; if he's been abusing these products, begin to wean him from them. As ordered, use a disposable glove and lubricant to remove impacted fecal contents. (Check if an oil-retention enema can be given first to soften the fecal mass.)

Pediatric pointers
The high content of casein and calcium in cow's milk can produce hard stools and possible constipation in bottle-fed infants. Other causes of constipation in infants include inadequate fluid intake, Hirschsprung's disease, and anal fissures.

In older children, constipation usually results from inadequate fiber intake and excessive intake of milk. However, it may also result from bowel spasm, mechanical obstruction, and hypothyroidism.

Corneal Reflex— Absent

The corneal reflex is tested bilaterally by drawing a fine-pointed wisp of sterile cotton from a corner of each eye to the cornea. Normally, even though only one eye is tested at a time, the patient blinks bilaterally each time either cornea is touched. This is the corneal reflex. When this reflex is absent, however, neither eyelid closes when the cornea of one is touched.

The site of the afferent fibers for this reflex is in the ophthalmic branch of the trigeminal nerve (cranial nerve V); the efferent fibers are located in the facial nerve (cranial nerve VII). Unilateral or bilateral absence of the corneal reflex may result from damage to these nerves.

Assessment
If you're unable to elicit the corneal reflex, assess the patient for other signs of trigeminal nerve dysfunction. To test the three sensory portions of the nerve, touch each side of the patient's face on the brow, cheek, and jaw with a cotton wisp, and ask him to compare the sensations.

If you suspect facial nerve involvement, note if both the upper face (brow and eyes) and lower face (cheek, mouth, and chin) are weak bilaterally. Lower motor neuron facial weakness affects the face on the same side as the

ELICITING THE CORNEAL REFLEX

To elicit the corneal reflex, have the patient turn the eyes away from you to avoid involuntary blinking during the procedure. Then approach the patient from the opposite side, out of the line of vision, and brush the cornea lightly with a fine wisp of sterile cotton. Repeat the procedure on the other eye.

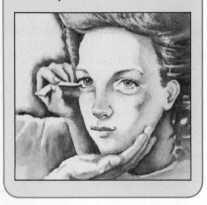

lesion, whereas upper motor neuron weakness affects the side opposite the lesion—and predominantly affects the lower facial muscles.

Because an absent corneal reflex may signify such progressive neurologic disorders as Guillain-Barré syndrome, ask the patient about associated symptoms—facial pain, dysphagia, and limb weakness.

Medical causes

• *Acoustic neuroma.* This tumor affects the trigeminal nerve, causing a diminished or absent corneal reflex, tinnitus, and unilateral hearing impairment. Facial palsy and anesthesia, palate weakness, and signs of cerebellar dysfunction (ataxia, nystagmus) may result if the tumor impinges on the adjacent cranial nerves, brain stem, and cerebellum.

• *Bell's palsy.* A common cause of diminished or absent corneal reflex, this disorder causes paralysis of cranial nerve VII. It can also produce complete hemifacial weakness or paralysis, and drooling on the affected side. The affected side also sags and appears masklike. The eye on this side can't be shut and tears constantly.

• *Brainstem infarction or injury.* Absent corneal reflex can occur on the side opposite the lesion when infarction or injury affects cranial nerve V or VII, or their connection in the central trigeminal tract. The patient's level of consciousness may be decreased, and he may have dysphagia, dysarthria, and contralateral limb weakness. He may also show such early signs of increased intracranial pressure as headache and vomiting.

In massive brainstem infarction or injury, the patient also displays respiratory changes, such as apneustic breathing or periods of apnea; bilateral pupillary dilation or constriction with decreased responsiveness to light; rising systolic blood pressure; widening pulse pressure; bradycardia; and coma.

• *Guillain-Barré syndrome.* In this polyneuropathic disorder, a diminished or absent corneal reflex accompanies ipsilateral loss of facial muscle control. The patient may also have dysarthria, nasality, and dysphagia. Muscle weakness, which is the dominant neurologic sign of this disorder, typically starts in the legs, then extends to the arms and facial nerves within 72 hours. Other findings may include paresthesias, respiratory muscle paralysis, respiratory insufficiency, postural hypotension, incontinence, diaphoresis, and tachycardia.

• *Trigeminal neuralgia (tic douloureux).* A diminished or absent corneal reflex may stem from a superior maxillary lesion that affects the ophthalmic branch. The patient characteristically experiences sudden bursts of intense pain or shooting sensations, lasting from 1 to 15 minutes, in one of the divisions of the trigeminal nerve, primarily the superior mandibular or maxillary division. Local stimulation, such as a light touch to the cheeks, may trigger an attack—or an attack may follow exposure to hot or cold temperatures or eating or drinking hot or cold beverages or food. Areas around the patient's nose and mouth may be hypersensitive.

Special considerations

When the corneal reflex is absent, you'll need to take measures to protect the patient's affected eye from injury. For example, lubricate the eye with artificial tears to prevent drying. Cover the cornea with a shield and avoid excessive corneal reflex testing.

As ordered, prepare the patient for cranial X-rays or a computed tomography scan.

Pediatric pointers

Brainstem lesions and injuries are the most common causes of absent corneal reflexes in children; Guillain-Barré syndrome occurs less commonly. Infants, especially those born prematurely, may have an absent corneal reflex due to anoxic damage to the brainstem.

Costovertebral Angle Tenderness

This elicited symptom indicates sudden distention of the renal capsule. It almost always accompanies unelicited, dull, constant flank pain in the costovertebral angle (CVA) just lateral to the sacrospinalis muscle and below the 12th rib. This associated pain typically travels anteriorly in the subcostal region toward the umbilicus.

Percussing the costovertebral angle elicits CVA tenderness. (See *Eliciting CVA Tenderness,* page 186.) A patient who doesn't have this symptom will perceive a thudding, jarring, or pressure-like sensation when tested, but no pain. A patient with a disorder that distends the renal capsule will expe-

rience intense pain as the renal capsule stretches and stimulates the afferent nerves, which emanate from the spinal cord at levels T11 through L2 and innervate the kidney.

Assessment

After detecting CVA tenderness, assess the possible extent of renal damage. First, find out if the patient has other symptoms of renal or urologic dysfunction. Ask about his voiding habits: How frequently does he urinate, and in what amounts? Has he noticed any change in intake or output? If so, when did he notice the change? (Be sure to ask about fluid intake before judging his output abnormal.) Is there any nocturia? Ask about pain or burning during urination or difficulty starting a stream. Does the patient strain to urinate without being able to do so (tenesmus)? Ask about urine color; brown or bright red urine may contain blood.

Explore other signs and symptoms. For example, if the patient's experiencing pain in his flank, abdomen, or back, when did he first notice the pain? How severe is it, and where is it located?

Find out if the patient or a family member has a history of urinary tract infections, congenital anomalies, calculi, or other obstructive nephropathies or uropathies. Ask about a history of renovascular disorders, such as occlusion of the renal arteries or veins.

Perform a brief physical examination. Begin by taking the patient's vital signs. Fever and chills in a patient with CVA tenderness may indicate acute pyelonephritis. If the patient has hypertension and bradycardia, be alert for other autonomic effects of renal pain, such as diaphoresis and pallor. Inspect, auscultate, and gently palpate the abdomen for clues to the underlying cause of CVA tenderness. Be alert for abdominal distention, hypoactive bowel sounds, or palpable masses.

Medical causes

- *Calculi.* Infundibular and ureteropel-

ELICITING C.V.A. TENDERNESS

To elicit CVA tenderness, have the patient sit upright facing away from you or have him lie prone. Place the palm of your left hand over the left costovertebral angle, then strike the back of your left hand with the ulnar surface of your right fist, as shown. Repeat this percussion technique over the right costovertebral angle. A patient with CVA tenderness will experience intense pain.

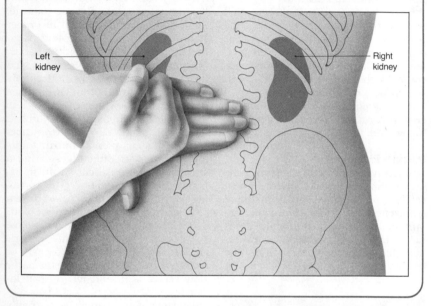

Left kidney

Right kidney

vic junction calculi produce CVA tenderness and flank pain. The patient may also have nausea, vomiting, severe abdominal pain, abdominal distention, and decreased bowel sounds.

• *Perirenal abscess.* Causing exquisite CVA tenderness, this disorder may also produce severe unilateral flank pain, dysuria, persistent high fever, chills, and sometimes a palpable abdominal mass.

• *Pyelonephritis (acute).* Perhaps the most common cause of CVA tenderness, acute pyelonephritis is often accompanied by persistent high fever, chills, flank pain, weakness, dysuria, hematuria, nocturia, and urinary urgency, frequency, and tenesmus.

• *Renal artery occlusion.* In this disorder, the patient experiences flank pain as well as CVA tenderness. Other findings may include severe, continuous

upper abdominal pain; nausea; vomiting; decreased bowel sounds; and high fever after 1 or 2 days.

• *Renal vein occlusion.* The patient with this disorder has CVA tenderness and flank pain. He also may have sudden, severe back pain, fever, and hematuria.

Special considerations

Administer pain medication, as ordered, and continue to monitor vital signs and intake and output. As ordered, collect serum and urine samples and prepare the patient for radiologic studies, such as intravenous pyelography, renal arteriography, and computed tomography.

Pediatric pointers

An infant with a disorder that distends the renal capsule won't have CVA tenderness. Instead, he'll display nonspecific signs, such as vomiting, diarrhea, and fever. In older children, however, CVA tenderness has the same diagnostic significance as in adults.

Cough—Barking

Resonant, brassy, and harsh, a barking cough is part of a complex of signs and symptoms that characterize croup syndrome—a group of pediatric disorders marked by varying degrees of respiratory distress. Croup syndrome is most common in boys and most prevalent in winter, and it may recur in the same child. Because infants' and children's airways are smaller in diameter than adults', pediatric patients can rapidly develop airway occlusion from edema.

A barking cough indicates edema of the larynx and surrounding tissue and may signal a life-threatening emergency.

Assessment

Quickly assess the child's respiratory status, and have another nurse notify the doctor. Then take the child's vital signs, being especially alert for tachycardia and signs of hypoxemia. Check for decreased level of consciousness.

Find out if the child has been playing with any small object that he may have aspirated. Check for cyanosis in the lips and nailbeds. Observe for sternal or intercostal retractions or nasal flaring. Next, note the depth and rate of his respirations—they may become increasingly shallow as respiratory distress increases. Observe the child's body position: Is he sitting up, leaning forward, struggling to breathe? Observe his activity level, facial expression, and level of consciousness. With increasing respiratory distress from airway edema, the child will become restless, with a frightened, wide-eyed expression. As air hunger continues,

he'll become lethargic and difficult to arouse.

If the child shows signs of severe respiratory distress, maintain airway patency and provide oxygen. Prepare to assist with endotracheal intubation or tracheotomy.

When the child's condition permits, ask his parents when the barking cough began, and find out what other signs and symptoms accompanied it. When did the child first appear to be ill? Has he had previous episodes of croup syndrome? Spasmodic croup and epiglottitis both typically occur in the middle of the night; the child with spasmodic croup has no fever, but the child with epiglottitis does—a high one. Laryngotracheobronchitis typically follows an upper respiratory infection.

Medical causes

• *Aspiration of foreign body.* Partial obstruction of the upper airway first produces sudden hoarseness, then a barking cough and inspiratory stridor. Other effects of this life-threatening condition include gagging, tachycardia, dyspnea, decreased breath sounds, wheezing, and possibly cyanosis.

• *Epiglottitis.* Typically, this life-threatening disorder arises during the night, heralded by barking cough and high fever. The child is hoarse, dysphagic, dyspneic, and restless and appears extremely ill and panicky. His barking cough may progress to severe respiratory distress with sternal and intercostal retractions, nasal flaring, cyanosis, and tachycardia. The child will struggle to get air as the epiglottic edema increases. Total airway occlusion may occur within 2 to 5 hours.

• *Laryngotracheobronchitis (acute).* Most common in children between the ages of 2 months and 3 years, this viral infection initially produces low to moderate fever, runny nose, poor appetite, and infrequent cough. When the infection descends into the laryngotracheal area, such signs as barking cough, hoarseness, and inspiratory stridor occur. As respiratory distress progresses, substernal and intercostal retractions occur along with tachycardia and shallow, rapid respirations. Sleeping in a dry room worsens these signs. The patient becomes restless and irritable, pale and cyanotic.

• *Spasmodic croup.* Acute spasmodic croup usually occurs during sleep with abrupt onset of a barking cough that awakens the child. Typically, he will not have a fever, but he may be hoarse, restless, and dyspneic. As his respiratory distress worsens, the child may exhibit sternal and intercostal retractions, nasal flaring, tachycardia, cyanosis, and an anxious, frantic appearance. The symptoms most often subside within a few hours, but attacks tend to recur.

Special considerations
If the child's respiratory distress isn't severe, a lateral neck X-ray may be done to visualize any epiglottal edema; a chest X-ray may also be done, to rule out lower respiratory tract infection. Depending on the child's age and his degree of respiratory distress, a mist tent, oxygen hood, or bedside humidifier may be used.

Observe the child frequently and check fluid levels in the mist tent to ensure continual delivery of humidified air, and monitor the oxygen level in the hood or mist tent. Provide periods of rest with minimal interruptions. Encourage the parents to stay with the child to help alleviate stress. For short periods of time, especially during a coughing attack, the child can be removed from the tent to be held and calmed.

Be sure the parents understand the importance of operating a humidifier at the child's bedside, to humidify the air and prevent a recurrence of croup syndrome. Teach the parents to assess and treat recurrent episodes, however, just in case. For example, creating steam by running hot water in a sink or shower and sitting with the child in the closed bathroom may help relieve subsequent attacks of croup syndrome.

Cough—Nonproductive

A nonproductive cough is a noisy, forceful expulsion of air from the lungs that doesn't yield sputum or blood. It's one of the most common complaints of patients with respiratory disorders.

Coughing is a necessary protective mechanism that clears airway passages. However, a nonproductive cough is not only ineffective but can also cause damage—such as airway collapse or rupture of alveoli or blebs. And a nonproductive cough that later becomes productive is a classic sign of progressive respiratory disease.

The cough reflex generally occurs when mechanical, chemical, thermal, inflammatory, or psychogenic stimuli activate cough receptors. (See *Reviewing the Cough Mechanism,* page 190.) But external pressure—for example, from subdiaphragmatic irritation or a mediastinal tumor—can also induce it. So can voluntary expiration of air, which occasionally occurs as a nervous habit.

Cough may occur once or several times, as in a paroxysm of coughing, and can worsen by becoming more frequent. An acute cough has a sudden onset and may be self-limiting; a cough that persists beyond 1 month is considered chronic and often results from cigarette smoking.

A patient may minimize or overlook a chronic nonproductive cough, or he may accept it as normal. In fact, such a patient generally won't seek medical attention unless he has other symptoms.

Assessment
Ask the patient when his cough began and whether any body position, time of day, or specific activity affects it. How does the cough sound—harsh, brassy, dry, hacking? Try to determine if the cough is related to smoking or a chemical irritant. If the patient smokes or has smoked, note the number of

packs smoked daily multiplied by years. Next, ask how often the patient coughs and if he has paroxysms of coughing. If he has pain associated with coughing, breathing, or activity, when did it begin? Where is it located?

Ask the patient about recent illness, surgery, or trauma, and find out if he's had any cardiovascular or pulmonary disorders. Also ask about hypersensitivity to drugs, foods, pets, dust, or pollen. Find out what medications the patient takes, if any, and ask about recent changes in schedule or dosages. Also find out about recent changes in his appetite, weight, exercise tolerance, or energy level and recent exposure to irritating fumes, chemicals, or smoke.

As you're taking his history, observe the patient's general appearance and manner: Is he agitated, restless, or lethargic; pale, diaphoretic, or flushed; anxious, confused, or nervous? Also note whether he's cyanotic or has clubbed fingers or peripheral edema.

Now perform a physical examination. Start by taking the patient's vital signs. Next, check the depth and rhythm of his respirations, and note if wheezing or "crowing" noises occur with breathing. Feel the patient's skin: Is it cold or warm, clammy or dry? Check his nose and mouth for congestion, inflammation, drainage, or signs of infection. Inspect his neck for distended veins and tracheal deviation, and palpate for masses or enlarged lymph nodes.

Examine the chest, observing its configuration and looking for abnormal chest wall motion. Do you note any retractions or use of accessory muscles? Percuss for dullness, tympany, or flatness. Auscultate for wheezes, crackles, rhonchi, pleural friction rubs, and decreased or absent breath sounds. Finally, examine the abdomen for distention, tenderness, masses, or abnormal bowel sounds.

Medical causes

● *Airway occlusion.* Partial occlusion of the upper airway produces sudden onset of dry, paroxysmal coughing. The patient is gagging, wheezing, and hoarse, with stridor, tachycardia, and decreased breath sounds.

● *Aortic aneurysm (thoracic).* This disorder causes a brassy cough with dyspnea, hoarseness, wheezing, and a substernal ache in the shoulders, lower back, or abdomen. The patient may also have facial or neck edema, neck vein distention, dysphagia, prominent veins over his chest, stridor, and possibly paresthesia or neuralgia.

● *Asthma.* An attack often occurs at night and starts with a nonproductive cough and mild wheezing; this progresses to severe dyspnea, audible wheezing, chest tightness, and cough that produces thick mucus. Other signs may include apprehension, rhonchi, prolonged expirations, intercostal and supraclavicular retractions on inspiration, accessory muscle use, flaring nostrils, tachypnea, tachycardia, diaphoresis, and flushing or cyanosis.

● *Atelectasis.* As lung tissue deflates, it stimulates cough receptors, causing a nonproductive cough. The patient may also have pleuritic chest pain, anxiety, dyspnea, tachypnea, and tachycardia. His skin may be cyanotic and diaphoretic, his breath sounds may be decreased, his chest may be dull on percussion, and he may exhibit inspiratory lag, substernal or intercostal retractions, decreased vocal fremitus, and tracheal deviation toward the affected side.

● *Bronchitis (chronic).* This disorder starts with a nonproductive, hacking cough that later becomes productive. It also causes prolonged expiration, wheezing, dyspnea, accessory muscle use, barrel chest, cyanosis, tachypnea, crackles, and scattered rhonchi. Clubbing can occur in late stages.

● *Bronchogenic carcinoma.* The earliest indicators of this disorder can be a chronic nonproductive cough, dyspnea, and vague chest pain. The patient may also be wheezing.

● *Common cold.* This disorder generally starts with a nonproductive, hacking

REVIEWING THE COUGH MECHANISM

Cough receptors are thought to be located in the nose, sinuses, auditory canals, nasopharynx, larynx, trachea, bronchi, pleurae, diaphragm, and possibly the pericardium and GI tract. Once a cough receptor is stimulated, the vagus and glossopharyngeal nerves transmit the impulse to the "cough center" in the medulla. From there, it's transmitted to the larynx and to the intercostal and abdominal muscles. Deep inspiration (1) is followed by closure of the glottis (2), relaxation of the diaphragm, and contraction of the abdominal and intercostal muscles. The resulting increased pressure in the lungs opens the glottis to release the forceful, noisy expiration known as a cough (3).

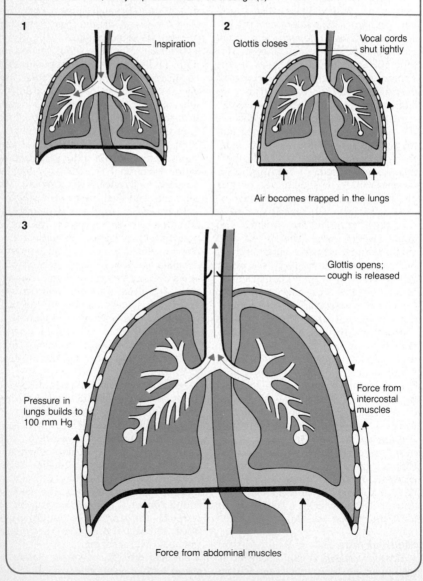

1

Inspiration

2

Glottis closes — Vocal cords shut tightly

Air becomes trapped in the lungs

3

Glottis opens; cough is released

Pressure in lungs builds to 100 mm Hg

Force from intercostal muscles

Force from abdominal muscles

cough and progresses to some mix of sneezing, headaches, malaise, fatigue, rhinorrhea, myalgia, arthralgia, nasal congestion, and sore throat.

• *Esophageal achalasia.* In this disorder, regurgitation produces a dry cough. The patient may also have recurrent pulmonary infections and dysphagia.

• *Esophageal cysts.* This disorder is typically asymptomatic, but it occasionally causes a nonproductive cough as well as dyspnea, dysphagia, cyanosis, and pressurelike chest pain.

• *Esophageal diverticula.* The patient with this disorder has a nocturnal nonproductive cough, regurgitation, dyspepsia, and dysphagia. His neck may appear swollen and have a gurgling sound. He may also have halitosis and weight loss.

• *Esophageal occlusion.* Immediate nonproductive coughing and gagging characterize this disorder. The patient has a sensation of something stuck in his throat. Other findings include neck or chest pain, dysphagia, and inability to swallow.

• *Esophagitis with reflux.* This disorder often causes a nonproductive nocturnal cough due to regurgitation while the patient's recumbent. He may have chest pain, which mimics angina pectoris, and heartburn that worsens if he lies down after eating. He may also have increased salivation, dysphagia, hematemesis, and melena.

• *Hodgkin's disease.* This disease may cause a crowing nonproductive cough. However, the earliest sign is usually painless swelling of one of the cervical lymph nodes or, occasionally, of the axillary, mediastinal, or inguinal lymph nodes. Another early sign is pruritus. Other findings depend on the degree and location of systemic involvement and may include dyspnea, dysphagia, hepatosplenomegaly, edema, jaundice, nerve pain, and hyperpigmentation.

• *Hypersensitivity pneumonitis.* In this disorder, acute nonproductive coughing, fever, dyspnea, and malaise usually occur 5 to 6 hours after exposure to an antigen.

• *Interstitial lung disease.* A patient with this disorder has a nonproductive cough and progressive dyspnea. He may also be cyanotic and have clubbing, fine crackles, fatigue, variable chest pain, and weight loss.

• *Laryngeal tumor.* Mild, nonproductive cough is an early sign of this disorder, along with minor throat discomfort and hoarseness. Later, dysphagia, dyspnea, cervical lymphadenodopathy, stridor, and earache may occur.

• *Laryngitis.* In its acute form, this disorder causes a nonproductive cough with localized pain (especially when the patient's swallowing or speaking) as well as fever and malaise. His hoarseness can range from mild to complete loss of voice.

• *Legionnaire's disease.* After a prodrome of malaise, headache, and possibly diarrhea, anorexia, diffuse myalgias, and general weakness, this disease causes a nonproductive cough that later becomes productive of mucoid, mucopurulent, possibly bloody sputum.

• *Lung abscess.* This disorder typically begins with nonproductive coughing, weakness, dyspnea, and pleuritic chest pain. The patient may also have diaphoresis, fever, headache, malaise, fatigue, crackles, decreased breath sounds, anorexia, and weight loss. Later, his cough becomes productive of large amounts of purulent, foul-smelling, possibly bloody sputum.

• *Mediastinal tumor.* A large mediastinal tumor produces a nonproductive cough, dyspnea, and retrosternal pain. The patient may also have stertorous respirations with suprasternal retraction on inspiration, hoarseness, dysphagia, tracheal shift or tug, neck vein distention, and facial or neck edema.

• *Pericardial effusion.* Rarely, this disorder causes a severe nonproductive cough. But its more common signs and symptoms include dysphagia, fever, pleuritic chest pain, and pericardial friction rub.

• *Pleural effusion.* A nonproductive cough is associated with this disorder along with dyspnea, pleuritic chest pain, and decreased chest motion. The patient also has a pleural friction rub, tachycardia, tachypnea, egophony, flatness on percussion, decreased or absent breath sounds, and decreased tactile fremitus.

● *Pneumonia.* Bacterial pneumonia usually starts with a nonproductive, hacking, painful cough that rapidly becomes productive. Other findings include shaking chills, headache, high fever, dyspnea, pleuritic chest pain, tachypnea, tachycardia, grunting respirations, nasal flaring, decreased breath sounds, fine crackles, rhonchi, and cyanosis. The patient's chest may be dull on percussion.

In *mycoplasma pneumonia,* a nonproductive cough arises 2 to 3 days after onset of malaise, headache, and sore throat. The cough can be paroxysmal, causing substernal chest pain. Fever commonly occurs, but the patient won't appear seriously ill.

Viral pneumonia causes a nonproductive, hacking cough and gradual onset of malaise, headache, anorexia, and low-grade fever.

● *Pneumothorax.* This life-threatening disorder causes a dry cough and signs of respiratory distress, such as severe dyspnea, tachycardia, tachypnea, and cyanosis. The patient experiences sudden, sharp chest pain that worsens with chest movement. He also has subcutaneous crepitation, hyperresonance or tympany, decreased vocal fremitus, and decreased or absent breath sounds on the affected side.

● *Psittacosis.* Initially, this disorder causes a dry, hacking cough that later becomes productive of small amounts of blood-streaked mucoid sputum. The disorder may begin abruptly with chills, fever, headache, myalgias, and prostration. The patient may also have tachypnea, fine crackles, epistaxis, and (rarely) chest pain.

● *Pulmonary edema.* Initially, this disorder causes a dry cough, exertional dyspnea, paroxysmal nocturnal dyspnea, orthopnea, tachycardia, tachypnea, dependent crackles, and ventricular gallop. If pulmonary edema is severe, the patient's respirations become more rapid and labored, with diffuse crackles and coughing that produces frothy, bloody sputum.

● *Pulmonary embolism.* Life-threatening pulmonary embolism may produce sudden onset of dry cough along with dyspnea and pleuritic or anginal chest pain. More often, though, the cough produces blood-tinged sputum. Tachycardia and low-grade fever are also common; less common signs and symptoms include massive hemoptysis, chest splinting, leg edema, and (with a large embolus) cyanosis, syncope, and distended neck veins. The patient may also have a pleural friction rub, diffuse wheezing, dullness on percussion, and decreased breath sounds.

● *Sarcoidosis.* In this disorder, a nonproductive cough is accompanied by dyspnea, substernal pain, and malaise. The patient may also have fatigue, arthralgia, myalgia, weight loss, tachypnea, crackles, lymphadenopathy, hepatosplenomegaly, skin lesions, visual impairment, difficulty swallowing, and dysrhythmias.

● *Sinusitis (chronic).* This disorder can cause a chronic nonproductive cough due to postnasal drip. The patient's nasal mucosa may appear inflamed, and he may have nasal congestion and profuse drainage. Usually, his breath smells musty.

● *Tracheobronchitis (acute).* Initially, this disorder produces a dry cough that later becomes productive as secretions increase. Chills, sore throat, slight fever, muscle and back pain, and substernal tightness generally precede the cough's onset. Rhonchi and wheezes are usually heard. Severe illness causes a fever of 101° to 102° F. (38.3° to 38.8° C.) and possibly bronchospasm, with severe wheezing and increased coughing.

Other causes

● *Diagnostic tests.* Pulmonary function tests and bronchoscopy may stimulate

cough receptors and trigger coughing.
• *Treatments.* Irritation of the carina during suctioning can trigger a paroxysmal or hacking cough. Intermittent positive pressure breathing or incentive spirometry can also cause nonproductive coughing.

Special considerations

A nonproductive, paroxysmal cough may induce life-threatening bronchospasm. You may be asked to give the patient a bronchodilator to relieve his bronchospasm and open his airways. Unless the patient has chronic obstructive pulmonary disease, you may be asked to administer antitussives and sedatives to suppress the cough.

To relieve mucous membrane inflammation and dryness, humidify the air in the patient's room, or instruct him to use a humidifier at home. Tell him to avoid using aerosols, powders, or other respiratory irritants—especially cigarettes. And make sure the patient receives adequate fluids and nutrition.

As indicated, prepare the patient for diagnostic tests, such as X-rays, a lung scan, bronchoscopy, and pulmonary function tests.

Pediatric pointers

A nonproductive cough can be difficult to evaluate in infants and young children, because it can't be voluntarily induced and must be observed.

Sudden onset of paroxysmal nonproductive coughing may indicate aspiration of a foreign body—a common danger in children, especially those between 6 months and 4 years old. Nonproductive coughing can also result from several disorders that affect infants and children. In *asthma,* a characteristic nonproductive "tight" cough can arise suddenly or insidiously as an attack begins. The cough usually becomes productive toward the end of the attack. In *bacterial pneumonia,* a nonproductive, hacking cough arises suddenly and becomes productive in two or three days. *Acute bronchiolitis* has a peak incidence at age 6, with paroxysms of nonproductive coughing that become more frequent as the disease progresses. *Acute otitis media* frequently occurs in infants and young children due to their short eustachian tubes; it also produces nonproductive coughing. Typically, a child with *measles* has a slight, nonproductive, hacking cough that increases in severity. The earliest sign of *cystic fibrosis* may be a nonproductive, paroxysmal cough from retained secretions. Life-threatening *pertussis* produces a cough that becomes paroxysmal, with an inspiratory "whoop" or crowing sound. *Airway hyperactivity* causes a chronic nonproductive cough that increases with exercise or exposure to cold air. And *psychogenic coughing* may occur when the child is under stress, emotionally stimulated, or seeking attention.

Cough—Productive

Productive coughing is the body's mechanism for clearing airway passages of accumulated secretions that normal mucociliary action doesn't remove. It's a sudden, forceful, noisy expulsion of air from the lungs that contains sputum or blood (or both). (The sputum's color, consistency, and odor provide important clues about the patient's condition.) It can occur as a single cough or as paroxysmal coughing, and it can be voluntarily induced—although it's usually a reflexive response to stimulation of the airway mucosa.

Usually due to a cardiovascular or respiratory disorder, productive coughing often results from an acute or chronic infection causing inflammation, edema, and increased mucus production in the airways. However, this sign can also result from inhalation of antigenic or irritating substances or foreign bodies. In fact, the most common cause of chronic productive coughing is cigarette smoking, which produces brownish, mucoid sputum.

Many patients minimize or overlook chronic productive coughing or accept it as normal. Such patients may not seek medical attention until an associated problem develops—such as dyspnea, hemoptysis, chest pain, weight loss, or recurrent respiratory infections. The delay can have serious consequences, because productive coughing is associated with several life-threatening disorders and can also herald airway occlusion from excessive secretions.

Assessment

A patient with a productive cough can develop acute respiratory distress from thick or excessive secretions, bronchospasm, or fatigue. So, because his cough may signal an emergency condition, examine him before you take his history. First, take his vital signs and check the rate, depth, and rhythm of his respirations. Keep his airway patent, and be prepared to provide supplemental oxygen if he becomes restless or confused or if his respirations become shallow, irregular, rapid, or slow. Also assess for stridor, wheezing, choking, or gurgling, and be alert for nasal flaring and cyanosis.

Remember that a productive cough typically occurs in several life-threatening disorders. For example, coughing due to pulmonary edema produces thin, frothy, pink sputum, and coughing due to an asthmatic attack produces thick, mucoid sputum.

When the patient's condition permits, ask when the cough began, and find out how much sputum he's coughing up each day. (Remember, the tracheobronchial tree can produce up to 3 oz [90 ml] of sputum per day.) At what time of day does the patient cough up the most sputum? Does his sputum production have any relationship to what or when he eats or to his activities or environment? Ask the patient if he's noticed an increase in sputum production since his coughing began. This may result from external stimuli or from such internal causes as chronic bronchial infection or a lung abscess. Also ask about the color, odor, and consistency of the sputum. Blood-tinged or rust-colored sputum may result from trauma due to coughing or from an underlying condition such as a pulmonary infection or a tumor. Foul-smelling sputum may result from an anaerobic infection, such as bronchitis or lung abscess.

How does the cough sound? A hacking cough results from laryngeal involvement, whereas a "brassy" cough indicates major airway involvement. Does the patient feel any pain associated with his productive cough? If so, ask about its location and severity and whether it radiates to other areas. Does coughing, changing body position, or inspiration increase or help relieve his pain?

Next, ask the patient about his cigarette, drug, and alcohol use and whether his weight or appetite has changed. Find out if he has a history of asthma, allergies, or respiratory disorders, and ask about recent illnesses, surgery, or trauma. What medications is he taking? Does he work around chemicals or respiratory irritants, such as silicone?

Now examine the patient's mouth and nose for congestion, drainage, or inflammation. Note his breath odor: Halitosis can be a sign of pulmonary infection. Inspect his neck for distended veins, and palpate for tenderness and masses or enlarged lymph nodes. Observe his chest for accessory muscle use, retractions, and uneven chest expansion, and percuss for dullness, tympany, or flatness. Finally, auscultate for pleural friction rub and abnormal breath sounds—rhonchi, crackles, or wheezes.

Medical causes

● *Actinomycosis.* This disorder begins with a cough that produces purulent sputum. Fever, weight loss, fatigue, weakness, dyspnea, night sweats, pleuritic chest pain, and hemoptysis may also occur.

• *Aspiration pneumonitis.* This disorder causes coughing productive of pink, frothy, possibly purulent sputum. The patient also has marked dyspnea, fever, tachypnea, tachycardia, wheezing, and cyanosis.

• *Asthma.* A severe asthmatic attack, which can be life-threatening, may produce mucoid, tenacious sputum and mucous plugs. Such an attack typically starts with a dry cough and mild wheezing, then progresses to severe dyspnea, audible wheezing, chest tightness, and productive cough. Other findings may include apprehension, prolonged expirations, intercostal and supraclavicular retraction on inspiration, accessory muscle use, rhonchi, crackles, flaring nostrils, tachypnea, tachycardia, diaphoresis, and flushing or cyanosis. Attacks often occur at night or during sleep.

• *Bronchiectasis.* The chronic cough of this disorder produces copious, mucopurulent sputum that has characteristic layering (top, frothy; middle, clear; bottom, dense with purulent particles). The patient has halitosis: His sputum may smell foul or sickeningly sweet. Other characteristic findings include hemoptysis; persistent, coarse crackles over the affected lung area; occasional wheezes; rhonchi; exertional dyspnea; weight loss; fatigue; malaise; weakness; recurrent fever; and late-stage finger clubbing.

• *Bronchitis (chronic).* This disorder causes a cough that may be nonproductive initially. Eventually, however, it produces mucoid sputum that becomes purulent. Secondary infection can also cause mucopurulent sputum, which may become blood-tinged and foul-smelling. The coughing, which may be paroxysmal during exercise, most often occurs when the patient is recumbent or rises from sleep.

The patient also has prolonged expirations, increased use of accessory muscles for breathing, barrel chest, tachypnea, cyanosis, wheezing, exer-

tional dyspnea, scattered rhonchi, coarse crackles (which can be precipitated by coughing), and late-stage clubbing.

• *Chemical pneumonitis.* This disorder causes coughing that produces purulent sputum. It can also cause dyspnea, wheezing, orthopnea, fever, malaise, and crackles; mucous membrane irritation of the conjunctivae, throat, and nose; laryngitis; or rhinitis. Signs and symptoms may increase for 24 to 48 hours after exposure, then resolve; if severe, however, they may recur 2 to 5 weeks later.

• *Common cold.* When this disorder causes productive coughing, the sputum is mucoid or mucopurulent. Early indications of the common cold include a dry, hacking cough, sneezing, headache, malaise, fatigue, rhinorrhea (watery to tenacious, mucopurulent secretions), nasal congestion, sore throat, myalgia, and arthralgia.

• *Legionnaire's disease.* This disorder causes cough productive of scant mucoid, nonpurulent, possibly blood-streaked sputum. Usually, prodromal signs and symptoms occur: malaise, fatigue, weakness, anorexia, diffuse myalgias, and possibly diarrhea. Then, within 48 hours, the patient develops a dry cough and a sudden high fever with chills. Many patients also have pleuritic chest pain, headache, tachypnea, tachycardia, nausea, vomiting, dyspnea, crackles, mild temporary amnesia, disorientation, confusion, flushing, mild diaphoresis, and prostration.

• *Lung abscess (ruptured).* The cardinal sign of ruptured lung abscess is coughing that produces copious amounts of purulent, foul-smelling, possibly blood-tinged sputum. A ruptured abscess can also cause diaphoresis, anorexia, clubbing, weight loss, weakness, fatigue, fever with chills, dyspnea, headache, malaise, pleuritic chest pain, halitosis, inspiratory crackles, and tubular or amphoric breath sounds. The patient's chest is dull on percussion on the affected side.

• *Lung cancer.* One of the earliest signs

PRODUCTIVE COUGH: CAUSES AND ASSOCIATED FINDINGS

S&S CAUSES	MAJOR ASSOCIATED SIGNS AND SYMPTOMS												
	Chest pain	Crackles	Cyanosis	Decreased breath sounds	Dyspnea	Fatigue	Fever	Rhonchi	Sore throat	Tachycardia	Tachypnea	Weight loss	Wheezes
Actinomycosis	●				●	●	●					●	
Aspiration pneumonitis			●		●		●			●	●		●
Asthma (acute)	●	●	●		●			●		●	●		●
Bronchiectasis		●			●	●	●	●				●	●
Bronchitis (chronic)		●	●		●			●			●		●
Chemical pneumonitis		●			●		●						●
Common cold						●			●				
Legionnaire's disease	●	●			●	●	●			●	●		
Lung abscess	●	●			●	●	●					●	
Lung cancer	●				●	●	●					●	●
Nocardiosis	●			●	●	●						●	
North American blastomycosis	●					●	●					●	
Pneumonia (bacterial)	●	●	●	●	●		●	●		●	●		
Pneumonia (mycoplasma)	●	●					●		●				
Psittacosis	●	●					●			●			
Pulmonary coccidioidomycosis	●						●	●	●				●
Pulmonary edema		●	●		●	●	●			●	●		

(continued)

PRODUCTIVE COUGH: CAUSES AND ASSOCIATED FINDINGS (continued)

CAUSES	Chest pain	Crackles	Cyanosis	Decreased breath sounds	Dyspnea	Fatigue	Fever	Rhonchi	Sore throat	Tachycardia	Tachypnea	Weight loss	Wheezes
Pulmonary embolism	●	●	●	●	●		●			●	●		●
Pulmonary emphysema				●	●		●				●	●	
Pulmonary tuberculosis	●	●			●	●						●	
Silicosis		●			●	●					●	●	
Tracheobronchitis	●	●						●	●	●			●

of bronchogenic carcinoma is a chronic cough that produces small amounts of purulent (or mucopurulent), blood-streaked sputum. In a patient with bronchioalveolar cancer, however, coughing produces large amounts of frothy sputum. Other signs and symptoms include dyspnea, anorexia, fatigue, weight loss, chest pain, fever, diaphoresis, wheezing, and clubbing.

• *Nocardiosis.* This disorder causes a productive cough (with purulent, thick, tenacious, and possibly blood-tinged sputum) and fever that may last several months. Other findings include night sweats, pleuritic pain, anorexia, malaise, fatigue, weight loss, and diminished or absent breath sounds. The patient's chest is dull on percussion.

• *North American blastomycosis.* In this chronic disorder, coughing is dry and hacking or productive of bloody or purulent sputum. Other findings are pleuritic chest pain, fever, chills, anorexia, weight loss, malaise, fatigue, night sweats, cutaneous lesions (small, painless, nonpruritic macules or papules), and prostration.

• *Pneumonia.* Bacterial pneumonias initially produce a dry cough that becomes productive. Rust-colored sputum occurs in pneumococcal pneumonia; "brick red" or "currant jelly" sputum in *Klebsiella* pneumonia; salmon-colored sputum in staphylococcal pneumonia; or mucopurulent sputum in streptococcal pneumonia. Associated signs and symptoms develop suddenly—there may be shaking chills, high fever, myalgias, headache, pleuritic chest pain that increases with chest movement, tachypnea, tachycardia, dyspnea, cyanosis, diaphoresis, decreased breath sounds, fine crackles, and rhonchi.

Mycoplasma pneumonia may cause a cough that produces scant, blood-flecked sputum. Most common, however, is a nonproductive cough that starts 2 to 3 days after the onset of malaise, headache, fever, and sore throat. Paroxysmal coughing causes substernal chest pain. Patients may have crackles, but generally don't appear seriously ill.

• **Psittacosis.** As this disorder progresses, the characteristic hacking cough, nonproductive at first, may later produce a small amount of mucoid, blood-streaked sputum. The infection may begin abruptly, with chills, fever, headache, myalgias, and prostration. Other signs and symptoms may include tachypnea, fine crackles, chest pain (rare), epistaxis, photophobia, abdominal distention and tenderness, nausea, vomiting, and a faint macular rash. Severe infection may produce stupor, delirium, and coma.

• **Pulmonary coccidioidomycosis.** This disorder causes a nonproductive or slightly productive cough with fever, occasional chills, pleuritic chest pain, sore throat, headache, backache, malaise, marked weakness, anorexia, hemoptysis, and an itchy macular rash. Rhonchi and wheezing may be heard. The disease may spread to other areas, causing arthralgia, swelling of the knees and ankles, and erythema nodosum or erythema multiforme.

• **Pulmonary edema.** When severe, this life-threatening disorder causes coughing productive of frothy, bloody sputum. Early signs and symptoms include dyspnea on exertion; paroxysmal nocturnal dyspnea, then orthopnea; and coughing, which may be initially nonproductive. Other clinical features include fever, fatigue, tachycardia, tachypnea, dependent crackles, and ventricular gallop. As the patient's respirations become increasingly rapid and labored, he develops more diffuse crackles and the productive cough, his tachycardia increases, and dysrhythmias may appear. His skin becomes cold, clammy, and cyanotic; his blood pressure falls; and his pulse becomes thready.

• **Pulmonary embolism.** This life-threatening disorder causes a cough that may be nonproductive or may produce blood-tinged sputum. Usually, the first symptom of pulmonary embolism is severe dyspnea, which may be accompanied by anginal or pleuritic chest pain. The patient has marked anxiety, a low-grade fever, tachycardia, tachypnea, and diaphoresis. Less common signs include massive hemoptysis, chest splinting, leg edema, and (with a large embolus) cyanosis, syncope, and distended neck veins. The patient may also have a pleural friction rub, diffuse wheezing, crackles, chest dullness on percussion, decreased breath sounds, and signs of circulatory collapse.

• **Pulmonary emphysema.** This disorder causes minimal chronic productive cough with scant, mucoid, translucent, grayish white sputum that can become mucopurulent. The patient is thin and has the characteristic "pink puffer" appearance with weight loss, increased accessory muscle use, tachypnea, grunting expirations through pursed lips, diminished breath sounds, exertional dyspnea, rhonchi, barrel chest, and anorexia. Clubbing is a late sign.

• **Pulmonary tuberculosis.** This disorder causes a mild-to-severe productive cough along with some combination of hemoptysis, malaise, dyspnea, and pleuritic chest pain. Sputum may be scant and mucoid or copious and purulent. Typically, the patient experiences night sweats, easy fatigability, and weight loss. His breath sounds are amphoric. He may have chest dullness on percussion and, after coughing, increased tactile fremitus with crackles.

• **Silicosis.** Productive cough with mucopurulent sputum is the earliest sign of this disorder. The patient also has exertional dyspnea, tachypnea, weight loss, fatigue, general weakness, and recurrent respiratory infections. Auscultation reveals end-inspiratory, fine crackles at the lung bases.

• **Tracheobronchitis.** Inflammation initially causes a nonproductive cough that later—following onset of chills, sore throat, slight fever, muscle and back pain, and substernal tightness—

becomes productive as secretions increase. Sputum is mucoid, mucopurulent, or purulent. The patient typically has rhonchi and wheezes; he may also have crackles. Severe tracheobronchitis may cause fever of 101° to 102° F. (38.3° to 38.8 °C.) and bronchospasm.

Other causes

• **Diagnostic tests.** Bronchoscopy and pulmonary function tests may increase productive coughing.
• **Drugs.** Expectorants, of course, increase productive coughing. These include ammonium chloride, calcium iodide, guaifenesin, iodinated glycerol, potassium iodide, and terpin hydrate.
• **Respiratory therapy.** Intermittent positive pressure breathing (IPPB) and incentive spirometry often loosen secretions and cause or increase productive cough.

Special considerations

Avoid taking measures to suppress a productive cough, because retention of sputum may interfere with alveolar aeration or impair pulmonary resistance to infection. Expect to give mucolytics and expectorants, and increase the patient's intake of oral fluids to thin his secretions and increase their flow. You may also give a bronchodilator to relieve bronchospasms and open airways. Antibiotics may be ordered to treat underlying infection.

Humidify the air around the patient; this will relieve mucous membrane inflammation and also help loosen dried secretions. As ordered, provide pulmonary physiotherapy, such as postural drainage with vibration and percussion to loosen secretions. You may also be asked to provide respiratory therapy, such as IPPB.

Provide the patient with uninterrupted rest periods. Keep him from using aerosols, powders, or other respiratory irritants. Also encourage the patient not to smoke, if possible, because it can aggravate his condition.

Teach the patient how to deep breathe, to cough effectively, and, if appropriate, to splint his incision when he coughs. Tell him to sit or stand upright when coughing, if possible, to facilitate maximum chest expansion. If he's confined to bed rest, change his position often to promote drainage of secretions. Tell the patient to cover his mouth and nose with a tissue when he coughs and to dispose of contaminated tissues properly, to protect himself and others from the cough and secretions. Provide a container for tissues and sputum.

Prepare the patient for diagnostic tests, such as chest X-ray, bronchoscopy, a lung scan, and pulmonary function tests. Collect sputum samples, as ordered, for culture and sensitivity testing.

Pediatric pointers

Because his airway is narrow, a child with a productive cough can quickly develop airway occlusion and respiratory distress from thick or excessive secretions. Causes of productive cough in children include asthma, bronchiectasis, bronchitis, acute bronchiolitis, cystic fibrosis, and pertussis.

When caring for a child with a productive cough, administer expectorants, as ordered, but don't expect to give cough suppressants. To soothe inflamed mucous membranes and prevent drying of secretions, provide humidified air or oxygen. Remember, high humidity can induce bronchospasm in a hyperactive child or overhydration in an infant.

Crackles

[Rales; crepitations]

A common finding in certain cardiovascular and pulmonary disorders, crackles are nonmusical clicking or rattling noises heard during auscultation of breath sounds. They usually occur during inspiration and recur con-

HOW CRACKLES OCCUR

Crackles occur when air passes through fluid-filled airways, causing collapsed alveoli to pop open as airway pressure equalizes. They can also occur when membranes lining the chest cavity and the lungs become inflamed. The illustrations below show a normal alveolus and two pathologic alveolar changes, which cause crackles.

Normal alveolus

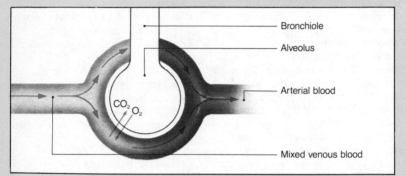

Bronchiole
Alveolus
Arterial blood
CO_2 O_2
Mixed venous blood

Alveolus in pulmonary edema

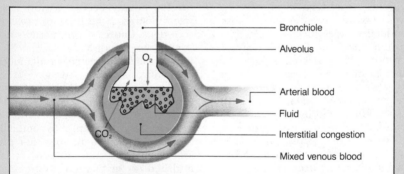

Bronchiole
Alveolus
O_2
Arterial blood
Fluid
CO_2
Interstitial congestion
Mixed venous blood

Alveolus in inflammation

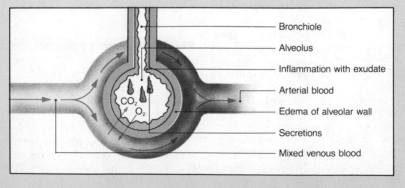

Bronchiole
Alveolus
Inflammation with exudate
Arterial blood
CO_2
Edema of alveolar wall
O_2
Secretions
Mixed venous blood

stantly from one respiratory cycle to the next. They can be unilateral or bilateral, moist or dry. They're characterized by their pitch, loudness, occurrence during the respiratory cycle, location, and persistence.

Crackles indicate abnormal movement of air through fluid-filled airways. They can be irregularly dispersed, as in pneumonia, or localized, as in bronchiectasis. (A few basilar crackles can be heard in normal lungs after prolonged shallow breathing. These normal crackles clear with a few deep breaths.) Usually, though, crackles indicate the degree of an underlying illness. When crackles result from a generalized disorder, they usually occur in the less distended and more dependent areas of the lungs, such as the lung bases when the patient is standing. Crackles due to air passing through inflammatory exudate may not be audible if the involved portion of the lung isn't being ventilated because of shallow respirations.

Assessment

Quickly take the patient's vital signs and assess for signs of respiratory distress or airway obstruction. Check the depth and rhythm of his respirations. Is he struggling to breathe? Check for increased accessory muscle use and chest wall motion, retractions, stridor, or nasal flaring. Provide supplemental oxygen, and be prepared to assist with endotracheal intubation, if necessary.

If the patient also has a cough, ask when it began and if it's constant or intermittent. Find out what the cough sounds like, too, and whether the patient is coughing up sputum or blood. If the cough is productive, determine the sputum's consistency, amount, odor, and color.

Ask the patient if he has any pain. If so, where is it located? When did he first notice it? Does it radiate to other areas? Also ask the patient if movement, coughing, or breathing worsens or helps relieve his pain. Note the pa-

tient's position: Is he lying still or moving about restlessly?

Obtain a brief medical history. Does the patient have cancer or any known respiratory or cardiovascular problems? Ask about recent surgery, trauma, or illness, and ask the patient if he has hoarseness or difficulty swallowing. Find out what medications the patient is taking, and ask about tobacco and alcohol use. Also ask about recent weight loss, anorexia, nausea, vomiting, fatigue, weakness, vertigo, and syncope. Has the patient been exposed to irritants, such as vapors, fumes, or smoke?

Now perform a physical examination. Examine the patient's nose and mouth for signs of infection, such as inflammation or increased secretions. Note his breath odor: Halitosis could indicate pulmonary infection. Check his neck for masses, tenderness, swelling, lymphadenopathy, or venous distention.

Inspect the patient's chest for abnormal configuration or uneven expansion. Percuss for dullness, tympany, or flatness. Auscultate his lungs for other abnormal, diminished, or absent breath sounds. Listen to his heart for abnormal sounds, and check his hands and feet for edema or clubbing.

Medical causes

• *Adult respiratory distress syndrome (ARDS).* A life-threatening disorder, ARDS causes diffuse, fine-to-coarse crackles usually heard in the dependent portions of the lungs. It also produces cyanosis, nasal flaring, tachypnea, tachycardia, grunting respirations, rhonchi, dyspnea, anxiety, and decreased level of consciousness.

• *Asthma.* A severe attack usually occurs at night or during sleep, causing dry, whistling crackles. An attack typically starts with a dry cough and mild wheezing, then progresses to severe dyspnea, audible wheezing, chest tightness, and productive cough. Other possible findings: apprehension, prolonged expirations, rhonchi, intercostal and supraclavicular retraction on inspiration, accessory muscle use, flaring nostrils, tachypnea, tachycardia, diaphoresis, and flushing or cyanosis.

● *Bronchiectasis.* In this disorder, persistent, coarse crackles are heard over the affected area of the lung. They're accompanied by a chronic cough that produces copious amounts of mucopurulent sputum. Other characteristics include halitosis, occasional wheezes, exertional dyspnea, rhonchi, weight loss, fatigue, malaise, weakness, recurrent fever, and late-stage clubbing.

● *Bronchitis (chronic).* This disorder causes coarse crackles that are usually heard at the lung bases. Prolonged expirations, wheezing, rhonchi, exertional dyspnea, tachypnea, and persistent, productive cough occur because of increased bronchial secretions. Clubbing and cyanosis may occur.

● *Chemical pneumonitis.* In acute chemical pneumonitis, diffuse, fine-to-coarse, moist crackles accompany a productive cough with purulent sputum, dyspnea, wheezing, orthopnea, fever, malaise, and mucous membrane irritation. Signs and symptoms may worsen for 24 to 48 hours after exposure, then resolve; if severe, however, they may recur 2 to 5 weeks later.

● *Interstitial fibrosis of the lungs.* In this disorder, cellophane-like crackles can be heard over all lobes. As the disease progresses, nonproductive cough, dyspnea, fatigue, weight loss, cyanosis, and pleuritic chest pain develop.

● *Legionnaire's disease.* This disorder produces diffuse moist crackles and cough productive of scant mucoid, nonpurulent, possibly blood-streaked sputum. Usually, prodromal signs and symptoms occur: malaise, fatigue, weakness, anorexia, diffuse myalgias, and possibly diarrhea. Within 12 to 48 hours, the patient develops a dry cough and a sudden high fever with chills. He may also have pleuritic chest pain, headache, tachypnea, tachycardia, nausea, vomiting, dyspnea, mild temporary amnesia, confusion, flushing, mild diaphoresis, and prostration.

● *Lung abscess.* This disorder produces fine-to-medium and moist inspiratory crackles. Onset is insidious; signs and symptoms include sweats, anorexia, weight loss, fever, fatigue, weakness, dyspnea, clubbing, pleuritic chest pain, pleural friction rub, and cough productive of copious amounts of foul-smelling, purulent sputum that may be blood-tinged. The patient's breath sounds are hollow and tubular or amphoric; the affected side of his chest is dull on percussion.

● *Pneumonia. Bacterial pneumonia* produces diffuse fine crackles, sudden onset of shaking chills, high fever, tachypnea, pleuritic chest pain, cyanosis, grunting respirations, nasal flaring, decreased breath sounds, myalgias, headache, tachycardia, dyspnea, cyanosis, diaphoresis, and rhonchi. The patient has a dry cough that later becomes productive.

Mycoplasma pneumonia produces medium-to-fine crackles together with a nonproductive cough, malaise, sore throat, headache, and fever. The patient may have blood-flecked sputum.

Viral pneumonia causes gradually developing, diffuse crackles. The patient may also have a nonproductive cough, malaise, headache, anorexia, low-grade fever, and decreased breath sounds.

● *Psittacosis.* As this disorder progresses, diffuse fine crackles may be heard. Accompanying findings include a characteristic hacking, productive cough, chills, fever, headache, myalgias, and prostration. Other features may include tachypnea, chest pain (rare), epistaxis, photophobia, abdominal distention and tenderness, nausea, vomiting, and a faint macular rash.

● *Pulmonary edema.* Moist, bubbling crackles on inspiration are one of the first signs of this life-threatening disorder. Other early findings include dyspnea on exertion; paroxysmal nocturnal dyspnea, then orthopnea; and coughing, which may be initially nonproductive but later produces frothy, bloody sputum. Related clinical effects

CRACKLES: CAUSES AND ASSOCIATED FINDINGS

CAUSES	Chest pain	Cough	Cyanosis	Dyspnea	Fatigue	Fever	Hemoptysis	Rhonchi	Tachycardia	Tachypnea	Vomiting	Weakness	Weight loss
ARDS			●	●				●	●	●			
Asthma (acute)	●	●	●	●				●	●	●			
Bronchiectasis		●		●	●	●		●				●	●
Bronchitis (chronic)		●	●	●				●		●			
Chemical pneumonitis		●		●		●							
Interstitial fibrosis	●	●	●	●	●								●
Legionnaire's disease	●	●		●	●	●	●		●	●	●	●	
Lung abscess	●	●		●	●	●	●					●	●
Pneumonia (bacterial)	●	●	●	●		●		●	●	●			
Pneumonia (mycoplasma)		●				●	●						
Pneumonia (viral)		●				●							
Psittacosis	●	●				●				●	●		
Pulmonary edema		●	●	●			●		●	●			
Pulmonary embolism	●	●	●	●		●	●		●	●			
Pulmonary tuberculosis	●	●		●	●		●					●	●
Sarcoidosis		●		●	●				●			●	●
Silicosis		●		●	●				●			●	●
Tracheobronchitis	●	●				●		●					

include tachycardia, tachypnea, and S_3 gallop. As the patient's respirations become increasingly rapid and labored, he develops more diffuse crackles, worsening tachycardia, hypotension, a rapid and thready pulse, cyanosis, and cold, clammy skin.

• *Pulmonary embolism.* This life-threatening disorder can cause fine-to-coarse crackles and a cough that may be dry or productive of blood-tinged sputum. Usually, the first sign of pulmonary embolism is severe dyspnea, which may be accompanied by anginal or pleuritic chest pain. The patient has marked anxiety, a low-grade fever, tachycardia, tachypnea, and diaphoresis. Less common signs include massive hemoptysis, chest splinting, leg edema, and (with a large embolus) cyanosis, syncope, and distended neck veins. The patient may also have a pleural friction rub, diffuse wheezing, chest dullness on percussion, decreased breath sounds, and signs of circulatory collapse.

• *Pulmonary tuberculosis.* In this disorder, fine crackles occur after coughing. The patient has some combination of hemoptysis, malaise, dyspnea, and pleuritic chest pain. Sputum may be scant and mucoid or copious and purulent. Typically, the patient experiences night sweats, easy fatigue, weakness, and weight loss. His breath sounds are amphoric.

• *Sarcoidosis.* This disorder produces fine, bibasilar, end-inspiratory crackles and (rarely) wheezes. The patient doesn't have a fever, but he does have malaise, fatigue, weakness, weight loss, cough, dyspnea, and tachypnea.

• *Silicosis.* This disorder produces end-inspiratory, fine crackles heard at the lung bases. It also causes a productive cough with mucopurulent sputum— the earliest sign of this disorder. The patient also has exertional dyspnea, tachypnea, weight loss, fatigue, general weakness, and recurrent respiratory infections.

• *Tracheobronchitis.* In its acute form, this disorder produces moist or coarse crackles along with a productive cough, chills, sore throat, slight fever, muscle and back pain, and substernal tightness. The patient typically has rhonchi and wheezes. Severe tracheobronchitis may cause moderate fever and bronchospasm.

Special considerations

To keep the patient's airway patent, elevate the head of his bed to facilitate his breathing. To liquefy thick secretions and relieve mucous membrane inflammation, administer fluids, humidified air, or oxygen, as ordered. Turn the patient every 1 to 2 hours, and encourage him to breathe deeply. Teach him how to cough effectively and to splint incision areas, if appropriate. Encourage him to avoid smoking and using aerosols, powders, or other products that might irritate his airway. Plan daily uninterrupted rest periods to help him relax and sleep. And check his vital signs frequently until his condition is stable.

Prepare the patient for diagnostic tests, such as chest X-rays, a lung scan, and sputum analysis.

Pediatric pointers

Infants and children can rapidly develop airway occlusion because of their narrow airways. They also develop fatigue from dyspnea sooner than adults and may have more rapid onset and progression of disease.

Crackles in an infant or child may indicate a serious cardiovascular or respiratory disorder. *Pneumonias* produce diffuse, sudden crackles in children. *Esophageal atresia* and *tracheoesophageal fistula* can cause bubbling, moist crackles due to aspiration of food or secretions into the lungs—especially in newborn infants. *Pulmonary edema* causes fine crackles at the bases of the lungs, and *bronchiectasis* produces moist crackles. *Cystic fibrosis* produces widespread, fine-to-coarse inspiratory crackles and wheezing in infants. And *sickle cell anemia* may produce crackles when it causes pulmonary infarction or infection.

Crepitation—Bony

[Bony crepitus]

Bony crepitation is a palpable vibration or an audible crunching sound that results when one bone grates against another. It often results from a fracture. Or it can happen when bones that have been stripped of their protective articular cartilage grind against each other as they articulate—for example, in advanced arthritic or degenerative joint disorders.

Eliciting bony crepitation can help confirm diagnosis of a fracture. But it can also cause further soft tissue, nerve, or vessel injury. What's more, rubbing fractured bone ends together can convert a closed fracture into an open one if a bone end penetrates the skin. So, after initial detection of crepitation in a patient with a fracture, avoid subsequent elicitation of this sign.

Assessment

If you detect bony crepitation in a patient with a suspected fracture, ask him if he feels any pain and if he can point to the painful area. Immobilize the affected area by applying a splint to prevent lacerating nerves, blood vessels, or other structures. Elevate the affected area, if possible, and apply cold packs. Ask the patient or his companion to describe how and when the injury occurred. Inspect the affected area for abrasions or lacerations. Palpate pulses distal to the injury site, and check the skin for pallor or coolness. Also test motor and sensory function distal to the injury site.

If the patient doesn't have a suspected fracture, ask about a history of osteoarthritis or rheumatoid arthritis. Ask what medications he takes: Has any medication helped ease arthritic discomfort? Take the patient's vital signs and test range of motion.

Medical causes

● *Fracture.* Besides bony crepitation, a fracture also causes acute local pain, edema, and decreased range of motion. Other findings may include deformity, point tenderness, discoloration of the limb, and loss of limb function. Neurovascular damage may cause prolonged capillary refill time, diminished or absent pulses, mottled cyanosis, paresthesias, and decreased sensation (all distal to the fracture site). An open fracture, of course, produces an obvious skin wound.

● *Osteoarthritis.* In advanced cases of this disorder, joint crepitation may be elicited during range-of-motion testing. The cardinal symptom of osteoarthritis is joint pain, especially during motion and weight bearing. Other findings include joint stiffness that typically occurs after resting and subsides within a few minutes after the patient begins moving.

● *Rheumatoid arthritis.* In advanced cases of this disorder, bony crepitation is heard when the affected joint is rotated. However, rheumatoid arthritis usually develops insidiously, producing nonspecific signs and symptoms such as fatigue, malaise, anorexia, a persistent low-grade fever, weight loss, lymphadenopathy, and vague arthralgias and myalgias. Then, more specific and localized articular signs develop, frequently at the proximal finger joints. These signs usually occur bilaterally and symmetrically and may extend to the wrists, knees, elbows, and ankles. The affected joints stiffen after inactivity. The patient also has increased warmth, swelling, and tenderness of affected joints, and limited range of motion.

Special considerations

If a fracture is suspected, prepare the patient for X-rays of the affected area, and reassess his neurovascular status frequently. Keep the affected part immobilized and elevated until treatment is begun. Give analgesics, as ordered, to relieve pain.

Pediatric pointers
Bony crepitation in a child usually occurs after a fracture. Obtain an accurate history of the injury, and be alert for the possibility of child abuse. In a teenager, bony crepitation and pain in the patellofemoral joint help diagnose chondromalacia of the patella.

Crepitation— Subcutaneous
[Subcutaneous crepitus]

When bubbles of air or other gases (such as carbon dioxide) are trapped in subcutaneous tissue, palpation or stroking of the skin produces a crackling sound called subcutaneous crepitation. The bubbles feel like small, unstable nodules and aren't painful, even though subcutaneous crepitation is often associated with painful disorders. Usually, the affected tissue is visibly edematous—this can lead to life-threatening airway occlusion if the edema affects the neck or upper chest.

The air or gas bubbles enter the tissues through open wounds, from the action of anaerobic microorganisms, or from traumatic or spontaneous rupture or perforation of pulmonary or gastrointestinal organs.

Assessment
Because subcutaneous crepitation can indicate a life-threatening disorder, you'll need to perform a rapid initial assessment. (See *Managing Subcutaneous Crepitation.*)

When the patient's condition permits, palpate the affected skin to evaluate the location and extent of subcutaneous crepitation and to obtain baseline information. Repalpate frequently to determine if the subcutaneous crepitation is increasing. Ask the patient if he's experiencing any pain. If he is, find out where the pain is located, how severe it is, and when it began. Ask about recent thoracic surgery, diagnostic tests, respiratory therapy, or a history of trauma or chronic pulmonary disease.

Medical causes
● *Gas gangrene.* Subcutaneous crepitation is the hallmark of this rare but often fatal infection. It's accompanied by local pain, swelling, and discoloration, with formation of bullae and necrosis. The skin over the wound may rupture, revealing dark red or black necrotic muscle and producing foul-smelling watery or frothy discharge. Related findings include tachycardia, tachypnea, moderate fever, cyanosis, and lassitude.

● *Orbital fracture.* This fracture allows air from the nasal sinuses to escape into subcutaneous tissue, causing subcutaneous crepitations of the eyelid and orbit. The most common sign of orbital fracture is periorbital ecchymosis. Visual acuity is usually normal, although a swollen lid may prevent accurate testing. The patient has facial edema, diplopia, a hyphema or, occasionally, a dilated or unreactive pupil on the affected side.

● *Pneumothorax.* Severe pneumothorax produces subcutaneous crepitation in the upper chest and neck. Often, the patient has chest pain that is unilateral, rarely localized initially, and increased on inspiration. Dyspnea, anxiety, restlessness, tachypnea, cyanosis, tachycardia, accessory muscle use, and asymmetrical chest expansion can also occur, as well as a nonproductive cough. On the affected side, breath sounds are absent or decreased, hyperresonance or tympany may be heard, and decreased vocal fremitus may be present.

● *Rupture of the esophagus.* A ruptured esophagus usually produces subcutaneous crepitation in the neck, chest wall, or supraclavicular fossa, although this sign doesn't always occur. In rupture of the *cervical esophagus*, the patient has excruciating pain in the neck or supraclavicular area, his neck is resistant to passive motion, and he has local tenderness, soft tissue swelling, dysphagia, odynophagia, and orthostatic vertigo.

Life-threatening rupture of the *intrathoracic esophagus* can produce mediastinal emphysema confirmed by a positive Hamman's sign. The patient has severe retrosternal, epigastric, neck, or scapular pain and edema of the chest wall and neck. He may also display dyspnea, tachypnea, asymmetrical chest expansion, nasal flaring, cyanosis, diaphoresis, tachycardia, hypotension, dysphagia, and fever.

● **Rupture of the trachea or major bronchus.** This life-threatening injury produces abrupt subcutaneous crepitation of the neck and anterior chest wall. The patient has severe dyspnea with nasal flaring, tachycardia, accessory muscle use, hypotension, cyanosis, extreme anxiety, and possibly hemoptysis and mediastinal emphysema, with a positive Hamman's sign.

Other causes

● *Diagnostic tests.* Endoscopic tests, such as bronchoscopy, can cause rupture or perforation of respiratory or GI organs, producing subcutaneous crepitation.

● *Respiratory treatments.* Mechanical ventilation and intermittent positive pressure breathing can rupture alveoli, producing subcutaneous crepitation.

● *Thoracic surgery.* If air escapes into the tissue in the area of the incision, subcutaneous crepitation can occur.

Special considerations

Monitor the patient's vital signs frequently, especially respirations. Because excessive edema from subcutaneous crepitation in the neck and upper chest can cause airway obstruction, be alert for signs of respiratory distress, such as dyspnea. Tell the patient that

EMERGENCY

MANAGING SUBCUTANEOUS CREPITATION

Subcutaneous crepitation occurs when air or gas bubbles escape into tissues. It may signal life-threatening rupture of an air-filled or gas-producing organ, or may indicate sepsis due to a fulminating anaerobic infection.

● *Organ rupture.* If the patient shows signs of respiratory distress—such as severe dyspnea, tachypnea, accessory muscle use, nasal flaring, air hunger, or tachycardia—have another nurse notify the doctor while you quickly test for Hamman's sign to detect trapped air bubbles in the mediastinum.

To test for Hamman's sign, help the patient assume a left-lateral recumbent position. Then, place your stethoscope over the precordium. If you hear a loud crunching sound that synchronizes with his heartbeat, the patient has a positive Hamman's sign. Depending on which organ is ruptured, be prepared to assist with endotracheal intubation, emergency tracheotomy, or chest tube insertion. Immediately start administering supplemental oxygen. Start an I.V. to administer fluids and medication, and connect the patient to a cardiac monitor.

● *Anaerobic infection.* If the patient has an open wound with a foul odor and local swelling and discoloration, you must act quickly. First, have another nurse immediately notify the doctor. Then, take the patient's vital signs, checking especially for fever, tachycardia, hypotension, and tachypnea. Next, start an I.V. to administer fluids and medication, provide supplemental oxygen, and be prepared to assist with emergency surgery to drain and debride the wound. If the patient's condition is life-threatening, you may need to prepare him for transfer to a facility with a hyperbaric chamber.

the affected tissues will eventually absorb the air or gas bubbles, so the subcutaneous crepitation will decrease.

Pediatric pointers

Children may develop subcutaneous crepitation in the neck from ingestion of corrosive substances that perforate the esophagus.

Cry—High-Pitched

[Cerebral cry]

A high-pitched cry is a brief, sharp, piercing vocal sound produced by a neonate or infant. Whether acute or chronic, this cry is a late sign of increased intracranial pressure (ICP). However, the acute onset of a high-pitched cry demands emergency treatment to prevent permanent brain damage or death.

Any change in the volume of one of the brain's components—brain tissue, cerebrospinal fluid, and blood—may cause increased ICP. In the neonate, increased ICP may result from intracranial bleeding associated with birth trauma or from congenital malformation, such as craniostenosis and Arnold-Chiari syndrome. In fact, a high-pitched cry may be an early sign of congenital malformation. In the infant, increased ICP may result from meningitis or head trauma.

Assessment

If an infant suddenly produces a high-pitched cry, have another nurse notify the doctor immediately. Take the infant's vital signs, then obtain a brief history. Has the infant fallen recently or experienced even minor head trauma? Ask the mother about any changes in his behavior during the past 24 hours. Has he seemed restless or unlike himself? Has his sucking reflex diminished? Does he cry when moved about?

Next perform a neurologic examination. Remember that neurologic responses in the neonate and young infant are primarily reflex responses. Assess the infant's level of consciousness. Is he awake, irritable, or lethargic? Does he reach for an attractive object or turn toward the sound of a rattle? Observe his posture. Is he in the normal flexed position or in extension or opisthotonos? Examine muscle tone and observe for signs of seizure, such as tremors and twitching.

Now examine the size and shape of the infant's head. Is the anterior fontanelle bulging? Measure head circumference and check pupillary size and response to light. Unilateral or bilateral dilation and sluggish response to light may accompany increased ICP. Also note setting sun sign. Finally, test reflexes; expect Moro's reflex to be diminished.

After completing your assessment, elevate the infant's head to promote cerebral venous drainage and decrease ICP. Start an I.V. and, if ordered, give diuretics and corticosteroids to decrease ICP. Keep endotracheal intubation equipment close by to secure an airway.

Medical cause

• *Increased ICP.* High-pitched cry is a late sign of increased ICP. Typically, the infant also displays bulging fontanelles, increased head circumference, and widened sutures. Earlier signs and symptoms of increasing pressure include seizures, bradycardia, possible vomiting, dilated pupils, decreased level of consciousness, increased systolic blood pressure, widened pulse pressure, and altered respiratory pattern.

Special considerations

The infant with increased ICP requires specialized care and monitoring in the intensive care unit. For example, you'll need to monitor his vital signs and neurologic status to detect subtle changes in his condition. Also monitor intake and output. If ordered, monitor ICP, restrict fluids, and administer diuretics and corticosteroids. For an infant with severely increased ICP, the doctor may order endotracheal intubation and mechanical hyperventilation to decrease serum carbon dioxide (PCO_2) and constrict cerebral blood vessels, or barbiturate coma or hypothermia therapy to decrease the infant's metabolic rate.

Remember to avoid jostling the infant, which may aggravate increased ICP. Comfort the infant and maintain a calm, quiet environment, since the infant's crying or exposure to environmental stimuli may also worsen increased ICP.

Cyanosis

Cyanosis—a bluish or bluish black discoloration of the skin and mucous membranes—results from excessive concentration of unoxygenated hemoglobin in the blood. This common sign may develop abruptly or gradually. It can be classified as central or peripheral, although the two types may exist together.

Central cyanosis reflects inadequate oxygenation of systemic arterial blood caused by right-to-left cardiac shunting or pulmonary disease, or by hematologic disorders. It may occur anywhere on the skin and also on the mucous membranes of the mouth, lips, and conjunctiva.

Peripheral cyanosis reflects sluggish peripheral circulation caused by vasoconstriction, reduced cardiac output, or vascular occlusion. It may be widespread or may occur locally in one extremity; however, it doesn't affect mucous membranes. Typically, peripheral cyanosis appears on exposed areas, such as the fingers, nail beds, feet, nose, and ears.

Although cyanosis is an important sign of cardiovascular and pulmonary disorders, it isn't always an accurate gauge of oxygenation. Several factors contribute to its development: hemoglobin concentration and oxygen saturation, cardiac output, and PO_2. Cyanosis is usually undetectable until the oxygen saturation of hemoglobin falls below 80%. Severe cyanosis is quite obvious, whereas mild cyanosis is more difficult to detect—even in natural, bright light. In dark-skinned patients, cyanosis is most apparent in the mucous membranes and nail beds.

A transient, nonpathologic cyanosis may result from environmental factors. For example, peripheral cyanosis may result from cutaneous vasoconstriction following brief exposure to cold air or water. Central cyanosis may result from reduced PO_2 at high altitudes.

Assessment

If the patient displays sudden, localized cyanosis and other signs of arterial occlusion, you'll need to protect the affected limb from injury; however, do not massage the limb. Or, if you see central cyanosis stemming from a pulmonary disorder or shock, perform a rapid assessment. Then take immediate steps to maintain an airway, assist breathing, and monitor circulation.

If cyanosis accompanies less acute conditions, perform a thorough assessment. First review the patient's history, focusing on cardiac, pulmonary, and hematologic disorders. Also ask about previous surgery. Then begin the physical examination by taking vital signs. Inspect the skin and mucous membranes to determine the extent of cyanosis. Ask the patient when he first noticed the cyanosis. Does it subside and recur? Is it aggravated by cold, smoking, or stress? Alleviated by massage or rewarming? Check for cool, pallid skin, redness, and ulceration. Also note clubbing.

Next assess the patient's level of consciousness. Ask about headache, dizziness, or blurred vision. Then test the patient's motor strength. Also ask about pain in the arms and legs (especially with walking) and about abnormal sensations (numbness, tingling, or coldness).

Ask about chest pain and its severity. Can the patient identify any aggravating and alleviating factors? Palpate peripheral pulses and test capillary refill time. Also note edema. Auscultate heart rate and rhythm, noting especially gallops and murmurs. Also auscultate the abdominal aorta and femoral arteries to allow detection of any bruits.

Ask about a cough. Is it productive? If so, have the patient describe the sputum. Assess respiratory rate and rhythm, and check for nasal flaring and use of accessory muscles. Ask about nocturnal dyspnea. Does the patient sleep with his head propped up on pillows? Inspect for asymmetrical chest expansion or barrel chest. Percuss the lungs for dullness or hyperresonance, and auscultate for decreased or adventitious breath sounds.

Inspect the abdomen for ascites, and test for shifting dullness or fluid wave. Percuss and palpate for liver enlargement and tenderness. Also ask about nausea, anorexia, and weight loss.

Medical causes

• *Arteriosclerotic occlusive disease (chronic).* In this disorder, peripheral cyanosis occurs in the legs whenever they're in a dependent position. Associated signs and symptoms include intermittent claudication and burning pain at rest, paresthesias, pallor, muscle atrophy, weak leg pulses, and impotence. Late signs are leg ulcers and gangrene.

• *Bronchiectasis.* This disorder produces chronic central cyanosis. Its classic sign, though, is chronic productive cough with copious, foul-smelling, mucopurulent sputum or hemoptysis. Auscultation reveals rhonchi and coarse rales during inspiration. Other features are dyspnea, recurrent fever and chills, weight loss, malaise, clubbing, and signs of anemia.

• *Buerger's disease.* In this disorder, exposure to cold initially causes the feet to become cold, cyanotic, and numb; later, they redden, become hot, and tingle. Intermittent claudication of the instep is characteristic; it's aggravated by exercise and relieved by rest. Associated clinical features include weak peripheral pulses and, in later stages, ulceration, muscle atrophy, and gangrene.

• *Chronic obstructive pulmonary disease (COPD).* Chronic central cyanosis oc-

curs with this disorder and may be aggravated by exertion. Associated signs and symptoms include exertional dyspnea, productive cough with thick sputum, anorexia, weight loss, purse-lipped breathing, tachypnea, and use of accessory muscles. Examination reveals wheezes and hyperresonant lung fields. Barrel chest and clubbing are late signs. Tachycardia, diaphoresis, and flushing may also accompany this disorder.

• *Congestive heart failure.* Acute or chronic cyanosis may occur. Typically, it's a late sign and may be central, peripheral, or both. In left heart failure, central cyanosis occurs with tachycardia, fatigue, dyspnea, cold intolerance, orthopnea, cough, ventricular or atrial gallop, bibasilar rales, and diffuse apical impulse. In right heart failure, peripheral cyanosis occurs with fatigue, peripheral edema, ascites, jugular vein distention, and hepatomegaly.

• *Deep-vein thrombosis.* In this disorder, acute peripheral cyanosis occurs in the affected extremity associated with tenderness, painful movement, edema, warmth, and prominent superficial veins. Also, Homans' sign can be elicited.

• *Lung cancer.* This disorder causes chronic central cyanosis accompanied by fever, weakness, weight loss, anorexia, dyspnea, chest pain, hemoptysis, and wheezing. Atelectasis causes mediastinal shift, decreased diaphragmatic excursion, asymmetrical chest expansion, a dull percussion note, and diminished breath sounds.

• *Methemoglobinemia.* Whether the result of toxicity or heredity, this disorder produces chronic central cyanosis. Its accompanying effects may also include headache, syncope, dyspnea, tachypnea, nausea, anorexia, and vomiting.

• *Peripheral arterial occlusion (acute).* This disorder produces acute cyanosis of one arm or leg or, occasionally, of both legs. The cyanosis is accompanied by sharp or aching pain that worsens when the patient moves. The affected extremity will also have paresthesias, weakness, and pale, cool skin. Examination reveals decreased or absent pulse and prolonged capillary refill time.

• *Pneumonia.* In this disorder, acute central cyanosis is usually preceded by fever, shaking chills, cough with purulent sputum, rales and rhonchi, and pleuritic chest pain that's exacerbated by deep inspiration. Associated signs and symptoms may include tachycardia, dyspnea, tachypnea, diminished breath sounds, diaphoresis, myalgias, fatigue, headache, and anorexia.

• *Pneumothorax.* A cardinal sign of pneumothorax, acute central cyanosis is accompanied by sharp chest pain that's exacerbated by movement, deep breathing, and coughing; asymmetrical chest wall expansion; and shortness of breath. There may also be rapid, shallow respirations; weak, rapid pulse; pallor; neck vein distention; anxiety; and absence of breath sounds over the affected lobe.

• *Polycythemia vera.* Chronic central cyanosis, often marked by a ruddy complexion, is characteristic in this chronic myeloproliferative disorder. Other findings are hepatosplenomegaly, headache, dizziness, fatigue, blurred vision, chest pain, intermittent claudication, and coagulation defects.

• *Pulmonary edema.* In this disorder, acute central cyanosis occurs with dyspnea; orthopnea; frothy, blood-tinged sputum; tachycardia; tachypnea; dependent rales; ventricular gallop; cold, clammy skin; hypotension; weak, thready pulse; and confusion.

• *Pulmonary embolism.* Acute central cyanosis occurs when a large embolus causes significant obstruction of the pulmonary circulation. Syncope and neck vein distention may also occur. Other common signs and symptoms include dyspnea, chest pain, tachycardia, dry cough or productive cough with blood-tinged sputum, low-grade fever, restlessness, and diaphoresis.

• *Raynaud's disease.* In this disorder, exposure to cold or stress causes the fingers or hands first to blanch and turn cold, then to become cyanotic, and finally to redden with return of normal temperature. Numbness and tingling may also occur.

• *Shock.* In this disorder, acute peripheral cyanosis develops in the hands and feet, which may also be cold, clammy, and pale. Other characteristic clinical features include lethargy, confusion, prolonged capillary refill time, and a rapid, weak pulse. Tachypnea, hyperpnea, and hypotension may also be present.

Special considerations

Prepare the patient for such tests as arterial blood gas analysis and complete blood count to determine the cause of cyanosis.

Provide supplemental oxygen to relieve shortness of breath and decrease cyanosis. However, deliver small doses (2 liters/minute) in patients with COPD, who may retain carbon dioxide. Position the patient comfortably to ease breathing. As ordered, administer diuretics, bronchodilators and antibiotics, or cardiac drugs. Ensure that the patient rests between activities to prevent dyspnea.

Pediatric pointers

Many pulmonary disorders responsible for cyanosis in adults also cause cyanosis in children. In addition, central cyanosis may result from cystic fibrosis, asthma, airway obstruction by a foreign body, acute laryngotracheobronchitis, and epiglottitis. It may also result from congenital heart defects, such as transposition of the great vessels, that cause right-to-left intracardiac shunting.

In children, circumoral cyanosis may precede generalized cyanosis. Acrocyanosis (also called "glove and bootee" cyanosis) may occur in infants due to excessive crying or exposure to cold. Exercise and agitation enhance cyanosis, so provide comfort and regular rest periods. Also, administer supplemental oxygen during cyanotic episodes.

decerebrate posture • decorticate posture • deep tendon reflexes—hyperactive
hypoactive • depression • diaphoresis • diarrhea • diplopia • dizziness • doll'
drooling • dysarthria • dysmenorrhea • dyspareunia • dyspepsia • dysphagia
dysuria • earache • edema—generalized • edema of the arms • edema of the
legs • enophthalmos • enuresis • epistaxis • eructation • erythema • exophtha
eye pain • facial pain • fasciculations • fatigue • fecal incontinence • fetor he
pain • flatulence • fontanelle bulging • fontanelle depression • footdrop • gag
gait—bizarre • gait—propulsive • gait—scissors • gait—spastic • gait—stepp
gallop—atrial • gallop—ventricular • genital lesions in the male • grunting re
bleeding • gum swelling • gynecomastia • halitosis • halo vision • headache •
intolerance • Heberden's nodes • hematemesis • hematochezia • hematuria •
hemoptysis • hepatomegaly • hiccups • hirsutism • hoarseness • Homans' sig
hyperpnea • hypopigmentation • impotence • insomnia • intermittent claudic
jaundice • jaw pain • jugular vein distention • Kehr's sign • Kernig's sign • k
consciousness—decreased • lid lag • light flashes • low birth weight • lymph
facies • McBurney's sign • McMurray's sign • melena • menorrhagia • metror
face • mouth lesions • murmurs • muscle atrophy • muscle flaccidity • muscl
spasticity • muscle weakness • mydriasis • myoclonus • nasal flaring • nause
blindness • nipple discharge • nipple retraction • nocturia • nuchal rigidity
deviation • oligomenorrhea • oliguria • opisthotonos • orofacial dyskinesia •
hypotension • Ortolani's sign • Osler's nodes • otorrhea • pallor • palpitation
paralysis • paresthesias • paroxysmal nocturnal dyspnea • peau d'orange • p
peristaltic waves—visible • photophobia • pica • pleural friction rub • polyd
polyuria • postnasal drip • priapism • pruritus • psoas sign • psychotic beha
absent or weak • pulse—bounding • pulse pressure—narrowed • pulse press
rhythm abnormality • pulsus alternans • pulsus bisferiens • pulsus paradoxu
pupils—sluggish • purple striae • purpura • pustular rash • pyrosis • raccoc
tenderness • rectal pain • retractions—costal and sternal • rhinorrhea • rhoi
salivation—decreased • salivation—increased • salt craving • scotoma • scro
absence • seizure—focal • seizure—generalized tonic-clonic • seizure—psyc
sign • shallow respirations • skin—bronze • skin—clammy • skin—mottled
turgor—decreased • spider angioma • splenomegaly • stertorous respirations
stridor • syncope • tachycardia • tachypnea • taste abnormalities • tearing—
tic • tinnitus • tracheal deviation • tracheal tugging • tremors • trismus • tu
frost • urethral discharge • urinary frequency • urinary hesitancy • urinary
urgency • urine cloudiness • urticaria • vaginal bleeding—postmenopausal •
venous hum • vertigo • vesicular rash • violent behavior • vision loss • visua
floaters • vomiting • vulvar lesions • weight gain—excessive • weight loss—
wristdrop• abdominal distention • abdominal mass • abdominal pain • abc
accessory muscle use • agitation • alopecia • amenorrhea • amnesia • analg
anorexia • anosmia • anuria • anxiety • aphasia • apnea • apneustic respira
pain • asterixis • ataxia • athetosis • aura • Babinski's reflex • back pain • I
sign • Biot's respirations • bladder distention • blood pressure decrease • bl
bowel sounds—absent • bowel sounds—hyperactive • bowel sounds—hypo
bradypnea • breast dimpling • breast nodule • breast pain • breast ulcer • I
odor • breath with fecal odor • breath with fruity odor • Brudzinski's sign
butterfly rash • café-au-lait spots • capillary refill time—prolonged • carpop
chest expansion—asymmetrical • chest pain • Cheyne-Stokes respirations •
sign • clubbing • cogwheel rigidity • cold intolerance • confusion • conjunc

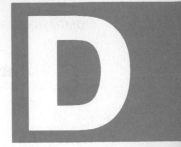

Decerebrate Posture

[Decerebrate rigidity, abnormal extensor reflex]

Usually, decerebrate posture heralds neurologic deterioration. It's characterized by adduction and extension of the arms, with the wrists pronated and the fingers flexed. The legs are stiffly extended, with plantar flexion of the feet. In severe cases, the back is acutely arched (opisthotonos). This sign indicates upper brain stem damage, which may result from primary lesions such as infarction, hemorrhage, or tumor; metabolic encephalopathy; head injury; or brain stem compression associated with increased intracranial pressure (ICP).

Decerebrate posture may be elicited by noxious stimuli or may occur spontaneously. It may be unilateral or bilateral. In concurrent brain stem and cerebral damage, decerebrate posture may affect only the arms, while the legs may remain flaccid. Or decerebrate posture may affect one side of the body and decorticate posture the other. The two postures may also alternate as the patient's neurologic status fluctuates. Generally, the duration of each posturing episode correlates with the severity of brain stem damage.

Assessment

When the patient displays decerebrate posture, notify the doctor immediately. As your first priority, ensure a patent airway. Insert an artificial airway, elevate the head of the bed, and turn the patient's head to the side to prevent aspiration (don't disrupt spinal alignment if you suspect spinal cord injury). Suction the patient, as necessary. Next, assess spontaneous respirations. Give supplemental oxygen and ventilate the patient with an Ambu bag, if necessary. Or prepare to assist with intubation and mechanical ventilation. Keep emergency resuscitation equipment handy. Be sure to check the patient's chart for a no-code order.

After taking vital signs, assess the patient's level of consciousness. Use the Glasgow Coma Scale as a reference. Then evaluate the pupils for size, equality, and response to light. Test deep tendon reflexes, cranial nerve reflexes, and for doll's eye sign.

Next, explore the history of the patient's coma. If you're unable to obtain this information, look for clues to the causative disorder, such as hepatomegaly, cyanosis, diabetic skin changes, needle tracks, or obvious trauma. If a family member is available, find out when the patient's level of consciousness began deteriorating.

COMPARING DECEREBRATE AND DECORTICATE POSTURES

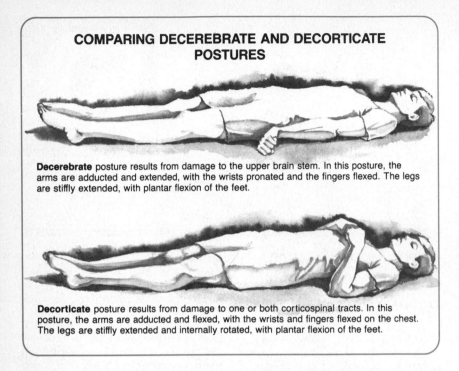

Decerebrate posture results from damage to the upper brain stem. In this posture, the arms are adducted and extended, with the wrists pronated and the fingers flexed. The legs are stiffly extended, with plantar flexion of the feet.

Decorticate posture results from damage to one or both corticospinal tracts. In this posture, the arms are adducted and flexed, with the wrists and fingers flexed on the chest. The legs are stiffly extended and internally rotated, with plantar flexion of the feet.

Did it occur abruptly? What did the patient complain of before he lost consciousness? Is there a history of diabetes, liver disease, cancer, blood clots, or aneurysm? Ask about any accident or trauma responsible for the coma.

Medical causes

• *Brain stem infarction.* When this primary lesion produces coma, decerebrate posture may also be elicited. Associated signs and symptoms vary with the severity of the infarct. There may be cranial nerve palsies, bilateral cerebellar ataxia, and sensory loss. In deep coma, all normal reflexes are usually lost, resulting in absence of doll's eye sign, a positive Babinski's reflex, and flaccidity.

• *Brain stem tumor.* In this disorder, decerebrate posture is a late sign that accompanies coma. Commonly, the posture is preceded by hemiparesis, cranial nerve palsies, vertigo, dizziness, ataxia, and vomiting.

• *Cerebral lesion.* Whether the etiology

is trauma, tumor, abscess, or infarction, any cerebral lesion that increases ICP may also produce decerebrate posture. Typically, this posture is a late sign. Associated findings vary with the lesion's site and extent but commonly include coma, abnormal pupil size and response to light, and the classic triad of increased ICP—bradycardia, increasing systolic blood pressure, and widening pulse pressure.

• *Hepatic encephalopathy.* A late sign in this disorder, decerebrate posture occurs with coma resulting from increased ICP and ammonia toxicity. Associated signs include fetor hepaticus, a positive Babinski's reflex, and hyperactive deep tendon reflexes.

• *Hypoglycemic encephalopathy.* Characterized by extremely low blood glucose levels, this disorder may produce decerebrate posture and coma. It also causes dilated pupils, slow respirations, and bradycardia. Muscle spasms, twitching, and convulsions eventually progress to flaccidity.

• *Hypoxic encephalopathy.* Severe hypoxia may produce decerebrate posture—the result of brain stem compression associated with anaerobic metabolism and increased ICP. Other findings include coma, a positive Babinski's reflex, absence of doll's eye sign, hypoactive deep tendon reflexes, and, possibly, fixed pupils and respiratory arrest.

• *Pontine hemorrhage.* Typically, this life-threatening disorder rapidly leads to decerebrate posture with coma. Accompanying signs include total paralysis, absence of doll's eye sign, a positive Babinski's reflex, and small, reactive pupils.

• *Posterior fossa hemorrhage.* This subtentorial lesion causes decerebrate posture. Its earlier effects include vomiting, vertigo, ataxia, stiff neck, drowsiness, and cranial nerve palsies. The patient eventually slips into coma and, possibly, suffers respiratory arrest.

Other causes

• *Diagnostic tests.* Rarely, certain neurologic tests may cause decerebrate posture. In this category are lumbar puncture, cisternography, and pneumoencephalography—which may increase ICP, leading to brain stem compression.

Special considerations

Help prepare the patient for diagnostic tests to determine the cause of decerebrate posture. These may include skull X-rays, computed tomography scan, cerebral angiography, digital subtraction angiography, electroencephalography, brain scan, and ICP monitoring.

Monitor neurologic status and vital signs every 30 minutes or hourly. Be alert for signs of increased ICP (bradycardia, increasing systolic blood pressure, and widening pulse pressure) and neurologic deterioration (altered respiratory pattern and abnormal temperature). Report subtle changes in the patient's condition to allow the doctor to intervene promptly and prevent further deterioration.

Inform the patient's family that decerebrate posture is a reflex response—not a voluntary response to pain or a sign of recovery. Offer emotional support.

Pediatric pointers

Children under age 2 may not display decerebrate posture because of nervous system immaturity. However, if the posture does occur, it's usually the more severe opisthotonos. In fact, opisthotonos is more common in infants and young children than in adults and is usually a terminal sign.

In children, the most common cause of decerebrate posture is head injury. It also occurs in Reye's syndrome—the result of increased ICP causing brain stem compression.

Decorticate Posture

[Decorticate rigidity, abnormal flexor response]

A sign of corticospinal damage, decorticate posture is characterized by adduction and flexion of the arms, with the wrists and fingers flexed on the chest. The legs are extended and internally rotated, with plantar flexion of the feet. This posture may occur unilaterally or bilaterally. Most often, it results from cerebrovascular accident (CVA) or head injury. It may be elicited by noxious stimuli or may occur spontaneously. The intensity of the required stimulus, the duration of the posture, and the frequency of spontaneous episodes vary with the severity of cerebral injury.

Although a serious sign, decorticate posture carries a more favorable prognosis than decerebrate posture. However, if the causative disorder extends lower in the brain stem, decorticate posture may progress to decerebrate posture.

Assessment

When the patient displays decorticate posture, notify the doctor and begin a neurologic assessment. First evaluate level of consciousness. If consciousness is impaired, insert an oropharyngeal airway, elevate the head of the bed 30°, and turn the patient's head to the side to prevent aspiration (unless spinal cord injury is suspected). Assess respiratory rate, rhythm, and depth. Prepare to assist respirations with an Ambu bag or intubation and mechanical ventilation, if necessary. Also, institute seizure precautions. Then record other vital signs.

Test the patient's motor and sensory functions. Evaluate pupil size, equality, and response to light. Then test cranial nerve and deep tendon reflexes. Ask about headache, dizziness, nausea, abnormal vision, or numbness and tingling. When did the patient first notice these symptoms? Is his family aware of any behavior changes? Also ask about a history of cerebrovascular disease, cancer, meningitis, encephalitis, upper respiratory infection, or recent trauma.

Medical causes

• **Brain abscess.** Decorticate posture may occur in this infection. Accompanying findings vary depending on the size and location of the abscess but may include aphasia, hemiparesis, headache, dizziness, seizures, nausea, and vomiting. Behavior changes, altered vital signs, and decreased level of consciousness may also occur.

• **Brain tumor.** This disorder may produce decorticate posture that's usually bilateral—the result of increased ICP associated with tumor growth. Related signs and symptoms include headache, behavior changes, memory loss, diplopia, blurred vision or vision loss, seizures, ataxia, dizziness, apraxia, aphasia, paresis, sensory loss, paresthesia, vomiting, papilledema, and signs of hormonal imbalance.

• **Cerebrovascular accident.** Typically, a CVA involving the cerebral cortex produces unilateral decorticate posture, also called spastic hemiplegia. Other clinical features are hemiplegia (contralateral to the lesion), dysarthria, dysphagia, unilateral sensory loss, apraxia, agnosia, aphasia, memory loss, decreased level of consciousness, urinary retention and incontinence, and constipation. Ocular effects include homonymous hemianopia, diplopia, and blurred vision.

• **Head injury.** Decorticate posture may be among the variable features of this disorder, depending on the site and severity of head injury. Associated signs and symptoms may include headache, nausea and vomiting, dizziness, irritability, decreased level of consciousness, aphasia, hemiparesis, unilateral numbness, seizures, and pupillary dilation.

Special considerations

Assess the patient frequently to detect subtle signs of neurologic deterioration. Also monitor neurologic status and vital signs every 30 minutes to 2 hours. Be alert for signs of increased ICP, including bradycardia, increasing systolic blood pressure, and widening pulse pressure.

Pediatric pointers

Decorticate posture is an unreliable sign before age 2 because of nervous system immaturity. In children, decorticate posture most commonly results from head injury. It also occurs in Reye's syndrome.

Deep Tendon Reflexes— Hyperactive

A hyperactive deep tendon reflex (DTR) is an abnormally brisk muscle contraction in response to a sudden stretch induced by sharply tapping the muscle's tendon of insertion. This elicited sign may be graded as brisk (+ + +) or hyperactive (+ + + +).

The corticospinal tract governs the reflex arc—the relay cycle that produces any reflex response. A corticospinal lesion above the level of the reflex arc being tested may result in a hyperactive DTR. Abnormal neuromuscular transmission at the end of the reflex arc may also cause a hyperactive DTR. For example, deficiency of calcium or magnesium may cause a hyperactive DTR because these electrolytes regulate neuromuscular excitability.

Hyperactive DTRs frequently accompany other neurologic findings but usually lack specific diagnostic value. An exception is hypocalcemia, in which hyperactive DTRs are an early, cardinal sign.

Assessment

After eliciting hyperactive DTRs, begin neurologic assessment with the patient's history. Ask about spinal cord injury or other trauma and about prolonged exposure to cold, wind, or water. Is there a possibility of pregnancy? A positive response to any of these questions requires prompt assessment to rule out life-threatening autonomic hyperreflexia, tetanus, preeclampsia, or hypothermia. Ask about the onset and progression of associated signs and symptoms. Next, evaluate the patient's level of consciousness. Test motor and sensory function in the limbs. Also ask about paresthesias. Check for ataxia or tremors and for speech and visual deficits. Test for Chvostek's and Trousseau's signs and for carpopedal spasm. Ask about vomiting or altered bladder habits. Finally, take vital signs.

Medical causes

• *Amyotrophic lateral sclerosis.* This disorder produces generalized hyperactive DTRs. Weakness of the hands and forearms and spasticity of the legs accompany these DTRs. Eventually, the patient develops atrophy of the neck and tongue muscles, fasciculations, occa-sional weakness of the legs, and possible bulbar signs (dysphagia, dysphonia, facial weakness, and dyspnea).

• *Brain tumor.* A cerebral tumor causes hyperactive DTRs on the side opposite the lesion. Associated signs and symptoms develop slowly and may include unilateral paresis or paralysis, anesthesia, visual field deficits, spasticity, and a positive Babinski's reflex.

• *Cerebrovascular accident (CVA).* Any CVA that affects the origin of the corticospinal tracts causes sudden onset of hyperactive DTRs on the side opposite the lesion. There may also be unilateral paresis or paralysis, anesthesia, visual field deficits, spasticity, and a positive Babinski's reflex.

• *Hepatic encephalopathy.* Generalized hyperactive DTRs occur late and are followed by a positive Babinski's reflex, fetor hepaticus, and coma.

• *Hypocalcemia.* This disorder may produce sudden or gradual onset of generalized hyperactive DTRs with paresthesia, muscle twitching and cramping, positive Chvostek's and Trousseau's signs, carpopedal spasm, and tetany.

• *Hypomagnesemia.* This disorder results in gradual onset of generalized hyperactive DTRs accompanied by muscle cramps, hypotension, tachycardia, paresthesia, ataxia, tetany, and possible convulsions.

• *Hypothermia.* Mild hypothermia (90° to 94° F., 32.2° to 34.4° C.) produces generalized hyperactive DTRs. Other signs and symptoms include shivering, fatigue, weakness, lethargy, slurred speech, ataxia, muscle stiffness, tachycardia, diuresis, bradypnea, hypotension, and cold, pale skin.

• *Multiple sclerosis.* Typically, hyperactive DTRs are preceded by weakness and paresthesia in one or both arms or legs. Associated signs include clonus and a positive Babinski's reflex. Passive flexion of the patient's neck may cause a tingling sensation down his back. Later, ataxia, diplopia, vertigo, vomiting, and urinary retention or incontinence may occur.

TRACING THE REFLEX ARC IN DEEP TENDON REFLEXES

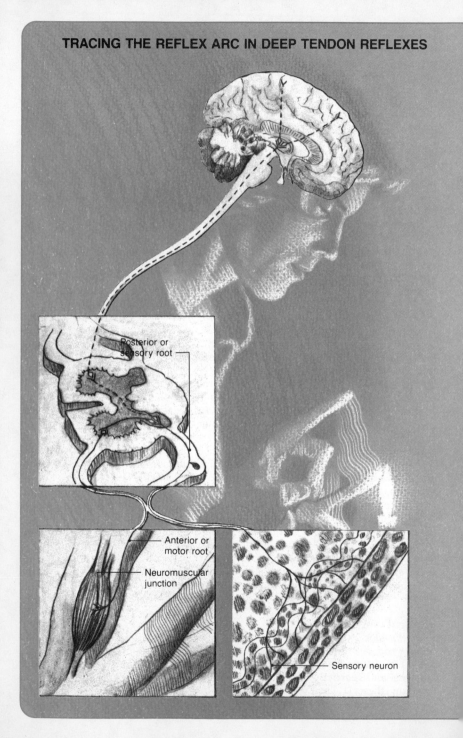

Posterior or sensory root

Anterior or motor root

Neuromuscular junction

Sensory neuron

Sharply tapping a tendon initiates a sensory (afferent) impulse that travels along a peripheral nerve to a spinal nerve and then to the spinal cord. The impulse enters the spinal cord through the posterior root, synapses with a motor (efferent) neuron in the anterior horn on the same side of the spinal cord, and then is transmitted through a motor nerve fiber back to the muscle. When the impulse crosses the neuromuscular junction, the muscle contracts, completing the reflex arc.

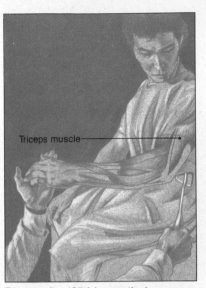

Triceps muscle

Triceps reflex (C7-8 innervation)

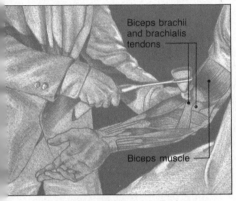

Biceps brachii and brachialis tendons

Biceps muscle

Biceps reflex (C5-6 innervation)

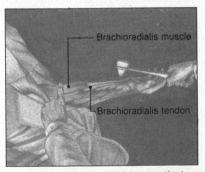

Brachioradialis muscle

Brachioradialis tendon

Brachioradialis reflex (C5-6 innervation)

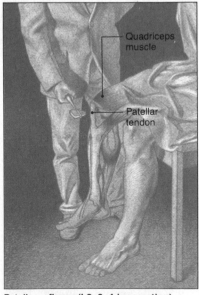

Quadriceps muscle

Patellar tendon

Patellar reflexes (L2, 3, 4 innervation)

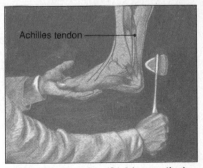

Achilles tendon

Achilles tendon reflex (S1-2 innervation)

• **Preeclampsia.** Occurring in pregnancy of at least 20 weeks' duration, preeclampsia may cause gradual onset of generalized hyperactive DTRs. Accompanying signs and symptoms include increased blood pressure; abnormal weight gain; edema of the face, fingers, and abdomen after bedrest; oliguria; severe headache; blurred or double vision; epigastric pain; nausea and vomiting; irritability; cyanosis; shortness of breath; and rales. If preeclampsia progresses to eclampsia, the patient will have seizures.

• **Spinal cord lesion.** Incomplete spinal cord lesions cause hyperactive DTRs below the level of the lesion. In a traumatic lesion, hyperactive DTRs follow resolution of spinal shock. In a neoplastic lesion, hyperactive DTRs gradually replace normal DTRs. Other signs and symptoms are paralysis and sensory loss below the level of the lesion, urinary retention and overflow incontinence, and alternating constipation and diarrhea. In a lesion above T6, there may also be autonomic hyperreflexia with diaphoresis and flushing above the level of the lesion, headache, nasal congestion, nausea, increased blood pressure, and bradycardia.

• **Tetanus.** In this disorder, sudden onset of generalized hyperactive DTRs accompanies tachycardia, diaphoresis, low-grade fever, painful and involuntary muscle contractions, trismus (lock-jaw), and risus sardonicus.

Special considerations

Prepare the patient for diagnostic tests to evaluate hyperactive DTRs. These may include laboratory tests for serum calcium and magnesium, spinal X-rays, computed tomography, lumbar puncture, and myelography.

If motor weakness accompanies hyperactive DTRs, perform or encourage range-of-motion exercises to preserve muscle integrity. Also reposition the patient frequently, provide a special mattress, and massage his back to prevent skin breakdown. Administer muscle relaxants and sedatives, if ordered, to relieve severe muscle contractions. Keep emergency resuscitation equipment on hand. Provide a quiet, calm atmosphere to decrease neuromuscular excitability.

Pediatric pointers

Hyperreflexia may be a normal sign in neonates. After age 6, reflex responses are similar to those of adults. However, when testing DTRs in small children, use distraction techniques to promote reliable results.

Cerebral palsy frequently causes hyperactive DTRs in children. Reye's syndrome causes generalized hyperactive DTRs in Stage II; in Stage V, DTRs are absent. Adult causes of hyperactive DTRs may also appear in children.

Deep Tendon Reflexes— Hypoactive

A hypoactive deep tendon reflex (DTR) is an abnormally diminished muscle contraction in response to a sudden stretch induced by sharply tapping the muscle's tendon of insertion. It may be graded as minimal (+) or absent (0).

Normally, a DTR operates via the reflex arc, which is governed by the corticospinal tract. A hypoactive DTR may result from damage to the reflex arc involving the specific muscle, the peripheral nerve, the nerve roots, or the spinal cord at that level. Hypoactive DTRs are an important sign of many disorders, especially when they appear with other neurologic signs and symptoms.

Assessment

After eliciting hypoactive DTRs, obtain a thorough history from the patient or a family member. Have him describe current signs and symptoms in detail. Then take a family and drug history.

Next, perform a physical examination. First assess the patient's level of consciousness. Test motor function in his limbs and palpate for muscle atrophy or increased mass. Test sensory function, including pain, touch, temperature, and vibration sense. Ask about paresthesia. Have the patient take several steps so that you can observe his gait and coordination. To check for Romberg's sign, ask him to stand with feet together and eyes closed. During conversation, assess the patient's speech. Also observe for signs of vision or hearing loss. Remember that abrupt onset of hypoactive DTRs accompanied by muscle weakness may occur in life-threatening Guillain-Barré syndrome, botulism, or spinal cord lesions with spinal shock.

Assess for autonomic nervous system effects by taking vital signs. Also inspect the patient's skin for pallor, dryness, flushing, or diaphoresis. Auscultate for hypoactive bowel sounds. Ask about nausea, vomiting, constipation, and incontinence. Palpate for bladder distention.

Medical causes

● *Botulism.* In this disorder, generalized hypoactive DTRs accompany progressive descending muscle weakness. Initially, the patient usually complains of blurred and double vision and, occasionally, of anorexia, nausea, and vomiting. Other early bulbar signs and symptoms include vertigo, hearing loss, dysarthria, and dysphagia. The patient may have signs of respiratory distress and severe constipation marked by hypoactive bowel sounds.

● *Eaton-Lambert syndrome.* This disorder produces generalized hypoactive (but not absent) DTRs. Early signs include difficulty in rising from a chair, climbing stairs, and walking. The patient may complain of achiness, paresthesia, and muscle weakness that's most severe in the morning. Weakness improves with mild exercise but worsens with strenuous exercise. Other signs and symptoms may include ptosis, diplopia, dysarthria, and dysphagia.

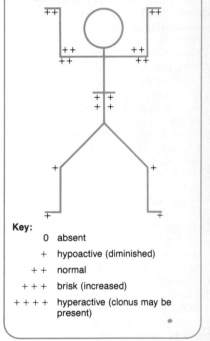

DOCUMENTING DEEP TENDON REFLEXES

Record the patient's deep tendon reflex scores by drawing a stick figure and entering the grades on this scale at the proper location. The figure shown here indicates hypoactive deep tendon reflexes in the legs; other reflexes are normal.

Key:

0	absent
+	hypoactive (diminished)
+ +	normal
+ + +	brisk (increased)
+ + + +	hyperactive (clonus may be present)

● *Guillain-Barré syndrome.* This disorder causes bilateral hypoactive DTRs that progress rapidly from hypotonia to areflexia in several days. Typically, this disorder causes muscle weakness that begins in the legs and then extends to the arms and, possibly, to the trunk and neck muscles. Occasionally, weakness may progress to total paralysis. Other clinical features include cranial nerve palsies, pain, paresthesia, and signs of brief autonomic dysfunction—sinus tachycardia or bradycardia, flushing, fluctuating blood pressure, and anhidrosis or episodic diaphoresis.

Usually, muscle weakness and hypoactive DTRs peak in severity within 10 to 14 days; then symptoms begin to clear. However, there may be residual hypoactive DTRs and motor weakness in severe cases.

• **Peripheral neuropathy.** Characteristic in end-stage diabetes mellitus, renal failure, and alcoholism, peripheral neuropathy results in progressive hypoactive DTRs. Other effects include motor weakness, sensory loss, paresthesia, tremors, and possible autonomic dysfunction, such as orthostatic hypotension and incontinence.

• **Polymyositis.** In this disorder, hypoactive DTRs accompany muscle weakness, pain, stiffness, spasms, and, possibly, increased size or atrophy. These effects are usually temporary; their location varies with the affected muscles.

• **Spinal cord lesions.** Spinal cord injury or complete transection produces spinal shock, resulting in hypoactive DTRs (areflexia) below the level of the lesion. Associated signs and symptoms may include quadriplegia or paraplegia, flaccidity, loss of sensation below the level of the lesion, and dry, pale skin. Also characteristic are urinary retention with overflow incontinence, hypoactive bowel sounds, constipation, and genital reflex loss. Hypoactive DTRs and flaccidity are usually transient; minimal reflex activity returns within several weeks.

• **Syringomyelia.** Permanent bilateral hypoactive DTRs occur early in this slowly progressive disorder. Other clinical features are muscle weakness and atrophy; loss of sensation, usually extending in a capelike fashion over the arms, shoulders, neck, back, and occasionally the legs; deep, boring pain (despite anesthesia) in the limbs; and signs of brain stem involvement (nystagmus, facial numbness, unilateral vocal cord paralysis or weakness, and unilateral tongue atrophy).

• **Tabes dorsalis.** This progressive disorder results in bilateral hypoactive DTRs in the legs and, occasionally, the arms. Associated signs and symptoms include sharp pain and paresthesia of the legs, face, or trunk; visceral pain with retching and vomiting; sensory loss in the legs; ataxic gait with a positive Romberg's sign; urinary retention and incontinence; and arthropathies.

Other causes

• **Drugs.** Barbiturates and paralyzing drugs, such as pancuronium and curare, may cause hypoactive DTRs.

Special considerations

Help the patient carry out his daily activities. Try to strike a balance between promoting independence and ensuring his safety. Encourage him to walk with assistance. Make sure personal care articles are within easy reach on a bedside stand, and provide an obstacle-free course from his bed to the bathroom. In sensory deficits, protect the patient from injury from heat or pressure. Test his bath water, and reposition him frequently, ensuring a soft, smooth bed surface. Also, keep his skin clean and dry to prevent breakdown. Perform or encourage range-of-motion exercises. Also encourage a balanced diet with increased protein.

Pediatric pointers

Hypoactive DTRs frequently occur in muscular dystrophy, Friedreich's ataxia, syringomyelia, and spinal cord injury. They also accompany progressive muscular atrophy, which affects preschoolers and adolescents.

Use distraction techniques to test DTRs; assess motor function by watching the infant or child at play.

Depression

Depression defies easy definition, often eluding diagnosis and treatment. Its character, intensity, and duration vary from periodic bouts of "the blues" to persistent thoughts of suicide.

Depression can be classified as mild, moderate, or severe. *Mild depression* is transient and characterized by down-heartedness, sadness, and dejection. *Moderate depression* is marked by noticeably disturbed thought processes, impaired communication and socialization, and sensory dysfunction. These factors intensify in *severe depression:* The patient may appear withdrawn, expressionless, or unaffected by his surroundings, and may exhibit delusional thinking, dramatic sensory dysfunction, and limited or agitated motor activity.

Depression is more common in women than men and is especially prevalent among adolescents. Among its causes are drugs and psychiatric and organic disorders.

Assessment

During assessment, try to determine how the patient feels about himself, his family, and his environment. Your goal is to explore the nature of his depression, the extent to which other factors affect it, and his coping mechanisms. Begin by asking the patient what's bothering him. How does his current mood differ from his usual mood? Then ask the patient to describe the way he feels about himself. What are his plans and dreams? How realistic are they? Is he generally satisfied with what he's accomplished in his work, relationships, and other interests? Ask about any changes in his social interactions, sleep patterns, ability to make decisions or concentrate, or normal activities. Explore drug and alcohol use.

Ask the patient about his family—its patterns of interaction and characteristic responses to success and failure. What part does he feel he plays in his family life? Find out if other family members have been depressed, and whether anyone important to the patient has been sick or has died in the past year. Finally, ask the patient about his environment. Has his life-style changed in the past month? Six months? Year? When he's feeling blue, where does he go and what does he do to feel better? Find out how he feels about his

role in the community and the resources that are available to him. Try to determine if the patient has an adequate support network to help him cope with his depression.

Medical causes

• *Organic disorders.* Various organic disorders and chronic illnesses produce mild, moderate, or severe depression. Among these are *metabolic and endocrine disorders,* such as hypothyroidism, hyperthyroidism, and diabetes; *infectious diseases,* such as influenza, hepatitis, and encephalitis; *degenerative diseases,* such as Alzheimer's disease, multiple sclerosis, and multi-infarct dementia; and *neoplastic disorders,* such as cancer of the pancreas.

• *Psychiatric disorders. Affective disorders* are often characterized by abrupt mood swings from depression to elation (mania) or by prolonged episodes of either mood. In fact, severe depression may last for weeks. More moderate depression occurs in *cyclothymic disorders* and usually alternates with moderate mania. Moderate depression that is more or less constant over a 2-year period often results from *dysthymic disorders.* In addition, *chronic anxiety disorders,* characterized by obsessive-compulsive behavior, may cause depression.

Other causes

• *Alcohol abuse.* Intoxication or withdrawal often produces depression.

• *Drugs.* Various drugs cause depression as a side effect. Among the more common are barbiturates; antineoplastic agents, such as asparaginase; anticonvulsants, such as diazepam; and antiarrhythmics, such as disopyramide. Other depression-inducing drugs include centrally acting antihypertensives, such as reserpine (common in high dosages), methyldopa, and clonidine; beta-adrenergic blockers, such as propranolol; levodopa; indomethacin; cycloserine; corticosteroids; and oral contraceptives.

SUICIDE: CARING FOR THE HIGH-RISK PATIENT

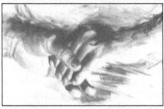

One of the most common factors contributing to suicide is hopelessness—an emotion that a depressed patient frequently experiences. As a result, you'll need to regularly assess him for suicidal tendencies. Usually, the patient will provide specific clues of his intentions. For example, you may notice the patient talking frequently about death or the futility of life, concealing potentially harmful items, giving away personal belongings, or getting legal and financial accounts in order. If you suspect that he's suicidal, follow these care guidelines:

• First, try to determine the patient's suicide potential. Find out how upset he is. Does he have a simple, straightforward suicide plan that's likely to succeed? Does he have any positive supports—family, friends, a therapist? A patient with low-to-moderate suicide potential is noticeably depressed but has some form of support system. He may have thoughts of suicide, but no specific plan. A patient with high suicide potential feels profoundly hopeless and has little or no support system. He thinks about suicide frequently and has a plan that's likely to succeed.

• Next, observe precautions. Ensure the patient's safety by removing any objects he could use to harm himself, such as razors, belts, and electrical cords. Know his whereabouts and what he's doing at all times—this may require one-to-one nursing surveillance. Place the patient in a room that's close to the nursing station. Always have someone accompany him off the unit.

• Be alert for in-hospital suicide attempts. Typically, they occur when there's a low staff-to-patient ratio—between shifts, during evening and night shifts, or when a critical event such as a code draws attention away from the patient.

• Finally, arrange for follow-up counseling. Recognize suicidal ideation and behavior as a desperate cry for help. Contact a mental health professional for a referral.

Special considerations

Caring for the depressed patient takes time, tact, and energy. It also requires an awareness of your own vulnerability to feelings of despair that can stem from your interactions with the patient. Help him set realistic goals; encourage him to promote feelings of self-worth by asserting his opinions and making decisions. Encourage him to talk about his emotions and feelings. Since anger typically underlies depression, help the patient acknowledge this emotion and express it safely. For example, plan physical activities that provide a controlled outlet for anger. To help him overcome feelings of helplessness, plan activities that he can succeed at and teach him to solve problems constructively. Help foster feelings of competency by focusing on past and present experiences in which the patient was successful. Try to determine his suicide potential, and take steps to help ensure his safety.

Make sure the patient receives adequate nourishment and rest, and keep his environment free from stress and excessive stimulation. Assist with diagnostic tests to determine if his depression has an organic cause, and administer drugs, as ordered. Also, arrange for follow-up counseling or contact a mental health professional for a referral.

Pediatric pointers

Because emotional lability is normal in adolescence, depression can be difficult to assess and diagnose in teenagers. Clues to underlying depression may include somatic complaints, sexual promiscuity, low academic achievement, and abuse of alcohol or drugs.

Use of a family systems model often helps determine the cause of depression in adolescents. Once family roles are determined, family therapy or group therapy with peers may help the patient overcome his depression.

Diaphoresis

Diaphoresis is profuse sweating—at times, amounting to more than 1 liter of sweat per hour. This sign represents an autonomic nervous system response to physical or psychogenic stress, or to fever or high environmental temperature. When caused by stress, diaphoresis may be generalized or limited to the palms of the hands, soles of the feet, and the forehead. When caused by fever or high environmental temperature, it's usually generalized.

Usually diaphoresis begins abruptly and may be accompanied by other autonomic system signs, such as tachycardia and increased blood pressure. However, it varies with age because sweat glands function immaturely in the infant and are less active in the elderly. As a result, these agegroups may fail to display diaphoresis associated with its common causes.

Intermittent diaphoresis may accompany chronic disorders characterized by recurrent fever; isolated diaphoresis may mark an episode of acute pain or fever. Night sweats may characterize intermittent fever because body temperature tends to return to normal between 2 and 4 a.m. before rising again.

When caused by excessive external temperature, diaphoresis is a normal response. Acclimatization usually requires several days of exposure to high temperatures; during this process, diaphoresis helps maintain normal body temperature. Diaphoresis also commonly occurs during menopause. It's preceded by a sensation of intense heat (a hot flash). Other causes include exercise or exertion that accelerates metabolism, creating internal heat, and mild-to-moderate anxiety that helps initiate the fight-or-flight response.

Assessment

If the patient is diaphoretic, quickly rule out the possibility of a life-threatening cause. (See *When Diaphoresis Spells Crisis,* page 229.) Begin the history by having the patient describe his chief complaint. Then explore associated signs and symptoms. Note general fatigue and weakness. Does the patient have insomnia, headache, and changes in vision or hearing? Is the patient often dizzy? Does he have palpitations? Ask about pleuritic pain, cough, sputum, and difficulty breathing; nausea, vomiting, altered bowel or bladder habits; and abdominal pain. Ask the female patient about amenorrhea. Is she menopausal? Note weight loss or gain. Ask about paresthesia, muscle cramps or stiffness, and joint pain.

Complete the history by asking about travel to tropical countries. Note recent exposure to high environmental temperatures or to pesticides. Was the patient recently bitten by a snake? Check for a history of partial gastrectomy or of drug or alcohol abuse. Finally, obtain a thorough drug history.

Now perform a physical examination. First, determine the extent of diaphoresis by inspecting the trunk and extremities as well as the palms, soles, and forehead. Also check the patient's clothing and bedding for dampness. Note whether diaphoresis occurs during the day or at night. Observe for flushing, abnormal skin texture or lesions, and increased coarse body hair. Note poor skin turgor and dry mucous membranes. Check for splinter hemorrhages and Plummer's nails. Then, evaluate the patient's mental status and take his vital signs. Observe for fasciculations and flaccid paralysis. Be alert for seizures. Note the patient's facial expression and examine the eyes for pupillary dilation or constriction, exophthalmos, and excessive tearing. Test visual fields. Also check for hearing loss and for tooth or gum disease. Percuss the lungs for dullness and auscultate for crackles, diminished or bronchial breath sounds, and increased vocal fremitus. Look for decreased respiratory excursion. Palpate for lymphadenopathy and hepatosplenomegaly.

UNDERSTANDING DIAPHORESIS

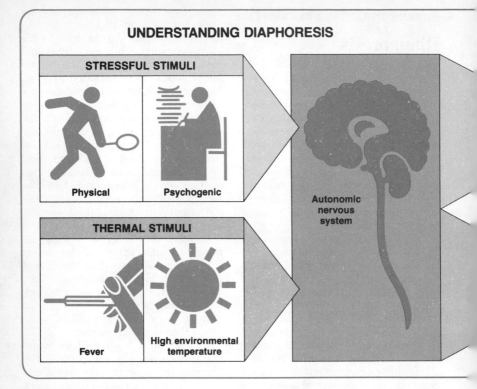

STRESSFUL STIMULI

Physical

Psychogenic

THERMAL STIMULI

Fever

High environmental
temperature

Autonomic
nervous
system

Medical causes

● *Acquired immunodeficiency syndrome.* Night sweats may be an early feature. The patient also displays fever, fatigue, lymphadenopathy, anorexia, dramatic and unexplained weight loss, diarrhea, and persistent cough.

● *Acromegaly.* In this slowly progressive disorder, diaphoresis is a sensitive gauge of disease activity, which involves hypersecretion of growth hormone and increased metabolic rate. The patient has a hulking appearance with an enlarged supraorbital ridge and thickened ears and nose. Other signs and symptoms include warm, oily, thickened skin; enlarged hands, feet, and jaw; joint pain; weight gain; hoarseness; and increased coarse body hair. Increased blood pressure, severe headache, and visual field deficits or blindness may also occur.

● *Anxiety disorders.* Acute anxiety characterizes panic, while chronic anxiety characterizes phobias, conversion disorders, obsessions, and compulsions. Whether acute or chronic, anxiety may cause sympathetic stimulation, resulting in diaphoresis. The diaphoresis is most dramatic on the palms, soles, and forehead. It's accompanied by palpitations, tachycardia, tachypnea, tremor, and gastrointestinal distress. Psychologic symptoms—fear, difficulty concentrating, and behavior changes—also occur.

● *Autonomic hyperreflexia.* Occurring after resolution of spinal shock in spinal cord injury above T6, hyperreflexia causes profuse diaphoresis, pounding headache, blurred vision, and dramatically elevated blood pressure. Diaphoresis occurs above the level of the injury, especially on the forehead, and is accompanied by flushing. Other findings may include restlessness, nausea, nasal congestion, and bradycardia.

● *Congestive heart failure.* Typically,

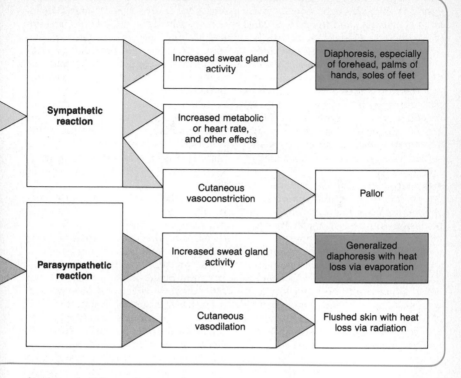

diaphoresis follows fatigue, dyspnea, orthopnea, and tachycardia in left heart failure and neck vein distention and dry cough in right heart failure. Other features include tachypnea, cyanosis, dependent edema, crackles, ventricular gallop, and anxiety.

• *Drug and alcohol withdrawal syndromes.* Withdrawal from alcohol and narcotic analgesics may cause generalized diaphoresis, dilated pupils, tachycardia, tremors, and altered mental status (confusion, delusions, hallucinations, agitation). Associated signs and symptoms may include severe muscle cramps, generalized paresthesia, tachypnea, increased or decreased blood pressure, and possibly seizures. Nausea and vomiting are common.

• *Empyema.* Pus accumulation in the pleural space leads to drenching night sweats and fever. The patient also complains of chest pain, cough, and weight loss. Examination reveals decreased

respiratory excursion on the affected side and absent or distant breath sounds.

• *Envenomation.* Depending on the type of snake bite, neurotoxic effects may include diaphoresis, chills (with or without fever), weakness, dizziness, blurred vision, increased salivation, nausea and vomiting, and possibly paresthesia and muscle fasciculations. Local features may include progressively severe pain and edema, and ecchymosis. Palpation reveals tender regional lymph nodes.

• *Heat exhaustion.* Initially, this condition causes profuse diaphoresis, fatigue, weakness, and anxiety. It may progress to circulatory collapse and shock—confusion, thready pulse, hypotension, tachycardia, and cold, clammy skin. Other features are an ashen-gray appearance, dilated pupils, and normal or subnormal temperature.

• *Hodgkin's disease.* Especially in the elderly, early features of Hodgkin's disease may include night sweats, fever, fatigue, pruritus, and weight loss. Most often, though, Hodgkin's disease initially causes painless swelling of a cervical lymph node. Occasionally, a Pel-Ebstein fever pattern is present—several days or weeks of fever and chills alternating with afebrile periods with no chills. Systemic symptoms indicate a poor prognosis. Progressive lymphadenopathy eventually causes widespread effects, such as hepatomegaly and dyspnea.

• *Hypoglycemia.* Rapidly induced hypoglycemia may cause diaphoresis accompanied by irritability, tremors, hypotension, blurred vision, tachycardia, hunger, and loss of consciousness.

• *Immunoblastic lymphadenopathy.* Resembling Hodgkin's disease but rarer, this disorder causes episodic diaphoresis, along with fever, weight loss, weakness, generalized lymphadenopathy, rash, and hepatosplenomegaly.

• *Infective endocarditis (subacute).* Generalized night sweats occur early in this disorder. Accompanying signs and symptoms include intermittent low-grade fever, weakness, fatigue, weight loss, anorexia, and arthralgia. A sudden change in a murmur or the discovery of a new murmur is a classic sign. Petechiae and splinter hemorrhages are also common.

• *Liver abscess.* Signs and symptoms vary, depending on the extent of the abscess. Common findings include diaphoresis, right upper quadrant pain, weight loss, fever, chills, nausea, vomiting, and signs of anemia.

• *Lung abscess.* Drenching night sweats are common in this disorder. Its chief sign, though, is a cough productive of copious purulent, foul-smelling, often bloody sputum. Associated findings are fever with chills, pleuritic chest pain, dyspnea, weakness, anorexia, weight loss, headache, malaise, clubbing, tubular or amphoric breath sounds, and dullness on percussion.

• *Malaria.* Profuse diaphoresis marks the third stage of the malarial paroxysm. It's preceded by chills (first stage) and high fever (second stage). Headache, arthralgia, and hepatosplenomegaly may also occur. These paroxysms alternate with periods of well-being in the benign form of malaria. However, its severe form may progress to delirium, convulsions, and coma.

• *Ménière's disease.* Characterized by severe vertigo, tinnitus, and hearing loss, this disorder may also cause diaphoresis, nausea, vomiting, and nystagmus. Hearing loss may be progressive, and tinnitus may persist between attacks.

• *Myocardial infarction.* Usually, diaphoresis accompanies acute, substernal, radiating chest pain in this life-threatening disorder. Associated signs and symptoms include anxiety, dyspnea, nausea, vomiting, tachycardia, irregular pulse, blood pressure change, fine crackles, pallor, and clammy skin.

• *Pesticide poisoning.* Among the toxic effects of pesticides are diaphoresis, nausea, vomiting, diarrhea, blurred vision, miosis, and excess lacrimation and salivation. The patient may display fasciculations, muscle weakness, and flaccid paralysis. Signs of respiratory depression and coma may also occur.

• *Pheochromocytoma.* This disorder commonly produces diaphoresis. Its cardinal sign, though, is persistent or paroxysmal hypertension. Other effects include headache, palpitations, tachycardia, anxiety, tremors, pallor, flushing, paresthesia, abdominal pain, tachypnea, nausea, vomiting, and orthostatic hypotension.

• *Pneumonia.* Intermittent, generalized diaphoresis accompanies fever and chills in pneumonia. The patient complains of pleuritic chest pain that increases with deep inspiration. Other features are tachypnea, dyspnea, productive cough (with scant and mucoid or copious and purulent sputum), headache, fatigue, myalgia, abdominal pain, anorexia, and cyanosis. Auscultation reveals bronchial breath sounds.

• *Relapsing fever.* Profuse diaphoresis marks resolution of the crisis stage in this disorder. Typically, the disorder produces attacks of high fever accompanied by severe myalgia, headache, arthralgia, diarrhea, vomiting, coughing, and eye or chest pain. Splenomegaly is common, but hepatomegaly and lymphadenopathy may also occur. The patient may develop a transient, macular rash. Three to 10 days after onset, the febrile attack abruptly terminates in a chill with increased pulse and respirations. Diaphoresis, flushing, and hypotension may then lead to circulatory collapse and death. Invariably, relapse occurs if the patient survives the initial attack.

• *Tetanus.* This disorder commonly causes profuse sweating accompanied by low-grade fever, tachycardia, and hyperactive deep tendon reflexes. Early restlessness and pain and stiffness in the jaw, abdomen, and back progress to spasms associated with lockjaw, risus sardonicus, and opisthotonos. Laryngospasm may result in cyanosis or sudden death by asphyxiation.

• *Thyrotoxicosis.* This disorder commonly produces diaphoresis accompanied by heat intolerance, weight loss despite increased appetite, tachycardia, palpitations, an enlarged thyroid, dyspnea, nervousness, diarrhea, tremors, Plummer's nails, and possibly exophthalmos. Gallops may also occur.

EMERGENCY

WHEN DIAPHORESIS SPELLS CRISIS

Diaphoresis is an early sign of certain life-threatening disorders. These guidelines will help you detect such disorders promptly and intervene to minimize patient harm.

If you observe diaphoresis in a patient who complains of blurred vision, ask about increased irritability and anxiety. Has the patient been unusually hungry? Does he have tremors? Take vital signs, noting hypotension and tachycardia. Then ask about a history of insulin-dependent diabetes. If you suspect *hypoglycemia*, notify the doctor immediately. Then assess the patient's blood glucose level using a glucose reagent strip, or send a serum sample to the lab. Administer I.V. glucose 50%, as ordered, to return the patient's glucose level to normal. Monitor vital signs and cardiac rhythm. Ensure a patent airway and be prepared to assist breathing and circulation if necessary.

If you observe profuse diaphoresis in a weak, tired, and apprehensive patient, suspect *heat stroke,* which can progress to circulatory collapse. Take vital signs, noting a normal or subnormal temperature. Check for ashen-gray skin and dilated pupils. Was the patient recently exposed to high temperatures and humidity? Was he wearing heavy clothing at the time? Also ask about use of diuretics, which interfere with normal sweating. Take the patient to a cool room, remove his clothing, and use a fan to direct cool air over his body. Insert an I.V. line and prepare for electrolyte and fluid replacement. Monitor for signs of shock.

If you observe diaphoresis in a patient with spinal cord injury above T6 or T7, ask about pounding headache, restlessness, blurred vision, and nasal congestion. Take vital signs, noting bradycardia and extremely elevated blood pressure. If you suspect *autonomic hyperreflexia*, quickly rule out its common complications. Assess for eye pain associated with intraocular hemorrhage and for facial paralysis, slurred speech, or limb weakness associated with intracerebral hemorrhage. Quickly reposition the patient to remove any pressure stimulus. Also check for a distended bladder or fecal impaction. Remove any kinks from the urinary catheter if necessary. Or administer a suppository or manually remove fecal impaction. If you can't locate and relieve the causative stimulus, start an I.V. and notify the doctor immediately. Prepare to administer hydralazine for hypertension, as ordered.

If the diaphoretic patient complains of chest pain and dyspnea, suspect *myocardial infarction* or *congestive heart failure.* Connect the patient to a cardiac monitor, ensure a patent airway, and administer supplemental oxygen. Start an I.V. and administer analgesics, as ordered. Be prepared to begin emergency resuscitation if cardiac or respiratory arrest occurs.

• *Tuberculosis.* Although often asymptomatic in primary infection, this disorder may cause night sweats, low-grade fever, fatigue, weakness, anorexia, and weight loss. In reactivation, there may be productive cough with mucopurulent sputum, occasional hemoptysis, and chest pain.

Other causes
• *Drugs.* Sympathomimetics, certain antipsychotics, thyroid hormone, and antipyretics may cause diaphoresis. Aspirin and acetaminophen poisoning also cause this sign.
• *Dumping syndrome.* The result of rapid emptying of gastric contents into the small intestine after partial gastrectomy, this syndrome causes diaphoresis, palpitations, profound weakness, epigastric distress, nausea, and explosive diarrhea. This syndrome occurs soon after eating.

Special considerations
After an episode of diaphoresis, sponge the patient's face and body and change wet clothes and sheets. Dust skin folds in the groin, axillae, and under pendulous breasts with cornstarch or powder to prevent skin irritation. Or tuck gauze or cloth into these folds. Encourage regular bathing.

Replace fluids and electrolytes. Regulate infusions of I.V. saline or Ringer's lactate, and monitor urine output. Encourage oral fluids high in electrolytes (such as Gatorade). Enforce bed rest, if ordered, and maintain a quiet environment. Keep the patient's room temperature moderate to prevent additional diaphoresis.

Explain to the patient and his family that diaphoresis signals a return to normal body temperature in an infection and occurs after taking an antipyretic. It may also be a sympathetic reaction to pain or stress.

Prepare the patient for diagnostic tests, such as blood tests, cultures, chest X-rays, immunologic studies, biopsy, computed tomography scan, and audiometry.

Pediatric pointers
Diaphoresis often results from environmental heat or overdressing an infant or child. Typically, it's most apparent around the head.

Other causes include drug withdrawal associated with maternal addiction, congestive heart failure, thyrotoxicosis, and the effects of drugs such as antihistamines, ephedrine, haloperidol, and thyroid hormone.

You'll need to assess fluid status carefully. Some fluid loss through diaphoresis may precipitate hypovolemia more rapidly in the child than in the adult. Monitor input and output, weigh the child daily, and note the duration of each episode of diaphoresis.

Diarrhea

Usually a chief sign of intestinal disorders, diarrhea is an increase in the frequency and fluidity of bowel movements compared to the patient's normal bowel habits. It varies in severity and may be acute or chronic. Acute diarrhea may result from acute infection, stress, fecal impaction, or the effects of drugs. Chronic diarrhea may result from chronic infection, obstructive and inflammatory bowel disease, malabsorption syndrome, certain endocrine disorders, and the effects of gastrointestinal surgery. Periodic diarrhea may result from food allergy or from ingestion of spicy or high-fiber foods or caffeine.

One or more pathophysiologic mechanisms may contribute to diarrhea (see *What Causes Diarrhea,* page 232). The fluid and electrolyte imbalances it produces may precipitate life-threatening dysrhythmias or hypovolemic shock.

Assessment
If the patient's diarrhea is profuse, check for signs of shock— tachycardia, hypotension, and cool, pale, clammy skin. If you detect

these signs, place the patient supine and elevate his legs 20°. Insert an I.V. line for fluid replacement. Also assess for electrolyte imbalance; in hypokalemia, look for an irregular pulse, muscle weakness, anorexia, and nausea and vomiting. Report these signs and symptoms at once. Keep emergency resuscitation equipment handy.

If the patient isn't in shock, proceed with a physical examination. Assess hydration first; check skin turgor and take blood pressure with the patient lying, sitting, and standing. Inspect the abdomen for distention and palpate for tenderness. Auscultate bowel sounds. Also, take the patient's temperature and note any chills.

Explore signs and symptoms associated with diarrhea. Does the patient have abdominal pain and cramps? Difficulty breathing? Is he weak or fatigued? Find out the patient's drug history. Has he had GI surgery or radiation therapy? Ask the patient to briefly describe his diet. Does he have any known food allergies? Lastly, find out if the patient is under unusual stress.

Medical causes

• *Carcinoid syndrome.* In this disorder, severe diarrhea occurs with flushing, abdominal cramps, dyspnea, and palpitations. Associated signs and symptoms include skin lesions, weight loss, anorexia, weakness, and depression.

• *Crohn's disease.* This recurring inflammatory disorder produces diarrhea accompanied by hyperactive bowel sounds, abdominal pain with guarding and tenderness, and nausea. The patient also displays fever, chills, weakness, anorexia, and weight loss.

• *Infections.* Acute viral, bacterial, and protozoal infections cause the sudden onset of extremely watery diarrhea. They also cause abdominal pain, cramps, nausea, vomiting, and fever. Occasionally, significant fluid and electrolyte loss causes signs of dehydration and shock. Chronic tuberculosis and fungal and parasitic infections cause less severe but more persistent diarrhea, accompanied by epigastric distress, vomiting, weight loss, and possibly passage of blood and mucus.

• *Intestinal obstruction.* Partial intestinal obstruction increases intestinal motility, resulting in diarrhea, abdominal pain with tenderness and guarding, nausea, and possibly distention.

• *Irritable bowel syndrome.* Diarrhea alternates with constipation or normal bowel function. Related findings: abdominal pain, tenderness, and distention; dyspepsia; and nausea.

• *Ischemic bowel disease.* In this life-threatening disorder, bloody diarrhea occurs with abdominal pain. In severe ischemia, there may be signs of shock.

• *Lactose intolerance.* Diarrhea occurs within several hours of ingesting milk or milk products. It's accompanied by cramps, abdominal pain, and flatus.

• *Large-bowel neoplasms.* In this disorder, bloody diarrhea alternates with pencil-thin stools. Other clinical findings: abdominal pain, anorexia, weight loss, weakness, and depression.

• *Lead poisoning.* Alternating diarrhea and constipation occur here. Other GI effects include abdominal pain, anorexia, nausea, and vomiting. The patient complains of a metallic taste, headache, and dizziness, and displays a lead line on his gums.

• *Malabsorption syndrome.* Occurring after meals, diarrhea is accompanied by steatorrhea, abdominal distention, and muscle cramps. The patient also displays anorexia, weight loss, bone pain, anemia, weakness, and fatigue.

• *Pseudomembranous enterocolitis.* This life-threatening disorder produces copious watery or bloody diarrhea that rapidly precipitates signs of shock. Other features include colicky abdominal pain and distention, fever, nausea, vomiting, and disorientation.

• *Thyrotoxicosis.* In this disorder, diarrhea is accompanied by nervousness, tremor, diaphoresis, weight loss despite increased appetite, dyspnea, palpitations, tachycardia, an enlarged thyroid, heat intolerance, and possibly exophthalmos.

• *Ulcerative colitis.* The hallmark of this disorder is recurrent bloody diarrhea with pus or mucus. Other features are tenesmus, hyperactive bowel sounds, cramping lower abdominal pain, low-grade fever, anorexia, and, at times, nausea and vomiting. Weight loss and weakness are late findings.

Other causes

• *Drugs.* Many antibiotics, such as ampicillin, cephalosporins, tetracyclines, and clindamycin, cause diarrhea. Other drugs that may cause diarrhea include magnesium-containing antacids, colchicine, guanethidine, lactulose, dantrolene, ethacrynic acid, mefenamic acid, methotrexate, metyrosine, and, in high doses, digitalis and quinidine. Laxative abuse can cause acute or chronic diarrhea.

• *Treatments.* Gastrectomy, gastroenterostomy, and pyloroplasty may produce diarrhea. High-dose radiation therapy may produce enteritis associated with diarrhea.

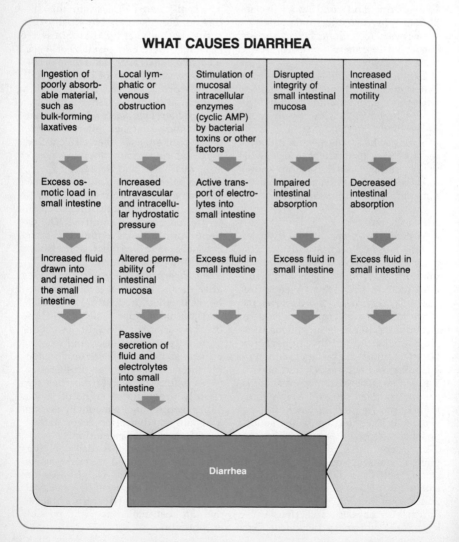

WHAT CAUSES DIARRHEA

Ingestion of poorly absorbable material, such as bulk-forming laxatives	Local lymphatic or venous obstruction	Stimulation of mucosal intracellular enzymes (cyclic AMP) by bacterial toxins or other factors	Disrupted integrity of small intestinal mucosa	Increased intestinal motility
Excess osmotic load in small intestine	Increased intravascular and intracellular hydrostatic pressure	Active transport of electrolytes into small intestine	Impaired intestinal absorption	Decreased intestinal absorption
Increased fluid drawn into and retained in the small intestine	Altered permeability of intestinal mucosa	Excess fluid in small intestine	Excess fluid in small intestine	Excess fluid in small intestine
	Passive secretion of fluid and electrolytes into small intestine			

Diarrhea

Special considerations

Explain the purpose and procedure of diagnostic tests to the patient. These tests may include blood studies, stool cultures, X-rays, and endoscopy.

Help the patient maintain adequate hydration. Remember that dehydration occurs rapidly in the elderly. Measure liquid stools and weigh the patient daily. Monitor electrolyte levels and hematocrit. Encourage oral fluids and accurately administer I.V. fluid replacements.

Administer analgesics for pain and an opiate to decrease intestinal motility, if ordered. Ensure the patient's privacy during defecation, and empty bedpans promptly. Cleanse the perineum thoroughly, and apply ointments to prevent skin breakdown.

Advise the patient to avoid spicy or high-fiber foods (such as fruits), caffeine, and milk. Suggest smaller, more frequent meals if he's had GI surgery or disease. If appropriate, teach the patient stress-reducing exercises, such as guided imagery and deep-breathing techniques, or recommend counseling.

In inflammatory bowel disease (particularly ulcerative colitis), stress the need for medical follow-up. The risk of colon cancer is greater in these patients.

Pediatric pointers

Diarrhea in children frequently results from infection, although chronic diarrhea may result from malabsorption syndrome, anatomic defects, or allergy. Because dehydration and electrolyte imbalance occur rapidly in children, diarrhea can be life-threatening. Diligently monitor all episodes of diarrhea and replace fluids immediately.

Diplopia

Diplopia is double vision—seeing one object as two. This symptom results when extraocular muscles fail to work together, causing images to fall on noncorresponding parts of the retinas. What causes this muscle incoordination? Orbital lesions, the effects of surgery, or impaired function of cranial nerves that supply extraocular muscles (oculomotor, CN III; trochlear, CN IV; abducens, CN VI) may be responsible.

Diplopia usually begins intermittently or affects near or far vision exclusively. It can be classified as monocular or binocular. More common binocular diplopia may result from ocular deviation or displacement, extraocular muscle palsies, or psychoneurosis. It may also follow retinal surgery. Monocular diplopia may result from an early cataract, retinal edema or scarring, iridodialysis, subluxated lens, poorly fitting contact lens, or uncorrected refractive error. Diplopia may also occur in hysteria or malingering.

Assessment

If the patient complains of double vision, first check his neurologic status. Evaluate his level of consciousness, pupil size and response to light, and motor and sensory functions. Then take his vital signs. Briefly ask about associated symptoms, especially severe headache. Find out about associated neurologic symptoms first because diplopia can accompany serious disorders.

Now continue with a more detailed assessment. Find out when the patient first noticed diplopia. Are the images side-by-side (horizontal), one above the other (vertical), or a combination? Does diplopia affect near or far vision? Does it affect certain directions of gaze? Ask if diplopia has worsened, remained the same, or subsided. Does its severity change throughout the day? Worsening of diplopia or its appearance by evening may indicate myasthenia gravis. Find out if the patient can correct diplopia by tilting his head. If so, ask him to show you. (If the patient has a fourth nerve lesion, tilting of his head toward the opposite shoulder causes compensatory tilting of the unaffected eye. If he has incomplete sixth nerve palsy, tilting of his head toward the side of the paralyzed muscle may relax the affected lateral rectus muscle.)

Explore associated symptoms, such as eye pain. Ask about hypertension, diabetes mellitus, allergies, and thyroid, neurologic, or muscular disorders. Also note a history of extraocular muscle disorders, trauma, or eye surgery.

Observe the patient for ocular deviation, ptosis, proptosis, lid edema, and conjunctival injection. Distinguish monocular and binocular diplopia by asking the patient to occlude one eye. If he still sees double, he has monocular diplopia. Test visual acuity and extraocular muscles. Check vital signs.

Medical causes

● *Alcohol intoxication.* Diplopia is a common symptom of this disorder. It's accompanied by confusion, slurred speech, halitosis, staggering gait, behavior changes, nausea, vomiting, and possible conjunctival injection.

● *Botulism.* Hallmark signs are diplopia, dysarthria, dysphagia, and ptosis. Early findings include dry mouth, sore throat, vomiting, and diarrhea. Later, descending weakness or paralysis of extremity and trunk muscles causes hyporeflexia and dyspnea.

● *Brain tumor.* In this disorder, diplopia may be an early symptom. Accompanying features vary with the tumor's size and location. There may be eye deviation, emotional lability, decreased level of consciousness, headache, vomiting, petit or grand mal seizures, hearing loss, visual field cuts, abnormal pupillary responses, nystagmus, motor weakness, and paralysis.

● *Cavernous sinus thrombosis.* This disorder may produce diplopia and limited eye movement. Associated signs and symptoms include proptosis, orbital and lid edema, diminished or absent pupillary responses, impaired visual acuity, papilledema, and fever.

● *Cerebrovascular accident.* Diplopia characterizes this life-threatening disorder when it affects the vertebrobasilar artery. Other clinical features may include unilateral motor weakness or paralysis, ataxia, decreased level of consciousness, dizziness, aphasia, visual field cuts, circumoral numbness, slurred speech, dysphagia, and amnesia.

● *Diabetes mellitus.* Among the long-term effects of this disorder may be diplopia—the result of isolated third cranial nerve palsy. Typically, diplopia begins suddenly and may be accompanied by pain.

● *Encephalitis.* Initially, this disorder may cause a brief episode of diplopia and eye deviation. Most commonly, though, it begins with sudden onset of high fever, severe headache, and vomiting. As the inflammation progresses, there may be signs of meningeal irritation, decreased level of consciousness, seizures, ataxia, and paralysis.

● *Head injury.* This potentially life-threatening disorder may cause diplopia, depending on the site and extent of the injury. Associated signs and symptoms may include eye deviation, pupillary changes, headache, decreased level of consciousness, altered vital signs, nausea, vomiting, and motor weakness or paralysis.

● *Intracranial aneurysm.* This life-threatening disorder initially produces diplopia and eye deviation, perhaps accompanied by ptosis and a dilated pupil on the affected side. The patient will complain of a recurrent, severe, unilateral, frontal headache. After rupture of the aneurysm, the headache becomes violent. Associated signs and symptoms include neck and spinal pain and rigidity, decreased level of consciousness, tinnitus, dizziness, nausea, vomiting, and unilateral muscle weakness or paralysis.

● *Multiple sclerosis.* Diplopia is commonly an early symptom in this disorder. It's usually accompanied by blurred vision and paresthesias. As the disorder progresses, its variable signs

TESTING EXTRAOCULAR MUSCLES

The coordinated action of six muscles controls eyeball movements. To test the function of each muscle and the cranial nerve (CN) that innervates it, ask the patient to look in the direction controlled by that muscle. The six directions you can test make up the *cardinal fields of gaze*. The patient's inability to turn the eye in the designated direction indicates muscle weakness or paralysis.

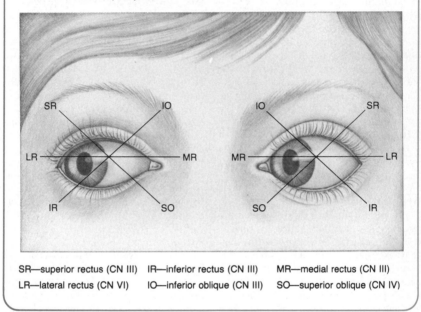

SR—superior rectus (CN III)   IR—inferior rectus (CN III)   MR—medial rectus (CN III)

LR—lateral rectus (CN VI)   IO—inferior oblique (CN III)   SO—superior oblique (CN IV)

and symptoms may include nystagmus, constipation, muscle weakness, paralysis, spasticity, hyperreflexia, intention tremor, gait ataxia, dysphagia, dysarthria, impotence, emotional lability, and urinary frequency, urgency, and incontinence.

• *Myasthenia gravis.* Initially, this disorder produces diplopia and ptosis that worsen throughout the day. It then progressively involves other muscles, resulting in blank facial expression; nasal voice; difficulty in chewing, swallowing, and making fine hand movements; and possibly signs of life-threatening respiratory muscle weakness.

• *Ophthalmoplegic migraine.* Occurring most often in young adults, this disorder results in diplopia that persists for days after the headache. Accom-

panying signs and symptoms are severe, unilateral pain, ptosis, and extraocular muscle palsies. Irritability, depression, or slight confusion may also occur.

• *Orbital blowout fracture.* This fracture usually causes monocular diplopia affecting the upward gaze. However, with marked periorbital edema, diplopia may affect other directions of gaze. Most commonly, this fracture causes periorbital ecchymosis. It usually doesn't affect visual acuity, although eyelid edema may prevent accurate testing. Subcutaneous crepitation of the eyelid and orbit is typical. Occasionally, the patient's pupil is dilated and unreactive, and he may have a hyphema.

• *Orbital cellulitis.* Inflammation of the orbital tissues and eyelids causes sudden diplopia. Other findings are eye deviation and pain, purulent drainage, lid edema, chemosis and redness, proptosis, nausea, and fever.

• **Orbital tumors.** Enlarging tumors can cause diplopia. Proptosis and possibly blurred vision may also occur.

• **Thyrotoxicosis.** Diplopia occurs when exophthalmos characterizes the disorder. It's accompanied by impaired eye movement, excessive tearing, lid edema, and possibly inability to close the lids. Other cardinal findings include tachycardia, palpitations, weight loss, diarrhea, tremors, an enlarged thyroid, dyspnea, nervousness, diaphoresis, and heat intolerance.

Other cause
• **Eye surgery.** Fibrosis associated with eye surgery may restrict eye movement, resulting in diplopia.

Special considerations
Continue to monitor vital signs and neurologic status if an acute neurologic disorder is suspected. Prepare the patient for neurologic tests, such as a computed tomography scan. Provide a safe environment. In severe diplopia, remove sharp obstacles and assist the patient with ambulation. Also institute seizure precautions, if indicated.

Pediatric pointers
Strabismus, a congenital disorder or one acquired at an early age, produces diplopia; however, in young children, the brain rapidly compensates for double vision by suppressing one image, so diplopia is a rare complaint. School-age children who complain of double vision require a careful examination to rule out serious disorders, such as brain tumor.

Dizziness

A common symptom, dizziness is a sensation of imbalance or faintness, sometimes associated with giddiness, weakness, confusion, and blurred or double vision. Usually, episodes of dizziness are brief; they may be mild or severe with abrupt or gradual onset. Dizziness may be aggravated by standing up quickly and alleviated by lying down and by rest.

Typically, dizziness results from inadequate blood flow and oxygen supply to the cerebrum and spinal cord. It may occur in anxiety, in respiratory and cardiovascular disorders, and in postconcussion syndrome. It's a key symptom in certain serious disorders such as hypertension and vertebrobasilar artery insufficiency.

Dizziness is often confused with vertigo—a sensation of revolving in space or of surroundings revolving about oneself. However, unlike dizziness, vertigo is often accompanied by nausea, vomiting, nystagmus, staggering gait, and tinnitus or hearing loss. Dizziness and vertigo may occur together, as in postconcussion syndrome.

Assessment
If the patient complains of dizziness, first assess its severity. When did it begin? Is it associated with headache or blurred vision? Next take the patient's vital signs and ask about a history of high blood pressure. If his diastolic pressure exceeds 100 mm Hg, notify the doctor immediately. Tell the patient to lie down, and recheck his vital signs every 15 minutes until the doctor arrives. Start an I.V. and prepare to administer an antihypertensive. While you wait, continue to gather assessment data. Ask about a history of diabetes and cardiovascular disease. Is the patient taking drugs prescribed for high blood pressure? If so, when was his last dose?

If the patient's blood pressure is normal, obtain a more complete history. Ask about myocardial infarction, congestive heart failure, or atherosclerosis—which may predispose the patient to cardiac dysrhythmias, hypertension, or transient ischemic attack (TIA). Is there a history of anemia, chronic obstructive pulmonary disease (COPD), anxiety disorders, or head injury? Obtain a complete drug history.

Next, explore the patient's dizziness fully. How often does it occur? How long does each episode last? Does his dizziness abate spontaneously? Or does it lead to loss of consciousness? Find out if dizziness is triggered by sitting up suddenly or stooping over. Does being in a crowd make the patient feel dizzy? Ask about emotional stress. Has the patient been irritable or anxious? Does he have insomnia or difficulty concentrating? During the interview, look for fidgeting and eyelid twitching. Does the patient startle easily? Also ask about palpitations, chest pain, diaphoresis, shortness of breath, and chronic cough.

Next perform a physical examination. Begin with a quick neurocheck, assessing level of consciousness, motor and sensory functions, and reflexes. Then inspect for poor skin turgor and dry mucous membranes—signs of dehydration. Auscultate heart rate and rhythm. Inspect for barrel chest, clubbing, cyanosis, and use of accessory muscles. Also auscultate breath sounds. Take the patient's blood pressure while he's lying, sitting, and standing to check for orthostatic hypotension. Test capillary refill time in the extremities, and palpate for edema.

Medical causes

● *Anemia.* Typically, this disorder causes dizziness that's aggravated by postural changes or exertion. Other clinical features include pallor, dyspnea, fatigue, tachycardia, and bounding pulse. Capillary refill time will be prolonged.

● *Cardiac dysrhythmias.* Dizziness lasts for several minutes or longer with this disorder, and may precede fainting. The patient may experience palpitations; irregular, rapid, or thready pulse; and possible hypotension. He may also experience weakness, blurred vision, paresthesias, and confusion.

● *Carotid sinus hypersensitivity.* Brief episodes of dizziness that usually terminate in fainting are characteristic. These episodes are precipitated by stimulation of one or both carotid arteries by wearing a tight collar, movement of the patient's head, or other seemingly minor sensations or actions. Associated signs and symptoms are sweating, nausea, and pallor.

● *Emphysema.* Dizziness may follow exertion or the chronic, productive cough in this disorder. Associated signs and symptoms include dyspnea, anorexia, weight loss, malaise, use of accessory muscles, pursed-lip breathing, tachypnea, peripheral cyanosis, and diminished breath sounds. Barrel chest and clubbing are late signs.

● *Generalized anxiety disorder.* This disorder produces continuous dizziness that may intensify as the disorder worsens. Associated signs and symptoms are persistent anxiety (for at least 1 month), insomnia, difficulty concentrating, and irritability. The patient may show signs of motor tension—for example, twitching or fidgeting, muscle aches, furrowed brow, and a tendency to be startled. He may also display signs of autonomic hyperactivity—for example, diaphoresis, palpitations, cold and clammy hands, dry mouth, paresthesia, indigestion, hot or cold flashes, frequent urination, diarrhea, a lump in the throat, pallor, and increased pulse and respirations.

● *Hypertension.* In this disorder, dizziness may precede fainting. However, it may also be relieved by rest. Other common signs and symptoms are elevated blood pressure, headache, and blurred vision. Retinal changes include hemorrhage, exudate, and papilledema.

● *Hyperventilation syndrome.* Episodes of hyperventilation cause dizziness that usually lasts a few minutes; however, if these episodes occur frequently, dizziness may persist between them. Other effects include apprehension, diaphoresis, pallor, dyspnea, chest tightness, palpitations, trembling, fatigue, and peripheral and circumoral paresthesia.

● *Orthostatic hypotension.* This condition produces dizziness that may terminate in fainting or disappear with rest. Related findings include dim vision, spots before the eyes, pallor, diaphoresis, hypotension, tachycardia, and possibly signs of dehydration.

• *Panic disorder.* Dizziness accompanies acute attacks of panic in this disorder. Other findings include anxiety, dyspnea, palpitations, chest pain, a choking or smothering sensation, vertigo, paresthesia, hot and cold flashes, sweating, and trembling or shaking. The patient may be troubled by a fear of dying or losing his mind.

• *Postconcussion syndrome.* Occurring 1 to 3 weeks after head injury, this syndrome is marked by dizziness, headache (throbbing, aching, bandlike, or stabbing), emotional lability, alcohol intolerance, fatigue, anxiety, and possibly vertigo. Dizziness and other symptoms are intensified by mental or physical stress. The syndrome may persist for years, but symptoms eventually abate.

• *Transient ischemic attack.* Lasting from a few seconds to 24 hours, an attack frequently signals impending stroke and may be triggered by turning the head to the side. Dizziness of varying severity occurs during an attack. It's accompanied by unilateral or bilateral diplopia, blindness or visual field deficits, ptosis, tinnitus, hearing loss, paresis, and numbness. Other findings: dysarthria, dysphagia, vomiting, hiccups, confusion, decreased level of consciousness, and pallor.

Other causes

• *Drugs.* Antianxiety drugs, central nervous system depressants, narcotics, decongestants, antihistamines, antihypertensives, and vasodilators frequently cause dizziness.

Special considerations

Prepare the patient for diagnostic tests, such as blood studies, arteriography, computed tomography, electroencephalography, and magnetic resonance imaging.

Help the patient control dizziness. If he's hyperventilating, have him breathe and rebreathe into his cupped hands or a paper bag. If the patient experiences dizziness in an upright position, tell him to lie down and to rest, then rise slowly. Advise the patient with carotid sinus hypersensitivity to avoid wearing garments that fit tightly at the neck. Instruct the patient who risks a TIA from vertebrobasilar insufficiency to avoid sharply turning his head to one side; have him turn his body instead.

Pediatric pointers

Dizziness is less common in a child than in an adult. Often the child has difficulty describing this symptom and will instead complain of tiredness, stomachache, or feeling sick. If you suspect dizziness, assess for vertigo as well. A more common symptom, vertigo may result from vision disorders, ear infections, and the effects of antibiotics.

Doll's Eye Sign—Absent
[Negative oculocephalic reflex]

An ominous indicator of brain stem dysfunction, the absence of the doll's eye sign is detected by rapid, but gentle, turning of the patient's head from side to side. The eyes remain fixed in midposition, instead of moving laterally toward the side opposite the direction the head is turned. Usually, this sign can't be elicited in the conscious patient because he voluntarily controls eye movements.

The absence of doll's eye sign indicates injury to the midbrain, pons, and cranial nerves III, VI, and VIII. Typically, it accompanies coma caused by lesions of the cerebellum and brain stem. In fact, when it's detected in deep coma, absent doll's eye sign is a mark of brain death.

A variant of absent doll's eye sign that develops gradually is known as abnormal doll's eye sign: conjugate eye movement is lost, so that one eye may move laterally while the other remains fixed or moves in the opposite direction. Usually, an abnormal doll's eye sign accompanies metabolic coma or increased intracranial pressure (ICP). The associated brain stem dysfunction may be reversible or may progress to deeper coma with absent doll's sign.

Assessment

After detecting an absent doll's eye sign, perform a neurologic assessment. First assess the patient's level of consciousness using the Glasgow Coma Scale. Look for lightening or deepening coma and note decerebrate or decorticate posture. Examine the pupils for size, equality, and response to light. Check for signs of increased ICP—increased blood pressure, increasing pulse pressure, and bradycardia.

Medical causes

• **Brain stem infarction.** This infarction causes absent doll's eye sign with coma. It also causes limb paralysis, cranial nerve palsies (facial weakness, diplopia, blindness or visual field deficits, nystagmus), bilateral cerebellar ataxia, and variable sensory loss. Late signs are a positive Babinski's reflex, decerebrate posture, and flaccidity.

• **Brain stem tumors.** Absent doll's eye sign accompanies coma with this disorder. This sign may be preceded by hemiparesis, nystagmus, extraocular nerve palsies, facial pain or sensory loss, facial paralysis, diminished corneal reflex, tinnitus, hearing loss, dysphagia, drooling, vertigo, dizziness, ataxia, and vomiting.

• **Central midbrain infarction.** Accompanying absent doll's eye sign are coma, Weber's syndrome (oculomotor palsy with contralateral hemiplegia), contralateral ataxic tremor, nystagmus, and pupillary abnormalities.

• **Cerebellar lesion.** Whether associated with abscess, hemorrhage, or tumor, a

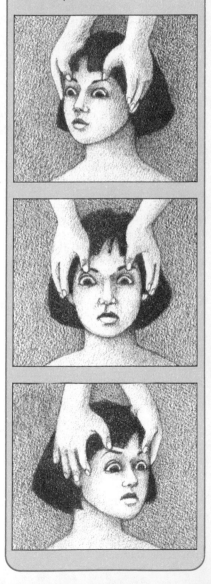

TESTING FOR ABSENT DOLL'S EYE SIGN

To evaluate the patient's oculocephalic reflex, hold her upper eyelids open and quickly (but gently) turn her head from side to side, noting eye movements with each head turn.

In *absent doll's eye sign*, the eyes remain fixed in midposition.

cerebellar lesion that progresses to coma may also cause an absent doll's eye sign. Coma may be preceded by headache, nystagmus, ocular deviation to the side of the lesion, unequal pupils, dysarthria, dysphagia, ipsilateral facial paresis, and cerebellar ataxia. Characteristic signs of increased ICP may also occur, including decreased level of consciousness, abnormal pupillary responses, increased systolic blood pressure, widening pulse pressure, bradycardia, altered respiratory pattern, papilledema, and vomiting.

• *Pontine hemorrhage.* Absent doll's eye sign and coma develop within minutes in this life-threatening disorder. Other ominous signs, such as complete paralysis, decerebrate posture, a positive Babinski's reflex, and small, reactive pupils, may then rapidly progress to death.

• *Posterior fossa hematoma.* A subdural hematoma at this location typically causes absent doll's eye sign and coma. These signs may be preceded by characteristic clinical features, such as headache, vomiting, drowsiness, confusion, unequal pupils, dysphagia, cranial nerve palsies, stiff neck, and cerebellar ataxia.

Other causes
• *Drugs.* Barbiturates may produce severe central nervous system depression, resulting in coma and absent doll's eye sign.

Special considerations
Do not attempt to elicit doll's eye sign in the comatose patient with suspected cervical spine injury; this risks spinal cord damage. Instead, evaluate the oculovestibular reflex with the cold caloric test. Normally, instillation of cold water in the ear causes the eyes to move slowly toward the irrigated ear, then rapidly away. Cold caloric testing may also be done to confirm absent doll's eye sign.

Continue to monitor vital signs and neurologic status in the patient with an absent doll's eye sign.

Pediatric pointers
Normally, the doll's eye sign is not present for the first 10 days after birth, and it may be irregular until age 2. After that, this sign reliably indicates brain stem function.

An absent doll's eye sign in children may accompany coma associated with head injury, near-drowning or suffocation, or brain stem astrocytoma.

Drooling

Drooling—the flow of saliva from the mouth—results from a failure to swallow or retain saliva, or from excess salivation. It may stem from facial muscle paralysis or weakness that prevents mouth closure, from neuromuscular disorders or local pain that causes dysphagia, or less commonly from the effects of drugs or toxins that induce salivation. Drooling may be scant or copious (up to 1 liter daily) and may cause circumoral irritation. Because it signals an inability to handle secretions, drooling warns of potential aspiration.

Assessment
If you observe the patient drooling, first assess its amount. Is it scant or copious? When did it begin? Ask the patient if his pillow is wet in the morning. Also inspect for circumoral irritation.

Then explore associated signs and symptoms. Ask about sore throat and difficulty in swallowing, chewing, speaking, or breathing. Have the patient describe any pain or stiffness in the face and neck and any muscle weakness in the face and extremities. Has he noticed any mental status changes such as drowsiness or agitation? Ask about changes in vision, hearing, and sense of taste. Also ask about anorexia, weight loss, fatigue, nausea, vomiting, and altered bowel or bladder habits. Has the patient recently had a cold or other infection? Was he bitten by an animal within the past few months? Was he exposed to pesticides? Finally, obtain a complete drug history.

Next perform a physical examination. Take vital signs. Inspect for signs of facial paralysis or abnormal expression. Examine the mouth and neck for swelling, the throat for edema and redness, and the tonsils for exudate. Note foul breath odor. Examine the tongue for bilateral furrowing (trident tongue). Look for pallor and skin lesions and for frontal baldness. Carefully assess any bite or puncture marks.

Assess cranial nerves II through VII, IX, and X. Then, check pupillary size and response to light. Assess the patient's speech. Evaluate muscle strength and palpate for tenderness or atrophy. Also palpate for lymphadenopathy, especially in the cervical area. Test for poor balance, hyperreflexia, and positive Babinski's reflex. Also assess sensory function for paresthesia.

Medical causes

• *Achalasia.* Progressively severe dysphagia may cause copious drooling late in this disorder. When the patient lies down, food and saliva in the dilated esophagus flow back to the pharynx and mouth, resulting in drooling. Coughing or choking and aspiration may follow regurgitation. Other findings are weight loss and possibly spasms or substernal pain after eating.

• *Acoustic neuroma.* When this malignant tumor involves the facial nerve, it produces facial weakness or paralysis with constant scant-to-copious drooling. The drooling follows with tinnitus, unilateral hearing loss, and vertigo. Other symptoms may include dysphagia, poor balance, and ear or eye pain.

• *Amyotrophic lateral sclerosis.* Brain stem involvement in this degenerative disorder weakens muscles of the face and tongue, resulting in constant scant-to-copious drooling. The drooling is accompanied by dysarthria and difficulty chewing, swallowing, and breathing. Fasciculations are common along with muscle atrophy and weakness, especially in the forearms and hands, and hyperreflexia and spasticity in the legs.

• *Bell's palsy.* In this disorder, constant drooling accompanies sudden onset of facial hemiplegia. The affected side of the face sags and is expressionless, the nasolabial fold flattens, and the palpebral fissure (distance between upper and lower eyelids) widens. The patient usually complains of pain in or behind the ear. Other cardinal signs and symptoms include unilateral diminished or absent corneal reflex, decreased lacrimation, Bell's phenomenon (upward deviation of the eye with attempt at lid closure), and partial loss of taste or abnormal taste sensation.

• *Cerebrovascular accident (CVA).* Facial paralysis associated with CVA results in scant-to-copious drooling. Other signs and symptoms may include diplopia, visual field deficits, dysarthria, hearing loss, paresthesia, paralysis, ataxia, headache, dizziness, confusion, nausea, vomiting, unilateral or bilateral hyperactive deep tendon reflexes, and a positive Babinski's reflex.

• *Diphtheria.* In this infection, moderate drooling results from dysphagia associated with sore throat. The hallmark of diphtheria, though, is a bluish white, gray, or black membrane over the mucous membranes of the tonsils, pharynx, larynx, soft palate, and nose. This membrane causes pooling of saliva, which aggravates drooling. Other signs and symptoms may include fever, pallor, tachycardia, foul breath, noisy respirations, cervical lymphadenopathy, purpuric skin lesions, drowsiness, and delirium.

• *Envenomation.* Some snake bites trigger excess salivation, resulting in drooling. The drooling is accompanied by other neurotoxic effects, such as diaphoresis, chills (with or without fever), weakness, dizziness, nausea, vomiting, paresthesia, fasciculations, and tender lymphadenopathy. Local swelling, pain, and ecchymoses may occur.

• *Esophageal tumor.* In this disorder, copious and persistent drooling is typically preceded by weight loss and progressively severe dysphagia. Other clinical features include substernal, back, or neck pain and blood-flecked regurgitation.

• *Glossopharyngeal neuralgia.* Drooling may accompany the sharp paroxysms of pain that characterize this rare disorder. The pain may be precipitated by swallowing, talking, chewing, or coughing, or by external pressure on the ear; it may affect the posterior pharynx, the ear, or the base of the tongue or jaw. Associated findings include hoarseness, soft palate deviation to the unaffected side, absent gag reflex, partial loss of taste, and trapezius and sternocleidomastoid muscle weakness.

• *Guillain-Barré syndrome.* The hallmark of this polyneuritis is ascending muscle weakness that typically starts in the legs and extends to the arms and face within 24 to 72 hours. Facial diplegia and dysphagia set the stage for scant-to-copious drooling. The drooling is accompanied by dysarthria, nasal voice tone, and a diminished or absent corneal reflex. Other clinical findings may include paresthesias, signs of respiratory distress, and signs of sympathetic dysfunction, such as postural hypotension, loss of bowel and bladder control, diaphoresis, and tachycardia.

• *Hypocalcemia.* The chief feature of this disorder is tetany, characterized by muscle twitching, cramps, and convulsions; carpopedal spasm; and a positive Chvostek's sign. Moderate-to-copious drooling may accompany the resultant dysphagia. In severe hypocalcemia, there may be laryngeal spasm with stridor, cyanosis, and grand mal seizures.

• *Ludwig's angina.* In this disorder, moderate-to-copious drooling stems from dysphagia and local swelling of the floor of the mouth, causing tongue displacement. Submandibular swelling of the neck and signs of respiratory distress may also occur.

• *Myasthenia gravis.* Facial and pharyngeal muscle weakness in this disorder causes scant-to-copious drooling. It's accompanied by difficulty swallowing, chewing, and speaking. Typically, drooling is preceded by diplopia and ptosis. The patient displays a masklike face and myasthenia snarl (smile with lips elevated but not retracted). Other features include a weak tongue with bilateral furrowing (trident tongue) and sagging jaw if masseter muscles are affected. Skeletal muscle weakness is characteristic; typically, muscles weaken throughout the day, especially after exercise.

• *Myotonic dystrophy.* Facial weakness and a sagging jaw account for constant drooling in this disorder. Other characteristic findings include myotonia (inability to relax a muscle after its contraction), muscle wasting, cataracts, testicular atrophy, frontal baldness, ptosis, and a nasal, monotone voice.

• *Paralytic poliomyelitis.* When this infection involves the brain stem, it may produce facial paralysis and dysphagia, resulting in scant-to-copious drooling. Typically, the drooling is preceded by fever, headache, nuchal rigidity, and intense muscle aches. The patient then develops fasciculations and usually asymmetrical paralysis in the lower legs and trunk, associated with transient urinary retention.

• *Parkinson's disease.* In this degenerative disorder, drooling occurs because saliva isn't directed to the back of the mouth. Other cardinal features include pill-rolling tremor, rigidity, bradykinesia, shuffling gait, stooped posture, masklike facies, dysarthria, and a high-pitched, monotone voice.

• *Peritonsillar abscess.* Severe sore throat causes dysphagia with moderate-to-copious drooling with this abscess. It's accompanied by high fever, rancid breath, and enlarged, reddened, edematous tonsils that may be covered by a soft, gray exudate. Palpation may reveal cervical lymphadenopathy.

• *Pesticide poisoning.* Toxic effects of pesticides may include excess salivation with drooling. Other effects are diaphoresis, nausea and vomiting, involuntary urination and defecation, blurred vision, miosis, increased lacrimation, fasciculations, weakness, flaccid paralysis, signs of respiratory distress, and coma.

• *Rabies.* When this acute central nervous system infection advances to the brain stem, it produces drooling, or "foaming at the mouth." Drooling stems from excessive salivation, facial palsy, and/or extremely painful pharyngeal spasms that prohibit swallowing. It's accompanied by hydrophobia in about 50% of patients. Seizures and hyperactive deep tendon reflexes may also occur before the patient displays generalized flaccid paralysis and coma.

• *Retropharyngeal abscess.* This disorder causes painful swallowing, resulting in moderate-to-copious drooling. The patient complains of a lump in his throat that he can't swallow and of dyspnea when he's sitting that disappears when he lies down. Other cardinal signs and symptoms include coughing, snoring, choking, noisy breathing, and a "cry of a duck" voice tone. Cervical lymphadenopathy, pharyngeal edema and redness, and a high fever may also occur.

• *Seizures (generalized).* This tonic-clonic muscular reaction causes excessive salivation and frothing at the mouth accompanied by loss of consciousness and cyanosis. In the unresponsive postictal state, the patient may also drool.

• *Tetanus.* This acute infection may produce scant-to-copious drooling associated with dysphagia. Typically, drooling is preceded by restlessness and pain and stiffness in the jaw, abdomen, and back that progress to tonic spasms. A locked jaw and a grotesque, grinning expression called risus sardonicus are characteristic of this disorder. Profuse sweating, low-grade fever, and tachycardia are also common.

Other causes
• *Drugs.* Excess salivation caused by drugs such as clonazepam, ethion-amide, and haloperidol may result in drooling.

Special considerations
Be alert for aspiration in the patient with drooling. Position him upright or on his side. Provide frequent mouth care and suction, as necessary, to control drooling. Be prepared to assist with tracheostomy and intubation, to administer oxygen, or to execute the Heimlich maneuver.

Help the patient cope with drooling by providing a covered, opaque collecting jar to decrease odor and prevent possible transmission of infection. Keep tissues handy and drape a towel across the patient's chest at mealtime. Encourage oral hygiene. Also, teach the patient exercises to help strengthen facial muscles, if appropriate.

Pediatric pointers
Normally, the infant can't control saliva flow until about age 1, when muscular reflexes that initiate swallowing and lip closure mature. Typically, salivation and drooling increase with teething, which begins about the fifth month and continues until about age 2. Excessive salivation and drooling may also occur in response to hunger or anticipation of feeding, and in association with nausea.

Common causes of drooling include epiglottitis, retropharyngeal abscess, severe tonsillitis, stomatitis, herpetic lesions, esophageal atresia, cerebral palsy, mental deficiency, and drug withdrawal in neonates of addicted mothers. It may also result from a foreign body in the esophagus, causing dysphagia.

Dysarthria

Dysarthria, or poorly articulated speech, is characterized by slurring and labored, irregular rhythm. It may be accompanied by nasal voice tone caused by palate weakness. Whether it occurs abruptly or gradually, dysarthria is usually evident in ordinary conversation. It's confirmed by asking the patient to produce a few simple sounds and words, such as "ba," "sh," and "cat." However, dysarthria is occasionally confused with aphasia, which involves loss of the ability to produce or comprehend speech.

Dysarthria results from damage to the brain stem that affects cranial

DYSARTHRIA: CAUSES AND ASSOCIATED FINDINGS

CAUSES	Aphasia	Ataxia	Bradykinesia	Diplopia	Drooling	Dysphagia	Dyspnea	Fasciculations	Gait—propulsive	Hyperreflexia	Hypotension	LOC-decreased	Masklike facies
Alcoholic cerebellar degeneration		•		•							•	•	
Amyotrophic lateral sclerosis					•	•	•	•		•			
Basilar artery insufficiency		•		•									
Botulism				•		•	•						
CVA (brain stem)					•	•	•						
CVA (cerebral)	•				•	•				•			
Manganese poisoning				•					•			•	
Mercury poisoning		•										•	
Multiple sclerosis		•		•		•				•			
Myasthenia gravis				•	•	•	•						
Olivopontocerebellar degeneration		•											
Parkinson's disease			•		•	•			•				•
Shy-Drager syndrome		•									•	•	•

nerves IX, X, or XI. Degenerative neurologic disorders commonly cause dysarthria. In fact, dysarthria is a chief sign of olivopontocerebellar degeneration. It may also result from ill-fitting dentures.

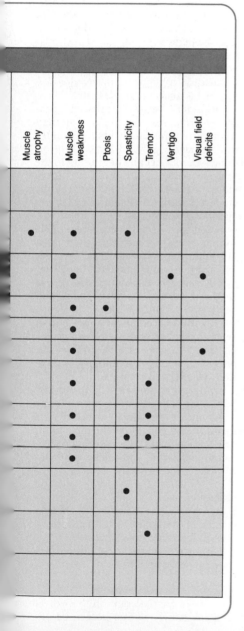

Assessment

If the patient displays dysarthria, ask him about associated difficulty in swallowing. Then assess respiratory rate and depth. Measure vital capacity with a Wright respirometer, if available. Next, obtain blood pressure and heart rate. Usually, tachycardia and slightly increased blood pressure are early signs of respiratory muscle weakness. Notify the doctor immediately if these signs accompany shortness of breath.

Ensure a patent airway. Place the patient in Fowler's position and suction him, if necessary. Administer oxygen, and keep emergency resuscitation equipment close by. Anticipate intubation and mechanical ventilation in progressive respiratory muscle weakness. Withhold oral fluids in the patient with associated dysphagia.

If the patient's dysarthria is not accompanied by respiratory muscle weakness and dysphagia, continue to assess for other neurologic deficits. Compare muscle strength and tone in the limbs. Then evaluate tactile sensation. Ask the patient about numbness or tingling. Test deep tendon reflexes. Also, note gait ataxia. Next, test visual fields and ask about double vision. Check for signs of facial weakness, such as ptosis. Finally, assess level of consciousness and mental status.

Next, explore dysarthria fully. When did it begin? Has it gotten better? Speech improves with resolution of a transient ischemic attack, but not in a completed stroke. Ask if dysarthria worsens during the day. Then obtain a drug and alcohol history. Also note a history of seizures.

Medical causes

• *Alcoholic cerebellar degeneration.* This disorder commonly causes chronic, progressive dysarthria along with ataxia, diplopia, ophthalmoplegia, hypotension, and altered mental status.
• *Amyotrophic lateral sclerosis.* Dysarthria occurs when this disorder affects the bulbar nuclei. It may worsen as the

disease progresses. Other signs and symptoms are dysphagia; difficulty breathing; muscle atrophy and weakness, especially of the hands and feet; fasciculations; spasticity; hyperactive deep tendon reflexes in the legs; and occasionally excessive drooling. Progressive bulbar palsy may cause crying spells or inappropriate laughter.

• *Basilar artery insufficiency.* This disorder causes random, brief episodes of bilateral brain stem dysfunction, resulting in dysarthria. Accompanying it are diplopia, vertigo, facial numbness, ataxia, paresis, and visual field loss, all of which last for minutes to hours.

• *Botulism.* The hallmark of this disorder is acute cranial nerve dysfunction causing dysarthria, dysphagia, diplopia, and ptosis. Early findings include dry mouth, sore throat, weakness, vomiting, and diarrhea. Later, descending weakness or paralysis of muscles in the extremities and trunk causes hyporeflexia and dyspnea.

• *Brain stem cerebrovascular accident (CVA).* This CVA is characterized by bulbar palsy, resulting in the triad of dysarthria, dysphonia, and dysphagia. The dysarthria is most severe at the onset of stroke; it may lessen or disappear with rehabilitation. Other findings may include facial weakness, hemiparesis, drooling, dyspnea, and decreased level of consciousness.

• *Cerebral CVA.* A massive bilateral CVA causes pseudobulbar palsy. Bilateral weakness produces dysarthria that is most severe at the onset of the stroke. It's accompanied by dysphagia, drooling, dysphonia, bilateral hemianopia, and aphasia. Sensory loss and hyperreflexia may also be present.

• *Multiple sclerosis.* When demyelination affects the brain stem and cerebellum, the patient displays dysarthria accompanied by nystagmus, blurred or double vision, dysphagia, ataxia, and intention tremor. These signs and symptoms worsen and subside with exacerbation and remission of the disorder. Other clinical features may include paresthesias, spasticity, hyper-

reflexia, muscle weakness or paralysis, constipation, and emotional lability. Urinary frequency, urgency, and incontinence may also occur.

• *Myasthenia gravis.* This neuromuscular disorder causes dysarthria associated with nasal voice tone. Typically, the dysarthria worsens during the day. Other findings are dysphagia, drooling, facial weakness, diplopia, dyspnea, and skeletal muscle weakness.

• *Olivopontocerebellar degeneration.* Dysarthria, a major sign, accompanies cerebellar ataxia and spasticity.

• *Parkinson's disease.* This disorder produces dysarthria and low-pitched monotonic speech. It also produces muscle rigidity, bradykinesia, involuntary tremor usually beginning in the fingers, difficulty in walking, and a stooped posture. Other features include a masklike facies, dysphagia, and occasionally drooling.

• *Poisoning.* Chronic *manganese* poisoning causes progressive dysarthria accompanied by weakness, fatigue, confusion, hallucinations, drooling, hand tremors, limb stiffness, gross rhythmic movements of the trunk and head, and propulsive gait.

Chronic *mercury* poisoning also causes progressive dysarthria. Accompanying it are weakness, fatigue, depression, lethargy, irritability, confusion, ataxia, and tremors.

• *Shy-Drager syndrome.* Characterized by chronic orthostatic hypotension, this syndrome eventually causes dysarthria. It also causes cerebellar ataxia, possible stooped posture and masklike facies, dementia, impotence, and occasionally incontinence.

Other causes

• *Anticonvulsants.* Usually, dysarthria occurs at the start of anticonvulsant therapy but then disappears.

• *Barbiturates.* Ingestion of large doses may cause dysarthria.

Special considerations

Encourage the patient with dysarthria to speak slowly so that he can be understood. Give him time to express himself, and encourage him to use gestures.

Pediatric pointers

Dysarthria most often results from brain stem glioma, a slow-growing tumor that occurs chiefly in children. It may also result from cerebral palsy.

Dysarthria may be difficult to detect, especially in the infant or young child who hasn't perfected speech. Be sure to assess for other neurologic deficits, too.

Encourage speech in the child with dysarthria; his potential for rehabilitation is typically greater than the adult's.

Dysmenorrhea

Dysmenorrhea—painful menstruation—affects over 50% of menstruating women. In fact, it's the leading cause of lost time from school and work among women of childbearing age. Dysmenorrhea may involve sharp, intermittent pain or dull, aching pain. Usually, it's characterized by mild-to-severe cramping or colicky pain in the pelvis or lower abdomen that may radiate to the thighs and lower sacrum. This pain may precede menstruation by several days or may accompany it. The pain gradually subsides as bleeding tapers off.

Dysmenorrhea may be idiopathic, as in premenstrual syndrome and primary dysmenorrhea. It commonly results from endometriosis and other pelvic disorders. It may also result from structural abnormalities, such as an imperforate hymen. Stress and poor health may aggravate dysmenorrhea, while rest and mild exercise may relieve it.

Assessment

If the patient complains of dysmenorrhea, have her describe it fully. Is it intermittent or continuous? Is the pain sharp, cramping, or aching? Ask where the pain is located. Is it bilateral? How long has she been experiencing it? Find out when the pain begins and ends and when it's severe. Does it radiate to the back? Next explore associated symptoms, such as nausea and vomiting, altered bowel habits, bloating, pelvic or rectal pressure, and unusual fatigue, irritability, or depression.

Then, obtain a menstrual and sexual history. Ask the patient if her menstrual flow is heavy or scant. Also have her describe any vaginal discharge between menses. Does she experience dyspareunia with menses? Find out what relieves her cramps. Does she take pain medication? Does it relieve cramping? Note her method of contraception and check for a history of pelvic infection. Does she have any signs and symptoms of urinary obstruction such as pyuria and urinary retention or incontinence? Determine how the patient copes with stress.

Next perform a focused physical examination. Take vital signs, noting fever and any accompanying chills. Inspect the abdomen for distention and palpate for tenderness and masses. Note costovertebral angle (CVA) tenderness.

Medical causes

● *Adenomyosis.* In this disorder, endometrial tissue invades the myometrium, resulting in severe dysmenorrhea with pain radiating to the back or rectum, menorrhagia, and an enlarged, globular uterus.

● *Cervical stenosis.* This structural disorder causes dysmenorrhea and scant menstrual flow.

● *Endometriosis.* Typically, this disorder produces steady, aching pain that begins before menses and peaks at the height of menstrual flow. However, the pain may also occur between menstrual periods. It may arise at the endometrial deposit site or may radiate to the perineum or rectum. Associated signs and symptoms include menorrhagia, irregular menses, dyspareunia,

RELIEF FOR DYSMENORRHEA

To relieve cramping and other symptoms caused by primary dysmenorrhea or an intrauterine device, a doctor may recommend prostaglandin inhibitors, such as aspirin, ibuprofen, indomethacin, and naproxen. These nonsteroidal anti-inflammatory drugs block prostaglandin synthesis early in the inflammatory reaction, thereby inhibiting prostaglandin action at receptor sites. These drugs also have analgesic and antipyretic effects.

NURSING CONSIDERATIONS

Point out side effects. Alert the patient to possible side effects of prostaglandin inhibitors. CNS effects include dizziness, headache, and visual disturbances. GI effects include nausea, vomiting, heartburn, and diarrhea. As a result, advise the patient to take the drug with milk or after meals to reduce gastric irritation.

Recognize contraindications. Because prostaglandin inhibitors are potentially teratogenic, be sure to rule out the possibility of pregnancy before the start of therapy. Advise any patient who suspects she's pregnant to delay therapy until menstruation begins.

Recognize cautions. Administer cautiously in patients with cardiac decompensation, hypertension, or renal dysfunction and in patients with coagulation defects or ongoing anticoagulant therapy. Because patients who are hypersensitive to aspirin may also be hypersensitive to other prostaglandin inhibitors, watch for signs of gastric ulceration and bleeding.

infertility, nausea and vomiting, painful defecation, and rectal bleeding and hematuria with menses.

• **Pelvic inflammatory disease.** Chronic infection produces dysmenorrhea accompanied by fever; malaise; foulsmelling, purulent vaginal discharge; menorrhagia; dyspareunia; soft, enlarged uterus; severe abdominal pain; nausea and vomiting; and diarrhea.

• **Premenstrual syndrome (PMS).** Usually, PMS follows an ovulatory cycle. As a result, it's rare during the first 12 months of menses, which may be anovulatory. The cramping pain usually begins with menstrual flow and persists for several hours or days, diminishing with decreasing flow. Common associated effects precede menses by several days to 2 weeks and include abdominal bloating, breast tenderness, palpitations, diaphoresis, flushing, depression, and irritability. Other effects: nausea, vomiting, diarrhea, and headache.

• **Primary (idiopathic) dysmenorrhea.** Increased prostaglandin secretion intensifies uterine contractions, apparently causing mild-to-severe spasmodic cramping pain in the lower abdomen, which radiates to the sacrum and inner thighs. Cramping abdominal pain peaks a few hours before menses.

• **Right ovarian vein syndrome.** Intermittent flank pain occurs before and early in menses, accompanied by signs of ureteral obstruction, such as chills, fever, CVA tenderness, and pyuria.

• **Uterine leiomyomas.** Tumors may cause lower abdominal pain that worsens with menses. The pain may be constant or intermittent. Associated findings include backache, constipation, and signs of ureteral obstruction. Palpation may reveal the tumor mass and an enlarged uterus.

• **Uterine prolapse.** Displacement of the uterus may produce dysmenorrhea and chronic lower back pain, pelvic pressure, fatigue, leukorrhea, dyspareunia, and urinary difficulties.

Other causes

• **Intrauterine devices.** These devices may cause severe cramping and heavy menstrual flow.

Special considerations

In the past, women with dysmenorrhea were considered neurotic. Although current research suggests that prostaglandins contribute to this symptom, old attitudes persist. Encourage the patient to view dysmenorrhea as a medical problem, not as a sign of maladjustment.

If dysmenorrhea is idiopathic, advise the patient to place a heating pad on her abdomen to relieve pain. This therapy reduces abdominal muscle tension and increases blood flow. Effleurage, a light circular massage with the fingertips, may also provide relief. Other comfort measures include drinking warm beverages, taking a warm shower, performing waist-bending and pelvic-rocking exercises, and walking.

Explain the action and side effects of oral contraceptives and prostaglandin inhibitors, if prescribed. Point out that these drugs also inhibit ovulation.

Pediatric pointers

Dysmenorrhea is rare during the first year before the menstrual cycle becomes ovulatory. However, the incidence of dysmenorrhea is generally higher among adolescents than older women. Teach the adolescent about dysmenorrhea. Dispel myths about its role in menstrual pain, and inform her that it's a common medical problem. Encourage good hygiene, nutrition, and exercise.

Dyspareunia

A major obstacle to sexual enjoyment, dyspareunia is painful or difficult coitus. Although most sexually active women occasionally experience mild dyspareunia, persistent or severe dyspareunia is cause for concern. Dyspareunia may occur with attempted penetration or during or after coitus. It may stem from friction of the penis against perineal tissue or from jarring of deeper adnexal structures. The location of pain helps determine its cause.

Dyspareunia frequently accompanies pelvic disorders. However, it may also result from diminished vaginal lubrication associated with aging, the effects of drugs, and psychological factors—most notably, fear of pain or injury. A fear-pain-tension cycle may become established in which repeated painful coitus conditions the patient to anticipate pain, causing fear that prevents sexual arousal and adequate vaginal lubrication. Contraction of the pubococcygeus muscle also occurs, making penetration still more difficult and traumatic. Other psychological factors include guilt feelings about sex, fear of pregnancy or of injury to the fetus during pregnancy, and anxiety caused by a disrupted sexual relationship or by a new sexual partner. Inadequate vaginal lubrication associated with insufficient foreplay and mental or physical fatigue may also cause dyspareunia.

Assessment

Begin by asking the patient to describe the dyspareunia. Does the pain occur with attempted penetration or deep thrusting? How long does it last? Is the pain intermittent or does it always accompany intercourse? Ask whether changing coital position relieves the pain.

Next ask about a history of pelvic, vaginal, or urinary infection. Does the patient have signs and symptoms of current infection? Have the patient describe any discharge. Also ask about malaise, headache, fatigue, abdominal or back pain, nausea and vomiting, and diarrhea or constipation.

Obtain a sexual and menstrual history. Determine whether dyspareunia is related to the patient's menstrual cycle. Are her cycles regular? Ask about dysmenorrhea and metrorrhagia. Has the patient had a baby? If so, did she have an episiotomy? Note if she's breastfeeding. Ask about previous abortion or pelvic surgery. Also find out what contraceptive method the patient uses. Then try to determine her attitude toward sexual intimacy. Does she feel tense during coitus? Is she satisfied with the length of foreplay? Does she usually achieve orgasm? Ask about a history of rape, incest, or sexual abuse as a child.

Next perform a physical examination. Take vital signs. Palpate the abdomen for tenderness, pain, or masses and for inguinal lymphadenopathy. Finally, inspect the genitalia for lesions and vaginal discharge.

Medical causes

● *Atrophic vaginitis.* In postmenopausal and lactating women, decreased estrogen secretion may lead to inadequate vaginal lubrication and dyspareunia, which intensifies as intercourse continues. Accompanying signs and symptoms are metrorrhagia, pruritus, burning, and vaginal tenderness.

● *Bartholinitis.* This inflammatory disorder may produce throbbing pain during intercourse accompanied by vulvar tenderness. The patient may also complain of pain with walking or sitting. Chronic inflammation causes purulent discharge from the infected cyst.

● *Cervicitis.* This inflammatory disorder causes pain with deep penetration. It may also cause dull, lower abdominal pain, purulent vaginal discharge, backache, and metrorrhagia.

● *Condylomata acuminata.* These warty growths occur on the vulva, vaginal and cervical walls, and perianal area. They may bleed, itch, and become tender during and after intercourse. A profuse discharge may also occur.

● *Cystitis.* Vulvar pain may occur during coitus. Associated findings include dysuria, urinary urgency and frequency or incontinence, pyuria, and, after coitus, hematuria.

● *Endometriosis.* This disorder causes intense pain during deep penetration, which jars endometrial deposits on the ovaries or cul-de-sac. Aching pain may also occur with gentle thrusting or during a pelvic examination. The pain is usually bilateral in the lower abdomen, although it may be worse on one side. It may be relieved by changing coital positions. Other clinical features may include dysmenorrhea, menorrhagia, irregular menses, infertility, painful defecation, and rectal bleeding and hematuria with menses.

● *Herpes genitalis.* During intercourse, friction against lesions on the labia, vulva, vagina, or perianal skin causes pain and itching. The lesions are fluid-filled and usually painless at first, but may rupture and form shallow, painful ulcers with erythema and edema. Related findings are leukorrhea, fever, malaise, headache, inguinal lymphadenopathy, and dysuria.

● *Occlusive or rigid hymen.* In this condition, dyspareunia may prevent penetration.

● *Ovarian cyst or tumor.* In this disorder, lower abdominal pain accompanies deep penetration during intercourse. Other clinical features are chronic low back pain; a tender, palpable abdominal mass; constipation or urinary frequency; and irregular menses.

● *Pelvic inflammatory disease.* Deep penetration causes the most severe pain. It's unrelieved by changing coital positions. Uterine tenderness may also occur with gentle thrusting or during a pelvic examination. This disorder also causes fever; malaise; foul-smelling, purulent vaginal discharge; menorrhagia; dysmenorrhea; soft, enlarged uterus; severe abdominal pain; nausea and vomiting; and diarrhea.

● *Uterine prolapse.* Sharp or aching pain occurs with uterine prolapse when the penis strikes the descended cervix. Other effects: dysmenorrhea, pelvic pressure, urinary retention or incontinence, and chronic low back pain.

● *Vaginitis.* Infection produces dyspareunia along with vulvar pain, burning, and itching during and for several hours following coitus. These symptoms may be aggravated by sexual arousal aside from intercourse. Vaginal discharge is typical and varies with the causative organism. *Candida albicans* produces a curdlike, odorless discharge, while *Trichomonas vaginalis, Gardnerella vaginalis,* and *Neisseria gonorrhoeae* produce a whitish-yellowish, foul-smelling, profuse discharge. Pruritus and dysuria may also occur.

Other causes

• *Contraceptive and hygienic products.* Some spermicidal jellies, douches, and vaginal creams and deodorants cause irritation and edema, resulting in dyspareunia.

• *Diaphragms and intrauterine devices.* An ill-fitting diaphragm may produce cramps with intercourse. An incorrectly placed intrauterine device may cause dyspareunia during orgasm.

• *Episiotomy.* If the episiotomy scar constricts the vaginal introitus or narrows the vaginal barrel, the patient may experience perineal pain with coitus.

• *Pelvic irradiation.* Therapy for pelvic cancer may cause pelvic and vaginal scarring, resulting in dyspareunia.

Special considerations

Encourage the patient to discuss dyspareunia openly. A woman may hesitate to report dyspareunia because of embarrassment and modesty.

To minimize dyspareunia, advise the patient to apply vaginal lubricants before intercourse, to attempt different coital positions, and to increase foreplay time. Teach her Kegel exercises to reduce muscle tension.

Prepare the patient for a pelvic examination. Explain that it involves inspection of the vagina and cervix and bimanual palpation of the uterus, fallopian tubes, and ovaries. Remind her to breathe deeply and evenly during the examination. If the doctor prescribes an antimicrobial or anti-inflammatory agent, teach her how to apply the cream or insert a vaginal suppository.

Pediatric pointers

Dyspareunia is an adolescent problem, too. Although about 40% of adolescents

are sexually active by the age of 19, most are reluctant to initiate a frank sexual discussion. Be sure to obtain a thorough sexual history by asking the patient direct but nonjudgmental questions.

HOW TO DO KEGEL EXERCISES

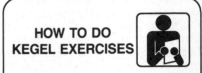

Dear Patient:

Repeated painful intercourse may cause involuntary contraction of a muscle called pubococcygeus (PC), which encircles your urinary opening and vagina. When this happens, intercourse becomes even more difficult.

Below are some isometric exercises—called Kegel exercises—that can strengthen and help you gain voluntary control of the PC muscle.

• Begin by sitting on the toilet with your legs spread. Then, without moving your legs, start and stop the flow of urine. The PC muscle is the one that contracts to help control urine flow.

• Now that you've identified the PC muscle, you can exercise it regularly. Like most isometric exercises, Kegel exercises can be performed almost anywhere—while sitting at your desk, lying in bed, standing in line, and especially while urinating. As you perform these exercises, remember to breathe naturally—don't hold your breath.

Now, periodically contract the PC muscle as you did to stop the urine flow. Count slowly to three, then relax the muscle.

• Next, contract and relax the PC muscle as quickly as possible, without using your stomach or buttock muscles.

• Finally, *slowly* contract the entire vaginal area. Then bear down, using your abdominal muscles as well as your PC muscle.

For the first week, repeat each exercise 10 times (1 set) for 5 sets daily. Then each week add 5 repetitions to each exercise (15, 20, and so forth). Keep doing 5 sets daily.

After a week or two of practice, you'll notice improvement. To monitor your progress, insert one or two well-lubricated fingers into your vagina so you can feel the PC muscle contract.

Dyspepsia

Dyspepsia may be described as an uncomfortable fullness after meals that's associated with nausea, belching, heartburn, and possibly cramping and abdominal distention. Frequently aggravated by spicy, fatty, or high-fiber foods and by excess caffeine consumption, dyspepsia indicates impaired digestive function.

Dyspepsia results from gastrointestinal (GI) disorders and, to a lesser extent, from cardiac, pulmonary, and renal disorders and the effects of drugs. This symptom may also result from emotional upset and overly rapid eating or improper chewing. Usually, it occurs a few hours after eating and lasts for a variable period of time. Its severity depends on the amount and type of food eaten and on gastrointestinal motility. Additional food or antacids may relieve the discomfort.

Dyspepsia apparently results when altered gastric secretions lead to excess stomach acidity.

Assessment

If the patient complains of dyspepsia, begin by asking him to describe it fully. How often and when does it occur? Do any drugs or activities relieve or aggravate it? Has he had nausea, vomiting, melena, hematemesis, cough, or chest pain? Ask what drugs he's currently taking. Also find out about any recent surgery. Does he have a history of renal, cardiovascular, or pulmonary disease? Has he noticed any change in the amount or color of his urine?

Focus the physical examination on the abdomen. Inspect for distention, ascites, scars, jaundice, uremic frost, or bruising. Then auscultate for bowel sounds and characterize their motility. Palpate and percuss the abdomen, noting any tenderness, pain, organ enlargement, or tympany.

Finally, assess other body systems. Ask about behavior changes and evaluate level of consciousness. Auscultate for gallops and crackles, and percuss the lungs to detect consolidation. Note peripheral edema.

Medical causes

● *Cholelithiasis.* Heavy or greasy meals can precipitate dyspepsia with bloating, flatulence, nausea, vomiting, belching, and biliary colic. Acute pain in the right upper quadrant may radiate to the back, shoulders, and chest. The patient may have diaphoresis, tachycardia, chills, low-grade fever, petechiae, and bleeding tendencies. Jaundice with pruritus, dark urine, and clay-colored stools may occur.

● *Cirrhosis.* Dyspepsia in this chronic disorder varies in intensity and duration and is relieved by antacids. Other GI effects are anorexia, nausea, vomiting, flatulence, diarrhea, constipation, abdominal distention, and epigastric or right upper quadrant pain. Weight loss, jaundice, hepatomegaly, ascites, dependent edema, fever, bleeding tendencies, and muscle weakness are also common. Skin changes include severe pruritus, extreme dryness, easy bruising, and lesions such as telangiectasis and palmar erythema.

● *Congestive heart failure.* Common in right heart failure, transient dyspepsia may be accompanied by chest tightness and a constant ache or sharp pain in the right upper quadrant. Typically, this disorder also causes hepatomegaly, anorexia, nausea, vomiting, bloating, tachycardia, distended neck veins, tachypnea, dyspnea, and orthopnea. Other findings include dependent edema, anxiety, fatigue, diaphoresis, hypotension, cough, rales, ventricular and atrial gallops, and cool, pale skin.

● *Duodenal ulcer.* A primary symptom of duodenal ulcer, dyspepsia ranges from a vague feeling of fullness or pressure to a boring or aching sensation in the middle or right epigastrium. It usually occurs 1½ to 3 hours after eating and is relieved by food or antacids. The pain may awaken the patient at night with heartburn and water brash (fluid regurgitation). Abdominal tenderness and weight gain may occur; vomiting and anorexia are rare.

• *Gastric dilatation (acute).* Epigastric fullness is an early symptom of this painless, yet life-threatening, disorder.

Accompanying this dyspepsia are nausea and vomiting, upper abdominal distention, succussion splash, and apathy. The patient may display signs and symptoms of dehydration, such as poor tissue turgor and dry mucous membranes, and of electrolyte imbalance,

DYSPEPSIA: CAUSES AND ASSOCIATED FINDINGS

CAUSES	Abdominal distention	Abdominal pain	Anorexia	Bruising, easy	Chest pain	Cough	Edema	Hepatomegaly	Jaundice	Nausea/vomiting	Oliguria	Tachycardia	Weight loss
Cholelithiasis		•							•	•		•	
Cirrhosis	•	•	•	•			•	•	•	•			•
Congestive heart failure		•	•		•	•	•	•		•		•	
Duodenal ulcer		•								•			
Gastric dilatation (acute)	•									•			
Gastric ulcer	•	•								•			•
Gastritis (chronic)		•	•							•			
Gastrointestinal neoplasms		•	•						•				
Hepatitis			•					•	•	•			
Pancreatitis (chronic)		•	•						•	•			•
Pulmonary embolus					•	•						•	
Pulmonary tuberculosis			•			•							•
Uremia		•	•				•			•	•		

such as irregular pulse and muscle weakness. Gastric bleeding may produce hematemesis and melena.

• *Gastric ulcer.* Typically, dyspepsia and heartburn after eating occur early in this disorder. The cardinal symptom, though, is epigastric pain that may not be relieved by food but that may occur with vomiting, fullness, and abdominal distention. Weight loss and GI bleeding are also characteristic.

• *Gastritis (chronic).* In this disorder, dyspepsia is relieved by antacids and aggravated by spicy foods or excessive caffeine. It occurs with anorexia, a feeling of fullness, vague epigastric pain, belching, nausea, and vomiting.

• *Gastrointestinal neoplasms.* These neoplasms usually produce chronic dyspepsia. Other features include anorexia, fatigue, jaundice, melena, hematemesis, constipation, and abdominal pain.

• *Hepatitis.* Dyspepsia occurs in two of the three stages in hepatitis. The preicteric phase produces moderate-to-severe dyspepsia, fever, malaise, arthralgia, coryza, myalgia, nausea, vomiting, an altered sense of taste or smell, and hepatomegaly. Jaundice then marks the onset of the icteric phase, along with continued dyspepsia and anorexia, irritability, and severe pruritus. As jaundice clears, the dyspepsia and other GI effects also diminish. In the recovery phase, only fatigue remains.

• *Pancreatitis (chronic).* A feeling of fullness or dyspepsia is usually accompanied by severe continuous or intermittent epigastric pain that radiates to the back or through the abdomen. Anorexia, nausea, vomiting, jaundice, dramatic weight loss, hyperglycemia, and steatorrhea may also occur.

• *Pulmonary embolus.* Sudden dyspnea characterizes this potentially fatal disorder; however, dyspepsia may occur as an oppressive, severe, substernal discomfort. Other findings include tachycardia, tachypnea, cough, pleuritic chest pain, hemoptysis, syncope, cyanosis, and hypotension.

• *Pulmonary tuberculosis.* Vague dyspepsia may occur, along with anorexia, malaise, and weight loss. Common associated findings include high fever, night sweats, palpitations on mild exertion, a productive cough, dyspnea, and occasional hemoptysis.

• *Uremia.* Of the many GI complaints associated with this condition, dyspepsia may be the earliest and most important. Others include anorexia, nausea, vomiting, bloating, diarrhea, abdominal cramps, epigastric pain, and weight gain. As the renal system deteriorates, findings may include edema, pruritus, pallor, hyperpigmentation, uremic frost, ecchymoses, sexual dysfunction, poor memory, irritability, headache, drowsiness, muscle twitching, convulsions, and oliguria.

Other causes

• *Drugs.* Nonsteroidal anti-inflammatory drugs, especially aspirin, commonly cause dyspepsia. Diuretics, antibiotics, antihypertensives, and many other drugs can cause dyspepsia, depending on the patient's tolerance of the dosage.

• *Surgery.* After GI or other surgery, postoperative gastritis can cause dyspepsia, which usually disappears in a few weeks.

Special considerations

Changing the patient's position usually doesn't relieve dyspepsia, but providing food or antacids may. So have food available at all times and give antacids, as ordered, 30 minutes before a meal or 1 hour after it. Because various drugs can cause dyspepsia, give these after meals, if possible. Provide a calm environment to reduce stress, and make sure the patient gets plenty of rest. Discuss other ways to deal with stress, such as deep breathing and guided imagery.

Prepare the patient for endoscopy, if ordered, to evaluate the cause of dyspepsia.

Pediatric pointers

Dyspepsia may occur in adolescents with peptic ulcer disease, but it isn't relieved by food. This symptom may occur in congenital pyloric stenosis, but projectile vomiting after meals is a more characteristic sign. It may also result from lactose intolerance.

Dysphagia

Dysphagia—swallowing difficulty—is a common symptom that's usually easy to localize. It may be constant or intermittent and is classified by the phase of swallowing it affects (see *Classifying Dysphagia by Phases of Swallowing*, page 257). Among the factors that interfere with swallowing are severe pain, obstruction, abnormal peristalsis, impaired gag reflex, and excessive, scanty, or thick oral secretions.

Dysphagia is the most common—and sometimes the *only*—symptom of esophageal disorders. However, it may also result from oropharyngeal, respiratory, neurologic, and collagen disorders and the effects of toxins and treatments. Dysphagia increases the risk of choking and aspiration and may lead to malnutrition and dehydration.

Assessment

If the patient suddenly complains of dysphagia and displays signs of respiratory distress, such as dyspnea and stridor, suspect an airway obstruction and quickly perform abdominal thrusts (Heimlich maneuver). Have another nurse notify the doctor immediately if this maneuver doesn't clear the patient's airway. Prepare to administer oxygen by mask or nasal cannula, or to assist with endotracheal intubation.

If the patient's dysphagia doesn't suggest airway obstruction, begin a health history. Ask the patient if it's painful to swallow. If so, is the pain constant or intermittent? Have the patient point to where dysphagia feels most intense. Does eating alleviate or aggravate the symptom? Is it more dif-

ficult for him to swallow solids than to swallow liquids? If he has dysphagia for liquids, ask if hot, cold, and lukewarm fluids affect him differently. Does the symptom disappear after he tries to swallow a few times? Is swallowing easier if he changes position? Ask if he's experienced vomiting, regurgitation, weight loss, anorexia, hoarseness, dyspnea, or cough.

To evaluate the patient's swallowing reflex, place your finger along his thyroid notch and instruct him to swallow. If you feel his larynx rise, this reflex is intact. Next, have him cough to assess his cough reflex. Check his gag reflex if you're sure he has a good swallow or cough reflex. Listen closely to his speech for signs of muscle weakness. Does he have aphasia or dysarthria? Is his voice nasal, hoarse, or breathy? Assess the patient's mouth carefully. Check for dry mucous membranes and thick, sticky secretions. Observe for tongue and facial weakness. Assess for disorientation, which may make him neglect to swallow.

Medical causes

● *Achalasia.* Most common in patients age 20 to 40, this disorder produces phase 3 dysphagia for solids and liquids. The dysphagia develops gradually and may be precipitated or exacerbated by stress. Occasionally, it's preceded by esophageal colic. Regurgitation of undigested food, especially at night, may cause wheezing, coughing, or choking as well as halitosis. Weight loss, cachexia, hematemesis, and, possibly, heartburn are late findings.

● *Airway obstruction.* Life-threatening upper airway obstruction is marked by signs of respiratory distress, such as crowing and stridor. Phase 2 dysphagia occurs with gagging and dysphonia. When hemorrhage obstructs the trachea, dysphagia's usually painless and rapid in onset. When inflammation causes the obstruction, dysphagia may be painful and develop slowly.

● *Amyotrophic lateral sclerosis (ALS).* Besides dysphagia, ALS causes muscle weakness and atrophy, fasciculations, dysarthria, dyspnea, shallow respirations, tachypnea, and emotional lability.

● *Botulism.* This type of food poisoning causes phase 1 dysphagia and dysuria usually within 36 hours of toxin ingestion. Other early findings include blurred or double vision, dry mouth, sore throat, nausea, vomiting, and diarrhea. Descending weakness or paralysis occurs gradually.

● *Bulbar paralysis.* Phase 1 dysphagia occurs along with drooling, difficulty chewing, dysarthria, and nasal regurgitation. Dysphagia, which occurs for both solids and liquids, is painful and progressive. Accompanying features may be arm and leg spasticity, hyperreflexia, and emotional lability.

● *Dysphagia lusoria.* The only symptom of this congenital anomaly is phase 3 dysphagia for solids, which may not occur until late adulthood.

● *Esophageal carcinoma.* Phase 2 and 3 dysphagia is the earliest and most common symptom of esophageal carcinoma. Typically, this painless, progressive symptom is accompanied by rapid weight loss. As carcinoma advances, dysphagia becomes painful and constant. The patient complains of steady chest pain, cough with hemoptysis, hoarseness, and sore throat. He may also have nausea and vomiting, fever, hiccups, hematemesis, melena, and halitosis.

● *Esophageal compression (external).* Most often caused by a dilated carotid or aortic aneurysm, this rare condition causes phase 3 dysphagia as the primary symptom. Other features depend on the cause of the compression.

● *Esophageal diverticulum.* This disorder causes phase 3 dysphagia when the enlarged diverticulum obstructs the esophagus. Associated findings: food regurgitation, chronic cough, hoarseness, and halitosis.

● *Esophageal leiomyoma.* This relatively rare benign tumor may cause phase 3 dysphagia with retrosternal pain or discomfort. The patient also has weight loss and a feeling of fullness.

● *Esophageal obstruction by foreign body.* Sudden onset of phase 2 or 3 dysphagia, gagging, coughing, and esophageal pain characterize this potentially life-threatening condition. Dyspnea may occur if the obstruction compresses the trachea.

● *Esophageal spasm.* The two most striking symptoms of this disorder are phase 2 dysphagia for solids and liquids and dull or squeezing substernal chest pain. Frequently the pain is relieved by drinking a glass of water. It may last up to an hour and may radiate to the neck, arm, back, or jaw. Bradycardia may also occur.

● *Esophagitis.* *Corrosive esophagitis*, resulting from ingestion of alkalies or acids, causes severe phase 3 dysphagia. It's accompanied by marked salivation, hematemesis, tachypnea, fever, and intense pain in the mouth and anterior chest that's aggravated by swallowing. Signs of shock, such as hypotension and tachycardia, may also occur.

Monilial esophagitis causes phase 2 dysphagia, sore throat, and possibly retrosternal pain on swallowing.

In *reflux esophagitis*, phase 3 dysphagia is a late symptom that usually accompanies stricture development. The patient complains of heartburn that's aggravated by strenuous exercise, bending over, or lying down and that's relieved by sitting up or taking antacids. Other features include regurgitation; frequent, effortless vomiting; a dry, nocturnal cough; and substernal chest pain that may mimic angina pectoris. If the esophagus ulcerates, signs of bleeding, such as melena and hematemesis, may occur along with weakness and fatigue.

● *Gastric carcinoma.* Infiltration of the cardia or esophagus by gastric carcinoma causes phase 3 dysphagia. It's accompanied by nausea, vomiting, and pain that may radiate to the neck, back, or retrosternum. Perforation causes massive bleeding with melena.

● *Hiatal hernia.* This common disorder

causes phase 3 dysphagia with retrosternal or substernal chest pain. The patient complains of dyspepsia associated with heartburn, belching, flatulence, and regurgitation that's aggravated by lying down or stooping over. Weight loss and halitosis may occur.

• *Hypocalcemia.* Although tetany is its primary sign, severe hypocalcemia may cause neuromuscular irritability, producing phase 1 dysphagia associated with numbness and tingling in the nose, ears, fingertips, and toes. Carpopedal spasms, muscle twitching, and laryngeal spasms may also occur.

• *Laryngeal carcinoma (extrinsic).* Phase 2 dysphagia and dyspnea develop late in this disorder. Accompanying fea-

---

CLASSIFYING DYSPHAGIA BY PHASES OF SWALLOWING

Swallowing occurs in three distinct phases and dysphagia can be classified by the phase that it affects. Each phase suggests a specific pathology for dysphagia.

Phase 1
Swallowing begins in the *transfer phase* with chewing and moistening of food with saliva. The tongue presses against the hard palate to transfer the chewed food to the back of the throat; the fifth cranial nerve then stimulates the swallowing reflex. Phase 1 dysphagia typically results from a neuromuscular disorder.

Phase 2
In the *transport phase,* the soft palate closes against the pharyngeal wall to prevent nasal regurgitation. At the same time, the larynx rises and the vocal cords close to keep food out of the lungs; breathing stops momentarily as the throat muscles constrict to move food into the esophagus. Phase 2 dysphagia usually indicates spasm or carcinoma.

Phase 3
Peristalsis and gravity work together in the *entrance phase* to move food through the esophageal sphincter and into the stomach. Phase 3 dysphagia results from lower esophageal narrowing by diverticula, esophagitis, and other disorders.

tures include muffled voice, stridor, pain, halitosis, weight loss, and cachexia. Palpation reveals enlarged cervical nodes.

• *Laryngeal nerve damage.* Often the result of radical neck surgery, superior laryngeal nerve damage may produce painless phase 2 dysphagia.

• *Lead poisoning.* Painless, progressive dysphagia may result from lead poisoning. Related findings include a lead line on the gums, papilledema, ocular palsy, foot- or wristdrop, and signs of hemolytic anemia, such as abdominal pain and fever. The patient may be depressed and display severe mental impairment and convulsions.

• *Lower esophageal ring.* Narrowing of the lower esophagus may cause an attack of phase 3 dysphagia that may recur several weeks or months later. During the attack, the patient complains of a foreign body in the lower esophagus—a sensation that may be relieved by drinking water or vomiting. Esophageal rupture produces severe lower chest pain followed by a feeling of something giving way.

• *Mediastinitis.* Varying with the extent of esophageal perforation, mediastinitis can cause insidious or rapid onset of phase 3 dysphagia. The patient displays chills, fever, and severe retrosternal chest pain that may radiate to the epigastrium, back, or shoulder. The pain may be aggravated by breathing, coughing, or sneezing. Other findings may include tachycardia, subcutaneous crepitation in the suprasternal notch, and falling blood pressure.

• *Myasthenia gravis.* Fatigue and progressive muscle weakness characterize this disorder and account for painless phase 1 dysphagia and possibly choking. Typically, dysphagia follows ptosis and diplopia. Other features may be masklike facies, nasal voice, frequent nasal regurgitation, and head bobbing. Shallow respirations and dyspnea may occur with respiratory muscle weakness. Signs and symptoms worsen during menses and with exposure to stress, cold, or infection.

• *Oral cavity tumor.* Painful phase 1 dysphagia develops along with hoarseness and ulcerating lesions.

• *Parkinson's disease.* Usually a late symptom, phase 1 dysphagia is painless but progressive and may cause choking. Other signs and symptoms include bradykinesia, tremors, muscle rigidity, dysarthria, an expressionless face, muffled voice, increased salivation and lacrimation, constipation, stooped posture, and propulsive gait.

• *Pharyngitis (chronic).* This condition causes painful phase 2 dysphagia for solids and liquids. Rarely serious, it's accompanied by a dry sore throat, cough, and thick mucus in the throat.

• *Plummer-Vinson syndrome.* Also known as sideropenic dysphagia, this syndrome causes phase 3 dysphagia for solids in some women with severe iron deficiency anemia. Related features include upper esophageal pain; atrophy of the oral or pharyngeal mucous membranes; tooth loss; smooth, red, sore tongue; dry mouth; chills; inflamed lips; spoon-shaped nails; pallor; and splenomegaly.

• *Progressive systemic sclerosis.* Typically, dysphagia is preceded by Raynaud's phenomenon in this disorder. The dysphagia may be mild at first and described as a feeling of food sticking behind the breastbone. The patient also complains of heartburn after meals that's aggravated by lying down. As the disease progresses, dysphagia worsens until only liquids can be swallowed. It may be accompanied by other GI effects, including weight loss, abdominal distention, diarrhea, and malodorous, floating stools. Other characteristic late features include joint pain and stiffness and thickening of the skin that progresses to taut, shiny skin. The patient usually has a masklike face.

• *Rabies.* Severe phase 2 dysphagia for liquids results from painful pharyngeal muscle spasms occurring late in this rare, life-threatening disorder. In fact, the patient may become dehydrated and possibly apneic. Dysphagia also causes drooling, and in 50% of patients it's responsible for hydrophobia. Eventually, this disorder causes progressive flaccid paralysis that leads to peripheral vascular collapse, coma, and death.

• *Syphilis.* Rarely, tertiary-stage syphilis causes ulceration and stricture of the upper esophagus, resulting in phase 3 dysphagia. The dysphagia may be accompanied by regurgitation after meals and heartburn that's aggravated by lying down or bending over.

• *Systemic lupus erythematosus.* This disorder may cause progressive phase 2 dysphagia. However, its primary clinical features include nondeforming arthritis, a characteristic "butterfly rash," and photosensitivity.

• *Tetanus.* About 1 week after receiving a puncture wound, phase 1 dysphagia usually develops. Other characteristics include marked muscle hypertonicity, hyperactive deep tendon reflexes, tachycardia, diaphoresis, and low-grade fever. Painful, involuntary muscle spasms account for locked jaw (trismus), risus sardonicus, opisthotonos, boardlike abdominal rigidity, and intermittent tonic convulsions.

Other causes

• *Radiation therapy.* When directed against oral cancer, this therapy may cause scant salivation and temporary dysphagia.

• *Surgery.* Recent tracheostomy may cause temporary dysphagia.

Special considerations

At mealtime, take measures to minimize the patient's risk of choking and aspiration. Place the patient in an upright position and have him flex his neck forward slightly and keep his chin at midline. Stimulate salivation by talking with the patient about food, adding a lemon slice or dill pickle to his tray, and providing mouth care before and after meals. Or administer an anticholinergic or antiemetic to control excess salivation, as ordered.

Consult with the dietician to select foods with distinct temperatures and textures. Avoid sticky foods, such as bananas and peanut butter. If the patient has mucus production, avoid uncooked milk products. During meals, separate solids from liquids, which are harder to swallow. If the patient has decreased saliva production, moisten his food with a little liquid. If he has trouble swallowing meat, instruct him to take several spoonfuls of a proteolytic enzyme, such as papain or meat tenderizer, mixed with water, to break down the meat. If the patient has a weak or absent cough reflex, begin tube feedings or esophageal drips of special formulas.

Prepare the patient for diagnostic evaluation to pinpoint the cause of dysphagia, including endoscopy, esophageal manometry, the acid perfusion test, and the esophageal acidity test.

Pediatric pointers

To assess for dysphagia in an infant or small child, pay close attention to his sucking and swallowing ability. Coughing, choking, or regurgitation during feeding suggest dysphagia. Corrosive esophagitis and esophageal obstruction by a foreign body are more common causes of dysphagia in children than in adults. However, dysphagia may also result from congenital anomalies, such as annular stenosis, dysphagia lusoria, and esophageal atresia.

Dyspnea

Often a symptom of cardiopulmonary dysfunction, dyspnea is the sensation of difficult or uncomfortable breathing. Usually, it's reported as shortness of breath. Its severity varies greatly but is often unrelated to the severity of the underlying cause. Dyspnea may arise suddenly or slowly and may subside rapidly or persist for years.

Most people normally experience dyspnea when they overexert themselves, and its severity depends on their physical condition. In the healthy person, dyspnea is quickly relieved by rest. Pathologic causes of dyspnea include pulmonary, cardiac, neuromuscular, and allergic disorders. In addition, anxiety may cause shortness of breath.

Assessment

After the patient complains of shortness of breath, quickly assess for signs of respiratory distress, such as tachypnea, cyanosis, restlessness, and accessory muscle use. If you detect these signs, notify the doctor immediately. Prepare to administer oxygen by nasal cannula, mask, or endotracheal tube. Start an intravenous infusion and begin cardiac monitoring to detect dysrhythmias, as ordered. Expect to assist with chest tube insertion for severe pneumothorax and application of rotating tourniquets for pulmonary edema.

If the patient can answer questions without increasing his distress, take a complete history. Ask if the shortness of breath began suddenly or gradually. Is it constant or intermittent? Does it occur with activity or while at rest? If he's had dyspneic attacks before, ask if they're increasing in severity. Can he identify what aggravates or alleviates these attacks? Does he have a productive or nonproductive cough or chest pain? Ask about recent trauma, and note a history of upper respiratory tract infections, deep vein phlebitis, or other disorders. Ask the patient if he smokes or is exposed to toxic fumes or irritants on the job. Find out if he also has orthopnea, paroxysmal nocturnal dyspnea, or progressive fatigue.

During the physical examination, look for signs of chronic dyspnea, such as accessory muscle hypertrophy (especially in the shoulders and neck). Also look for pursed-lip exhalation, clubbing, peripheral edema, barrel chest, diaphoresis, and distended neck veins. Check blood pressure and auscultate for rales, abnormal heart sounds or rhythms, egophony, bronchophony, and whispered pectoriloquy. Finally, palpate the abdomen for hepatomegaly.

Medical causes

● *Adult respiratory distress syndrome (ARDS).* This life-threatening form of noncardiogenic pulmonary edema usually produces acute dyspnea as the first complaint. Progressive respiratory distress then develops with restlessness, anxiety, decreased mental acuity, tachycardia, and rales and rhonchi in both lung fields. Other findings may include cyanosis, tachypnea, motor dysfunction, and intercostal and suprasternal retractions. Severe ARDS can produce signs of shock, such as hypotension and cool, clammy skin.

● *Amyotrophic lateral sclerosis.* Also known as Lou Gehrig's disease, this disorder causes slow onset of dyspnea that worsens with time. Other features include dysphagia, dysarthria, muscle weakness and atrophy, fasciculations, shallow respirations, tachypnea, and emotional lability.

● *Anemia.* Usually, dyspnea develops gradually in this disorder. Anemia commonly causes fatigue, weakness, and syncope; if severe, it may also cause tachycardia, tachypnea, restlessness, anxiety, and thirst.

● *Aspiration of a foreign body.* Acute dyspnea marks this life-threatening condition, along with paroxysmal intercostal, suprasternal, and substernal retractions. The patient may also display accessory muscle use, inspiratory stridor, tachypnea, decreased or absent breath sounds, possibly asymmetrical chest expansion, anxiety, cyanosis, diaphoresis, and hypotension.

● *Asthma.* Acute dyspneic attacks occur in this chronic disorder, along with audible wheezing, dry cough, accessory muscle use, nasal flaring, intercostal and supraclavicular retractions, tachypnea, tachycardia, diaphoresis, prolonged expiration, flushing or cyanosis, and apprehension.

● *Cardiac dysrhythmias.* In dysrhythmias, acute or gradual dyspnea can result from decreased cardiac output. The pulse rate may be rapid, slow, or irregular, with frequent premature or escape beats. Pulsus alternans may be present. Other symptoms may include palpitations, chest pain, diaphoresis, light-headedness, weakness, or vertigo.

• *Congestive heart failure.* Here, dyspnea usually develops gradually. Chronic paroxysmal nocturnal dyspnea, orthopnea, tachypnea, tachycardia, palpitations, ventricular gallop, fatigue, dependent peripheral edema, hepatomegaly, dry cough, weight gain, and loss of mental acuity may occur. With acute onset, congestive heart failure may produce distended neck veins, bibasilar rales, oliguria, and hypotension.

• *Cor pulmonale.* Chronic dyspnea begins gradually with exertion and progressively worsens until it occurs even at rest. Underlying cardiac or pulmonary disease is usually present. The patient may have a chronic productive cough, wheezing, tachypnea, distended neck veins, dependent edema, and hepatomegaly. He may also experience increasing fatigue, weakness, and light-headedness.

• *Emphysema.* This chronic disorder gradually causes progressive exertional dyspnea. A history of smoking or exposure to an occupational irritant usually accompanies barrel chest, accessory muscle hypertrophy, diminished breath sounds, anorexia, weight loss, malaise, peripheral cyanosis, tachypnea, pursed-lip breathing, prolonged expiration, and possibly a chronic productive cough. Clubbing is a late sign.

• *Flail chest.* Sudden dyspnea results from multiple rib fractures, along with paradoxical chest movement, severe chest pain, hypotension, tachypnea, tachycardia, and cyanosis. Bruising and decreased or absent breath sounds occur over the affected side.

• *Guillain-Barré syndrome.* Usually following a fever and upper respiratory infection, this syndrome causes slowly worsening dyspnea. It characteristically causes fatigue, ascending muscle weakness, and eventually paralysis.

• *Inhalation injury.* Dyspnea may develop suddenly or gradually over several hours, following inhalation of chemicals or hot gases. Increasing hoarseness, persistent cough, sooty or bloody sputum, and oropharyngeal edema may also occur. Thermal burns, singed nasal hairs, and orofacial burns may occur, along with rales, rhonchi, and wheezes. Signs of respiratory distress may develop.

• *Interstitial fibrosis.* Besides dyspnea, this disorder causes chest pain, dry cough, rales, weight loss and, possibly, cyanosis and pleural friction rub.

• *Lung cancer.* Dyspnea that develops slowly and progressively worsens occurs with late-stage cancer. Other findings include fever, hemoptysis, productive cough, wheezing, clubbing, chest pain, and pleural friction rub.

• *Myasthenia gravis.* This neuromuscular disorder causes bouts of dyspnea as the respiratory muscles weaken. With myasthenic crisis, acute respiratory distress may occur, with shallow respiration and tachypnea.

• *Myocardial infarction.* Sudden dyspnea occurs with crushing substernal chest pain that may radiate to the back, neck, jaw, and arms. Other signs and symptoms include nausea, vomiting, diaphoresis, vertigo, hypertension or hypotension, tachycardia, anxiety, and pale, cool, clammy skin.

• *Pleural effusion.* Dyspnea develops slowly and becomes progressively worse with this disorder. Initially, a pleural friction rub occurs, accompanied by pleuritic pain that worsens with coughing or deep breathing. Other findings include dry cough; dullness to percussion; egophony, bronchophony, or whispered pectoriloquy; tachycardia; tachypnea; weight loss; and decreased chest motion, tactile fremitus, and breath sounds. With infection, fever may occur.

• *Pneumonia.* Dyspnea occurs suddenly, usually accompanied by fever, shaking chills, pleuritic chest pain that worsens with deep inspiration, and a

DYSPNEA: CAUSES AND ASSOCIATED FINDINGS

CHIEF CAUSES	Accessory muscle use	Blood pressure decrease	Breath sounds—decreased	Chest pain	Cough—nonproductive	Cough—productive	Cyanosis	Diaphoresis	Edema	Fasciculations	Fever	
Adult respiratory distress syndrome		•					•					
Amyotrophic lateral sclerosis										•		
Aspiration of a foreign body	•	•	•				•	•				
Asthma	•				•		•	•				
Congestive heart failure		•			•				•			
Cor pulmonale						•			•			
Emphysema	•		•			•	•					
Flail chest		•	•	•			•					
Inhalation injury						•			•			
Lung cancer				•		•					•	
Myasthenia gravis												
Myocardial infarction		•		•				•				
Pleural effusion			•	•	•						•	
Pneumonia			•	•		•	•	•			•	
Pneumothorax	•	•	•	•	•		•					
Pulmonary edema		•			•	•	•	•				
Pulmonary embolism		•	•	•	•	•		•			•	
Shock		•										

MAJOR ASSOCIATED SIGNS AND SYMPTOMS

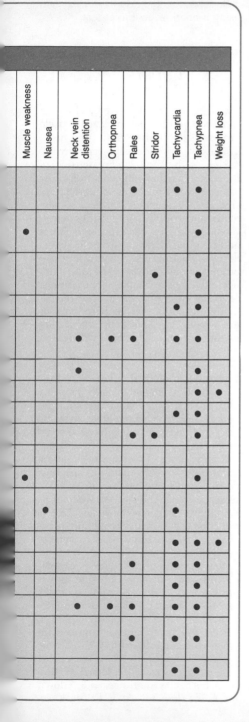

productive cough. Fatigue, headache, myalgias, anorexia, abdominal pain, rales, rhonchi, tachycardia, tachypnea, cyanosis, decreased breath sounds, and diaphoresis may also occur.

• *Pneumothorax.* This life-threatening disorder causes acute dyspnea unrelated to the severity of pain. Sudden, stabbing chest pain may radiate to the arms, face, back, or abdomen. Other signs include anxiety, restlessness, dry cough, cyanosis, decreased vocal fremitus, tachypnea, tympany, decreased or absent breath sounds on the affected side, asymmetrical chest expansion, splinting, and accessory muscle use. With *tension pneumothorax,* tracheal deviation occurs in addition to these typical findings. Decreased blood pressure and tachycardia may occur.

• *Poliomyelitis (bulbar).* Dyspnea develops gradually and progressively worsens. Additional signs and symptoms include fever, facial weakness, dysphasia, hypoactive deep tendon reflexes, decreased mental acuity, dysphagia, nasal regurgitation, and hypopnea.

• *Pulmonary edema.* Often preceded by signs of congestive heart failure, such as distended neck veins and orthopnea, this life-threatening disorder causes acute dyspnea. Other features include tachycardia, tachypnea, rales in both lung fields, S₃ gallop, oliguria, thready pulse, hypotension, diaphoresis, cyanosis, and marked anxiety. The patient's cough may be dry or may produce copious amounts of pink, frothy sputum.

• *Pulmonary embolism.* Acute dyspnea usually accompanied by sudden pleuritic chest pain characterizes this life-threatening disorder. Related findings may include tachycardia, low-grade fever, tachypnea, nonproductive or productive cough with blood-tinged sputum, pleural friction rub, rales, diffuse wheezing, dullness to percussion, decreased breath sounds, diaphoresis, restlessness, and acute anxiety. If massive, the embolism may cause signs of shock, such as hypotension and cool, clammy skin.

• **Sepsis.** This potentially fatal disorder gradually causes dyspnea along with chills and sudden fever. As dyspnea worsens, it may be accompanied by tachycardia, tachypnea, restlessness, anxiety, decreased mental acuity, and warm, flushed, dry skin. Late findings: hypotension, oliguria, cool and clammy skin, and rapid, thready pulse.

• **Shock.** Dyspnea arises suddenly and worsens progressively in this life-threatening disorder. Related findings include severe hypotension, tachypnea, tachycardia, decreased peripheral pulses, cool, clammy skin, decreased mental acuity, restlessness, and anxiety.

• **Tuberculosis.** Dyspnea commonly occurs with chest pain, crackles, and productive cough. Other findings: night sweats, fever, anorexia and weight loss, vague dyspepsia, palpitations on mild exertion, and dullness to percussion.

Special considerations
Monitor the dyspneic patient closely. Be as calm and reassuring as possible to reduce his anxiety, and help him into a comfortable position—usually high Fowler's or forward-leaning. Support him with pillows, loosen his clothing, and administer oxygen, as ordered.

Prepare the patient for diagnostic studies, such as arterial blood gas analysis and chest X-rays. As ordered, administer bronchodilators, antiarrhythmics, diuretics, and analgesics to dilate bronchioles, correct cardiac dysrhythmias, promote fluid excretion, and relieve pain.

Pediatric pointers
Normally, an infant's respirations are abdominal, gradually changing to costal by age 7. Suspect dyspnea in an infant who breathes costally, in an older child who breathes abdominally, or in any child who uses his neck or shoulder muscles to help him breathe.

Both acute epiglottitis and laryngotracheobronchitis (croup) can cause severe dyspnea in a child and may even lead to respiratory or cardiovascular collapse. Expect to administer oxygen, using a hood or cool mist tent.

Dystonia

Dystonia is characterized by slow involuntary movements of large muscle groups of the limbs, trunk, and neck. This extrapyramidal sign may involve flexion of the foot, hyperextension of the legs, extension and pronation of the arms, arching of the back, and extension and rotation of the neck (spasmodic torticollis). It's typically aggravated by walking and emotional stress and relieved by sleep. It may be intermittent—lasting just a few minutes—or continuous and painful. Occasionally, it causes permanent contractures, resulting in a grotesque posture. Although dystonia may be hereditary or idiopathic, it results more often from extrapyramidal disorders or drugs.

Assessment
If possible, include the patient's family in history taking—they may be more aware of behavior changes than the patient is. Begin by asking when dystonia occurs. Is it aggravated by emotional upset? Does it disappear during sleep? Ask about a family history of dystonia. Then, take a drug history, especially noting use of phenothiazines and antipsychotics. If you suspect dystonia is drug-induced, notify the doctor. Expect to adjust the causative drug and to administer diphenhydramine to reverse the dystonia.

Next, examine the patient's coordination and voluntary muscle movement. Observe his gait as he walks across the room; then have him squeeze your fingers to assess muscle strength. Check coordination by having him touch your fingertip and then his nose repeatedly. Follow this by testing gross motor movement of the leg: have him place his heel on one knee, slide it down his shin, then return it to his knee.

Finally, assess fine motor movement by asking him to touch each finger to his thumb in succession.

Medical causes

- **Alzheimer's disease.** Dystonia is a late sign of this disorder, which is marked by slowly progressive dementia. The patient typically displays decreased attention span, amnesia, agitation, an inability to carry out activities of daily living, dysarthria, and emotional lability.
- **Dystonia musculorum deformans.** Prolonged, generalized dystonia is the hallmark of this disorder, which usually develops in childhood and worsens with age. Initially, it causes foot inversion followed by growth retardation and scoliosis. Late signs include twisted, bizarre postures, limb contractures, and dysarthria.
- **Hallervorden-Spatz disease.** This degenerative disease causes dystonic trunk movements accompanied by choreoathetosis, ataxia, myoclonus, and generalized rigidity. The patient also shows progressive intellectual decline and dysarthria.
- **Huntington's chorea.** Dystonic movements mark the preterminal stage of Huntington's chorea. Characterized by progressive intellectual decline, this disorder leads to dementia and emotional lability. The patient displays choreoathetosis accompanied by dysarthria, dysphagia, facial grimacing, and wide-based prancing gait.
- **Olivopontocerebellar atrophy.** Ataxia— an early sign in this rare disorder— slowly progresses to dystonia. Other signs include dysarthria, action tremor, bradykinesia, and visual deterioration.
- **Parkinson's disease.** Here, dystonic spasms are common. Other classic features include uniform or jerky rigidity, "pill-rolling" tremor, bradykinesia, dysarthria, dysphagia, drooling, masklike facies, monotone voice, stooped posture, and propulsive gait.
- **Pick's disease.** Dystonia appears as a late sign in this rare disorder, which resembles Alzheimer's disease.

RECOGNIZING DYSTONIA

Dystonia, chorea, and athetosis may occur simultaneously. To differentiate these three, keep these points in mind:
- *Dystonic* movements are slow and twisting and involve large-muscle groups in the head, neck (as shown below), trunk, and limbs. They may be intermittent or continuous.
- *Choreiform* movements are rapid, highly complex, and jerky.
- *Athetoid* movements are slow, sinuous, and writhing, but *always* continuous; they typically affect the hands and extremities.

**Dystonia of the neck
(Spasmodic torticollis)**

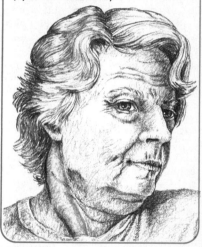

- **Supranuclear ophthalmoplegia (Steele-Richardson-Olszewski syndrome).** This rare disorder affects mainly the middle-aged, causing intermittent dystonia with extreme neck flexion or extension. Other signs include impaired extraocular movement, diminished voice volume, dysarthria, truncal rigidity, dementia, ataxia, masklike facies, and dysphagia.
- **Wilson's disease.** Progressive dystonia and chorea of the arms and legs mark this disorder. Other common signs include hoarseness, bradykinesia, be-

havior changes, dysphagia, drooling, dysarthria, tremors, and Kayser-Fleischer rings (rusty-brown rings at the periphery of the cornea).

Other causes
● *Drugs.* All three types of phenothiazines may cause dystonia. Piperazine phenothiazines, such as acetophenazine and carphenazine, produce this sign most frequently; aliphatics, such as chlorpromazine, cause it less often; and piperidines rarely cause it.

Haloperidol, loxapine, and other antipsychotics usually produce acute facial dystonia. So do antiemetic doses of metoclopramide, excessive doses of L-dopa, and metyrosine.

Special considerations
Encourage the patient to obtain adequate sleep and avoid emotional upset. Avoid range-of-motion exercises, which can aggravate dystonia.

If dystonia is severe, protect the patient from injury by raising and padding his bed rails. Provide an uncluttered environment if he's ambulatory.

Pediatric pointers
Children don't exhibit dystonia until after they can walk. Even so, it rarely occurs until after age 10. Common causes include Fahr's syndrome, dystonia musculorum deformans, athetoid cerebral palsy, and the residual effects of anoxia at birth.

Dysuria

Dysuria refers to painful or difficult urination. It's often accompanied by urinary frequency, urgency, or hesitancy. Usually, this symptom reflects lower urinary tract infection—a common disorder, especially in women.

Dysuria results from lower urinary tract irritation or inflammation, which stimulates nerve endings in the bladder and urethra. The pain's onset provides clues to its cause: for example, pain just *before* voiding usually indicates bladder irritation or distention, while pain at the *start* of urination typically results from bladder outlet irritation. Pain at the *end* of voiding may signal bladder spasms.

Assessment
If the patient complains of dysuria, have him describe its severity and location. When did the patient first notice it? Did anything precipitate it? Does anything aggravate or alleviate it?

Next, ask about previous urinary or genital tract infections. Has the patient recently undergone invasive procedures, such as cystoscopy or urethral dilatation? Also ask if he has a history of intestinal disease. In the female patient, ask about menstrual disorders and use of products that irritate the urinary tract, such as bubble bath salts, feminine deodorants, contraceptive gels, or perineal lotions.

During the physical examination, inspect the urethral meatus for discharge, irritation, or other abnormalities. Assist the doctor with a pelvic or rectal examination, as ordered.

Medical causes
● *Appendicitis.* Occasionally, this disorder causes dysuria that persists throughout voiding and is accompanied by bladder tenderness. However, it's characterized by right upper quadrant pain that shifts to McBurney's point. The patient also has anorexia, nausea, vomiting, constipation, slight fever, abdominal rigidity and rebound tenderness, and tachycardia.
● *Bladder tumor.* In this predominantly male disorder, dysuria throughout voiding is a late symptom associated with urinary frequency and urgency, nocturia, hematuria, and perineal, back, or flank pain.
● *Chemical irritants.* Dysuria may result from irritating substances such as bubble bath salts and feminine deodorants; it's usually most intense at the end of voiding. Other findings may include

PREVENTING URINARY TRACT INFECTIONS

Dear Patient:

To prevent recurrent urinary tract infections:
• Drink at least 10 glasses of fluid—especially water—daily. This helps flush bacteria from the urinary tract.
• Empty your bladder completely every 2 to 3 hours, or as soon as you feel the urge to urinate.
• Wipe your perineum from front to back after urinating or defecating to prevent contamination with fecal material.
• Wear cotton underpants, which allow better ventilation and absorption than synthetic ones.
• Take showers instead of baths. If you must bathe, don't use bubble bath salts,

bath oil, perfume, or other chemical irritants in the water. Also, avoid using feminine deodorants, douches, and similar irritants.
• Urinate before and after intercourse.
• Eat a high-acid ash diet. Include meats, eggs, cheese, nuts, prunes, plums, whole grains, and especially cranberry juice in your daily intake. These foods acidify the urine, which helps decrease bacterial growth. Avoid foods containing baking soda or powder, such as most baked goods.
• Avoid coffee, tea, and alcohol, which tend to irritate the bladder.
• Seek medical help for any unusual vaginal discharge, which suggests infection.

urinary frequency and urgency, a diminished urinary stream, and, possibly, hematuria.

• **Cystitis.** Dysuria throughout voiding is common in all types of cystitis, as are urinary frequency, nocturia, straining to void, and hematuria. *Bacterial cystitis*—the most common cause of dysuria in women—may also produce urinary urgency, perineal and low back pain, suprapubic discomfort, fatigue, and, possibly, low-grade fever. In *chronic interstitial cystitis*, the dysuria is accentuated at the end of voiding. In *tubercular cystitis*, there may also be urinary urgency, flank pain, fatigue, and anorexia. In *viral cystitis*, severe dysuria occurs with gross hematuria, urinary urgency, and fever.

• **Diverticulitis.** Inflammation near the bladder may cause dysuria throughout voiding. Other effects are urinary frequency and urgency, nocturia, hematuria, fever, abdominal pain and tenderness, perineal pain, constipation, and, possibly, an abdominal mass.

• *Paraurethral gland inflammation.* Here, dysuria throughout voiding occurs with

urinary frequency and urgency, diminished urinary stream, mild perineal pain, and, occasionally, hematuria.

• *Prostatitis. Acute prostatitis* commonly causes dysuria throughout or toward the end of voiding. It's accompanied by diminished urinary stream, urinary frequency and urgency, hematuria, perineal fullness, fever, chills, fatigue, myalgia, nausea, vomiting, and constipation. In *chronic prostatitis*, urethral narrowing causes dysuria throughout voiding. Related effects are urinary frequency and urgency; diminished urinary stream; perineal, back, and buttock pain; urethral discharge; and, at times, hematospermia.

• *Pyelonephritis (acute).* More common in females, this disorder causes dysuria throughout voiding. Other features include persistent high fever with chills, costovertebral angle tenderness, flank pain, weakness, urinary urgency and frequency, nocturia, straining on urination, and hematuria. Nausea, vomiting, and anorexia may also occur.

• *Reiter's syndrome.* In this male disorder, dysuria occurs 1 to 2 weeks after

DYSURIA: CAUSES AND ASSOCIATED FINDINGS

S&S CAUSES	MAJOR ASSOCIATED SIGNS AND SYMPTOMS													
	Abdominal pain	Anorexia	Back pain	Constipation	CVA tenderness	Erythema of meatus	Fatigue	Fever	Flank pain	Hematuria	Nausea	Nocturia	Perineal pain	Straining to void
Appendicitis	●	●		●				●			●			
Bladder tumor			●						●	●			●	●
Chemical irritants										●				
Cystitis (bacterial)			●				●	●		●		●	●	●
Cystitis (chronic interstitial)										●		●		●
Cystitis (tubercular)		●					●		●	●		●		●
Cystitis (viral)								●		●		●		●
Diverticulitis	●			●				●		●		●	●	
Paraurethral gland inflammation										●			●	
Prostatitis (acute)				●			●	●		●	●		●	
Prostatitis (chronic)			●										●	
Pyelonephritis		●			●			●	●	●	●	●		●
Reiter's syndrome		●				●		●		●				
Urethral syndrome			●							●				●
Urethritis						●								
Urinary obstruction														
Vaginitis										●		●	●	

Suprapubic pain	Urethral discharge	Urinary frequency	Urinary stream—diminished	Urinary urgency	Vaginal discharge	Vomiting	Weakness
						●	
		●		●			
		●	●	●			
●		●		●			
		●					
		●		●			
		●		●			
		●	●	●			
		●	●	●	●		
	●	●	●	●			
		●		●		●	●
●	●	●		●			
●		●	●				
	●						
		●	●	●			
		●		●	●		

sexual contact. Initially, it's accompanied by mucopurulent discharge, urinary urgency and frequency, meatal swelling and redness, suprapubic pain, anorexia, weight loss, and low-grade fever. Hematuria, conjunctivitis, arthritic symptoms, a papular skin rash, and penile lesions may follow.

● *Urethral syndrome.* Occurring in women, this syndrome mimics urethritis. Dysuria throughout voiding may occur with urinary frequency, diminished urinary stream, suprapubic aching and cramping, tenesmus, and low back and unilateral flank pain.

● *Urethritis.* Primarily found in males, this infection causes dysuria throughout voiding. It's accompanied by a reddened meatus and copious, yellow, purulent discharge (gonorrheal infection) or white or clear mucoid discharge (nongonorrheal infection).

● *Urinary obstruction.* Outflow obstruction by urethral strictures or calculi produces dysuria throughout voiding. (In complete obstruction, bladder distention will develop and dysuria will precede voiding.) Other features are diminished urinary stream and urinary frequency and urgency.

● *Vaginitis.* Characteristically, dysuria occurs throughout voiding as urine touches inflamed or ulcerated labia. Other findings: urinary frequency and urgency, nocturia, hematuria, perineal pain, and vaginal discharge.

Other causes
● *Drugs.* Dysuria can result from monoamine oxidase inhibitors. Metyrosine can also cause transient dysuria.

Special considerations
Monitor vital signs, intake, and output. Administer drugs, as ordered, and prepare the patient for such tests as urinalysis and cystoscopy.

Pediatric pointers
If an infant or toddler cries during voiding, use a collection bag to obtain an uncontaminated specimen. Most often, bacterial cystitis causes the dysuria.

earache • edema—generalized • edema of the arms • edema of the face • ede
enophthalmos • enuresis • epistaxis • eructation • erythema • exophthalmos
pain • facial pain • fasciculations • fatigue • fecal incontinence • fetor hepati
flatulence • fontanelle bulging • fontanelle depression • footdrop • gag reflex
bizarre • gait—propulsive • gait—scissors • gait—spastic • gait—steppage •
gallop—atrial • gallop—ventricular • genital lesions in the male • grunting r
bleeding • gum swelling • gynecomastia • halitosis • halo vision • headache
intolerance • Heberden's nodes • hematemesis • hematochezia • hematuria •
hemoptysis • hepatomegaly • hiccups • hirsutism • hoarseness • Homans' sig
hyperpnea • hypopigmentation • impotence • insomnia • intermittent claudic
jaundice • jaw pain • jugular vein distention • Kehr's sign • Kernig's sign • l
consciousness—decreased • lid lag • light flashes • low birth weight • lymph
facies • McBurney's sign • McMurray's sign • melena • menorrhagia • metro
face • mouth lesions • murmurs • muscle atrophy • muscle flaccidity • musc
spasticity • muscle weakness • mydriasis • myoclonus • nasal flaring • nause
blindness • nipple discharge • nipple retraction • nocturia • nuchal rigidity
deviation • oligomenorrhea • oliguria • opisthotonos • orofacial dyskinesia •
hypotension • Ortolani's sign • Osler's nodes • otorrhea • pallor • palpitation
paralysis • paresthesias • paroxysmal nocturnal dyspnea • peau d'orange •
peristaltic waves—visible • photophobia • pica • pleural friction rub • polyd
polyuria • postnasal drip • priapism • pruritus • psoas sign • psychotic beh
absent or weak • pulse—bounding • pulse pressure—narrowed • pulse pres
rhythm abnormality • pulsus alternans • pulsus bisferiens • pulsus paradox
pupils—sluggish • purple striae • purpura • pustular rash • pyrosis • raccoo
tenderness • rectal pain • retractions—costal and sternal • rhinorrhea • rho
salivation—decreased • salivation—increased • salt craving • scotoma • scro
absence • seizure—focal • seizure—generalized tonic-clonic • seizure—psyc
sign • shallow respirations • skin—bronze • skin—clammy • skin—mottled
turgor—decreased • spider angioma • splenomegaly • stertorous respiration
stridor • syncope • tachycardia • tachypnea • taste abnormalities • tearing—
tic • tinnitus • tracheal deviation • tracheal tugging • tremors • trismus • tu
frost • urethral discharge • urinary frequency • urinary hesitancy • urinary
urgency • urine cloudiness • urticaria • vaginal bleeding—postmenopausal
venous hum • vertigo • vesicular rash • violent behavior • vision loss • visua
floaters • vomiting • vulvar lesions • weight gain—excessive • weight loss—
wristdrop • abdominal distention • abdominal mass • abdominal pain • ab
accessory muscle use • agitation • alopecia • amenorrhea • amnesia • anal
anorexia • anosmia • anuria • anxiety • aphasia • apnea • apneustic respir
pain • asterixis • ataxia • athetosis • aura • Babinski's reflex • back pain •
sign • Biot's respirations • bladder distention • blood pressure decrease • bl
bowel sounds—absent • bowel sounds—hyperactive • bowel sounds—hypo
bradypnea • breast dimpling • breast nodule • breast pain • breast ulcer •
odor • breath with fecal odor • breath with fruity odor • Brudzinski's sign
butterfly rash • café-au-lait spots • capillary refill time—prolonged • carpo
chest expansion—asymmetrical • chest pain • Cheyne-Stokes respirations •
sign • clubbing • cogwheel rigidity • cold intolerance • confusion • conjun
constipation • corneal reflex—absent • costovertebral angle tenderness • co
nonproductive • cough—productive • crackles • crepitation—bony • crepita
cry—high-pitched • cyanosis • decerebrate posture • decorticate posture •
hyperactive • deep tendon reflexes—hypoactive • depression • diaphoresis

Earache

[Otalgia]

Usually, earache results from disorders of the external and middle ear associated with infection, obstruction, or trauma. Its severity ranges from a feeling of fullness or blockage to deep, boring pain; at times, it may be difficult to localize precisely. This common symptom may be intermittent or continuous and may develop suddenly or gradually.

Assessment

Ask the patient to characterize his earache. How long has he had it? Is it intermittent or continuous? Is it painful or slightly annoying? Is the patient able to localize the site of ear pain? Does he have pain in any other areas, such as the jaw?

Ask about ear injury or other trauma. Does swimming or showering trigger ear discomfort? Is discomfort associated with itching? If so, find out where itching is most intense and when it began. Ask about ear drainage and, if present, have the patient characterize it. Does he hear ringing or noise in his ears? Ask about dizziness or vertigo. Does it worsen when the patient changes position? Does he have difficulty swallowing, hoarseness, neck pain, or pain from opening the mouth?

Find out if the patient's recently had a head cold or problems with his eyes, mouth, teeth, jaws, sinuses, or throat. Disorders in these areas may refer pain to the ear along the cranial nerves.

Begin your physical examination by inspecting the external ear for redness, drainage, swelling, or deformity. Then apply pressure to the mastoid process and tragus to elicit any tenderness. Using an otoscope, examine the external auditory canal for lesions, bleeding or discharge, impacted cerumen, foreign bodies, tenderness, or swelling. Examine the tympanic membrane: Is it intact? Is it pearly gray (normal)? Look for tympanic membrane landmarks: the cone of light, umbo, pars tensa, and the handle and short process of the malleus. Perform the watch tick, whispered voice, Rinne, and Weber's tests to assess for hearing loss.

Medical causes

● **Barotrauma (acute).** Earache associated with this trauma ranges from mild pressure to severe pain. Tympanic membrane ecchymosis or bleeding into the tympanic cavity may occur, producing a blue drumhead; usually, the eardrum isn't perforated.

● **Cerumen impaction.** Impacted cerumen (earwax) may cause a plugged, blocked, or full sensation in the ear.

USING AN OTOSCOPE CORRECTLY

When the patient reports an earache, use an otoscope to inspect ear structures closely. Follow these techniques to obtain the best view and ensure patient safety.

CHILD

To inspect an infant's or young child's ear, grasp the *lower* part of the auricle and pull it *down and back* to straighten the upward S-curve of the external canal. Then gently insert the speculum into the canal no more than 1.2 cm (½").

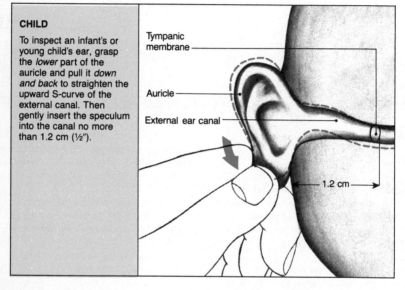

ADULT

To inspect an adult's ear, grasp the *upper* part of the auricle and pull it *up and back* to straighten the external canal. Then insert the speculum about 2.5 cm (1"). Also use this technique for children over age 3.

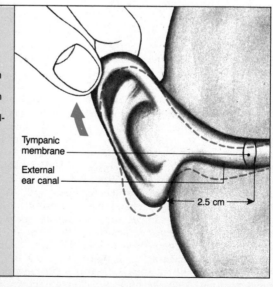

Additional features: partial hearing loss, itching, and, possibly, dizziness.

• *Chondrodermatitis nodularis chronica helicis.* This disorder produces small, painful, indurated areas along the auricle's upper rim.

• *Ear canal obstruction by an insect.* An insect lodged in the ear canal may cause severe pain and distressing noise.

• *Extradural abscess.* Severe earache accompanied by persistent ipsilateral headache, malaise, and recurrent mild fever characterizes this serious complication of middle ear infection.

• *Frostbite.* Prolonged exposure to cold may cause burning or tingling pain in the ear, followed by numbness. The ear appears mottled and gray or white; it turns purplish-blue as it's warmed.

• *Furunculosis.* Infected hair follicles in the outer ear canal may produce severe, localized ear pain associated with a pus-filled furuncle (boil). The pain is aggravated by jaw movement and relieved by rupture or incision of the furuncle. Pinna tenderness, swelling of the auditory meatus, partial hearing loss, and a feeling of fullness in the ear canal may also occur.

• *Herpes zoster oticus (Ramsay Hunt syndrome).* This disorder causes burning or stabbing ear pain, often associated with ear vesicles. The patient also complains of hearing loss and vertigo. Associated signs and symptoms include transitory, ipsilateral, facial paralysis; partial loss of taste; tongue vesicles; and nausea and vomiting.

• *Keratosis obturans.* Mild ear pain occurs here, along with otorrhea and tinnitus. Inspection reveals a white glistening plug obstructing the external meatus.

• *Mastoiditis (acute).* This bacterial infection causes a dull ache behind the ear accompanied by low-grade fever (99° to 100° F., or 37.2° to 37.8° C.) and thick, purulent discharge in the external canal. The eardrum appears dull and edematous and may be perforated; soft tissue near the eardrum may sag.

• *Ménière's disease.* This inner ear disorder can produce a sensation of fullness in the affected ear. Its classic effects, though, include severe vertigo, tinnitus, and sensorineural hearing loss. The patient may also experience nausea and vomiting, diaphoresis, and nystagmus.

• *Middle ear tumor.* Deep, boring ear pain and facial paralysis are late signs of a malignant tumor.

• *Myringitis bullosa.* This rare viral infection causes sudden, severe ear pain that radiates over the mastoid and lasts for up to 48 hours. Small serous- or blood-filled vesicles may dot the reddened tympanic membrane. Transient hearing loss and a serosanguineous discharge may also occur.

• *Otitis externa.* Earache characterizes both types of otitis externa. *Acute otitis externa* begins with mild-to-moderate ear pain that occurs with tragus manipulation. The pain may be accompanied by low-grade fever, sticky yellow or purulent ear discharge, partial hearing loss, and a feeling of blockage. Later, ear pain intensifies, causing the entire side of the head to ache and throb. Fever may reach 104° F. (40° C.). Examination reveals swelling of the tragus, external meatus, and external canal; eardrum erythema; and lymphadenopathy. The patient also complains of dizziness and malaise.

Malignant otitis externa abruptly causes ear pain that's aggravated by moving the auricle or tragus. The pain is accompanied by intense itching, purulent ear discharge, fever, parotid gland swelling, and trismus. Examination reveals a swollen external canal with exposed cartilage and temporal bone. Cranial nerve palsy may occur.

• *Otitis media (acute).* This middle ear inflammation may be serous or suppurative.

Acute serous otitis media may cause a feeling of fullness in the ear, hearing loss, and a vague sensation of top-heaviness. The eardrum may be slightly retracted, amber colored, and marked by air bubbles and a meniscus, or it may be blue-black from hemorrhage.

Severe, deep, throbbing ear pain and

fever that may reach 102° F. (38.9° C.) characterize *acute suppurative otitis media.* The pain increases steadily over several hours or days and may be aggravated by pressure on the mastoid antrum. Typically, the patient experiences mild hearing loss, slight dizziness, nausea, and vomiting. Before rupture, the eardrum appears bulging and fiery red. Rupture causes purulent drainage and relieves the pain.

• *Perichondritis.* This infection may cause ear pain accompanied by warmth and tenderness in the outer ear and a reddened, dough-like auricle.

• *Petrositis.* The result of acute otitis media, this infection produces deep ear pain with headache and pain behind the eye. Other findings are diplopia, loss of lateral gaze, vomiting, sensorineural hearing loss, vertigo, and, possibly, nuchal rigidity.

• *Temporomandibular joint infection.* Typically unilateral, this infection produces ear pain that's referred from the jaw joint. The pain is aggravated by pressure on the joint with jaw movement; commonly, it radiates to the temporal area or the entire side of the head.

Special considerations

Administer analgesics and apply heat to relieve discomfort, as ordered. Instill eardrops, if necessary. Teach the patient how to instill drops if they're prescribed for home use.

Pediatric pointers

Common causes of earache in children are acute otitis media and insertion of foreign bodies that become lodged or infected. Be alert for crying or ear-tugging in a young child—nonverbal clues to earache. To examine the child's ears, place him supine with his arms extended and held securely by his parent. Then hold the otoscope with the handle pointing toward the top of the child's head, and brace it against him with one or two fingers. Because an ear examination may upset the child with an earache, save it for the end of your physical examination.

Edema—Generalized

A common sign in severely ill patients, generalized edema is the excessive accumulation of interstitial fluid throughout the body. Its severity varies widely; slight edema may be difficult to detect, especially if the patient's obese, while massive edema is immediately apparent.

Typically, generalized edema is chronic and progressive. It may result from cardiac, renal, endocrine, or hepatic disorders. However, this sign may also result from severe burns, malnutrition, or the effects of certain drugs and treatments.

Common factors responsible for edema are hypoalbuminemia and excess sodium ingestion or retention—both of which influence plasma osmotic pressure (see *Understanding Fluid Balance*). Also, cyclic edema associated with increased aldosterone secretion may occur in premenopausal women.

Assessment

Quickly assess the edema's severity, including the degree of pitting. (See *Edema: Pitting or Nonpitting?*, page 277.) If the patient has severe edema, promptly take his vital signs, and check for distended neck veins and cyanotic lips. Auscultate the lungs and heart. If you detect signs of cardiac failure or pulmonary congestion, such as rales or ventricular gallop, have another nurse notify the doctor immediately. Place the patient in Fowler's position to promote lung expansion, unless he's hypotensive. Prepare to administer oxygen and intravenous diuretics. Have emergency resuscitation equipment nearby.

When the patient's condition permits, obtain a complete medical history. First, note when the edema began. Is it affected by position changes? Accompanied by shortness of breath or pain in the arms or legs? Find out how much weight the patient has gained. Has his urine output changed?

Next, ask about previous burns or cardiac, renal, hepatic, endocrine, or gastrointestinal disorders. Also, have the patient describe his diet so you can assess for protein malnutrition. Explore his drug history and note recent I.V. therapy.

Begin the physical examination by comparing the arms and legs for symmetrical edema. Also note ecchymoses

and cyanosis. Assess the back, sacrum, and hips of the bedridden patient for dependent edema. Palpate peripheral pulses, noting whether hands and feet feel cold. Finally, perform a complete cardiac and respiratory assessment.

Medical causes

● *Angioneurotic edema.* Recurrent attacks of acute, painless, pitting edema affect the skin and mucous membranes, especially those of the respiratory tract. Abdominal pain, nausea, vomiting,

UNDERSTANDING FLUID BALANCE

Normally, fluid moves freely between the interstitial and intravascular spaces to maintain homeostasis. Four basic pressures control fluid shifts across the capillary membrane that separates these spaces:
● capillary hydrostatic pressure (the internal fluid pressure on the capillary membrane)
● interstitial fluid pressure (the external fluid pressure on the capillary membrane)
● plasma osmotic pressure (the fluid-attracting pressure from protein concentration within the capillary)
● interstitial osmotic pressure (the fluid-attracting pressure from protein concentration outside the capillary).

Here's how these pressures maintain

homeostasis. Normally, capillary hydrostatic pressure is greater than plasma osmotic pressure at the capillary's arterial end, forcing fluid out of the capillary. At the capillary's venous end, the reverse is true: the plasma osmotic pressure is greater than the capillary hydrostatic pressure, drawing fluid into the capillary. Normally, the lymphatic system transports excess interstitial fluid back to the intravascular space. Edema results when this balance is upset by increased capillary permeability, lymphatic obstruction, persistently increased capillary hydrostatic pressure, decreased plasma osmotic or interstitial fluid pressure, or dilation of precapillary sphincters.

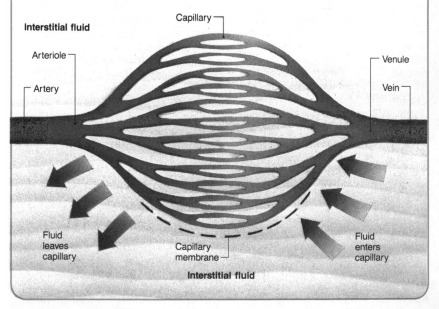

Interstitial fluid

Capillary

Arteriole

Venule

Artery

Vein

Fluid leaves capillary

Capillary membrane

Fluid enters capillary

Interstitial fluid

and diarrhea accompany visceral edema; dyspnea and stridor accompany life-threatening laryngeal edema.

• **Burns.** Edema and associated tissue damage vary with the severity of the burn. Severe generalized edema (4 +) may occur within 2 days of a major burn, while localized edema may occur with a less severe burn.

• **Cirrhosis.** Progressive anasarca is a late sign of this chronic disorder. Accompanying features may include abdominal pain, anorexia, nausea and vomiting, hepatomegaly, ascites, jaundice, pruritus, bleeding tendencies, musty breath, lethargy, mental changes, and asterixis.

• **Congestive heart failure.** Severe, pitting generalized edema—occasionally anasarca—may follow leg edema late in this disorder. The edema may improve with exercise or elevation of the limbs. Among other classic late findings are hemoptysis, cyanosis, marked hepatomegaly, clubbing, crackles, and a ventricular gallop. Typically, the patient has tachypnea, palpitations, hypotension, weight gain despite anorexia, nausea, slowed mental response, diaphoresis, and pallor. Dyspnea, orthopnea, tachycardia, and fatigue typify left heart failure, while distended neck veins typify right heart failure.

• **Malnutrition.** Anasarca in this disorder may mask dramatic muscle wasting. Malnutrition also typically causes muscle weakness; lethargy; anorexia; diarrhea; apathy; dry, wrinkled skin; and signs of anemia, such as dizziness and pallor.

• **Myxedema.** In this severe form of hypothyroidism, nonpitting generalized edema is accompanied by dry, waxy, pale skin. Observation also reveals masklike facies, hair loss or coarsening, and psychomotor slowing. Associated findings include hoarseness, weight gain, fatigue, cold intolerance, bradycardia, hypoventilation, constipation, abdominal distention, menorrhagia, impotence, and infertility.

• **Nephrotic syndrome.** Pitting generalized edema characterizes this syndrome. In severe cases, anasarca develops—increasing body weight by up to 50%. Other common signs and symptoms are ascites, anorexia, fatigue, malaise, depression, and pallor.

• **Pericardial effusion.** Generalized pitting edema may be most prominent in the arms and legs. It may be accompanied by chest pain, dyspnea, orthopnea, nonproductive cough, pericardial friction rub, dysphagia, and fever.

• **Pericarditis (chronic constrictive).** Resembling right heart failure, this disorder usually begins with pitting edema of the arms and legs that may progress to generalized edema. Other signs and symptoms may include ascites, Kussmaul's sign, dyspnea, fatigue, weakness, abdominal distention, and hepatomegaly.

• **Protein-losing enteropathy.** Progressive, pitting generalized edema occurs in this disorder. The patient may also have mild fever and abdominal pain with bloody diarrhea and steatorrhea.

• **Renal failure.** In *acute renal failure,* generalized pitting edema occurs as a late sign. In *chronic renal failure,* though, generalized edema is less likely; its severity depends on the degree of fluid overload. Both forms of renal failure cause oliguria, anorexia, nausea and vomiting, drowsiness, confusion, hypertension, dyspnea, rales, dizziness, and pallor.

• **Septic shock.** A late sign of this life-threatening disorder, generalized edema typically develops rapidly. The edema is pitting and moderately severe. Accompanying it may be cool skin, hypotension, oliguria, tachycardia, cyanosis, thirst, anxiety, and signs of respiratory failure.

Other causes

• **Drugs.** Any drug that causes sodium retention may aggravate or cause generalized edema. Some examples are antihypertensives, corticosteroids, androgenic and anabolic steroids, estrogens, and nonsteroidal anti-inflam-

EDEMA: PITTING OR NONPITTING?

To differentiate pitting from nonpitting edema, press your finger against a swollen area for five seconds, then remove it quickly. In pitting edema, pressure forces fluid into the underlying tissues, causing an indentation that slowly fills. To determine the severity of pitting edema, estimate the indentation's depth in centimeters: 1+ (1 cm), 2+ (2 cm), 3+ (3 cm), or 4+ (4 cm).

In nonpitting edema, pressure leaves no indentation because fluid has coagulated in the tissues. Typically, the skin feels unusually firm.

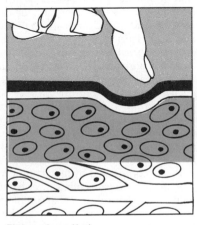

Pitting edema (4 +)

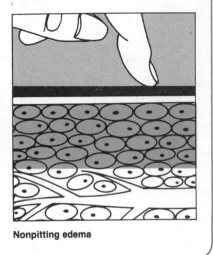

Nonpitting edema

matory agents such as phenylbutazone, ibuprofen, and naproxen.

• **I.V. infusions and feedings.** Intravenous saline administration or internal feedings may cause sodium and fluid overload, resulting in generalized edema.

Special considerations

Position the patient with his limbs above heart level to promote drainage. Periodically reposition him to avoid pressure sores. If the patient develops dyspnea, lower his limbs, elevate the head of the bed, and administer oxygen. Massage reddened areas, especially where dependent edema has formed (back, sacrum, hips, buttocks). Prevent skin breakdown in these areas by placing a pressure mattress, lamb's wool pad, or flotation ring on the pa-

tient's bed. Restrict fluids and sodium, and administer diuretics or intravenous albumin, as ordered. Monitor intake, output, and daily weight.

Monitor serum electrolytes—especially sodium—and albumin levels. Prepare the patient for blood and urine tests, X-rays, echocardiography, or electrocardiography, as ordered.

Pediatric pointers

Renal failure in children commonly causes generalized edema. Monitor fluid balance closely. Notify the doctor of fever or diaphoresis, which can lead to fluid loss, and promote fluid intake.

Kwashiorkor—protein deficiency malnutrition—occurs more frequently in children than in adults and causes anasarca.

Edema of the Arm

The result of excess interstitial fluid in the arm, this edema may be unilateral or bilateral and may develop gradually or abruptly. It may be aggravated by immobility and alleviated by arm elevation and exercise.

Arm edema signals localized fluid imbalance between vascular and interstitial spaces (see *Understanding Fluid Balance*, page 275). Commonly, it results from trauma, venous disorders, toxins, and treatments.

Assessment

When taking the patient's history, one of the first questions to ask is "How long has your arm been swollen?" Then find out if the patient also has arm pain, numbness, or tingling. Does exercise or arm elevation decrease the edema? Ask about recent arm injury, such as burns or insect stings. Also note recent intravenous therapy or surgery for breast cancer.

Assess the edema's severity by comparing the size and symmetry of both arms. Use a tape measure to determine the exact girth. Note whether the edema's unilateral or bilateral, and test for pitting. (See *Edema: Pitting or Nonpitting?*, page 277.) Next, assess and compare the color and temperature of both arms. Look for erythema and for ecchymoses or wounds that suggest injury. Palpate and compare radial and brachial pulses. Finally, assess for arm tenderness and decreased mobility. If you detect signs of neurovascular compromise, elevate the arm and notify the doctor immediately.

Medical causes

• *Angioneurotic edema.* This common reaction is characterized by sudden onset of painless, nonpruritic edema affecting the hands, feet, eyelids, lips, face, neck, genitalia, or viscera. Although these swellings usually don't itch, they may burn and tingle. If edema spreads to the larynx, signs of respiratory distress may occur.

• *Arm trauma.* Shortly after a crush injury, severe edema may affect the entire arm. Ecchymoses or superficial bleeding, pain or numbness, and, possibly, paralysis may occur.

• *Burns.* Two days or less after injury, arm burns may cause mild-to-severe edema, pain, and tissue damage.

• *Envenomation.* Initially, envenomation by snakes, aquatic animals, or insects may cause edema around the bite or sting that quickly spreads to the entire arm. Pain at the site is common, as are erythema, pruritus, and, occasionally, paresthesia. Later, there may be generalized signs and symptoms such as nausea, vomiting, weakness, muscle cramps, fever, chills, hypotension, headache, and, in severe cases, dyspnea, seizures, and paralysis.

• *Superior vena cava syndrome.* Usually, bilateral arm edema progresses slowly and is accompanied by facial and neck edema. Dilated veins mark these edematous areas. The patient also complains of headache, vertigo, and visual disturbances.

• *Thrombophlebitis.* This disorder may cause arm edema, pain, and warmth. *Deep vein thrombophlebitis* can also produce cyanosis, fever, chills, and malaise, while *superficial thrombophlebitis* also causes redness, tenderness, and induration along the vein.

Other causes

• *Treatments.* Localized arm edema may result from infiltration of I.V. fluid into the interstitial tissue. A radical or modified radical mastectomy that disrupts lymphatic drainage may cause edema of the entire arm. Also, radiation therapy for breast cancer may produce arm edema immediately after treatment or months later.

Special considerations

Treatment of the patient with arm edema depends on the underlying cause. However, general care measures include elevation of the arm, frequent repositioning, and appropriate use of bandages and dressings to promote drainage and circulation. Of course, you'll need to provide meticulous skin care to prevent breakdown and decubiti formation. You'll also need to give prescribed drugs, such as analgesics and anticoagulants, as ordered.

Pediatric pointers

Arm edema rarely occurs in children, except as part of generalized edema. But it may result from arm trauma, such as burns and crush injuries.

Edema of the Face

Facial edema refers to localized swelling—around the eyes, for instance—or more generalized facial swelling that may extend to the neck and upper arms. Occasionally painful, this sign may develop gradually or abruptly. At times, it precedes onset of peripheral or generalized edema. Mild edema may be difficult to detect; the patient or someone who's familiar with the patient's appearance may report it before it's noticed during assessment.

Facial edema results from disruption of the hydrostatic and osmotic pressures that govern fluid movement between the arteries, veins, and lymphatics. (See *Understanding Fluid Balance*, page 275.) It may result from venous, inflammatory, and certain systemic disorders; trauma; allergy; malnutrition; or the effects of drugs, tests, and treatments.

Assessment

If the patient has facial edema associated with burns or if he reports recent exposure to an allergen, quickly assess his respiratory status: Edema may also affect his upper airway, causing life-threatening obstruction. If you detect audible wheezes, inspiratory stridor, or other signs of respiratory distress, notify the doctor immediately and give epinephrine, as ordered. In severe distress— with absent breath sounds and cyanosis—assist with tracheal intubation, cricothyroidotomy, or tracheotomy. Administer oxygen, as ordered.

If the patient isn't in severe distress, take his health history. Ask if facial edema developed suddenly or gradually. Is it more prominent in the early morning, or does it worsen throughout the day? Has the patient noticed any weight gain? If so, how much and over what length of time? Has he noticed a change in his urine color or output? In his appetite? Take a drug history and ask about recent facial trauma.

Begin the physical examination by characterizing the edema. Is it localized to one part of the face, or does it affect other parts of the body? Determine if it's pitting or nonpitting and grade its severity. Next, take vital signs and assess neurologic status.

Medical causes

• *Allergic reaction.* Facial edema may characterize both local allergic reactions and anaphylaxis. In life-threatening *anaphylaxis*, angioneurotic facial edema may occur with urticaria and flushing. Airway edema causes hoarseness, stridor, and bronchospasm with dyspnea and tachypnea. Signs of shock, such as hypotension and cool, clammy skin, may also occur. A localized reaction produces facial edema, erythema, and urticaria.

• *Cavernous sinus thrombosis.* This rare disorder may begin with unilateral edema that quickly progresses to bilateral edema of the forehead, base of the nose, and eyelids. It may also produce chills, fever, headache, nausea, lethargy, exophthalmos, and eye pain.

• *Chalazion.* A chalazion causes localized swelling and tenderness of the affected eyelid, accompanied by a small red lump on the conjunctival surface.

• *Conjunctivitis.* This inflammation causes eyelid edema, excessive tearing, and itchy, burning eyes. Inspection re-

RECOGNIZING ANGIONEUROTIC EDEMA

Most dramatic in the lips, eyelids, and tongue, angioneurotic edema frequently results from an allergic reaction. It's characterized by rapid onset of painless, nonpitting, subcutaneous swelling that usually resolves in 1 to 2 days. This edema may also involve the hands, feet, genitalia, and viscera; laryngeal edema may cause life-threatening airway obstruction.

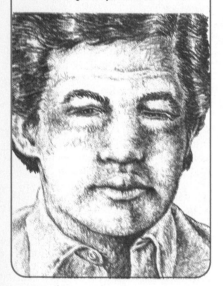

veals a thick purulent discharge, crusty eyelids, and conjunctival injection. Corneal involvement causes photophobia and pain.

• **Corneal ulcers (fungal).** Accompanying red, edematous eyelids in this disorder are conjunctival injection, intense pain, photophobia, and severely impaired visual acuity. Copious, purulent eye discharge makes eyelids sticky and crusted. The characteristic dense, central ulcer grows slowly, appears whitish-gray, and is surrounded by progressively clearer rings.

• **Dacryoadenitis.** Severe periorbital swelling characterizes this disorder, which may also cause conjunctival injection, purulent discharge, and temporal pain.

• **Dacryocystitis.** Lacrimal sac inflammation causes prominent eyelid edema and constant tearing. In acute cases, pain and tenderness near the tear sac accompany purulent discharge.

• **Dermatomyositis.** Periorbital edema and heliotropic rash develop gradually in this rare disease. An itchy, lilac-colored rash appears on the bridge of the nose, cheeks, and forehead. Localized or diffuse erythema, eye pain, and fever may also occur.

• **Facial burns.** These may cause extensive edema that impairs respiration. Additional findings may include singed nasal hairs, red mucosa, sooty sputum, and signs of respiratory distress, such as inspiratory stridor.

• **Facial trauma.** In this disorder, edema depends on the type of injury. For example, contusion may cause localized edema, whereas nasal or maxillary fracture causes more generalized edema. Associated features also depend on the injury.

• **Frontal sinus carcinoma.** This rare disorder causes cheek edema on the affected side, reddened skin over the sinus, unilateral nasal bleeding or discharge, and exophthalmos. Pain over the forehead and unilateral hypoesthesia or anesthesia may occur later.

• **Herpes zoster ophthalmicus (shingles).** In this disorder, edematous and red eyelids are usually accompanied by excessive tearing and a serous discharge. Severe unilateral facial pain may occur several days before vesicles erupt.

• **Hordeolum (stye).** Typically, localized eyelid edema, erythema, and pain occur with a hordeolum.

• **Malnutrition.** Severe malnutrition causes facial edema followed by swelling of the feet and legs. Associated signs and symptoms include muscle atrophy and weakness; anorexia; diarrhea; lethargy; dry, wrinkled skin; sparse, brittle, easily plucked hair; and slowed pulse and respirations.

• **Melkersson's syndrome.** Facial edema—especially of the lips—is one of three characteristic signs of this rare disorder, along with facial paralysis and folds in the patient's tongue.

• *Myxedema.* This disorder eventually causes generalized facial edema, waxy dry skin, hair loss or coarsening, and other signs of hypothyroidism.

• *Nephrotic syndrome.* Often the first sign of nephrotic syndrome, periorbital edema precedes dependent and abdominal edema. Associated findings include weight gain, nausea, anorexia, lethargy, fatigue, and pallor.

• *Orbital cellulitis.* Sudden onset of periorbital edema marks this inflammatory disorder. It may be accompanied by a unilateral purulent discharge, hyperemia, exophthalmos, conjunctival injection, fever, and extreme orbital pain.

• *Osteomyelitis.* When this disorder affects the frontal bone, it may cause forehead edema, as well as fever, chills, headache, and cool, pallid skin.

• *Peritonsillar abscess.* This complication of tonsillitis may cause unilateral facial edema. Other key signs and symptoms include severe throat pain, neck swelling, drooling, cervical adenopathy, fever, chills, and malaise.

• *Preeclampsia.* Edema of the face, hands, and ankles is an early sign of this disorder of pregnancy. Other characteristics include excessive weight gain, severe headache, blurred vision, hypertension, and midepigastric pain.

• *Rhinitis (allergic).* In this disorder, red and edematous eyelids are accompanied by paroxysmal sneezing, itchy nose and eyes, and profuse, watery rhinorrhea. The patient may also have nasal congestion, excessive tearing, headache, sinus pain, and, sometimes, malaise and fever.

• *Sinusitis. Frontal sinusitis* causes edema of the forehead and eyelids. *Maxillary sinusitis* produces edema in the maxillary area. In addition, it causes malaise, gingival swelling, and trismus. Both types are also accompanied by facial pain, fever, nasal congestion, purulent nasal discharge, and red, swollen nasal mucosa.

• *Superior vena cava syndrome.* This disorder gradually produces facial and neck edema accompanied by thoracic or neck vein distention. It also causes CNS symptoms, such as headache, visual disturbances, and vertigo.

• *Trachoma.* In this disorder, edema affects the eyelid and conjunctiva and is accompanied by eye pain, excessive tearing, photophobia, and eye discharge. Examination reveals an inflamed preauricular node and visible conjunctival follicles.

• *Trichinosis.* This relatively rare disorder causes sudden onset of eyelid edema with fever (102° to 104° F., or 38.9° to 40° C.), conjunctivitis, muscle pain, itching and burning skin, sweating, skin lesions, and delirium.

Other causes

• *Diagnostic tests.* An allergic reaction to contrast media used in radiologic tests may produce facial edema.

• *Drugs.* Long-term use of glucocorticoids may produce facial edema. Any drug that causes an allergic reaction (aspirin, antipyretics, penicillin, and sulfa preparations, for example) may have the same effect.

• *Surgery and transfusion.* Cranial, nasal, or jaw surgery may cause facial edema, as may a blood transfusion that causes an allergic reaction.

Special considerations

Administer pain medications for facial edema and apply creams to reduce itching, as ordered. Unless contraindicated, apply cold compresses to the patient's eyes to decrease edema. Elevate the head of his bed to help drain the accumulated fluid. Commonly, urine and blood tests are ordered to help diagnose the cause of facial edema.

Pediatric pointers

Normally, the pressure in the child's periorbital tissue is lower than in the adult's. As a result, the child is more likely to develop periorbital edema. In fact, periorbital edema is more common than peripheral edema in children with such disorders as heart failure and acute glomerulonephritis. Pertussis may also cause periorbital edema.

Edema of the Leg

This edema results when excess interstitial fluid accumulates in one or both legs. It may affect just the foot and ankle or extend to the thigh. This common sign may be slight or dramatic, pitting or nonpitting.

Leg edema may result from venous disorders, trauma, and certain bone and cardiac disorders that disturb normal fluid balance. (See *Understanding Fluid Balance,* page 275.) However, several nonpathologic mechanisms may also cause it. For example, prolonged sitting, standing, or immobility may cause bilateral orthostatic edema. Usually, this pitting edema affects the foot and disappears with rest and leg elevation. Increased venous pressure late in pregnancy may also cause ankle edema.

Assessment

To assess the patient with leg edema, first ask how long he's had it. Did the edema develop suddenly or gradually? Does it decrease if he elevates his legs? Is it painful when touched? When he walks? Ask about recent surgery or illness that may have immobilized the patient. Does he have a history of cardiovascular disease? Also ask about recent leg injury. Finally, obtain a drug history.

Begin the physical examination by assessing each leg for pitting edema. (See *Edema: Pitting or Nonpitting?,* page 277.) Because leg edema may compromise arterial blood flow, palpate peripheral pulses to detect any insufficiency. Observe leg color and look for unusual vein patterns. Then, palpate for warmth, tenderness, or cords, and gently squeeze the calf muscle against the tibia to check for deep pain. If leg edema is unilateral, dorsiflex the foot to assess for Homans' sign. Finally, note skin thickening or ulceration in the edematous areas.

Medical causes

● *Burns.* Two days or less after injury, leg burns may cause mild-to-severe edema, pain, and tissue damage.

● *Congestive heart failure.* Bilateral leg edema is an early sign in right heart failure. Other effects may be weight gain despite anorexia, nausea, chest tightness, hypotension, pallor, tachypnea, palpitations, ventricular gallop, and inspiratory rales. Pitting ankle edema signals more advanced heart failure, as do hepatomegaly, hemoptysis, and cyanosis.

● *Envenomation.* Mild-to-severe localized edema may develop suddenly at the site of a bite or sting, along with erythema, pain, urticaria, pruritus, and a burning sensation.

● *Leg trauma.* Mild-to-severe localized edema may form around the trauma site.

● *Osteomyelitis.* When this bone infection affects the lower leg, it usually produces localized, mild-to-moderate edema, which may spread to the adjacent joint. Typically, edema follows fever, localized tenderness, and pain that increases with leg movement.

● *Phlegmasia cerulea dolens.* Severe unilateral leg edema and cyanosis may spread to the abdomen and flank in this rare form of venous thrombosis. Other features: pain, cold skin, absent pulse in the affected leg, and signs of shock, such as hypotension and tachycardia.

● *Thrombophlebitis.* Both deep and superficial vein thrombosis may cause sudden onset of unilateral mild-to-moderate edema. *Deep vein thrombophlebitis* may be asymptomatic or may cause mild-to-severe pain, warmth, and cyanosis in the affected leg as well as fever, chills, and malaise. *Superficial thrombophlebitis* typically causes pain, warmth, redness, tenderness, and induration along the affected vein.

● *Venous insufficiency (chronic).* Unilateral or bilateral leg edema occurs and is moderate to severe in this disorder. Initially, the edema is soft and pitting; later, it becomes hard as tissues thicken. Other signs include darkened skin and painless, easily infected stasis ulcers that develop around the ankle.

Other causes
- *Diagnostic tests.* Venography is a rare cause of leg edema.
- *I.V. therapy.* Infiltration of the I.V. site can cause leg edema.

Special considerations
Show the patient with leg edema how to apply antiembolism stockings or bandages to promote venous return. Also encourage leg exercises; provide analgesics as necessary. If ordered, apply a zinc-gelatin compression boot (Unna's boot) to help reduce the edema. Have the patient avoid prolonged sitting or standing, and elevate his legs as necessary.

Monitor the patient's intake and output, and check his weight and leg circumference daily to detect any change in the edema. As ordered, prepare him for diagnostic tests, such as blood and urine studies and X-rays.

Pediatric pointers
Uncommon in children, leg edema may result from osteomyelitis, leg trauma, or, rarely, congestive heart failure.

Enophthalmos

Enophthalmos is the backward displacement of the eye into the orbit. This sign may develop suddenly or gradually. It may be severe or mild enough to go unnoticed by the patient. Most often, enophthalmos results from trauma. It may also result from severe dehydration and eye disorders. In the elderly, senile atrophy of orbital fat may produce physiologic enophthalmos.

Because enophthalmos allows the upper lid to droop over the sunken eye, it's often mistaken for ptosis. However, exophthalmometry can differentiate these signs (see *Differentiating Enophthalmos from Ptosis*, page 284).

Assessment
Begin by asking the patient how long he's had enophthalmos. Is it accompanied by headache or eye pain? If so, ask him to describe its severity and location. Next, ask about a history of trauma, cancer, or other eye disorders.

If you suspect an orbital fracture, do *not* open the patient's eye or place any pressure on the eyeball; this risks ocular laceration. Apply a metal (Fox) or plastic eye shield until the ophthalmologist can perform a complete exam.

Otherwise, perform a visual acuity test, with and without correction. Then evaluate extraocular movements and assess intraocular pressure with a Schiøtz tonometer. Using a direct ophthalmoscope, check for papilledema and other abnormalities. Next, check pupil response to light. Also note eyelid drooping.

Medical causes
- *Dehydration.* Mild-to-severe enophthalmos may accompany severe dehydration. Typically, the patient also displays poor skin turgor, dry mucous membranes, extreme thirst, weight loss, fatigue, tachycardia, hypotension, nausea, vomiting, and diarrhea.
- *Duane's syndrome.* In this congenital syndrome, transient enophthalmos occurs when the patient looks to the side. Visual acuity is usually normal, but horizontal eye movement is impaired.
- *Greig's syndrome (craniofacial dystosis).* Typically, enophthalmos is accompanied by an abnormally wide distance between the pupils in this syndrome. Other common findings include mental deficiency, astigmatism, epicanthal folds, skull deformity, and, occasionally, ocular deviation.
- *Orbital fracture.* Here, enophthalmos may not be apparent until edema subsides. The affected eyeball is displaced down and in, and is surrounded by ecchymosis. Other findings include diplopia in the affected eye, eye or head pain, subconjunctival hemorrhage, and a dilated or unreactive pupil.
- *Parinaud's syndrome.* In this form of

DIFFERENTIATING ENOPHTHALMOS FROM PTOSIS

In enophthalmos, the eye is displaced backward in its socket, causing the upper eyelid to droop. In ptosis, eyelid drooping is also characteristic but results from muscle weakness or cranial nerve paralysis.

To differentiate enophthalmos from ptosis, use a Hertel exophthalmometer to measure the distance between the orbital rim and the tip of the cornea. Have the patient stand against the wall and look into your eyes. Place the device on the patient's face like a pair of glasses, adjust it to fit snugly at the orbital rims, and note the bar reading. Then look into the 45° angle mirrors and measure the corneal apex by lining it up visually against the millimeter scale. Normally, the corneal apex is 12 to 24 mm in front of the orbital rim, and the difference between the eyes is less than 2 mm. In ptosis, the readings are within the normal range; in enophthalmos, the reading in one or both eyes may be less than 12 mm.

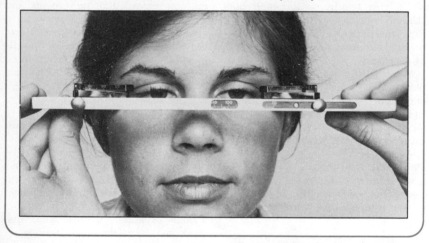

ophthalmoplegia, enophthalmos is accompanied by nystagmus when the patient tries to look up. Ocular muscles show absent voluntary movement but normal conjugate movement. Other signs include lid retraction, ptosis, dilated pupils with poor or absent light response, and papilledema.

• *Parry-Romberg syndrome.* This syndrome produces enophthalmos and, possibly, irises of different color. The patient may have facial hemiatrophy, miotic pupils with a sluggish response to dim light, nystagmus, ocular muscle paralysis, and ptosis.

Special considerations
Regularly monitor vital signs and assess pupillary response to light. As or-

dered, prepare the trauma patient for skull X-rays and eye examination.

Pediatric pointers
Enophthalmos usually results from microphthalmos—abnormally small eyes—in the newborn. Later, its causes resemble those found in adults.

Enuresis

Usually, enuresis refers to nighttime urinary incontinence in a girl over age 5 or a boy over age 6. Rarely, this sign may continue into adulthood. It's most common in boys and may be classified as primary or secondary. *Primary enuresis* describes the child who has never achieved bladder control; *secondary enuresis* describes the child who achieved bladder control for at least 3 months but has lost it.

Among factors that may contribute to enuresis are delayed development of detrusor muscle control, unusually deep or sound sleep, organic disorders such as urinary tract infection or obstruction, and psychological stress. Probably the most important factor, psychological stress commonly results from the birth of a sibling, the death of a parent or loved one, or premature, rigorous toilet training. The child may be too embarrassed or ashamed to discuss his enuresis, which intensifies psychological stress and makes enuresis more likely—thus creating a vicious cycle.

Assessment

When taking a history, include the parents as well as the child. First, determine the number of nights each week or month that the child wets the bed. Is there a family history of enuresis? Ask about the child's daily fluid intake. Does he drink much after supper? What are his typical sleep and voiding patterns? Find out if the child's ever had control of his bladder. If so, try to pinpoint what may have precipitated enuresis, such as an organic disorder or psychological stress. Does the bed-wetting occur at home and away from home? Ask the parents how they have tried to manage the problem and have them describe the child's toilet training. Observe the child's and parents' attitudes toward bed-wetting. Finally, ask the child if it hurts when he urinates.

Next, perform a physical examination to detect signs of neurologic or urinary tract disorders. Observe the child's gait to assess for motor dysfunction. Also test sensory function in the legs. Inspect the urethral meatus for erythema and obtain a urine specimen. Assist the doctor with a rectal examination to assess sphincter control.

Medical causes

● *Detrusor muscle hyperactivity.* Involuntary detrusor muscle contractions may cause primary or secondary enuresis associated with urinary urgency, frequency, and incontinence. Signs and symptoms of urinary tract infection are also common.

● *Urinary tract infection.* In children, most urinary tract infections produce secondary enuresis. Associated features include urinary frequency and urgency, dysuria, straining to urinate, and hematuria. Lower back pain, fatigue, and suprapubic discomfort may also occur.

● *Urinary tract obstruction.* Although

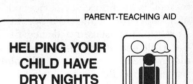

PARENT-TEACHING AID

HELPING YOUR CHILD HAVE DRY NIGHTS

Dear Parent:

Although no single treatment for bedwetting is always effective, following these recommendations can help your child achieve bladder control.
● Restrict your child's fluid intake—especially of cola drinks—after supper.
● Make sure your child urinates before bedtime. In addition, wake him once during the night to go to the bathroom.
● Reward your child after each dry night with praise and encouragement.
● Keep a progress chart, marking each dry night with a sticker. Reward a certain number of consecutive dry nights with a book, small toy, or special activity.
● Always give your child emotional support. Never punish him if he wets the bed, but reassure him that he will learn to achieve bladder control. Remember that most children simply "outgrow" bed-wetting. However, periods of wet and dry nights will occur before your child develops a constant pattern of dryness.

daytime incontinence occurs more frequently, this disorder may produce primary or secondary enuresis. It may also cause flank and lower back pain; upper abdominal distention; urinary frequency, urgency, hesitancy, and dribbling; dysuria; diminished urinary stream; hematuria; and variable urinary output.

Special considerations

Provide emotional support for the child and his family. Encourage the parents to accept and support the child, and tell them how to manage enuresis at home. (See *Helping Your Child Have Dry Nights,* page 285.)

If the child has detrusor muscle hyperactivity, bladder training may help control enuresis. Another treatment method is the Enuretone device, which may be useful for the child over age 8. This moisture-sensitive device fits in the child's mattress and triggers an alarm when it becomes wet. The alarm wakes the child immediately, conditioning him to avoid bed-wetting.

Epistaxis

A common sign, epistaxis can be spontaneous or induced from the front or back of the nose. Most nosebleeds occur in the anterior-inferior nasal septum (Kiesselbach's plexus), but they may also occur at the point where the inferior turbinates meet the nasopharynx. Usually unilateral, they may seem bilateral when blood runs from the bleeding side behind the nasal septum and out the opposite side. Epistaxis ranges from mild oozing to severe— possibly life-threatening—blood loss.

A rich supply of fragile blood vessels makes the nose particularly vulnerable to bleeding. Air moving through the nose can dry and irritate the mucous membranes, forming crusts that bleed when they're removed; dry mucous membranes are also more susceptible to infections, which can produce epistaxis as well. Trauma is another common cause of epistaxis. Additional causes include hematologic, coagulation, renal, and gastrointestinal disorders, and certain drugs and treatments.

Assessment

If your patient has severe epistaxis, quickly take his vital signs. If you detect tachypnea, hypotension, or other signs of hypovolemic shock, have another nurse notify the doctor immediately. Insert a large-gauge I.V. for rapid fluid and blood replacement, and attempt to control bleeding by pinching the nares closed. (However, if you suspect a nasal fracture, *don't* pinch the nares. Instead, place gauze under the nose to absorb the blood.) Have the hypovolemic patient lie down and turn his head to the side to prevent blood from draining down the back of his throat, which could cause aspiration or vomiting of swallowed blood. Or, if the patient isn't hypovolemic, have him sit upright and tilt his head forward. Constantly check airway patency. If the patient's condition is unstable, begin cardiac monitoring and give supplemental oxygen by mask, as ordered.

If your patient isn't in distress, take a history. Does he have a history of recent trauma? How often has he had nosebleeds in the past? Have they been long or unusually severe? Has he recently had surgery in the sinus area? Ask about a history of hypertension, bleeding disorders, liver diseases, and other recent illnesses, and ask if he bruises easily. Find out what drugs he uses, especially anti-inflammatories, such as aspirin, and anticoagulants, such as warfarin sodium.

Continue the physical examination by inspecting the patient's skin for other signs of bleeding, such as ecchymoses and petechiae, and noting any jaundice, pallor, or other abnormalities. For a trauma patient, assess for associated injuries, such as eye trauma or facial fractures. Be prepared to assist the doctor with a nasal examination to visualize the bleeding site.

Medical causes

• *Aplastic anemia.* This disorder develops insidiously, eventually producing nosebleeds as well as ecchymoses, retinal hemorrhages, menorrhagia, petechiae, bleeding from the mouth, and signs of gastrointestinal bleeding. Fatigue, dyspnea, headache, tachycardia, and pallor may also occur.

• *Barotrauma.* Commonly seen in airline passengers and scuba divers, barotrauma may cause severe, painful epistaxis when the patient has an upper respiratory infection.

• *Biliary obstruction.* This disorder produces bleeding tendencies, including epistaxis. Typical features are colicky right upper quadrant pain after eating fatty food, nausea, vomiting, fever, flatulence, and, possibly, jaundice.

• *Chemical irritants.* Some chemicals, including phosphorus, sulfuric acid, ammonia, printer's ink, and chromates, irritate the nasal mucosa, producing epistaxis.

• *Cirrhosis.* In this disorder, epistaxis is a late sign that occurs with a tendency to bleed in other areas (bleeding gums, easy bruising, hematemesis, melena). Other typical late findings include ascites, abdominal pain, shallow respirations, hepatomegaly or splenomegaly, and fever of 101° to 103° F. (38.3° to 39.4° C.). The patient may also have muscle atrophy, enlarged superficial abdominal veins, severe pruritus, extremely dry skin, poor tissue turgor, abnormal pigmentation, spider angiomas, palmar erythema, and possibly jaundice and central nervous system disturbances.

• *Coagulation disorders.* Such disorders as hemophilia and thrombocytopenic purpura can cause epistaxis along with ecchymoses, petechiae, and bleeding from the gums, mouth, and I.V. puncture sites. Menorrhagia and signs of GI bleeding, such as melena and hematemesis, can occur.

• *Glomerulonephritis (chronic).* This disorder insidiously produces nosebleeds as well as hypertension, proteinuria, hematuria, headache, edema, oliguria, hemoptysis, nausea, vomiting, pruritus, dyspnea, malaise, and fatigue.

• *Hepatitis.* When this disorder interferes with the clotting mechanism, epistaxis and abnormal bleeding tendencies can result. Associated signs and symptoms typically include jaundice, clay-colored stools, pruritus, hepatomegaly, abdominal pain, fever, fatigue, weakness, dark amber urine, anorexia, nausea, and vomiting.

• *Hereditary hemorrhagic telangiectasia (Rendu-Osler-Weber disease).* This disease causes frequent, sometimes daily, epistaxis, as well as hemoptysis and gastrointestinal bleeding. Telangiectases appear as bright red or purple skin lesions on the face, scalp, ears, palms, and soles; they range in size from a pinpoint to 3 mm in diameter.

• *Hypertension.* If severe, hypertension can produce extreme epistaxis, usually in the posterior nose, with pulsation above the middle turbinate. Blood pressure exceeds 140/90 mm Hg, and dizziness, a throbbing headache, anxiety, peripheral edema, nocturia, nausea, vomiting, drowsiness, and mental impairment may occur.

• *Infectious mononucleosis.* Blood may ooze from the nose in this infectious disorder. Hallmarks are sore throat, cervical lymphadenopathy, and a fluctuating fever with an evening peak up to 101° to 102° F. (38.3° to 38.9° C.).

• *Influenza.* When influenza affects the capillaries, a slow, oozing nosebleed results. Other findings include dry cough, chills, fever, malaise, myalgia, sore throat, hoarseness or loss of voice, conjunctivitis, facial flushing, headache, rhinitis, and rhinorrhea.

• *Juvenile angiofibroma.* This rare disorder usually occurs in males and is characterized by severe recurrent epistaxis and nasal obstruction.

• *Leukemia.* In *acute leukemia,* sudden epistaxis is accompanied by a high fever and other abnormal bleeding, such as bleeding gums, ecchymoses, petechiae, easy bruising, and prolonged menses. These may follow less noticeable signs, such as weakness, lassitude, pallor, chills, recurrent infections, and low-grade fever. In addition, acute leukemia may cause dyspnea, fatigue, malaise, tachycardia, palpitations, a systolic ejection murmur, and abdominal or bone pain.

In *chronic leukemia,* epistaxis is a late sign that may be accompanied by other abnormal bleeding, extreme fatigue, weight loss, hepatosplenomegaly, bone tenderness, edema, macular or nodular skin lesions, pallor, weakness, dyspnea, tachycardia, palpitations, and headache.

● *Maxillofacial injury.* With this type of injury, a pumping arterial bleed usually causes severe epistaxis. Associated features may include facial pain, numbness, swelling, asymmetry, open bite malocclusion or inability to open the mouth, diplopia, conjunctival hemorrhage, lip edema, and buccal, mucosal, and soft palatal ecchymoses.

● *Nasal fracture.* Bilateral epistaxis is accompanied by nasal swelling, periorbital ecchymoses and edema, pain, nasal deformity and displacement, and crepitation of the nasal bones.

● *Nasal tumors.* Blood may ooze from the nose when a tumor disrupts the nasal vasculature. Benign tumors usually bleed when touched, but malignant tumors produce spontaneous unilateral epistaxis, along with a foul discharge, cheek swelling, and—in the late stage—pain and polyps.

● *Orbital floor fracture.* This type of trauma may damage the maxillary sinus mucosa and—on rare occasions—cause epistaxis. More typical features include periorbital edema and ecchymoses, diplopia, infraorbital numbness, enophthalmos, limited eye movement, and facial asymmetry.

● *Polycythemia vera.* A common sign of polycythemia vera, spontaneous epistaxis may be accompanied by bleeding gums; ecchymoses; ruddy cyanosis of the face, nose, ears, and lips; and congestion of the conjunctiva, retina, and oral mucous membranes. Other signs and symptoms depend on the body system affected but may include headache, dizziness, tinnitus, visual disturbances, hypertension, chest pain, intermittent claudication, early satiety and fullness, marked splenomegaly, epigastric pain, pruritus, and dyspnea.

● *Renal failure.* Chronic renal failure is more likely than acute renal failure to cause epistaxis and a tendency to bruise easily. More common signs and symptoms are oliguria or anuria, weight loss, anorexia, abdominal pain, diarrhea, nausea, vomiting, tissue wasting, dry mucous membranes, uremic breath, Kussmaul's respirations, deteriorating mental status, and tachycardia. Skin changes include pruritus, pallor, yellow-bronze pigmentation, purpura, excoriation, uremic frost, and brown arcs under the nail margins. Neurologic signs and symptoms may include muscle twitches, fasciculations, asterixis, paresthesias, and footdrop. Cardiovascular effects include hypertension, dysrhythmias, signs of congestive heart failure, signs of pericarditis, and peripheral edema.

● *Sarcoidosis.* An oozing epistaxis may occur in this disorder, along with a nonproductive cough, substernal pain, malaise, and weight loss. Related findings: tachycardia, dysrhythmias, parotid enlargement, cervical lymphadenopathy, skin lesions, hepatosplenomegaly, and arthritis in the ankles, knees, and wrists.

● *Scleroma.* In this disorder, oozing epistaxis occurs with a watery nasal discharge that becomes foul-smelling and crusty. Progressive anosmia and turbinate atrophy may also occur.

● *Scurvy.* This disorder causes capillary fragility that leads to epistaxis, large subcutaneous hematomas, and petechiae, especially around the hair follicles, inner thighs, and buttocks. Other signs and symptoms include pallor, weakness, swollen or bleeding gums, loose teeth, hemoptysis, and melena.

● *Sinusitis (acute).* In this disorder, a

CONTROLLING EPISTAXIS WITH NASAL PACKING

When direct pressure and cautery fail to control epistaxis, assist with nasal packing. Prepare for *anterior packing* if the patient has severe bleeding in the anterior nose. In this procedure, the doctor inserts horizontal layers of petrolatum gauze strips into the nostrils near the turbinates.

If the patient has severe bleeding in the posterior nose or if anterior bleeding starts flowing backward, prepare for *posterior packing*. This consists of a gauze pack secured by three strong silk sutures. After anesthetizing the nose, the doctor pulls the sutures through the nostrils with a soft catheter, positioning the pack behind the soft palate. He ties two of the sutures to a gauze roll under the patient's nose, which keeps the pack in place, and tapes the third suture to the patient's cheek. (Anterior packing may also be inserted for extra traction and to avoid pressure on the nostrils.)

If the patient has nasal packing, remember these important nursing considerations:
• Watch for signs of respiratory distress, such as dyspnea, which may occur if the packing slips and obstructs the airway.
• Keep emergency equipment (flashlights, scissors, and hemostat) at the patient's bedside. Be prepared to cut the cheek suture and remove the pack at the first sign of airway obstruction.
• Avoid tension on the cheek suture, which could cause the posterior pack to slip out of place.
• Keep the call bell within easy reach.
• Monitor the patient's vital signs frequently. Notify the doctor if you detect signs of

hypoxia, such as tachycardia and restlessness.
• Elevate the head of the patient's bed, and remind him to breathe through his mouth.
• Administer humidified oxygen, as ordered.
• Instruct the patient *not* to blow his nose for 48 hours after the packing's removed.

bloody or blood-tinged nasal discharge may become purulent and copious after 24 to 48 hours. Associated signs and symptoms include nasal congestion, pain, tenderness, malaise, headache, low-grade fever, and red, edematous nasal mucosa.

• *Skull fracture.* Depending on the type of fracture, epistaxis can be direct—when blood flows directly down the nares—or indirect—when blood drains through the eustachian tube and into the nose. Abrasions, contusions, lacerations, or avulsions are common. A severe skull fracture may cause severe headache, decreased level of con-

sciousness, hemiparesis, dizziness, convulsions, projectile vomiting, and decreased pulse and respirations.

A *basilar fracture* may also cause bleeding from the pharynx, ears, and conjunctiva, along with raccoon's eyes and Battle's sign. Cerebrospinal fluid or even brain tissue may leak from the nose or ears. A *sphenoid fracture* may also cause blindness, while a *temporal fracture* may also cause unilateral deafness or facial paralysis.

• *Syphilis.* Epistaxis occurs most frequently in tertiary syphilis as posterior septum ulcerations produce a foul, bloody nasal discharge. It may be accompanied by a painful nasal obstruction and nasal deformity. Occasionally, primary syphilis causes painful nasal crusting and bleeding accompanied by the characteristic chancre sores.

• *Systemic lupus erythematosus (SLE).* Commonly affecting women under age 50, SLE causes oozing epistaxis. More characteristic signs and symptoms include butterfly rash, lymphadenopathy, joint pain and stiffness, anorexia, nausea, vomiting, myalgia, and weight loss.

• *Typhoid fever.* Oozing epistaxis and dry cough are common. In addition, typhoid fever may cause abrupt onset of chills and high fever, vomiting, abdominal distention, constipation or diarrhea, splenomegaly, hepatomegaly, "rose-spot" rash, jaundice, anorexia, weight loss, and profound fatigue.

Other causes
• *Drugs.* Anticoagulants, such as coumadin, and anti-inflammatories, such as aspirin, can cause epistaxis.

• *Surgery and procedures.* Rarely, epistaxis results from facial and nasal surgery, including septoplasty, rhinoplasty, Caldwell-Luc, antrostomy, and sinus procedures, as well as orbital decompression and dental extraction.

Special considerations
Until the bleeding's completely under control, continue to monitor the patient for signs of hypovolemic shock, such as tachycardia and clammy skin. If external pressure doesn't control the bleeding, help the doctor insert cotton impregnated with a vasoconstrictor and local anesthetic into the patient's nose. If bleeding persists, expect to assist with anterior or posterior nasal packing. (See *Controlling Epistaxis with Nasal Packing*, page 289.) Administer humidified oxygen by face mask to a patient with posterior packing, as ordered.

A complete blood count may be ordered to assess blood loss and detect anemia. The doctor may also order clotting studies, such as prothrombin time and activated partial thromboplastin time, to test coagulation time. Prepare the patient for X-rays if he's had a recent trauma.

Pediatric pointers
In children, a foreign body that causes nasal trauma is the most common cause of epistaxis. Nose-picking is also a common cause. Biliary atresia, cystic fibrosis, and hereditary afibrinogenemia can also cause epistaxis. Rubeola may cause an oozing nosebleed along with the characteristic maculopapular rash. Two rare childhood diseases— pertussis and diphtheria—can also cause oozing epistaxis.

Suspect a bleeding disorder if you see excess umbilical cord bleeding at birth or profuse bleeding during circumcision. Epistaxis frequently begins at puberty with hereditary hemorrhagic telangiectasia.

Eructation

Eructation (belching) occurs when gas or acidic fluid rises from the stomach, producing a characteristic sound. Depending on the cause, it may vary in duration and intensity. Occasionally, this sign results from GI disorders. More often, though, it results from aerophagia—the unconscious swallowing of air—or from ingestion of gas-producing food. Eructation may relieve associated symptoms, most notably nausea, heartburn, or dyspepsia.

Assessment
Focus your history to help decipher the cause of eructation. Ask if belching occurs after drinking carbonated beverages. Does it occur immediately after eating or several hours later? Is it relieved by vomiting or antacids? By changing position? Find out if the patient has associated abdominal pain. If so, ask him to describe its location,

duration, and intensity. Also ask about recent weight loss, lack of appetite, heartburn, nausea, or vomiting. Has the patient noticed a change in his bowel habits? Does he have trouble breathing when he's lying down?

Begin the physical examination by taking the patient's vital signs. As you do so, note his facial expression and posture. Does he appear to guard his abdomen? Is he sitting still or moving about? Check for foul-smelling breath. Next, inspect his abdomen for distention or visible peristalsis. Auscultate for bowel sounds and characterize their motility. Then palpate or percuss for abdominal tenderness, rigidity, distention, and masses.

Medical causes

• *Abdominal lymphadenopathy.* The result of infectious or neoplastic disorders, enlarged abdominal lymph nodes may cause belching and other digestive effects, such as abdominal discomfort and distention, constipation, and jaundice. Edema, backache, and fever may also occur.

• *Gastric outlet obstruction.* This common complication of duodenal ulcer disease causes eructation, epigastric fullness and discomfort, anorexia, nausea, and vomiting.

• *Hiatal hernia.* In this disorder, eructation occurs after eating and is accompanied by heartburn, regurgitation of sour-tasting fluid, and abdominal distention. The patient complains of dull substernal or epigastric pain that may radiate to the shoulder. Other features include dysphagia, nausea, weight loss, dyspnea, tachypnea, cough, and halitosis.

• *Peptic ulcer.* This common disorder may cause eructation. Its classic symptoms, though, are heartburn and gnawing or burning stomach pain that's relieved by food or antacids. Associated signs and symptoms may include nausea, vomiting, abdominal distention, and epigastric tenderness.

• *Superior mesenteric artery syndrome (acute).* Eructation and halitosis are late signs of this uncommon syndrome. Typically, the eructation occurs after eating and is accompanied by regurgitation.

Special considerations

Place the patient in a side-lying or knee-chest position to help relieve eructation. To prevent aerophagia, advise him not to chew gum or smoke. If he's sensitive to gas-producing food, such as onions and cucumbers, adjust his diet as necessary.

Pediatric pointers

Aerophagia is a common cause of eructation in children, who often swallow air when eating or crying. Organic causes are rare and usually result from a congenital anomaly, such as aganglionic megaduodenum.

Erythema

[Erythroderma]

Dilated or congested blood vessels produce red skin, or erythema, the most common sign of skin inflammation or irritation. Erythema may be localized or generalized and may occur suddenly or gradually. Skin color can range from bright red in acute conditions to pale violet or brown in chronic problems. Erythema must be differentiated from purpura, which causes redness from bleeding into the skin. When pressure's applied directly to the skin, erythema blanches momentarily, but purpura does not.

Usually, erythema results from changes in the arteries, veins, and small vessels, which lead to increased small-vessel perfusion. Drugs and neurogenic mechanisms may also allow extra blood to enter the small vessels. In addition, erythema can result from trauma and tissue damage as well as from changes in supporting tissues, which increase vessel visibility.

RARE CAUSES OF ERYTHEMA

In exceptional cases, your patient's erythema may be caused by one of these rare disorders:
- *acute febrile neutrophilic dermatosis,* which produces erythematous lesions on the face, neck, and extremities following a high fever
- *erythema ab igne,* which produces lacy erythema and telangiectases after exposure to radiant heat
- *erythema chronicum migrans,* which produces erythematous macules and papules on the trunk, upper arms, or thighs after a tick bite
- *erythema gyratum repens,* which produces wavy bands of erythema and is often associated with internal malignancy
- *toxic epidermal necrolysis,* which causes severe, widespread erythema, tenderness, and skin loss, related to *Staphylococci* or, possibly, drugs.

Assessment

If your patient has sudden progressive erythema along with rapid pulse, dyspnea, hoarseness, and agitation, quickly take his vital signs and have another nurse contact the doctor immediately—these may be signs of anaphylactic shock. Provide emergency respiratory support and give epinephrine, as ordered.

If the patient's erythema isn't associated with anaphylaxis, obtain a detailed health history. Find out how long he's had the erythema and where it first began. Ask if he's had any associated pain or itching. Has he recently had a fever, upper respiratory infection, or joint pain? Does he have a history of skin disease or other illness? Does he or anyone in his family have allergies, asthma, or eczema? Has he been exposed to someone who's had a similar rash or who's now ill?

Obtain a complete drug history, including recent immunizations. Ask about the patient's food intake and any exposure to chemicals.

Begin the physical examination by assessing the extent, distribution, and intensity of erythema. Look for edema and other skin lesions, such as hives, scales, papules, and purpura. Examine the affected area for warmth, and gently palpate it to check for tenderness.

Medical causes

- **Allergic reactions.** Foods, drugs, chemicals, and other allergens can cause a mild-to-severe allergic reaction and erythema. A *localized allergic reaction* also produces hivelike eruptions and edema.

Anaphylaxis, a life-threatening condition, produces relatively sudden erythema in the form of urticaria. It also produces flushing; facial edema; diaphoresis; weakness; sneezing; possibly, airway edema with hoarseness and stridor; bronchospasm with dyspnea and tachypnea; and shock with hypotension and cool, clammy skin.

- **Burns.** With *thermal burns,* erythema and swelling appear first, possibly followed by deep or superficial blisters and other signs of damage that depend on the severity of the burn. *Burns from ultraviolet rays,* such as sunburn, cause delayed erythema and tenderness on exposed areas of the skin.
- **Candidiasis.** When this fungal infection affects the skin, it produces erythema and a scaly, papular rash under the breasts and at the axillae, neck, umbilicus, and groin.
- **Dermatitis.** Erythema commonly occurs with this family of inflammatory disorders. In *atopic dermatitis,* erythema and intense pruritus precede the development of small papules that may redden, weep, scale, and lichenify.

Contact dermatitis occurs after exposure to an irritant. It quickly produces erythema and vesicles, blisters, or ulcerations on exposed skin.

In *seborrheic dermatitis,* erythema appears with dull red or yellow lesions. Sharply marginated, these lesions are sometimes ring-shaped and covered with greasy scales. Usually, they occur on the scalp, eyebrows, ears, and nasolabial folds, but they may form a butterfly rash on the face or move to the chest or to skin folds on the trunk.

● *Dermatomyositis.* This disorder, most common in women over age 50, produces a dusky lilac rash on the face, neck, upper torso, and nail beds. Grotton's papules (violet, flat-topped lesions) may appear on finger joints.

● *Erysipelas.* This infection suddenly causes rosy or crimson swollen lesions, mainly on the head and neck. If severe, it may cause hemorrhagic pus-filled blisters. Other signs and symptoms may include fever, chills, cervical lymphadenopathy, vomiting, headache, sore throat, warmth and tenderness in the affected area, and, possibly, alopecia.

● *Erythema annulare centrifugum.* Small pink infiltrated papules appear on the trunk, buttocks, and inner thighs, slowly spreading at the margins and clearing in the center. Itching, scaling, and tissue hardening may occur.

● *Erythema marginatum rheumaticum.* Associated with rheumatic fever, this disorder causes erythematous lesions that are superficial, flat, and slightly hardened. They shift, spread rapidly, and may last for hours or days, recurring after a time.

● *Erythema multiforme.* Often occurring in the spring and fall, *erythema multiforme major* (Stevens-Johnson syndrome) produces sudden hivelike erythema with blisters, and pathognomonic petechial or "iris" lesions that usually appear symmetrically and bilaterally on the face, hands, and feet. Erythema is characteristically preceded by blisters on the lips, tongue, and buccal mucosa; a thick, gray film over the mucous membranes; increased salivation; and an extremely sore throat. Other early signs may include cough, vomiting, diarrhea, corneal ulcers, conjunctival injection with a copious purulent discharge, coryza, epistaxis, and severe inflammation of the urethra, vagina, and anus. Fever may range from 102° to 104° F. (39° to 40° C.). Tachypnea, a rapid, weak pulse, chest pain, malaise, and muscle and joint pain may also occur.

With *erythema multiforme minor,*

erythematous macules and papules, purpura, and occasional blisters occur. Characteristic urticarial "iris" lesions may burn or itch slightly; they usually appear in crops and last for 2 to 3 weeks. After 1 week, individual lesions become flat or hyperpigmented. Early signs and symptoms may include a mild fever, cough, and sore throat.

● *Erythema nodosum.* Sudden bilateral eruption of tender erythematous nodules characterizes this disorder. These firm, round, protruding lesions usually appear in crops on the shins, knees, and ankles but may occur on the buttocks, arms, calves, and trunk as well. Other effects are mild fever, chills, malaise, muscle and joint pain, and, possibly, swollen feet and ankles.

● *Frostbite.* First-degree frostbite turns the affected body part a lifeless gray, followed by an intense bluish red flush on rewarming. Blisters, lack of feeling, and tissue necrosis may follow.

● *Intertrigo.* In this disorder, skin friction usually causes symmetrical erythema that may be accompanied by soreness or itching. Typically, erythema occurs in skin folds, such as in the groin; in severe cases, the skin may become bright red with erosion and maceration.

● *Liver disease (chronic).* Any chronic liver disease, such as cirrhosis, can cause local vasodilation and palmar erythema, with jaundice, pruritus, spider angiomas, xanthomas, and characteristic systemic signs.

● *Lupus erythematosus.* Both discoid and systemic lupus erythematosus can produce a characteristic butterfly rash. This erythematous eruption may range from a blush with swelling to a scaly, sharply demarcated, macular rash with plaques that may spread to the forehead, chin, ears, chest, and other sun-exposed parts of the body.

In *discoid lupus erythematosus,* telangiectasia, hyperpigmentation, ear and nose deformity, and mouth, tongue, and eyelid lesions may occur.

In *systemic lupus erythematosus,* acute onset of erythema may also be

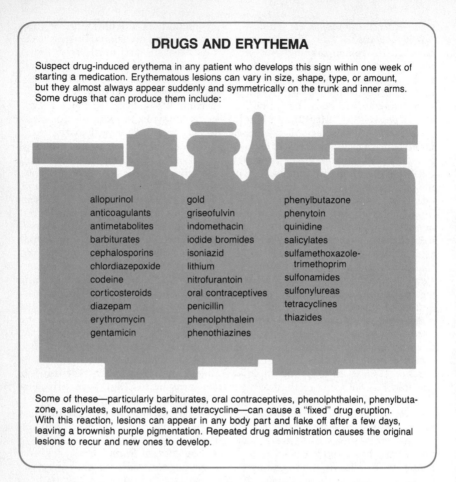

DRUGS AND ERYTHEMA

Suspect drug-induced erythema in any patient who develops this sign within one week of starting a medication. Erythematous lesions can vary in size, shape, type, or amount, but they almost always appear suddenly and symmetrically on the trunk and inner arms. Some drugs that can produce them include:

allopurinol	gold	phenylbutazone
anticoagulants	griseofulvin	phenytoin
antimetabolites	indomethacin	quinidine
barbiturates	iodide bromides	salicylates
cephalosporins	isoniazid	sulfamethoxazole-
chlordiazepoxide	lithium	trimethoprim
codeine	nitrofurantoin	sulfonamides
corticosteroids	oral contraceptives	sulfonylureas
diazepam	penicillin	tetracyclines
erythromycin	phenolphthalein	thiazides
gentamicin	phenothiazines	

Some of these—particularly barbiturates, oral contraceptives, phenolphthalein, phenylbutazone, salicylates, sulfonamides, and tetracycline—can cause a "fixed" drug eruption. With this reaction, lesions can appear in any body part and flake off after a few days, leaving a brownish purple pigmentation. Repeated drug administration causes the original lesions to recur and new ones to develop.

accompanied by photosensitivity and mucous membrane ulcers, especially in the nose and mouth. Mottled erythema may occur on the hands, with edema around the nails and macular reddish purple lesions on the fingers. Telangiectasia occurs at the base of the nails or eyelids, along with purpura, petechiae, ecchymoses, and urticaria. Joint pain and stiffness are common. Other findings depend on the body systems affected but typically include low-grade fever, malaise, weakness, headache, depression, lymphadenopathy, fatigue, weight loss, anorexia, nausea, vomiting, diarrhea, and constipation.

• *Polymorphous light eruption (PLE).* PLE produces erythema, vesicles, plaques, and multiple small papules on sun-exposed areas, which may later eczematize, lichenify, and excoriate. Pruritus may also occur.

• *Psoriasis.* Silvery white scales over a thickened erythematous base usually affect the elbows, knees, chest, scalp, and intergluteal folds. The fingernails may become thick and pitted.

• *Raynaud's disease.* Typically, the skin on hands and feet blanches and cools after exposure to cold or stress. Later, it becomes warm and purplish red.

• *Rheumatoid arthritis.* In a flare-up of this disorder, erythema over the affected joints occurs with heat, swelling, pain, and stiffness. Earlier symptoms include malaise, fatigue, myalgias, prolonged morning stiffness, and clumsiness. As the disease progresses, muscle atrophy, palmar erythema, generalized edema, mottled skin, and structural deformities occur.

• *Rosacea.* Scattered erythema across the center of the face characterizes this disorder initially, followed by superficial telangiectases, papules, pustules, and nodules. Rhinophyma may occur on the lower half of the nose.

• *Rubella.* Typically, flat solitary lesions join to form a blotchy pink erythematous rash that spreads rapidly to the trunk and extremities in this disorder. Occasionally, small red lesions (Forschheimer's spots) occur on the soft palate. Lesions clear in 4 to 5 days. The rash usually follows fever (up to 102° F., 39° C.), headache, malaise, sore throat, a gritty eye sensation, lymphadenopathy, and coryza.

• *Thrombophlebitis.* Although this disorder is sometimes asymptomatic, it can produce erythema over the inflamed vein. Fever, chills, and malaise may accompany severe localized pain, warmth, and induration; distal edema; and a positive Homans' sign.

• *Toxic shock syndrome.* This disorder, which usually affects young women, causes sudden, diffuse erythema in the form of a macular rash. It's accompanied by a sudden high fever, myalgia, vomiting, severe diarrhea, and sudden hypotension that may lead to shock. Desquamation occurs after 1 to 2 weeks, especially on palms and soles.

Other causes

• *Drugs.* Many drugs commonly cause erythema. (See *Drugs and Erythema.*)
• *Radiation and other treatments.* Radiation therapy may produce dull erythema and edema within 24 hours. As the erythema fades, the skin becomes light brown and mildly scaly. In addition, any treatment that causes an allergic reaction, such as a blood transfusion, can cause erythema.

Special considerations

Because erythema can cause fluid loss, closely monitor and replace fluids and electrolytes, especially in patients with burns or widespread erythema. Withhold all medications until the cause of the erythema has been identified. Then expect to administer antibiotics and topical or systemic corticosteroids. For the patient with itching skin, expect to give soothing baths or apply open wet dressings containing starch, bran, or sodium bicarbonate. Administer antihistamines and analgesics as ordered. Advise a patient with leg erythema to keep his legs elevated above heart level. For a burn patient with erythema, immerse the affected area in cold water or apply towels soaked in cold water to reduce pain, edema, and erythema.

As ordered, prepare the patient for diagnostic tests, such as skin biopsy to detect cancerous lesions, cultures to identify infectious organisms, and sensitivity studies to confirm allergies.

Pediatric pointers

Normally, newborn rash (erythema neonatorum toxicum)—a pink papular rash—develops in the first 4 days after birth and spontaneously disappears by the 10th day. Newborns and infants can also develop erythema from infections and other disorders. For instance, candidiasis can produce thick white lesions over an erythematous base on the oral mucosa, as well as diaper rash with beefy red erythema.

Roseola, rubeola, scarlet fever, granuloma annulare, and cutis marmorata also cause erythema in pediatric patients.

Exophthalmos

[Proptosis]

Exophthalmos—the abnormal protrusion of one or both eyeballs—may result from hemorrhage, edema, or inflammation behind the eye; extraocular muscle relaxation; or space-occupying

ASSESSMENT TIP

DETECTING UNILATERAL EXOPHTHALMOS

If one of the patient's eyes seems more prominent than the other, assess them from above the patient's head. Look down across his face, gently draw his lids up, and compare the relationship of the corneas to the lower lids. Abnormal protrusion of one eye suggests unilateral exophthalmos. *Remember:* If you suspect eye trauma, don't do this test.

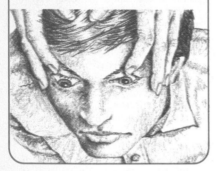

intraorbital lesions. This sign may occur suddenly or gradually, causing mild-to-dramatic protrusion. Occasionally, the affected eye also pulsates.

Usually, exophthalmos is easily observed. However, lid retraction may mimic exophthalmos even though protrusion is absent. Similarly, ptosis in one eye may make the other eye appear exophthalmic by comparison. Fortunately, an exophthalmometer can differentiate these signs by measuring ocular protrusion.

Assessment

Begin your assessment by asking when the patient first noticed exophthalmos. Is it associated with pain in or around the eye? If so, ask him how severe it is and how long he's had it. Then ask about recent sinus infection or vision problems. Take the patient's vital signs, noting fever, which may accompany eye infection. Next, evaluate the severity of exophthalmos with an exophthalmometer. If the eyes bulge severely, look for

cloudiness on the cornea, which may indicate ulcer formation. Describe any eye discharge and observe for ptosis. Then check visual acuity, with and without correction, and evaluate extraocular movements.

Medical causes

• *Cavernous sinus thrombosis.* Usually, this disorder causes sudden onset of pulsating, unilateral exophthalmos. Accompanying it may be eyelid edema, decreased or absent pupillary reflexes, and impaired extraocular movement and visual acuity. Other features may include high fever with chills, papilledema, headache, nausea, vomiting, somnolence, and, rarely, seizures.

• *Dacryoadenitis.* Unilateral, slowly progressive exophthalmos is the most common sign of dacryoadenitis. Assessment may also reveal limited extraocular movements (especially on elevation and abduction), ptosis, eyelid edema and erythema, conjunctival injection, eye pain, and diplopia.

• *Foreign body in the eye.* Although rare, exophthalmos may accompany other signs and symptoms of ocular trauma, such as eye pain, redness, and tearing.

• *Hemangioma.* Most common in young adults, this orbital tumor produces progressive exophthalmos, which may be mild or severe, unilateral or bilateral. Other signs and symptoms may include ptosis, limited extraocular movements, and blurred vision.

• *Hodgkin's disease.* In this disorder, unilateral exophthalmos may develop gradually, along with eyelid edema, diplopia, and a palpable eyelid mass. More characteristic findings are painless swelling of one or more lymph nodes, intermittent fever, weight loss, fatigue, malaise, night sweats, hepatosplenomegaly, and pruritus.

• *Lacrimal gland tumor.* Exophthalmos usually develops slowly in one eye, causing its downward displacement toward the nose. The patient may also have ptosis and eye deviation and pain.

• *Leiomyosarcoma.* Most common in people over age 45, this tumor is characterized by slowly developing, unilateral exophthalmos. Other effects include diplopia, impaired vision, and intermittent eye pain.

• *Leukemia.* When leukemia causes intraorbital hemorrhage, mild-to-moderate bilateral exophthalmos and lacrimal gland enlargement also result. Associated signs and symptoms include bleeding tendency, fever, joint pain, pallor, weakness, hepatosplenomegaly, and, possibly, lymphadenopathy.

• *Lymphangioma.* Hemorrhage of this congenital tumor causes unilateral or bilateral exophthalmos, among other signs.

• *Ocular tuberculosis.* Occasionally, this rare disease causes progressive exophthalmos. It's accompanied by ptosis, painless eyelid edema and erythema, and enlarged lacrimal glands. Examination may reveal yellow or white fat deposits on the cornea and small white nodules in the iris.

• *Optic nerve meningioma.* Usually, this tumor produces unilateral exophthalmos and a swollen temple. Impaired visual acuity, visual field deficits, and headache may occur.

• *Orbital cellulitis.* Often the result of sinusitis, this ocular emergency causes sudden onset of unilateral exophthalmos, which may be mild or severe. It may also produce fever, eye pain, headache, malaise, conjunctival injection, tearing, eyelid edema and erythema, purulent discharge, and impaired extraocular movements.

• *Orbital choristoma.* A common sign of this benign tumor, progressive exophthalmos may be associated with diplopia and blurred vision.

• *Orbital emphysema.* Air leaking from the sinus into the orbit usually causes unilateral exophthalmos. Palpation of the globe elicits crepitation.

• *Orbital pseudotumor.* Progressive unilateral exophthalmos characterizes this uncommon disorder. Limited extraocular movements, eyelid edema, eye pain, and diplopia may also occur.

• *Parasite infestation.* Usually, this disorder causes painless, progressive exophthalmos in one eye that may spread to the other eye. Associated signs and symptoms include limited extraocular movements, diplopia, eye pain, and impaired visual acuity.

• *Scleritis (posterior).* Gradual onset of mild-to-severe unilateral exophthalmos is common with scleritis. Other findings: severe eye pain, diplopia, papilledema, limited extraocular movements, and impaired visual acuity.

• *Thyrotoxicosis.* Although a classic sign of this disorder, exophthalmos is absent in many patients. It's usually bilateral, progressive, and severe. Associated ocular features include ptosis, increased tearing, lid lag and edema, photophobia, conjunctival injection, diplopia, and decreased visual acuity.

Elsewhere in the body, characteristic signs and symptoms include an enlarged thyroid, nervousness, heat intolerance, weight loss despite increased appetite, sweating, diarrhea, tremors, palpitations, and tachycardia.

Special considerations
Because exophthalmos usually makes the patient self-conscious, provide privacy and emotional support. Protect the exophthalmic eye from infection and other trauma, especially drying of the cornea. However, *never* place a gauze eye pad or other object over this eye; damage to the corneal epithelium may result when the pad's removed.

If a slit lamp examination is ordered, explain the procedure to the patient. If necessary, refer him to an ophthalmologist for a complete examination.

Pediatric pointers
In children around age 5, a rare tumor—optic nerve glioma—may cause exophthalmos. Rhabdomyosarcoma, a more common tumor, usually affects children between ages 4 and 12 and produces rapid onset of exophthalmos. In Hand-Schüller-Christian syndrome, exophthalmos typically accompanies signs of diabetes insipidus and bone destruction.

Eye Discharge

Usually associated with conjunctivitis, eye discharge refers to the excretion of any substance other than tears. This common sign may occur in one or both eyes, producing scant-to-copious discharge. The discharge may be purulent, frothy, mucoid, cheesy, or ropey. Sometimes, discharge can be expressed by applying pressure to the tear sac, punctum, meibomian glands, or canaliculus.

Eye discharge commonly results from inflammatory and infectious eye disorders but may also result from certain systemic disorders. Because this sign may accompany a disorder that threatens vision, it must be assessed and treated immediately.

Assessment

Begin your assessment by finding out when the discharge began. Does it occur at certain times of day or in connection with certain activities? If the patient complains of pain, ask him to show you its exact location and describe its character. Is it dull, continuous, sharp, or stabbing? Ask the patient if his eyes itch or burn. Do they tear excessively? Are they sensitive to light? Does he feel like something is in them?

After taking vital signs, carefully inspect the eye discharge. Note its amount and consistency. Then test visual acuity, with and without correction. Examine external eye structures, beginning with the unaffected eye to prevent cross-contamination. Observe for eyelid edema, entropion, crusts, lesions, or trichiasis. Next, ask the patient to blink as you watch for impaired lid movement. If the eyes seem to bulge, measure them with an exophthalmometer. Test the six cardinal fields of gaze. Examine for conjunctival injection and follicles, and for corneal cloudiness or white lesions.

Medical causes

● *Canaliculitis.* This uncommon, chronic disorder causes scant purulent discharge, usually from one eye's lower canaliculus. The eye is red and irritated, and its punctum bulges a bit.

● *Conjunctivitis.* Four types of conjunctivitis may cause eye discharge with redness and hyperemia.

In *allergic conjunctivitis,* bilateral ropey discharge is accompanied by itching and tearing.

Bacterial conjunctivitis causes moderate purulent discharge that may form sticky crusts on the eyelids during sleep. Itching, burning, excessive tearing, and the sensation of a foreign body in the eye may also occur. Eye pain indicates corneal involvement.

Fungal conjunctivitis produces copious, thick, purulent discharge that makes eyelids crusty and sticky. Also characteristic are eyelid edema, itching, burning, and tearing. Pain and photophobia occur only with corneal involvement.

Inclusion conjunctivitis causes scant mucoid discharge—especially in the morning—in both eyes, accompanied by pseudoptosis and conjunctival follicles.

● *Corneal ulcers.* Both bacterial and fungal ulcers produce copious, purulent, unilateral eye discharge. Related findings are crusty, sticky eyelids, and, possibly, severe pain, photophobia, and impaired visual acuity.

A *bacterial corneal ulcer* is also characterized by an irregular gray-white area on the cornea, blurred vision, unilateral pupil constriction, and conjunctival injection.

A *fungal corneal ulcer* is also characterized by conjunctival injection and eyelid edema and erythema. A painless, dense, whitish gray central ulcer develops slowly and may be surrounded by progressively clearer rings.

● *Dacryoadenitis.* This disorder may cause moderate purulent discharge associated with temporal eye pain, conjunctival injection, and severe eyelid edema and erythema. However, its

SOURCES OF EYE DISCHARGE

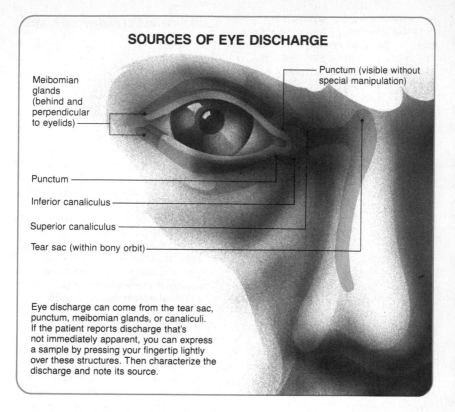

Meibomian glands (behind and perpendicular to eyelids) —

Punctum (visible without special manipulation)

Punctum —

Inferior canaliculus —

Superior canaliculus —

Tear sac (within bony orbit) —

Eye discharge can come from the tear sac, punctum, meibomian glands, or canaliculi. If the patient reports discharge that's not immediately apparent, you can express a sample by pressing your fingertip lightly over these structures. Then characterize the discharge and note its source.

most characteristic sign is unilateral exophthalmos.

• *Dacryocystitis.* Lacrimal sac infection may produce scant but continuous purulent discharge that's easily expressed from the tear sac. Additional signs and symptoms include excessive tearing, pain, and tenderness near the tear sac. Eyelid inflammation and edema are most noticeable around the lacrimal punctum.

• *Erythema multiforme major (Stevens-Johnson syndrome).* A purulent discharge characterizes this disorder. Other ocular effects may include severe eye pain, entropion, trichiasis, photophobia, and decreased tear formation. Also typical are erythematous, urticarial, bullous lesions that suddenly erupt over the skin.

• *Herpes zoster ophthalmicus.* This disorder yields moderate-to-copious serous eye discharge accompanied by excessive tearing. Examination reveals eyelid edema and erythema, conjunctival injection, and a white, cloudy cornea. The patient also complains of eye pain and severe unilateral facial pain that occurs several days before vesicles erupt.

• *Keratoconjunctivitis sicca.* Better known as dry eye syndrome, this disorder typically causes excessive, continuous mucoid discharge and insufficient tearing. Accompanying signs and symptoms may include eye pain, itching, burning, a foreign-body sensation, and dramatic conjunctival injection. The patient may also have difficulty closing his eyes.

• *Meibomianitis.* This disorder may produce continuous frothy eye discharge. The application of pressure on the meibomian glands yields a soft, foul-smelling, cheesy yellow discharge. The eyes also appear chronically red, with inflamed lid margins.

• *Orbital cellulitis.* Although exophthalmos is the most obvious sign of this disorder, unilateral purulent eye discharge may also be present. Related findings: eyelid edema, conjunctival injection, headache, orbital pain, impaired visual acuity, limited extraocular movement, and fever.

• *Pemphigus.* This rare disorder may cause thick, mucuslike discharge. Initially, it may cause unilateral or bilateral conjunctivitis that's unrelieved by treatment, followed by entropion and, occasionally, corneal ulceration. Other symptoms include eye pain, burning, irritation, and blurred vision.

• *Psoriasis vulgaris.* Usually, psoriasis vulgaris causes substantial mucus discharge in both eyes, accompanied by redness. The characteristic lesions it produces on the eyelids may extend into the conjunctiva, causing irritation, excessive tearing, and a foreign-body sensation.

• *Trachoma.* A bilateral eye discharge occurs in this disorder, with severe pain, excessive tearing, photophobia, eyelid edema, redness, and visible conjunctival follicles.

Special considerations

Apply warm soaks to soften crusts on eyelids and lashes. Then gently wipe the eyes with a soft gauze pad. Carefully dispose of all used dressings, tissues, and cotton swabs to prevent possible spread of infection. Teach the patient how to avoid contaminating the unaffected eye. Also be sure to sterilize ophthalmic equipment after use.

Explain the diagnostic tests that may be ordered, including culture and sensitivity studies to identify infectious organisms.

Pediatric pointers

In infants, prophylactic eye medication (silver nitrate) frequently causes eye irritation and discharge. However, in children, discharge most often results from eye trauma and eye or upper respiratory infection.

Eye Pain
[Ophthalmalgia]

Eye pain may be described as a burning, throbbing, aching, or stabbing sensation in or around the eye. It may also be characterized as a foreign-body sensation. This sign varies from mild to severe; its duration and exact location provide clues to the causative disorder.

Most commonly, eye pain results from corneal abrasion. It may also result from glaucoma and other eye disorders, trauma, and neurologic and systemic disorders. Any of these may stimulate nerve endings in the cornea or external eye, producing pain.

Assessment

If the patient's eye pain results from a chemical burn, have another nurse notify the doctor immediately. Remove contact lenses, if present, and irrigate the eye with at least 1 liter of normal saline solution over 10 minutes. Evert the lids and wipe the fornices with a cotton-tipped applicator to remove any particles or chemicals.

If the patient's eye pain *doesn't* result from a chemical burn, take a complete history. Have the patient describe the eye pain fully. Is it an ache or a sharp pain? How long does it last? Is it accompanied by burning or itching? Find out when it began. Is it worse in the morning or late in the evening? Ask about recent trauma or surgery, especially if the patient complains of sudden, severe pain. Does he have headaches? If so, find out how often and at what time of day they occur.

During the physical examination, *don't* manipulate the eye if you suspect trauma. Carefully assess the lids and conjunctiva for redness, inflammation, and swelling. Then examine the eyes for ptosis or exophthalmos. Finally, test

EXAMINING THE EXTERNAL EYE

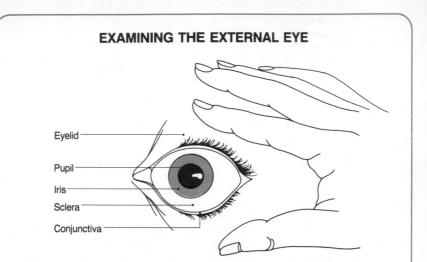

Eyelid
Pupil
Iris
Sclera
Conjunctiva

For the patient with eye pain or other ocular symptoms, examination of the external eye forms an important part of the ocular assessment. Here's how to examine the external eye.

First, inspect the eyelids for ptosis and incomplete closure of the lids. Also observe the lids for edema, erythema, cyanosis, hematoma, and masses. Are the lids everted or inverted? Do the eyelashes turn inward? Have some of them been lost? Do the lashes adhere to one another or contain discharge? Next, examine the lid margins, noting especially any debris, scaling, lesions, or unusual secretions. Also watch for eyelid spasms.

Now gently retract the eyelid with your thumb and forefinger, and assess the conjunctiva for redness, cloudiness, follicles, and blisters or other lesions. Check for chemosis by pressing the lower lid against the eyeball and noting any bulging above this compression point. Observe the sclera, noting any changes from its normal white color.

Next, shine a light across the cornea to detect scars, abrasions, or ulcers. Note any color changes, dots, or opaque or cloudy areas. Also assess the anterior eye chamber, which should be clean, deep, shadow-free, and filled with clear aqueous humor.

Inspect the color, shape, texture, and pattern of the iris. Then assess the pupils' size, shape, and equality. Finally, evaluate their response to light. Are they sluggish, fixed, or unresponsive? Does pupil dilation or constriction occur only on one side?

---

visual acuity with and without correction, and assess extraocular movements. Characterize any discharge.

Medical causes

• *Acute closed-angle glaucoma.* Blurred vision and sudden, excruciating pain in and around the eye characterize this disorder; the pain may be so severe that it causes nausea and vomiting. Other findings are halo vision, a fixed, nonreactive, moderately dilated pupil, and rapidly decreasing visual acuity.

• *Astigmatism.* Uncorrected astigmatism frequently causes headache and eye fatigue, aching, and redness.

• *Blepharitis.* Burning pain in both eyelids is accompanied by itching, sticky discharge, and conjunctival injection. Related findings include foreign-body sensation, lid ulcerations, and loss of eyelashes.

• *Burns.* In *chemical burns,* sudden and severe eye pain may occur with erythema and blistering of the face and lids, photophobia, miosis, conjunctival injection, blurring, and inability to keep the eyelids open. In *ultraviolet radiation burns,* moderate-to-severe pain occurs about 12 hours after exposure along with photophobia and vision changes.

• *Chalazion.* A chalazion causes localized tenderness and swelling on the upper or lower eyelid. Eversion of the lid reveals conjunctival injection and a small red lump.

• *Conjunctivitis.* Some degree of eye pain and excessive tearing occurs with four types of conjunctivitis. *Allergic conjunctivitis* causes mild, burning, bilateral pain accompanied by itching, conjunctival injection, and a characteristic ropey discharge. *Bacterial conjunctivitis* causes pain only when it affects the cornea. Otherwise, it produces burning and a foreign-body sensation. A purulent discharge and conjunctival injection are also typical. If it affects the cornea, *fungal conjunctivitis* may cause pain and photophobia. Even without corneal involvement, it produces itching, burning eyes; a thick, purulent discharge; and conjunctival injection. *Viral conjunctivitis* produces itching, red eyes accompanied by a foreign-body sensation, visible conjunctival follicles, and eyelid edema.

• *Corneal abrasions.* In this type of injury, eye pain is characterized by a foreign-body sensation. Excessive tearing, photophobia, and conjunctival injection are also common.

• *Corneal erosion (recurrent).* Severe pain occurs on waking and continues throughout the day. Accompanying the pain are conjunctival injection and photophobia.

• *Corneal ulcers.* Both bacterial and fungal corneal ulcers cause severe eye pain. They may also cause a purulent eye discharge, sticky eyelids, photophobia, and impaired visual acuity. In addition, a *bacterial corneal ulcer* produces a grayish white, irregularly shaped ulcer on the cornea, unilateral pupil constriction, and conjunctival injection. A *fungal corneal ulcer* produces conjunctival injection, eyelid edema and erythema, and a dense, cloudy, central ulcer surrounded by progressively clearer rings.

• *Dacryoadenitis.* Temporal pain may affect both eyes in this disorder. Associated features include exophthalmos, conjunctival injection, severe eyelid erythema and edema, and a purulent eye discharge.

• *Dacryocystitis.* Pain and tenderness near the tear sac characterize acute dacryocystitis. Additional signs include excessive tearing, a purulent discharge, eyelid erythema, and swelling in the lacrimal punctum area.

• *Episcleritis.* Deep eye pain occurs as tissues over sclera become inflamed. Related effects: photophobia, excessive tearing, conjunctival edema, and a red or purplish sclera.

• *Erythema multiforme major.* This disorder commonly produces severe eye pain, entropion, trichiasis, purulent conjunctivitis, photophobia, and decreased tear formation.

• *Foreign bodies in the cornea and conjunctiva.* Sudden severe pain is common but vision usually remains intact. Other findings: excessive tearing, photophobia, miosis, a foreign body sensation, a dark speck on the cornea, and dramatic conjunctival injection.

• *Herpes zoster ophthalmicus.* Eye pain occurs with severe unilateral facial pain, usually several days before vesicles erupt. Other signs include red, swollen eyelids, excessive tearing, a serous eye discharge, conjunctival injection, and a white, cloudy cornea.

• *Hordeolum (stye).* Generally, this lesion produces localized eye pain that increases as the stye grows. Eyelid erythema and edema are also common.

• *Hyphema.* Occurring after eye injury or surgery, hyphema accompanies sudden pain in and around the eye. Orbital and lid edema, conjunctival injection, and visual impairment may occur.

• *Interstitial keratitis.* Associated with congenital syphilis, this corneal inflammation produces eye pain with photophobia, blurred vision, prominent conjunctival injection, and grayish pink corneas.

• *Iritis (acute).* Moderate-to-severe eye pain occurs with severe photophobia, dramatic conjunctival injection, and blurred vision. The constricted pupil may respond poorly to light.

• *Keratoconjunctivitis sicca.* This condition—known as dry eye syndrome—causes chronic burning pain in both eyes, itching, a foreign-body sensation, photophobia, dramatic conjunctival injection, and difficulty moving the eyelids. Excessive mucoid discharge and inadequate tearing are typical.

• *Lacrimal gland tumor.* This neoplastic lesion usually produces unilateral eye pain, impaired visual acuity, and some degree of exophthalmos.

• *Migraine headache.* Here, pain may be so severe that the eyes also ache. Nausea, vomiting, blurred vision, and light and noise sensitivity may occur.

• *Ocular laceration and intraocular foreign bodies.* Penetrating eye injuries usually cause mild-to-severe unilateral eye pain and impaired visual acuity. Eyelid edema, conjunctival injection, and an abnormal pupillary response may also occur.

• *Optic neuritis.* Here, pain in and around the eye occurs with eye movement. Severe visual loss and tunnel vision develop but improve in 2 to 3 weeks. Pupils respond sluggishly to direct light but normally to consensual light.

• *Orbital cellulitis.* This disorder causes dull, aching pain in the affected eye, some degree of exophthalmos, eyelid edema and erythema, purulent discharge, impaired extraocular movement, and, occasionally, decreased visual acuity and fever.

• *Orbital floor fracture.* Sometimes called a blow-out fracture, this injury causes eye pain, dramatic eyelid edema, and, possibly, enophthalmos and diplopia.

• *Orbital pseudotumor.* This disorder causes deep, boring eye pain and diplopia in about 50% of all patients. However, prominent exophthalmos and lateral ocular deviation are more characteristic. Eyelid edema and restricted extraocular movement may also occur.

• *Pemphigus.* In this disorder, bilateral eye pain and irritation may be accompanied by blurred vision and a thick discharge. Blisters may develop on the conjunctiva alone or may extend to the nasal, oral, and vulvar mucous membranes as well as the skin.

• *Scleritis.* This inflammation produces severe eye pain and tenderness, along with conjunctival injection, bluish purple sclera, and, possibly, photophobia and excessive tearing.

• *Sclerokeratitis.* Inflammation of the sclera and cornea causes pain, burning, irritation, and photophobia.

• *Subdural hematoma.* Following head trauma, a subdural hematoma commonly causes severe eyeache and headache. Related neurologic signs depend on the hematoma's location and size.

• *Trachoma.* Along with pain in the affected eye, trachoma causes excessive tearing, photophobia, eye discharge, eyelid edema and redness, and visible conjunctival follicles.

• *Uveitis. Anterior uveitis* causes sudden onset of severe pain, dramatic conjunctival injection, photophobia, and a small, nonreactive pupil. *Posterior uveitis* causes insidious onset of similar features, plus gradual blurring of vision and distorted pupil shape. *Lens-induced uveitis* causes moderate eye pain, conjunctival injection, pupil constriction, and severely impaired visual acuity. In fact, the patient usually has light perception alone.

Other causes

• *Treatments.* Contact lenses may cause eye pain and a foreign-body sensation. Ocular surgery may also produce eye pain, ranging from a mild ache to a severe pounding or stabbing sensation.

Special considerations

To help ease eye pain, have the patient lie down in a darkened, quiet environment and close his eyes. As ordered, prepare him for diagnostic studies, including tonometry and orbital X-rays.

Pediatric pointers

Trauma and infection are the most common causes of eye pain in children. Be alert for nonverbal clues to pain, such as tightly shutting or frequently rubbing the eyes.

facial pain • fasciculations • fatigue • fecal incontinence • fetor hepaticus • fev
flatulence • fontanelle bulging • fontanelle depression • footdrop • gag reflex a
bizarre • gait—propulsive • gait—scissors • gait—spastic • gait—steppage • g
gallop—atrial • gallop—ventricular • genital lesions in the male • grunting re
bleeding • gum swelling • gynecomastia • halitosis • halo vision • headache •
intolerance • Heberden's nodes • hematemesis • hematochezia • hematuria • l
hemoptysis • hepatomegaly • hiccups • hirsutism • hoarseness • Homans' sig
hyperpnea • hypopigmentation • impotence • insomnia • intermittent claudica
jaundice • jaw pain • jugular vein distention • Kehr's sign • Kernig's sign • le
consciousness—decreased • lid lag • light flashes • low birth weight • lympha
facies • McBurney's sign • McMurray's sign • melena • menorrhagia • metror
face • mouth lesions • murmurs • muscle atrophy • muscle flaccidity • muscl
spasticity • muscle weakness • mydriasis • myoclonus • nasal flaring • nause
blindness • nipple discharge • nipple retraction • nocturia • nuchal rigidity •
deviation • oligomenorrhea • oliguria • opisthotonos • orofacial dyskinesia •
hypotension • Ortolani's sign • Osler's nodes • otorrhea • pallor • palpitation
paralysis • paresthesias • paroxysmal nocturnal dyspnea • peau d'orange • p
peristaltic waves—visible • photophobia • pica • pleural friction rub • polydi
polyuria • postnasal drip • priapism • pruritus • psoas sign • psychotic beha
absent or weak • pulse—bounding • pulse pressure—narrowed • pulse press
rhythm abnormality • pulsus alternans • pulsus bisferiens • pulsus paradoxu
pupils—sluggish • purple striae • purpura • pustular rash • pyrosis • raccoo
tenderness • rectal pain • retractions—costal and sternal • rhinorrhea • rhon
salivation—decreased • salivation—increased • salt craving • scotoma • scro
absence • seizure—focal • seizure—generalized tonic-clonic • seizure—psycl
sign • shallow respirations • skin—bronze • skin—clammy • skin—mottled
turgor—decreased • spider angioma • splenomegaly • stertorous respirations
stridor • syncope • tachycardia • tachypnea • taste abnormalities • tearing—
tic • tinnitus • tracheal deviation • tracheal tugging • tremors • trismus • tu
frost • urethral discharge • urinary frequency • urinary hesitancy • urinary
urgency • urine cloudiness • urticaria • vaginal bleeding—postmenopausal •
venous hum • vertigo • vesicular rash • violent behavior • vision loss • visua
floaters • vomiting • vulvar lesions • weight gain—excessive • weight loss—
wristdrop• abdominal distention • abdominal mass • abdominal pain • abd
accessory muscle use • agitation • alopecia • amenorrhea • amnesia • analg
anorexia • anosmia • anuria • anxiety • aphasia • apnea • apneustic respira
pain • asterixis • ataxia • athetosis • aura • Babinski's reflex • back pain • l
sign • Biot's respirations • bladder distention • blood pressure decrease • bl
bowel sounds—absent • bowel sounds—hyperactive • bowel sounds—hypoa
bradypnea • breast dimpling • breast nodule • breast pain • breast ulcer • l
odor • breath with fecal odor • breath with fruity odor • Brudzinski's sign •
butterfly rash • café-au-lait spots • capillary refill time—prolonged • carpop
chest expansion—asymmetrical • chest pain • Cheyne-Stokes respirations • c
sign • clubbing • cogwheel rigidity • cold intolerance • confusion • conjunc
constipation • corneal reflex—absent • costovertebral angle tenderness • cou
nonproductive • cough—productive • crackles • crepitation—bony • crepita
cry—high-pitched • cyanosis • decerebrate posture • decorticate posture • c
hyperactive • deep tendon reflexes—hypoactive • depression • diaphoresis •
dizziness • doll's eye sign—absent • drooling • dysarthria • dysmenorrhea •
dyspepsia • dysphagia • dyspnea • dystonia • dysuria • earache • edema—

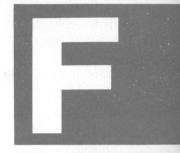

Facial Pain

This symptom may result from various neurologic, vascular, or infectious disorders. It can also be referred to the face in disorders of the ear, nose, paranasal sinuses, teeth, neck, and jaw. Its most common cause is trigeminal neuralgia, or tic douloureux.

Typically paroxysmal and intense, facial pain may occur along the pathway of a specific facial nerve or nerve branch, usually cranial nerve V (trigeminal nerve) or cranial nerve VII (facial nerve). Differentiating facial pain from the more diffuse pain of headache is sometimes difficult, since many patients refer to all head and facial pain as headache.

Assessment

Begin by characterizing the patient's facial pain. Is it stabbing, throbbing, or dull? When did it begin? How long has it lasted? What relieves it? Worsens it? Ask the patient to point to the painful area. If his facial pain is recurrent, have him describe a typical episode. Review his medical and dental history, noting especially previous head trauma, dental disease, and infection.

Carefully examine the patient's face and head. Inspect the ear for vesicles and changes in the tympanic membrane to rule out referred ear pain. Inspect the nose for deformity or asymmetry. Assess the condition of the mucous membranes and septum, and the size and shape of the turbinates. Characterize any secretions. Palpate the frontal and maxillary sinuses for tenderness and swelling.

Evaluate oral hygiene by inspecting the teeth for caries, percussing any diseased teeth for pain, and asking the patient about any sensitivity to hot, cold, or sweet liquids or foods. Have him open and close his mouth as you palpate the temporomandibular joint for tenderness, spasm, or crepitus.

Assess function in cranial nerves V and VII. To assess cranial nerve V, instruct the patient to clench his teeth. Then palpate the temporal and masseter muscles and evaluate muscle contraction. Test pain and touch sensation on his forehead, cheeks, and jaw. Next test the corneal reflex by lightly touching the cornea with a piece of cotton.

To assess cranial nerve VII, inspect the face for symmetry and then have the patient perform facial movements—raise his eyebrows, frown, show his teeth, and puff his cheeks—to demonstrate facial muscle strength.

Medical causes

• *Dental caries.* Caries in the mandibular molars can produce ear, preauricular, and temporal pain. In contrast,

MAJOR NERVE PATHWAYS OF THE FACE

Cranial nerve V

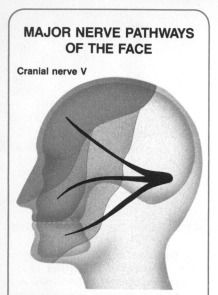

Cranial nerve V has three branches. The *ophthalmic branch* supplies sensation to the anterior scalp, forehead, upper nose, and cornea. The *maxillary branch* supplies sensation to the midportion of the face, lower nose, upper lip, and mucous membrane of the anterior palate. The *mandibular branch* supplies the lower face, lower jaw, mucous membrane of the cheek, and base of the tongue.

Cranial nerve VII

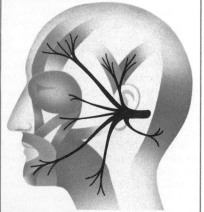

Cranial nerve VII innervates the facial muscles. Its motor branch controls the muscles of the forehead, eye orbit, and mouth.

caries in the maxillary teeth can produce orbital, retroorbital, and parietal pain.

● *Herpes zoster oticus.* Severe pain localizes around the ear, followed by the appearance of vesicles in the ear and on the oral mucosa, tonsils, and posterior tongue. Eye pain may occur with corneal and scleral damage and possibly impaired vision. The patient may also have ageusia, decreased salivation, ipsilateral facial palsy, hearing loss, vertigo, nausea, and vomiting.

● *Multiple sclerosis.* Facial pain may resemble that of trigeminal neuralgia accompanied by jaw and facial weakness. Other common findings include visual blurring, diplopia, and nystagmus; sensory impairment, such as paresthesia; generalized muscle weakness and gait abnormalities; urinary disturbances; and emotional lability.

● *Postherpetic neuralgia.* Burning, itching, prickly pain persists along any of the three trigeminal nerve divisions and worsens with contact or movement. Mild hypoesthesia or paresthesia and vesicles (with possible scarring) affect the area before the onset of pain.

● *Sinus carcinoma.* In *ethmoid sinus carcinoma,* facial pain is a late symptom, preceded by exophthalmos. In rare *frontal sinus carcinoma,* late-stage forehead pain may be accompanied by local erythema, unilateral epistaxis or purulent discharge, exophthalmos, and swelling and hypoesthesia in the cheek. In *maxillary sinus carcinoma,* persistent pain along the second division of cranial nerve V is a late symptom. Associated findings may include exophthalmos and loose maxillary teeth.

● *Sinusitis. Acute maxillary sinusitis* produces unilateral or bilateral pressure, fullness, or burning pain behind the eyes and over the cheek, nose, and upper teeth. Bending or stooping increases the pain. Other findings include nasal congestion and purulent discharge; red, swollen nasal mucosa and turbinates; facial and gingival swelling; trismus; fever; and malaise.

Frontal sinusitis commonly produces dull, aching pain above or around the eyes, which worsens with bending or stooping. It also causes nasal obstruction; red, swollen nasal mucosa; rhinorrhea; fever; and edema of the eyelids and face.

In *sphenoid sinusitis*, dull pain persists behind the eyes and nose. Related findings include swelling of the forehead and eye, blurred vision, diplopia, fever, and chills.

• *Sphenopalatine neuralgia.* Unilateral, deep, boring pain occurs below the ear and may radiate to the eye, ear, cheek, nose, palate, maxillary teeth, temple, back of the head, neck, or shoulder. Attacks bring increased tearing and salivation, rhinorrhea, a sensation of fullness in the ear, tinnitus, vertigo, taste disturbances, pruritus, and shoulder stiffness or weakness.

• *Temporal arteritis.* Unilateral pain occurs behind the eye or in the scalp, jaw, tongue, or neck. A typical episode consists of a severe throbbing or boring temporal headache with redness, swelling, and nodulation of the temporal artery. The patient may have low-grade fever, malaise, diaphoresis, and possibly ipsilateral vision loss.

• *Temporomandibular joint syndrome.* Intermittent pain, usually unilateral, is described as a severe, dull ache or intense spasm that radiates to the cheek, temple, lower jaw, ear, or mastoid area. Associated findings include trismus; malocclusion; and clicking, crepitus, and tenderness in the temporomandibular joint. Earache occurs without involvement of the tympanic membrane or external auditory canal.

• *Trigeminal neuralgia.* Paroxysms of intense pain, lasting up to 15 minutes, shoot along the superior maxillary or mandibular division of the trigeminal nerve. The pain can be triggered by touching the nose, cheek, or mouth; by hot or cold weather; by consuming hot or cold foods and beverages; or even by smiling or talking. Between attacks, the pain may diminish to a dull ache or may disappear.

• *Trotter's syndrome.* Unilateral mandibular pain follows hearing loss and precedes lower jaw anesthesia and trismus.

Special considerations
If ordered, prepare the patient for diagnostic tests, such as sinus, skull, or dental X-rays; sinus transillumination; and intracranial computed tomography. As ordered, give pain medications, and apply direct heat or administer a muscle relaxant to ease muscle spasms. Provide a humidifier, vaporizer, or decongestant to relieve nasal or sinus congestion. If appropriate, teach the patient to avoid stressful situations, hot or cold foods, or sudden jarring movements, which could trigger painful attacks.

Pediatric pointers
Facial pain may be difficult to assess in a young child if his language skills aren't developed sufficiently for him to describe the pain. Be alert for subtle signs of pain, such as facial rubbing, irritability, or poor eating habits.

Fasciculations

Fasciculations are minor local muscle contractions representing the spontaneous discharge of a muscle fiber bundle innervated by a single motor nerve filament. These contractions cause visible dimpling or wavelike twitching of the skin, but aren't strong enough to produce joint movement. They occur irregularly at frequencies ranging from once every several seconds to two or three times per second; infrequently, myokymia—continuous, rapid fasciculations that cause a rippling effect—may occur. Because fasciculations are brief and painless, they often go undetected or are ignored.

Benign, nonpathologic fasciculations are common and normal. They often occur in tense, anxious, or overtired persons and typically affect the eyelid, thumb, or calf. However, fasciculations may also indicate a severe neurologic disorder, most notably a diffuse motor neuron disorder that causes loss of control over muscle fiber discharge. They're also an early sign of pesticide poisoning.

Assessment

Begin your assessment by asking the patient about the nature, onset, and duration of his fasciculations. If onset is acute, ask about any precipitating events, such as exposure to pesticides. *Remember that pesticide poisoning, although uncommon, represents a medical emergency requiring prompt and vigorous intervention.* You may need to maintain airway patency, monitor vital signs, administer oxygen, and perform gastric lavage or induce vomiting.

If the patient isn't in severe distress, find out about any sensory changes, such as paresthesias, and any difficulty in speaking, swallowing, breathing, or controlling bowel or bladder function. Ask the patient if he's in pain.

Explore the patient's medical history for neurologic disorders, malignancies, and recent infections. Also explore the patient's life-style, asking especially about stress at home, on the job, or at school.

Perform a physical examination, looking for fasciculations while the affected muscle is at rest. Observe and test for motor and sensory abnormalities, particularly muscle atrophy and weakness, and decreased deep tendon reflexes. If you note these signs, suspect motor neuron disease, and perform a comprehensive neurologic exam.

Medical causes

• *Amyotrophic lateral sclerosis.* Coarse fasciculations usually begin in the small muscles of the hands and feet, then spread to the forearms and legs. Widespread, symmetrical muscle atrophy and weakness may result in dysarthria; difficulty chewing, swallowing, and breathing; and occasionally choking and drooling.

• *Bulbar palsy.* Fasciculations of the face and tongue commonly appear early. Progressive signs include dysarthria, dysphagia, hoarseness, and drooling. Eventually, weakness spreads to the respiratory muscles.

• *Guillain-Barré syndrome.* Fasciculations may occur, but the dominant neurologic sign is muscle weakness, which typically begins in the legs and spreads quickly to the arms and face. Other findings include paresthesias, incontinence, footdrop, tachycardia, dysphagia, and respiratory insufficiency.

• *Herniated disk.* Fasciculations of the muscles innervated by compressed nerve roots may be widespread and profound, but the overriding symptom is severe low back pain that may radiate unilaterally to the leg. Coughing, sneezing, bending, and straining exacerbate the pain. Related effects include muscle weakness, atrophy, and spasms; paresthesias; footdrop; steppage gait; and hypoactive deep tendon reflexes in the leg.

• *Pesticide poisoning.* Ingestion of organophosphate or carbamate pesticides commonly produces acute onset of long, wavelike fasciculations and muscle weakness that rapidly progresses to flaccid paralysis. Other common effects include nausea, vomiting, diarrhea, loss of bowel and bladder control, hyperactive bowel sounds, and abdominal cramping. Cardiopulmonary findings may include bradycardia, dyspnea or bradypnea, and pallor or cyanosis. Other possible signs and symptoms include seizures, visual disturbances (pupillary constriction or blurred vision), and increased secretions (tearing, salivation, pulmonary secretions, or diaphoresis).

• *Poliomyelitis (spinal paralytic).* Coarse fasciculations, usually transient but occasionally persistent, accompany progressive muscle weakness, spasms, and atrophy. The patient may have decreased reflexes, paresthesias, and coldness and cyanosis in the affected limbs. He may also display bladder paralysis, dyspnea, elevated blood pressure, and tachycardia.

• *Spinal cord tumors.* Fasciculations may develop, along with muscle atrophy and cramps, asymmetrically at first and then bilaterally as cord compression progresses. Motor and sensory changes distal to the tumor include weakness or paralysis, areflexia, paresthesias, and a tightening band of pain. Bowel and bladder control may also be lost.

• *Syringomyelia.* Fasciculations may occur along with Charcot's joints, deep aching pain, areflexia, and muscle atrophy. Additional findings may include thoracic scoliosis and loss of pain and temperature sensation over the neck, shoulders, and arms.

Special considerations

Prepare the patient for diagnostic studies, such as spinal X-rays, myelography, computed tomography, and electromyography with nerve conduction velocity tests.

For the patient with progressive neuromuscular degeneration, focus your care on helping him cope with activities of daily living. Also provide appropriate assistive devices.

Teach effective stress management techniques to the patient with stress-induced fasciculations.

Pediatric pointers

Fasciculations, particularly of the tongue, are an important early sign of Werdnig-Hoffmann disease.

Fatigue

Fatigue is a feeling of excessive tiredness, lack of energy, or exhaustion accompanied by a strong desire to rest or sleep. This common symptom is distinct from weakness, which involves the muscles, but may occur with it.

Fatigue represents a normal and important response to physical overexertion, prolonged emotional stress, and sleep deprivation. However, it can also be a nonspecific symptom of a psychological or physiologic disorder—especially viral infections and endocrine, cardiovascular, or neurologic disease.

Fatigue reflects both hypermetabolic and hypometabolic states in which nutrients needed for cellular energy and growth are lacking because of overly rapid depletion, impaired replacement mechanisms, insufficient hormone production, or inadequate nutrient intake or metabolism.

Assessment

Obtain a careful history to identify the patient's fatigue pattern. Fatigue that worsens with activity and improves with rest generally indicates a physical disorder; the opposite pattern, a psychological disorder. Also associated with psychological disorders are fatigue lasting longer than 4 months, constant fatigue that's unrelieved by rest, and transient exhaustion that quickly gives way to bursts of energy.

Ask the patient about related symptoms and explore any recent stressful changes in his life-style. Also explore his nutritional habits and any appetite or weight changes. Carefully review his medical and psychiatric history for any chronic disorders that commonly produce fatigue. Also ask about a family history of such disorders.

Observe the patient's general appearance for overt signs of depression or organic illness. Is he unkempt or expressionless? Does he appear tired or sickly, or have a slumped posture? If warranted, assess the patient's mental status, noting especially mental clouding, attention deficits, agitation, or psychomotor retardation.

Medical causes

• *Adrenocortical insufficiency.* Mild fatigue, the hallmark of this disorder, initially appears after exertion and stress but later becomes more severe and persistent. Typically, weakness and weight loss accompany gastrointestinal disturbances such as nausea, vomiting, anorexia, abdominal pain, and chronic diarrhea; hyperpigmentation; orthostatic hypotension; and a weak, irregular pulse.

• *Anemia.* Fatigue following mild activity is often the first symptom of this disorder. Associated signs and symptoms vary but generally include pallor, tachycardia, and dyspnea. Cardiopulmonary signs may include rales, bounding pulse, atrial gallop, and a systolic bruit over the carotid arteries.

• *Anxiety.* Chronic, unremitting anxiety invariably produces fatigue, often characterized as nervous exhaustion. Other persistent signs and symptoms include apprehension, indecisiveness, restlessness, insomnia, trembling, and increased muscle tension. The patient may also experience autonomic effects such as diaphoresis, palpitations, dry mouth, cold and clammy hands, frequent urination, diarrhea, flushing or pallor, tachycardia, and tachypnea.

• *Cancer.* Unexplained fatigue is often the earliest sign of cancer. Related signs and symptoms reflect the type, location, and stage of the tumor, and often include pain, nausea, vomiting, anorexia, weight loss, abnormal bleeding, and a palpable mass.

• *Chronic obstructive pulmonary disease.* The earliest and most persistent symptoms of this disease are progressive fatigue and dyspnea. The patient may also have a chronic and usually productive cough, weight loss, barrel chest, cyanosis, and slight dependent edema.

• *Cirrhosis.* Severe fatigue typically occurs late in this disorder, accompanied by weight loss, bleeding tendencies, jaundice, hepatomegaly, ascites, dependent edema, severe pruritus, and decreased level of consciousness.

• *Congestive heart failure.* Persistent fatigue and lethargy characterize this disorder. Left heart failure produces exertional and paroxysmal nocturnal dyspnea, orthopnea, and tachycardia. Right heart failure produces distended neck veins and possibly slight but persistent nonproductive cough. In both types, slowed mental response appears with later signs and symptoms, including nausea, anorexia, unexplained weight gain, and possible oliguria. Cardiopulmonary findings include tachypnea, inspiratory rales, palpitations and chest tightness, hypotension, narrowed pulse pressure, ventricular gallop, pallor, diaphoresis, clubbing, and dependent edema.

• *Depression.* Persistent fatigue, unrelated to exertion, nearly always accompanies chronic depression. Associated somatic complaints include headache, anorexia (occasionally, increased appetite), constipation, and sexual dysfunction. The patient may have insomnia, slowed speech, agitation or bradykinesia, irritability, loss of concentration, feelings of worthlessness, and persistent thoughts of death.

• *Diabetes mellitus.* Fatigue, the most common symptom in this disorder, may begin insidiously or abruptly. Related findings include weight loss, polyuria, polydipsia, and polyphagia.

• *Hypercortisolism.* This disorder typically causes fatigue, related in part to accompanying sleep disturbances. Unmistakable signs include truncal obesity with slender extremities, buffalo hump, and moon face; purple striae; acne; hirsutism; increased blood pressure; and muscle weakness.

• *Hypopituitarism.* Fatigue, lethargy, and weakness usually develop slowly. Other insidious effects may include irritability, anorexia, amenorrhea or impotence, decreased libido, hypotension, dizziness, headache, visual disturbances, and cold intolerance.

• *Hypothyroidism.* Fatigue begins early, along with forgetfulness, cold intolerance, weight gain, and constipation.

• *Infection.* In *chronic infection,* fatigue is often the most prominent symptom— and sometimes the only one. Low-grade fever and weight loss may accompany symptoms that reflect the type and location of infection, such as burning upon urination or swollen, painful gums. In *acute infection,* brief fatigue typically accompanies headache, anorexia, arthralgia, chills, high fever, and such infection-specific signs as cough, vomiting, or diarrhea.

● *Malnutrition.* Easy fatigability frequently occurs in protein-calorie malnutrition, along with lethargy and apathy. The patient may also have weight loss, muscle wasting, sensations of coldness, pallor, and edema. His skin may be dry and flaky.

● *Myasthenia gravis.* The cardinal symptoms of this disorder are easy fatigability and muscle weakness, which worsen with exertion and abate with rest. Depending on the specific muscles affected, related findings may include diplopia, ptosis, difficulty chewing, dysarthria, dysphagia, and possibly respiratory distress.

● *Myocardial infarction.* Fatigue can be severe, but is typically overshadowed by chest pain. Related findings may include dyspnea, anxiety, pallor, cold sweats, increased or decreased blood pressure, and abnormal heart sounds.

● *Renal failure.* Acute renal failure commonly causes sudden fatigue, drowsiness, and lethargy. Oliguria is an early sign, followed by severe systemic effects: ammonia breath, nausea, vomiting, diarrhea or constipation, and dry skin and mucous membranes. Neurologic signs include muscle twitching and changes in personality and level of consciousness, possibly progressing to convulsions and coma. In *chronic renal failure,* insidious fatigue and lethargy are accompanied by marked changes in all body systems. These include gastrointestinal disturbances, ammonia breath and Kussmaul's respirations, bleeding tendencies, poor skin turgor and severe pruritus, paresthesias, visual disturbances, confusion, convulsions, and coma.

● *Restrictive lung disease.* Chronic fatigue may accompany characteristic signs: dyspnea, cough, and rapid, shallow respirations. Cyanosis first appears with exertion; later, even at rest.

● *Rheumatoid arthritis.* Fatigue, weakness, and anorexia precede localized articular signs and symptoms: joint pain, tenderness, warmth, and swelling; morning stiffness; and possibly paresthesias in the hands and feet.

● *Systemic lupus erythematosus.* Fatigue usually occurs along with generalized aching, malaise, low-grade fever, headache, and irritability. Primary clinical features include joint pain and stiffness, butterfly rash, and photosensitivity. Also common are Raynaud's phenomenon, patchy alopecia, and mucous membrane ulcers.

● *Thyrotoxicosis.* In this disorder, fatigue may occur with characterisitic signs and symptoms. These include an enlarged thyroid, tachycardia and palpitations, tremors, weight loss despite increased appetite, diarrhea, dyspnea, nervousness, diaphoresis, heat intolerance, and possible exophthalmos. Auscultation may also detect an atrial or ventricular gallop.

● *Valvular heart disease.* All types of valvular heart disease commonly produce progressive fatigue and a cardiac murmur. Additional signs and symptoms vary but generally include exertional dyspnea, cough, and hemoptysis.

Other causes

● *Drugs.* Fatigue may result from various drugs, notably antihypertensives and sedatives. In cardiac glycoside therapy, it may indicate toxicity.

● *Surgery.* Most types of surgery cause temporary fatigue, probably due to the combined effects of hunger, anesthesia, and sleep deprivation.

Special considerations

No matter what's causing the patient's fatigue, you may need to help him alter his life-style to achieve a balanced diet, a program of regular exercise (within prescribed limits), and adequate rest. Counsel the patient about setting priorities, maintaining a reasonable schedule, and developing good sleep habits. Teach stress management techniques as appropriate.

If fatigue results from organic illness, help the patient determine what activities he must accomplish, which of these he may need help with, and how to pace himself to ensure sufficient rest. Also, you can often help reduce chronic fatigue by alleviating pain, which may interfere with rest, or nausea, which may lead to malnutrition. The patient may also benefit from referral to a community health nurse or housekeeping service.

If fatigue results from a psychogenic cause, refer the patient for psychological counseling.

Pediatric pointers
When assessing a child for fatigue, ask his parents if they've noticed any change in his activity level. Fatigue without an organic cause occurs normally during accelerated growth phases in preschool-age and prepubescent children. However, psychological causes of fatigue must be considered; for instance, a depressed child may try to escape problems at home or school by taking refuge in sleep. Also, in the pubescent child, consider the possibility of drug abuse, particularly of hypnotics and tranquilizers.

Fecal Incontinence

Fecal incontinence, the involuntary passage of feces, follows any loss or impairment of external anal sphincter control. It can result from various gastrointestinal (GI), neurologic, and psychological disorders, the effects of drugs, and surgery. In some patients, it may even be a purposeful manipulative behavior.

Fecal incontinence may be temporary or permanent; its onset may be gradual, as in dementia, or sudden, as in spinal cord trauma. Although usually not a sign of severe illness, it can greatly affect the patient's physical and psychological well-being.

Assessment
Ask the patient with fecal incontinence about its onset, duration, severity, and any discernible pattern—for instance, at night or with diarrhea. Note the frequency, consistency, and volume of stool passed within the last 24 hours and obtain a stool sample. Focus your history-taking on GI, neurologic, and psychological disorders.

Let the history guide your physical assessment. If you suspect a brain or spinal cord lesion, perform a complete neurologic examination. If a GI disturbance seems likely, inspect the abdomen for distention, auscultate for bowel sounds, percuss, and palpate for a mass. Inspect the anal area for signs of excoriation or infection. If not contraindicated, check for fecal impaction, which may be associated with incontinence.

Medical causes
• *Cerebrovascular accident.* Temporary fecal incontinence occasionally occurs but usually disappears with the restoration of muscle tone and deep tendon reflexes. Persistent fecal incontinence may reflect extensive neurologic damage. Other findings reflect the location and extent of damage and may include urinary incontinence, hemiplegia, dysarthria, aphasia, sensory losses, reflex changes, and visual field deficits. Typical generalized signs and symptoms include headache, vomiting, nuchal rigidity, fever, disorientation, mental impairment, convulsions, and coma.
• *Dementias.* Any of these chronic degenerative brain diseases can produce fecal incontinence. Associated signs and symptoms include impaired judgment and abstract thinking, amnesia, emotional lability, hyperactive deep tendon reflexes, aphasia or dysarthria, and possibly diffuse choreoathetotic movements.
• *Gastroenteritis.* Severe gastroenteritis may result in temporary fecal incontinence manifested by explosive diarrhea. Nausea, vomiting, and colicky abdominal pain are typical. Other possible findings include headache, myalgia, and hyperactive bowel sounds.
• *Head trauma.* Disruption of the neu-

NEUROLOGIC CONTROL OF DEFECATION

From conscious cortex

Afferent nerves

Skeletal motor nerve

Parasympathetic nerves

Three neurologic mechanisms normally regulate defecation: the intrinsic defecation reflex in the colon, the parasympathetic defecation reflex involving sacral segments of the spinal cord, and voluntary control. Here's how they interact:

Fecal distention of the rectum activates the relatively weak intrinsic reflex, causing afferent impulses to spread through the myenteric plexus, initiating peristalsis in the descending and sigmoid colons and in the rectum. Subsequent movement of feces toward the anus causes receptive relaxation of the internal anal sphincter.

To ensure defecation, the parasympathetic reflex magnifies the intrinsic reflex. Stimulation of afferent nerves in the rectal wall circles impulses through the spinal cord and back to the descending and sigmoid colons, rectum, and anus to intensify peristalsis (see illustration).

However, fecal movement and internal sphincter relaxation cause immediate contraction of the external anal sphincter and temporary fecal retention. At this point, conscious control of the external sphincter either prevents or permits defecation. Except in the infant or the neurologically impaired patient, this voluntary mechanism further contracts the sphincter to prevent defecation at inappropriate times, or relaxes it and allows defecation to occur.

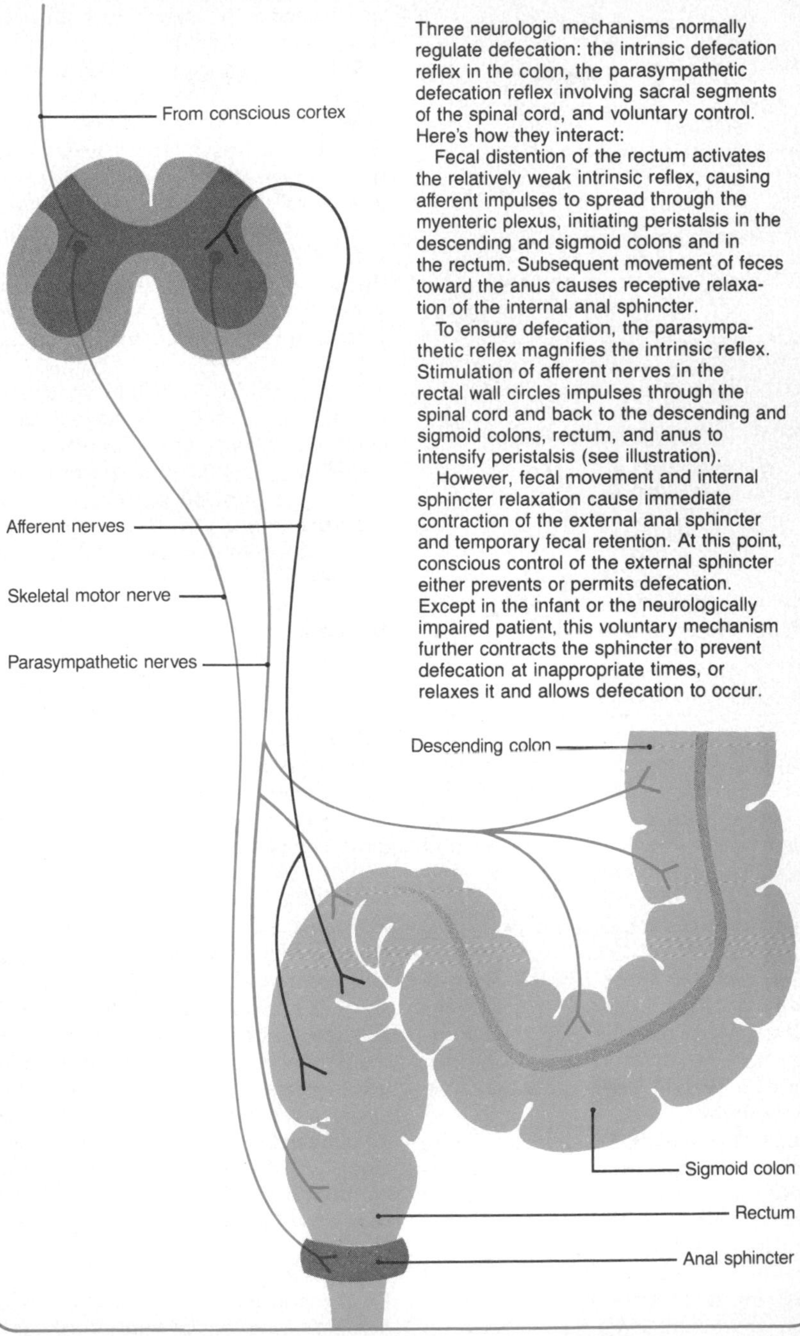

Descending colon

Sigmoid colon

Rectum

Anal sphincter

BOWEL RETRAINING TIPS

You can help your patient control fecal incontinence by instituting a bowel retraining program. Here's how:
• Begin by establishing a specific time for defecation. A typical schedule: once a day or once every other day after a meal, usually breakfast. However, be flexible when establishing this schedule, and consider the patient's normal habits and preferences.
• If necessary, help ensure regularity by administering a suppository, either glycerin or bisacodyl, about 30 minutes before the time scheduled for defecation. Avoid the routine use of enemas or laxatives, as they can cause dependence.
• Provide privacy and a relaxed environment to encourage regularity. If "accidents" occur, assure the patient that they're normal and don't represent a failure of the program.
• Adjust the patient's diet to provide adequate bulk and fiber; encourage him to eat more raw fruits and vegetables and whole grains. Ensure a fluid intake of at least 1,000 ml/day.
• If appropriate, encourage the patient to exercise regularly to help stimulate peristalsis.
• Be sure to keep accurate intake and elimination records.

rologic pathways that control defecation can cause fecal incontinence. Additional findings depend on the location and severity of the injury and may include decreased level of consciousness, seizures, vomiting, and a wide range of motor and sensory impairments.

• *Inflammatory bowel disease.* Nocturnal fecal incontinence occurs occasionally with diarrhea. Related findings may include abdominal pain, anorexia, weight loss, and hyperactive bowel sounds.

• *Multiple sclerosis.* Fecal incontinence occasionally appears as one of this disorder's extremely variable signs. Other effects depend on the area of demyelination, and may include muscle weakness, ataxia, and paralysis; gait disturbances; sensory impairment, such as paresthesias; visual blurring,

diplopia, or nystagmus; urinary disturbances; and emotional lability.

• *Rectovaginal fistula.* Fecal incontinence occurs in tandem with uninhibited passage of flatus.

• *Spinal cord lesions.* Any lesion that causes compression or transection of sensorimotor spinal tracts can lead to fecal incontinence. Incontinence may be permanent, especially with severe lesions of the sacral segments. Other signs and symptoms reflect motor and sensory disturbances below the level of the lesion, such as urinary incontinence, weakness or paralysis, paresthesias, and analgesia and thermanesthesia.

• *Tabes dorsalis.* This late sequela of syphilis occasionally results in fecal incontinence. It also produces urinary incontinence; ataxic gait; paresthesias; loss of position, deep pain, and temperature sensation; Charcot's joints; Argyll Robertson pupils; and possibly impotence.

Other causes

• *Drugs.* Chronic laxative abuse may cause insensitivity to a fecal mass or loss of the colonic defecation reflex.

• *Surgery.* Pelvic, prostate, or rectal surgery occasionally produces temporary fecal incontinence. Colostomy or ileostomy causes permanent or temporary fecal incontinence.

Special considerations

Maintain effective hygienic care, including control of foul odors. Also provide emotional support for the patient, since he may feel deep embarrassment. For the patient with intermittent or temporary incontinence, encourage Kegel exercises to strengthen abdominal and perirectal muscles (see *How to Do Kegel Exercises*, page 251). For the neurologically capable patient with chronic incontinence, provide bowel retraining (see *Bowel Retraining Tips*).

Pediatric pointers

Fecal incontinence is normal in an infant and may occur temporarily in a young child who experiences stress-related psychological regression or physical illness with diarrhea. Pediatric fecal incontinence can also result from myelomeningocele.

Fetor Hepaticus

Fetor hepaticus—a distinctive musty-sweet breath odor—characterizes hepatic encephalopathy, a life-threatening complication of severe liver disease. The odor results from the damaged liver's inability to metabolize and detoxify mercaptans produced by bacterial degradation of methionine, a sulfurous amino acid. These substances circulate in the blood, are expelled by the lungs, and flavor the breath.

Assessment

If you detect fetor hepaticus, quickly assess the patient's level of consciousness. If he's comatose, have another nurse notify the doctor while you assess respiratory status. Prepare to assist with intubation and provide ventilatory support, if necessary. As ordered, start a peripheral I.V. for fluid administration, begin cardiac monitoring, and insert an indwelling (Foley) catheter to monitor output. Obtain arterial and venous samples for analysis of blood gases, ammonia, and electrolytes.

If the patient is conscious, closely observe him for signs of impending coma. Assess deep tendon reflexes, and attempt to elicit Babinski's sign. Be alert for signs of gastrointestinal (GI) bleeding and shock, common complications of end-stage liver failure. Inform the doctor immediately if you note increased anxiety; restlessness; tachycardia; tachypnea; cool, moist, pale skin; hypotension; oliguria; hematemesis; or melena. Place the patient supine with his legs elevated 20°, administer oxygen, and increase the infusion rate of I.V. fluids, as ordered. Draw blood samples for a complete blood count, typing, cross matching, and clotting profile. Be prepared to assist with intubation and ventilation or to begin cardiopulmonary resuscitation.

Continue your physical examination by assessing the degree of jaundice and abdominal distention and by palpating the liver for degree of enlargement.

Obtain a complete medical history, relying on the patient's family if necessary. Focus on any factors that may have precipitated hepatic disease or coma, such as recent severe infection; overuse of sedatives, analgesics, or diuretics; excessive protein intake; and recent blood transfusion or surgery.

Medical cause

• *Hepatic encephalopathy.* Fetor hepaticus usually occurs in the final, comatose stage of this disorder but may occur earlier. Tremors progress to asterixis in the impending stage, along with lethargy, aberrant behavior, and apraxia. Hyperventilation and stupor mark the stuporous stage, and the patient acts agitated when aroused. Seizures and coma herald the final stage, along with decreased pulse and respiratory rates, positive Babinski's sign, hyperactive reflexes, decerebrate posture, and opisthotonos.

Special considerations

Effective treatment of hepatic encephalopathy reduces blood ammonia levels by eliminating ammonia from the GI tract. You may be asked to administer neomycin or lactulose to suppress bacterial production of ammonia, give sorbitol solution to induce osmotic diuresis, give potassium supplements to correct alkalosis, provide continuous gastric aspiration of blood, or maintain the patient on a low-protein diet. If these methods aren't successful, hemodialysis or exchange transfusions may be employed.

During treatment, closely monitor the patient's level of consciousness, intake and output, and fluid and electrolyte balance.

Pediatric pointers
The child slipping into hepatic coma may cry, show disobedience, or become preoccupied with an activity.

Fever

[Pyrexia]

This common sign can arise from disorders affecting virtually every body system. As a result, fever in the absence of other signs usually has little diagnostic significance. Persistent high fever, though, represents an emergency.

Fever can be classified as low (oral reading of 99° to 100.4° F., or 37.2° to 38° C.), moderate (100.5° to 104° F., or 38° to 40° C.), or high (above 104° F.). Fever over 108° F. (42.2° C.) causes unconsciousness and, if sustained, leads to permanent brain damage.

Fever may also be classified as remittent, intermittent, sustained, or relapsing. *Remittent fever,* the most common type, is characterized by daily temperature fluctuations above the normal range. *Intermittent fever* comprises a daily temperature drop into the normal range, then a rise back to above normal. An intermittent fever that fluctuates widely, typically producing chills and sweating, is called *hectic* or *septic fever. Sustained fever* involves persistent temperature elevation with little fluctuation. *Relapsing fever* consists of alternating feverish and afebrile periods.

Further classification involves duration—either brief (less than 3 weeks) or prolonged. Prolonged fevers include fever of unknown origin, a classification used when careful examination fails to detect an underlying cause.

Assessment
If you detect fever greater than 106° F. (41.1° C.), notify the doctor immediately. Take the patient's other vital signs and assess his level of consciousness. Administer antipyretic drugs and begin rapid cooling measures: apply ice packs to the axillae and groin, give tepid sponge baths, or apply a hypothermia blanket. Remember that these methods may evoke a *hypothermic* response—to prevent this, constantly monitor the patient's rectal temperature.

If the patient's fever is only mild to moderate, ask him when it began and how high his temperature reached. Did the fever disappear, only to reappear later? Did the patient experience any other symptoms, such as chills, fatigue, pain?

Obtain a complete medical history, noting especially immunosuppressive treatments or disorders; infection; trauma, surgery, or diagnostic testing; and use of anesthesia or other medications. Ask about recent travel, since certain diseases are endemic.

Let the history findings direct your physical examination. Since fever can accompany diverse disorders, this examination may range from a brief evaluation of one body system to a comprehensive review of all systems.

Medical causes
• *Immune complex dysfunction.* When present, fever usually remains low, although moderate elevations may accompany erythema multiforme. Fever may be remittent or intermittent, as in acquired immunodeficiency syndrome (AIDS) or systemic lupus erythematosus, or sustained, as in polyarteritis. As one of several vague prodromal complaints (such as fatigue, anorexia, and weight loss), fever produces nocturnal diaphoresis and accompanies such associated signs as diarrhea and persistent cough in AIDS, and morning stiffness in rheumatoid arthritis. Other disease-specific findings include headache and possible vision loss (temporal arteritis); pain and stiffness in the neck, shoulders, back, or pelvis (ankylosing spondylitis and polymyalgia rheumatica); skin and mucous membrane lesions (erythema multiforme);

and urethritis with urethral discharge and conjunctivitis (Reiter's syndrome).

• *Infectious and inflammatory disorders.* Fever ranges from low (in Crohn's disease and ulcerative colitis) to extremely high (in bacterial pneumonia). It may be remittent, as in infectious mononucleosis and otitis media; hectic, as in lung abscess, influenza, and endocarditis; sustained, as in meningitis; or relapsing, as in malaria. Fever may arise abruptly, as in toxic shock syndrome and Rocky Mountain spotted fever, or insidiously, as in mycoplasmal pneumonia. In hepatitis, fever may represent a disease prodrome; in appendicitis, it follows the acute stage. Its sudden late appearance with tachycardia, tachypnea, and confusion heralds life-threatening septic shock in peritonitis and gram-negative bacteremia.

Associated signs and symptoms involve every system. The cyclic variations of hectic fever typically produce alternating chills and diaphoresis. General systemic complaints include fatigue, weakness, anorexia, and malaise.

• *Neoplasms.* Primary neoplasms and metastases can produce prolonged fever of varying elevations. For instance, acute leukemia may present insidiously with low fever, pallor, and bleeding tendencies, or more abruptly with high fever, frank bleeding, and prostration. Occasionally, Hodgkin's lymphoma produces Pel-Ebstein fever, an irregularly relapsing fever.

Besides fever and nocturnal diaphoresis, neoplastic disease often causes anorexia, fatigue, malaise, and weight loss. Examination may reveal palmar, plantar, or mucous membrane lesions; lymphadenopathy; palpable masses; and hepatosplenomegaly.

• *Thermoregulatory dysfunction.* Sudden onset of fever that rises rapidly and remains as high as 107° F. (41.7° C.) typically occurs in life-threatening disorders such as heatstroke, thyroid storm, and malignant hyperthermia, and with lesions of the central nervous system (CNS). Low or moderate fever appears

with dehydration.

Prolonged high fever commonly produces vomiting; anhidrosis; hot, flushed skin; and decreased level of consciousness. Related cardiovascular effects may include tachycardia, tachypnea, or hypotension. Other disease-specific findings may include skin changes—dry skin and mucous membranes and poor skin turgor in dehydration; mottled cyanosis in malignant hyperthermia; diarrhea in thyroid storm; oliguria in dehydration; and ominous signs of increased intracranial pressure (decreased level of consciousness with bradycardia, widened pulse pressure, and increased systolic pressure) in CNS tumor, trauma, or hemorrhage.

Other causes

• *Diagnostic tests.* Immediate or delayed fever infrequently follows radiographic tests that use contrast medium.

• *Drugs.* Fever and skin rash commonly result from hypersensitivity to antifungals, sulfonamides, penicillins, cephalosporins, tetracyclines, barbiturates, phenytoin, quinidine, iodides, phenolphthalein, methyldopa, procainamide, and some antitoxins. Fever can accompany chemotherapy, especially with bleomycin, vincristine, and asparaginase. It can result from drugs that impair sweating, such as anticholinergics, phenothiazines, and monoamine oxidase inhibitors. Fever can also stem from toxic doses of salicylates, amphetamines, and tricyclic antidepressants.

Inhalant anesthetics and muscle relaxants can trigger malignant hyperthermia in patients with this inherited trait.

• *Treatments.* After surgery, remittent or intermittent low fever may occur for several days. Transfusion reactions characteristically produce abrupt onset of fever and chills.

Special considerations

Regularly monitor the patient's temperature. Provide increased fluid and nutritional intake, as ordered. When administering prescribed antipyretic drugs, minimize resultant chills and diaphoresis by following a regular dosage schedule. Promote patient comfort by maintaining a stable room temperature and providing frequent changes of bedding and clothing.

Pediatric pointers
Infants and young children experience higher and more prolonged fevers, more rapid temperature increases, and greater temperature fluctuations than older children and adults.

Keep in mind that seizures commonly accompany extremely high fe-

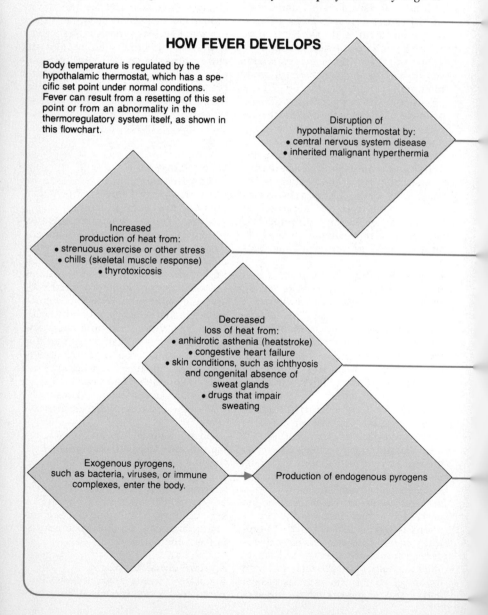

HOW FEVER DEVELOPS

Body temperature is regulated by the hypothalamic thermostat, which has a specific set point under normal conditions. Fever can result from a resetting of this set point or from an abnormality in the thermoregulatory system itself, as shown in this flowchart.

Disruption of hypothalamic thermostat by:
• central nervous system disease
• inherited malignant hyperthermia

Increased production of heat from:
• strenuous exercise or other stress
• chills (skeletal muscle response)
• thyrotoxicosis

Decreased loss of heat from:
• anhidrotic asthenia (heatstroke)
• congestive heart failure
• skin conditions, such as ichthyosis and congenital absence of sweat glands
• drugs that impair sweating

Exogenous pyrogens, such as bacteria, viruses, or immune complexes, enter the body.

Production of endogenous pyrogens

ver, so take appropriate precautions. Also, instruct parents not to give aspirin to a child with varicella or flulike symptoms, because of the risk of precipitating Reye's syndrome.

Common pediatric causes of fever include varicella, croup syndrome, dehydration, meningitis, mumps, otitis media, pertussis, roseola infantum, rubella, rubeola, and tonsillitis. Fever can also occur as a reaction to immunizations and antibiotics.

Flank Pain

Pain in the flank, the area extending from the ribs to the ilium, is a leading indicator of renal and upper urinary tract disease or trauma. Depending on the cause, this symptom may vary from a dull ache to severe stabbing or throbbing pain, and may be unilateral or bilateral and constant or intermittent. It's aggravated by costovertebral angle (CVA) percussion and, in patients with renal or urinary tract obstruction, by increased fluid intake or ingestion of alcohol, caffeine, and diuretic drugs. Unaffected by position changes, flank pain typically responds only to analgesics or, of course, to treatment of the underlying disorder.

Assessment

If the patient's suffered trauma, quickly assess for a visible or palpable flank mass, associated injuries, CVA pain, hematuria, Grey Turner's sign, and signs of shock (such as tachycardia and cool, clammy skin). If you find any of these signs and symptoms, notify the doctor immediately, and insert an I.V. line to enable fluid or drug infusion. As ordered, insert an indwelling (Foley) catheter to monitor urinary output and assess hematuria. Obtain blood samples for typing and cross matching, complete blood count, and electrolyte levels.

If the patient's condition isn't critical, take a thorough history. Ask about the onset of the flank pain and apparent precipitating events. Have the patient describe the location, intensity, pattern, and duration of the pain. Find out if anything aggravates or alleviates it.

Ask the patient about any changes in his normal pattern of fluid intake and

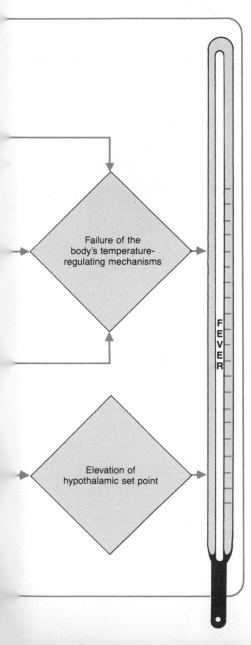

Failure of the body's temperature-regulating mechanisms

Elevation of hypothalamic set point

FEVER

FLANK PAIN: CAUSES AND ASSOCIATED FINDINGS

S&S CAUSES	\[MAJOR ASSOCIATED SIGNS AND SYMPTOMS\] Abdominal distention	Abdominal mass	Abdominal pain	Anuria	Back pain	Bladder distention	Blood pressure—decreased	Blood pressure—increased	Bowel sounds—hypoactive	Chills	CVA tenderness	
Bladder neoplasm					●	●						
Calculi			●		●				●		●	
Cortical necrosis (acute)				●								
Cystitis (bacterial)					●							
Glomerulonephritis (acute)				●				●				
Obstructive uropathy	●	●	●	●		●			●		●	
Pancreatitis (acute)			●		●		●		●			
Papillary necrosis (acute)			●	●					●	●	●	
Perirenal abscess		●								●	●	
Polycystic kidney disease					●			●				
Pyelonephritis (acute)			●							●	●	
Renal infarction			●	●					●		●	
Renal neoplasm								●				
Renal trauma	●		●						●		●	
Renal vein thrombosis					●						●	

Dysuria	Edema—generalized	Fatigue	Fever	Flank mass	Groin pain	Hematuria	Leg pain	Nausea	Nocturia	Oliguria	Perineal pain	Polyuria	Pyuria	Suprapubic pain	Tenesmus	Urinary frequency	Urinary retention	Urinary urgency	Vomiting
•						•	•		•		•		•			•		•	•
•		•	•		•	•		•	•					•	•	•		•	•
			•			•													
•		•	•			•			•		•			•	•	•		•	
	•	•	•			•		•		•									•
					•			•		•	•								•
			•					•											•
			•			•				•			•						•
•			•																
						•					•		•	•	•	•		•	
•		•	•			•			•						•	•		•	
			•				•		•										•
			•	•		•	•										•		•
				•	•	•	•		•										•
			•			•	•		•										•

urinary output. Explore his history for urinary tract infection or obstruction, renal disease, or recent streptococcal infection.

During the physical examination, palpate the patient's flank area and percuss the CVA to determine the extent of pain.

Medical causes

● *Bladder neoplasm.* Dull, constant flank pain may be unilateral or bilateral and may radiate to the leg, back, and perineum. Commonly, the first sign of this neoplasm is gross, painless, intermittent hematuria, often with clots. Related effects may include urinary frequency and urgency, nocturia, dysuria, pyuria, bladder distention, diarrhea, vomiting, and sleep disturbances.

● *Calculi.* Renal and ureteral calculi produce intense unilateral, colicky flank pain. Typically, initial CVA pain radiates to the flank, suprapubic region, and perhaps the genitalia, with abdominal and low back pain also possible. Nausea and vomiting often accompany severe pain. Associated findings include CVA tenderness, hematuria, hypoactive bowel sounds, and possibly signs of urinary tract infection (urinary frequency and urgency, dysuria, nocturia, fatigue, low-grade fever, and tenesmus).

● *Cortical necrosis (acute).* Unilateral flank pain is usually severe. Accompanying findings include gross hematuria, anuria, and fever.

● *Cystitis (bacterial).* Unilateral or bilateral flank pain occurs secondarily to an ascending urinary tract infection. The patient may also report perineal, low back, and suprapubic pain. Other effects include dysuria, nocturia, hematuria, frequency, urgency, tenesmus, fatigue, and low-grade fever.

● *Glomerulonephritis (acute).* Flank pain is bilateral, constant, and of moderate intensity. The most common findings in this disorder are moderate facial and generalized edema, hematuria, oliguria or anuria, and fatigue. Other effects include slightly increased blood pressure, low-grade fever, malaise, headache, nausea, and vomiting. Accompanying signs of pulmonary congestion include dyspnea, tachypnea, and crackles.

● *Obstructive uropathy.* In acute obstruction, flank pain may be excruciating; in gradual obstruction, it's typically a dull ache. In both, the pain may also localize in the upper abdomen and may radiate to the groin. Nausea and vomiting, abdominal distention, anuria alternating with periods of oliguria and polyuria, and hypoactive bowel sounds may also occur. Additional findings— a palpable abdominal mass, CVA tenderness, and bladder distention—depend on the site and cause of the obstruction.

● *Pancreatitis (acute).* Bilateral flank pain may develop as severe epigastric or left upper quadrant pain radiates to the back. A severe attack causes extreme pain, nausea and persistent vomiting, abdominal tenderness and rigidity, hypoactive bowel sounds, and possibly restlessness, low-grade fever, tachycardia, hypotension, and positive Grey Turner's and Cullen's signs.

● *Papillary necrosis (acute).* Intense bilateral flank pain occurs along with renal colic, CVA tenderness, and abdominal pain and rigidity. Possible urinary signs include oliguria or anuria, hematuria, and pyuria, with associated high fever, chills, vomiting, and hypoactive bowel sounds.

● *Perirenal abscess.* Intense unilateral flank pain and CVA tenderness accompany dysuria, persistent high fever, chills, and, in some patients, a palpable abdominal mass.

● *Polycystic kidney disease.* Dull, aching, bilateral flank pain is often the earliest symptom. The pain can become severe and colicky if cysts rupture and clots migrate or cause obstruction. Nonspecific early findings may include polyuria, increased blood pressure, and signs of urinary tract infection. Later findings include hematuria and perineal, low back, and suprapubic pain.

● *Pyelonephritis (acute).* Intense, constant, unilateral or bilateral flank pain develops over a few hours or days along with typical urinary features: dysuria, nocturia, hematuria, urgency, frequency, and tenesmus. Other common findings include persistent high fever, chills, anorexia, weakness, fatigue, generalized myalgia, abdominal pain, and marked CVA tenderness.

• *Renal infarction.* Unilateral, constant, severe flank pain and tenderness typically accompany persistent, severe upper abdominal pain. The patient may also have CVA tenderness, anorexia, nausea, and vomiting. Fever, hypoactive bowel sounds, hematuria, and oliguria or anuria may also develop.

• *Renal neoplasm.* Unilateral flank pain, gross hematuria, and a palpable flank mass form the classic clinical triad. Flank pain is usually dull and vague, although severe colicky pain can occur during bleeding or passage of clots. Possible associated signs and symptoms include fever, increased blood pressure, and urinary retention. Weight loss, leg edema, nausea, and vomiting point to advanced disease.

• *Renal trauma.* Variable bilateral or unilateral flank pain is a common symptom. A visible or palpable flank mass may also exist, along with CVA or abdominal pain—possibly severe and radiating to the groin. Other findings may include hematuria, oliguria, abdominal distention, positive Grey Turner's sign, hypoactive bowel sounds, and nausea or vomiting. Severe injury may produce signs of shock, such as tachycardia and cool, clammy skin.

• *Renal vein thrombosis.* Severe unilateral flank and low back pain with CVA and epigastric tenderness typify the rapid onset of venous obstruction. Other features may include fever, hematuria, and leg edema. Bilateral flank pain, oliguria, and other uremic signs (nausea, vomiting, and uremic fetor) typify bilateral obstruction.

Special considerations
Administer pain medication, as ordered. Continue to monitor the pa-

tient's vital signs, and maintain precise intake and output records.

Diagnostic evaluation may involve serial urine and serum analysis, I.V. pyelography, flank ultrasonography, computed tomography scan, voiding cystourethrography, cystoscopy, and retrograde ureteropyelography, urethrography, and cystography.

Pediatric pointers
Assessment of flank pain can be difficult if the child can't describe the pain. In such cases, transillumination of the abdomen and flanks may help assess bladder distention and identify masses. Common causes of flank pain in children include obstructive uropathy, acute poststreptococcal glomerulonephritis, infantile polycystic kidney disease, and nephroblastoma.

Flatulence

A sensation of gaseous abdominal fullness, flatulence can result from GI disorders, abdominal surgery, and excessive intake of certain foods. It can also stem from stress, and can be accompanied by belching, discomfort, and excessive passage of flatus. This symptom reflects slowed intestinal motility, which hampers the passage of gas; excessive swallowing of air (aerophagia), often brought on by stress; or increased intraluminal gas production due to an excess of fermentable substrates, such as digested, unabsorbed carbohydrates and proteins.

Although usually not a serious symptom, flatulence and accompanying expulsion of flatus may cause the patient embarrassment and discomfort.

Assessment
Find out how long the patient's noticed the flatulence, and if he also passes an excessive amount of flatus. Ask about frequent belching or snoring, and observe for overly rapid speech—all pos-

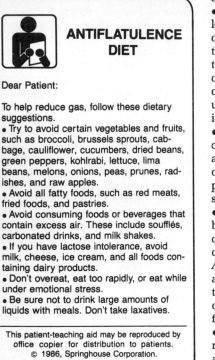

sible clues to aerophagia. Ask if he's undergoing unusual emotional stress—a possible cause of aerophagia or of irritable bowel syndrome. Obtain a medical history, focusing on GI disorders and on systemic illnesses such as scleroderma or congestive heart failure, which can cause malabsorption syndrome.

Inspect the abdomen for distention and auscultate for abnormal bowel sounds. Percuss for increased tympany due to gas accumulation, and palpate for tenderness and masses.

Medical causes

- **Cholecystitis.** Both acute and chronic cholecystitis commonly produce flatulence with frequent passage of flatus. Accompanying colicky pain in the right upper quadrant becomes persistent and severe in an acute attack. Nausea and vomiting may also occur, and fever is common within 48 hours of an attack.

- **Cholelithiasis.** Complaints of flatulence and belching are common in this disorder. Abdominal pain develops in the right upper quadrant, usually after the patient eats fatty foods. With cystic duct obstruction, excruciating pain radiates to the back or the right shoulder, usually accompanied by nausea, vomiting, and fever.

- **Cirrhosis.** Typically, flatulence develops early and insidiously, along with anorexia, dyspepsia, nausea, vomiting, diarrhea or constipation, dull right upper quadrant pain, hepatomegaly, and splenomegaly.

- **Colon cancer.** Obstruction of the colon by a tumor may cause flatulence; acute obstruction also produces abdominal distention and tympany on percussion. Abdominal pain may be present, with anorexia, weight loss, malaise, and altered bowel habits—constipation, diarrhea, or a change in the timing, frequency, or consistency of stools.

- **Crohn's disease.** Flatulence accompanies other acute inflammatory signs and symptoms that mimic appendicitis: right lower quadrant pain, cramps, and tenderness; diarrhea; low-grade fever; nausea; and melena.

- **Irritable bowel syndrome.** Effects include chronic flatulence, belching, and excessive flatus. Chronic constipation is typical, but diurnal diarrhea may also occur. Intermittent lower abdominal pain characteristically abates with defecation or passage of flatus.

- **Lactose intolerance.** Flatulence, cramping abdominal pain, and possibly diarrhea develop within several hours of ingesting dairy products.

- **Malabsorption syndromes.** This group of syndromes may cause flatulence. Associated findings vary considerably, depending on which dietary constituent isn't absorbed, but may include passage of bulky, oily, malodorous, or slightly watery stools; abdominal pain; anorexia; and weight loss. Severe malabsorption may cause muscle wasting and weakness, skeletal pain, edema, ecchymoses, and tongue ulceration.

Other cause

• *Abdominal surgery.* With the return of peristalsis after postoperative paralytic ileus, gas accumulation in hypomotile areas produces flatulence.

Special considerations

If ordered, prepare the patient for diagnostic studies, such as blood tests, stool analysis, upper GI series, barium enema, and endoscopy. To aid expulsion of excessive flatus, position the patient on his left side; to prevent gas buildup, encourage frequent repositioning, ambulation, and normal fluid intake, as permitted. If these measures aren't effective, try inserting a rectal tube into the anus to relieve flatus or administering enemas, suppositories, antiflatulents, or anticholinergics, as ordered.

As appropriate, provide the patient with a dietary plan that excludes gaseous foods.

Pediatric pointers

The common childhood complaint of stomachache often results from flatulence. Children may also be more sensitive than adults to flatus-producing foods and are generally more prone to aerophagia, especially during eating.

Fontanelle Bulging

In a normal infant, the anterior fontanelle, or "soft spot," is flat, soft yet firm, and well demarcated against surrounding skull bones. (The posterior fontanelle, if not fused at birth, usually closes by age 2 months.) Subtle pulsations may be visible, reflecting the arterial pulse. A bulging fontanelle— widened, tense, and with marked pulsations—is a cardinal sign of potentially life-threatening increased intracranial pressure (ICP), a medical emergency. Since prolonged coughing, crying, or lying down can cause transient, physiologic bulging, the infant's head should be observed and palpated while he's upright and relaxed to detect pathologic bulging.

Assessment

If you detect a bulging fontanelle, notify the doctor immediately. Measure fontanelle size and head circumference, and note the overall shape of the head. Take vital signs, and assess level of consciousness by observing spontaneous activity, postural reflex activity, and sensory responses. Note whether the infant assumes a normal, flexed posture or one of extreme extension, opisthotonos, or hypotonia. Observe movements of his arms and legs—excessive tremulousness or frequent twitching may herald the onset of a seizure. Look for other signs of increased ICP—abnormal respiratory patterns and a distinctive, high-pitched cry.

Ensure airway patency, and have size-appropriate emergency equipment on hand. Provide oxygen, establish I.V. access, and, if the infant is having a seizure, stay with him to prevent injury. As ordered, administer anticonvulsants and antipyretics, osmotic diuretics to help reduce cerebral edema and ICP, and dexamethasone for edema secondary to head trauma. If the infant has an extremely high fever, give him a tepid sponge bath. If these measures fail to reduce ICP, neuromuscular blockage, intubation, mechanical ventilation, and, in rare cases, barbiturate coma and total body hypothermia may be necessary.

Once the infant's condition is stabilized, you can begin investigating the underlying cause of increased ICP. Obtain his medical history from a parent or caretaker, paying particular attention to any recent infection or trauma, including birth trauma. Has the infant or any family member had a recent rash or fever? Ask about any changes in the infant's behavior, such as frequent vomiting, lethargy, or disinterest in feeding.

LOCATING FONTANELLES

Lambdoidal suture —

Posterior fontanelle —

Sagittal suture —

Anterior fontanelle —
Coronal suture —
Frontal suture —

The anterior fontanelle lies at the junction of the sagittal, coronal, and frontal sutures. It normally measures about 2.5 cm by 4 to 5 cm at birth and usually closes by age 18 to 20 months.

The posterior fontanelle lies at the junction of the sagittal and lambdoidal sutures. If it hasn't already fused by the time of birth, it measures 1 to 2 cm and normally closes by age 2 months.

Medical cause

• *Increased ICP.* Besides a bulging fontanelle and increased head circumference, other early signs and symptoms are often subtle and difficult to discern. They may include behavioral changes, irritability, and fatigue.

As intracranial pressure rises, the infant's pupils may dilate and his level of consciousness may decrease to drowsiness and eventual coma. Seizures commonly occur.

Special considerations

Closely monitor the infant's condition, including urinary output (via an indwelling catheter, if necessary), and continue to observe for seizures. Restrict fluids, as ordered, and position the infant supine at a 30° head-up tilt to enhance cerebral venous drainage and reduce intracranial blood volume.

Explain the purpose and procedure of diagnostic tests to the infant's parents or caretaker. Such tests may include intracranial computed tomography or skull X-ray, cerebral angiog-raphy, and a full sepsis workup, including blood and urine cultures.

Fontanelle Depression

Depression of the anterior fontanelle below the surrounding bony ridges of the skull is a sign of dehydration. A common disorder of infancy and early childhood, dehydration can result from insufficient intake, but typically reflects excessive fluid loss from severe vomiting or diarrhea. It may also reflect insensible water loss, pyloric stenosis, or tracheoesophageal fistula.

Assessment

If you detect a markedly depressed fontanelle, call the doctor immediately. Take the infant's vital signs, weigh him, and check for signs of shock—tachycardia, tachypnea, and cool, clammy skin. If these signs are present, insert an I.V. line and administer fluids, as ordered. Have size-appropriate emergency equipment at hand, and prepare to administer oxygen, as ordered. Apply a pediatric urine collection bag (or insert an indwelling catheter, if necessary) to enable accurate output measurement.

Obtain a thorough patient history from a parent or caretaker, focusing on recent fever, vomiting, diarrhea, and behavioral changes. Determine the infant's fluid intake and urine output over the last 24 hours. Ask about his preillness weight, and compare it with his current weight; weight loss in an infant virtually equals water loss.

Medical cause

• *Dehydration.* In *mild dehydration* (5% weight loss), the anterior fontanelle appears slightly depressed. The infant has pale, dry skin and mucous membranes, decreased urine output, a normal or slightly elevated pulse rate, and possibly a decreased level of activity.

Moderate dehydration (10% weight loss) causes slightly more pronounced fontanelle depression, along with gray skin with poor turgor, dry mucous membranes, and decreased urine output. The infant has normal or decreased blood pressure, an increased pulse rate, and possibly lethargy.

Severe dehydration (15% or greater weight loss) may result in a markedly depressed fontanelle, along with extremely poor skin turgor, parched mucous membranes, marked oliguria, lethargy, and signs of shock.

Special considerations

Continue to monitor the infant's vital signs, intake, and output, and watch for signs of worsening dehydration. In mild dehydration, frequently provide small amounts of clear fluids. If the infant's unable to ingest sufficient fluid, begin I.V. hyperalimentation.

In moderate and severe dehydration, your first priority is rapid restoration of extracellular fluid volume to treat or prevent shock. Continue to administer I.V. solution with sodium bicarbonate added, as ordered, to combat acidosis. As renal function improves, administer I.V. potassium replacements. Once the infant's fluid status stabilizes, begin to replace depleted fat and protein stores through diet. If the infant can't eat or if feeding aggravates diarrhea, provide I.V. hyperalimentation to prevent severe malnourishment.

Tests to evaluate dehydration include urinalysis for specific gravity and possibly blood tests to determine electrolyte concentrations, blood urea nitrogen and serum creatinine levels, osmolality, and acid-base status.

Footdrop

Footdrop—plantar flexion of the foot with the toes bent toward the instep—results from weakness or paralysis of the dorsiflexor muscles of the foot and ankle. A characteristic and important sign of certain peripheral nerve or motor neuron disorders, it may also stem from prolonged immobility when inadequate support, improper positioning, or infrequent passive exercise produces shortening of the Achilles tendon. Unilateral footdrop can result from compression of the common peroneal nerve against the head of the fibula.

Footdrop can range in severity from slight to complete, depending on the extent of muscle weakness or paralysis. It develops slowly in progressive muscle degeneration, or suddenly in spinal cord injury.

Assessment

Ask the patient about the sign's onset, duration, and character. Does the footdrop fluctuate in severity or remain constant? Does it worsen with fatigue? Improve with rest? Ask the patient if he feels weak or tires easily.

During the physical examination, assess muscle tone and strength in the patient's feet and legs, and compare findings on both sides. Assess deep tendon reflexes (DTRs) in both legs as well. Have the patient walk while you observe for steppage gait—a compensatory response to footdrop.

Medical causes

- **Cerebrovascular accident.** Unilateral footdrop often appears with arm and leg weakness or paralysis. Other effects depend on the site and severity of vascular damage. Sensorimotor disturbances may include paresthesias, dysphagia, visual field deficits, diplopia, and bowel and bladder dysfunction. Personality changes, amnesia, aphasia, dysarthria, and decreased level of consciousness (LOC) may also occur.

- **Guillain-Barré syndrome.** Unilateral or bilateral footdrop and steppage gait may result from profound muscle weakness. This weakness usually begins in the legs and extends to the arms and face within 72 hours. It can progress to total motor paralysis with respiratory failure. The patient may also have transient paresthesias, hypernasality, dysphagia, diaphoresis, tachycardia, orthostatic hypotension, and incontinence.

- **Herniated lumbar disk.** Footdrop and steppage gait may result from leg muscle weakness and atrophy. However, the most pronounced symptom is severe low back pain, which may radiate to the buttocks, legs, and feet, usually unilaterally. Sciatic pain follows, often accompanied by muscle spasms and sensorimotor loss. Paresthesias and fasciculations may occur.

- **Multiple sclerosis.** Footdrop may develop suddenly or slowly, producing steppage gait; it typically fluctuates in severity with this disorder's cycle of periodic exacerbation and remission. Muscle weakness most commonly affects the legs and ranges from minor fatigability to paraparesis with urinary urgency and constipation. Related findings include facial pain, visual disturbances, paresthesias, incoordination, and loss of vibration and position sensation in the ankle and toes.

- **Myasthenia gravis.** Footdrop and related limb weakness are common manifestations of this disorder, which is often heralded by weak eye closure, ptosis, and diplopia. Skeletal muscle weakness and fatigability may progress to paralysis. Typically, muscle function worsens through the day and with exercise, and improves with rest. Involvement of respiratory muscles can cause breathing difficulty.

- **Peroneal muscle atrophy.** Bilateral footdrop, ankle instability, and steppage gait occur early in this chronic disorder. Foot, peroneal, and ankle dorsiflexor muscles are affected first. Other early signs and symptoms include paresthesias, aching, and cramping in the feet and legs, along with coldness, swelling, and cyanosis. As the disease progresses, all leg muscles become weak and atrophic, with hypoactive or absent DTRs. Later, atrophy and sensory losses spread to the hands and forearms.

- **Peroneal nerve trauma.** Footdrop may occur suddenly—but it's temporary, resolving with the release of peroneal nerve compression. It's associated with ipsilateral steppage gait, muscle weakness, and sensory loss over the lateral surface of the calf and foot.

- **Poliomyelitis.** Unilateral or bilateral footdrop may develop, producing a steppage gait. Initially, fever precedes asymmetrical muscle weakness, coarse fasciculations, paresthesias, hypoactive or absent DTRs, and permanent muscle paralysis and atrophy. Dysphagia, urinary retention, and respiratory difficulty may occur.

- **Polyneuropathy.** Footdrop and steppage gait may accompany muscle weakness, which usually affects distal areas of the extremities and can progress to flaccid paralysis. Muscle atrophy and hypoactive or absent DTRs may occur, along with paresthesia, hyperesthesia, or anesthesia, and loss of vibration sensation in the hands and feet. Cutaneous manifestations include glossy red skin and anhidrosis.

- **Spinal cord trauma.** Unilateral or bilateral footdrop can occur suddenly and

FOOTDROP: CAUSES AND ASSOCIATED FINDINGS

CAUSES	Bowel and bladder dysfunction	DTRs—hypoactive	Gait—steppage	LOC—altered	Muscle atrophy	Muscle weakness	Pain	Paralysis	Paresthesias	Respiratory difficulty	Sensory loss	Visual disturbances
Cerebrovascular accident	•			•		•		•	•			•
Guillain-Barré syndrome	•		•			•		•	•	•		
Herniated lumbar disk			•		•	•	•		•		•	
Multiple sclerosis	•		•			•			•		•	•
Myasthenia gravis						•		•		•		•
Peroneal muscle atrophy		•	•		•	•	•		•		•	
Peroneal nerve trauma			•			•					•	
Poliomyelitis	•	•	•		•	•		•	•	•		
Polyneuropathy		•	•		•	•	•	•	•		•	
Spinal cord trauma	•	•	•			•	•	•	•	•	•	

may be permanent. In the ambulatory patient, it also produces steppage gait. Additional findings vary, and may include neck and back pain; paresthesias, sensory loss, and muscle weakness or paralysis distal to the injury; asymmetrical or absent DTRs; and fecal and urinary incontinence.

Special considerations
Prepare the patient for electromyography, as ordered, to evaluate nerve damage. If appropriate, refer the patient to a physical therapist for gait retraining and possible in-shoe splints or leg braces to maintain correct foot alignment for walking and standing.

Pediatric pointers
Common causes of footdrop in children include spinal birth defects (such as spina bifida) and degenerative disorders (such as muscular dystrophy). To aid ambulation, the child should be fitted with supportive shoes and possibly in-shoe splints or braces.

gag reflex abnormalities • gait—bizarre • gait—propulsive • gait—scissors • g
steppage • gait—waddling • gallop—atrial • gallop—ventricular • genital lesio
grunting respirations • gum bleeding • gum swelling • gynecomastia • halitos
headache • hearing loss • heat intolerance • Heberden's nodes • hematemesis •
hematuria • hemianopia • hemoptysis • hepatomegaly • hiccups • hirsutism •
sign • hyperpigmentation • hyperpnea • hypopigmentation • impotence • inso
claudication • Janeway's spots • jaundice • jaw pain • jugular vein distention
sign • leg pain • level of consciousness—decreased • lid lag • light flashes • lo
lymphadenopathy • masklike facies • McBurney's sign • McMurray's sign • m
metrorrhagia • miosis • moon face • mouth lesions • murmurs • muscle atroj
muscle spasms • muscle spasticity • muscle weakness • mydriasis • myoclonu
nausea • neck pain • night blindness • nipple discharge • nipple retraction •
rigidity • nystagmus • ocular deviation • oligomenorrhea • oliguria • opisthot
dyskinesia • orthopnea • orthostatic hypotension • Ortolani's sign • Osler's no
palpitations • papular rash • paralysis • paresthesias • paroxysmal nocturnal
d'orange • pericardial friction rub • peristaltic waves—visible • photophobia
rub • polydipsia • polyphagia • polyuria • postnasal drip • priapism • prurit
psychotic behavior • ptosis • pulse—absent or weak • pulse—bounding • pul
pulse pressure—widened • pulse rhythm abnormality • pulsus alternans • pi
paradoxus • pupils—nonreactive • pupils—sluggish • purple striae • purpura
pyrosis • raccoon's eyes • rebound tenderness • rectal pain • retractions—cos
rhinorrhea • rhonchi • Romberg's sign • salivation—decreased • salivation—
scotoma • scrotal swelling • seizure—absence • seizure—focal • seizure—ger
seizure—psychomotor • setting-sun sign • shallow respirations • skin—bron
skin—mottled • skin—scaly • skin turgor—decreased • spider angioma • spl
respirations • stool—clay-colored • stridor • syncope • tachycardia • tachypn
tearing—increased • throat pain • tic • tinnitus • tracheal deviation • trache
trismus • tunnel vision • uremic frost • urethral discharge • urinary frequen
urinary incontinence • urinary urgency • urine cloudiness • urticaria • vagin
postmenopausal • vaginal discharge • venous hum • vertigo • vesicular rash
loss • visual blurring • visual floaters • vomiting • vulvar lesions • weight ga
loss—excessive • wheezing • wristdrop• abdominal distention • abdominal j
abdominal rigidity • accessory muscle use • agitation • alopecia • amenorrh
analgesia • anhidrosis • anorexia • anosmia • anuria • anxiety • aphasia • a
respirations • apraxia • arm pain • asterixis • ataxia • athetosis • aura • Ba
pain • barrel chest • Battle's sign • Biot's respirations • bladder distention •
blood pressure increase • bowel sounds—absent • bowel sounds—hyperacti
hypoactive • bradycardia • bradypnea • breast dimpling • breast nodule • b
breath with ammonia odor • breath with fecal odor • breath with fruity od
bruits • buffalo hump • butterfly rash • café-au-lait spots • capillary refill ti
carpopedal spasm • cat cry • chest expansion—asymmetrical • chest pain •
respirations • chills • chorea • Chvostek's sign • clubbing • cogwheel rigidit
confusion • conjunctival injection • constipation • corneal reflex—absent • c
tenderness • cough—barking • cough—nonproductive • cough—productive
bony • crepitation—subcutaneous • cry—high-pitched • cyanosis • decerebr
posture • deep tendon reflexes—hyperactive • deep tendon reflexes—hypoac
diaphoresis • diarrhea • diplopia • dizziness • doll's eye sign—absent • dro
dysmenorrhea • dyspareunia • dyspepsia • dysphagia • dyspnea • dystonia
edema—generalized • edema of the arms • edema of the face • edema of th
enuresis • epistaxis • eructation • erythema • exophthalmos • eye discharge

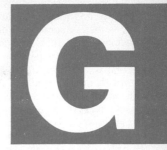

Gag Reflex Abnormalities

[Pharyngeal reflex abnormalities]

The gag reflex—a protective mechanism that prevents aspiration of food, fluid, and vomitus—normally can be elicited by touching the posterior wall of the oropharynx with a tongue depressor or by suctioning the throat. Prompt elevation of the palate, constriction of the pharyngeal musculature, and a sensation of gagging indicate a normal gag reflex. An abnormal gag reflex—either decreased or absent—interferes with the ability to swallow and, more importantly, increases susceptibility to life-threatening aspiration. An impaired gag reflex can result from any lesion affecting its mediators—cranial nerves IX (glossopharyngeal) and X (vagus) or the pons or medulla. It can also occur in coma or temporarily as a result of anesthesia.

Assessment

If you detect an abnormal gag reflex, immediately stop the patient's oral intake to prevent aspiration. Quickly evaluate his level of consciousness. If it's decreased, place him in a side-lying position to prevent aspiration; if not, place him in Fowler's position. Make sure you have suction equipment at hand.

Ask the patient (or a family member, if the patient's unable to communicate) about the onset and duration of his swallowing difficulties. Determine if he has more difficulty swallowing liquids than solids, and if swallowing is more difficult at certain times of the day, as occurs in the bulbar palsy associated with myasthenia gravis. If the patient also has trouble chewing, suspect more widespread neurologic involvement, since chewing involves different cranial nerves.

Explore the patient's medical history for vascular and degenerative disorders. Then assess his respiratory status for evidence of aspiration, and perform a neurologic examination.

Medical causes

• **Basilar artery occlusion.** This disorder may suddenly diminish or obliterate the gag reflex. It also causes diffuse sensory loss, dysarthria, facial weakness, extraocular muscle palsies, quadriplegia, and decreased level of consciousness.

• **Brain stem glioma.** This lesion causes gradual loss of the gag reflex. Related symptoms reflect bilateral brain stem involvement and include diplopia and facial weakness. Common involvement of the corticospinal pathways causes spasticity and paresis of the arms and legs, as well as gait disturbances.

• *Bulbar palsy.* Loss of the gag reflex reflects temporary or permanent paralysis of muscles supplied by cranial nerves IX and X. Similar indicators of this paralysis include jaw and facial muscle weakness, dysphagia, loss of sensation at the base of the tongue, increased salivation, possible difficulty articulating and breathing, and fasciculations.

• *Wallenberg's syndrome.* Paresis of the palate and an impaired gag reflex usually develop within hours to days of thrombosis. The patient may have analgesia and thermanesthesia, occurring ipsilaterally on the face and contralaterally on the body, and vertigo. He may also display nystagmus, ipsilateral ataxia of the arm and leg, and signs of Horner's syndrome (unilateral ptosis and miosis, and hemifacial anhidrosis).

Other cause

• *Anesthesia.* General and local (throat) anesthesia can produce temporary loss of the gag reflex.

Special considerations

Continually assess the patient's ability to swallow. If his gag reflex is absent, provide tube feedings; if it's merely diminished, try pureed foods. Advise the patient to take small amounts and eat slowly, while in a high Fowler's or sitting position. Stay with him while he eats and observe for choking. Remember to keep suction equipment handy in case of aspiration. Keep accurate intake and output records, and assess the patient's nutritional status daily.

If ordered, prepare the patient for diagnostic studies, such as computed tomography, electroencephalography, lumbar puncture, and arteriography.

Pediatric pointers

Brain stem glioma is an important cause of abnormal gag reflex in children.

Gait—Bizarre

[Hysterical gait]

A bizarre gait has no obvious organic basis—rather, it's produced unconsciously by a person with a somatoform disorder (hysterical neurosis), or consciously by a malingerer. The gait has no consistent pattern. It may mimic an organic impairment, but characteristically has a more theatrical or bizarre quality with key elements missing—such as a spastic gait without hip circumduction, or leg "paralysis" with normal reflexes and motor strength. Its manifestations may include wild gyrations, exaggerated stepping, leg dragging, or mimicking unusual walks, such as that of a tightrope walker.

Assessment

If you suspect that the patient's gait impairment has no organic cause, begin to investigate other possibilities. Ask the patient when he first developed the impairment and whether it coincided with any stressful period or event, such as the death of a loved one or loss of a job. Ask about associated symptoms, and explore any reports of frequent unexplained illnesses and multiple doctor's visits. Subtly try to determine if he'll achieve any gain from malingering—added attention, a lawsuit, or insurance settlement, for instance.

Begin the physical examination by testing the patient's reflexes and sensorimotor function, noting any abnormal response patterns. To quickly check his reports of leg weakness or paralysis, perform Hoover's test: position the patient supine and stand at his feet. Cradle a heel in each of your palms and rest your hands on the table. Ask the patient to raise the affected leg. In the presence of true motor weakness, the heel of the other leg will press downward; in hysteria, this movement will be absent. As a further check, observe the patient for normal movements when he's unaware of being watched.

Medical causes

- *Conversion disorder.* In this rare somatoform disorder, bizarre gait usually develops suddenly after severe stress and isn't accompanied by other symptoms. The patient typically shows indifference toward his impairment.
- *Malingering.* In this rare cause of bizarre gait, the patient may also complain of headache and chest and back pain.
- *Somatization disorder.* Bizarre gait is one of many possible somatic complaints. The patient may exhibit any combination of pseudoneurologic signs and symptoms—fainting, weakness, memory loss, dysphagia, visual problems (diplopia, vision loss, blurred vision), loss of voice, seizures, and bladder dysfunction. He may also report pain in the back, joints, and extremities (most commonly the legs) and perhaps complaints in almost any body system. For example, characteristic gastrointestinal complaints include pain and bloating, nausea and vomiting.

The patient's reflexes and motor strength remain normal, but peculiar contractures and arm or leg rigidity may occur. His reputed sensory loss doesn't conform to any known sensory dermatome. In some cases, he won't stand or walk (astasia/abasia), remaining bedridden although still able to move his legs in bed.

Special considerations

A full neurologic workup may be necessary to completely rule out an organic cause of the patient's abnormal gait.

Remember, even though bizarre gait has no organic basis, it's real to the patient (unless, of course, he's malingering). Avoid expressing judgment on the patient's actions or motives; be supportive and reinforce positive progress. Because muscle atrophy and bone demineralization can develop in the bedridden patient, encourage ambulation

and resumption of normal activities. Report your observations to the doctor, and suggest that appropriate referrals be made for psychiatric counseling.

Pediatric pointers

Bizarre gait is rare before age 8. More common in prepubescence, it usually results from a conversion disorder.

Gait—Propulsive

[Festinating gait]

Propulsive gait is characterized by a stooped, rigid posture—the patient's head and neck are bent forward, his flexed, stiffened arms are held away from the body, his fingers are extended, and his knees and hips are stiffly bent. During ambulation, this posture results in a forward shifting of the body's center of gravity and consequent impairment of balance, causing increasingly rapid, short, shuffling steps with involuntary acceleration (festination) and lack of control over forward motion (propulsion) or backward motion (retropulsion). (See *Identifying Gait Abnormalities*, pages 334 and 335.)

Propulsive gait is a cardinal sign of advanced Parkinson's disease, resulting from progressive degeneration of the ganglia, which are primarily responsible for smooth muscle movement. Because this sign develops gradually and its accompanying effects are often wrongly attributed to aging, propulsive gait often goes unnoticed or unreported until severe disability results.

Assessment

Ask the patient when his gait impairment first developed, and whether it's recently worsened. Since he may have difficulty remembering, having attributed the gait to "old age," you may gain information from family members or friends, especially those who see the patient only sporadically.

IDENTIFYING GAIT ABNORMALITIES

Spastic gait   Scissors gait

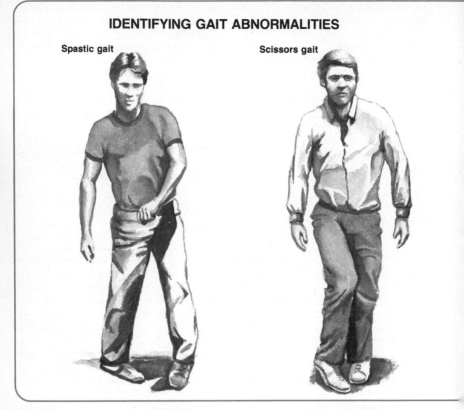

Also obtain a thorough drug history, including both medication type and dosage. Ask the patient if he's been taking any tranquilizers, especially phenothiazines. If the patient knows he has Parkinson's disease and has been taking L-dopa, pay particular attention to the dosage, since an overdose can cause acute exacerbation of signs and symptoms.

If Parkinson's disease isn't a known or suspected diagnosis, ask the patient if he's been acutely or routinely exposed to carbon monoxide or manganese.

Medical causes

● *Carbon monoxide poisoning.* Propulsive gait often appears several weeks after acute carbon monoxide intoxication. Earlier effects include muscle rigidity, choreoathetotic movements, generalized seizures, myoclonic jerks,

masklike facies, and dementia.

● *Manganese poisoning.* Chronic overexposure to manganese can cause an insidious, usually permanent, propulsive gait. Typical early findings include fatigue, muscle weakness and rigidity, dystonia, resting tremor, choreoathetotic movements, masklike facies, and personality changes.

● *Parkinson's disease.* The characteristic and permanent propulsive gait begins early as a shuffle. As the disease progresses, the gait slows. Cardinal signs of the disease are progressive muscle rigidity, which may be uniform (leadpipe rigidity) or jerky (cogwheel rigidity); akinesia; and an insidious tremor that begins in the fingers, increases during stress or anxiety, and decreases with purposeful movement and sleep. Besides the gait, akinesia produces a high-pitched, monotone

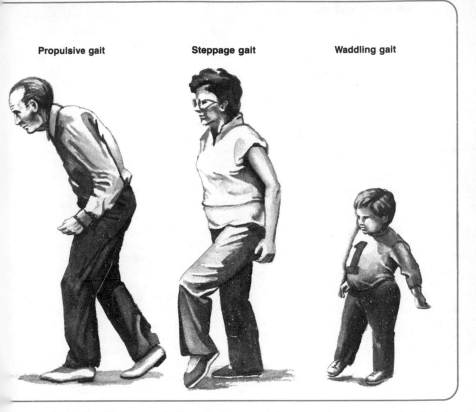

Propulsive gait   **Steppage gait**   **Waddling gait**

voice; drooling; masklike facies; stooped posture; and dysarthria, dysphagia, or both. Occasionally, it also causes oculogyric crises or blepharospasm.

Other causes

• *Drugs.* Propulsive gait and possibly other extrapyramidal effects can also result from use of phenothiazines, other antipsychotics (notably haloperidol, thiothixene, and loxapine) and, infrequently, metoclopramide and metyrosine. Such effects are usually temporary, disappearing within 1 to 2 weeks after cessation of therapy.

Special considerations

Because of his gait and associated motor impairment, the patient may have problems performing activities of daily living. Assist him as appropriate, while at the same time encouraging his independence and self-reliance. Instruct the patient and his family to allow plenty of time for these activities, especially walking, since he's particularly susceptible to falls due to festination and poor balance. Encourage the patient to maintain ambulation; for safety reasons, remember to stay with him while he's walking, especially if he's on unfamiliar or uneven ground. You may need to refer the patient to a physical therapist for exercise therapy and gait retraining.

Pediatric pointers

Propulsive gait, usually with severe tremors, typically occurs in juvenile parkinsonism, a rare familial form of Parkinson's disease. Other rare congenital causes include Hallervorden-Spatz syndrome and kernicterus.

Gait—Scissors

Resulting from spastic hemiparesis (diplegia), a scissors gait affects both legs and has little or no effect on the arms. The patient's legs flex slightly at the hips and knees, giving the appearance of crouching. With each step, his thighs adduct and his knees hit or cross in a scissors-like movement. His steps are short, regular, and laborious, as if he were wading through waist-deep water. His feet may be plantar-flexed and turned inward (equinovarus position), with a shortened Achilles tendon—as a result, he walks on his toes or the balls of his feet and may scrape his toes on the ground.

Assessment

Ask the patient (or a family member, if the patient can't answer) about the onset and duration of the gait. Has it progressively worsened or remained constant? Ask about a history of trauma, including birth trauma, and neurologic disorders. Thoroughly evaluate motor and sensory function and deep tendon reflexes in the legs.

Medical causes

• *Cerebrovascular accident.* Rarely, scissors gait develops during the late recovery stage of bilateral occlusion of the anterior cerebral artery. The patient may also display leg muscle paraparesis and atrophy, incoordination, numbness, urinary incontinence, confusion, and personality changes.

• *Cervical spondylosis with myelopathy.* Scissors gait develops in the late stages of this degenerative disease and steadily worsens. Associated signs and symptoms mimic those of a herniated disk: severe low back pain, which may radiate to the buttocks, legs, and feet; muscle spasms; sensorimotor loss; and muscle weakness and atrophy.

• *Hepatic failure.* Scissors gait may appear several months before the onset of hepatic encephalopathy. Other findings may include asterixis, generalized seizures, jaundice, purpura, dementia, and fetor hepaticus.

• *Multiple sclerosis.* Progressive scissors gait usually develops gradually, with infrequent remissions. Characteristic muscle weakness, most often in the legs, ranges from minor fatigability to paraparesis with urinary urgency and constipation. Related findings include facial pain, visual disturbances, paresthesias, incoordination, and loss of proprioception and vibration sensation in the ankle and toes.

• *Pernicious anemia.* Scissors gait sometimes occurs as a late sign in untreated anemia. Besides this disorder's classic triad of symptoms—weakness, sore tongue, and numbness and tingling in the extremities—the patient may exhibit pale lips, gums, and tongue; faintly jaundiced sclera and pale to bright yellow skin; disturbed proprioception; incoordination; and altered vision (diplopia, blurring).

• *Spinal cord trauma.* Scissors gait may develop during recovery from partial spinal cord compression, particularly with injury below C6. Associated signs and symptoms depend on the site and severity of injury but may include sensory loss or paresthesias, muscle weakness or paralysis distal to the injury, and bladder and bowel dysfunction.

• *Spinal cord tumor.* Scissors gait can develop gradually from a thoracic or lumbar tumor. Other findings reflect the location of the tumor and may include radicular, subscapular, shoulder, groin, leg, or flank pain; muscle spasms or fasciculations; muscle atrophy; sensory deficits, such as paresthesias and a girdle sensation of the abdomen and chest; hyperactive deep tendon reflexes; bilateral Babinski's reflex; spastic, neurogenic bladder; and sexual dysfunction.

• *Syphilitic meningomyelitis.* Scissors gait appears late in this disorder and may improve with treatment. The patient may have sensory ataxia, changes in proprioception and vibration sensation, optic atrophy, and dementia.

● *Syringomyelia.* Scissors gait usually occurs late, along with analgesia and thermanesthesia, muscle atrophy and weakness, and Charcot's joints. Other musculoskeletal effects may include loss of fingernails, fingers, or toes; Dupuytren's contracture of the palms; scoliosis; and clubfoot. Skin in the affected areas is often dry, scaly, and grooved. Autonomic disturbances may include anhidrosis, hyperkeratosis, trophic ulcers, hypoactive bowel sounds, and poor bowel and bladder control.

Special considerations

Because of the sensory loss associated with scissors gait, provide meticulous skin care to prevent skin breakdown and decubiti formation. Also give the patient and his family complete skin care instructions. If appropriate, provide bladder and bowel retraining.

Provide daily active and passive range-of-motion exercises. As appropriate, refer the patient to a physical therapist for gait retraining and for possible in-shoe splints or leg braces to maintain proper foot alignment for standing and walking.

Pediatric pointers

The major causes of scissors gait in children are cerebral palsy, hereditary spastic paraplegia, and spinal injury at birth. If spastic paraparesis is present at birth, scissors gait becomes apparent when the child begins to walk, which is usually later than normal.

Gait—Spastic

[Hemiplegic gait]

Spastic gait—a stiff, foot-dragging walk caused by unilateral leg muscle hypertonicity—indicates focal damage to the corticospinal tract. The affected leg becomes rigid, with a marked decrease in flexion at the hip and knee and possibly plantar flexion and equinovarus deformity of the foot. Because the patient's leg doesn't swing normally at the hip or knee, his foot tends to drag or shuffle, scraping his toes on the ground. To compensate, the pelvis of the affected side tilts upward in an attempt to lift the toes, causing the patient's leg to abduct and circumduct. In addition, arm swing is hindered on the same side as the affected leg.

Spastic gait usually develops after a period of flaccidity (hypotonicity) in the affected leg. Once the gait develops, it's usually permanent—regardless of the cause.

Assessment

Find out when the patient first noticed the gait impairment and whether it developed suddenly or gradually. Ask him if it waxes and wanes or if it has worsened progressively. Do fatigue, hot weather, or warm baths or showers worsen the gait? Such exacerbation typically occurs in multiple sclerosis.

Focus your medical history questions on neurologic disorders, recent head trauma, and degenerative diseases.

During the physical examination, test and compare strength, range of motion, and sensory function in all limbs. Also observe and palpate for muscle flaccidity or atrophy.

Medical causes

● *Brain abscess.* In this disorder, spastic gait generally develops slowly after a period of muscle flaccidity and fever. Early signs and symptoms of abscess reflect increased intracranial pressure: headache, nausea, vomiting, and focal or generalized seizures. Later, site-specific features may include hemiparesis, tremors, visual disturbances, nystagmus, and pupillary inequality. The patient's level of consciousness may range from drowsiness to stupor.

● *Brain tumor.* Depending on the site and type of tumor, spastic gait usually develops gradually and worsens over time. Accompanying effects may include signs of increased intracranial pressure (headache, nausea, vomiting, and focal or generalized seizures), papilledema, sensory loss on the affected side, dysarthria, ocular palsies, aphasia, and personality changes.

• **Cerebrovascular accident.** Spastic gait usually appears after a period of muscle weakness and hypotonicity on the affected side. Associated effects may include unilateral muscle atrophy, sensory loss, and footdrop; aphasia; dysarthria; dysphagia; visual field deficits; diplopia; and ocular palsies.

• **Head trauma.** Spastic gait typically follows the acute stage of head trauma. The patient may also have focal or generalized seizures, personality changes, headache, and focal neurologic signs, such as aphasia and visual field deficits.

• **Multiple sclerosis.** Spastic gait begins insidiously and follows this disorder's characteristic cycle of remission and exacerbation. The gait, as well as other signs and symptoms, often worsens in warm weather or after a warm bath or shower. Characteristic weakness, most often affecting the legs, ranges from minor fatigability to paraparesis with urinary urgency and constipation. Other effects: facial pain, paresthesias, incoordination, loss of proprioception and vibration sensation in the ankle and toes, and visual disturbances.

Special considerations

Because leg muscle contractures are commonly associated with spastic gait, promote daily exercise—both active and passive. As appropriate, refer the patient to a physical therapist for gait retraining and possible in-shoe splints or leg braces to maintain proper foot alignment for standing and walking.

The patient may have poor balance and a tendency to fall to the paralyzed side, so stay with him while he's walking. Provide a cane or a walker, as indicated.

Pediatric pointers

Causes of spastic gait in children include sickle cell crisis, cerebral palsy, porencephalic cysts, and arteriovenous malformation that causes hemorrhage or ischemia.

Gait—Steppage

[Equine gait, prancing gait]

Steppage gait typically results from footdrop caused by weakness or paralysis of pretibial and peroneal muscles, usually from lower motor neuron lesions. Footdrop causes the foot to hang with the toes pointing down, causing the toes to scrape the ground during ambulation. To compensate, the hip rotates outward and the hip and knee flex in an exaggerated fashion to lift the advancing leg off the ground. The foot is thrown forward and the toes hit the ground first, producing an audible slap. The rhythm of the gait is usually regular, with even steps and normal upper body posture and arm swing.

Steppage gait can be unilateral or bilateral and permanent or transient, depending on the site and type of neural damage.

Assessment

Begin by asking the patient about the onset of the gait and any recent changes in its character. Find out if any family member has a similar gait. Also find out if the patient has had any traumatic injury to the buttocks, hips, legs, or knees. Ask about a history of chronic disorders that may be associated with polyneuropathy, such as diabetes mellitus, polyarteritis nodosa, or alcoholism. While you're taking the history, observe whether the patient crosses his legs while sitting, since this may put pressure on the peroneal nerve.

Inspect and palpate the patient's calves and feet for muscle atrophy and wasting. Using a pin, test for sensory deficits along the entire length of both legs.

Medical causes

• *Guillain-Barré syndrome.* Typically occurring after recovery from the acute stage of this disorder, steppage gait can be mild or severe, and unilateral or bilateral; it's invariably permanent. Muscle weakness usually begins in the legs, extends to the arms and face within 72 hours, and can progress to total motor paralysis and respiratory failure. Other effects include footdrop, transient paresthesias, hypernasality, dysphagia, diaphoresis, tachycardia, orthostatic hypotension, and incontinence.

• *Herniated lumbar disk.* Unilateral steppage gait and footdrop commonly occur with late-stage weakness and atrophy of leg muscles. However, the most pronounced symptom is severe low back pain, which may radiate to the buttocks, legs, and feet, usually unilaterally. Sciatic pain follows, often accompanied by muscle spasms and sensorimotor loss. Paresthesias and fasciculations may occur.

• *Multiple sclerosis.* Steppage gait and footdrop typically fluctuate in severity with this disorder's cycle of periodic exacerbation and remission. Muscle weakness, most often affecting the legs, can range from minor fatigability to paraparesis with urinary urgency and constipation. Related findings include facial pain, visual disturbances, paresthesias, incoordination, and sensory loss in the ankle and toes.

• *Peroneal muscle atrophy.* Bilateral steppage gait and footdrop begin insidiously in this disorder. Foot, peroneal, and ankle dorsiflexor muscles are affected first. Other early signs and symptoms include paresthesias, aching, and cramping in the feet and legs, along with coldness, swelling, and cyanosis. As the disorder progresses, all leg muscles become weak and atrophic, with hypoactive or absent deep tendon reflexes. Later, atrophy and sensory losses spread to the hands and arms.

• *Peroneal nerve trauma.* Temporary ipsilateral steppage gait occurs suddenly, but resolves with the release of peroneal nerve pressure. It's associated with footdrop and muscle weakness and sensory loss over the lateral surface of the calf and foot.

• *Poliomyelitis.* Steppage gait, usually permanent and unilateral, often develops after the acute stage. It's typically preceded by fever, asymmetrical muscle weakness, coarse fasciculations, paresthesias, hypoactive or absent deep tendon reflexes, and permanent muscle paralysis and atrophy. Dysphagia, urinary retention, and respiratory difficulty may occur.

• *Polyneuropathy.* Diabetic polyneuropathy is a rare cause of bilateral steppage gait, which appears as a late but permanent effect. It's preceded by burning pain in the feet and accompanied by leg weakness, sensory loss, and skin ulcers.

In *polyarteritis nodosa with polyneuropathy,* unilateral or bilateral steppage gait is a late finding. Related findings include vague leg pain, abdominal pain, hematuria, fever, and increased blood pressure.

In *alcoholic polyneuropathy,* steppage gait appears 2 to 3 months after onset of vitamin B deficiency. The gait may be bilateral, and it resolves with treatment of the deficiency. Early findings include paresthesias in the feet, leg muscle weakness, and possibly sensory ataxia.

• *Spinal cord trauma.* In the ambulatory patient, spinal cord trauma may cause steppage gait. Its other effects depend on the severity of injury and may include unilateral or bilateral footdrop, neck and back pain, and vertebral tenderness and deformity. Paresthesias, sensory loss, asymmetrical or absent deep tendon reflexes, and muscle weakness or paralysis may develop distal to the injury. The patient may also have fecal and urinary incontinence.

Special considerations

The patient with steppage gait may tire rapidly when walking because of the extra effort he must expend to lift his feet off the ground. And when he tires, he may stub his toes, causing a fall. To

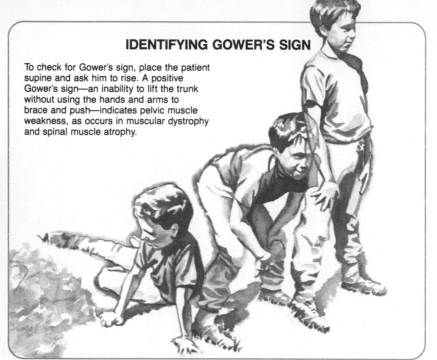

IDENTIFYING GOWER'S SIGN

To check for Gower's sign, place the patient supine and ask him to rise. A positive Gower's sign—an inability to lift the trunk without using the hands and arms to brace and push—indicates pelvic muscle weakness, as occurs in muscular dystrophy and spinal muscle atrophy.

prevent this, help the patient recognize his exercise limits, and encourage him to get adequate rest. Refer him to a physical therapist, if appropriate, for gait retraining and possible application of in-shoe splints or leg braces to maintain correct foot alignment.

Pediatric pointers
Bilateral steppage gait may result from Jering-Soppof disease, a rare progressive neuritis.

Gait—Waddling

Waddling gait, a distinctive ducklike walk, is an important sign of muscular dystrophy, spinal muscle atrophy, or, rarely, congenital hip displacement. It may be present when the child begins to walk or may appear only later in life. The gait results from deterioration of the pelvic girdle muscles—primarily the gluteus medius, hip flexors, and hip extensors. Weakness in these muscles hinders stabilization of the weight-bearing hip during walking, causing the opposite hip to drop and the trunk to lean toward that side in an attempt to maintain balance. Typically, the legs assume a wide stance and the trunk is thrown back to further improve stability, exaggerating lordosis and abdominal protrusion. In severe cases, leg and foot muscle contractures may cause equinovarus deformity of the foot combined with circumduction or bowing of the legs.

Assessment
Ask the patient (or a family member, if the patient's a young child) when the gait first appeared and if it has recently worsened. To determine the extent of pelvic girdle and leg muscle weakness, ask if the patient falls frequently or has difficulty climbing stairs, rising from a chair, or walking. Also find out if the patient was late in learning to walk or

holding his head upright. Obtain a family history, focusing on problems of muscle weakness and gait and on congenital motor disorders.

Inspect and palpate leg muscles, especially in the calves, for size and tone. Check for a positive Gower's sign. Next, assess motor strength and function in the shoulders, arms, and hands, looking for weakness or asymmetrical movements.

Medical causes

● *Congenital hip dysplasia.* Bilateral hip dislocation produces waddling gait with lordosis and pain.

● *Muscular dystrophy.* In *Duchenne's muscular dystrophy*, waddling gait gradually appears at ages 3 to 4 and becomes pronounced by age 6. The gait worsens as the disease progresses, until the child loses the ability to walk and becomes wheelchair-bound—usually by age 12. Early signs are usually subtle: delay in learning to walk, frequent falls, or intermittent calf pain. Common later findings include lordosis with abdominal protrusion, a positive Gower's sign, and equinovarus foot position. As the disease progresses, its effects become more prominent; they commonly include rapid muscle wasting beginning in the legs and spreading to the arms (although calf and upper arm muscles may become hypertrophied, firm, and rubbery), muscle contractures, limited dorsiflexion of the feet and extension of the knees and elbows, obesity, and possibly mild mental retardation.

In *Becker's muscular dystrophy*, waddling gait typically becomes apparent in late adolescence, slowly worsens during the third decade, and culminates in total loss of ambulation. Muscle weakness first appears in the pelvic and upper arm muscles. Progressive wasting with selected muscle hypertrophy produces lordosis with abdominal protrusion, poor balance, a positive Gower's sign, and possibly mental retardation.

In *facioscapulohumeral muscular dystrophy,* waddling gait appears late, after muscle wasting has spread downward from the face and shoulder girdle to the pelvic girdle and legs. Earlier effects include progressive weakness and atrophy of facial, shoulder, and arm muscles, and slight lordosis and pelvic instability.

● *Spinal muscle atrophy.* In *Kugelberg-Welander disease,* waddling gait occurs early and usually progresses slowly, with loss of ambulation occurring up to 20 years later. Related findings may include muscle atrophy in the legs and pelvis, progressing to the shoulders; a positive Gower's sign; ophthalmoplegia; and tongue fasciculations.

In *Werdnig-Hoffmann disease,* waddling gait typically begins when the child learns to walk. The gait progressively worsens, culminating in complete loss of ambulation by adolescence. Associated findings include lordosis with abdominal protrusion and muscle weakness in the hips and thighs.

Special considerations

Perform daily passive and active muscle stretching exercises for both the arms and legs. If possible, have the patient walk at least 3 hours each day (with leg braces, if necessary) to maintain muscle strength, reduce contractures, and delay further gait deterioration. Stay near the patient while he's walking, especially if he's on unfamiliar or uneven ground. Caution him against long, unbroken periods of bed rest, which accelerate muscle deterioration. Provide a balanced diet to maintain energy levels and prevent obesity.

Because of the grim prognosis associated with muscular dystrophy and spinal muscle atrophy, provide emotional support for the patient and his family. As indicated, refer him to a local Muscular Dystrophy Association chapter. Suggest genetic testing and counseling for the parents, if they're considering having another child.

Gallop—Atrial

[S₄]

An atrial or presystolic gallop (S₄) is an extra heart sound that's heard or often palpated immediately before the first heart sound. This low-pitched sound is best heard with the bell of the stethoscope pressed lightly against the cardiac apex. Some clinicians say an S₄ has the cadence of the "Ten" in Tennessee (Ten = S₄; nes = S₁; see = S₂).

Typically, this gallop results from hypertension, conduction defects, valvular disorders, and other cardiac abnormalities. Occasionally, it helps differentiate angina from other causes of chest pain. It results from abnormally forceful atrial contraction caused by augmented ventricular filling or by decreased left ventricular compliance. Usually, an S₄ originates from left atrial contraction, is heard at the apex, and doesn't vary with inspiration. It may also originate from right atrial contraction. Here, it's best heard at the lower left sternal border and intensifies with inspiration.

An S₄ seldom occurs in normal hearts; however, it may occur in the elderly, in athletes with physiologic hypertrophy of the left ventricle, or during pregnancy because of augmented ventricular filling.

Assessment

If you auscultate an S₄ in a patient with chest pain, suspect myocardial ischemia and have another nurse notify the doctor immediately. Take the patient's vital signs and quickly assess for signs of heart failure, such as dyspnea, crackles (rales), and distended neck veins. If you detect these signs, connect the patient to a cardiac monitor and obtain an EKG. Administer antianginal drugs, as ordered. If the patient has dyspnea, elevate the head of the bed. Then auscultate for abnormal breath sounds. If you detect coarse crackles, start an I.V. and give oxygen and diuretics, as ordered. If the patient has bradycardia, administer atropine and assist with pacemaker insertion, if ordered.

When the patient's condition permits, ask about a history of hypertension, angina, valvular stenosis, or cardiomyopathy. If appropriate, have him describe the frequency and severity of anginal attacks.

Medical causes

• *Anemia.* In this disorder, an S₄ may accompany increased cardiac output. Associated findings may include fatigue, pallor, dyspnea, tachycardia, bounding pulse, crackles, and a systolic bruit over the carotid arteries.

• *Angina.* An intermittent S₄ is characteristic here, occurring during an anginal attack and disappearing when it subsides. This gallop may be accompanied by a paradoxical S₂ or a new murmur. Typically, the patient complains of anginal chest pain—a feeling of tightness, pressure, achiness, or burning that usually radiates from the retrosternal area to the neck, jaws, left shoulder, and arm. He may also have dyspnea, tachycardia, palpitations, increased blood pressure, dizziness, diaphoresis, belching, nausea, and vomiting.

• *Aortic insufficiency (acute).* This disorder causes an S₄ accompanied by a soft, short diastolic murmur along the left sternal border. S₂ may be soft or absent. Sometimes, a soft, short midsystolic murmur may be heard over the second intercostal space. Related cardiopulmonary findings may include tachycardia, S₃, dyspnea, neck vein distention, and crackles. The patient may have fatigue and cool extremities.

• *Aortic stenosis.* This disorder usually causes an S₄, especially when valvular obstruction is severe. Auscultation reveals a harsh, crescendo-decrescendo, systolic ejection murmur that's loudest at the right sternal border near the second intercostal space. Dyspnea, an-

LOCATING HEART SOUNDS

When auscultating heart sounds, remember that certain sounds are best heard in specific areas. Use these auscultatory points to locate heart sounds quickly and accurately. Then expand your auscultation to nearby areas. Note that the numbers indicate pertinent intercostal spaces.

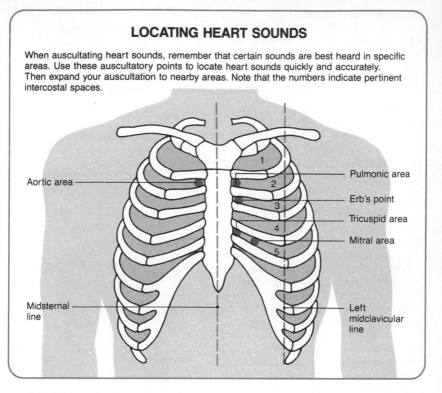

Aortic area

Midsternal line

Pulmonic area

Erb's point

Tricuspid area

Mitral area

Left midclavicular line

ginal chest pain, and syncope are cardinal associated findings. There may also be crackles, palpitations, fatigue, and diminished carotid pulses.

• *Atrioventricular (AV) block. First-degree AV block* may cause an S_4 accompanied by a faint first heart sound (S_1). Although the patient may have bradycardia, he's usually asymptomatic. In *second-degree AV block*, an S_4 is easily heard. If bradycardia develops, the patient may also have hypotension, light-headedness, dizziness, and fatigue. An S_4 is also common in *third-degree AV block*. It varies in intensity with S_1 and is loudest when atrial systole coincides with early, rapid ventricular filling during diastole. The patient may be asymptomatic or have hypotension, light-headedness, dizziness, or syncope, depending on the ventricular rate. Bradycardia may also aggravate or provoke angina or symptoms of congestive heart failure, such as dyspnea.

• *Cardiomyopathy.* In this disorder, an S_4 becomes progressively louder with advancing disease. However, in some patients, it may become faint or occasionally disappear. Additional signs and symptoms may include dyspnea, orthopnea, crackles, fatigue, syncope, chest pain, palpitations, edema, neck vein distention, and S_3.

• *Hypertension.* One of the earliest findings in systemic arterial hypertension is an S_4. The patient may be asymptomatic or may experience headache, weakness, epistaxis, tinnitus, dizziness, syncope, fatigue, facial flushing, and nervousness.

• *Mitral insufficiency.* In acute mitral insufficiency, auscultation may reveal an S_4 accompanied by an S_3, a harsh holosystolic murmur that's heard best at the apex or over the precordium. This murmur radiates to the axilla and back and along the left sternal border. Other features may include fatigue, dyspnea, tachypnea, orthopnea, tachycardia, crackles, and neck vein distention.

• **Mitral stenosis.** When associated with a normal sinus rhythm, mitral stenosis commonly causes an S_4. Initially, the patient may report exertional dyspnea, fatigue, and possibly palpitations. As the disorder progresses, he may report paroxysmal nocturnal dyspnea, orthopnea, dyspnea at rest, and weakness. Cardinal findings include a loud apical first sound and an opening snap with a diastolic murmur heard at the apex.

• **Myocardial infarction (MI).** An S_4 is a classic sign of life-threatening MI; in fact, it may persist even after the infarction heals. Typically, the patient reports crushing substernal chest pain that may radiate to the back, neck, jaw, shoulder, and left arm. Associated signs and symptoms include dyspnea, restlessness, anxiety, a feeling of impending doom, diaphoresis, pallor, clammy skin, nausea, vomiting, and increased or decreased blood pressure.

• **Pulmonary embolism.** This life-threatening disorder causes a right-sided S_4 that's usually heard along the lower left sternal border with a loud pulmonic closure sound. Other features include tachycardia, tachypnea, chest pain, dyspnea, decreased breath sounds, crackles, apprehension, diaphoresis, syncope, and cyanosis. The patient may have a productive cough with blood-tinged sputum or a nonproductive cough.

• **Thyrotoxicosis.** An S_4 and an S_3 may both be auscultated in thyroid hormone overproduction. Other cardinal features include tachycardia, palpitations, weight loss despite increased appetite, diarrhea, tremors, an enlarged thyroid, dyspnea, nervousness, diaphoresis, and heat intolerance. Exophthalmos may be present.

Special considerations
If ordered, prepare the patient for diagnostic tests, such as electro- and echocardiography, cardiac catheterization, and possibly a lung scan.

INTERPRETING HEART SOUNDS

HEART SOUND AND ITS CAUSE

First heart sound (S_1)

Vibrations associated with mitral and tricuspid valve closure

Second heart sound (S_2)

Vibrations associated with aortic and pulmonic valve closure

Ventricular gallop (S_3)

Vibrations produced by rapid blood flow into the ventricles

Atrial gallop (S_4)

Vibrations produced by an increased resistance to sudden, forceful ejection of atrial blood

Summation gallop

Vibrations produced in middiastole by simultaneous ventricular and atrial gallops, usually caused by tachycardia

Detecting subtle variations in heart sounds requires both concentration and practice. Once you recognize normal heart sounds, the abnormal gallops become more obvious.

TIMING AND CADENCE	AUSCULTATION TIPS

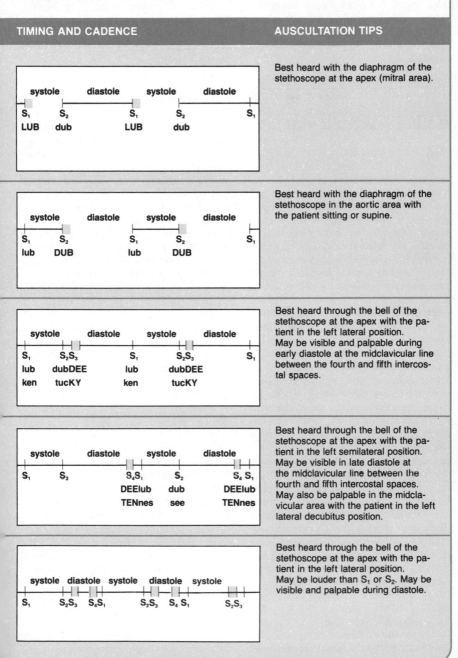

Best heard with the diaphragm of the stethoscope at the apex (mitral area).

Best heard with the diaphragm of the stethoscope in the aortic area with the patient sitting or supine.

Best heard through the bell of the stethoscope at the apex with the patient in the left lateral position.
May be visible and palpable during early diastole at the midclavicular line between the fourth and fifth intercostal spaces.

Best heard through the bell of the stethoscope at the apex with the patient in the left semilateral position.
May be visible in late diastole at the midclavicular line between the fourth and fifth intercostal spaces.
May also be palpable in the midclavicular area with the patient in the left lateral decubitus position.

Best heard through the bell of the stethoscope at the apex with the patient in the left lateral position.
May be louder than S_1 or S_2. May be visible and palpable during diastole.

Pediatric pointers

An atrial gallop may occur in children, especially after exercise. However, it may also result from congenital heart diseases, such as atrial septal defect, ventricular septal defect, patent ductus arteriosus, and severe pulmonary valvular stenosis.

Gallop—Ventricular

[S₃]

A ventricular gallop is an extra heart sound associated with rapid ventricular filling in early diastole. Usually palpable, this low-frequency sound occurs about .15 second after the second heart sound (S_2). It may originate in either the left or right ventricle. A right-sided gallop usually sounds louder on inspiration and is best heard along the lower left sternal border or over the xiphoid region. A left-sided gallop usually sounds louder on expiration and is best heard at the apex.

Ventricular gallops are easily overlooked because they're usually faint. Fortunately, certain techniques make their detection more likely. These include auscultating in a quiet environment; examining the patient in the supine, left lateral, and semi-Fowler's positions; and having the patient cough or raise his legs to augment the sound.

A physiologic ventricular gallop occurs in children and young adults; however, most people lose this third heart sound by age 40. This gallop may also occur during the third trimester of pregnancy. Although the physiologic S_3 has the same timing as the pathologic S_3, its intensity waxes and wanes with respiration. It's also heard more faintly if the patient is sitting or standing.

A pathologic ventricular gallop may be one of the earliest signs of ventricular failure. It may result from one of two mechanisms: rapid deceleration of blood entering a stiff, noncompliant ventricle or rapid acceleration of blood associated with increased flow into the ventricle. The gallop's intensity correlates with the patient's prognosis. Generally, the louder the gallop, the more ominous the prognosis. A gallop that persists despite therapy is also more significant.

Assessment

After auscultating a ventricular gallop, focus your assessment on the cardiovascular system. Begin the history by asking the patient if he's had any chest pain. If so, have him describe its character, location, frequency, duration, and any alleviating or aggravating factors. Also ask about palpitations, dizziness, or syncope. Does the patient have difficulty breathing after exertion? While lying down? At rest? Does he have a productive cough? Ask about a history of cardiac disorders. Is the patient currently receiving treatment for heart failure? If so, what drugs is he taking?

During the physical examination, carefully auscultate for murmurs or abnormalities in the first and second heart sounds. Then listen for pulmonary crackles (rales). Next, assess peripheral pulses, noting pulsus alternans—an alternating strong and weak pulse. Finally, palpate the liver for enlargement or tenderness, and assess for neck vein distention and peripheral edema.

Medical causes

• *Aortic insufficiency.* Both acute and chronic aortic insufficiency may produce an S_3. Typically, *acute aortic insufficiency* also causes an S_4 and a soft, short diastolic murmur over the left sternal border. S_2 may be soft or absent. At times, a soft, short midsystolic murmur may be heard over the second right intercostal space. Related cardiopulmonary findings include tachycardia, dyspnea, neck vein distention, and crackles. The patient may also have fatigue and pale, cool extremities.

Chronic aortic insufficiency produces an S_3 and a high-pitched blowing, decrescendo diastolic murmur that's best heard over the second or third right intercostal space or the left sternal border. An Austin Flint murmur—an apical, rumbling, middle-to-late diastolic murmur—may also occur. Typical related signs and symptoms include palpitations, tachycardia, anginal chest pain, fatigue, dyspnea, orthopnea, and crackles.

• *Cardiomyopathy.* A ventricular gallop is characteristic. When accompanied by pulsus alternans and altered first and second heart sounds, this gallop usually signals advanced heart disease. Other effects may include fatigue, dyspnea, orthopnea, chest pain, palpitations, syncope, crackles, peripheral edema, neck vein distention, and S_4.

• *Congestive heart failure.* A cardinal sign of congestive heart failure (CHF) is a ventricular gallop. When it's loud and accompanied by sinus tachycardia, this gallop may indicate severe heart failure. The patient with left heart failure will also have fatigue, exertional dyspnea, paroxysmal nocturnal dyspnea, orthopnea, and possibly a dry cough; with right heart failure, neck vein distention. Other late features include tachypnea, chest tightness, palpitations, anorexia, nausea, dependent edema, weight gain, slowed mental response, diaphoresis, pallor, hypotension, narrowed pulse pressure, and possibly oliguria. In some patients, inspiratory crackles, clubbing, and a tender, palpable liver may be present. As CHF progresses, hemoptysis, cyanosis, severe pitting edema, and marked hepatomegaly may develop.

• *Mitral insufficiency.* Both acute and chronic mitral insufficiency may produce a ventricular gallop. In *acute mitral insufficiency,* auscultation may also reveal an early or holosystolic decrescendo murmur at the apex, an S_4, and a widely split second heart sound. Typically, the patient will have sinus tachycardia, tachypnea, orthopnea, dyspnea, crackles, distended neck veins, and fatigue.

SUMMATION GALLOP: TWO GALLOPS IN ONE

When atrial and ventricular gallops occur simultaneously, they produce a short, low-pitched sound known as a summation gallop. This relatively uncommon gallop occurs during middiastole (between S_2 and S_1) and is best heard with the bell of the stethoscope pressed lightly against the cardiac apex. It may be louder than either S_1 or S_2 and may cause visible apical movement during diastole.

A summation gallop may result from tachycardia or from delayed or blocked atrioventricular (AV) conduction. Tachycardia shortens ventricular filling time during diastole, causing it to coincide with atrial contraction. When heart rate slows, the summation gallop is replaced by separate atrial and ventricular gallops, producing a quadruple rhythm much like the canter of a horse. Delayed AV conduction also brings atrial contraction closer to ventricular filling, creating a summation gallop. Most commonly, a summation gallop results from congestive heart failure and dilated congestive cardiomyopathy; it may also accompany other cardiac disorders. Occasionally, it signals further cardiac deterioration. For example, consider the hypertensive patient with a chronic atrial gallop who develops tachycardia and a superimposed ventricular gallop. If this patient abruptly displays a summation gallop, heart failure is the likely cause.

In *chronic mitral insufficiency*, a progressively severe ventricular gallop is typical. Auscultation will also reveal a holosystolic, blowing, high-pitched apical murmur. The patient may report fatigue, exertional dyspnea, and palpitations, or he may be asymptomatic.

• *Thyrotoxicosis.* This disorder may produce ventricular and atrial gallops. Its cardinal features, though, are an enlarged thyroid gland, weight loss despite increased appetite, heat intolerance, diaphoresis, nervousness, tremors, tachycardia, palpitations, diarrhea, and dyspnea. Exophthalmos may be present.

Special considerations

Carefully monitor the patient with an S_3; watch for and report such changes as tachycardia, dyspnea, crackles, or neck vein distention. As ordered, administer oxygen, diuretics, and other drugs, such as digitalis, to prevent pulmonary edema.

As ordered, prepare the patient for echocardiography, gated blood pool imaging, and cardiac catheterization.

Pediatric pointers

A ventricular gallop is normally heard in children. However, it may accompany congenital abnormalities—such as large ventricular septal defect and patent ductus arteriosus—associated with congestive heart failure. It may also result from sickle cell anemia. Clearly, this gallop must be correlated with the patient's associated signs and symptoms to be of diagnostic value.

Genital Lesions in the Male

Among the diverse lesions that may affect the male genitalia are warts, papules, ulcers, scales, and pustules. These common lesions may be painful or painless, singular or multiple. They may be limited to the genitalia or may also occur elsewhere on the body.

Genital lesions may result from infection, neoplasms, parasites, allergy, or the effects of drugs. Frequently, these lesions profoundly affect the patient's self-image. In fact, he may hesitate to seek medical attention, fearing malignancy or sexually transmitted disease. Unfortunately, self-treatment may alter the lesions, making differential diagnosis especially difficult.

Assessment

Begin by asking the patient when he first noticed the lesion. Did it erupt after he began taking a new drug or after a trip out of the country? Has he had similar lesions before? If so, did he get medical treatment for them? Find out if he's been treating the lesion himself. If so, what measures is he using? Does he have any itching? Is it constant or does it bother him only at night? Note if the lesion is painful. Next, take a complete sexual history, noting the frequency of relations and the number of sexual partners.

Before you examine the patient, observe his clothing. Do his pants fit properly? Tight pants or underwear, especially in nonabsorbent fabrics, may promote the growth of bacteria and fungi. Examine his entire skin, noting the location, size, color, and pattern of the lesions. Do genital lesions resemble those on other parts of the body? Palpate for nodules, masses, and tenderness. Also look for bleeding, edema, or signs of infection, such as erythema. Finally, take the patient's vital signs.

Medical causes

• *Balanitis and balanoposthitis.* Typically, balanitis (glans infection) and posthitis (prepuce infection) occur together (balanoposthitis), causing painful ulceration on the glans, foreskin, or penile shaft. Ulceration is usually preceded by 2 to 3 days of prepuce irritation and soreness, followed by foul discharge and edema. The patient may then develop features of acute infection, such as fever with chills, malaise, and dysuria. Without treatment, the ulcers may deepen and multiply. Eventually, the entire penis and scrotum may become gangrenous, resulting in life-threatening sepsis.

• *Bowen's disease.* This painless, premalignant lesion commonly occurs on the penis or scrotum but may also appear elsewhere. It appears as a brownish red, raised, scaly, indurated plaque, which may ulcerate at its center.

• *Candidiasis.* When this infection involves the anogenital area, it produces erythematous, weepy, circumscribed lesions, usually under the prepuce. Sometimes, vesicles and pustules also develop.

• *Chancroid.* In this sexually transmitted disease, one or more lesions erupt, usually on the groin, inner thigh, or penis. Within 24 hours, the lesion changes from a reddened area to a small papule. (A similar papule may erupt on the tongue, lip, breast, or umbilicus.) It then becomes an inflamed pustule that rapidly ulcerates. This painful—usually deep—ulcer bleeds easily and frequently has a purulent gray or yellow exudate covering its base. Rarely more than 2 cm in diameter, it's typically irregular in shape. Accompanying the ulcer may be a headache, malaise, and a fever that reaches 102.2° F. (39° C.). The inguinal lymph nodes also enlarge, become very tender, and may drain pus. Phimosis may develop as the ulcer heals.

• *Erythroplasia of Queyrat.* This premalignant lesion may occur on the penis, glans, or corona. Typically, it appears as a red, raised, indurated plaque, which may have an ulcerated center.

• *Folliculitis and furunculosis.* Hair follicle infection may cause red, sharply pointed lesions that are tender and swollen with central pustules. If folliculitis progresses to furunculosis, these lesions become hard, painful nodules that may gradually enlarge and rupture, discharging pus and necrotic material. Rupture relieves the pain, but erythema and edema may persist for days or weeks.

• *Fournier's gangrene.* In this life-threatening cellulitis, the scrotum suddenly becomes tense, swollen, painful, red, warm, and glossy. As gangrene develops, the scrotum also becomes moist. Fever and malaise may accompany these scrotal changes.

• *Genital herpes.* Caused by herpesvirus Type II, this infection produces fluid-filled vesicles on the glans penis, foreskin, or penile shaft and, occasionally, on the mouth or anus. Usually painless at first, these vesicles may rupture and become extensive, shallow, painful ulcers accompanied by redness, marked edema, and tender, inguinal lymph nodes. Other findings may include fever, malaise, and dysuria. If the vesicles recur in the same area, the patient will usually feel localized numbness and tingling before they erupt. Typically, associated inflammation is less marked.

• *Genital warts.* Most common in uncircumcised, sexually active males, genital warts initially develop on the subpreputial sac, urethral meatus, and less commonly the penile shaft and then spread to the perineum and the perianal area. These painless warts start as tiny red or pink swellings that may grow to 4″ (10.2 cm) and become pedunculated. Multiple swellings are common, giving the warts a cauliflower appearance. Infected warts are also malodorous.

• *Granuloma inguinale.* Initially, this rare, chronic venereal infection causes a single, painless macule or papule on the external genitalia that ulcerates and becomes a raised, beefy-red lesion with a granulated, friable border. Then other painless lesions may erupt and blend together on the glans penis, foreskin, or penile shaft. Sometimes lesions develop on the nose, mouth, or pharynx, too. Eventually, these lesions become infected, foul-smelling, and painful and may be accompanied by pseudobuboes, fever, weight loss, malaise, and signs of anemia, such as weakness. Later, lesions are marked by fibrosis, keloidal scarring, and depigmentation.

• *Leukoplakia.* This precancerous disorder is characterized by white, scaly patches on the glans and prepuce accompanied by skin thickening and occasionally fissures.

• *Lichen planus.* Small, polygonal, violet papules develop on the glans penis in this disorder. Usually, they're shiny and less than 3 cm in diameter and have milky striations. They may be linear or coalesce into plaques. Occasionally, oral lesions precede genital lesions. Also, lesions may affect the lower back, ankles, and lower legs. Accompanying findings may include pruritus, distorted nails, and alopecia.

RECOGNIZING COMMON MALE GENITAL LESIONS

A wide variety of lesions may affect the male genitalia. Some of the more common ones and their causes appear below.

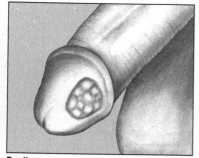

Penile cancer causes a painless ulcerative lesion on the glans or foreskin, possibly accompanied by a foul-smelling discharge.

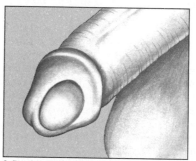

A fixed drug eruption causes a bright red-to-purplish lesion on the glans penis.

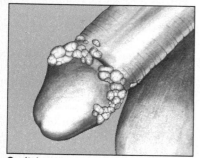

Genital warts are marked by clusters of flesh-colored papillary growths that may be barely visible or several inches in diameter.

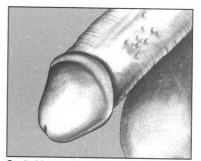

Genital herpes begins as a swollen, slightly pruritic wheal and becomes a group of small vesicles or blisters on the foreskin, glans, or penile shaft.

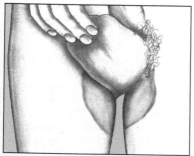

Tinea cruris, or "jock itch," produces itchy patches of well-defined, slightly raised, scaly lesions that usually affect the inner thighs and groin.

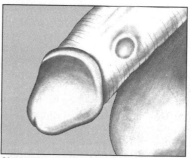

Chancroid causes a painful ulcer that's usually less than 2 cm in diameter and bleeds easily. The lesion may be deep and covered by a gray or yellow exudate at its base.

• *Lymphogranuloma venereum.* One to three weeks after sexual exposure, this disorder may produce a penile erosion or papule that heals rapidly and spontaneously; in fact, it often goes unnoticed. A few days or weeks later, the inguinal and subinguinal nodes enlarge, becoming painful, fluctuant masses. If these nodes become infected, they rupture and form sinus tracts, discharging a thick, yellow, granular secretion. Eventually, a scar or chronic indurated mass forms in the inguinal area. Systemic signs and symptoms are a skin rash, fever with chills, headache, joint and muscle pain, malaise, and weight loss.

• *Pediculosis pubis.* This parasitic infestation is characterized by erythematous, itching papules in the pubic area and around the anus, abdomen, and thigh. Inspection may detect grayish white specks (lice eggs) attached to hair shafts. Skin irritation from scratching in these areas is common.

• *Penile cancer.* Usually, this cancer produces a painless, ulcerative lesion or enlarging "wart" on the glans or foreskin. It may be accompanied by localized pain, though, if the foreskin becomes unretractable. Examination may reveal a foul-smelling discharge from the prepuce, a firm lump in the glans, and enlarged lymph nodes. Late signs and symptoms may include dysuria, pain, bleeding from the lesion, and urinary retention and bladder distention associated with obstruction of the urinary tract.

• *Psoriasis.* Red, raised, scaly plaques typically affect the scalp, chest, knees, elbows, and lower back. When they occur on the groin or on the shaft and glans of the penis, the plaques are usually redder and lack the characteristic silver scale. Commonly, the patient reports itching and, occasionally, pain from dry, cracked, encrusted lesions. Nail pitting and joint stiffness may also occur.

• *Scabies.* Mites burrow under the skin in this disorder, possibly causing crusted lesions on the glans and shaft of the penis and on the scrotum. Lesions may also occur on the wrists, elbows, axillae, and waist. Usually, they're threadlike and 1 to 10 cm long and have a swollen nodule or red papule that contains the mite. Nocturnal itching is typical and commonly causes excoriation.

• *Seborrheic dermatitis.* Initially, this disorder causes erythematous, scaling papules that enlarge to form annular plaques. These itchy plaques may affect the glans and shaft of the penis, scrotum, and groin as well as the scalp, chest, eyebrows, back, axillae, and umbilicus.

• *Syphilis.* Two to four weeks after exposure to *Treponema pallidum*, one or more primary lesions, or chancres, may erupt on the genitalia; occasionally, they also erupt elsewhere on the body. The chancre usually starts as a small, red, fluid-filled papule and then erodes to form a painless, firm, indurated, shallow ulcer with a clear base or, less commonly, a hard papule. This lesion gradually involutes and disappears. Painless, unilateral regional lymphadenopathy is also typical.

• *Tinea cruris.* Also called "jock itch," this fungal infection usually causes sharply defined, slightly raised, scaling patches on the inner thigh or groin and, less commonly, on the scrotum and penis. Pruritus may be severe.

• *Urticaria.* This common allergic reaction is characterized by intensely pruritic hives, which may appear on the genitalia, especially on the foreskin or shaft of the penis. These distinct, raised, evanescent wheals are surrounded by an erythematous flare.

Other causes
• *Drugs.* Phenolphthalein, barbiturates, and certain broad-spectrum antibiotics, like tetracycline and sulfonamides, may cause a fixed drug eruption and a genital lesion.

Special considerations
Many disorders produce penile lesions that resemble those of syphilis. Expect

to screen every patient with penile lesions for sexually transmitted disease, using the dark-field examination and the Venereal Disease Research Laboratory (VDRL) test. Also prepare the patient for biopsy to confirm or rule out penile cancer, as ordered. Provide emotional support, especially if cancer is suspected.

Explain to the patient how to use prescribed ointments or creams. Use a heat lamp to dry moist lesions, or advise sitz baths to relieve crusting and itching. Also instruct the patient to report any changes in the lesions.

To prevent cross-contamination, wash your hands before and after every patient contact. Wear gloves when handling urine or performing catheter care. Dispose of all needles carefully. Also double-bag all material contaminated by secretions.

Pediatric pointers
In infants, contact dermatitis or "diaper rash" is common; it may produce minor irritation or bright red, weepy, excoriated lesions. Use of disposable diapers and careful cleaning of the penis and scrotum are two measures to help reduce diaper rash.

In children, impetigo may cause pustules with thick, yellow, weepy crusts. Like adults, children may also develop genital warts, but they will need more reassurance that the treatment (excision) won't hurt or castrate them.

In adolescents ages 15 to 19, the incidence of sexually transmitted disease—and related genital lesions—is high. Syphilis, however, may also be congenital.

Grunting Respirations

Characterized by a deep, low-pitched grunting sound at the end of each breath, these respirations are a chief sign of respiratory distress in infants and children. They may be soft and heard only on auscultation, or loud and clearly audible without a stethoscope. Typically, the intensity of grunting respirations reflects the severity of respiratory distress. The grunting sound coincides with closure of the glottis—an effort to increase end-expiratory pressure in the lungs and prolong alveolar gas exchange, thereby enhancing ventilation and perfusion.

Grunting respirations indicate intrathoracic disease with lower respiratory involvement. Although they may also occur in adults with severe respiratory distress, they're not as common. Whether they occur in children or adults, grunting respirations demand immediate medical attention.

Assessment
If the patient has grunting respirations, quickly check for other signs of respiratory distress. These include tachypnea (a respiratory rate of 60 breaths/minute in infants, 40 breaths/minute in children ages 1 to 5, or 30 breaths/minute in children over age 5); accessory muscle use; substernal, subcostal, or intercostal retractions; nasal flaring; tachycardia (160 beats/minute in infants, 120 to 140 beats/minute in children ages 1 to 5, or 120 beats/minute in children over age 5); cyanotic lips or nail beds; hypotension (< 80/40 in infants, < 80/50 in children ages 1 to 5, or < 90/55 in children over age 5); and decreased level of consciousness. If you detect any of these signs, have another nurse notify the doctor while you gather emergency equipment, such as suction apparatus, an airway, and oxygen setup. If the patient's a premature infant, assist with intubation and mechanical ventilation.

After addressing the patient's respiratory status, ask his parents when the grunting respirations began. If the patient is a premature infant, find out his gestational age. Ask the parents if anyone in the home has had an upper respiratory infection (URI) recently. Has the patient had signs of a URI, such as a runny nose, cough, low-grade fever, or anorexia? Does he have a history of frequent colds or URIs? Ask the parents to describe changes in the infant's activity level. Is he lethargic or less alert than usual?

Begin the physical examination by auscultating the lungs, especially the lower lobes. Note diminished or abnormal sounds, such as crackles or sibilant rhonchi, which may indicate mucous or fluid buildup. If the patient has a cough, note whether it's productive or nonproductive. Also characterize the color, amount, and consistency of any nasal discharge or sputum.

Medical causes

• *Congestive heart failure.* A late sign of left heart failure, grunting respirations accompany increasing pulmonary edema. Associated features include productive cough, crackles, and chest wall retractions. Typically, the child has anorexia, is lethargic, and tires easily. Cyanosis may also be present, depending on the underlying congenital cardiac defect.

• *Respiratory distress syndrome.* The result of lung immaturity in a premature infant (< 37 weeks gestation), this syndrome initially causes audible expiratory grunts along with intercostal, subcostal, or substernal retractions; tachycardia; and tachypnea. Later, as respiratory distress tires the infant, apnea or irregular respirations replace the grunting. Severe respiratory distress is characterized by cyanosis, dramatic nasal flaring, lethargy, bradycardia, and hypotension. Eventually, the infant becomes unresponsive. Auscultation reveals harsh, diminished breath sounds and crackles over the base of the lungs on deep inspiration. Oliguria and peripheral edema may also occur.

• *Staphylococcus aureus pneumonia.* Life-threatening bacterial pneumonia primarily affects infants under age 1 and often follows URIs or colds. It causes grunting respirations accompanied by high fever, tachypnea, productive

cough, anorexia, and lethargy. Auscultation reveals diminished breath sounds, scattered crackles, and sibilant rhonchi over the affected lung. As the disorder progresses, there may also be severe dyspnea, substernal and subcostal retractions, nasal flaring, cyanosis, and increasing lethargy. Some infants display gastrointestinal signs, such as vomiting, diarrhea, and abdominal distention.

Special considerations

Closely monitor the patient's condition. Keep emergency equipment nearby in case respiratory distress worsens. Prepare to administer oxygen using an oxygen hood or tent, as ordered. To help prevent oxygen-induced retrolental fibroplasia—retina and lens damage resulting in permanent blindness—continually monitor arterial blood gases (ABGs) and deliver the minimum amount of oxygen possible. Whenever ABGs are drawn, record the amount of oxygen being given, the patient's temperature, and whether he was crying.

Begin inhalation therapy with bronchodilators, or antimicrobials, as ordered. Follow this with chest physical therapy (CPT), as needed. (See *Positioning the Infant for Chest Physical Therapy,* pages 354 and 355). Schedule CPT before meals to help prevent severe or spasmodic coughing and resultant vomiting. Try to group CPT with other treatments or activities, such as bathing, to ensure regular 2- to 4-hour rest periods.

Prepare the patient for chest X-rays, as ordered. Because sedatives are contraindicated in respiratory distress, help restrain the restless child during testing, as necessary. To prevent exposure to radiation, wear a lead apron and cover the child's genital area with a lead shield. If the doctor also orders a blood culture, make sure to record any current antibiotic treatment on the laboratory slip.

Remember to explain all procedures to the patient's parents and to provide emotional support.

POSITIONING THE INFANT FOR CHEST PHYSICAL THERAPY

The infant with grunting respirations may need chest physical therapy to mobilize and drain excess lung secretions. Auscultate first to locate congested areas and determine the best drainage position. Then review the illustrations here, which show the various drainage positions and where to place your hands for percussion. When you percuss the infant, use the fingers of one hand. You'll also vibrate these fingers and move them toward the infant's head to facilitate drainage.

Place the infant supine to percuss and drain the anterior segments of the upper lobes.

Hold the infant upright and about 30° forward to percuss and drain the apical segments of the upper lobes.

Use this position to percuss and drain the posterior segments of the upper lobes.

Hold the infant at a 45° angle on his side with his head down about 15° to percuss and drain the right middle lobe.

Place the infant in a supine position with his head 30° lower than his feet to percuss and drain the anterior segments of the lower lobes.

Place the infant on his side with his head down 30° to percuss and drain the lateral basal segments of the lower lobes. Repeat this on the other side.

Position the infant prone with his head down 30° to percuss and drain the posterior basal segments of the lower lobes.

Use a prone position to percuss and drain the superior segments of the lower lobes.

Gum Bleeding
[Gingival bleeding]

Bleeding gums usually result from dental disorders or, less often, from blood dyscrasias or the effects of certain drugs. Physiologic causes of this common sign include pregnancy, which can produce gum swelling in the first or second trimester (pregnancy epulis); atmospheric pressure changes, which most commonly affect divers and aviators; and oral trauma. Bleeding ranges from slight oozing to life-threatening hemorrhage. It may be spontaneous or may follow trauma. Occasionally, direct pressure can control it.

Assessment

If you detect profuse, spontaneous bleeding in the oral cavity, quickly check the patient's airway and assess for signs of cardiovascular collapse, such as tachycardia and hypotension. Have another nurse notify the doctor as you suction the patient. Apply direct pressure to the bleeding site. Expect to assist with airway insertion, to administer intravenous fluids, and to collect serum samples for diagnostic evaluation.

If gum bleeding isn't an emergency, obtain a history. Find out when the bleeding began. Has it been continuous or intermittent? Does it occur spontaneously or when the patient brushes his teeth? Have the patient show you the site of the bleeding, if possible.

Determine if the patient or his family has bleeding tendencies; for example, ask about easy bruising and frequent nosebleeds. How much does the patient bleed after a tooth extraction? Does he have a history of liver or spleen disease? Next, check the patient's dental history. Find out how often he brushes his teeth and goes to the dentist. Has he seen a dentist recently? To evaluate nutritional status, have the patient describe his normal diet and intake of alcohol. Finally, note any prescription and over-the-counter drugs the patient takes.

Next, perform a complete oral examination. If the patient wears dentures, have him remove them. Examine the gums to determine the site and amount of bleeding. Gums normally appear pink and rippled with their margins snugly against the teeth. Check for inflammation, pockets around the teeth, swelling, retraction, hypertrophy, discoloration, and gum hyperplasia. Note obvious decay; discoloration; foreign material, such as food; and absence of any teeth.

Medical causes

• **Agranulocytosis.** Spontaneous gum bleeding and other systemic hemorrhages may occur in this hematologic disorder. Typically, the disorder causes progressive fatigue and weakness followed by signs of infection, such as fever and chills. Inspection may reveal oral and perianal lesions, which are usually rough-edged with a gray or black membrane.

• **Aplastic anemia.** In this disorder, profuse or scant gum bleeding may follow trauma. Other signs of bleeding—such as epistaxis and ecchymoses—are also characteristic. The patient has progressive weakness and fatigue, shortness of breath, headache, pallor, and possibly fever. Eventually, tachycardia and signs of congestive heart failure, such as neck vein distention and dyspnea, also develop.

• **Chemical irritants.** Occupational exposure to benzene may irritate the gums, resulting in bleeding. Other signs of abnormal bleeding may accompany limb weakness and sensory changes.

• **Cirrhosis.** Gum bleeding is a late sign of cirrhosis that occurs with epistaxis and other bleeding tendencies. Many other late effects occur, such as ascites, hepatomegaly, pruritus, and jaundice.

• **Ehlers-Danlos syndrome.** In this congenital syndrome, gums bleed easily after toothbrushing. Easy bruising and other signs of abnormal bleeding are also typical. Skin is fragile and hyperelastic; joints are hyperextendible.

• *Familial thrombasthenia.* This hereditary blood platelet disorder causes spontaneous bleeding from the oral cavity, especially the gums. Commonly, the patient will have purpura, epistaxis, hemarthrosis, and signs of gastrointestinal bleeding, such as hematemesis and melena.

• *Giant cell epulis.* This pedunculated granuloma occurs on the gums or alveolar process in front of the molars. It's dark red and vascular, resembling a surface ulcer. Gums bleed easily with slight trauma.

• *Gingivitis.* In this disorder, reddened and edematous gums are characteristic. The gingivae between the teeth become bulbous and bleed easily with slight trauma. However, in *acute necrotizing ulcerative gingivitis*, bleeding is spontaneous. The gums also become so painful that the patient may be unable to eat. A characteristic grayish yellow pseudomembrane develops over punched-out gum erosions. Offensive halitosis is typical and may be accompanied by headache, malaise, fever, and cervical adenopathy.

• *Hemophilia.* Here, hemorrhage occurs from many sites in the oral cavity, especially the gums. *Mild hemophilia* causes easy bruising, hematomas, epistaxis, bleeding gums, and prolonged bleeding during and up to 8 days after even minor surgery. *Moderate hemophilia* produces more frequent episodes of abnormal bleeding and occasional bleeding into the joints, which may cause swelling and pain. *Severe hemophilia* causes spontaneous or severe bleeding after minor trauma, possibly resulting in large subcutaneous and intramuscular hematomas. Bleeding into joints and muscles causes pain, swelling, extreme tenderness, and possibly permanent deformity. Bleeding near peripheral nerves causes peripheral neuropathies, pain, paresthesias, and muscle atrophy. Signs of anemia and fever may follow bleeding. Severe blood loss may lead to shock and death.

• *Hereditary hemorrhagic telangiectasia.* This disorder is characterized by red to violet spiderlike hemorrhagic areas on the gums, which blanch on pressure and bleed spontaneously. These telangiectases may also occur on the lips, buccal mucosa, and palate as well as the face, ears, scalp, hands, arms, feet, and under the nails. Epistaxis commonly occurs early and is difficult to control. Hemoptysis and signs of gastrointestinal bleeding may also occur.

• *Hypofibrinogenemia.* In this rare disorder, the patient has frequent, spontaneous episodes of severe gum bleeding. Hematomas, ecchymoses, and epistaxis are also common. Signs of gastrointestinal bleeding, such as hematemesis, and of central nervous system bleeding, such as focal neurologic deficits, may also occur.

• *Leukemia.* Easy gum bleeding is an early sign of acute monocytic, lymphocytic, or myelocytic leukemia. It's accompanied by gum swelling, necrosis, and petechiae. The soft, tender gums appear glossy and bluish. *Acute leukemia* causes severe prostration marked by high fever and bleeding tendencies, such as epistaxis and prolonged menses. Sometimes, it also causes dyspnea, tachycardia, palpitations, and abdominal or bone pain. Later effects may include confusion, headaches, vomiting, seizures, papilledema, and nuchal rigidity.

Chronic leukemia usually develops insidiously, producing less severe bleeding tendencies. Other effects may include anorexia, weight loss, low-grade fever, chills, skin eruptions, and enlarged spleen, tonsils, and lymph nodes. Signs of anemia, such as fatigue and pallor, may occur.

• *Pemphigoid (benign mucosal).* Most common in women between ages 40 and 50, this autoimmune disorder typically causes thick-walled gum lesions that rupture, desquamate, and then bleed easily. Extensive scars form with healing, and the gums remain red for months. Lesions may also develop on

PREVENTING BLEEDING GUMS

Dear Patient,

Follow these tips to improve oral hygiene and prevent your gums from bleeding:
- Eliminate between-meal snacks and reduce carbohydrate intake to help prevent plaque formation on your teeth.
- Visit the dentist once every 6 months for thorough plaque removal.
- Avoid citrus fruits and juices, rough or spicy food, alcohol, and tobacco if they irritate mouth ulcers or sore gums and cause bleeding. Be sure to take vitamin C supplements if you can't consume citrus fruits and juices.
- If dentures make your gums bleed, wear them *only* during meals.
- Avoid using toothpicks, which may cause gum injury and infection.

- Brush your teeth gently after every meal, using a soft-bristle toothbrush held at a 45° angle to the gum line.
- If the doctor tells you not to brush your teeth, rinse your mouth with salt water or hydrogen peroxide and water. Avoid using commercial mouthwashes which contain irritating alcohol.
- Floss your teeth daily to remove plaque, unless flossing causes pain or bleeding.
- Use a water pik on the low pressure setting to massage your gums.
- Use aspirin *sparingly* for toothaches or general pain relief.
- Control gum bleeding by applying direct pressure to the area with a gauze pad soaked in ice water.

other parts of the oral mucosa, conjunctiva and, less often, the skin. Secondary fibrous bands may lead to dysphagia, hoarseness, or blindness.

- **Periodontal disease.** Typically, chewing, toothbrushing, or gum probing initiates gum bleeding, or bleeding occurs spontaneously. As gingivae separate from the bone, pus-filled pockets develop around the teeth and, occasionally, pus can be expressed. Other findings include unpleasant taste with halitosis, facial pain, loose teeth, and dental calculus and plaque.

- **Pernicious anemia.** Gum bleeding and a sore tongue often make eating painful in this disorder. Among other cardinal symptoms are weakness and paresthesias. The patient's lips, gums, and tongue appear markedly pale, and his sclera and skin are jaundiced. Other features are typically widespread, affect the gastrointestinal, cardiovascular, and central nervous systems, and include altered bowel and bladder habits, personality changes, ataxia, tinnitus, dyspnea, and tachycardia.

- **Polycythemia vera.** In this disorder, engorged gums ooze blood following slight trauma. Usually, polycythemia vera turns the oral mucosa—especially the gums and tongue—a deep red-violet. Among associated findings are headache, dyspnea, dizziness, fatigue, paresthesias, tinnitus, double or blurred vision, pruritus, epigastric distress, weight loss, increased blood pressure, ruddy cyanosis, ecchymosis, and hepatosplenomegaly.

- **Pyogenic granuloma.** Frequently affecting the gums, lips, tongue, and buccal mucosa, this granuloma may ulcerate and bleed spontaneously or with slight trauma. The lesion is pedunculated with a smooth or warty surface.

- **Thrombocytopenia.** Blood usually oozes between the teeth and gums; however, severe bleeding may follow minor trauma. Associated signs of hemorrhage include large blood-filled bullae in the mouth, petechiae, ecchymosis, epistaxis, hematuria, and others. Malaise, fatigue, weakness, and lethargy eventually develop.

• **Thrombocytopenic purpura (idiopathic).** Profuse gum bleeding occurs in this disorder. Its classic feature, though, is spontaneous hemorrhagic skin lesions that range from pinpoint petechiae to massive hemorrhages. The patient has a tendency to bruise easily, petechiae on the oral mucosa, and possibly melena, epistaxis, or hematuria.

• **Vitamin C deficiency.** This deficiency causes swollen, spongy, tender gums that bleed easily. Between the teeth, the gums are red or purple. The teeth themselves become loose and may be surrounded by pockets filled with clotted blood. Other findings include muscle and joint pain, petechiae, ecchymoses, splinter hemorrhages in the nail beds, and ocular hemorrhages. Associated effects are anorexia, dry mouth, pallor, weakness, lethargy, insomnia, scaly skin, and psychological disturbances, such as depression or hysteria.

• **Vitamin K deficiency.** Usually, gums that bleed after toothbrushing are the first sign of vitamin K deficiency. Other signs of abnormal bleeding, such as ecchymosis, epistaxis, and hematuria, may occur. Gastrointestinal bleeding may produce hematemesis and melena, while intracranial bleeding may cause decreased level of consciousness and focal neurologic deficits.

Other causes

• **Drugs.** Coumadin and heparin interfere with blood clotting and may cause prolonged gum bleeding. Aspirin abuse may alter platelets, producing bleeding gums. Localized gum bleeding may also occur with mucosal "aspirin burn" caused by dissolving aspirin near an aching tooth.

Special considerations

When providing mouth care, avoid using lemon-glycerin swabs, which may burn or dry the gums. Teach the patient about mouth and gum care. (See *Preventing Bleeding Gums.*)

Prepare the patient for diagnostic tests, such as blood studies or facial X-rays.

Pediatric pointers

In newborns, bleeding gums may result from vitamin K deficiency, associated with a lack of normal intestinal flora or poor maternal nutrition. In infants who primarily drink cow's milk and don't receive vitamin supplements, bleeding gums can result from vitamin C deficiency.

Encourage parents to instill good oral hygiene habits early. Daily toothbrushing in the morning and before bedtime should begin with eruption of the first tooth. When the child has all of his baby teeth, he should begin receiving regular dental checkups.

Gum Swelling

[Gingival swelling]

Gum swelling may result from one of two mechanisms: an increase in the size of existing gum cells (hypertrophy) or an increase in their number (hyperplasia). This common sign may involve one or many papillae—the triangular-shaped bits of gum between adjacent teeth. Occasionally, the gums swell markedly, obscuring the teeth altogether. Usually, the swelling is most prominent on the labia and bucca.

Most commonly, gum swelling results from the effects of phenytoin. It may also result from nutritional deficiency and certain systemic disorders. Physiologic gum swelling and bleeding may occur during the first or second trimester of pregnancy when hormonal changes make the gums highly vascular; even slight irritation causes swelling and gives the papillae a characteristic raspberry hue (pregnancy epulis). Irritating dentures may also cause swelling associated with red, soft, moveable masses on the gums.

Assessment

After ruling out pregnancy or the use of phenytoin or similar prescription drugs as the cause of gum swelling, take a history. Have the patient describe the swelling fully. Has he had it before? Is it localized or generalized? Find out when the swelling began and ask about any aggravating or alleviating factors. Note if the swelling is painful. Then explore the patient's medical history, focusing on major illnesses, bleeding disorders, and pregnancies. Also check his dental history. Does he wear dentures? If so, are they new? Ask about use of alcohol and tobacco, which are gum irritants. Then have the patient describe his diet to assess nutritional status. Be sure to ask about his intake of citrus fruits and vegetables.

Next, inspect the patient's mouth in a good light. If he wears dentures, ask him to remove them before you begin. As you examine the gums, characterize their color and texture, and note any ulcers, lesions, masses, lumps, or debris-filled pockets around the teeth. Then inspect the teeth for discoloration, obvious decay, and looseness.

Medical causes

• **Crohn's disease.** Granular or cobblestone gum swelling occurs in this disorder, which is characterized by cramping abdominal pain and diarrhea. In *acute* Crohn's disease, the patient may also have nausea, fever, tachycardia, abdominal tenderness and guarding, hyperactive bowel sounds, and abdominal distention. *Chronic* effects are anorexia, weight loss, a palpable lower quadrant mass, perianal lesions, and occasionally constipation.

• **Fibrous hyperplasia (idiopathic).** In this disorder, the gums become diffusely enlarged and may even cover the teeth. Large, firm, painless masses of fibrous tissue form on the gums and may prevent tooth eruption and cause lip protrusion and difficulty chewing.

• **Leukemia.** Gum swelling is frequently an early sign—especially in acute monocytic, lymphocytic, or myelocytic leukemia. Usually, the swelling is localized and accompanied by necrosis. The tender gums appear blue and

glossy and bleed easily. *Acute leukemia* also causes severe prostration, high fever, and signs of abnormal bleeding, such as ecchymoses and prolonged menses. Sometimes it produces dyspnea, tachycardia, palpitations, and abdominal or bone pain. Late effects may include confusion, headache, vomiting, seizures, papilledema, and nuchal rigidity. In *chronic leukemia,* signs and symptoms develop insidiously such as malaise, pallor, low-grade fever, chills, and minor bleeding tendencies. Enlarged tonsils, lymph nodes, and spleen are also common.

• **Vitamin C deficiency.** The gums are spongy, tender, and edematous, and the papillae appear red or purple. The gums bleed easily, and inspection may reveal pockets filled with clotted blood around loose teeth. Associated findings include anorexia, pallor, dry mouth, scaly dermatitis, weakness, lethargy, insomnia, and signs of abnormal bleeding, such as myalgia and arthralgia (possibly with swelling), from hemorrhage into joints and muscles. Occasionally, psychological changes, such as depression and hysteria, occur.

Other causes

• **Drugs.** A common side effect of phenytoin is gum swelling. Cyclosporine, a drug used to prevent rejection of transplanted organs, also produces this sign in about 15% of patients.

Special considerations

Because gum swelling may affect the patient's appearance, offer emotional support and reassure him that swelling usually resolves with treatment. For phenytoin-induced swelling, substitute another anticonvulsant, such as ethotoin, and prepare the patient for surgery, as ordered.

When providing mouth care, avoid using lemon-glycerin swabs, which can irritate the gums. Instead, use a soft toothbrush or one that's padded with sponge or gauze. To prevent further swelling, teach the patient the basics of good nutrition. Remind him to eat foods high in vitamin C daily. Also encourage him to avoid gum irritants, such as commercial mouthwashes, alcohol, and tobacco. Advise him to see a periodontist at least every 6 months.

Pediatric pointers
Gum swelling in children commonly results from nutritional deficiency. It may also accompany phenytoin therapy; in fact, drug-induced gum swelling is more common in children than in adults. Fortunately, this dramatic swelling is usually painless and limited to one or two papillae. Gum swelling may also result from idiopathic fibrous hyperplasia and from inflammatory gum hyperplasia, which is especially common in pubertal girls.

Good nutrition and oral hygiene help control gum swelling in children. So encourage parents to make toothbrushing as much fun as possible.

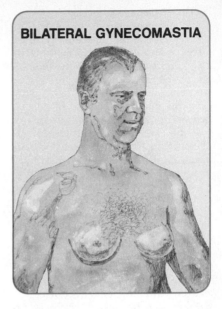

BILATERAL GYNECOMASTIA

Gynecomastia

Occurring only in males, gynecomastia refers to excessive mammary gland development, resulting in increased breast size. This size change may be barely palpable or immediately obvious. Usually bilateral, gynecomastia may be associated with breast tenderness and milk secretion.

Normally, several hormones regulate breast development. Estrogens, growth hormone, and corticosteroids stimulate ductal growth, while progesterone and prolactin stimulate growth of the alveolar lobules. Although the pathophysiology of gynecomastia isn't fully understood, hormonal imbalance—particularly a change in the estrogen-androgen ratio and an increase in prolactin—is a likely contributing factor. This explains why gynecomastia commonly results from the effects of estrogens and other drugs. It may also result from hormone-secreting tumors and from endocrine, genetic, hepatic, and renal disorders. Physiologic gynecomastia may occur in neonatal, pubertal, and geriatric males due to normal fluctuations in hormone levels.

Assessment
Begin the assessment by asking the patient when he first noticed his breast enlargement. How old was he at the time? Since then have his breasts gotten progressively larger, smaller, or stayed the same? Is gynecomastia accompanied by breast tenderness or discharge? Next, take a thorough drug history, including prescription, over-the-counter, and street drugs. Then explore associated signs and symptoms, such as a testicular mass or pain, loss of libido, decreased potency, or loss of chest, axillary, and facial hair.

Focus the physical examination on the breasts, testicles, and penis. As you examine the breasts, note any asymmetry, dimpling, abnormal pigmentation, or ulceration. Observe the testicles for size and symmetry. Then palpate them to detect nodules, tenderness, or unusual consistency. Look for normal penile development after puberty, and note hypospadias.

Medical causes

• **Adrenal carcinoma.** Estrogen production by an adrenal tumor may produce a feminizing syndrome in males characterized by bilateral gynecomastia, loss of libido, impotence, testicular atrophy, and reduced facial hair growth. Cushingoid signs, like moon face and purple striae, may occur.

• **Breast cancer.** Painful unilateral gynecomastia develops rapidly in this disorder. Palpation may reveal a hard or stony breast lump suggesting malignancy. Breast examination may also detect changes in breast symmetry; thickening, dimpling, peau d'orange, or ulceration of the skin; and a warm, reddened area. The patient's nipples may produce a watery, bloody, or purulent discharge and may itch or burn. He may also have nipple erosion, deviation, flattening, or retraction.

• **Cirrhosis.** A late sign of cirrhosis, bilateral gynecomastia results from failure of the liver to inactivate circulating estrogens. It's often accompanied by testicular atrophy, decreased libido, impotence, and loss of facial, chest, and axillary hair. Other late signs and symptoms include mental changes, bleeding tendencies, spider angiomas, palmar erythema, severe pruritus and dry skin, fetor hepaticus, enlarged superficial abdominal veins, and possibly jaundice and hepatomegaly.

• **Hepatic carcinoma.** This carcinoma may produce bilateral gynecomastia and other characteristics of feminization, such as testicular atrophy, impotence, and reduced facial hair growth. The patient may complain of severe epigastric or right upper quadrant pain that's associated with a right upper quadrant mass. A large tumor may also produce a bruit on auscultation. Related findings may include anorexia, weight loss, dependent edema, fever, cachexia, and possibly jaundice or ascites.

• **Hermaphroditism.** In true hermaphroditism, ovarian and testicular tissues coexist, resulting in external genitalia with both feminine and masculine characteristics. At puberty, the patient typically develops marked bilateral gynecomastia. About half of these patients also display male menstruation in the form of cyclic hematuria.

• **Hypothyroidism.** Typically, this disorder produces bilateral gynecomastia along with bradycardia, cold intolerance, weight gain despite anorexia, and mental dullness. The patient may display periorbital edema and puffiness in the face, hands, and feet. His hair appears brittle and sparse and his skin is dry, pale, cool, and doughy.

• **Klinefelter's syndrome.** Painless bilateral gynecomastia first appears during adolescence in this genetic disorder. Before puberty, the patient also has abnormally small testicles and slight mental deficiency; after puberty, he has sparse facial hair, a small penis, decreased libido, and impotence.

• **Lung cancer.** Bronchogenic carcinoma or metastasis to the lung from testicular choriocarcinoma may result in bilateral gynecomastia. Other effects depend on the tumor's primary site but usually include weight loss, anorexia, fatigue, chronic cough, hemoptysis, clubbing, dyspnea, and diffuse chest pain. Fever and wheezing may occur.

• **Malnutrition.** Painful unilateral gynecomastia—known as refeeding gynecomastia—may occur when the patient begins to take nourishment again. Other effects of malnutrition include apathy, muscle wasting, weakness, limb paresthesias, anorexia, nausea, vomiting, and diarrhea. Inspection may reveal dull, sparse, dry hair; brittle nails; dark, swollen cheeks and lips; dry, flaky skin; and, occasionally, edema and hepatomegaly.

• **Pituitary tumor.** This hormone-secreting tumor causes bilateral gynecomastia accompanied by galactorrhea, impotence, and decreased libido. Other hormonal effects may include enlarged hands and feet, coarse facial features with prognathism, voice deepening, weight gain, increased blood pressure, diaphoresis, heat intolerance, hyperpigmentation, and thickened, oily skin. Paresthesia or sensory loss and muscle weakness commonly affect the limbs. If the tumor expands, it may cause blurred vision, diplopia, headache, or partial bitemporal hemianopia that may progress to blindness.

● *Reifenstein's syndrome.* This genetic disorder produces painless bilateral gynecomastia that appears at puberty. Associated signs may include hypospadias, testicular atrophy, and an underdeveloped penis.

● *Renal failure (chronic).* This disorder may produce bilateral gynecomastia accompanied by decreased libido and impotence. Among its more characteristic features, though, are ammonia breath odor, oliguria, fatigue, decreased mental acuity, convulsions, muscle cramps, and peripheral neuropathy. Common gastrointestinal effects include anorexia, nausea, vomiting, and constipation or diarrhea. The patient also typically has bleeding tendencies, pruritus, yellow-brown or bronze skin, and, occasionally, uremic frost and increased blood pressure.

● *Testicular failure (secondary).* Commonly associated with mumps or other infectious disorders, secondary testicular failure produces bilateral gynecomastia that appears after normal puberty. This disorder may also cause sparse facial hair, decreased libido, impotence, and testicular atrophy.

● *Testicular tumor.* Choriocarcinomas, Leydig's cell tumors, and other testicular tumors typically cause bilateral gynecomastia, nipple tenderness, and decreased libido. Because these tumors are usually painless, testicular swelling may be the patient's initial complaint. A firm mass and a heavy sensation in the scrotum may occur.

● *Thyrotoxicosis.* Bilateral gynecomastia may occur with loss of libido and impotence. Cardinal findings include tachycardia, palpitations, weight loss despite increased appetite, diarrhea, tremors, an enlarged thyroid, dyspnea, nervousness, diaphoresis, heat intolerance, and possibly exophthalmos. An S_3 or S_4 gallop may also occur.

Other causes

● *Drugs.* Typically, drugs produce painful unilateral gynecomastia. Estrogens used to treat prostatic cancer, including diethylstilbestrol (DES), estramustine, and chlorotrianisene, directly affect the estrogen-androgen ratio. Drugs that have an estrogen-like effect, such as digitalis and human chorionic gonadotropin, may do the same. Regular marijuana or heroin use reduces plasma testosterone, causing gynecomastia. Other drugs—such as spironolactone, cimetidine, and ketoconazole—produce this sign by interfering with androgen production or action. Some common drugs, including phenothiazines, tricyclic antidepressants, and antihypertensives, produce gynecomastia in an unknown way.

● *Treatments.* Gynecomastia may develop within weeks of starting hemodialysis for chronic renal failure. It may also follow major surgery or testicular irradiation.

Special considerations

To make the patient as comfortable as possible, apply cold compresses to his breasts and administer analgesics, as ordered.

Because gynecomastia may alter the patient's body image, provide emotional support. Reassure the patient that treatment can reduce the gynecomastia and that surgical removal of breast tissue can be done, if necessary.

Prepare the patient for diagnostic tests, including chest and skull X-rays and blood hormone levels.

Pediatric pointers

In newborns, gynecomastia may be associated with galactorrhea ("witch's milk"). They usually disappear in a few weeks but may persist until age 2.

Most males have physiologic gynecomastia at some time during adolescence, usually around age 14. This gynecomastia is usually asymmetrical and tender; it commonly resolves within 2 years and rarely persists beyond age 20.

halitosis • halo vision • headache • hearing loss • heat intolerance • Heberder
hematochezia • hematuria • hemianopia • hemoptysis • hepatomegaly • hiccu
hoarseness • Homans' sign • hyperpigmentation • hyperpnea • hypopigmenta
insomnia • intermittent claudication • Janeway's spots • jaundice • jaw pain •
distention • Kehr's sign • Kernig's sign • leg pain • level of consciousness—de
flashes • low birth weight • lymphadenopathy • masklike facies • McBurney's
sign • melena • menorrhagia • metrorrhagia • miosis • moon face • mouth le
muscle atrophy • muscle flaccidity • muscle spasms • muscle spasticity • mus
mydriasis • myoclonus • nasal flaring • nausea • neck pain • night blindness
nipple retraction • nocturia • nuchal rigidity • nystagmus • ocular deviation •
oliguria • opisthotonos • orofacial dyskinesia • orthopnea • orthostatic hypote
Osler's nodes • otorrhea • pallor • palpitations • papular rash • paralysis • pa
nocturnal dyspnea • peau d'orange • pericardial friction rub • peristaltic wa
photophobia • pica • pleural friction rub • polydipsia • polyphagia • polyuri
priapism • pruritus • psoas sign • psychotic behavior • ptosis • pulse—abser
bounding • pulse pressure—narrowed • pulse pressure—widened • pulse rh
pulsus alternans • pulsus bisferiens • pulsus paradoxus • pupils—nonreactiv
purple striae • purpura • pustular rash • pyrosis • raccoon's eyes • rebound
retractions—costal and sternal • rhinorrhea • rhonchi • Romberg's sign • sa
salivation—increased • salt craving • scotoma • scrotal swelling • seizure—a
seizure—generalized tonic-clonic • seizure—psychomotor • setting-sun sign •
skin—bronze • skin—clammy • skin—mottled • skin—scaly • skin turgor—
angioma • splenomegaly • stertorous respirations • stool—clay-colored • stri
tachycardia • tachypnea • taste abnormalities • tearing—increased • throat p
tracheal deviation • tracheal tugging • tremors • trismus • tunnel vision • ur
discharge • urinary frequency • urinary hesitancy • urinary incontinence • u
cloudiness • urticaria • vaginal bleeding—postmenopausal • vaginal dischar
vertigo • vesicular rash • violent behavior • vision loss • visual blurring • vis
vulvar lesions • weight gain—excessive • weight loss—excessive • wheezing
distention • abdominal mass • abdominal pain • abdominal rigidity • acces
agitation • alopecia • amenorrhea • amnesia • analgesia • anhidrosis • anor
anxiety • aphasia • apnea • apneustic respirations • apraxia • arm pain • a
athetosis • aura • Babinski's reflex • back pain • barrel chest • Battle's sign
bladder distention • blood pressure decrease • blood pressure increase • bov
bowel sounds—hyperactive • bowel sounds—hypoactive • bradycardia • br
dimpling • breast nodule • breast pain • breast ulcer • breath with ammoni
odor • breath with fruity odor • Brudzinski's sign • bruits • buffalo hump •
lait spots • capillary refill time—prolonged • carpopedal spasm • cat cry • c
asymmetrical • chest pain • Cheyne-Stokes respirations • chills • chorea • Cl
cogwheel rigidity • cold intolerance • confusion • conjunctival injection • cc
reflex—absent • costovertebral angle tenderness • cough—barking • cough—
productive • crackles • crepitation—bony • crepitation—subcutaneous • cry
cyanosis • decerebrate posture • decorticate posture • deep tendon reflexes—
reflexes—hypoactive • depression • diaphoresis • diarrhea • diplopia • dizz
absent • drooling • dysarthria • dysmenorrhea • dyspareunia • dyspepsia •
dystonia • dysuria • earache • edema—generalized • edema of the arms • e
of the legs • enophthalmos • enuresis • epistaxis • eructation • erythema • e
discharge • eye pain • facial pain • fasciculations • fatigue • fecal incontine
ever • flank pain • flatulence • fontanelle bulging • fontanelle depression •
bnormalities • gait—bizarre • gait—propulsive • gait—scissors • gait—spa

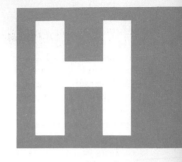

Halitosis

Halitosis describes any breath odor that's unpleasant, disagreeable, or offensive. Usually, it's easy to detect, but an embarrassed patient may take measures to hide it. Occasionally, the patient isn't aware of halitosis, although he may complain of a bad taste in his mouth. Or he may believe he has halitosis, but no one else can detect it (psychogenic halitosis).

Certain types of halitosis characterize specific disorders; for example, a fruity breath odor typifies ketoacidosis. (See "Breath with Ammonia Odor," "Breath with Fecal Odor," "Breath with Fruity Odor," and "Fetor Hepaticus.") Other types of halitosis include putrid, foul, fetid, and musty breath odors.

This common sign may result from disorders of the oral cavity, nasal passages, sinuses, or respiratory tract. Halitosis may also stem from gastrointestinal disorders associated with belching, regurgitation, or vomiting. It may be a side effect of oral or inhalant drugs.

Usually, halitosis results from cigarette smoking and ingestion of alcohol and certain foods, such as garlic and onions. Poor oral hygiene—especially in the patient with an orthodontic device, dentures, or dental caries—commonly causes halitosis. Surprisingly, offensive skin odors—for example, from foot perspiration—may be absorbed locally and later expelled by the lungs, resulting in halitosis.

Assessment

If you detect halitosis, try to characterize the odor. Does it smell fruity? Fecal? Musty? If the patient is aware of the halitosis, find out how long he's had it. Does he also have a bad taste in his mouth? Does he have difficulty swallowing or chewing? Any pain or tenderness?

Find out if the patient smokes or chews tobacco. Have him describe his diet and daily oral hygiene. Does he wear dentures? Complete the history by asking about chronic disorders and recent respiratory infection. If the patient reports a cough, find out if it's productive.

Begin the physical examination by assessing the patient's mouth, throat, and nose. Look for lesions, bleeding, drainage, obstruction, or signs of infection, such as redness and swelling. Assess for tenderness by percussing and palpating over the sinuses. Then auscultate the lungs for abnormal breath sounds. Finally, take vital signs.

Medical causes

- **Bowel obstruction.** Halitosis is a late sign of both small- and large-bowel obstruction. In *small-bowel obstruction,* vomiting of gastric, bilious, and then feculent material produces a related breath odor. Other findings include diarrhea or constipation, abdominal distention, and intermittent periumbilical cramping pain. Auscultation may initially reveal borborygmi and hyperactive bowel sounds; later, hypoactive or absent sounds signal complete obstruction. In *large-bowel obstruction,* fecal vomiting produces fecal breath odor. Unlike small-bowel obstruction, abdominal pain is milder, more constant, and usually located lower in the abdomen. Abdominal distention may be dramatic and loops of the large bowel may be visible.

● *Bronchiectasis.* Usually, this disorder produces foul or putrid halitosis; however, some patients may have a sickeningly sweet breath odor. Typically, the patient also has a chronic productive cough with copious, foul-smelling, mucopurulent sputum. The cough is aggravated by lying down and is most productive in the morning. Associated signs and symptoms frequently include exertional dyspnea, fatigue, malaise, weakness, and weight loss. Auscultation reveals coarse crackles over the affected lung areas during inspiration. Clubbing is a late sign.

● *Common cold.* A musty breath odor may accompany the common cold. Usually, this disorder also causes a dry, hacking cough with sore throat, sneezing, nasal congestion with rhinorrhea, headache, malaise, fatigue, and aching joints and muscles.

● *Esophageal cancer.* In this disorder, halitosis may accompany classic findings of dysphagia, hoarseness, chest pain, and weight loss. Nocturnal regurgitation and cachexia are late signs.

● *Gastric carcinoma.* Halitosis is a late sign of this uncommon malignancy. Accompanying findings include chronic dyspepsia, a vague feeling of fullness, nausea, anorexia, fatigue, pallor, weakness, altered bowel habits, weight loss, and muscle wasting. Hematemesis and melena reflect associated gastric bleeding.

● *Gastrojejunocolic fistula.* In this disorder, fecal vomiting is responsible for fecal breath odor. Typically, halitosis is preceded by intermittent diarrhea. Other signs and symptoms may include anorexia, weight loss, and abdominal pain and distention.

● *Gingivitis.* Characterized by red, edematous gums, this disorder may also cause halitosis. The gingivae between the teeth become bulbous and bleed easily with slight trauma.

Acute necrotizing ulcerative gingivitis also causes fetid breath, a bad taste in the mouth, and ulcers—especially between the teeth—that may become covered with a gray exudate. Severe ulceration may be accompanied by fever, cervical adenopathy, headache, and malaise.

● *Hepatic encephalopathy.* A characteristic late sign of this disorder is a musty, sweet, or mousy (new-mown hay) breath odor called fetor hepaticus. Other major late effects include coma, asterixis (flapping tremor), hyperactive reflexes, and positive Babinski's reflex.

● *Ketoacidosis.* Both diabetic and starvation ketoacidosis produce a fruity breath odor. Other common effects of these life-threatening conditions include orthostatic hypotension, generalized weakness, anorexia, abdominal pain, and altered level of consciousness.

Diabetic ketoacidosis also produces a rapid, thready pulse, nausea, and vomiting. Its early features are the triad of polydipsia, polyphagia, and polyuria. *Starvation ketoacidosis* also produces rapid, deep respirations (Kussmaul's respirations); weight loss; bradycardia; dry, scaly skin; sore tongue; muscle and tissue wasting; and abdominal distention. The patient displays signs of dehydration, such as oliguria and poor skin turgor.

● *Lung abscess.* This disorder typically causes putrid halitosis. Its major sign, though, is a productive cough with copious, purulent, often bloody sputum.

Other signs and symptoms include fever with chills, dyspnea, headache, anorexia, malaise, pleuritic chest pain, weight loss, and temporary clubbing. Auscultation may reveal crackles and amphoric breath sounds; percussion reveals dullness on the affected side.

• *Necrotizing ulcerative mucositis (acute).* A strong, putrid breath odor is characteristic here. Initially, this uncommon disorder causes slight cheek inflammation, which is rapidly followed by tooth loss and extensive bone sloughing in the mandible or maxilla.

• *Ozena.* This severe, chronic form of rhinitis causes a musty or fetid breath odor. It also produces thick, green mucus and progressive anosmia.

• *Periodontal disease.* In this disorder, halitosis is accompanied by an unpleasant taste. Typically, the patient's gums bleed spontaneously or with slight trauma and are marked by pus-filled pockets around the teeth. Related findings include facial pain, headache, and loose teeth covered by calculus and plaque.

• *Pharyngitis (gangrenous).* Halitosis is a chief sign of this disorder. The patient also complains of a foul taste in the mouth, an extremely sore throat, and a choking sensation. Examination will reveal a swollen, red, ulcerated pharynx, possibly with a grayish membrane. Fever and cervical lymphadenopathy are also common.

• *Renal failure (chronic).* This disorder produces a urinous or ammonia breath odor. Among its widespread effects are lethargy, irritability, decreased mental acuity, coarse muscular twitches, peripheral neuropathies, muscle wasting, anorexia, signs of GI bleeding, ecchymoses, yellow-brown or bronze skin, pruritus, anuria, increased blood pressure, and others.

• *Sinusitis.* Acute sinusitis causes a purulent nasal discharge that leads to halitosis. Besides characteristic postnasal drip, the patient may have nasal congestion, sore throat, cough, malaise, headache, facial pain and tenderness, and fever.

Chronic sinusitis causes continuous mucopurulent discharge that leads to a musty breath odor. Postnasal drip, nasal congestion, and a chronic, nonproductive cough may accompany this musty odor.

• *Zenker's diverticulum.* This esophageal disorder causes halitosis and a bad taste in the mouth associated with regurgitation. The patient may also have a chronic cough that's most pronounced at night, hoarseness, and "gurgling" sounds in the throat when he swallows liquids.

Other causes

• *Drugs.* Triamterene and inhaled anesthetics can cause halitosis. So can paraldehyde, which is excreted through the lungs.

Special considerations

If mouth and sinus examination doesn't reveal the cause of halitosis, prepare the patient for upper GI and chest X-rays or endoscopy, as ordered.

To help control halitosis, encourage good oral hygiene. If halitosis is drug-induced, reassure the patient that it will disappear as soon as his body eliminates the drug completely.

Pediatric pointers

In children, halitosis commonly results from physiologic causes, such as continual mouth breathing and thumb or blanket sucking. However, phenylketonuria—a metabolic disorder that affects infants—may produce a musty or mousy breath odor.

Halo Vision

[Halos]

Halo vision refers to seeing rainbow-like, colored rings around lights or bright objects. The rainbowlike effect can be explained by this physical principle: as light passes through water (in the eye, through tears or the cells of various anteretinal media), it breaks up into spectral colors.

Usually, halo vision develops suddenly; its duration depends on the causative disorder. This symptom may occur in disorders associated with excessive tearing and corneal epithelial edema. Among these causes, the most common and significant is acute closed-angle glaucoma, which can lead to blindness. Here, increased intraocular pressure forces fluid into corneal tissues anterior to Bowman's membrane, causing edema. Halos are also an early symptom of cataracts and result from dispersion of light by abnormal opacities on the lens.

Nonpathologic causes of excessive tearing associated with halos include poorly fitted or overworn contact lenses, emotional extremes, and exposure to intense light, as in snow blindness.

Assessment

One of the first history questions to ask the patient is "How long have you been seeing halos around lights?" Find out when halos are most frequently seen. Patients with glaucoma typically see halos most frequently in the morning, when intraocular pressure is most severely elevated. Ask the patient if light bothers his eyes. Does he have any eye pain? If so, have him describe it. Remember that halos associated with excruciating eye pain or severe headache may point to acute closed-angle glaucoma—an ocular emergency. Note a history of glaucoma or cataracts.

Next, examine the patient's eyes, noting conjunctival injection, excessive tearing, and lens changes. Assess pupil size, shape, and response to light. Then test visual acuity and assist the doctor with an ophthalmoscopic examination.

Medical causes

• *Cataract.* Halos may be an early symptom of painless, progressive cataract formation. The glare of headlights may blind the patient, making nighttime driving impossible. Other features include blurred vision, impaired visual acuity, and lens opacity, all of which develop gradually.

• *Corneal endothelial dystrophy.* Typically, halos are a late symptom. Impaired visual acuity may also occur.

• *Glaucoma.* Halos characterize all types of glaucoma. *Acute closed-angle glaucoma*—an ophthalmic emergency—also causes blurred vision followed by severe headache or excruciating pain in and around the affected eye. Examination will reveal a moderately dilated fixed pupil that doesn't respond to light, conjunctival injection, a cloudy cornea, and impaired visual acuity. Nausea and vomiting may also occur. Usually, *chronic closed-angle glaucoma* is asymptomatic until pain and blindness occur in advanced disease. Sometimes, halos and blurred vision develop slowly.

In *chronic open-angle glaucoma,* halos are a late symptom accompanied by mild eye ache, peripheral vision loss, and impaired visual acuity.

Special considerations

To help minimize halos, remind the patient not to look directly at bright lights.

Pediatric pointers

A young child's limited verbal ability may make halos difficult to assess. Usually, halo vision in a child results from congenital cataracts or glaucoma.

Headache

The most common neurologic symptom, a headache may be localized or generalized, producing mild-to-severe pain. About 90% of all headaches are benign and can be described as vascular, muscle-contraction, or a combination of both (see *Comparing Benign Headaches.*). Occasionally,

COMPARING BENIGN HEADACHES

Of the many patients who report headaches, only about 10% have an underlying medical disorder. The other 90% suffer from benign headaches, which may be muscle-contraction (tension), vascular (migraine and cluster), or a combination of both.

As you review the chart below, you'll see that the two major types—muscle-contraction and vascular headaches—are quite different. In a combined headache, features of both appear. This headache may affect the patient with a severe muscle-contraction headache or a late-stage migraine. Treatment of a combined headache requires analgesics and sedatives.

CHARACTER-ISTICS	MUSCLE-CONTRACTION HEADACHES	VASCULAR HEADACHES
Incidence	• Most common type, accounting for 80% of *all* headaches	• More common in women and those with a family history of migraines • Onset after puberty
Precipitating factors	• Stress, anxiety, or tension • Prolonged muscle contraction without structural damage • Eye, ear, and paranasal sinus disorders that produce reflex muscle contractions	• Hormone fluctuations • Alcohol • Emotional upset • Too little or too much sleep • Foods, such as chocolate, cheese, monosodium glutamate, and cured meats • Weather changes, such as shifts in barometric pressure
Intensity and duration	• Produce an aching tightness or a band of pain around the head, especially in the neck, occipital, and temporal areas • Occur frequently and usually last for several hours	• May begin with an awareness of an impending migraine or a 5- to 15-minute prodrome of neurologic deficits such as visual disturbances; tingling of the face, lips, or hands; dizziness; or unsteady gait • Produce severe, constant, throbbing pain that's typically unilateral and may be incapacitating • Last for 4 to 6 hours
Associated signs and symptoms	• Tense neck and facial muscles	• Anorexia, nausea, and vomiting • Occasionally, photophobia, sensitivity to loud noises, weakness, and fatigue • Depending on the type (classic, common, or hemiplegic migraine; or cluster headache), there may be chills, depression, eye pain, ptosis, tearing, rhinorrhea, diaphoresis, and facial flushing
Alleviating factors	• Mild analgesics, muscle relaxants, or other drugs during an attack • Measures to reduce stress, such as biofeedback, relaxation techniques and counseling, and posture correction to prevent attacks	• Methysergide and propranolol to prevent vascular headache • Ergot drugs at the first sign of a migraine • Rest in a quiet, darkened room • Elimination of irritating foods from diet

though, this symptom indicates a severe neurologic disorder. A pathologic headache may result from disorders associated with intracranial inflammation, increased intracranial pressure, or meningeal irritation. It may also result from ocular or sinus disorders and the effects of drugs, tests, and treatments. In certain metabolic disturbances—hypoxemia, hypercapnia, hyperglycemia, and hypoglycemia—headache may occur, but it's not a diagnostic or prominent symptom.

Among the many other causes of headache are fever, eyestrain, and dehydration. Some individuals get headaches from coughing, sneezing, heavy lifting, or stooping. Others experience headaches after seizures.

Assessment

If the patient reports a headache, ask him to describe its character and location. How often does he get a headache? How long does a typical headache last? Try to identify precipitating factors, such as certain foods and exposure to bright lights. Is the patient under stress? Has he been unable to sleep?

Take a drug history and ask about head trauma within the last 4 weeks. Has the patient had nausea, vomiting, photophobia, or any visual changes? Does he feel drowsy, confused, or dizzy? Has he recently developed seizures, or does he have a history of seizures?

Begin the physical examination by assessing the patient's level of consciousness (LOC). Then check his vital signs. Be alert for signs of increased intracranial pressure—widened pulse pressure, bradycardia, altered respiratory pattern, or increased blood pressure. Check pupil size and response to light. Also note any neck stiffness.

Medical causes

• *Brain abscess.* Here, headache is localized to the abscess site. Usually, it intensifies over a few days and is aggravated by straining. Accompanying the headache may be nausea, vomiting, and focal or generalized seizures. The patient's LOC will vary from drowsiness to deep stupor. Depending on the abscess site, associated signs and symptoms may include aphasia, impaired visual acuity, hemiparesis, ataxia, tremors, and personality changes. Signs of infection, such as fever and pallor, usually develop late; however, if the abscess remains encapsulated, these signs may not appear.

• *Brain tumor.* Initially, this disorder causes a localized headache near the tumor site. The headache eventually becomes generalized as the tumor grows. Usually, it's intermittent, deep-seated and dull, and most intense in the morning. It's aggravated by coughing, stooping, Valsalva's maneuver, and changes in head position; it's relieved by sitting and rest. Associated signs and symptoms may include personality changes, altered LOC, motor and sensory dysfunction, and eventual signs of increased intracranial pressure, such as vomiting, increased systolic blood pressure, and widened pulse pressure.

• *Cerebral aneurysm (ruptured).* Sudden, excruciating headache characterizes this life-threatening disorder. The headache may be unilateral and usually peaks within minutes of aneurysmal rupture. The patient may lose consciousness immediately or display a variably altered LOC. Depending on the severity and location of the bleeding, he may also have nausea and vomiting; signs of meningeal irritation, such as nuchal rigidity and blurred vision; hemiparesis; and other features.

• *Encephalitis.* A severe, generalized headache is characteristic here. Typically, the patient's LOC then deteriorates within 48 hours—perhaps from lethargy to coma. Associated signs and symptoms include fever, nuchal rigidity, irritability, seizures, nausea, vomiting, photophobia, focal neurologic deficits, such as hemiparesis and hemiplegia, and cranial nerve palsies, such as ptosis.

• *Epidural hemorrhage (acute).* Usually,

head trauma and immediate, brief loss of consciousness precede this hemorrhage, which causes a progressively severe headache. It's accompanied by nausea and vomiting, bladder distention, confusion, and then a rapid decrease in LOC. Other signs and symptoms may include unilateral seizures, hemiparesis, hemiplegia, high fever, decreased pulse rate and bounding pulse, widened pulse pressure, and increased blood pressure. In addition, a positive Babinski's reflex and decerebrate posture may occur.

If the patient slips into coma, his respirations deepen and become stertorous, then become shallow and irregular, and eventually cease. Pupil dilation may occur on the same side as the hemorrhage.

● *Glaucoma (acute closed-angle).* This ophthalmic emergency may cause an excruciating headache. It also causes acute eye pain, blurred vision, halo vision, nausea, and vomiting. Assessment will reveal a conjunctival injection, a cloudy cornea, and a moderately dilated, fixed pupil.

● *Hypertension.* This disorder may cause a slightly throbbing occipital headache on awakening that decreases in severity during the day. However, if the patient's diastolic blood pressure exceeds 120 mm Hg, the headache remains constant. Associated signs and symptoms may include an S_4, restlessness, confusion, nausea, vomiting, blurred vision, seizures, and altered LOC.

● *Influenza.* A severe generalized or frontal headache usually begins suddenly with the flu. Accompanying signs and symptoms may last for 3 to 5 days and include stabbing retroorbital pain, weakness, diffuse myalgia, fever, chills, coughing, rhinorrhea, and occasionally hoarseness. However, cough and weakness may persist.

● *Intracerebral hemorrhage.* In some patients, this hemorrhage produces a severe generalized headache. Clinical features vary with the hemorrhage's size and location. A large hemorrhage may produce a rapid, steady decrease in LOC, perhaps resulting in coma. Other common findings may include hemiplegia, hemiparesis, abnormal pupil size and response, aphasia, dizziness, nausea, vomiting, seizures, decreased sensations, irregular respirations, positive Babinski's reflex, decorticate or decerebrate posture, and increased blood pressure.

● *Meningitis.* Sudden onset of a severe, constant, generalized headache that worsens with movement typifies this disorder. Associated signs include nuchal rigidity, positive Kernig's and Brudzinski's signs, hyperreflexia, and possibly opisthotonos. Fever occurs early in meningitis and may be accompanied by chills. As intracranial pressure increases, vomiting and, occasionally, papilledema develop. Other features may include altered LOC, seizures, ocular palsies, facial weakness, and hearing loss.

● *Postconcussional syndrome.* One to thirty days after head trauma, a generalized or localized headache may develop and last for 2 to 3 weeks. This characteristic symptom may be described as an aching, pounding, pressing, stabbing, or throbbing pain. The patient's neurologic examination will be normal, but he may have giddiness or dizziness, blurred vision, fatigue, insomnia, inability to concentrate, and noise and alcohol intolerance.

● *Psittacosis.* Abrupt onset of an excruciating headache marks the beginning of this disorder. It's accompanied by fever, chills, malaise, and myalgia. An early dry cough later produces small amounts of mucoid sputum with blood streaks. Auscultation may reveal tachypnea and crackles. The patient may also have epistaxis, photophobia, abdominal distention and tenderness, nausea, vomiting, a faint macular rash, and, rarely, chest pain. Severe infection may produce stupor, delirium, or even coma.

● *Sinusitis (acute).* Usually, a dull periorbital headache occurs in this disorder. The aching is typically aggravated by bending over or touching the face and relieved by sinus drainage. Fever, sinus tenderness, nasal turbinate edema, sore throat, malaise, cough, and nasal discharge may accompany the headache.

• *Subarachnoid hemorrhage.* Commonly, this hemorrhage produces a sudden, violent headache. Related signs and symptoms include nuchal rigidity, altered LOC that may rapidly progress to coma, nausea, vomiting, seizures, dizziness, and ipsilateral pupil dilation. The patient will also have positive Kernig's and Brudzinski's signs, photophobia, blurred vision, and possibly fever. Focal signs and symptoms, such as hemiparesis, hemiplegia, sensory or vision disturbances, and aphasia, may occur. Signs of elevated intracranial pressure—such as bradycardia and increased blood pressure—may also occur.

• *Subdural hematoma.* Typically associated with head trauma, both acute and chronic subdural hematomas may cause headache and decreased LOC. In *acute subdural hematoma*, head trauma produces immediate loss of consciousness followed by a latent period with headache, drowsiness, confusion, and agitation that may progress to coma. Later findings may include signs of increased intracranial pressure and focal neurologic deficits, such as hemiparesis.

Chronic subdural hematoma produces a dull, pounding headache that fluctuates in severity and is located over the hematoma. Weeks or months after head trauma, this disorder may cause giddiness, personality changes, confusion, seizures, and altered LOC that progressively worsens. Late signs may include unilateral pupil dilation, sluggish pupil reaction to light, and ptosis.

• *Temporal arteritis.* Here, a throbbing unilateral headache in the temporal or frontotemporal region is typical. It may be accompanied by vision loss, hearing loss, confusion, and fever. The temporal arteries are tender, swollen, nodular, and sometimes erythematous.

• *Typhoid fever.* Initially, this disorder causes a severe frontal headache, steadily increasing fever, abdominal discomfort, and constipation. After about a week, splenomegaly develops, followed by pathognomonic rose spots. These deep red macules, which blanch on pressure, mark the upper abdomen and chest and last for 2 to 3 days. Commonly, the patient has a dry cough and epistaxis. Later signs and symptoms include mental dullness or delirium, marked abdominal distention, diarrhea, weight loss, and profound fatigue.

Other causes

• *Diagnostic tests.* A pneumoencephalogram may produce a severe generalized headache, whereas a lumbar puncture or myelogram may produce a throbbing frontal headache.

• *Drugs.* A wide variety of drugs may cause headaches. For example, indomethacin produces headaches—usually in the morning—in about half of all patients. Vasodilators and drugs with a vasodilating effect, such as nitrates, typically cause a throbbing headache. This symptom may also follow withdrawal from vasopressors, such as caffeine, ergotamine, or sympathomimetic drugs.

• *Traction.* Cervical traction with pins commonly causes a headache, which may be generalized or localized to pin insertion sites.

Special considerations

Continue to monitor the patient's vital signs and LOC. Watch for any change in the headache's severity or location.

As ordered, prepare the patient for diagnostic tests, such as skull X-rays, computed tomography, lumbar puncture, or cerebral arteriography.

To help ease the headache, administer analgesics, as ordered. Also darken the patient's room and minimize other stimuli.

Pediatric pointers

If the child's too young to describe his symptom, suspect headache if you see him banging or holding his head. In an infant, a shrill cry or bulging fontanelles may indicate increased intracranial pressure and headache. In a school-age child, ask the parents about the child's recent scholastic performance and about any problems at home that may produce a tension headache.

Young boys have migraine headaches twice as often as girls. In children over age 3, headache is the most common symptom of a brain tumor.

Hearing Loss

Affecting nearly 16 million Americans, hearing loss may be temporary or permanent, partial or complete. This common symptom may involve reception of low-, middle-, or high-frequency tones. If the hearing loss doesn't affect speech frequencies, the patient may be unaware of it.

Normally, sound waves enter the external auditory canal, then travel to the middle ear's tympanic membrane and ossicles (incus, malleus, and stapes) and into the inner ear's cochlea. The cochlear division of the eighth cranial (auditory) nerve carries the sound impulse to the brain. This type of sound transmission, called *air conduction*, is normally better than *bone conduction*—sound transmission through bone to the inner ear.

Hearing loss can be classified as conductive, sensorineural, mixed, and functional. *Conductive hearing loss* results from disorders of the external and middle ear that block sound transmission. *Sensorineural hearing loss*—also known as nerve deafness, perceptive deafness, or inner ear deafness—results from disorders of the inner ear, or the eighth cranial nerve. *Mixed hearing loss* combines aspects of both conductive and sensorineural hearing loss. *Functional hearing loss* results from psychological factors; no identifiable organic damage exists.

Hearing loss may result from trauma, infection, allergy, tumors, certain systemic and hereditary disorders, and the effects of ototoxic drugs and treatments. Most commonly, though, it results from presbycusis—a sensorineural hearing loss that usually affects those older than age 50. Other physiologic causes of hearing loss include cerumen (ear wax) impaction; barotitis media—unequal pressure on the eardrum—associated with descent in an airplane or elevator, diving, or close proximity to an explosion; and chronic exposure to noise over 90 decibels. This noise exposure can occur on the job, at a hobby, or from listening to live or recorded music.

Assessment

If the patient reports hearing loss, ask him to describe it fully. Is it unilateral or bilateral? Continuous or intermittent? Ask about a family history of hearing loss. Then obtain the patient's medical history, noting chronic ear infections, ear surgery, and ear or head trauma. Has the patient recently had an upper respiratory infection? After taking a drug history, have the patient describe his occupation and work environment.

Next, explore associated signs and symptoms. Does he have any ear pain? If so, is it unilateral or bilateral? Continuous or intermittent? Ask the patient if he's noticed any discharge from one or both ears. If so, have him describe its color and consistency and note when it began. Does he hear ringing, buzzing, hissing, or other unusual noises in one or both ears? If so, when did he first notice it? Is the tinnitus constant or intermittent?

Begin the physical examination by inspecting the external ear for inflammation, boils, foreign bodies, or discharge. Then apply pressure to the tragus and mastoid to elicit tenderness. If you detect tenderness or external ear abnormalities, notify the doctor to discuss whether an otoscopic examination should be done. (See *Using an Otoscope*

DIFFERENTIATING CONDUCTIVE AND SENSORINEURAL HEARING LOSS

The Weber and Rinne tests can help determine whether the patient's hearing loss is conductive or sensorineural. The Weber test evaluates bone conduction; the Rinne test, bone and air conduction. Using a 512 Hz tuning fork, perform these preliminary tests as described below.

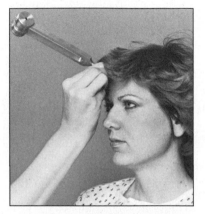

Weber test
Place the base of a vibrating tuning fork firmly against the midline of the patient's skull at the forehead. Ask her if she hears the tone equally well in both ears. If she does, the Weber test is graded *midline*—a normal finding. In an abnormal Weber test (graded *right* or *left*), sound is *louder* in one ear, suggesting a conductive hearing loss in that ear or a sensorineural loss in the opposite ear.

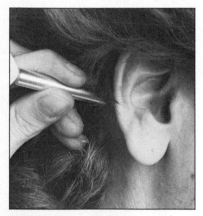

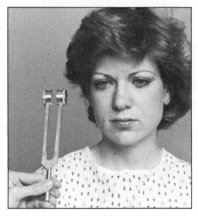

Rinne test
Hold the base of a vibrating tuning fork against the patient's mastoid process to test bone conduction. Then quickly move the vibrating fork in front of her ear canal to test air conduction. Ask her to tell you which location has the louder or longer sound. Repeat the procedure for the other ear. In a positive Rinne test, air conduction lasts longer or sounds louder than bone conduction—a normal finding. In a negative test the opposite is true: bone conduction lasts longer or sounds louder than air conduction.

After performing both tests, correlate the results with other assessment data.

Conductive hearing loss produces:
- Abnormal Weber test
- Negative Rinne test
- Improved hearing in noisy areas
- Normal ability to discriminate sounds
- Difficulty hearing when chewing
- A quiet speaking voice

Sensorineural hearing loss produces:
- Abnormal Weber test
- Positive Rinne test
- Poor hearing in noisy areas
- Difficulty hearing high-frequency sounds
- Complaints that others mumble or shout
- Tinnitus

Correctly, page 272.) During the otoscopic examination, note any color change, perforation, bulging, or retraction of the tympanic membrane—it normally looks like a shiny, pearl gray cone.

Next, evaluate hearing acuity. Use the ticking watch and whispered voice tests to assess gross hearing. Make a preliminary evaluation of the type and degree of hearing loss with the Weber and Rinne tests. (See *Differentiating Conductive and Sensorineural Hearing Loss.*)

Medical causes

• *Acoustic neuroma.* This eighth cranial nerve tumor causes unilateral, progressive, sensorineural hearing loss. The patient may also have tinnitus, vertigo, and—with cranial nerve compression—facial paralysis.

• *Adenoid hypertrophy.* Eustachian tube dysfunction gradually causes conductive hearing loss accompanied by intermittent ear discharge. The patient also tends to mouth breathe and may complain of a sensation of ear fullness.

• *Allergies.* Conductive hearing loss may result when an allergy produces eustachian tube and middle ear congestion. Among other features are ear pain or a feeling of fullness, nasal congestion, and conjunctivitis.

• *Aural polyps.* If a polyp occludes the external auditory canal, partial hearing loss may occur. Typically, the polyp bleeds easily and is covered by a purulent discharge.

• *Cholesteatoma.* Gradual hearing loss characterizes this disorder. It's accompanied by vertigo and, occasionally, facial paralysis. Examination reveals tympanic membrane perforation and pearly white balls in the ear canal.

• *Cyst.* Ear canal obstruction by a sebaceous or dermoid cyst causes progressive conductive hearing loss. On inspection, the cyst appears like a soft mass.

• *External ear canal tumor (malignant).* Progressive conductive hearing loss is characteristic. It's accompanied by deep, boring ear pain, purulent discharge, and eventually facial paralysis. Examination may detect the granular, bleeding tumor.

• *Furuncle.* A reversible conductive hearing loss may occur when one of these painful, hard nodules, or boils, forms in the ear. The patient may report a sense of fullness in the ear and pain on palpation of the tragus or auricle. Boil rupture relieves the pain and produces a purulent, necrotic discharge.

• *Glomus jugulare tumor.* Initially, this benign tumor causes a mild unilateral conductive hearing loss that becomes progressively more severe. The patient may report tinnitus that sounds like his heartbeat. Associated signs and symptoms include gradual congestion in the affected ear, throbbing or pulsating discomfort, bloody otorrhea, facial nerve paralysis, and vertigo. Although the tympanic membrane is normal, a reddened mass appears behind it.

• *Glomus tympanium.* This middle ear tumor causes slowly progressive hearing loss and throbbing or pulsating tinnitus. Usually, it bleeds easily when manipulated. Late features include ear pain, dizziness, and total unilateral deafness.

• *Granuloma.* A rare cause of conductive hearing loss, a granuloma may also produce fullness in the ear, deep-seated pain, and bloody discharge.

• *Head trauma.* Sudden conductive or sensorineural hearing loss may result from ossicle disruption, ear canal fracture, or tympanic membrane perforation associated with head trauma. Typically, the patient will report a headache and have bleeding from his ear. Neurologic features vary and may include impaired vision and altered level of consciousness.

• *Hypothyroidism.* This disorder may produce reversible sensorineural hearing loss. Other effects include bradycardia, weight gain despite anorexia, mental dullness, cold intolerance, facial edema, brittle hair, and dry skin that's pale, cool, and doughy.

• *Ménière's disease.* Initially, this inner

ear disorder produces intermittent, unilateral sensorineural hearing loss that involves only low tones. Later, hearing loss becomes constant and affects other tones. Associated signs and symptoms include intermittent severe vertigo, nausea, vomiting, a feeling of fullness in the ear, a roaring or hollow-seashell tinnitus, diaphoresis, and nystagmus.

● *Multiple sclerosis.* Rarely, this disorder causes sensorineural hearing loss associated with myelin destruction of the central auditory pathways. The hearing loss may be sudden and unilateral or intermittent and bilateral. Among other characteristics are impaired vision, paresthesias, muscle weakness, gait ataxia, intention tremor, urinary disturbances, and emotional lability.

● *Myringitis.* Rarely, *acute infectious myringitis* produces conductive hearing loss when fluid accumulates in the middle ear or a large bleb totally obstructs the ear canal. Associated findings may include severe ear pain, mastoid tenderness, and fever. Small, reddened inflamed blebs may develop in the canal, on the tympanic membrane, or in the middle ear and may produce a bloody discharge if they rupture.

Chronic granular myringitis produces a gradual hearing loss accompanied by pruritus and purulent discharge.

● *Nasopharyngeal cancer.* This tumor causes mild unilateral mixed hearing loss when it compresses the eustachian tube. Bone conduction is normal, and inspection reveals a retracted tympanic membrane backed by fluid. When this tumor obstructs the nasal airway, the patient may have bloody nasal and postnasal discharge, and nasal speech. Cranial nerve involvement produces other findings, such as diplopia and rectus muscle paralysis.

● *Osteoma.* Commonly affecting women or swimmers, osteoma may cause sudden or intermittent conductive hearing loss. Typically, bony projections are visible in the ear canal, but the tympanic membrane appears normal.

● *Otitis externa.* Conductive hearing loss characterizes both acute and malignant otitis externa and results from debris in the ear canal. In *acute otitis externa,* ear canal inflammation produces pain, itching, and a foul-smelling, sticky yellow discharge. Typically, severe tenderness is elicited by chewing, opening the mouth, and pressing on the tragus or mastoid. The patient may also have a low-grade fever, regional lymphadenopathy, headache on the affected side, and mild-to-moderate pain around the ear that may later intensify. Examination may reveal greenish white debris in the canal.

In *malignant otitis externa,* debris is also visible in the canal. This life-threatening disorder causes sensorineural hearing loss, pruritus, tinnitus, and severe ear pain.

● *Otitis media.* Typically, this middle ear inflammation produces unilateral conductive hearing loss. In *acute suppurative otitis media,* the hearing loss develops gradually over a few hours. It's usually accompanied by an upper respiratory infection with sore throat, cough, nasal discharge, and headache. Related signs and symptoms may include dizziness, a sensation of fullness in the ear, intermittent or constant ear pain, fever, nausea, and vomiting. Rupture of the bulging, swollen tympanic membrane relieves the pain and produces a brief, bloody, purulent discharge. Hearing will return after the infection subsides.

Also in *chronic otitis media,* hearing loss develops gradually. Assessment may reveal a perforated tympanic membrane, purulent ear drainage, earache, nausea, and vertigo.

Often associated with an upper respiratory infection or nasopharyngeal carcinoma, *serous otitis media* commonly produces a stuffy feeling in the ear and pain that worsens at night. Examination will reveal a retracted—and perhaps discolored—tympanic membrane; air bubbles may be visible behind the membrane.

● *Otosclerosis.* In this hereditary disorder, unilateral conductive hearing loss usually begins in the early twenties and may gradually progress to bilateral mixed loss. The patient may report tinnitus and an ability to hear better in a noisy environment.

● *Ramsay Hunt syndrome.* Associated with herpes infection, this syndrome causes sudden onset of severe unilateral mixed hearing loss. Vesicles appear in the external ear. Other features include tinnitus, vertigo, ear pain, malaise, and transient, ipsilateral facial paralysis.

● *Skull fracture.* Auditory nerve injury causes sudden unilateral sensorineural hearing loss. Accompanying signs and symptoms may include ringing tinnitus, blood behind the tympanic membrane, scalp wounds, and other findings.

● *Syphilis.* In tertiary syphilis, sensorineural hearing loss may develop suddenly or gradually and usually affects one ear more than the other. It's usually accompanied by a gumma lesion—a chronic, superficial nodule or a deep, granulomatous lesion on the skin or mucous membranes. The lesion is solitary, asymmetrical, painless, and indurated. The patient may also exhibit signs of liver, respiratory, cardiovascular, or neurologic dysfunction.

● *Temporal arteritis.* This disorder may produce unilateral sensorineural hearing loss accompanied by throbbing unilateral facial pain, pain behind the eye, temporal or frontotemporal headache, and, occasionally, vision loss. Usually, the hearing loss is preceded by a prodrome of malaise, anorexia, weight loss, weakness, and myalgia that lasts for several days. Examination may reveal a nodular, swollen temporal artery. Low-grade fever, confusion, and disorientation may also occur.

● *Temporal bone fracture.* This fracture causes sudden unilateral sensorineural hearing loss accompanied by hissing tinnitus. The tympanic membrane may be perforated, depending on the fracture's location. Loss of consciousness, Battle's sign, and facial paralysis may also occur.

● *Tuberculosis.* This pulmonary infection may spread to the ear, resulting in eardrum perforation, mild conductive hearing loss, and cervical lymphadenopathy.

● *Tympanic membrane perforation.* Often caused by trauma from sharp objects or rapid pressure changes, perforation of the tympanic membrane causes abrupt hearing loss. Associated symptoms include ear pain, tinnitus, vertigo, and a sensation of fullness in the ear.

● *Wegener's granulomatosis.* Conductive hearing loss develops slowly in this rare necrotizing, granulomatous vasculitis. Affecting various body systems, this disorder may also cause cough, pleuritic chest pain, epistaxis, hemorrhagic skin lesions, oliguria, nasal discharge, and other findings.

Other causes

● *Drugs.* Typically, ototoxic drugs produce ringing or buzzing tinnitus and a feeling of fullness in the ear. Chloroquine, cisplatin, vancomycin, and aminoglycosides—especially neomycin, kanamycin, and amikacin—may cause irreversible hearing loss. Loop diuretics, such as furosemide, ethacrynic acid, and bumetanide, usually produce a brief, reversible hearing loss. Quinine, quinidine, or high doses of erythromycin or salicylates such as aspirin may also cause reversible hearing loss.

● *Radiation therapy.* Irradiation of the middle ear, thyroid, face, skull, or nasopharynx may cause eustachian tube dysfunction, resulting in hearing loss.

● *Surgery.* Myringotomy, myringoplasty, simple or radical mastoidectomy, or fenestrations may cause scarring that interferes with hearing.

Special considerations

When talking with the patient, remember to face him and speak slowly. Don't shout, smoke, eat, or chew gum when talking.

As ordered, prepare the patient for audiometry and auditory evoked-response testing. After careful testing, the patient may require a hearing aid or cochlear implant to improve his hearing. Instruct the patient to avoid exposure to loud noises to prevent further hearing loss.

Pediatric pointers
Each year about 3,000 profoundly deaf infants are born in the United States. In about half of these infants, hereditary disorders cause the typically sensorineural hearing loss. Disorders associated with congenital sensorineural hearing loss include Usher's disease, albinism, onychodystrophy, and Pendred's, Waardenburg's, and Jervell and Lange-Nielsen syndromes. This type of hearing loss may also result from maternal use of ototoxic drugs, birth trauma, and anoxia during or after birth.

Hereditary disorders associated with sensorineural hearing loss in childhood and adolescence include Alport's and Paget's diseases and Hurler's and Klippel-Feil syndromes. But mumps is the most common pediatric cause of sensorineural hearing loss, and meningitis, measles, influenza, and acute febrile illness may also cause it.

Disorders associated with congenital conductive hearing loss include atresia, ossicle malformation, and other abnormalities. Unlike its effect in adults, serous otitis media commonly causes bilateral conductive hearing loss in children. Conductive hearing loss may also occur in children who put foreign objects in their ears.

Hearing disorders in children may lead to speech, language, and learning problems. Early identification and treatment of hearing loss is thus crucial—before the child is incorrectly labeled as mentally retarded, brain damaged, or a slow learner.

When assessing an infant or young child for hearing loss, remember that you can't use a tuning fork. Instead, test the startle reflex in infants under age 6 months or have an audiologist test brain stem evoked response in neonates, infants, and young children. Also obtain a gestational, perinatal, and family history from the parents.

Heat Intolerance

Heat intolerance refers to the inability to withstand high temperatures or to maintain a comfortable body temperature. It produces a continuous feeling of being overheated and, at times, profuse diaphoresis. Usually, this symptom develops gradually and is chronic.

Most often, heat intolerance results from thyrotoxicosis. In this disorder, excess thyroid hormone stimulates peripheral tissues, increasing basal metabolism and producing excess heat. Although rare, hypothalamic disease may also cause heat—and cold—intolerance by disrupting normal temperature control.

Assessment
As you begin the assessment, notice how much clothing the patient is wearing. Then ask him when he first noticed his heat intolerance. Did he gradually use fewer blankets at night? Does he have to turn up the air conditioning to keep cool? Is it hard for him to adjust to warm weather? Find out if the patient's appetite or weight has changed. Also ask about unusual nervousness or other personality changes. Then take a drug history, especially noting use of amphetamines or amphetamine-like drugs. Ask the patient if he takes prescribed thyroid drugs. If so, what is the daily dose? When did he last take it? After taking vital signs, inspect the patient's skin for flushing and diaphoresis. Also note tremors and lid lag.

Medical causes
• *Hypothalamic disease.* Among the common causes of this rare disease are pituitary adenoma and hypothalamic

and pineal tumors. Here, body temperature fluctuates dramatically, causing alternating heat and cold intolerance. Related features include amenorrhea, disturbed sleep patterns, increased thirst and urination, increased appetite with weight gain, impaired visual acuity, headache, and personality changes, such as bursts of rage or laughter.

• *Thyrotoxicosis.* A classic symptom of thyrotoxicosis, heat intolerance may be accompanied by an enlarged thyroid, nervousness, weight loss despite increased appetite, diaphoresis, diarrhea, tremor, and palpitations. Although exophthalmos is characteristic, many patients don't display this sign. Associated findings may affect virtually every body system. Some common findings include irritability, difficulty concentrating, mood swings, muscle weakness, fatigue, lid lag, tachycardia, full and bounding pulse, widened pulse pressure, dyspnea, and amenorrhea or gynecomastia. Typically, the patient's skin is warm and flushed; premature graying and alopecia occur in both sexes.

Other causes
• *Drugs.* Amphetamines and amphetamine-like appetite suppressants may increase basal metabolism, resulting in heat intolerance. Excessive doses of thyroid hormone may also cause heat intolerance.

Special considerations
Adjust room temperature to make the patient comfortable. If the patient has diaphoresis, change his clothing and bed linens, as necessary, and encourage fluids.

Pediatric pointers
Rarely, maternal thyrotoxicosis may be passed to the neonate, resulting in heat intolerance. More commonly, acquired thyrotoxicosis appears between ages 12 and 14, although this, too, is infrequent. Also, dehydration may make a child sensitive to heat.

Heberden's Nodes

Heberden's nodes are painless, irregular, bony enlargements of the distal finger joints. Approximately 2 to 3 mm in diameter, they develop on one or both sides of the dorsal midline. Usually, the dominant hand has larger nodes, which affect one or more fingers but not the thumb.

Repeated fingertip trauma may cause Heberden's nodes in only one joint ("baseball finger"). However, osteoarthritis is the most common cause; in fact, Heberden's nodes occur in more than half of all osteoarthritic patients. Because the nodes aren't associated with pain or loss of function, they're not a primary indicator of osteoarthritis but are a helpful adjunct to diagnosis.

Heberden's nodes reflect degeneration of articular cartilage, which irritates the bone and stimulates osteoblasts, causing bony enlargement.

Assessment
Begin by asking the patient if anyone else in his family has had Heberden's nodes or osteoarthritis. Also ask about repeated fingertip trauma on the job or associated with sports. Are the patient's joints stiff? Does stiffness disappear with movement? Ask him which hand is dominant.

Carefully palpate the nodes, noting any signs of inflammation, such as redness and tenderness. Then assess range of motion in the fingers of each hand. As you do so, listen and feel for crepitation.

Medical cause
• *Osteoarthritis.* This disorder commonly causes Heberden's nodes and, possibly, nodes in the proximal interphalangeal joints (Bouchard's nodes). Its chief symptom, though, is joint pain that's aggravated by movement or weight bearing. Joints may also be ten-

HEBERDEN'S NODES

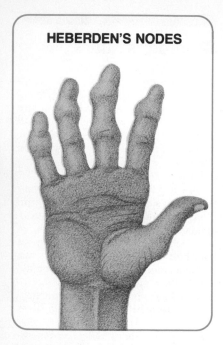

der and display restricted range of motion. Typically, joint stiffness is triggered by disuse and is relieved by brief exercise. Stiffness may be accompanied by bony enlargement and crepitus.

Special considerations
Remind the patient to take anti-inflammatory drugs, as ordered, and to exercise regularly. Encourage him to avoid joint strain, for example, by maintaining a healthy weight.

Pediatric pointers
Heberden's nodes don't occur in children, as they don't suffer from osteoarthritis.

Hematemesis

Hematemesis, or vomiting of blood, usually indicates gastrointestinal (GI) bleeding above the ligament of Treitz, which suspends the duodenum at its junction with the jejunum. Bright red or blood-streaked vomitus indicates fresh or recent bleeding. Dark red, brown, or black vomitus—about the color and consistency of coffee grounds—indicates that blood has been retained in the stomach and partially digested.

Most often, hematemesis results from GI disorders. It may also result from coagulation disorders and from treatments that irritate the GI tract. Swallowed blood from epistaxis or oropharyngeal erosions may also cause bloody vomitus.

Hematemesis is always an important sign, but its severity depends on the amount and source of the bleeding. Massive hematemesis (vomiting of 500 to 1,000 ml of blood) may rapidly be life-threatening. Hematemesis may be aggravated by straining, emotional stress, anti-inflammatory drugs, and alcohol ingestion.

Assessment
If the patient has massive hematemesis, quickly check his vital signs. If you detect signs of shock, such as tachypnea, hypotension, and tachycardia, have another nurse notify the doctor immediately. Place the patient in a supine position and elevate his feet 20° to 30°. Start a large bore I.V. for emergency fluid replacement. Also, send a blood specimen for typing and cross matching, and begin oxygen administration. As ordered, assist with emergency endoscopy to locate the source of bleeding. Prepare to insert a nasogastric or Sengstaken-Blakemore tube to perform suction or iced lavage or to compress bleeding sites.

If the patient's hematemesis isn't immediately life-threatening, begin with a thorough history. First, have the patient describe the amount, color, and consistency of the vomitus. When did he first notice this sign? Has he ever had hematemesis before? Find out if he also has bloody or black tarry stools. Note whether hematemesis is usually preceded by nausea, flatulence, diarrhea, or weakness. Has he recently had bouts of retching with or without vomiting?

Next, ask about a history of ulcers or of liver or coagulation disorders. Find out how much alcohol the patient drinks, if any. Is he taking aspirin or another nonsteroidal anti-inflammatory drug, such as phenylbutazone or indomethacin? These drugs may cause erosive gastritis.

Begin the physical examination by checking for postural hypotension, an early warning sign of hypovolemia. Take blood pressure and pulse with the patient supine, sitting, then standing. A decrease of 10 mm Hg or more in systolic pressure or an increase of 10 beats/minute or more in pulse rate indicates volume depletion. After obtaining other vital signs, inspect the mucous membranes, nasopharynx, and skin for any signs of bleeding or other abnormalities. Finally, palpate the abdomen for tenderness, pain, or masses. Note lymphadenopathy.

Medical causes

● *Achalasia.* Rarely, this disorder produces hematemesis; passive regurgitation is much more common. Achalasia also causes hoarseness or coughing that may be accompanied by aspiration and recurrent pulmonary infection. Usually painless, dysphagia commonly occurs early.

● *Coagulation disorders.* Any disorder that disrupts normal clotting may cause gastrointestinal bleeding and moderate-to-severe hematemesis. Bleeding may also occur in other body systems, resulting in such signs as epistaxis and ecchymosis. In addition, the specific coagulation disorder, such as thrombocytopenia or hemophilia, has distinct associated effects.

● *Esophageal carcinoma.* A late sign of this disorder, hematemesis may be accompanied by steady chest pain that radiates to the back. Other features include substernal fullness, severe dysphagia, nausea, vomiting with nocturnal regurgitation and aspiration,

---

RARE CAUSES OF HEMATEMESIS

Two relatively common disorders rarely cause hematemesis. When *acute diverticulitis* affects the duodenum, gastrointestinal bleeding and resultant hematemesis occur with abdominal pain and fever. With GI involvement, *secondary syphilis* can cause hematemesis. More characteristic signs and symptoms include a primary chancre, rash, fever, weight loss, malaise, anorexia, and headache.

Two rare disorders commonly cause hematemesis. *Malaria* produces this and other GI signs, but its most characteristic effects are chills, fever, headache, muscle pain, and splenomegaly. *Yellow fever* also causes hematemesis as well as sudden fever, bradycardia, jaundice, and severe prostration.

---

hemoptysis, fever, hiccups, sore throat, melena, and halitosis.

● *Esophageal injury by caustics.* Ingestion of corrosive acids or alkalies produces esophageal injury associated with grossly bloody or "coffee ground" vomitus. This hematemesis is accompanied by epigastric and anterior or retrosternal chest pain that's intensified by swallowing. In 3 to 4 weeks, dysphagia, marked salivation, and fever may develop and worsen as strictures form.

● *Esophageal rupture.* Here, the severity of hematemesis depends on the cause of the rupture. When instrumentation damages the esophagus, hematemesis is usually slight. However, rupture from Boerhaave's syndrome—increased esophageal pressure from vomiting or retching—or other esophageal disorders typically causes more severe hematemesis. This life-threatening disorder may also produce severe retrosternal, epigastric, neck, or scapular pain accompanied by chest and neck edema. Examination reveals subcutaneous crepitation in the chest wall, supraclavicular fossa, and neck. The patient may also show signs of respiratory distress, such as dyspnea and cyanosis.

MANAGING HEMATEMESIS WITH INTUBATION

When your patient has hematemesis, you'll need to assist with GI tube insertion to allow blood drainage, to aspirate gastric contents, or to perform gastric lavage. Here are some of the most common tubes and their uses.

NASOGASTRIC TUBES

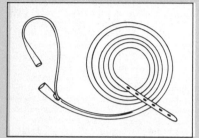

The *Salem-Sump tube* (above), a double-lumen nasogastric tube, is used to remove stomach fluid and gas or to aspirate gastric contents. It may also be used for gastric lavage, drug administration, or feeding. Its main advantage over the *Levin tube*—a single-lumen nasogastric device—is that it allows atmospheric air to enter the patient's stomach so the tube can float freely instead of risking adhesion and damage to the gastric mucosa.

WIDE-BORE GASTRIC TUBES

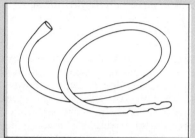

The *Ewald tube,* a wide-bore tube that allows passage of a large amount of fluid and clots quickly, is especially useful for gastric lavage in patients with profuse GI bleeding or poison ingestion. Another wide-bore tube, the double-lumen *Levacuator,* has a large lumen for evacuation of gastric contents and a small one for lavage. The *Edlich tube* (above) has one wide-bore lumen with four openings near the closed distal tip. A funnel or syringe can be connected at the proximal end. Like the others, the Edlich can aspirate a large volume of gastric contents quickly.

• **Esophageal varices (ruptured).** Life-threatening rupture of esophageal varices may produce "coffee ground" or massive, bright red vomitus. Signs of shock, such as hypotension or tachycardia, may follow or even precede hematemesis if the stomach fills with blood before vomiting occurs. Melena or painless hematochezia, ranging from slight oozing to massive rectal hemorrhage, may also occur.

• **Gastric carcinoma.** Painless bright red or dark brown hematemesis is a late sign of this uncommon cancer. Usually, gastric carcinoma begins insidiously with upper abdominal discomfort. The patient then develops chronic dyspepsia, anorexia, and slight nausea. Later, he may have fatigue, weakness, weight loss, feelings of fullness, melena, altered bowel habits, and signs of malnutrition, such as muscle wasting and dry skin.

• **Gastritis (acute).** Hematemesis and melena are the most common signs of this gastritis. In fact, they may be the only signs, although mild epigastric discomfort, nausea, fever, and malaise may also occur. Massive blood loss will precipitate signs of shock. Typically, the patient has a history of alcohol abuse, hospitalization for severe illness, or use of aspirin or some other nonsteroidal anti-inflammatory drug.

• **Gastroesophageal reflux disease.** Although rare in this disorder, hematemesis may occur and even may lead to signs of shock, such as hypotension and tachycardia. It's accompanied by pyrosis, flatulence, dyspepsia, and postural regurgitation that's aggravated by lying down or stooping over. Related

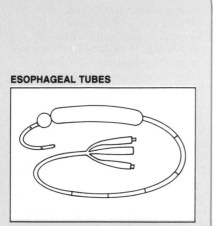

ESOPHAGEAL TUBES

The *Sengstaken-Blakemore tube* (above), a triple-lumen double-balloon esophageal tube, provides a gastric aspiration port that allows drainage from below the gastric balloon. It can also be used for instilling medication. A similar tube, the *Linton,* can aspirate esophageal and gastric contents without risking necrosis, because it has no esophageal balloon. The *Minnesota esophagogastric tamponade tube,* which has four lumens and two balloons, provides pressure monitoring ports for both balloons without the need for Y connectors.

effects include dysphagia, retrosternal pain, weight loss, halitosis, and signs of aspiration, such as dyspnea and recurrent pulmonary infection.

● *Gastrointestinal leiomyoma.* Rarely, this benign tumor may involve the gastrointestinal tract, eroding the mucosa or vascular supply to produce hematemesis. Other features vary with the tumor's size and location. For example, esophageal involvement may cause dysphagia and weight loss.

● *Mallory-Weiss syndrome.* Characterized by a mucosal tear of the cardia or lower esophagus, this syndrome may produce hematemesis and melena. Commonly, it's triggered by severe vomiting, retching, or straining (as from coughing). Severe bleeding may precipitate signs of shock, such as tachycardia, hypotension, dyspnea,

and cool, clammy skin.

● *Peptic ulcers.* Hematemesis may occur here when a peptic ulcer penetrates an artery, vein, or highly vascular tissue. Massive—and possibly life-threatening—hematemesis is typical with penetration of an artery. Other features include melena or hematochezia, chills, fever, and signs of shock and dehydration, such as tachycardia, hypotension, poor skin turgor, and thirst. Usually, the patient will have a history of epigastric pain that's relieved by foods or antacids and of nausea, vomiting, and epigastric tenderness.

Other causes
● *Treatments.* Traumatic nasogastric or endotracheal intubation may cause hematemesis associated with swallowed blood. Nose or throat surgery may also cause this sign in the same way.

Special considerations
Closely monitor the patient's vital signs every 15 minutes and watch for signs of shock. Also keep accurate intake and output records. Place the patient on bed rest in a low or semi-Fowler's position to prevent aspiration of emesis. Keep suctioning equipment nearby and use it, as needed. Provide frequent oral hygiene and emotional support—the sight of bloody vomitus can be very frightening. As ordered, administer epinephrine or vasopressin to control bleeding. As the bleeding tapers off, give hourly doses of antacids by nasogastric tube, as ordered.

Explain diagnostic tests, such as serum electrolyte studies, endoscopy, and barium swallow. Check the patient's stools regularly for occult blood, using guaiac.

Pediatric pointers
Hematemesis occurs much less frequently in children than in adults. Occasionally, neonates have hematemesis caused by swallowing maternal blood during delivery or nursing from a cracked nipple. Hemorrhagic disease of the newborn and esophageal erosion

may also cause hematemesis in infants, requiring immediate fluid replacement.

Hematochezia

[Rectal bleeding]

The passage of bloody stools—or hematochezia—usually indicates gastrointestinal (GI) bleeding below the ligament of Treitz. In fact, it may be the first sign of lower GI bleeding. However, hematochezia—usually preceded by hematemesis—may also accompany rapid hemorrhage of one liter or more from the upper GI tract.

Hematochezia ranges from formed, blood-streaked stools to liquid, bloody stools that may be bright red, dark mahogany, or maroon in color. Usually, hematochezia develops abruptly and is heralded by abdominal pain.

Although hematochezia commonly results from GI disorders, it may also result from coagulation disorders, the effects of toxins, and certain diagnostic tests. Always a significant sign, hematochezia may precipitate life-threatening hypovolemia.

Assessment

If the patient has severe hematochezia, quickly check his vital signs. If you detect signs of shock, such as hypotension and tachycardia, have another nurse notify the doctor. Place the patient in a supine position and elevate his feet 20° to 30°.

Prepare to administer oxygen, and start a large-bore I.V. for emergency fluid replacement. Next, obtain a blood sample for typing and cross matching. As ordered, assist with nasogastric intubation. To control bleeding, suction the patient and perform iced lavage, as ordered. Also assist with emergency endoscopy to detect the source of the bleeding, as ordered.

If the patient's hematochezia isn't immediately life-threatening, ask him to fully describe the amount, color, and consistency of his bloody stools. (If possible, also inspect and characterize the stool yourself.) How long have his stools been this way? Do they always look the same or does the amount of blood seem to vary? Ask about associated signs and symptoms.

Next, explore the patient's medical history, focusing on GI and coagulation disorders. Ask about use of gastrointestinal irritants, such as alcohol, aspirin, and other nonsteroidal anti-inflammatory drugs.

Begin the physical examination by checking for postural hypotension, an early sign of shock. Take the patient's blood pressure and pulse while he's lying down, sitting, and standing. If systolic pressure decreases by 10 mm Hg or more, or pulse rate increases by 10 beats/minute or more when he changes position, suspect volume depletion and impending shock.

Then assess the skin for petechiae or spider angiomas. Palpate the abdomen for tenderness, pain, or masses. Also note lymphadenopathy. Finally, assist the doctor with a digital rectal examination, as ordered.

Medical causes

● *Amyloidosis.* Rarely, hematochezia occurs when this disorder affects the GI tract. Massive, rapid hematochezia may precipitate signs of shock, such as hypotension and tachycardia. Other features include hypoactive or absent bowel sounds, abdominal pain, constipation, and diarrhea. The patient may also have a stiff, enlarged tongue, resulting in dysarthria.

● *Anal fissure.* Slight hematochezia characterizes this disorder; blood may streak the stool or appear on toilet tissue. Accompanying hematochezia is severe rectal pain that may make the patient reluctant to defecate, thereby causing constipation.

● *Angiodysplastic lesions.* Most common in the elderly, these arteriovenous lesions of the ascending colon typically cause chronic, bright red rectal bleeding. Occasionally, this painless hematochezia may result in life-threatening blood loss and signs of shock, such as tachycardia and hypotension.

• *Anorectal fistula.* Blood, pus, mucus, and occasionally stool may drain from this fistula. Other effects include rectal pain and pruritus.

• *Celiac disease.* Rarely, this malabsorption syndrome causes bright red, liquid stools. More typically, it produces frothy, foul-smelling, fatty stools (steatorrhea) with diarrhea. Other features include weight loss, abdominal distention, anorexia, and others.

• *Coagulation disorders.* Gastrointestinal bleeding marked by moderate-to-severe hematochezia may occur. Bleeding may also occur in other body systems, producing such signs as epistaxis and purpura. Specific coagulation disorders, such as thrombocytopenia and disseminated intravascular coagulation (DIC), also produce characteristic associated findings.

• *Colitis.* Ischemic colitis often causes bloody diarrhea, especially in the elderly. The hematochezia may be slight or massive and is usually accompanied by severe cramping lower abdominal pain and hypotension. Other effects: abdominal tenderness, distention, and absent bowel sounds. Severe colitis may cause signs of life-threatening hypovolemic shock and peritonitis.

Ulcerative colitis typically causes bloody diarrhea that may also contain mucus. Occasionally, the hematochezia occurs at night. It's preceded by mild-to-severe abdominal cramps and may cause slight-to-massive blood loss. Related features include fever, tenesmus, anorexia, nausea, vomiting, hyperactive bowel sounds, and occasionally tachycardia. Weight loss and weakness occur late.

• *Colon cancer.* Although pain is the most common symptom here, bright red hematochezia is also a telling sign—especially in cancer of the left colon. Early tumor growth in the right colon may cause melena, abdominal

aching, pressure, and dull cramps. As the disease progresses, the patient develops weakness, fatigue, exertional dyspnea, and vertigo. Later, there may also be diarrhea, anorexia, weight loss, vomiting, abdominal mass, and signs of obstruction, such as abdominal distention and abnormal bowel sounds.

Usually, a left colon tumor causes early signs of obstruction: commonly, rectal pressure, bleeding, and intermittent fullness or cramping. As the disease progresses, the patient develops obstipation, diarrhea, or ribbon-shaped stools. Passage of stool or flatus typically relieves the pain. Stools are grossly bloody or black and tarry.

• *Colorectal polyps.* These polyps are the most common cause of intermittent hematochezia in adults under age 60; however, they may be asymptomatic. When located high in the colon, polyps may cause blood-streaked stools; when closer to the rectum, they may bleed freely. Large polyps may also cause recurrent bowel obstruction marked by constipation and colicky abdominal pain.

• *Crohn's disease.* Although hematochezia isn't a common sign of this disorder, it's usually associated with massive, life-threatening blood loss when it does occur. The chief features of Crohn's disease are fever, abdominal distention and pain with guarding, diarrhea, hyperactive bowel sounds, anorexia, nausea, and fatigue.

• *Diverticulitis.* Most common in the elderly, this disorder can suddenly cause mild-to-moderate rectal bleeding after the patient feels the urge to defecate. The bleeding may end abruptly or lead to life-threatening blood loss with signs of shock. Associated findings may include left lower quadrant pain that's relieved by defecation and alternating constipation and diarrhea.

• *Dysentery.* Bloody diarrhea is common in infection with *Shigella, Ameba,* and *Campylobacter,* but rare with *Salmonella.* Abdominal pain or cramps, tenesmus, fever, and nausea may also occur.

• *Esophageal varices (ruptured).* In this life-threatening disorder, hematochezia may range from slight rectal oozing to grossly bloody stools. It may be accompanied by mild-to-severe hematemesis or melena. This painless—but massive—hemorrhage may precipitate signs of shock, such as tachycardia and hypotension. In fact, signs of shock occasionally precede overt signs of bleeding. Typically, the patient will have a history of chronic liver disease.

• *Food poisoning (staphylococcal).* One to six hours after ingesting food toxins, the patient may have bloody diarrhea. Accompanying signs and symptoms include severe, cramping abdominal pain, nausea and vomiting, and prostration, all of which last a few hours.

• *Heavy metal poisoning.* Here, bloody diarrhea is accompanied by cramping abdominal pain, nausea, and vomiting. Other signs may include tachycardia, hypotension, convulsions, and an altered level of consciousness.

• *Hemorrhoids.* Hematochezia may accompany external hemorrhoids, which typically cause painful defecation, resulting in constipation. Less painful internal hemorrhoids usually produce a constant oozing hematochezia that may eventually lead to signs of anemia, such as weakness and fatigue.

• *Leptospirosis.* The severe form of this infection—Weil's syndrome—produces hematochezia or melena along with other signs of bleeding, such as epistaxis and hemoptysis. Typically, the bleeding is preceded by a sudden frontal headache and severe thigh and lumbar myalgia that may be accompanied by cutaneous hyperesthesia. Chills and a rapidly rising fever then follow, perhaps with nausea and vomiting. Usually, fever, headache, and myalgia intensify and persist for weeks. Other findings may include right upper quadrant tenderness, hepatomegaly, and jaundice.

• *Peptic ulcers.* Upper GI bleeding is a frequent complication here. The patient may display hematochezia, hematemesis, or melena, depending on the rapidity and amount of bleeding. If the peptic ulcer penetrates an artery or vein, massive bleeding may precipitate signs of shock, such as hypotension and tachycardia. Other findings may include chills, fever, and signs of dehydration, such as dry mucous membranes, poor skin turgor, or thirst. Typically, the patient will have a history of epigastric pain that's relieved by foods or antacids; he may also complain of nausea and vomiting.

• *Rectal melanoma (malignant).* This rare rectal carcinoma typically causes recurrent rectal bleeding that arises from a painless, asymptomatic mass.

• *Small-intestine cancer.* Rarely, this disorder produces slight hematochezia, or blood-streaked stools. Its characteristic features include colicky pain and postprandial vomiting. Other common signs and symptoms include weight loss, anorexia, and fever. Palpation may reveal abdominal masses.

• *Typhoid fever.* About 10% of patients with this disorder develop hematochezia, which is occasionally massive. However, melena is more common. Both signs of bleeding occur late and may be accompanied by mental dullness, marked abdominal distention, diarrhea, significant weight loss, and profound fatigue. Among earlier signs and symptoms are pathognomonic rose spots, headache, chills, fever, constipation, dry cough, and epistaxis.

• *Ulcerative proctitis.* Typically, this disorder causes an intense urge to defecate, but the patient passes only bright red blood, pus, or mucus. Other common signs and symptoms include acute constipation and tenesmus.

Other causes

• *Tests.* Certain procedures, such as colonoscopy and proctosigmoidoscopy, may cause bowel perforation and lead to rectal bleeding.

Special considerations

Place the patient on bed rest and check his vital signs every 15 minutes, watching for signs of shock, such as hypotension and tachycardia. Monitor the patient's intake and output hourly. Remember to provide emotional support because hematochezia may frighten the patient.

Prepare the patient for blood tests, endoscopy, and GI X-rays, as ordered. Visually examine the patient's stools and test them for occult blood. If necessary, send a stool sample to the laboratory to check for parasites.

Pediatric pointers

Hematochezia is much less common in children than in adults. It may result from structural disorders, such as intussusception and Meckel's diverticulum, and from inflammatory disorders, such as peptic ulcer disease and ulcerative colitis.

In children, ulcerative colitis typically produces chronic, rather than acute, signs and symptoms and may also cause slow growth and maturation related to malnutrition.

Hematuria

A cardinal sign of renal and urinary tract disorders, hematuria is the abnormal presence of blood in the urine. By strict definition, it means three or more red blood cells per high-power microscopic field in the urine. Microscopic hematuria is confirmed by an occult blood indicator, whereas macroscopic hematuria is immediately visible. However, macroscopic hematuria must be distinguished from pseudohematuria (see *Confirming Hematuria.*). This common sign may be continuous or intermittent, is often accompanied by pain, and may be aggravated by prolonged standing or walking.

Hematuria may be classified by the stage of urination it predominantly affects. Bleeding at the start of urination—*initial hematuria*—usually indicates urethral pathology; bleeding at

---

CONFIRMING HEMATURIA

If the patient's urine appears blood-tinged, be sure to rule out pseudohematuria—red- or pink-colored urine caused by urinary pigments. First, carefully observe the urine specimen. If it contains a red sediment, it's probably *true* hematuria.

Then check the patient's history for use of drugs associated with pseudohematuria, including rifampin, chlorzoxazone, phenazopyridine, phenothiazines, doxorubicin, phensuximide, phenytoin, daunomycin, or laxatives with phenolphthalein.	Ask about the patient's intake of beets, berries, or foods with red dyes, which may color the urine red. Recognize that porphyrinuria or excess urate excretion may also cause pseudohematuria.	Finally, test the urine, using a chemical reagent strip, or "dip stick." This test can confirm hematuria—even if it's microscopic—and can also estimate the amount of blood present.

the end of urination—*terminal hematuria*—usually indicates pathology of the bladder neck, posterior urethra, or prostate. Bleeding throughout urination—*total hematuria*—usually indicates pathology above the bladder neck. Another clue to the source of the bleeding is the color of hematuria. Generally, dark or brownish blood indicates renal or upper urinary tract bleeding, whereas bright red blood indicates lower urinary tract bleeding.

Hematuria may result from one of two mechanisms: rupture or perforation of vessels in the renal system or urinary tract, or impaired glomerular filtration, which allows red blood cells to seep into the urine. Although it usually results from renal and urinary tract disorders, hematuria may also result from certain gastrointestinal, prostate, vaginal, or coagulation disorders, or from the effects of drugs. Invasive therapy or diagnostic tests that involve manipulative instrumentation of the renal and urologic systems may also cause hematuria. Nonpathologic hematuria may result from fever and hypercatabolic states. Transient hematuria may also follow strenuous exercise.

Assessment

After detecting hematuria, take a pertinent health history. Ask the patient when the macroscopic hematuria began. Does it vary in severity between voidings? Is it worse at the beginning, middle, or end of urination? Is the patient passing any clots? Find out if hematuria has occurred before. To rule out artifactitious hematuria, ask about bleeding hemorrhoids or the onset of menses, if appropriate.

Ask about recent abdominal or flank trauma. Has the patient been exercising strenuously? Note a history of renal, urinary, prostatic, or coagulation disorders. Then obtain a drug history.

Begin the physical examination by palpating and percussing the abdomen and flanks. Next, percuss the costovertebral angle (CVA) to elicit tenderness. Check the urinary meatus for bleeding or other abnormalities. Using a chemical reagent strip, test a urine sample for protein. Finally, assist the doctor with a vaginal or digital rectal examination, as ordered.

Medical causes

- **Appendicitis.** About 15% of these patients have either microscopic or macroscopic hematuria accompanied by bladder tenderness, dysuria, and urinary urgency. More typical findings include constant right lower quadrant pain (especially over McBurney's point), nausea, vomiting, anorexia, abdominal rigidity, rebound tenderness, constipation, tachycardia, and low-grade fever.
- **Bladder neoplasm.** A primary cause of gross hematuria in men, this disorder may also produce pain in the bladder, rectum, pelvis, flank, back, or leg. Other common features are nocturia, vomiting, diarrhea, and insomnia. Signs of urinary tract infection, such as dysuria and urinary frequency and urgency, may also occur.
- **Bladder trauma.** Gross hematuria is characteristic in traumatic rupture or perforation of the bladder. Typically, the hematuria is accompanied by lower abdominal pain and, occasionally, anuria despite a strong urge to void. The patient may also have swelling of the scrotum, buttocks, or perineum, and signs of shock, such as tachycardia and hypotension.
- **Calculi.** Both bladder and renal calculi produce hematuria, which may be associated with signs of urinary tract infection, such as dysuria and urinary frequency and urgency. *Bladder calculi* usually cause gross hematuria, referred pain to the penile or vulvar area, and, in some patients, bladder distention. *Renal calculi* may produce microscopic or gross hematuria. The cardinal symptom, though, is colicky pain that travels from the costovertebral angle to the flank, the suprapubic region, and the external genitalia. This pain occurs with passage of a stone and may be excruciating at its peak. Nausea and

vomiting are common. Other signs and symptoms may include restlessness, fever, chills, abdominal distention, and, possibly, decreased bowel sounds.

• *Coagulation disorders.* Macroscopic hematuria is often the first sign of hemorrhage in coagulation disorders, such as thrombocytopenia or disseminated intravascular coagulation. Among other features are epistaxis, purpura (petechiae and ecchymoses), and signs of gastrointestinal bleeding.

• *Cortical necrosis (acute).* Accompanying gross hematuria in this renal disorder are intense flank pain, anuria, and fever.

• *Cystitis.* Hematuria is a telling sign in all four types of cystitis. *Bacterial cystitis* usually produces macroscopic hematuria accompanied by urinary urgency and frequency, dysuria, nocturia, and tenesmus. The patient complains of perineal and lumbar pain, suprapubic discomfort, and fatigue and occasionally has a low-grade fever.

More common in women, *chronic interstitial cystitis* also causes grossly bloody hematuria. Associated features include urinary frequency, dysuria, nocturia, and tenesmus. Both microscopic and macroscopic hematuria may occur in *tubercular cystitis,* which may also cause urinary urgency and frequency, dysuria, tenesmus, flank pain, fatigue, and anorexia. Usually, *viral cystitis* produces hematuria, urinary urgency and frequency, dysuria, nocturia, tenesmus, and fever.

• *Diverticulitis.* When this disorder involves the bladder, it usually causes microscopic hematuria as well as urinary frequency and urgency, dysuria, and nocturia. Its characteristic findings include left lower abdominal pain, abdominal tenderness, constipation, and a palpable abdominal mass. The patient may also have mild nausea, flatulence, and a low-grade fever.

• *Endocarditis (subacute infective).* Occasionally, this disorder produces embolization, resulting in renal infarction and microscopic or gross hematuria. Among common related findings are constant fever, chills, fatigue, pallor, anorexia, weight loss, polyarthralgia, petechiae, flank pain, cardiac murmurs, tachycardia, and splenomegaly.

• *Glomerulonephritis.* Usually, *acute glomerulonephritis* begins with gross hematuria that eventually tapers off to microscopic hematuria, which may persist for months. It may also produce oliguria or anuria, proteinuria, mild fever, fatigue, flank and abdominal pain, generalized edema, increased blood pressure, nausea, vomiting, and signs of lung congestion, such as crackles and productive cough.

Chronic glomerulonephritis usually causes microscopic hematuria accompanied by proteinuria, generalized edema, and increased blood pressure. Signs and symptoms of uremia may also occur in advanced disease.

• *Nephritis (interstitial).* Typically, this infection causes microscopic hematuria. However, some patients with *acute interstitial nephritis* may develop gross hematuria. It also causes fever, maculopapular skin rash, and oliguria or anuria.

In *chronic interstitial nephritis*, the patient will have dilute—almost colorless—urine that may be accompanied by polyuria and increased blood pressure.

• *Obstructive nephropathy.* This disorder may cause microscopic or macroscopic hematuria; however, it's rarely grossly bloody. The patient may have colicky flank and abdominal pain, costovertebral angle tenderness, and anuria or oliguria that alternates with polyuria.

• *Polycystic kidney disease.* This hereditary disorder may cause recurrent microscopic or gross hematuria. Although often asymptomatic before age 40, it may cause increased blood pressure, polyuria, dull flank pain, and signs of urinary tract infection, such as dysuria and urinary frequency and urgency.

Later, the patient develops a swollen, tender abdomen and lumbar pain that's aggravated by exertion and relieved by lying down. There may also be proteinuria and colicky abdominal pain

HEMATURIA: CAUSES AND ASSOCIATED FINDINGS

S&S CHIEF CAUSES	MAJOR ASSOCIATED SIGNS AND SYMPTOMS												
	Abdominal distention	Abdominal pain	Anuria	Bladder distention	Blood pressure increase	Bowel sounds—hypoactive	Colicky pain	CVA tenderness	Dysuria	Edema—generalized	Edema of the legs	Fever	
Bladder neoplasm									•				
Bladder trauma		•	•										
Calculi (bladder)				•					•				
Calculi (renal)	•	•				•	•	•	•			•	
Coagulation disorders													
Cortical necrosis (acute)			•									•	
Cystitis (bacterial)									•			•	
Cystitis (chronic interstitial)									•				
Cystitis (tubercular)									•				
Cystitis (viral)									•			•	
Endocarditis (subacute infective)												•	
Glomerulonephritis (acute)		•	•		•					•		•	
Glomerulonephritis (chronic)					•					•			
Nephritis (acute interstitial)			•									•	
Nephritis (chronic interstitial)					•								

Flank mass	Flank pain	Lumbar pain	Murmurs	Nausea	Nocturia	Oliguria	Perineal pain	Polyarthralgia	Polyuria	Proteinuria	Purpura	Skin rash	Urethral discharge	Urinary frequency	Urinary hesitancy	Urinary stream—diminished	Urinary urgency	Vomiting
	•				•		•							•			•	•
							•							•			•	
	•			•										•			•	•
											•							
	•																	
		•			•		•							•			•	
					•									•				
	•													•			•	
					•									•				
	•		•					•										
	•			•		•				•								•
										•								
						•						•						
									•									

(continued)

HEMATURIA: CAUSES AND ASSOCIATED FINDINGS *(continued)*

CHIEF CAUSES	Abdominal distention	Abdominal pain	Anuria	Bladder distention	Blood pressure increase	Bowel sounds—hypoactive	Colicky pain	CVA tenderness	Dysuria	Edema—generalized	Edema of the legs	Fever	
Obstructive nephropathy		•	•				•	•					
Polycystic kidney disease		•			•		•		•				
Prostatic hypertrophy (benign)				•									
Prostatitis (acute)				•					•			•	
Prostatitis (chronic)				•					•				
Pyelonephritis (acute)	•					•		•	•			•	
Renal infarction		•	•		•	•		•				•	
Renal neoplasm					•		•	•			•	•	
Renal papillary necrosis (acute)		•	•			•	•	•				•	
Renal trauma						•							
Renal tuberculosis		•					•		•				
Renal vein thrombosis			•					•			•	•	
Schistosomiasis						•			•				
Sickle cell anemia													
Vasculitis			•		•							•	

Flank mass	Flank pain	Lumbar pain	Murmurs	Nausea	Nocturia	Oliguria	Perineal pain	Polyarthralgia	Polyuria	Proteinuria	Purpura	Skin rash	Urethral discharge	Urinary frequency	Urinary hesitancy	Urinary stream—diminished	Urinary urgency	Vomiting
	•					•			•									
	•	•							•	•				•			•	
					•		•							•	•	•		
		•		•			•	•						•			•	•
							•						•	•			•	
	•			•	•									•			•	•
	•			•		•				•								•
•	•			•														•
	•					•												•
•	•			•		•					•							•
		•								•				•				
	•	•				•				•								
			•			•												
						•					•	•						

from the ureteral passage of clots or stones.

● **Prostatic hypertrophy (benign).** About 20% of these patients have macroscopic hematuria, usually when prostatic hypertrophy causes significant obstruction. Typically, the hematuria is preceded by diminished urinary stream, tenesmus, and a feeling of incomplete voiding. It may be accompanied by urinary hesitancy, frequency, and incontinence; nocturia; perineal pain; and constipation. Inspection reveals a midline mass representing the distended bladder while rectal palpation discloses an enlarged prostate.

● **Prostatitis.** Whether it's acute or chronic, prostatitis may cause macroscopic hematuria, usually at the end of urination. It may also produce urinary frequency and urgency and dysuria followed by visible bladder distention. *Acute prostatitis* also produces fatigue, malaise, myalgia, polyarthralgia, fever with chills, nausea, vomiting, perineal and low back pain, and decreased libido. Rectal palpation will reveal a tender, swollen, firm prostate.

Chronic prostatitis often follows an acute attack. It may cause persistent urethral discharge, dull perineal pain, and decreased libido.

● **Pyelonephritis (acute).** This infection typically produces microscopic or macroscopic hematuria that progresses to grossly bloody hematuria. After the infection resolves, microscopic hematuria may persist for a few months. Related signs and symptoms include persistent high fever, flank pain, costovertebral angle tenderness, shaking chills, weakness, fatigue, dysuria, urinary frequency and urgency, tenesmus, and nocturia. The patient may also have nausea, anorexia, vomiting, and signs of paralytic ileus, such as hypoactive or absent bowel sounds and abdominal distention.

● **Renal infarction.** Typically, this disorder produces gross hematuria. The patient may complain of constant, severe flank and upper abdominal pain

accompanied by costovertebral angle tenderness, anorexia, and nausea and vomiting. Other findings include oliguria or anuria, proteinuria, hypoactive bowel sounds, and, a day or two after infarction, fever and increased blood pressure.

● **Renal neoplasm.** Here, the classic triad of signs and symptoms is macroscopic, grossly bloody hematuria; dull, aching flank pain; and a smooth, firm, palpable flank mass. Colicky pain may accompany the passage of clots. Other findings include fever, CVA tenderness, and increased blood pressure. In the advanced disease, the patient may have weight loss, nausea, vomiting, and leg edema with varicoceles.

● **Renal papillary necrosis (acute).** In this disorder, hematuria is usually macroscopic and grossly bloody. It may be accompanied by intense flank pain, costovertebral angle tenderness, abdominal rigidity and colicky pain, oliguria or anuria, fever, chills, vomiting, and hypoactive bowel sounds.

● **Renal trauma.** About 80% of patients with renal trauma will have microscopic or gross hematuria. Accompanying signs and symptoms may include flank pain, a palpable flank mass, oliguria, hematoma or ecchymoses over the upper abdomen or flank, nausea and vomiting, and hypoactive bowel sounds. Severe trauma may precipitate signs of shock, such as tachycardia and hypotension.

● **Renal tuberculosis.** Gross hematuria is often the first sign of this disorder. It may be accompanied by urinary frequency, dysuria, tenesmus, colicky abdominal pain, lumbar pain, and proteinuria.

● **Renal vein thrombosis.** Macroscopic, grossly bloody hematuria usually occurs with this thrombosis. In abrupt venous obstruction, the patient has severe flank and lumbar pain and epigastric and CVA tenderness. Other features include fever, pallor, proteinuria, peripheral edema, and, when the obstruction is bilateral, oliguria or anuria and other uremic signs. The kidneys are easily palpable. Gradual venous obstruction causes signs of nephrotic syndrome, proteinuria, and, occasionally, peripheral edema.

• *Schistosomiasis.* This infection usually causes intermittent hematuria at the end of urination. It may be accompanied by dysuria and colicky renal and bladder pain.

• *Sickle cell anemia.* In this hereditary disorder, gross hematuria may result from congestion of the renal papillae. Associated signs and symptoms may include pallor, chronic fatigue, polyarthralgia, leg ulcers, dyspnea, chest pain, impaired growth and development, hepatomegaly, and, possibly, jaundice. Auscultation also reveals tachycardia and systolic and diastolic murmurs.

• *Systemic lupus erythematosus.* Gross hematuria and proteinuria may occur when this disorder involves the kidneys. Cardinal associated features include nondeforming joint pain and stiffness, a butterfly rash, photosensitivity, Raynaud's phenomenon, convulsions or psychoses, recurrent fever, lymphadenopathy, anorexia, and weight loss.

• *Urethral trauma.* Initial hematuria may occur here, possibly with blood at the urinary meatus, local pain, and penile or vulvar ecchymoses.

• *Vaginitis.* When this infection spreads to the urinary tract, it may produce macroscopic hematuria. Related signs and symptoms may include urinary frequency and urgency, dysuria, nocturia, perineal pain, pruritus, and a malodorous vaginal discharge.

• *Vasculitis.* Hematuria is usually microscopic in this disorder. Associated signs and symptoms include malaise, myalgia, polyarthralgia, fever, increased blood pressure, pallor, and, occasionally, anuria. Other features—such as urticaria and purpura—may reflect the etiology of vasculitis.

Other causes
• *Diagnostic tests.* Renal biopsy is the diagnostic test most commonly associated with hematuria. This sign may also result from biopsy or manipulative instrumentation of the urinary tract, as in cystoscopy.

• *Drugs.* Among common drugs that may cause hematuria are anticoagulants, cyclophosphamide (Cytoxan), metyrosine, phenylbutazone, oxyphenbutazone, and thiabendazole.

• *Treatments.* Any therapy that involves manipulative instrumentation of the urinary tract, such as transurethral prostatectomy, may cause microscopic or macroscopic hematuria.

Special considerations
Because hematuria may frighten and upset the patient, be sure to provide emotional support. Check his vital signs at least every 4 hours and monitor intake and output, including the amount and pattern of hematuria. Administer prescribed pain drugs, as ordered, and encourage bed rest.

Prepare the patient for diagnostic tests, such as blood and urine studies, cystoscopy, and renal X-rays or biopsy. As ordered, teach the patient how to collect serial urine specimens using the three-glass technique. This technique helps determine whether hematuria marks the beginning, end, or course of urination.

Pediatric pointers
Many of the causes described above also produce hematuria in pediatric patients. However, cyclophosphamide is more likely to cause hematuria in children than in adults.

Common causes of hematuria chiefly affecting pediatric patients include congenital anomalies, such as obstructive uropathy and renal dysplasia; birth trauma; hematologic disorders, such as vitamin K deficiency, hemophilia, and hemolytic-uremic syndrome; certain neoplasms, such as Wilms' tumor, bladder leukemias, and rhabdomyosarcomas; allergies; and foreign bodies in the urinary tract. Artifactual hematuria may result from recent circumcision.

Hemianopia

Hemianopia is loss of vision in half the visual field (usually the vertical half) of one or both eyes. Its cause? A lesion affecting the optic chiasm, tract, or radiation. However, if the field defects are identical in both eyes but affect less than half the field of vision in each eye (incomplete homonymous hemianopia), the lesion may be in the occipital lobe; otherwise, it probably involves the parietal or temporal lobe. (See *Recognizing Types of Hemianopia.*)

Defects in visual perception due to cerebral lesions are usually associated with impaired color vision.

Assessment

Suspect a visual field defect if the patient seems startled when you approach him from one side or if he fails to see objects placed directly in front of him. To help determine the type of defect, compare the patient's visual fields to your own—assuming yours are normal. First, ask the patient to cover his right eye while you cover your left eye. Then, move a pen or similar-shaped object from the periphery of his (and your) uncovered eye into his field of vision. Ask the patient to indicate when he first sees the object. Does he see it at the same time you do? After you do? Repeat this test in each quadrant of both eyes. Then, for each eye, plot the defect by shading the area of a circle that corresponds to the area of vision loss.

Now evaluate the patient's level of consciousness, take his vital signs, and check his pupillary reaction and motor response. Ask if he's experienced headache, dysarthria, or seizures. Does he have ptosis or facial or extremity weakness? Hallucinations or loss of color vision? When did neurologic symptoms start? Obtain a medical history, noting especially eye disorders, hypertension, and diabetes mellitus.

Medical causes

• *Carotid artery aneurysm.* An aneurysm in the internal carotid artery can cause contralateral or bilateral defects in the visual fields. It can also cause hemiplegia, decreased level of consciousness, headache, aphasia, behavior disturbances, and unilateral hypoesthesia.

• *Cerebrovascular accident (CVA).* Hemianopia can result when a hemorrhagic, thrombotic, or embolic CVA affects any part of the optic pathway. Associated signs and symptoms depend on the location and size of the CVA but may include decreased level of consciousness; intellectual deficits, such as memory loss and poor judgment; personality changes; emotional lability; headache; and seizures. The patient may have contralateral hemiplegia, dysarthria, dysphagia, ataxia, a unilateral sensory loss, apraxia, agnosia, aphasia, blurred vision, decreased visual acuity, and diplopia. He may also have urinary retention or incontinence, constipation, and vomiting.

• *Occipital lobe lesion.* The most common symptoms arising from a lesion of one occipital lobe include incomplete homonymous hemianopia, scotomas, and impaired color vision. The patient may also experience visual hallucinations: flashes of light or color or visions of objects, people, animals, or geometric forms. These may appear in the defective field or may move toward it from the intact field.

• *Parietal lobe lesion.* This disorder produces homonymous hemianopia and sensory deficits, such as an inability to perceive body position or passive movement or to localize tactile, thermal, or vibratory stimuli. It may also cause apraxia and visual or tactile agnosia.

• *Pituitary tumor.* A tumor that compresses nerve fibers supplying the nasal half of both retinas causes complete or partial bitemporal hemianopia that occurs first in the upper visual fields but later can progress to blindness. Related findings include blurred vision, diplopia, headache, and (rarely) somno-

RECOGNIZING TYPES OF HEMIANOPIA

Lesions of the optic pathways cause visual field defects. The lesion's site determines the type of defect. For example, a lesion of the optic chiasm involving only those fibers that cross over to the opposite side causes *bitemporal hemianopia*—visual loss in the temporal half of each field. However, a lesion of the optic tract or a complete lesion of the optic radiation produces visual loss in the same half of each field—either left or right *homonymous hemianopia*.

Left visual field

Right visual field

Bitemporal hemianopia

Right homonymous hemianopia

Left homonymous hemianopia

Optic tract

Optic chiasm

BRAIN

Optic radiation

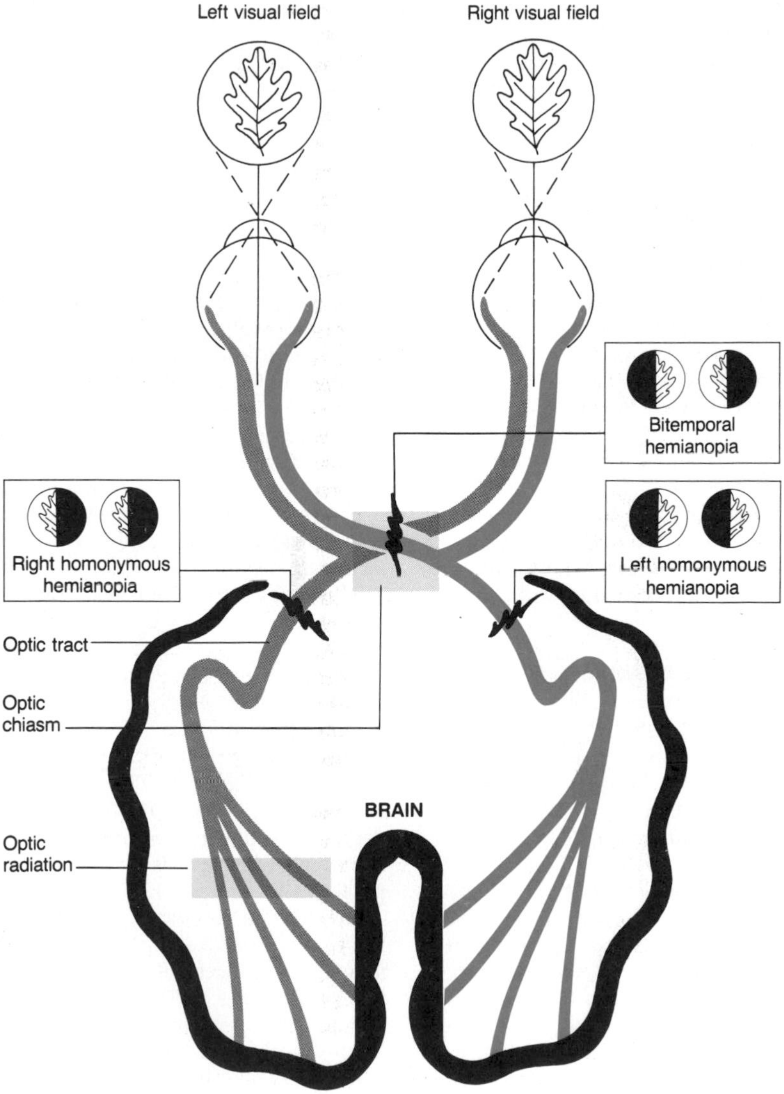

lence, hypothermia, or seizures.

Special considerations

If the patient's visual field defect is significant, prepare him for further visual field testing, such as perimetry or a tangent screen examination.

Tell the patient the extent of his defect so that he learns to compensate for it. Advise him to scan his surroundings frequently, turning his head in the direction of the defective visual field so he can directly view objects he'd normally notice peripherally. Also, approach him from the unaffected side. Position his bed so his unaffected side faces the door; if he's ambulatory, remove objects that could cause falls and alert him to other possible hazards. Place his clock and other objects within his field of vision, and avoid putting dangerous objects (such as hot dishes) where he can't see them.

Pediatric pointers

In children, a brain tumor is the most common cause of hemianopia. To help detect this sign, look for nonverbal clues—for example, the child may reach for a toy but miss it. To help the child compensate for hemianopia, place objects within his visual field and teach his parents to do this as well.

Hemoptysis

Frightening to the patient and often ominous, hemoptysis is the expectoration of blood or bloody sputum from the lungs or tracheobronchial tree. It's sometimes confused with bleeding from the mouth, throat, nasopharynx, or gastrointestinal tract. (See *Identifying Hemoptysis*.) Expectoration of 200 ml of blood in a single episode suggests severe bleeding, whereas expectoration of 400 ml in 3 hours or more than 600 ml in 16 hours signals life-threatening crisis.

Hemoptysis most commonly results from chronic bronchitis, bronchogenic carcinoma, or bronchiectasis. However, it may also result from inflammatory, infectious, cardiovascular, or coagulation disorders—or, in up to 15% of patients, from unknown causes. Rarely, it stems from a ruptured aortic aneurysm. The most common causes of *massive hemoptysis* are lung cancer, bronchiectasis, active tuberculosis, and cavitary pulmonary disease from necrotic infections or tuberculosis.

A number of pathophysiologic processes can cause hemoptysis. (See *What Happens in Hemoptysis,* page 401.)

Assessment

If the patient coughs up copious amounts of blood, prepare to assist with endotracheal intubation, and suction the patient frequently to remove blood. Remember, *massive hemoptysis* can cause airway obstruction and asphyxiation. Insert an I.V. line to allow fluid replacement, drug administration, and blood transfusions, if needed. Also be prepared to assist with emergency bronchoscopy to identify the bleeding site. Monitor blood pressure and pulse to detect hypotension and tachycardia, and draw an arterial blood sample for laboratory analysis to monitor respiratory status.

If the hemoptysis is mild, ask the patient when the current episode began. Has he ever coughed up blood before? About how much blood is he coughing up now? And how often? Ask about a history of cardiac, pulmonary, or bleeding disorders. If he's receiving anticoagulant therapy, find out the drug, its dosage and schedule, and the duration of therapy. Is he taking other prescription drugs? Does he smoke?

Take the patient's vital signs and examine his nose, mouth, and pharynx for sources of bleeding. Inspect the configuration of his chest and look for abnormal movement during breathing, use of accessory muscles, or retractions. Observe his respiratory rate, depth, and rhythm. Finally, examine his skin for lesions.

IDENTIFYING HEMOPTYSIS

These guidelines will help you distinguish hemoptysis from epistaxis, hematemesis, and brown, red, or pink sputum.

HEMOPTYSIS	HEMATEMESIS	BROWN, RED, OR PINK SPUTUM
Often frothy because it's mixed with air, hemoptysis is typically bright red with an alkaline pH (tested with nitrazine paper). It's strongly suggested by the presence of respiratory signs and symptoms— including a cough, a tickling sensation in the throat, and blood produced from repeated coughing episodes. (You can rule out epistaxis because the patient's nasal passages and posterior pharynx are usually clear.)	The usual site of hematemesis is the gastrointestinal tract; the patient vomits or regurgitates coffee-ground material that contains food particles, tests positive for occult blood, and has an acid pH. But he may vomit bright-red blood or swallowed blood from the oral cavity and nasopharynx. After an episode of hematemesis, the patient may have stools with traces of blood. Many patients with hematemesis also complain of dyspepsia.	Brown, red, or pink sputum can result from oxidation of inhaled bronchodilators. Sputum that looks like old blood may result from rupture of an amebic abscess into the bronchus. Red or brown sputum may occur in a patient with pneumonia caused by the enterobacterium *Serratia marcescens.*

Next, palpate the patient's chest for diaphragm level and for tenderness, respiratory excursion, fremitus, and abnormal pulsations; then percuss for flatness, dullness, resonance, hyperresonance, or tympany. Finally, auscultate the lungs, noting especially the quality and intensity of breath sounds. Also auscultate for heart murmurs, bruits, and pleural friction rubs.

Obtain a sputum sample and examine it for overall quantity, for the amount of blood it contains, and for its color, odor, and consistency.

Medical causes

● *Aortic aneurysm (ruptured).* Rarely, an aortic aneurysm ruptures into the tracheobronchial tree, causing hemoptysis and sudden death.

● *Bronchial adenoma.* This insidious disorder causes recurring hemoptysis in up to 30% of patients, along with a chronic cough and local wheezing.

● *Bronchiectasis.* Inflamed bronchial surfaces and eroded bronchial blood vessels cause hemoptysis, which can vary from blood-tinged sputum to blood (in about 20% of patients). The patient's sputum may also be copious, foul-smelling, and purulent. He may have a chronic cough, coarse crackles, clubbing (a late sign), fever, weight loss, fatigue, weakness, malaise, and dyspnea on exertion.

● *Bronchitis (chronic).* The first sign of this disorder is typically a productive cough lasting at least 3 months. Eventually this leads to production of blood-streaked sputum; massive hemorrhage is unusual. Other respiratory effects include dyspnea, prolonged expirations, wheezes, scattered rhonchi, accessory muscle use, barrel chest, tachypnea, and clubbing (a late sign).

● *Coagulation disorders.* Such disorders as thrombocytopenia and disseminated intravascular coagulation can cause hemoptysis. Besides their specific related findings, these disorders may share such general signs as multisystem hemorrhaging (for example, gastrointestinal bleeding or epistaxis) and purpuric lesions.

• *Laryngeal cancer.* Hemoptysis occurs here, but hoarseness is the usual early sign. Other findings may include dysphagia, dyspnea, stridor, cervical lymphadenopathy, and neck pain.

• *Lung abscess.* In about 50% of patients, this disorder produces blood-streaked sputum resulting from bronchial ulceration, necrosis, and granulation tissue. Common associated findings include a cough with large amounts of purulent, foul-smelling sputum; fever with chills; diaphoresis; anorexia; weight loss; headache; weakness; dyspnea; pleuritic or dull chest pain; and clubbing. Auscultation reveals tubular or cavernous breath sounds and crackles. Percussion reveals dullness on the affected side.

• *Lung cancer.* Ulceration of the bronchus commonly causes recurring hemoptysis (an early sign), which can vary from blood-streaked sputum to blood. Related findings include a productive cough, dyspnea, fever, anorexia, weight loss, wheezing, and chest pain (a late symptom).

• *Pneumonia.* In up to 50% of patients, *Klebsiella pneumonia* produces dark brown or red (currant-jelly) sputum, which is so tenacious the patient has difficulty expelling it from his mouth. The disorder begins abruptly with chills, fever, dyspnea, productive cough, and severe pleuritic chest pain. Associated findings may include cyanosis, prostration, tachycardia, decreased breath sounds, and crackles.

Pneumococcal pneumonia causes pinkish or rusty mucoid sputum. It begins with a sudden, shaking chill; a rapidly rising temperature; and, in over 80% of patients, tachycardia and tachypnea. Within a few hours, the patient typically experiences a productive cough along with severe, stabbing, pleuritic pain. The agonizing chest pain leads to rapid, shallow, grunting respirations with splinting. Examination reveals respiratory distress with dyspnea and accessory muscle use, crackles, and dullness on percussion over the affected lung. Malaise, weakness, myalgia, and prostration accompany high fever.

• *Pulmonary arteriovenous fistula.* Occurring in young adults, this genetic disorder causes intermittent hemoptysis. Associated signs and symptoms include cyanosis, clubbing, mild dyspnea, fatigue, vertigo, syncope, confusion, and speech and visual impairments. The patient may bleed from his nose, mouth, or lips. Ruby-red patches appear on his face, tongue, skin, mucous membranes, or nail beds.

• *Pulmonary contusion.* Blunt chest trauma commonly causes a cough with hemoptysis. Other signs and symptoms appear gradually within several hours after the injury. These include dyspnea, tachypnea, chest pain, tachycardia, hypotension, crackles, and decreased or absent breath sounds over the affected area. Severe respiratory distress—with oppressive dyspnea, nasal flaring, use of accessory muscles, extreme anxiety, cyanosis, and diaphoresis—may develop at any time.

• *Pulmonary edema.* Severe cardiogenic or noncardiogenic pulmonary edema commonly causes frothy, blood-tinged pink sputum, which accompanies severe dyspnea, orthopnea, gasping, anxiety, cyanosis, diffuse crackles, a ventricular gallop, and cold, clammy skin. This life-threatening condition may also cause tachycardia, lethargy, cardiac dysrhythmias, tachypnea, hypotension, and a thready pulse.

• *Pulmonary embolism with infarction.* Hemoptysis is a common finding in this life-threatening disorder, although massive hemoptysis is less common. Typical initial symptoms are dyspnea and anginal or pleuritic chest pain. Other common clinical features include tachycardia, tachypnea, low-grade fever, and diaphoresis. Less commonly, splinting of the chest, leg edema, and—with a large embolus—cyanosis, syncope, and distended neck veins may occur. Examination reveals decreased breath sounds, pleural friction rub, crackles, diffuse wheezing, dullness to percussion, and signs of circulatory collapse (weak, rapid pulse; hypotension), cerebral ischemia (transient loss of consciousness, convulsions), and hypoxemia (restlessness and—particularly in the elderly—hemiplegia and other focal neurologic deficits).

• *Pulmonary hypertension (primary).* Features generally develop late. Hemoptysis, exertional dyspnea, and fatigue are common. Anginalike pain usually occurs with exertion and may radiate to the neck but not to the arms. Other findings include dysrhythmias, syncope, cough, and hoarseness.

• *Pulmonary tuberculosis.* Blood-streaked or -tinged sputum commonly occurs in this disorder; massive hemoptysis may occur in advanced cavitary tuberculosis. Accompanying respiratory findings include a chronic productive cough, fine crackles after coughing, dyspnea, dullness to percussion, increased tactile fremitus, and possible amphoric breath sounds. The patient may also have night sweats, malaise, fatigue, fever, anorexia, weight loss, and pleuritic chest pain.

• *Silicosis.* Initially, this chronic disorder causes a productive cough with mucopurulent sputum. Subsequently, the sputum becomes blood-streaked and, occasionally, massive hemoptysis may occur. Other findings: fine, end-inspiratory crackles at lung bases, exertional dyspnea, tachypnea, weight loss, fatigue, and weakness.

• *Systemic lupus erythematosus.* In 50% of patients with this disorder, pleuritis and pneumonitis cause hemoptysis, cough, dyspnea, pleuritic chest pain, and crackles. Related findings are a butterfly rash in the acute phase, nondeforming joint pain and stiffness, photosensitivity, Raynaud's phenomenon, convulsions or psychoses, and such general features as fever, anorexia with weight loss, and lymphadenopathy.

WHAT HAPPENS IN HEMOPTYSIS

Hemoptysis results from bleeding into the respiratory tract by bronchial or pulmonary vessels. Bleeding reflects alterations in the vascular walls and in blood-clotting mechanisms. It can reflect any of the following pathophysiologic processes.

Hemorrhage and diapedesis of red blood cells from the pulmonary microvasculature into the alveoli

Necrosis of lung tissue that causes inflammation and rupture of blood vessels or hemorrhage into the alveolar spaces

Rupture of an aortic aneurysm into the tracheobronchial tree

Rupture of distended endobronchial blood vessels from pulmonary hypertension due to mitral stenosis

Rupture of a pulmonary arteriovenous fistula or of bronchial or pulmonary artery/pulmonary venous collateral channels

Sloughing of a caseous lesion into the tracheobronchial tree

Ulceration and erosion of the bronchial epithelium

• *Tracheal trauma.* Torn tracheal mucosa may cause hemoptysis, hoarseness, dysphagia, neck pain, airway occlusion, and respiratory distress.

• *Wegener's granulomatosis.* This multisystem disorder is characterized by necrotizing, granulomatous vasculitis. Pulmonary findings include hemoptysis, chest pain, cough, wheezing, dyspnea, epistaxis, severe sinusitis, and hemorrhagic skin lesions.

Other causes

• *Diagnostic tests.* Lung or airway injury from bronchoscopy, laryngoscopy, mediastinoscopy, or lung biopsy can cause bleeding and hemoptysis.

Special considerations

Expect the patient to react to this alarming sign with anxiety and apprehension. Comfort and reassure him, and place him in a slight Trendelenburg position to promote drainage of blood from the lung. If necessary to protect the nonbleeding lung, place the patient in the lateral decubitus position, with the suspected bleeding lung facing down. Cough suppression may or may not be desirable: cough suppressants can prevent blood from spreading throughout the lungs, but they can also lead to airway obstruction from accumulated blood.

Prepare the patient for diagnostic tests to determine the cause of bleeding. These may include a complete blood count, a sputum culture and smear, chest X-rays, coagulation studies, bronchoscopy, lung biopsy, pulmonary arteriography, or a lung scan.

Hemoptysis generally stops (but not abruptly) during treatment of the causative disorder. Many chronic disorders, however, cause recurrent hemoptysis. Instruct the patient to report recurring episodes and to bring a sputum sample containing blood if he returns for treatment or reevaluation.

Pediatric pointers

Sometimes no cause can be found for pulmonary hemorrhage occurring within the first 2 weeks of life; prognosis is poor. Hemoptysis in children may stem from Goodpasture's syndrome, Heiner syndrome, cystic fibrosis, or (rarely) idiopathic primary pulmonary hemosiderosis.

Hepatomegaly

[Liver enlargement]

This sign indicates potentially reversible primary or secondary liver disease. It may stem from diverse pathophysiologic mechanisms: dilated hepatic sinusoids (in congestive heart failure), persistently high venous pressure leading to liver congestion (in chronic constrictive pericarditis), dysfunction and engorgement of hepatocytes (in hepatitis), fatty infiltration of parenchymal cells causing fibrous tissue (in cirrhosis), distention of liver cells with glycogen (in diabetes), and infiltration of amyloid (in amyloidosis).

Hepatomegaly may be confirmed by palpation, percussion, or radiologic tests. It may be mistaken for displacement of the liver by the diaphragm, in a respiratory disorder; by an abdominal tumor; by a spinal deformity such as kyphosis; by the gallbladder; or by fecal material or a neoplasm in the colon.

Assessment

Hepatomegaly is seldom a patient's major complaint. It usually comes to light during palpation and percussion of the GI system.

If you suspect hepatomegaly, ask the patient about his use of alcohol and exposure to hepatitis. Also ask if he's currently ill or taking any prescribed drugs. If he complains of abdominal pain, ask him to locate and describe it.

Inspect the patient's skin and sclera for jaundice, dilated veins (suggesting generalized congestion), scars from previous surgery, and spider angiomas (often occurring in cirrhosis). Next, inspect the contour of his abdomen. Is it protuberant over the liver or distended (possibly from ascites)? Measure the patient's abdominal girth.

Percuss the liver, but be careful to identify structures and conditions that can obscure dull percussion notes—such as the sternum, ribs, breast tissue, pleural effusions, and gas in the colon. (See *Percussing for Liver Size and Position.*) Next, during the patient's deep inspiration, palpate the liver's edge (tender and rounded in hepatitis and cardiac decompensation, rocklike in carcinoma, or firm in cirrhosis).

Take the patient's vital signs for baseline data and assess his nutritional status. An enlarged liver that's functioning poorly will cause muscle wasting, exaggerated skeletal prominences, weight loss, thin hair, and edema.

Evaluate the patient's level of consciousness. When an enlarged liver loses its ability to detoxify waste products, the result is accumulation of metabolic substances toxic to brain cells. As a result, watch for personality changes, irritability, agitation, memory loss, inability to concentrate, and—in a severely ill patient—coma.

Medical causes

● *Amyloidosis.* This rare disorder can cause hepatomegaly and mild jaundice. It may also cause renal, cardiac, and other GI effects.

● *Cirrhosis.* Late in this disorder, the liver becomes enlarged, nodular, and hard. Other late signs and symptoms affect the entire body. *Respiratory* findings include limited thoracic expansion due to abdominal ascites, leading to hypoxia. *Central nervous system* findings include signs and symptoms of hepatic encephalopathy, such as lethargy, slurred speech, asterixis, peripheral neuritis, paranoia, hallucinations, extreme obtundation, and coma. *Hematologic* signs include epistaxis, easy bruising, and bleeding gums. *Endocrine* findings include testicular atrophy, gynecomastia, loss of chest and axillary hair, or menstrual irregularities. *Integumentary* effects include abnormal pigmentation, severe pruritus, extreme dryness, poor tissue turgor, spider angiomas, and palmar erythema. The patient may also have fetor hepaticus, enlarged superficial abdominal veins, muscle atrophy, right upper quadrant pain that worsens when he sits up or leans forward, a palpable spleen, and a temperature of 101° to 103° F. (38.3° to 39.4 °C.). Portal hypertension causes bleeding from esophageal varices.

● *Congestive heart failure.* This disorder produces hepatomegaly along with jugular vein distention, cyanosis, dependent edema of the legs and sacrum, steady weight gain, confusion, and possible nausea, vomiting, abdominal

PERCUSSING FOR LIVER SIZE AND POSITION

With your patient supine, begin at the right iliac crest to percuss up the right midclavicular line (MCL), as shown below. The percussion note becomes dull when you reach the liver's inferior border—usually at the costal margin but sometimes at a lower point in a patient with liver disease. Mark this point and then percuss down from the right clavicle, again along the right MCL. The liver's superior border usually lies between the fifth and seventh intercostal spaces. Mark the superior border.

The distance between the two marked points represents the approximate span of the liver's right lobe, which normally ranges from 2⅜″ to 4¾″ (6 to 12 cm).

Now assess the liver's left lobe similarly, percussing along the sternal midline. Again, mark the points where you hear dull percussion notes. Also measure the span of the left lobe, which normally ranges from 1½″ to 3⅛″ (4 to 8 cm). Record your findings for use as a baseline.

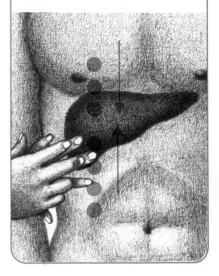

discomfort, and anorexia due to visceral edema. Ascites is a late sign. Massive right heart failure may cause anasarca, oliguria, severe weakness, and anxiety. If left heart failure precedes right heart failure, the patient will have dyspnea, orthopnea, paroxysmal nocturnal dyspnea, tachypnea, dysrhythmias, tachycardia, and fatigue.

● **Diabetes mellitus.** Poorly controlled diabetes in overweight patients often produces fatty infiltration of the liver, hepatomegaly, and right upper quadrant tenderness along with polydipsia, polyphagia, and polyuria. These features are more common in Type II than in Type I diabetes. The chronically enlarged fatty liver is typically asymptomatic except for slight tenderness.

● **Granulomatous disorders.** Sarcoidosis, histoplasmosis, and other such disorders commonly produce a slightly enlarged, firm liver.

● **Hepatic abscess.** Hepatomegaly may accompany fever (a primary sign), nausea, vomiting, chills, weakness, diarrhea, anorexia, and right upper quadrant pain and tenderness.

● **Hepatic neoplasms.** Primary tumors commonly cause hepatomegaly, with pain or tenderness in the right upper quadrant and a friction rub or bruit over the liver. Common related findings are weight loss, anorexia, nausea, and vomiting. Peripheral edema, ascites, jaundice, and a palpable right upper quadrant mass may also be present.

Metastatic liver tumors also cause hepatomegaly, but the patient's accompanying signs and symptoms reflect his primary cancer.

● **Hepatitis.** In viral hepatitis, early signs and symptoms include nausea, anorexia, vomiting, fatigue, malaise, photophobia, sore throat, cough, and headache. Hepatomegaly occurs in the icteric phase and continues during the recovery phase. Also, during the icteric phase, the early signs and symptoms diminish and others appear: liver tenderness, slight weight loss, dark urine, clay-colored stools, jaundice, pruritus, right upper quadrant pain, splenomegaly, and cervical adenopathy.

● **Infectious mononucleosis.** Occasionally, this disorder causes hepatomegaly. Prodromal symptoms include headache, malaise, and fatigue. After 3 to 5 days, the patient typically develops sore throat, cervical lymphadenopathy, and temperature fluctuations. He may also develop stomatitis, splenomegaly, exudative tonsillitis, pharyngitis, and, possibly, a maculopapular rash.

● **Leukemia and lymphomas.** These proliferative blood cell disorders frequently cause moderate-to-massive hepatomegaly and splenomegaly as well as abdominal discomfort. General signs and symptoms include malaise, low-grade fever, fatigue, weakness, tachycardia, weight loss, and anorexia.

● **Obesity.** Hepatomegaly can result from fatty infiltration of the liver. Weight reduction reduces liver size.

● **Pancreatic cancer.** In this disorder, hepatomegaly accompanies such classic signs and symptoms as anorexia, weight loss, abdominal or back pain, and jaundice. Other findings: nausea, vomiting, fever, fatigue, weakness, and skin lesions (usually on the legs).

● **Pericarditis.** In chronic constrictive pericarditis, an increase in systemic venous pressure produces marked congestive hepatomegaly. Distended neck veins (more prominent on inspiration) are a common finding. The patient typically doesn't have the usual signs of cardiac disease; other clinical features include peripheral edema, ascites, and decreased muscle mass.

Special considerations

Prepare the patient for hepatic enzyme, alkaline phosphatase, bilirubin, albumin, and globulin studies to evaluate liver function and for X-rays, liver scan, celiac arteriography, and ultrasonography to confirm hepatomegaly.

Bed rest, relief from stress, and adequate nutrition are important for the patient with hepatomegaly to help protect liver cells from further damage and to allow the liver to regenerate functioning cells. Hepatotoxic drugs or drugs metabolized by the liver should be given in very small doses, if at all.

Pediatric pointers

Assess hepatomegaly in children the same way you do in adults. Childhood hepatomegaly may stem from Reye's syndrome; biliary atresia; rare disorders such as Wilson's disease, Gaucher's disease, and Niemann-Pick disease; or poorly controlled Type I diabetes mellitus.

Hiccups

[Singultus]

Hiccups occur as a two-stage process: an involuntary, spasmodic contraction of the diaphragm followed by sudden closure of the glottis. Their characteristic sound reflects the vibration of closed vocal cords as air suddenly rushes into the lungs.

Usually benign and transient, hiccups are common and most often subside spontaneously or with simple treatment. However, in a patient with a neurologic disorder, they may indicate increasing intracranial pressure or extension of a brain stem lesion. They may also occur after ingestion of hot or cold liquids or other irritants, after exposure to cold, or with irritation from a drainage tube. Persistent hiccups cause considerable distress and may lead to vomiting.

Increased serum levels of carbon dioxide may inhibit hiccups; decreased levels may accentuate them.

Assessment

Find out when the patient's hiccups began. If he's also vomiting and unconscious, turn him on his side to prevent aspiration. Then notify the doctor.

If he's conscious, find out if the hiccups are tiring him. Ask if he's had hiccups before, what caused them, and what made them stop. Also note if he has a history of abdominal or thoracic disorders.

Medical causes

● *Abdominal distention.* The most common cause of hiccups, abdominal distention also causes a feeling of fullness and, depending on the cause, abdom-

inal pain, nausea, and vomiting.

● *Brain stem lesion.* Producing persistent hiccups, this lesion causes decreased level of consciousness, dysphagia, dysarthria, an absent corneal reflex on the side opposite the lesion, altered respiratory patterns, abnormal pupillary response, and ocular deviation.

● *Chronic renal failure.* Hiccups may occur in the late stages of this disorder. Associated signs and symptoms affect every body system and include fatigue, oliguria or anuria, nausea, vomiting, confusion, yellow-brown or bronze skin, uremic frost, ammonia breath odor, bleeding tendencies, gum ulcerations, and Kussmaul's respirations.

● *Gastric dilatation.* Besides hiccups, possible clinical features include a sense of fullness, epigastric pain, and regurgitation or persistent vomiting.

● *Gastritis.* This disorder can cause hiccups along with mild epigastric discomfort (sometimes the only symptom). The patient may have upper abdominal pain, eructation, fever, malaise, nausea, vomiting, hematemesis, and melena.

● *Increased intracranial pressure.* Early findings may include hiccups, drowsiness, and headache. Classic later signs include changes in pupillary reactions and respiratory pattern, increased systolic pressure, and bradycardia.

● *Pancreatitis.* Hiccups, vomiting, and sudden and steady epigastric pain (often radiating to the back) may occur in this disorder. A severe attack may also cause persistent vomiting, extreme restlessness, fever, and abdominal tenderness and rigidity.

● *Pleural irritation.* Besides hiccups, this condition may cause cough, dyspnea, or chest pain.

Other cause

● *Surgery.* Occasionally, mild and transient attacks of hiccups may follow abdominal surgery.

Special considerations

Teach the patient simple methods of relieving hiccups, such as increasing his

HOW HICCUPS OCCUR

Hiccups may result from irritations in the chest or abdomen that trigger transmission of impulses through the vagus (afferent) and the phrenic (efferent) nerves to the diaphragm. Upon completion of this reflex arc, the diaphragm contracts. The resulting abrupt intake of air is promptly cut off as the glottis snaps shut.

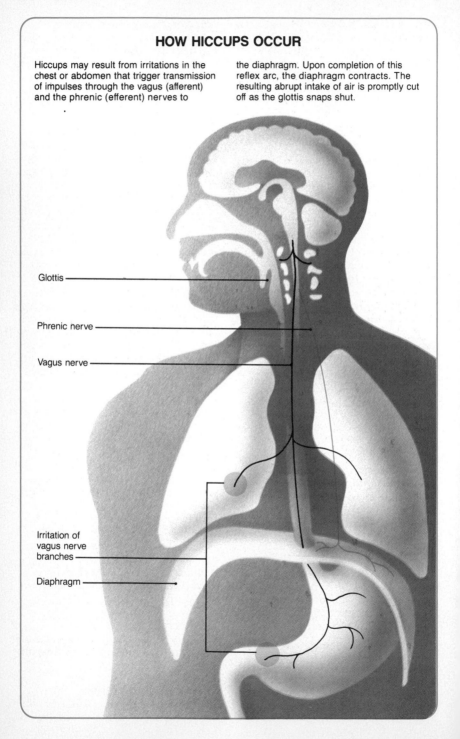

Glottis

Phrenic nerve

Vagus nerve

Irritation of vagus nerve branches

Diaphragm

serum carbon dioxide level by holding his breath repeatedly or by rebreathing into a paper bag. Other treatments include gastric lavage or finger pressure on the eyeballs (applied through closed lids). If hiccups persist, a phenothiazine (especially chlorpromazine) or nasogastric intubation may provide relief. (*Caution*: The tube may cause vomiting.) If simpler methods fail, treatment may include a phrenic nerve block.

Pediatric pointers
In an infant, hiccups most often result from rapid ingestion of liquids without adequate burping. Tell parents to hold the infant upright during feedings.

Hirsutism

Hirsutism is the excessive growth of dark, coarse body hair in females. Excessive androgen production stimulates hair growth on the pubic region, axilla, chin, upper lip, cheeks, anterior neck, sternum, linea alba, forearms, abdomen, back, and upper arms. In *mild hirsutism,* fine and pigmented hair appears on the sides of the face and the chin (but doesn't form a complete beard) and on the extremities, chest, abdomen, and perineum. In *moderate hirsutism,* coarse and pigmented hair appears on the same areas. In *severe hirsutism,* coarse hair also covers the whole beard area, the proximal interphalangeal joints, and the ears and nose.

Depending on the degree of excess androgen production, hirsutism may be associated with acne and increased skin oiliness, menstrual irregularity, and increased libido. Extremely high androgen levels cause further virilization (see *Recognizing Signs of Virilization,* page 408). Defeminization may also occur, producing signs such as amenorrhea, breast atrophy, and loss of female body contour.

Hirsutism may result from endocrine abnormalities and idiopathic causes. It may also occur in pregnancy due to transient androgen production by the placenta or corpus luteum, and in menopause due to increased androgen and decreased estrogen production.

Assessment
Begin with the patient history. Where did the patient first notice growth of excessive hair? How old was she then? Where—and how quickly—did other hirsute areas develop? Ask what hair removal technique she uses (if any), how often she uses it, and when she used it last. Next, obtain a menstrual history: the patient's age at menarche, the duration of her periods, the usual amount of blood flow, and the number of days between periods.

Ask about medications, too. If the patient is taking a drug containing an androgen or progestin compound, or another drug that can cause hirsutism, find out its name, dosage, schedule, and therapeutic aim. Does she sometimes miss doses or take extra ones?

Now examine the areas of excessive hair growth. Does it appear only on her upper lip or on other body parts as well? Is it mild but pigmented or dense and coarse? Is the patient obese? Observe for signs of virilization.

Medical causes
• *Acromegaly.* About 15% of patients with this chronic, progressive disorder display hirsutism. Acromegaly also causes enlarged hands and feet, coarsened facial features, prognathism, increased diaphoresis and need for sleep, skin oiliness, fatigue, weight gain, heat intolerance, and lethargy.
• *Adrenocortical carcinoma.* This disorder produces rapidly progressive hirsutism along with truncal obesity, buffalo hump, moon face, oligomenorrhea, amenorrhea, muscle wasting, and thin skin with purple striae. The patient also has muscle weakness, excessive diaphoresis, poor wound healing, weakness, fatigue, hypertension, hy-

RECOGNIZING SIGNS OF VIRILIZATION

Excessive androgen levels produce severe hirsutism and other marked signs of virilization, as shown in the figure below.

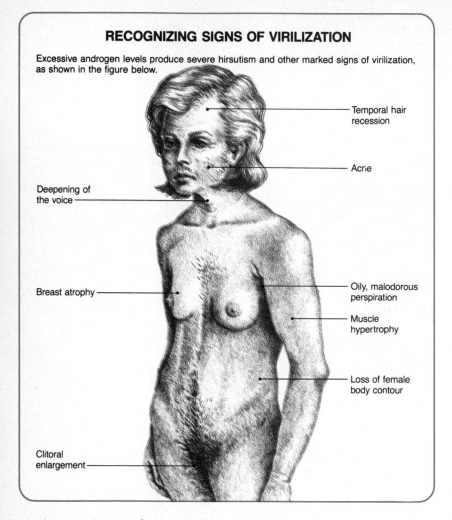

Temporal hair recession

Acne

Deepening of the voice

Breast atrophy

Oily, malodorous perspiration

Muscle hypertrophy

Loss of female body contour

Clitoral enlargement

perpigmentation, and personality changes.

• *Cushing's disease.* Facial hirsutism is a common finding. This disorder also causes increased hair growth on the abdomen, breasts, chest, or upper thighs. Other findings: truncal obesity, buffalo hump, moon face, thin skin, purple striae, ecchymoses, petechiae, muscle wasting and weakness, poor wound healing, hypertension, weakness, fatigue, excessive diaphoresis, hyperpigmentation, menstrual irregularities, and personality changes.

• *Hyperprolactinemia.* This disorder produces hirsutism, hypogonadism, galactorrhea, amenorrhea, and acne.

• *Idiopathic hirsutism.* In patients with normal-sized ovaries and no evidence of adrenal hyperplasia or adrenal or ovarian tumors, excess hair appears at puberty and increases into early adulthood. It's accompanied by thick, oily skin; acne; obesity; and infrequent or anovulatory menses. Idiopathic hirsutism with regular ovulation and no menstrual abnormalities may be hereditary or related to certain geographic areas and ethnic groups who are hypersensitive to androgens.

• *Ovarian overproduction of androgens.* The most common cause of hirsutism, this condition is associated with anovulation progressing slowly over several years.

• *Ovarian tumor.* Sometimes asymptomatic, this disorder can cause rapidly progressing hirsutism—but only if the tumor produces androgens. Amenorrhea and rapidly developing virilization are additional findings.

• *Polycystic ovary disease.* Ovarian cysts—particularly chronic ones—can cause hirsutism. This usually occurs after the onset of menstrual irregularities, which may begin at puberty. The patient may also have amenorrhea, oligomenorrhea, menometrorrhagia, infertility, acne, or obesity.

Other causes

• *Drugs.* Hirsutism can result from drugs containing androgens or progestins, aminoglutethimide, glucocorticoids, metoclopramide, cyclosporine, and minoxidil.

Special considerations

Prepare the patient for tests to determine blood levels of luteinizing hormone, follicle-stimulating hormone, prolactin, and other hormones. Other tests may include computed tomography scan and ultrasonography.

Help relieve the patient's anxiety by explaining the cause of excessive hair growth and by encouraging her to talk about her self-image problems or fears. Involve the family in your discussions.

At the patient's request, provide information on methods for eliminating excess hair—bleaching, tweezing, hot wax treatments, chemical depilatories, shaving, and electrolysis.

Pediatric pointers

Childhood hirsutism can stem from congenital adrenal hyperplasia. It's almost always detected at birth in females because of ambiguous genitalia. Rarely, a mild form becomes apparent after puberty when hirsutism, irregular bleeding or amenorrhea, and signs of virilization appear. Hirsutism occurring at or after puberty often results from polycystic ovary disease.

Give the parents, as well as the child, emotional support and clear explanations about the cause of hirsutism. Allow the parents and child to express their concerns separately.

Hoarseness

Hoarseness—a rough or harsh sound to the voice—can result from infections or inflammatory lesions or exudates of the larynx, from laryngeal edema, and from compression or disruption of the vocal cords or recurrent laryngeal nerve. This common sign can also result from a thoracic aortic aneurysm, vocal cord paralysis, and systemic disorders, such as Sjögren's syndrome and rheumatoid arthritis. It's characteristically worsened by excessive alcohol intake, smoking, inhalation of noxious fumes, cheering, and shouting.

Hoarseness can be acute or chronic. For example, chronic hoarseness and laryngitis (an occupational hazard of clergymen and singers) result when irritating polyps form on the vocal cords. It may also result from progressive atrophy of the laryngeal muscles and mucosa due to aging, leading to diminished control of the vocal cords.

Assessment

Obtain a patient history. First consider his age and sex; laryngeal cancer is most common in men between the ages of 50 and 70. Ask about the onset of hoarseness. Has the patient been overusing his voice? Has he experienced shortness of breath, a sore throat, dry mouth, a cough, or difficulty swallowing dry food? Has he been in or near a fire within the past 48 hours? Inhalation injury can cause sudden airway obstruction, so notify the doctor promptly and prepare to give oxygen and assist with other treatments.

Next, explore associated symptoms. Does the patient have a history of cancer, rheumatoid arthritis, or aortic aneurysm? Does he regularly drink alcohol or smoke?

Inspect the oral cavity and pharynx for redness or exudate, possibly indicating an upper respiratory infection. Palpate the neck for masses and the cervical lymph nodes and the thyroid for enlargement. Palpate the trachea—is it midline? Ask the patient to stick out his tongue: if he can't, he may have paralysis from cranial nerve involvement. Examine the eyes for corneal ulcers and enlarged lacrimal ducts (signs of Sjögren's syndrome). Dilated neck and chest veins may indicate compression by an aortic aneurysm.

Take the patient's vital signs, noting especially fever and bradycardia. Inspect for asymmetrical chest expansion or signs of respiratory distress—nasal flaring, stridor, and intercostal retractions. Then auscultate for crackles, rhonchi, wheezes, or tubular sounds, and percuss for dullness.

Medical causes

• *Hypothyroidism.* In this disorder, hoarseness may be an early sign. Others include fatigue, cold intolerance, weight gain despite anorexia, and menorrhagia.

• *Inhalation injury.* Inhalation injury from a fire or explosion produces hoarseness and coughing, singed nasal hairs, orofacial burns, and soot-stained sputum. Signs and symptoms that subsequently appear include crackles, rhonchi, and wheezes as well as rapid deterioration to respiratory distress.

• *Laryngeal cancer.* Hoarseness is an early sign of vocal cord cancer, but may not occur until later in cancer of other laryngeal areas. Other common findings: a mild, dry cough and minor throat discomfort.

• *Laryngitis.* Persistent hoarseness may be the only sign of *chronic laryngitis.* In *acute laryngitis,* hoarseness or a complete loss of voice develops suddenly. Related findings include pain (especially during swallowing or speaking), cough, fever, profuse diaphoresis, sore throat, and rhinorrhea.

• *Pulmonary tuberculosis.* In this disorder, hoarseness may be present if treatment has been delayed, but it isn't an early finding. Other signs and symptoms include pleuritic chest pain, productive cough, fine crackles after coughing, occasionally hemoptysis, night sweats, anorexia, weight loss, fever, malaise, dyspnea, and fatigue. Examination reveals dullness to percussion, increased tactile fremitus, and amphoric breath sounds.

• *Rheumatoid arthritis.* Hoarseness may signal laryngeal involvement. Other findings: pain, dysphagia, a sensation of fullness or tension in the throat, dyspnea on exertion, and stridor.

• *Sjögren's syndrome.* This rheumatic disorder produces hoarseness, but its cardinal signs are dry eyes and mouth. Initially, the patient complains of gritty, burning pain around the eyes and under the lids. Ocular dryness also leads to redness, photosensitivity, impaired vision, itching, and eye fatigue. Examination reveals enlarged lacrimal glands and corneal ulcers.

The patient may also complain of a dry, sore mouth and difficulty in chewing, talking, and swallowing. He may also have nasal crusting, epistaxis, enlarged parotid and submaxillary glands, dry and scaly skin, nonproductive cough, abdominal discomfort, and polyuria.

• *Thoracic aortic aneurysm.* Although typically asymptomatic, this aneurysm may cause hoarseness. Its most common symptom is penetrating pain that's especially severe when the patient's supine. Other clinical features include a brassy cough; dyspnea; wheezing; a substernal aching in the shoulders, lower back, or abdomen; a tracheal tug; facial and neck edema; jugular vein distention; dysphagia; prominent chest veins; stridor; and possibly paresthesia or neuralgia.

• *Tracheal trauma.* Torn tracheal mucosa may cause hoarseness, hemoptysis, dysphagia, neck pain, airway occlusion, and respiratory distress.

• *Vocal cord paralysis.* Unilateral vocal cord paralysis causes hoarseness and vocal weakness. Paralysis may accompany signs of trauma, such as pain and swelling of the head and neck.

• *Vocal cord polyps.* Raspy hoarseness, the chief complaint, accompanies a chronic cough and a crackling voice.

Other causes

• *Treatments.* Occasionally, surgical severing of the recurrent laryngeal nerve results in permanent unilateral vocal cord paralysis, leading to hoarseness. Prolonged intubation or a tracheostomy may cause temporary hoarseness.

Special considerations

Carefully observe the patient for stridor, which may indicate bilateral vocal cord paralysis. If the patient has laryngitis, advise him to use a humidifier. Stress the importance of resting his voice: talking—even whispering—further traumatizes the vocal cords. Suggest other ways to communicate (such as using pen and paper or body language). Urge the patient to avoid alcohol, smoking, and the company of smokers. Tell him to report hoarseness that lasts more than 2 weeks. The doctor may perform indirect laryngoscopy, observing the larynx at rest and during phonation.

Pediatric pointers

In children, hoarseness may result from congenital anomalies, such as laryngocele and dysphonia plicae ventricularis. In prepubescent boys, it can stem from juvenile papillomatosis of the upper respiratory tract.

In infants and young children, hoarseness commonly stems from acute laryngotracheobronchitis (croup). Temporary hoarseness frequently results from laryngeal irritation due to aspiration of liquids, foreign bodies, or stomach contents. Hoarseness may also stem from diphtheria, although immunization has made this disease rare.

Help the child with hoarseness rest his voice. Comfort an infant to minimize crying, play quiet games with him, and humidify his environment.

Homans' Sign

Homans' sign is positive when deep calf pain results from strong and abrupt dorsiflexion of the ankle. This pain results from venous thrombosis or inflammation of the calf muscles. However, because a positive Homans' sign appears in only 35% of patients with these conditions, it's an unreliable indicator. Even when accurate, a positive Homans' sign doesn't indicate the extent of the venous disorder.

This elicited sign may be confused with continuous calf pain, which can result from strains, contusions, cellulitis, or arterial occlusion; or with pain in the posterior ankle or Achilles tendon (for example, in a woman with Achilles tendons shortened from wearing high heels).

Assessment

When you detect a positive Homans' sign, focus your patient history on signs and symptoms that can accompany deep vein thrombosis (DVT) or thrombophlebitis: throbbing, aching, heavy, or tight sensations in the calf and leg pain during or after exercise or routine activity. Ask about predisposing events, such as leg injury, recent surgery, childbirth, and prolonged bed rest.

Next, inspect and palpate the patient's calf for warmth, tenderness, redness, swelling, and the presence of a palpable vein. Measure the circumferences of both calves. The one with the positive Homans' sign may be larger due to edema and swelling.

Medical causes

• *Deep vein thrombophlebitis.* A positive Homans' sign and calf tenderness may

ELICITING HOMANS' SIGN

To elicit this sign, first support the patient's thigh with one hand and his foot with the other. Bend his leg slightly at the knee, then firmly and abruptly dorsiflex the ankle. Resulting deep calf pain indicates a positive Homans' sign. (The patient may also resist ankle dorsiflexion or flex the knee involuntarily if Homans' sign is positive.)

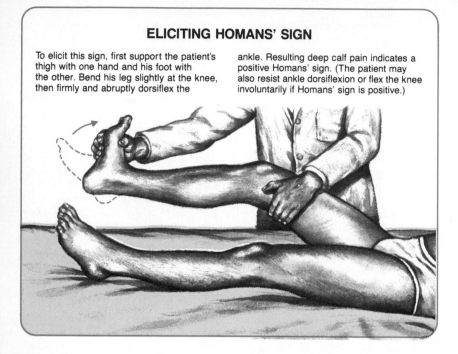

be the only clinical features of this disorder. But the patient may also have severe pain, heaviness, warmth, and swelling of the affected leg; visible, engorged superficial veins or palpable, cordlike veins; and fever, chills, and malaise.

• *Deep vein thrombosis.* DVT causes a positive Homans' sign along with tenderness over the deep calf veins, slight edema of the calves and thighs, a low-grade fever, and tachycardia. If DVT affects the femoral and iliac veins, you'll notice marked local swelling and tenderness. If it's causing venous obstruction, you'll notice cyanosis and, possibly, cool skin in the affected leg.

Special considerations

If you detect a positive Homans' sign in a patient whose calf is tender and feels warm, notify the doctor. Place the patient on bed rest with the affected leg elevated above the heart level. Apply warm, moist compresses to the affected area, and administer mild oral analgesics, as ordered.

For further assessment, you may be asked to slowly inflate a blood pressure cuff that's wrapped around each calf and then to compare the pressures at which the patient first reports pain. Pain occurring at a cuff pressure of less than 180 mm Hg indicates DVT or thrombophlebitis. However, because this test may dislodge a clot, you'll need to closely monitor the patient for sudden onset of signs and symptoms of pulmonary embolism—dyspnea, cough, pleural pain, and tachycardia. If any of these occurs, notify the doctor immediately.

Once the patient's ambulatory, advise him to wear elastic support stockings after his discomfort decreases (usually in 5 to 10 days) and to continue wearing them for at least 3 months. Instruct him to keep the affected leg elevated while sitting and to avoid crossing his legs at the knees. Why? Because this may impair circulation to the popliteal area. (Crossing at the ankles is acceptable.)

If the patient's put on long-term anticoagulant therapy with a coumadin compound such as warfarin, instruct him to report any signs of prolonged clotting time. These include black, tarry stools; brown or red urine; bleeding gums; and bruises. Stress the importance of keeping follow-up appointments so his prothrombin time can be monitored.

Pediatric pointers

Homans' sign is seldom assessed in children, who rarely have deep vein thrombosis or thrombophlebitis.

Hyperpigmentation

[Hypermelanosis]

Hyperpigmentation, or excessive skin coloring, usually reflects overproduction, abnormal location, or maldistribution of melanin—the dominant brown or black pigment found in skin, hair, mucous membranes, nails, brain tissue, cardiac muscle, and parts of the eye. This sign can also reflect abnormalities of other skin pigments: carotenoids (yellow), oxyhemoglobin (red), and hemoglobin (blue).

Hyperpigmentation most commonly results from exposure to sunlight. However, it can also result from metabolic, endocrine, neoplastic, and inflammatory disorders; chemical poisoning; drugs; genetic defects; thermal burns; ionizing radiation; and localized activation by sunlight of certain photosensitizing chemicals on the skin.

Many types of benign hyperpigmented lesions occur normally. Some—such as acanthosis nigricans and carotenemia—may also accompany certain disorders, but their significance is unproven. Chronic nutritional insufficiency may lead to dyspigmentation—increased pigmentation in some areas and decreased pigmentation in others.

Typically asymptomatic and chronic, hyperpigmentation is a common problem that can have distressing psychological and social implications. It varies in location and intensity and may fade over time.

Assessment

Hyperpigmentation isn't an acute process, of course, but an end result of another process—the main target of your assessment. Begin with a detailed patient history. Do any other family members have the same problem? Was the patient's hyperpigmentation present at birth? Did other signs or symptoms, such as skin rash, accompany or precede it? Obtain a history of medical disorders (particularly endocrine), as well as contact with or ingestion of chemicals, metals, plants, vegetables, or citrus fruits. Was the appearance of hyperpigmentation related to exposure to sunlight or a change of season? Is the patient pregnant or taking prescription or over-the-counter drugs?

Explore any other signs and symptoms, too. Ask about fatigue, weakness, muscle aches, chills, irritability, fainting, and itching. Does the patient have any cardiopulmonary signs or symptoms, such as cough, shortness of breath, or swelling of the ankles, hands, or other areas? Any gastrointestinal complaints, such as anorexia, nausea, vomiting, weight loss, abdominal pain, diarrhea, constipation, or epigastric fullness? Also ask about genitourinary signs and symptoms, such as dark or pink urine, increased or decreased urination, menstrual irregularities, and loss of libido.

Now examine the patient's skin. Note the color of hyperpigmented areas: brown suggests excess melanin in the epidermis; slate gray or a bluish tone suggests excess pigment in the dermis. Inspect for other changes, too—thickening and leatherlike texture and changes in hair distribution. Check the patient's skin and sclera for jaundice, and note any spider angiomas, palmar erythema, or purpura.

Take the patient's vital signs, noting

any fever, hypotension, or pulse irregularities. Evaluate the patient's general appearance. Do you note exophthalmos or an enlarged jaw, nose, or hands? Palpate for an enlarged thyroid and auscultate for a bruit over the gland. Palpate muscles for atrophy and joints for swelling and tenderness. Assess the abdomen for ascites and edema, and palpate and percuss the liver and spleen to evaluate their size and position. Check the male patient for testicular atrophy and gynecomastia.

Medical causes

• *Acromegaly.* This disorder results from a pituitary tumor that secretes excessive amounts of growth hormone after puberty. Hyperpigmentation (possibly acanthosis nigricans) may affect the face, neck, genitalia, axillae, palmar creases, and new scars. The patient's skin appears oily, sweaty, thick, and leathery, with burrows and ridges formed over the face, neck, and scalp. His tongue is enlarged and furrowed, his lips are thick, and his nose is large. His body hair is markedly increased and his hands are broad and spadelike. His marked prognathism interferes with chewing.

• *Adrenocortical insufficiency.* This disorder produces diffuse tan, brown, or bronze-to-black hyperpigmentation of both exposed and unexposed areas— the face, knees, knuckles, elbows, beltline, palmar creases, lips, gums, tongue, and buccal mucosa (where hyperpigmentation may be bluish black). Normally pigmented areas, moles, and scars become darker. Early in the disorder, hyperpigmentation occurs as persistent tanning after exposure to the sun. Some patients (usually female) lose axillary and pubic hair, and about 15% of patients have vitiligo. Patients may have slowly progressive fatigue, weakness, anorexia, nausea, vomiting, weight loss, postural hypotension, abdominal pain, irritability, and weak, irregular pulse. They may also have diarrhea or constipation, decreased libido, amenorrhea, syncope, and some-

times an enhanced sense of taste, smell, and hearing.

• *Arsenic poisoning.* Chronic arsenic poisoning can cause diffuse hyperpigmentation with scattered freckle-sized areas of normal or depigmented skin. Other clinical features may include weakness, muscle aches, peripheral neuropathy, headache, drowsiness, confusion, convulsions, and mucous membrane involvement (conjunctivitis, photophobia, pharyngitis, or irritating cough).

• *Biliary cirrhosis.* Hyperpigmentation is a classic feature of this disorder, which primarily affects women between the ages of 40 and 60. A widespread and accentuated brown hyperpigmentation appears on areas exposed to sunlight, but not on the mucosa. Pruritus that worsens at bedtime may be the earliest symptom. Weakness, fatigue, weight loss, and vague abdominal pain may appear years before the onset of jaundice. Malabsorption may cause nocturnal diarrhea, frothy and bulky stools, weight loss, purpura, and osteomalacia with bone and back pain. The patient may also have hematemesis from esophageal varices, xanthomas and xanthelasmas, hepatosplenomegaly, ascites, edema, spider angiomas, and palmar erythema.

• *Hemochromatosis.* In this inherited disorder (also called bronzed diabetes), most common in men between the ages of 40 and 60, early and progressive hyperpigmentation results from melanin (and possibly iron) deposits in the skin. Hyperpigmentation develops as generalized bronzing and metallic gray areas accentuated over sun-exposed areas, genitalia, and scars. Early related effects include weakness, lassitude, weight loss, abdominal pain, loss of libido, and signs of diabetes, such as polydipsia and polyuria. Later, signs of liver and cardiac involvement become prominent.

• *Laennec's cirrhosis.* After about 10 years of excessive alcohol ingestion, progressive liver dysfunction causes diffuse, generalized hyperpigmentation on sun-exposed areas. Early in the disorder, the patient may complain of increasing weakness, fatigue, anorexia, slight weight loss, nausea and vomiting, indigestion, constipation or diarrhea, and a dull abdominal ache. As the disorder progresses, the patient may display major signs and symptoms in every body system. These result from hepatic insufficiency and portal hypertension and may include hepatosplenomegaly, ascites, muscle wasting, spider angiomas, gynecomastia, enlarged superficial abdominal veins, testicular atrophy, menstrual irregularities, and palmar erythema. Other findings include loss of body hair, parotid gland enlargement, jaundice, pruritus, extreme skin dryness, purpura and other bleeding tendencies, ankle edema, and fetor hepaticus.

• *Malignant melanoma.* This form of cancer causes malignant lesions of pigmented skin, commonly moles. Common sites include the head and neck in men, the legs in women, and the backs in both men and women who are exposed to excessive sunlight; it rarely appears in the conjunctiva, choroid, pharynx, mouth, vagina, or anus. Up to 70% of lesions arise from a preexisting nevus.

The cardinal sign of malignant melanoma is a skin lesion or nevus that enlarges, changes color, becomes inflamed, itches, ulcerates, bleeds, changes texture, or develops associated halo nevus or vitiligo. Coloring of lesions varies: brown or black around the edges and red, blue, black, or gray in the central raised area. Bleeding and ulceration may occur.

• *Porphyria cutanea tarda.* Primarily affecting men between the ages of 40 and 60, this disorder produces generalized brownish hyperpigmentation on sun-exposed areas and extreme skin fragility (particularly on a bald scalp and on the face and hands). It also causes pink or brownish urine (from porphyrin excretion) and anorexia, jaundice, and hepatomegaly.

• *Scleroderma.* Localized and systemic scleroderma produce generalized dark brown hyperpigmentation that's unrelated to sun exposure. Other skin findings include areas of depigmentation and spider angiomas. Earlier signs and symptoms include those of Raynaud's phenomenon—blanching, cyanosis, and erythema of the fingers and toes when exposed to cold or stress, and possible finger shortening, fingertip ulcerations, and gangrene of the fingers and toes. Later findings include pain, stiffness, and swelling of the fingers and joints. Skin thickening progresses to taut, shiny, leathery skin over the entire hands and forearms, then over the arms, chest, abdomen, and back; contractures may develop. Tight, inelastic facial skin becomes masklike, pinching the mouth.

Systemic scleroderma also involves the GI, cardiovascular, and other body systems.

• *Thyrotoxicosis.* This disorder can cause hyperpigmentation on the face, neck, genitalia, axillae, and palmar creases as well as in new scars. Vitiligo may also develop. Other findings may include warm, moist skin; erythematous palms; fine scalp hair with premature graying; and Plummer's nails.

Classic signs and symptoms of Graves' disease, the most common form of thyrotoxicosis, include an enlarged thyroid, nervousness, heat intolerance, weight loss despite increased appetite, profuse diaphoresis, diarrhea, tremor, and palpitations. Exophthalmos, although characteristic, is absent in many patients. Other findings reflect involvement of every body system.

Other causes

• *Drugs.* Hyperpigmentation can stem from use of barbiturates, phenolphthalein, and salicylates; chemotherapeutic agents such as busulfan, cyclophosphamide, procarbazine, and nitrogen mustard; chlorpromazine; antimalarial drugs such as hydroxychloroquine; hydantoin; minocycline; metals such as silver (in argyria) and gold (in chrysiasis); adrenocorticotropic hormone;

and phenothiazines.

Special considerations
Wood's lamp, a special ultraviolet light, helps enhance the contrast between normal and hyperpigmented epidermis. A skin biopsy can help confirm the cause of hyperpigmentation.

Hyperpigmentation may persist even after treatment of the underlying disorder or withdrawal of the drug. Bleaching creams may not be effective if most of the excess melanin lies in subepidermal skin layers. Over-the-counter bleaching creams tend to be ineffective because they contain less than 2% hydroquinone.

Advise patients to use corrective cosmetics, to avoid excessive sun exposure, and to apply a sunscreen or sun-blocker, such as zinc oxide cream. Advise patients who stop using bleaching agents to continue using sunblockers, because rebound hyperpigmentation can occur.

Warn every patient with a benign hyperpigmented area to consult his doctor if the lesion's size, shape, or color changes; this may signal a developing malignancy.

Pediatric pointers
Most moles that are found in children are junctional nevi—flat, well demarcated, brown-to-black, and appearing anywhere on the skin. Although they're considered benign, recent evidence suggests that some of these may become malignant in later life. Some doctors recommend removal of junctional nevi; others advise regular inspection. If congenital melanocytic nevi are present at birth, they should be removed.

Bizarre arrangements of linear or streaky hyperpigmented lesions on a child's sun-exposed lower legs suggest phytophotodermatitis. Advise parents to protect the child's skin with long pants and socks. Congenital hyperpigmented lesions include mongolian spots (which are benign) and sharply defined or diffuse lesions occurring in such disorders as neurofibromatosis, xeroderma pigmentosum, Albright's syndrome, Fanconi's syndrome, Gaucher's disease, Niemann-Pick disease, Peutz-Jeghers syndrome, phenylketonuria, and Wilson's disease.

Hyperpnea

Hyperpnea indicates increased respiratory effort for a sustained period—a normal rate (at least 12 breaths/minute) with increased depth (a tidal volume greater than 500 ml), an increased rate (over 20 breaths/minute) with normal depth, or increased rate and depth. Hyperpnea differs from sighing (intermittent deep inspirations). However, it's also correctly called *tachypnea* (increased respiratory rate) when the depth of respirations remains normal, thereby increasing minute volume.

The typical patient with hyperpnea breathes at a normal or an increased rate and inhales deeply, displaying marked chest expansion. He may complain of shortness of breath if he has a respiratory disorder causing hypoxemia, or he may not be aware of his breathing if he has a metabolic or neurologic disorder causing involuntary hyperpnea. Other causes of hyperpnea include profuse diarrhea or dehydration, ureterosigmoidostomy, and loss of pancreatic juice or bile from gastrointestinal drainage. All these conditions cause a loss of bicarbonate ions, resulting in metabolic acidosis. Of course, hyperpnea may also accompany strenuous exercise, and voluntary hyperpnea can aid relaxation in patients experiencing stress or pain—as in labor.

Hyperventilation, a form of hyperpnea associated with respiratory alkalosis, results in excessive exhalation of carbon dioxide (indicated by an arterial pH above 7.45 and a PCO_2 below 35). In central neurogenic hyperventilation, brain stem dysfunction (as in severe head injury) increases the rate

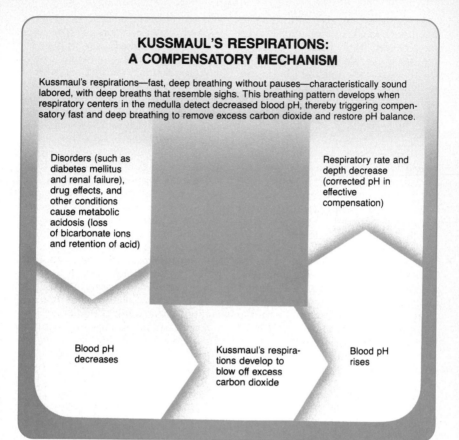

KUSSMAUL'S RESPIRATIONS: A COMPENSATORY MECHANISM

Kussmaul's respirations—fast, deep breathing without pauses—characteristically sound labored, with deep breaths that resemble sighs. This breathing pattern develops when respiratory centers in the medulla detect decreased blood pH, thereby triggering compensatory fast and deep breathing to remove excess carbon dioxide and restore pH balance.

Disorders (such as diabetes mellitus and renal failure), drug effects, and other conditions cause metabolic acidosis (loss of bicarbonate ions and retention of acid)

Respiratory rate and depth decrease (corrected pH in effective compensation)

Blood pH decreases

Kussmaul's respirations develop to blow off excess carbon dioxide

Blood pH rises

and depth of respirations. In acute intermittent hyperventilation, the respiratory pattern may be a response to hypoxemia, anxiety, fear, pain, or excitement. It may also be a compensatory mechanism to metabolic acidosis.

Kussmaul's respirations, another form of hyperpnea, occur as a compensatory response to excessive carbon dioxide levels.

Assessment

If you observe hyperpnea in a patient whose other signs and symptoms signal a life-threatening emergency, you'll need to intervene quickly and effectively. (See *Managing Hyperpnea*, page 419.) However, if the patient's condition isn't grave, first assess his level of consciousness. If he's alert (and if his hyperpnea isn't interfering with speaking), ask about any recent illnesses, infections, and ingestion of aspirin or other drugs or chemicals. Find out if he has diabetes mellitus or renal disease. Is he excessively thirsty or hungry? Has he recently had severe diarrhea or an upper respiratory infection?

Next, observe the patient for clues to his abnormal breathing pattern. Is he unable to speak, or does he speak only in brief, choppy phrases? Is his breathing abnormally rapid? Assess for cyanosis (especially of the mouth, lips, mucous membranes, and earlobes), restlessness, and anxiety—all signs of decreased tissue oxygenation, as in shock. Observe for intercostal and abdominal retractions, use of accessory muscles, and diaphoresis: these signs and symptoms may also indicate deep breathing related to an insufficient supply of oxygen. Next, inspect for draining wounds or signs of infection, and ask about nausea and vomiting. Take the patient's vital signs, noting fever, and examine his skin and mucous membranes for turgor, possibly indicating dehydration.

Medical causes

● **Head injury.** Hyperpnea that results from severe head injury is called central neurogenic hyperventilation. Whether its onset is acute or gradual, this type of hyperpnea indicates damage to the lower midbrain or upper pons. Accompanying signs of head injury reflect the site and extent of injury but can include loss of consciousness; soft tissue injury or bony deformity of the face, head, or neck; facial edema; clear or bloody drainage from the mouth, nose, or ears; raccoon's eyes; Battle's sign; an absent doll's eye sign; and motor and sensory disturbances.

Signs of increased intracranial pressure include decreased response to painful stimulation, loss of pupillary reaction, bradycardia, increased systolic pressure, and widening pulse pressure.

● **Hyperventilation syndrome.** Acute anxiety triggers episodic hyperpnea, resulting in respiratory alkalosis. Other findings may include agitation, vertigo, syncope, pallor, circumoral and peripheral paresthesia, muscle twitching, carpopedal spasm, weakness, and dysrhythmias.

● **Hypoxemia.** Many pulmonary disorders that cause hypoxemia—for example, pneumonia, pulmonary edema, chronic obstructive pulmonary disease, and pneumothorax—may cause hyperpnea and episodes of hyperventilation with chest pain, dizziness, and paresthesia. Other effects: dyspnea, cough, crackles, rhonchi, wheezes, and decreased breath sounds.

● **Ketoacidosis.** Alcoholic ketoacidosis (occurring most often in females with a history of alcohol abuse) typically follows cessation of drinking after a marked increase in alcohol consumption has caused severe vomiting. Kussmaul's respirations begin abruptly; they accompany vomiting for several days, slight dehydration, abdominal pain and distention, and absent bowel sounds. The patient is alert and has a normal blood glucose level, unlike the patient with diabetic ketoacidosis.

Diabetic ketoacidosis is potentially life-threatening and typically produces Kussmaul's respirations. Usually the patient has polydipsia, polyphagia, and polyuria before the onset of acidosis; he may or may not have a history of diabetes mellitus. Other clinical features include a fruity breath odor; orthostatic hypotension; rapid, thready pulse; generalized weakness; decreased level of consciousness (lethargic to comatose); nausea; vomiting; anorexia; and abdominal pain.

Starvation ketoacidosis is also potentially life-threatening and can cause Kussmaul's respirations. Its onset is gradual; typical findings include signs of cachexia and dehydration, decreased level of consciousness, bradycardia, and a history of severely limited food intake.

● **Renal failure.** Acute or chronic renal failure can cause life-threatening acidosis with Kussmaul's respirations. Signs and symptoms of severe renal failure include oliguria or anuria, uremic fetor, and yellow, dry, scaly skin. Other cutaneous signs are severe pruritus, uremic frost, purpura, and ecchymoses. The patient may complain of nausea and vomiting, weakness, burning pain in the legs and feet, and diarrhea or constipation.

As acidosis progresses, corresponding clinical features include frothy sputum, pleuritic chest pain, and signs of congestive heart failure and pleural or pericardial effusion. Neurologic signs include altered level of consciousness (lethargic to comatose), twitching, or seizures. Hyperkalemia and hypertension, if present, require rapid intervention to prevent cardiovascular collapse.

MANAGING HYPERPNEA

Carefully assess the patient with hyperpnea for related signs of such life-threatening conditions as increased intracranial pressure (ICP), metabolic acidosis, diabetic ketoacidosis, and uremia. Be prepared for rapid intervention.

In increased ICP

If you observe hyperpnea in a patient who has signs of head trauma from a recent accident (soft tissue injury, edema, or ecchymoses on the face or head) and has lost consciousness, act quickly to prevent further brain stem injury and irreversible deterioration. First notify the doctor. Then take the patient's vital signs, noting bradycardia, increased systolic blood pressure, or widening pulse pressure—signs of increased ICP. Examine his pupillary reaction. Elevate the head of the bed 30° (unless you suspect spinal cord injury), and insert an artificial airway. Connect the patient to a cardiac monitor, and continuously observe his respiratory pattern. (Irregular respirations signal deterioration.) As ordered, start an I.V. at a slow infusion rate and prepare to administer an osmotic diuretic, such as mannitol, to decrease cerebral edema. Catheterize the patient to measure output, administer supplemental oxygen, and keep emergency resuscitation equipment close by.

In metabolic acidosis

If the patient with hyperpnea doesn't have a head injury, his increased respirations probably indicate metabolic acidosis. If his level of consciousness is decreased, check his chart for history data to help you determine the cause of his metabolic acidosis and intervene appropriately. Suspect shock if he has cold, clammy skin. Palpate for a rapid, thready pulse and take his blood pressure, noting hypotension. Elevate the patient's legs 30°, apply pressure dressings to any obvious hemorrhage, start several large-bore I.V.s as ordered, and prepare to administer fluids, vasopressors, and blood transfusions.

A patient with hyperpnea who has a history of alcohol abuse, is vomiting profusely, has diarrhea or profuse abdominal drainage, has ingested an overdose of aspirin, or is cachectic with a history of starvation may also have metabolic acidosis. Inspect his skin for dryness and poor turgor, indicating dehydration. Take his vital signs, looking for low-grade fever and hypotension. Start an I.V. for fluid replacement, as ordered. Draw blood for electrolyte studies, and prepare to administer sodium bicarbonate.

In diabetic ketoacidosis

If the patient has a history of diabetes mellitus, is vomiting, and has a fruity breath odor (acetone breath), suspect diabetic ketoacidosis. Catheterize him to monitor increased output, and infuse saline solution as ordered. Perform a finger stick to estimate blood glucose levels with a reagent strip. Obtain a urine specimen to test for glucose and acetone, and draw blood for glucose and ketone tests, as ordered. Administer fluids, insulin, potassium, and sodium bicarbonate I.V., if ordered.

In uremia

If the patient has a history of renal disease, an ammonia odor on his breath (uremic fetor), and a fine, white powder on his skin (uremic frost), suspect uremia. Start an I.V. at a slow rate, and prepare to administer sodium bicarbonate. Monitor his EKG for dysrhythmias due to hyperkalemia. Monitor his serum electrolyte, blood urea nitrogen, and creatinine levels, too, until hemodialysis or peritoneal dialysis begins.

• *Sepsis.* A severe infection may cause lactic acidosis, resulting in Kussmaul's respirations. Other findings: tachycardia, fever, chills, headache, lethargy, profuse diaphoresis, anorexia, cough, wound drainage, urinary burning, or other signs of local infection.

• *Shock.* Potentially life-threatening metabolic acidosis produces Kussmaul's respirations, hypotension, tachycardia, narrowed pulse pressure, weak pulse, dyspnea, oliguria, anxiety, restlessness, stupor that can progress to coma, and cool, clammy skin. Other clinical features may include external or internal bleeding (in hypovolemic shock); chest pain or dysrhythmias and signs of congestive heart failure (in cardiogenic shock); high fever, chills and, rarely, hypothermia (in septic shock); or stridor due to laryngeal edema (in anaphylactic shock). Onset is usually acute in hypovolemic, cardiogenic, or anaphylactic shock, but it may be gradual in septic shock.

Other causes

• *Drugs.* Toxic levels of salicylates, acetazolamide and other carbonic anhydrase inhibitors, and ammonium chloride cause Kussmaul's respirations. So can ingestion of methanol and ethylene glycol, found in antifreeze solutions.

Special considerations

Monitor vital signs in all patients with hyperpnea, and observe for increasing respiratory distress or an irregular respiratory pattern signaling deterioration. Prepare for immediate intervention to prevent cardiovascular collapse: start an I.V. for administration of fluids, blood transfusions, and vasopressor drugs for hemodynamic stabilization, as ordered, and prepare to give ventilatory support. Prepare the patient for arterial blood gas analysis and blood chemistry studies.

Pediatric pointers

Hyperpnea in children indicates the same metabolic or neurologic causes as in adults and requires the same prompt intervention. The most common cause of metabolic acidosis in children is diarrhea, which can cause life-threatening crisis.

In infants, Kussmaul's respirations may accompany acidosis due to inborn errors of metabolism.

Hypopigmentation
[Hypomelanosis]

Hypopigmentation is a decrease in normal skin, hair, mucous membrane, or nail color resulting from deficiency, absence, or abnormal degradation of the pigment melanin. This sign may be congenital or acquired, asymptomatic or associated with other findings. Its causes include genetic disorders, nutritional deficiency, chemicals and drugs, inflammation, infection, and physical trauma. Typically chronic, hypopigmentation can be difficult to identify if the patient is light-skinned or has only slightly decreased coloring.

Assessment

Begin with a detailed patient history. Ask if any other family member has the same problem and if it was present from birth or followed skin lesions or a rash. Were the lesions painful? Does the patient have any medical problems or a history of burns, physical injury, or physical contact with chemicals? Is he taking prescription or over-the-counter drugs? Find out if he's noticed other skin changes—such as erythema, scaling, ulceration, or hyperpigmentation—or if sun exposure causes unusually severe burning.

Now examine the patient's skin, noting any erythema, scaling, ulceration, areas of hyperpigmentation, and other findings.

Medical causes

• *Burns.* Thermal and radiation burns can cause transient or permanent hypopigmentation.

• *Discoid lupus erythematosus.* This form of lupus erythematosus may produce hypopigmentation following inflammatory skin eruptions. Lesions are sharply defined, separate or fused macules, papules, or plaques; they vary from pink to purple, with a yellowish or brown crust and scaly, enlarged hair follicles. Telangiectasia may occur. After the inflammatory eruptive stage, noncontractile scarring and atrophy often affect the face and may also involve sun-exposed areas of the neck, ears, scalp (with possible alopecia), lips, and mucosa of the mouth.

• *Idiopathic guttate hypomelanosis.* Common in lightly pigmented people over age 30, this skin disorder produces sharply marginated, angular white spots on sun-exposed extremities. In blacks, hypopigmentation occurs mainly on the upper arms.

• *Inflammatory and infectious disorders.* Skin disorders, such as psoriasis, and infectious disorders, such as viral exanthems or syphilis, can cause transient or permanent hypopigmentation.

• *Leprosy.* This chronic disorder affects the skin and peripheral nervous system. Erythematous or hypopigmented macules have decreased or absent sensation for light, touch, and warmth. The lesions don't sweat, so the skin feels dry and rough; it may be scaly. Associated effects may include severely painful, palpable peripheral nerves; muscle atrophy and contractures; and ulcers of the fingers and toes.

• *Tinea versicolor.* This benign fungal skin infection produces scaly, sharply defined hypopigmented lesions, usually on the upper trunk, neck, and arms.

• *Vitiligo.* This common skin disorder produces sharply defined, flat white macules and patches ranging in diameter from 1 to over 20 cm. Usually bilaterally symmetrical, lesions appear on sun-exposed areas; in body folds; around the eyes, nose, mouth, and rectum; and over bony prominences. They're typically asymptomatic but may be pruritic. Hypopigmented patches (halo nevi) may surround pigmented moles.

Other causes

• *Chemicals.* Most phenolic compounds—for example, amylphenol and paratertiary butylphenol (PTBP), germicides used in many household and industrial products—can cause hypopigmentation. Monobenzyl ether of hydroquinone—contained in rubber products—produces permanent hypopigmented spots, resembling vitiligo, at the contact site (but they may spread).

• *Drugs.* Topical or intralesional administration of corticosteroids causes hypopigmentation at the treatment site. Chloroquine, an antimalarial drug, may cause hair depigmentation (including eyebrows and lashes) and poor tanning. These effects occur 2 to 5 months after therapy begins.

Special considerations

In fair-skinned patients, a special ultraviolet light (Wood's lamp) can help differentiate hypopigmented lesions, which appear pale, from depigmented lesions, which appear white.

Advise patients to use corrective cosmetics to help hide skin lesions, and to use a sunblock because hypopigmented areas may sunburn easily. Encourage regular examinations for early detection and treatment of lesions that may become premalignant or malignant. The doctor may prescribe repigmentation therapy, combining a photosensitizing drug (psoralen) and ultraviolet light, wavelength A. Advise patients with associated eye problems, such as albinism, to avoid the midday sun and to wear sunglasses. Refer patients for counseling if lesions cause stress.

Pediatric pointers

In children, hypopigmentation results from genetic or acquired disorders, including albinism, phenylketonuria, and tuberous sclerosis. In neonates, hypopigmentation may indicate a metabolic or nervous system disorder.

…potence • insomnia • intermittent claudication • Janeway's spots • jaundice • …in distention • Kehr's sign • Kernig's sign • leg pain • level of consciousness— …ght flashes • low birth weight • lymphadenopathy • masklike facies • McBurne… …gn • melena • menorrhagia • metrorrhagia • miosis • moon face • mouth lesio… …uscle atrophy • muscle flaccidity • muscle spasms • muscle spasticity • muscl… …ydriasis • myoclonus • nasal flaring • nausea • neck pain • night blindness • …pple retraction • nocturia • nuchal rigidity • nystagmus • ocular deviation • o… …iguria • opisthotonos • orofacial dyskinesia • orthopnea • orthostatic hypotens… …sler's nodes • otorrhea • pallor • palpitations • papular rash • paralysis • par… …octurnal dyspnea • peau d'orange • pericardial friction rub • peristaltic wave… …hotophobia • pica • pleural friction rub • polydipsia • polyphagia • polyuria • …riapism • pruritus • psoas sign • psychotic behavior • ptosis • pulse—absent • …ounding • pulse pressure—narrowed • pulse pressure—widened • pulse rhyt… …ulsus alternans • pulsus bisferiens • pulsus paradoxus • pupils—nonreactive • …urple striae • purpura • pustular rash • pyrosis • raccoon's eyes • rebound ten… …tractions—costal and sternal • rhinorrhea • rhonchi • Romberg's sign • saliv… …alivation—increased • salt craving • scotoma • scrotal swelling • seizure—abs… …eizure—generalized tonic-clonic • seizure—psychomotor • setting-sun sign • s… …in—bronze • skin—clammy • skin—mottled • skin—scaly • skin turgor—de… …ngioma • splenomegaly • stertorous respirations • stool—clay-colored • strido… …chycardia • tachypnea • taste abnormalities • tearing—increased • throat pai… …acheal deviation • tracheal tugging • tremors • trismus • tunnel vision • ure… …ischarge • urinary frequency • urinary hesitancy • urinary incontinence • uri… …oudiness • urticaria • vaginal bleeding—postmenopausal • vaginal discharge… …rtigo • vesicular rash • violent behavior • vision loss • visual blurring • visu… …lvar lesions • weight gain—excessive • weight loss—excessive • wheezing • …istention • abdominal mass • abdominal pain • abdominal rigidity • accesso… …gitation • alopecia • amenorrhea • amnesia • analgesia • anhidrosis • anore… …nxiety • aphasia • apnea • apneustic respirations • apraxia • arm pain • ast… …hetosis • aura • Babinski's reflex • back pain • barrel chest • Battle's sign • … …ladder distention • blood pressure decrease • blood pressure increase • bow… …owel sounds—hyperactive • bowel sounds—hypoactive • bradycardia • brad… …impling • breast nodule • breast pain • breast ulcer • breath with ammonia … …dor • breath with fruity odor • Brudzinski's sign • bruits • buffalo hump • … …it spots • capillary refill time—prolonged • carpopedal spasm • cat cry • ch… …symmetrical • chest pain • Cheyne-Stokes respirations • chills • chorea • Ch… …ogwheel rigidity • cold intolerance • confusion • conjunctival injection • con… …flex—absent • costovertebral angle tenderness • cough—barking • cough—… …roductive • crackles • crepitation—bony • crepitation—subcutaneous • cry… …anosis • decerebrate posture • decorticate posture • deep tendon reflexes—… …flexes—hypoactive • depression • diaphoresis • diarrhea • diplopia • dizzi… …sent • drooling • dysarthria • dysmenorrhea • dyspareunia • dyspepsia • d… …ystonia • dysuria • earache • edema—generalized • edema of the arms • ed… …f the legs • enophthalmos • enuresis • epistaxis • eructation • erythema • e… …ischarge • eye pain • facial pain • fasciculations • fatigue • fecal incontinen… …ver • flank pain • flatulence • fontanelle bulging • fontanelle depression • f… …onormalities • gait—bizarre • gait—propulsive • gait—scissors • gait—spas… …it—waddling • gallop—atrial • gallop—ventricular • genital lesions in the … …spirations • gum bleeding • gum swelling • gynecomastia • halitosis • hal… …earing loss • heat intolerance • Heberden's nodes • hematemesis • hematoc…

Impotence

Impotence is the inability to achieve and maintain penile erection sufficient to complete satisfactory intercourse; ejaculation may or may not be affected. Impotence varies from occasional and minimal to permanent and complete. Occasional impotence occurs in about half of adult American men, while chronic impotence affects about 10 million American men.

Impotence can also be classified as primary or secondary. A man with *primary impotence* has never been potent with a woman but may achieve normal erections in other situations. This uncommon condition is difficult to treat. *Secondary impotence* carries a more favorable prognosis because, despite present erectile dysfunction, the patient has succeeded in completing intercourse in the past.

Penile erection involves increased arterial blood flow secondary to psychological, tactile, or other sensory stimulation. Trapping of blood within the penis produces increased length, circumference, and rigidity. Impotence results when any component of this process—psychological, vascular, neurologic, or hormonal—malfunctions.

Organic causes of impotence may include vascular disease, diabetes mellitus, hypogonadism, a spinal cord lesion, alcohol and drug abuse, and surgical complications. (The incidence of organic impotence associated with other medical problems increases after age 50.) Psychogenic causes range from performance anxiety and marital discord to moral or religious conflicts.

Assessment

If the patient complains of impotence or of a condition that may be causing it, let him describe his problem without interruption. Then begin your assessment in a systematic way, moving from less sensitive to more sensitive matters. Begin with a psychosocial history. Is the patient married, single, or widowed? How long has he been married or had a sexual relationship? What's the age and health status of his sexual partner? Find out about past marriages, if any, and ask him why he thinks they ended. If you can do so discreetly, ask about sexual activity outside marriage or his primary sexual relationship. Also ask about his job history, his typical daily activities, and his living situation. How well does he get along with others in his household?

Focus your medical history on the causes of erectile dysfunction. Does the patient have Type II diabetes mellitus, hypertension, or heart disease? Ask about its onset and treatment. Also ask about neurologic diseases, such as multiple sclerosis. Get a surgical history, emphasizing neurologic, vascular, and urologic surgery. If trauma may be causing the patient's impotence, get information on the date of injury, its severity, associated effects, and treatment. Ask about intake of alcohol, drug use or abuse, smoking, diet, and exercise. Get a urologic history, including voiding problems and any past injury.

Next, ask when his impotence began. How did it progress? What's its current status? Make your questions specific but remember, patients often have difficulty discussing sexual problems, and many don't understand the physiology involved. These sample questions may yield helpful data:

When was the first time you remember not being able to initiate or maintain an erection? How often do you wake in the morning or at night with an erection? Do you have wet dreams? Has your sexual drive changed? How often do you try to have intercourse with your partner? How often would you *like* to? Can you ejaculate with or without an erection? Do you experience orgasm with ejaculation?

Ask the patient to rate the quality of a typical erection on a scale of 0 to 10, with 0 being completely flaccid and 10 being completely erect. Using the same scale, also ask him to rate his ability to ejaculate during sexual activity, with 0 being never and 10 being always.

Now perform a brief physical examination. Inspect and palpate the genitalia and prostate for structural abnormalities. Assess the patient's sensory function, concentrating on the perineal area. Next, test motor strength and deep tendon reflexes in all extremities, and note other neurologic deficits. Take the patient's vital signs and palpate his pulses for quality. Note any signs of peripheral vascular disease, such as cyanosis and cool extremities. Auscultate for abdominal aortic, femoral, or iliac bruits, and palpate the thyroid gland for enlargement.

Medical causes

● *Central nervous system disorders.* Spinal cord lesions from trauma produce sudden impotence. A complete lesion above S2 (upper motor neuron lesion) disrupts descending motor tracts to the genital area, causing loss of voluntary erectile control but not the reflexive ability for erection and ejaculation. But a complete lesion in the lumbosacral spinal cord (lower motor neuron lesions) causes loss of reflex ejaculation and reflex erection. Spinal cord tumors and degenerative diseases of the brain and spinal cord (such as multiple sclerosis and amyotrophic lateral sclerosis) cause progressive impotence.

● *Endocrine disorders.* Hypogonadism from testicular or pituitary dysfunction may lead to impotence from deficient secretion of androgens (primarily testosterone). Adrenocortical and thyroid dysfunction and chronic hepatic disease may also cause impotence due to these organs' roles (although minor) in sex hormone regulation.

● *Penile disorders.* Peyronie's disease makes erection painful because the penis is bent, and may make penetration difficult and eventually impossible. Phimosis prevents erection until circumcision releases constricted foreskin. Other inflammatory, infectious, or destructive diseases of the penis may also cause impotence.

● *Peripheral neuropathy.* Systemic diseases, such as chronic renal failure and diabetes mellitus, can cause progressive impotence if they progress to peripheral neuropathy. This occurs in about 50% of male diabetics. Associated signs and symptoms in diabetic neuropathy include bladder distention with overflow incontinence, orthostatic hypotension, syncope, paresthesias and other sensory disturbances, muscle weakness, and leg atrophy.

● *Psychological distress.* Impotence can result from diverse psychological causes, including depression, performance anxiety, memories of previous traumatic sexual experiences, moral or religious conflicts, and troubled emotional or sexual relationships.

• **Trauma.** Traumatic injury involving the penis, urethra, prostate, perineum, or pelvis may cause sudden impotence. This can result from structural alteration, nerve damage, or interrupted blood supply.

• **Vascular disorders.** Various vascular disorders can cause impotence. These include advanced arteriosclerosis affecting both major and peripheral blood vessels; Leriche's syndrome—slowly developing occlusion of the terminal abdominal aorta; and arteriosclerosis, thrombosis, or embolization of smaller vessels supplying the penis.

Other causes

• **Alcohol and drugs.** Alcohol and drug abuse are associated with impotence, as are many prescription drugs, especially antihypertensives. (See *Impotence: An Unsought Effect.*)

• **Surgery.** Surgical injury to the penis, bladder neck, urinary sphincter, rectum, or perineum can cause impotence. So can injury to local nerves or blood vessels.

Special considerations

Nursing care begins by establishing rapport with the patient. Probably no other medical condition in the male is as potentially frustrating, humiliating, even devastating to self-esteem and significant relationships as impotence. Help the patient feel comfortable about discussing his sexuality. This begins with feeling comfortable about your own sexuality and adopting an accepting attitude about the sexual experiences and preferences of others.

Prepare the patient for screening tests for hormonal irregularities and for Doppler readings of penile blood pressure to rule out vascular insufficiency. Other possible tests include voiding studies, nerve conduction tests, evaluation of nocturnal penile tumescence, and psychological screening.

Treatment for psychogenic impotence may include counseling of both the patient and his sexual partner;

IMPOTENCE: AN UNSOUGHT EFFECT

Many commonly used drugs—especially antihypertensives—can cause impotence that may be reversible if the drug is discontinued or the dosage reduced. Here are some examples.

amitriptyline	methyldopa
atenolol	naproxen
cimetidine	nortriptyline
clonidine	perphenazine
desipramine	prazosin
digoxin	propranolol
hydralazine	thiazide diuretics
imipramine	
methantheline bromide	thioridazine
	tranylcypromine

---

treatment for organic impotence focuses on reversing the cause, if possible. Other forms of treatment include surgical revascularization, drug-induced erection, surgical repair of venous leak, and penile prostheses. Encourage the patient to maintain follow-up appointments and treatment for underlying medical disorders.

Pediatric pointers

None.

Insomnia

Insomnia is the inability to fall asleep, remain asleep, or feel refreshed by sleep. Acute and transient during periods of stress, insomnia may become chronic and cause constant fatigue, extreme anxiety as the bedtime hour approaches, or even psychiatric disorders. A common complaint, it's experienced occasionally by about 25% of Americans and chronically by another 10%.

Physiologic causes of insomnia include jet lag, arguing, and lack of exercise. Its pathophysiologic causes range from medical and psychiatric disorders to pain, drug side effects, and idiopathic factors. Complaints of insomnia are subjective and require close investigation; the patient may mistakenly attribute to insomnia his fatigue from an organic cause, such as anemia.

Assessment

Take a thorough sleep and health history. Find out when the patient's insomnia began and the attending circumstances. Is the patient trying to stop using sedatives? Does he use stimulants, such as amphetamines, or pseudoephedrine? What about caffeine-containing drugs and beverages?

Find out if the patient has any chronic or acute conditions whose effects may be disturbing his sleep, particularly cardiac or respiratory disease, or painful or pruritic conditions. What about endocrine or neurologic disorders, or a history of drug or alcohol abuse? Is he a frequent traveler who suffers from jet lag? Does he use his legs a lot during the day, then feel restless at night? Ask about daytime fatigue and regular exercise. Also, ask about periods of gasping for air, periods of apnea, and frequent body repositioning. If possible, consult the patient's spouse or sleep partner, since the patient may not be aware of his behavior.

Assess the patient's emotional status, and try to estimate his level of self-esteem. Ask about personal and professional problems and psychological stress. Also ask about hallucinations, and note behavior that may indicate alcohol withdrawal.

After reviewing any complaints that suggest an undiagnosed disorder, perform a physical examination.

Medical causes

● *Affective disorders. Depression* commonly causes chronic insomnia with difficulty falling asleep, waking and being unable to fall back to sleep, or waking early in the morning. Typical adjuncts include dysphoria (a primary symptom), decreased appetite with weight loss or increased appetite with weight gain, and psychomotor agitation or retardation. The patient experiences loss of interest in his usual activities, feelings of worthlessness and guilt, fatigue, difficulty in concentrating, indecisiveness, and recurrent thoughts of death.

Episodes of *mania* produce a decreased need for sleep with an elevated mood and irritability. Related findings include increased activity, restlessness, loquacity, inflated self-esteem, easy distractibility, and involvement in high-risk activities, such as reckless driving.

● *Alcohol withdrawal syndrome.* Abrupt cessation of alcohol after long-term use causes insomnia that may persist for up to 2 years. Other early effects of this acute syndrome include excessive diaphoresis, tachycardia, increased blood pressure, tremor, restlessness, irritability, headache, nausea, flushing, and nightmares. Progression to delirium tremens produces confusion, disorientation, paranoia, delusions, hallucinations, and seizures.

● *Generalized anxiety disorder.* Hyperattentiveness due to anxiety can cause chronic insomnia. Related findings include signs of tension, such as fatigue and restlessness; of autonomic hyperactivity, such as diaphoresis, dyspepsia, and high resting pulse and respiratory rates; and of apprehension.

● *Nocturnal myoclonus.* In this seizure disorder, involuntary and fleeting muscle jerks of the legs occur every 20 to 40 seconds, disturbing sleep.

● *Pain.* Almost any condition that causes pain may cause insomnia. Related findings reflect the specific cause.

● *Pheochromocytoma.* This rare disorder causes paroxysms of acute hyper-

TIPS FOR RELIEVING INSOMNIA

COMMON PROBLEMS	WHAT PREVENTS OR DISTURBS SLEEP	NURSING INTERVENTIONS
Acroparesthesia	Improper positioning may compress superficial (ulnar, radial, peroneal) nerves, disrupting circulation to the compressed nerve. This causes numbness and tingling in an arm or leg.	Teach the patient to assume a comfortable position in bed, with his limbs unrestricted. If he tends to awaken with a numb leg or arm, teach him to massage and move it until sensation completely returns, and then to assume an unrestricted position.
Anxiety	Physical and emotional stress produces anxiety, which causes autonomic stimulation.	Encourage the patient to discuss his fears and concerns, and teach him such relaxation techniques as guided imagery and deep breathing. If ordered, administer a mild sedative, such as diazepam, before bedtime.
Dyspnea	In many cardiac and pulmonary disorders, a recumbent position and inactivity cause restricted chest expansion, secretion pooling, and pulmonary vascular congestion, leading to coughing and shortness of breath.	Elevate the head of the bed, or provide at least two pillows or a reclining chair to help the patient sleep. Suction him when he awakes, and encourage deep breathing every 2 to 4 hours. Also provide supplementary oxygen via nasal cannula.
Pain	Chronic or acute pain from any cause can prevent or disrupt sleep.	Administer pain medication, as ordered, 20 minutes before bedtime. Also teach deep, even, slow breathing to promote relaxation. Help the patient with back pain lie on his side with his legs flexed. Encourage the patient with epigastric pain to take an antacid before bedtime and to sleep with the head of the bed elevated.
Pruritus	A localized skin infection or a systemic disorder, such as liver failure, may produce intensely annoying itching.	Wash the patient's skin with a mild soap and water, and dry the skin thoroughly. Apply moisturizing lotion on dry, unbroken skin and an antipruritic, such as calamine lotion, on pruritic areas.
Restless leg movement	Excessive exercise during the day may cause tired, aching legs at night, requiring movement for relief.	Help the patient exercise his legs gently by slowly walking with him around the room and down the hall. If ordered, administer a muscle relaxant, such as diazepam.

metabolic activity, which can prevent or interrupt sleep. Its cardinal sign is severe hypertension, often sustained between attacks. Other effects: headache, palpitations, and anxiety.

• *Pruritic conditions.* Localized skin infections and systemic disorders, such as liver failure, can cause pruritus with resultant insomnia.

• *Sleep apnea syndrome.* Apneic periods begin with the onset of sleep, continue for 10 to 90 seconds, then end with a series of gasps and arousal. In *central sleep apnea,* respiratory movement ceases for the apneic period; in *obstructive sleep apnea,* upper airway obstruction blocks incoming air, although breathing movements continue. Some patients display both types of apnea. Repeated possibly hundreds of times during the night, this cycle alternates with bradycardia and tachycardia. Associated findings include morning headache, daytime fatigue, hypertension, ankle edema, and such personality changes as hostility, paranoia, and agitated depression.

• *Thyrotoxicosis.* Chronic signs and symptoms of hypermetabolism include insomnia, in which the patient has difficulty falling asleep and sleeps for only a brief time. Cardiopulmonary features include dyspnea, tachycardia, palpitations, and atrial or ventricular gallop. Other findings include weight loss despite increased appetite, diarrhea, tremors, nervousness, diaphoresis, hypersensitivity to heat, an enlarged thyroid, and exophthalmos.

Other causes

• *Drugs.* Use or abuse of, or withdrawal from, sedatives or hypnotics may produce insomnia. Central nervous system stimulants—including amphetamines, theophylline derivatives, ephedrine, phenylpropanolamine, cocaine, and caffeine-containing beverages—may also produce insomnia.

Special considerations

Prepare the patient for tests to evaluate his insomnia, such as blood and urine studies for 17-hydroxycorticosteroids and catecholamines; sleep EEG; or polysomnography (including an EEG, electrooculography, and electrocardiography).

Teach the patient comfort and relaxation techniques to promote natural sleep. Advise him to awaken and retire at the same time each day and to exercise regularly. Suggest that when he can't sleep, he should get up but remain inactive. Urge him to use his bed only for sleeping, not to relax.

Advise him to use tranquilizers or sedatives for acute insomnia only when relaxation techniques fail. If appropriate, refer the patient for counseling or to a sleep disorder clinic for biofeedback training or other interventions.

Pediatric pointers

Insomnia in early childhood may develop with separation anxiety at age 2 or 3, after a stressful or tiring day, or during illness or teething. In children ages 6 to 11, insomnia usually reflects residual excitement from the day's activities; a few children continue to have bedtime fears. Foster children often display sleep problems.

Intermittent Claudication

Most common in the legs, intermittent claudication is cramping limb pain brought on by exercise and relieved by 1 or 2 minutes of rest. It may be acute or chronic—when acute, it may signal acute arterial occlusion. Intermittent claudication occurs most often in men between the ages of 50 and 60; without treatment, it may progress to pain at rest. In chronic arterial occlusion, limb loss is uncommon because collateral circulation usually develops.

In occlusive artery disease, intermittent claudication results from an inadequate blood supply. Pain in the calf (the most common area) or foot indicates disease of the femoral or popliteal arteries; pain in the buttocks and upper thigh, disease of the aortoiliac arteries. During exercise, the pain typically results from the release of lactic acid due to anaerobic metabolism in the ischemic segment, secondary to atherosclerosis. When the patient stops exercising, the lactic acid clears and the pain subsides.

Intermittent claudication may also have a neurologic cause: narrowing of the vertebral column at the level of the cauda equina. This creates pressure on the nerve roots to the lower extremities. Walking stimulates circulation to the cauda equina, causing increased pressure on those nerves and pain.

Assessment

If the patient experiences *sudden intermittent claudication* along with severe or aching leg pain at rest, check the leg's temperature and palpate pulses. Check its color, too, and ask about numbness and tingling. If pulses are absent and the leg feels cold and looks pale, cyanotic, or mottled, and if paresthesias and pain are present, suspect acute arterial occlusion. Notify the doctor immediately.

Don't elevate the leg; instead, protect it and let nothing press on it. Prepare the patient for preoperative blood tests, urinalysis, electrocardiography, and chest X-rays. Start an I.V., and administer an anticoagulant and pain medication, as ordered.

If the patient has *chronic intermittent claudication,* gather history data first. Ask the patient how far he can walk before the pain occurs and how long he must rest before it subsides. Can he walk less far now than before, or does he need to rest longer? Is the pain-rest pattern variable? Has this symptom affected his life-style?

Get a history of risk factors for atherosclerosis, such as smoking, diabetes, heart disease, or cerebrovascular disease. Next, ask about associated signs and symptoms, such as pares-

thesias in the affected limb and changes in the color of the patient's fingers when he's smoking (white to blue to pink), exposed to cold, or under stress. If the patient's male, does he complain of impotence?

Focus the physical examination on the cardiovascular system. Palpate for femoral, popliteal, dorsalis pedis, and posterior tibial pulses. Diminished or absent popliteal and pedal pulses with the femoral pulse present may indicate atherosclerotic disease of the femoral artery. Diminished femoral and distal pulses may indicate disease of the terminal aorta or iliac branches. Absent pedal pulses with normal femoral and popliteal pulses may indicate Buerger's disease. An absent or diminished radial pulse indicates hand involvement.

Listen for bruits over the major arteries. Note color and temperature differences between the legs or as compared with the arms; also note the leg level where changes in temperature and color occur. Elevate the affected leg for 2 minutes; if it becomes pale or white, blood flow is severely decreased. When the leg hangs down, how long does it take for color to return? (Thirty seconds or longer indicates severe disease.) Check the patient's deep tendon reflexes after exercise; note if they're diminished in his lower extremities.

Examine the feet, toes, and fingers for ulceration, and inspect the hands and lower legs for small, tender nodules and erythema along blood vessels.

In the patient with arm pain, inspect the arms for color change (to white on elevation). Next, palpate for changes in temperature, for muscle wasting, and for a pulsating mass in the subclavian area. Palpate and compare the radial, ulnar, brachial, axillary, and subclavian pulses to identify obstructed areas.

Medical causes

• *Acute arterial occlusion.* This disorder produces intense intermittent claudication—sudden severe or aching leg pain aggravated by exercise. A saddle embolus may affect both legs. Associated findings include paresthesias, paresis, and sensations of cold in the affected limb. The limb is cool, pale, and cyanotic (mottled) with absent pulses below the occlusion. Capillary refill time is prolonged.

• *Aortic arteriosclerotic occlusive disease.* In this disorder, intermittent claudication occurs in the buttock, hip, thigh, and calf, along with absent or diminished femoral pulses. Bruits can be auscultated over the femoral and iliac arteries. Examination reveals pallor of the affected limb on elevation and profound limb weakness. The leg may be cool to the touch.

• *Arteriosclerosis obliterans.* This disorder usually affects the femoral and popliteal arteries, causing intermittent claudication (the most common symptom) in the calf. Typical associated findings include diminished or absent popliteal and pedal pulses, coolness in the affected limb, pallor on elevation, and profound limb weakness with continuing exercise. Other possible findings include numbness, paresthesias, and—in severe disease—pain at rest in the toes or foot, ulceration, and gangrene.

• *Buerger's disease.* Typically, this disorder produces intermittent claudication of the instep. Early signs include migratory superficial nodules and erythema along extremity blood vessels (nodular phlebitis). With exposure to cold, the feet initially become cold, cyanotic, and numb; later, they redden, become hot, and tingle. Occasionally, Buerger's disease also affects the hands and can cause painful fingertip ulcerations. Other characteristic findings include impaired peripheral pulses, paresthesias of the hands and feet, and migratory superficial thrombophlebitis.

• *Leriche's syndrome.* Arterial occlusion causes intermittent claudication of the hip, thigh, and buttocks. It also causes impotence in men. Examination reveals bruits, global atrophy, and absent or diminished pulses. The leg becomes cool and pale when elevated.

• *Neurogenic claudication.* Neurospinal disease causes pain from intermittent claudication that requires a longer rest time than the 2 to 3 minutes needed in vascular claudication. Associated findings include paresthesias, weakness and clumsiness when walking, and hypoactive deep tendon reflexes after walking. However, in this disorder, pulses are not affected.

• *Thoracic outlet syndrome.* Activity that requires raising the hands above the shoulders, lifting a weight, or abducting the arm can cause intermittent pain along the ulnar distribution of the arm and forearm along with paresthesias and weakness. This isn't true claudication pain because it's position-related, not exercise-related. Signs and symptoms disappear when the arm is lowered. Other features may include asymmetrical blood pressure and cool, pale skin.

Special considerations

Counsel the patient with intermittent claudication about risk factors. Encourage him to stop smoking, and refer him to a support group, if appropriate.

Promote exercise to improve collateral circulation and increase venous return, and advise him to avoid prolonged sitting or standing as well as crossing his legs at the knees.

Teach him to inspect his legs and feet for ulcers; to keep his extremities warm, clean, and dry; and to avoid injury.

Urge the patient to immediately report skin breakdown that doesn't heal. Also urge him to report any chest discomfort. Why? Because, when circulation is restored to his legs, increased exercise tolerance may lead to angina if he has coronary artery disease that was previously asymptomatic as a result of exercise limitations.

If intermittent claudication interferes with the patient's life-style, he may undergo diagnostic tests (Doppler flow studies, arteriography, and digital subtraction angiography) to determine the location and degree of occlusion.

Pediatric pointers

Intermittent claudication rarely occurs in children. Although it sometimes develops in coarctation of the aorta, extensive compensatory collateral circulation typically occurs and prevents manifestation of this sign.

Muscle cramps from exercise and growing pains may be mistaken for intermittent claudication.

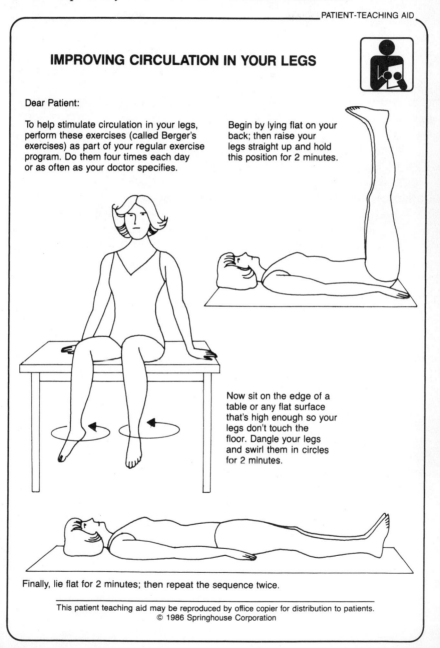

IMPROVING CIRCULATION IN YOUR LEGS

Dear Patient:

To help stimulate circulation in your legs, perform these exercises (called Berger's exercises) as part of your regular exercise program. Do them four times each day or as often as your doctor specifies.

Begin by lying flat on your back; then raise your legs straight up and hold this position for 2 minutes.

Now sit on the edge of a table or any flat surface that's high enough so your legs don't touch the floor. Dangle your legs and swirl them in circles for 2 minutes.

Finally, lie flat for 2 minutes; then repeat the sequence twice.

Janeway's spots • jaundice • jaw pain • jugular vein distention • Kehr's sign •
pain • level of consciousness—decreased • lid lag • light flashes • low birth w
lymphadenopathy • masklike facies • McBurney's sign • McMurray's sign • m
metrorrhagia • miosis • moon face • mouth lesions • murmurs • muscle atrop
muscle spasms • muscle spasticity • muscle weakness • mydriasis • myoclon
nausea • neck pain • night blindness • nipple discharge • nipple retraction •
rigidity • nystagmus • ocular deviation • oligomenorrhea • oliguria • opisthot
dyskinesia • orthopnea • orthostatic hypotension • Ortolani's sign • Osler's no
palpitations • papular rash • paralysis • paresthesias • paroxysmal nocturnal
d'orange • pericardial friction rub • peristaltic waves—visible • photophobia
rub • polydipsia • polyphagia • polyuria • postnasal drip • priapism • prurit
psychotic behavior • ptosis • pulse—absent or weak • pulse—bounding • pul
pulse pressure—widened • pulse rhythm abnormality • pulsus alternans • pu
paradoxus • pupils—nonreactive • pupils—sluggish • purple striae • purpur
pyrosis • raccoon's eyes • rebound tenderness • rectal pain • retractions—cos
rhinorrhea • rhonchi • Romberg's sign • salivation—decreased • salivation—
scotoma • scrotal swelling • seizure—absence • seizure—focal • seizure—ge
seizure—psychomotor • setting-sun sign • shallow respirations • skin—bron
skin—mottled • skin—scaly • skin turgor—decreased • spider angioma • spl
respirations • stool—clay-colored • stridor • syncope • tachycardia • tachypn
tearing—increased • throat pain • tic • tinnitus • tracheal deviation • trache
trismus • tunnel vision • uremic frost • urethral discharge • urinary frequen
urinary incontinence • urinary urgency • urine cloudiness • urticaria • vagir
postmenopausal • vaginal discharge • venous hum • vertigo • vesicular rash
loss • visual blurring • visual floaters • vomiting • vulvar lesions • weight ga
loss—excessive • wheezing • wristdrop• abdominal distention • abdominal
abdominal rigidity • accessory muscle use • agitation • alopecia • amenorrh
analgesia • anhidrosis • anorexia • anosmia • anuria • anxiety • aphasia • a
respirations • apraxia • arm pain • asterixis • ataxia • athetosis • aura • Ba
pain • barrel chest • Battle's sign • Biot's respirations • bladder distention •
blood pressure increase • bowel sounds—absent • bowel sounds—hyperacti
hypoactive • bradycardia • bradypnea • breast dimpling • breast nodule • b
breath with ammonia odor • breath with fecal odor • breath with fruity od
bruits • buffalo hump • butterfly rash • café-au-lait spots • capillary refill ti
carpopedal spasm • cat cry • chest expansion—asymmetrical • chest pain •
respirations • chills • chorea • Chvostek's sign • clubbing • cogwheel rigidi
confusion • conjunctival injection • constipation • corneal reflex—absent •
tenderness • cough—barking • cough—nonproductive • cough—productive
bony • crepitation—subcutaneous • cry—high-pitched • cyanosis • decereb
posture • deep tendon reflexes—hyperactive • deep tendon reflexes—hypoa
diaphoresis • diarrhea • diplopia • dizziness • doll's eye sign—absent • dro
dysmenorrhea • dyspareunia • dyspepsia • dysphagia • dyspnea • dystonia
edema—generalized • edema of the arms • edema of the face • edema of th
enuresis • epistaxis • eructation • erythema • exophthalmos • eye discharg
fasciculations • fatigue • fecal incontinence • fetor hepaticus • fever • flank
fontanelle bulging • fontanelle depression • footdrop • gag reflex abnormali
propulsive • gait—scissors • gait—spastic • gait—steppage • gait—waddlir
gallop—ventricular • genital lesions in the male • grunting respirations • g
swelling • gynecomastia • halitosis • halo vision • headache • hearing loss
Heberden's nodes • hematemesis • hematochezia • hematuria • hemianopi

J

Janeway's Spots

Slightly raised, irregular, and nontender, Janeway's spots are small, erythematous lesions (1 to 4 mm in diameter) on the palms and soles. They blanch with pressure and with elevation of the affected extremity; rarely, they form a diffuse rash over the trunk and extremities. They disappear spontaneously.

Janeway's spots are a common finding in infective endocarditis and may reflect an immunologic reaction to the infecting organism. They're a telltale sign of this disorder if other lesions (such as petechiae and Osler's nodes) and signs and symptoms of infection (such as fever) are present.

Assessment

If you observe Janeway's spots, obtain a medical history from your patient, noting especially valvular or rheumatic heart disease. If the patient has had valvular or rheumatic disease, ask about recent dental procedures or invasive diagnostic tests. Does he have a prosthetic replacement valve? Find out about recent meningitis and any skin, bone, or respiratory infections. Does the patient have renal disease requiring an arteriovenous shunt, or has he had recent long-term intravenous therapy, such as hyperalimentation?

Obtain a medication history, too. If the patient has had rheumatic fever or valvular disease, find out if his doctor's advised him to take prophylactic antibiotics. Ask the patient to describe how he feels. Does he have weakness, fatigue, chills, anorexia, or night sweats, possibly indicating an infection? Does he have other complaints?

Now perform a physical examination. Inspect the skin for other lesions, such as petechiae on his trunk or mucous membranes or Osler's nodes on his palms, soles, or finger or toe pads. Inspect the fingers for clubbing and splinter hemorrhages.

Take the patient's vital signs, noting fever and tachycardia—which may indicate heart failure if it persists after fever disappears. Inspect and palpate his extremities for edema. Auscultate for gallops and murmurs. Assess other body systems for embolic complications of infective endocarditis, such as acute abdominal pain and hematuria. Examining his eyes with an ophthalmoscope may reveal Roth's spots.

Medical causes

● *Acute infective endocarditis.* Janeway's spots are a late sign. Early effects include sudden onset of shaking chills and fever, peripheral edema and dyspnea, petechiae, Osler's nodes, Roth's spots, and hematuria.

• *Subacute infective endocarditis.* Janeway's spots may appear late in this disorder, which has an insidious onset. Early findings may include weakness, fatigue, weight loss, fever, night sweats, anorexia, and arthralgia. Other clinical features: elevated pulse, pale skin, Osler's nodes, splinter hemorrhages under the fingernails, petechiae, Roth's spots, clubbing of the fingers (in long-standing disease), splenomegaly, and murmurs. Embolization may produce acute signs and symptoms, such as chest, abdominal, and extremity pain; paralysis; hematuria; or blindness.

Special considerations

Tell the patient that the spots will disappear without damaging his skin. Treatment for infective endocarditis includes antibiotics and (with complications such as heart failure) diuretics and cardiac glycosides. Monitor the patient's intake, output, and cardiac status, and be alert for embolic complications. Notify the doctor immediately if the patient develops acute chest pain, abdominal pain, or paralysis.

Pediatric pointers

In children, Janeway's spots also result from infective endocarditis, which commonly stems from congenital heart defects and rheumatic fever.

Jaundice

[Icterus]

Jaundice is the yellow discoloration of the skin or mucous membranes, indicating excessive levels of conjugated or unconjugated bilirubin in the blood. In fair-skinned patients, it's most noticeable on the face, trunk, and sclera. In dark-skinned patients, it's most noticeable on the hard palate, sclera, and conjunctiva.

Jaundice is most apparent in natural sunlight. In fact, it may be undetectable in artificial or poor light. It's commonly accompanied by pruritus (because bile pigment damages sensory nerves), dark urine, and clay-colored stools.

Jaundice may result from any of three pathophysiologic processes. (See *Jaundice: Impaired Bilirubin Metabolism,* page 437.) It may be the only warning sign of certain disorders, such as pancreatic carcinoma.

Assessment

A history of the patient's jaundice is critical in determining its cause. Begin the history by asking the patient when he first noted the jaundice. Does he also have pruritus? Clay-colored stools or dark urine? Ask about past episodes or a family history of jaundice. Does he have any nonspecific signs or symptoms, such as fatigue, fever, or chills; GI signs or symptoms, such as anorexia, abdominal pain, nausea, or vomiting; or cardiopulmonary symptoms, such as shortness of breath or palpitations? Ask about alcohol use and any history of cancer, or liver or gallbladder disease. Has the patient lost weight? Obtain a medication history.

Perform the physical examination in a room with natural light. Inspect the skin for texture and dryness and for hyperpigmentation and xanthomas. Look for spider angiomas or petechiae, clubbed fingers, or gynecomastia. If the patient has congestive heart failure, auscultate for dysrhythmias, murmurs, and gallops. For all patients, auscultate for crackles and abnormal bowel sounds. Palpate the lymph nodes for swelling and the abdomen for tenderness, pain, or swelling. Palpate and percuss the liver and spleen for enlargement, and test for ascites with the shifting dullness and fluid wave techniques. Obtain baseline data on the patient's mental status: slight changes in sensorium may be early signs of deteriorating hepatic function.

Medical causes

• *Agnogenic myeloid metaplasia.* This myeloproliferative disorder of the bone marrow may cause jaundice. Its typical effects, however, are associated with anemia: fatigue, weakness, anorexia, massive splenomegaly, hepatomegaly, purpura, and bleeding tendencies.

• **Carcinoma.** *Carcinoma of the ampulla of Vater* initially produces fluctuating jaundice, mild abdominal pain, recurrent fever, and chills. Occult bleeding may be its first sign. Other findings include weight loss, pruritus, and back pain.

Hepatic carcinoma is usually metastatic; the resulting bile duct obstruction may cause jaundice. Even advanced cancer causes nonspecific signs and symptoms, such as right upper quadrant discomfort and tenderness, nausea, and slight fever. Examination may reveal hepatomegaly, ascites, peripheral edema, a bruit heard over the liver, and a right upper quadrant mass.

In *pancreatic carcinoma,* progressive jaundice—possibly with pruritus—may be the only sign. Related early findings are nonspecific, such as weight loss and back or abdominal pain. Other clinical features include anorexia, nausea, vomiting, fever, steatorrhea, fatigue, weakness, diarrhea, and skin lesions (usually on the legs).

• **Cholangitis.** Increased pressure and infection in the common bile duct cause Charcot's triad: jaundice, right upper quadrant pain, and high fever with chills.

• **Cholecystitis.** This disorder produces jaundice (without pruritus) in about 25% of patients. Typically, biliary colic occurs and peaks abruptly, and persists for 2 to 4 hours. This midepigastric or right upper quadrant pain frequently radiates to the right scapula or back, may be constant or intermittent, and worsens after meals. Other findings: nausea, vomiting (usually indicating the presence of a stone), fever, profuse diaphoresis, chills, tenderness on palpation, and possibly abdominal distention and rigidity.

• **Cholelithiasis.** This disorder commonly causes jaundice and biliary colic—the primary symptom. It's characterized by severe, steady pain in the right upper quadrant or epigastrium radiating to the right scapula or shoulder and intensifying over several hours. Accompanying signs and symptoms include nausea, vomiting, tachycardia, and restlessness. Occlusion of the common bile duct causes fever, chills, jaundice, clay-colored stools, and abdominal tenderness. After a fatty meal, the patient may experience vague epigastric fullness, dyspepsia, eructation, or flatulence.

• **Cholestasis.** In benign recurrent intrahepatic cholestasis, attacks of severe, prolonged jaundice occur (sometimes several years apart) with pruritus. Signs and symptoms of this disorder are similar to those of hepatitis—fatigue, nausea, weight loss, anorexia, and right upper quadrant pain.

• **Cirrhosis.** In *Laennec's cirrhosis,* mild-to-moderate jaundice with pruritus usually signals hepatocellular necrosis. Common early findings include ascites, weakness, leg edema, nausea, vomiting, diarrhea or constipation, anorexia, weight loss, and right upper quadrant pain. Massive hematemesis and other bleeding tendencies may occur. Gynecomastia, scanty chest and axillary hair, and testicular atrophy occur in the male patient, whereas menstrual irregularities affect the female patient. The liver and parotid gland may be enlarged, the fingers clubbed, and Dupuytren's contracture present. Other findings include purpura, fever of 101° to 102° F. (38.3° to 38.9° C.), mental changes, asterixis, fetor hepaticus, spider angiomas, and palmar erythema.

In *primary biliary cirrhosis,* fluctuating jaundice may appear years after the onset of other signs and symptoms, such as pruritus that worsens at bedtime (often the first sign), weakness, fatigue, weight loss, and vague abdominal pain. Itching frequently leads to skin excoriation. Associated findings include hyperpigmentation; indications of malabsorption, such as nocturnal diarrhea, steatorrhea, purpura, and osteomalacia; hematemesis from esophageal varices; ascites; edema; xanthelasmas; xanthomas on the palms, soles, and elbows; and hepatomegaly.

• **Congestive heart failure.** Jaundice due to liver dysfunction occurs in severe right heart failure. Other effects may include jugular vein distention, cyanosis, dependent edema of the legs and sacrum, steady weight gain, confusion, hepatomegaly, nausea, vomiting, abdominal discomfort, and anorexia due to visceral edema. Ascites is a late sign. Oliguria and marked weakness and anxiety may also occur. If left heart failure develops first, other findings may include fatigue, dyspnea, orthopnea, paroxysmal nocturnal dyspnea, tachypnea, dysrhythmias, and tachycardia.

• **Dubin-Johnson syndrome.** In this inherited syndrome, fluctuating jaundice—increasing with stress—is the major sign, appearing as late as age 40. Related findings include slight hepatic enlargement and tenderness, upper abdominal pain, nausea, and vomiting.

• **Glucose-6-phosphate dehydrogenase (G6PD) deficiency.** Acute intravascular hemolysis following ingestion of such drugs as quinine or aspirin causes jaundice, pallor, dyspnea, tachycardia, and malaise. Palpation may reveal splenomegaly and hepatomegaly.

• **Hemolytic anemia (acquired).** This disorder may produce prominent jaundice along with dyspnea, fatigue, pallor, tachycardia, and palpitations. Rapid hemolysis causes chills, fever, irritability, headache, and abdominal pain; severe hemolysis causes signs of shock.

• **Hepatic abscess.** Multiple abscesses may cause jaundice, but the primary effects are persistent fever with chills and sweating. Other, but possibly misleading, findings include steady, severe pain in the right upper quadrant or midepigastrium that may be referred to the shoulder; vomiting, nausea, and anorexia; hepatomegaly; and ascites.

• **Hepatitis.** Dark urine and clay-colored stools usually develop before jaundice in the late stages of acute viral hepatitis. Early systemic signs and symptoms vary and include fatigue, nausea, vomiting, malaise, arthralgias, myalgias, headache, anorexia, photophobia, pharyngitis, cough, diarrhea or constipation, and a low-grade fever associated with liver and lymph node enlargement. During the icteric phase (which subsides in 2 or 3 weeks unless complications occur), systemic signs subside, but an enlarged, palpable liver may be present along with weight loss, anorexia, and right upper quadrant pain and tenderness.

• **Leptospirosis.** Severe leptospirosis (Weil's disease) may cause jaundice. It begins suddenly with frontal headache and severe muscle aches in the thighs and lumbar area along with cutaneous hyperesthesia, abdominal pain, nausea, and vomiting. Chills and a rapidly rising fever follow. Signs of meningeal irritation include drowsiness, decreased mentation, stiff neck, and positive Kernig's and Brudzinski's signs. Right upper quadrant tenderness, hepatomegaly, and jaundice indicate hepatic involvement; proteinuria, pyuria, and hematuria indicate renal involvement. Epistaxis, hematemesis, melena, or hemoptysis may occur.

• **Pancreatitis (acute).** Edema of the head of the pancreas and obstruction of the common bile duct can cause jaundice. Usually, this disorder's primary symptom is severe epigastric pain that often radiates to the back. Lying with the knees flexed on the chest or sitting up and leaning forward brings relief. Early associated signs and symptoms include nausea, persistent vomiting, and abdominal distention. Other findings include fever, tachycardia, abdominal rigidity and tenderness, hypoactive bowel sounds, and crackles.

Severe pancreatitis produces extreme restlessness; mottled skin; cold, diaphoretic extremities; and paresthesias and tetany—signs of hypocalcemia. Fulminant pancreatitis causes massive hemorrhage.

• **Sickle cell anemia.** Hemolysis produces

JAUNDICE: IMPAIRED BILIRUBIN METABOLISM

Jaundice occurs in three forms: prehepatic, hepatic, and posthepatic. In all three, bilirubin levels in the blood increase.

In *prehepatic jaundice,* certain conditions and disorders—such as transfusion reactions and sickle cell anemia—cause massive hemolysis. Red blood cells rupture faster than the liver can conjugate bilirubin, so large amounts of unconjugated bilirubin pass into the blood, causing increased intestinal conversion of this bilirubin to water-soluble urobilinogen for excretion in urine and stools. (Unconjugated bilirubin is insoluble in water, so it can't be directly excreted in urine.)

Hepatic jaundice results from the liver's inability to conjugate or transport bilirubin, leading to increased blood levels of unconjugated bilirubin. This occurs in such disorders as hepatitis, cirrhosis, and metastatic cancer, and during prolonged use of drugs metabolized by the liver.

In *posthepatic jaundice,* occurring in biliary and pancreatic disorders, bilirubin forms at its normal rate; however, inflammation, scar tissue, a tumor, or gallstones block the flow of bile into the intestine. This causes an accumulation of conjugated bilirubin in the blood. Water-soluble, the bilirubin is excreted in the urine.

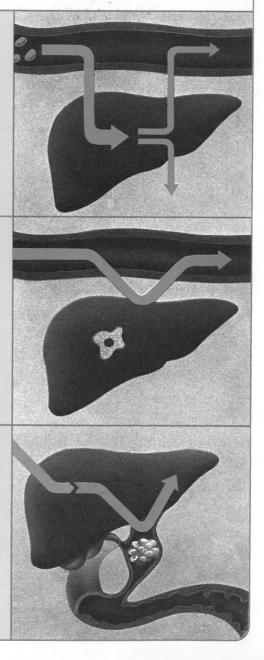

jaundice in this disorder. Other findings include impaired growth and development and increased susceptibility to infection; life-threatening thrombotic complications; and, commonly, leg ulcers and painful, swollen joints with fever and chills. Bone aches and chest pain may also occur. Severe hemolysis may cause hematuria and pallor, chronic fatigue, dyspnea (or dyspnea on exertion), and tachycardia. During sickle cell crisis, the patient may have severe bone, abdominal, thoracic, and muscular pain; low-grade fever; and increased weakness, jaundice, and dyspnea.

• **Zieve syndrome.** Caused by alcohol abuse, this relatively rare disorder produces abdominal pain and sudden onset of severe jaundice. However, spider angiomas, ascites, and other signs of advanced liver disease are absent.

Other causes
• **Drugs.** Many drugs may cause hepatic injury and resultant jaundice. Some examples include phenylbutazone, I.V. tetracycline, isoniazid, oral contraceptives, sulfonamides, mercaptopurine, erythromycin estolate, niacin, troleandomycin, androgenic steroids, and phenothiazines.
• **Treatments.** Upper abdominal surgery may cause postoperative jaundice. It occurs secondary to hepatocellular damage from manipulation of organs, leading to edema and obstructed bile flow; from administration of tetracyclines or halothane; or from prolonged surgery with shock, blood loss, or blood transfusion.

A surgical shunt used to reduce portal hypertension (such as a portacaval shunt) may also produce jaundice.

Special considerations
Encourage the patient with a hepatic disorder to decrease protein intake sharply and increase intake of carbohydrates. If he has obstructive jaundice, encourage a balanced, nutritious diet (avoiding high-fat foods) and frequent small meals. To help decrease the itching of pruritus, bathe the patient frequently, and apply an antipruritic lotion, such as calamine.

Prepare the patient for diagnostic tests to evaluate biliary and hepatic function. Laboratory studies may include urine and fecal urobilinogen, serum bilirubin, hepatic enzymes and cholesterol, prothrombin time, and a complete blood count. Other tests may include ultrasonography, cholangiography, liver biopsy, and exploratory laparotomy.

Pediatric pointers
Physiologic jaundice in the newborn is common; it develops about 3 to 5 days after birth. In infants, obstructive jaundice usually results from congenital biliary atresia. Choledochal cyst—a congenital cystic dilatation of the common bile duct—may also cause jaundice in children, particularly of Japanese descent.

Other causes of jaundice include Crigler-Najjar syndrome, Gilbert's disease, Rotor's syndrome, thalassemia major, hereditary spherocytosis, erythroblastosis fetalis, Hodgkin's disease, and infectious mononucleosis.

Jaw Pain

Jaw pain may arise from either or both of the bones that hold the teeth in the jaw—the maxilla, or upper jaw, and the mandible, or lower jaw. Jaw pain also includes pain in the temporomandibular joint (TMJ), where the mandible meets the temporal bone.

Jaw pain may develop gradually or abruptly and may range from barely noticeable to excruciating, depending on its cause. It usually results from disorders of the teeth, soft tissue, or glands of the mouth or throat, or from local trauma or infections. Systemic causes include musculoskeletal, neurologic, cardiovascular, endocrine, immunologic, metabolic, or infectious disorders. Such life-threatening disorders as myocardial infarction (MI) or tetany also produce jaw pain, as do drugs (especially phenothiazines) and dental or surgical procedures.

Jaw pain is seldom a primary indicator of any one disorder—but some of its causes represent medical emergencies.

Assessment

Begin your assessment by asking the patient to describe the pain's character, intensity, and frequency. When did he first notice the jaw pain? Where on the jaw does he feel pain? Does the pain radiate to other areas? Sharp or burning pain arises from the skin or subcutaneous tissues. Causalgia, an intense burning sensation, usually results from damage to the fifth cranial or trigeminal nerve. This type of superficial pain is easily localized, unlike dull, aching, boring, or throbbing pain, which originates in muscle, bone, or joints. Also ask about aggravating or alleviating factors.

Explore associated signs and symptoms. Ask about joint or chest pain, fatigue, headache, malaise, anorexia, weight loss, intermittent claudication, diplopia, and hearing loss. (Keep in mind that jaw pain may accompany more characteristic signs and symptoms of life-threatening disorders, such as chest pain in MI.)

Focus your physical examination on the jaw. Inspect the painful area for redness, and palpate for edema or warmth. Facing the patient directly, look for facial asymmetry indicating swelling. Check the TMJs by placing your fingertips just anterior to the external auditory meatus and asking the patient to open and close, and to thrust out and retract his jaw. Note the presence of crepitus, an abnormal scraping or grinding sensation in the joint. (Clicks heard when the jaw is widely spread apart are normal.) How wide can the patient open his mouth? Less than 3 cm or more than 6 cm between upper and lower teeth is abnormal. Next, palpate the parotid area for pain and swelling, and inspect and palpate the oral cavity for lesions, elevation of the tongue, or masses.

Medical causes

• **Angina pectoris.** Angina may produce jaw pain (usually radiating from the substernal area) and left arm pain. Unlike MI, anginal pain is less severe, often triggered by exertion or emotional stress or following a heavy meal. It usually subsides with rest and administration of nitroglycerin. Other signs and symptoms may include shortness of breath, nausea and vomiting, tachycardia, dizziness, diaphoresis, belching, and palpitations.

• **Arthritis.** In *osteoarthritis,* which usually affects the small hand joints, aching jaw pain increases with activity (talking, eating) and subsides with rest. Other features are crepitus heard and felt over the TMJ, enlarged joints with a restricted range of motion, and stiffness on awakening that improves with a few minutes of activity. Usually, redness and warmth are absent.

Rheumatoid arthritis causes symmetrical pain in all the joints, including the jaw (frequently affecting proximal finger joints first). Joints display limited range of motion and are tender, warm, swollen, and stiff after inactivity, especially in the morning. Myalgia is common. Systemic signs and symptoms include fatigue, weight loss, malaise, anorexia, lymphadenopathy, and mild fever. Painless, movable rheumatoid nodules may appear on the elbows, knees, and knuckles. Progressive disease causes deformities, crepitation with joint rotation, muscle weakness and atrophy around the involved joint, and multiple systemic complications.

• **Head and neck cancer.** Many types of head and neck cancer, especially of the oral cavity and nasopharynx, produce aching jaw pain of insidious onset. Other findings include a history of leukoplakia ulcers of the mucous membranes; palpable masses in the jaw, mouth, and neck; dysphagia; bloody discharges; drooling; and lymphadenopathy.

• *Hypocalcemic tetany.* Besides painful muscle contractions of the jaw and mouth, this life-threatening disorder produces paresthesias and carpopedal spasms. The patient may complain of weakness, fatigue, and palpitations. Examination reveals hyperreflexia and positive Chvostek's and Trousseau's signs. Muscle twitching, choreiform movements, and muscle cramps may also occur. In severe hypocalcemia, laryngeal spasm may occur with stridor, cyanosis, convulsions, and cardiac dysrhythmias.

• *Ludwig's angina.* Infection of the sublingual and submandibular spaces produces severe jaw pain in the mandibular area with tongue elevation, sublingual edema, and drooling. Fever is a common sign. Progressive disease produces dysphagia, dysphonia, and stridor and dyspnea due to laryngeal edema and obstruction by an elevated tongue.

• *Myocardial infarction.* Initially, this life-threatening disorder causes intense, crushing substernal pain unrelieved by rest or nitroglycerin. It may radiate to the lower jaw, left arm, neck, back, or shoulder blades. (Rarely, jaw pain occurs without chest pain.) The patient may have pallor, clammy skin, dyspnea, excessive diaphoresis, nausea and vomiting, anxiety, restlessness, and a feeling of impending doom. Associated findings may include a low-grade fever, decreased or increased blood pressure, dysrhythmias, an atrial gallop, new murmurs (frequently from mitral insufficiency), and crackles.

• *Osteomyelitis.* Bone infection following trauma, sinus infection, or dental injury may produce diffuse, aching jaw pain along with warmth, swelling, tenderness, erythema, and restricted jaw movement. Acute osteomyelitis may also cause tachycardia, sudden fever, nausea, and malaise. Chronic osteomyelitis may recur after minor trauma.

• *Sialolithiasis.* In this disorder, stones form in the salivary glands and cause painful swelling that makes chewing uncomfortable. Jaw pain occurs in the lower jaw, the floor of the mouth, and the TMJ. It may also radiate to the ear or neck.

• *Sinusitis.* Maxillary sinusitis produces intense boring pain in the maxilla and cheek that may radiate to the eye. This type of sinusitis also causes a feeling of fullness, increased pain on percussion of the first and second molars, and—in nasal obstruction—loss of the sense of smell. Sphenoid sinusitis causes chronic pain at the mandibular ramus, vertex of the head, and temporal area, and a scanty nasal discharge. Other signs and symptoms of both types of sinusitis include fever, halitosis, headache, malaise, cough, sore throat, and fever.

• *Suppurative parotitis.* Bacterial infection of the parotid gland by *Staphylococcus aureus* tends to develop in debilitated patients with dry mouth or poor oral hygiene. Besides abrupt onset of jaw pain, high fever, and chills, findings include redness and edema of the overlying skin; a tender, swollen gland; and pus at the second top molar (Stensen's ducts). Infection often leads to disorientation; shock and death are common.

• *Temporal arteritis.* Common in patients over age 60, this disorder produces sharp jaw pain after chewing or talking. Nonspecific signs and symptoms include low-grade fever, generalized muscle pain, malaise, fatigue, anorexia, and weight loss. Vascular lesions produce jaw pain; throbbing, unilateral headache in the frontotemporal region; swollen, nodular, tender temporal arteries; and, at times, erythema of the overlying skin.

• *Temporomandibular joint (TMJ) syndrome.* This common syndrome produces jaw pain at the TMJ; spasm and pain of the masticating muscle; clicking, popping, or crepitus of the TMJ; and restricted jaw movement. Unilateral, localized pain may radiate to other head and neck areas. The patient typically reports teeth clenching, bruxism, and emotional stress. He may also experience ear pain, headache, deviation of the jaw to the affected side upon opening the mouth, and jaw subluxation or dislocation, especially after yawning.

• *Tetanus.* A rare life-threatening disorder caused by a bacterial toxin, tetanus produces stiffness and pain in the jaw and difficulty opening the mouth. Early nonspecific signs and symptoms (often unnoticed or mistaken for influenza) include headache, irritability, restlessness, low-grade fever, and chills. Examination reveals tachycardia, profuse diaphoresis, and hyperreflexia. Progressive disease leads to painful, involuntary muscle spasms that spread to the abdomen, back, or face. The slightest stimulus may produce reflex spasms of any muscle group. Ultimately, laryngospasms, respiratory distress, and convulsions may occur.

• *Trauma.* Injury to the face, head, or neck, and particularly fracture of the maxilla or mandible, may produce jaw pain and swelling and decreased jaw mobility. Associated findings may include hypotension and tachycardia (indicating shock), lacerations, ecchymoses, and hematomas. Rhinorrhea or otorrhea indicates leakage of cerebrospinal fluid; blurred vision indicates orbital involvement.

• *Trigeminal neuralgia.* This disorder causes paroxysmal attacks of intense unilateral jaw pain (stopping at the facial midline) or rapid-fire shooting sensations in one of the divisions of the trigeminal nerve (usually the superior mandibular or maxillary division). This superficial pain, felt mainly over the lips and chin and in the teeth, lasts from 1 to 15 minutes. Mouth and nose areas may be hypersensitive. Involvement of the ophthalmic branch of the trigeminal nerve causes a diminished or absent corneal reflex on the same side. Stimulating the nerve—for example, by lightly touching the cheeks—

triggers an attack. Exposure to heat or cold and consuming hot or cold foods or beverages can also spur an attack.

Other causes
• *Drugs.* Some drugs, such as phenothiazines, affect the extrapyramidal tract, causing dyskinesias; others cause tetany of the jaw secondary to hypocalcemia.

Special considerations
If the patient is in severe pain, withhold food, liquids, and normally taken drugs until the diagnosis is confirmed. Administer pain medications, as ordered. Prepare the patient for diagnostic tests, such as jaw X-rays. Apply an ice pack if the jaw's swollen, and discourage the patient from talking or moving his jaws.

Pediatric pointers
Be alert for nonverbal signs of jaw pain, such as rubbing the affected area or wincing while talking or swallowing. In infants, initial signs of tetany from hypocalcemia may include episodes of apnea and generalized jitteriness progressing to facial grimaces and generalized rigidity. Finally, convulsions may occur.

Jaw pain in children sometimes stems from disorders not common in adults. Mumps, for example, causes unilateral or bilateral swelling from the lower mandible to the zygomatic arch. Parotiditis due to cystic fibrosis also causes jaw pain.

When trauma causes jaw pain in children, always consider the possibility of abuse.

Jugular Vein Distention

Jugular vein distention is the abnormal fullness and height of the pulse waves in the internal or external jugular veins. When the supine patient's head is elevated 45°, a pulse wave height greater

ASSESSING JUGULAR VEIN DISTENTION

First, position the supine patient so that you can visualize pulsations reflected from the right atrium. Elevate the head of the bed from 45° to 90°. (In the normal patient, veins distend only when the patient lies flat.) Next, locate the angle of Louis, or sternal notch—the reference point for measuring venous pressure. To do so, palpate the clavicles where they join the sternum (the suprasternal notch). Place your first two fingers on the suprasternal notch. Then, without lifting them from the skin, slide them down the sternum until you feel a bony protuberance—the angle of Louis.

Now find the internal jugular vein. (This indicates venous pressure more reliably than the external jugular vein.) Shine a flashlight across the patient's neck to create shadows that highlight his venous pulse. Be sure to distinguish jugular venous pulsations from carotid arterial pulsations. One way to do this is to palpate the vessel: arterial pulsations continue, whereas venous pulsations disappear with light finger pressure. Also, with changes in body position, venous pulsations increase or decrease, but arterial pulsations remain constant.

Next, locate the highest point along the vein where you can see pulsations. Using a centimeter ruler, measure the distance between that high point and the sternal notch. Record this finding as well as the angle at which the patient was lying. A finding greater than 4 cm above the sternal notch, with the head of the bed at a 45° angle, indicates jugular vein distention.

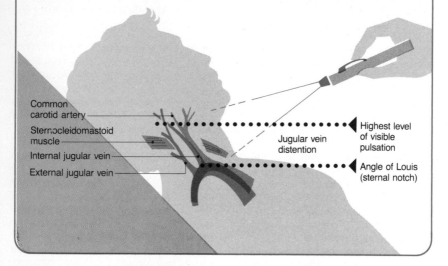

Common carotid artery

Sternocleidomastoid muscle

Internal jugular vein

External jugular vein

Jugular vein distention

Highest level of visible pulsation

Angle of Louis (sternal notch)

than 4 cm above the angle of Louis indicates distention. Engorged, distended veins reflect increased venous pressure in the right side of the heart. This common sign characteristically occurs in congestive heart failure and other cardiovascular disorders.

Assessment

Assessing jugular vein distention involves visualizing and evaluating venous pulsations. (See *Assessing Jugular Vein Distention.*) If you detect jugular vein disten-

tion in a patient with pale, clammy skin who suddenly appears anxious and dyspneic, take his blood pressure. If you note hypotension and pulsus paradoxus, suspect cardiac tamponade and notify the doctor immediately. Elevate the foot of the bed 20° to 30°, give supplemental oxygen, and monitor cardiac status. Start an I.V. for fluid administration, and keep cardiopulmonary resuscitation equipment close by. Assemble equipment for emergency pericardiocentesis to relieve pressure on the heart. Throughout the procedure, monitor the patient's blood pressure, heart rhythm, and respirations.

If the patient isn't in severe distress, begin your assessment with a personal history. Has the patient gained weight recently? Does he have difficulty putting on shoes? Are his ankles swollen? Ask about chest pain, shortness of breath, paroxysmal nocturnal dyspnea, anorexia, nausea, vomiting, and any history of cancer or heart, pulmonary, or renal disease.

Next, perform a physical examination. Take vital signs. Tachycardia, tachypnea, and increased blood pressure indicate fluid overload that's stressing the heart. Inspect and palpate the extremities and face for edema. Then weigh the patient.

Now auscultate the lungs for crackles and the heart for gallops and a pericardial friction rub. Inspect the abdomen for distention, and palpate and percuss for an enlarged liver. Finally monitor urinary output and note any decrease.

Medical causes

• *Cardiac tamponade.* This life-threatening condition produces jugular vein distention along with anxiety, restlessness, cyanosis, chest pain, and clammy skin. Cardiac tamponade also causes tachycardia, hypotension, dyspnea, tachypnea, pulsus paradoxus, and muffled heart sounds.

• *Congestive heart failure.* Sudden or gradual development of right heart failure commonly causes jugular vein distention along with possible weakness and anxiety, cyanosis, dependent edema of the legs and sacrum, steady weight gain, confusion, and hepatomegaly. Other findings may include nausea, vomiting, abdominal discomfort, and anorexia due to visceral edema. Ascites is a late sign. Massive right heart failure may produce anasarca and oliguria.

If left heart failure precedes right heart failure, jugular vein distention is a late sign. Other clinical features include fatigue, dyspnea, orthopnea, paroxysmal nocturnal dyspnea, tachypnea, tachycardia, and dysrhythmias. Auscultation reveals crackles and a ventricular gallop.

• *Hypervolemia.* Markedly increased intravascular fluid volume causes jugular vein distention along with rapid weight gain, elevated blood pressure, bounding pulse, peripheral edema, dyspnea, and crackles.

• *Pericarditis (chronic constrictive).* Progressive signs and symptoms of restricted heart filling cause jugular vein distention that's more prominent on inspiration (Kussmaul's sign). The patient usually complains of chest pain. Other clinical features typically include fluid retention with dependent edema; hepatomegaly; ascites; and pericardial friction rub.

• *Superior vena cava obstruction.* A tumor or, rarely, thrombosis may gradually lead to jugular vein distention when the veins of the head, neck, and arms fail to empty effectively, causing facial, neck, and upper-arm edema. Metastasis to the mediastinum may cause dyspnea, cough, substernal chest pain, and hoarseness.

Special considerations

If ordered, monitor central venous pressure to assess right heart function and administer pain medication and diuretics. Restrict fluids and monitor intake and output. Routinely change the patient's position to avoid skin breakdown from peripheral edema.

Teach the patient about treatment, including diet restrictions (such as a low-sodium diet) and possible side effects of drug therapy.

Pediatric pointers

Jugular vein distention is difficult (sometimes impossible) to assess in most infants and toddlers because of their short, fat necks. Even in school-age children, measurement of jugular vein distention can be unreliable, because the sternal angle may not be the same distance (5 to 7 cm) above the right atrium as in adults.

Kehr's sign • Kernig's sign • leg pain • level of consciousness—decreased • lid
birth weight • lymphadenopathy • masklike facies • McBurney's sign • McMur
menorrhagia • metrorrhagia • miosis • moon face • mouth lesions • murmurs
muscle flaccidity • muscle spasms • muscle spasticity • muscle weakness • my
nasal flaring • nausea • neck pain • night blindness • nipple discharge • nippl
nuchal rigidity • nystagmus • ocular deviation • oligomenorrhea • oliguria • o
dyskinesia • orthopnea • orthostatic hypotension • Ortolani's sign • Osler's nod
palpitations • papular rash • paralysis • paresthesias • paroxysmal nocturnal d
l'orange • pericardial friction rub • peristaltic waves—visible • photophobia •
rub • polydipsia • polyphagia • polyuria • postnasal drip • priapism • pruritu
psychotic behavior • ptosis • pulse—absent or weak • pulse—bounding • puls
pulse pressure—widened • pulse rhythm abnormality • pulsus alternans • pul
paradoxus • pupils—nonreactive • pupils—sluggish • purple striae • purpura
pyrosis • raccoon's eyes • rebound tenderness • rectal pain • retractions—costa
rhinorrhea • rhonchi • Romberg's sign • salivation—decreased • salivation—in
scotoma • scrotal swelling • seizure—absence • seizure—focal • seizure—gene
seizure—psychomotor • setting-sun sign • shallow respirations • skin—bronze
skin—mottled • skin—scaly • skin turgor—decreased • spider angioma • sple
respirations • stool—clay-colored • stridor • syncope • tachycardia • tachypne
tearing—increased • throat pain • tic • tinnitus • tracheal deviation • tracheal
trismus • tunnel vision • uremic frost • urethral discharge • urinary frequency
urinary incontinence • urinary urgency • urine cloudiness • urticaria • vagina
postmenopausal • vaginal discharge • venous hum • vertigo • vesicular rash •
loss • visual blurring • visual floaters • vomiting • vulvar lesions • weight gai
loss—excessive • wheezing • wristdrop• abdominal distention • abdominal m
abdominal rigidity • accessory muscle use • agitation • alopecia • amenorrhe
analgesia • anhidrosis • anorexia • anosmia • anuria • anxiety • aphasia • ap
respirations • apraxia • arm pain • asterixis • ataxia • athetosis • aura • Babi
pain • barrel chest • Battle's sign • Biot's respirations • bladder distention • b
blood pressure increase • bowel sounds—absent • bowel sounds—hyperactive
hypoactive • bradycardia • bradypnea • breast dimpling • breast nodule • bre
breath with ammonia odor • breath with fecal odor • breath with fruity odor
bruits • buffalo hump • butterfly rash • café-au-lait spots • capillary refill tim
carpopedal spasm • cat cry • chest expansion—asymmetrical • chest pain • C
respirations • chills • chorea • Chvostek's sign • clubbing • cogwheel rigidity
confusion • conjunctival injection • constipation • corneal reflex—absent • co
tenderness • cough—barking • cough—nonproductive • cough—productive •
pony • crepitation—subcutaneous • cry—high-pitched • cyanosis • decerebra
posture • deep tendon reflexes—hyperactive • deep tendon reflexes—hypoacti
diaphoresis • diarrhea • diplopia • dizziness • doll's eye sign—absent • drool
dysmenorrhea • dyspareunia • dyspepsia • dysphagia • dyspnea • dystonia •
edema—generalized • edema of the arms • edema of the face • edema of the
diuresis • epistaxis • eructation • erythema • exophthalmos • eye discharge •
fasciculations • fatigue • fecal incontinence • fetor hepaticus • fever • flank pa
fontanelle bulging • fontanelle depression • footdrop • gag reflex abnormalitie
propulsive • gait—scissors • gait—spastic • gait—steppage • gait—waddling
gallop—ventricular • genital lesions in the male • grunting respirations • gur
swelling • gynecomastia • halitosis • halo vision • headache • hearing loss •
Heberden's nodes • hematemesis • hematochezia • hematuria • hemianopia •
hepatomegaly • hiccups • hirsutism • hoarseness • Homans' sign • hyperpig

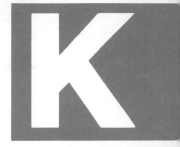

Kehr's Sign

A cardinal sign of hemorrhage within the peritoneal cavity, Kehr's sign is referred left shoulder pain due to diaphragmatic irritation by intraperitoneal blood. Usually, the pain arises when the patient assumes the supine position or lowers his head. Such positioning increases the contact of free blood or clots with the left diaphragm, involving the phrenic nerve.

Kehr's sign usually develops right after the hemorrhage, although onset is sometimes delayed up to 48 hours. It's a classic sign of a ruptured spleen, and also occurs with a ruptured ectopic pregnancy.

Assessment

After you detect Kehr's sign, quickly take the patient's vital signs and have another nurse immediately notify the doctor. If the patient shows signs of hypovolemia, elevate his feet 30°. Insert a large-bore I.V. for fluid and blood replacement and an indwelling (Foley) catheter; begin monitoring intake and output. Draw blood to determine hematocrit, and give supplemental oxygen.

Inspect the patient's abdomen for bruises and distention, and palpate for tenderness. Percuss for Ballance's sign—an indicator of massive peri-splenic clotting and free blood in the peritoneal cavity from a ruptured spleen.

Medical cause

● *Intraabdominal hemorrhage.* Kehr's sign usually accompanies intense abdominal pain, abdominal rigidity, and muscle spasm. Other findings vary with the cause of bleeding.

Special considerations

In anticipation of surgery, withhold oral intake, and prepare the patient for abdominal X-rays, computed tomography and ultrasound scans, and possibly paracentesis, peritoneal lavage, and culdocentesis. Give analgesics as prescribed.

Pediatric pointers

Since a child may have difficulty describing pain, watch for nonverbal clues, such as rubbing the shoulder.

Kernig's Sign

A reliable early indicator of meningeal irritation, Kernig's sign is combined resistance and hamstring muscle pain that's elicited when the examiner attempts to extend the supine patient's

ELICITING KERNIG'S SIGN

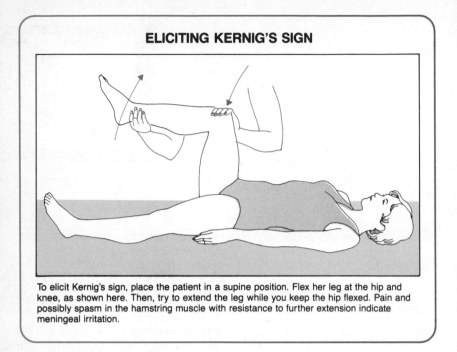

To elicit Kernig's sign, place the patient in a supine position. Flex her leg at the hip and knee, as shown here. Then, try to extend the leg while you keep the hip flexed. Pain and possibly spasm in the hamstring muscle with resistance to further extension indicate meningeal irritation.

flexed leg. This sign is usually elicited in meningitis or subarachnoid hemorrhage. In these potentially life-threatening disorders, hamstring muscle pain results from stretching the blood- or exudate-irritated meninges surrounding spinal nerve roots.

Kernig's sign can also indicate herniated disk and spinal tumor. In these disorders, the pain results from disk or tumor pressure on spinal nerve roots.

Assessment

If you elicit a positive Kernig's sign and suspect life-threatening meningitis or subarachnoid hemorrhage, immediately inform the doctor and prepare for emergency intervention. (See *When Kernig's Sign Signals CNS Crisis*.)

If meningeal irritation isn't suspected, ask the patient if he feels any back pain that radiates down one or both legs. Does he also feel leg numbness, tingling, or weakness? Ask about other signs and symptoms, and find out if he has a history of cancer or back

injury. Then, perform a physical examination, concentrating on motor and sensory function.

Medical causes

● *Lumbosacral herniated disk.* A positive Kernig's sign may be elicited in this disorder, but the cardinal and earliest feature is sciatic pain on the affected side or on both sides. Associated findings include postural deformity (lumbar lordosis or scoliosis), paresthesias, hypoactive deep tendon reflexes in the involved leg, and dorsiflexor muscle weakness.

● *Meningitis.* Usually, Kernig's sign is positive early in meningitis. Fever also occurs early, possibly with chills. Other signs and symptoms of meningeal irritation may include nuchal rigidity, hyperreflexia, Brudzinski's sign, and opisthotonos. As intracranial pressure (ICP) increases, headache and vomiting may occur. In severe meningitis, the patient may experience stupor, coma, and seizures. Cranial nerve involvement may produce ocular palsies, facial weakness, deafness, and photophobia. An erythematous maculopapular rash may occur in viral meningitis; a purpuric rash may be seen in meningococcal meningitis.

• **Spinal cord tumor.** Kernig's sign can be elicited occasionally, but the earliest symptom is often pain felt locally or along the spinal nerve, frequently in the leg. Associated findings may include weakness or paralysis distal to the tumor, paresthesias, urinary retention or incontinence, fecal incontinence, and sexual dysfunction.

• **Subarachnoid hemorrhage.** Kernig's sign and Brudzinski's sign can both be elicited within minutes after the initial bleed. The patient experiences sudden onset of severe headache, nuchal rigidity, and decreased level of consciousness. Photophobia, fever, nausea, vomiting, dizziness, and seizures are possible. Focal signs may include hemiparesis or hemiplegia, aphasia, and sensory or visual disturbances. Increasing ICP may produce bradycardia, increased blood pressure, respiratory pattern change, and rapid progression to coma.

Special considerations

Prepare the patient for diagnostic tests, such as computed tomography, spinal X-ray, and myelography. Closely monitor his vital signs, ICP, and cardiopulmonary and neurologic status. Ensure bed rest, quiet, and minimal stress.

If the patient has subarachnoid hemorrhage, darken the room and elevate the head of the bed at least 30° to reduce ICP. If he has a herniated disk or spinal tumor, he may require pelvic traction.

Pediatric pointers

Kernig's sign is considered ominous in children because of their greater potential for rapid deterioration.

EMERGENCY

WHEN KERNIG'S SIGN SIGNALS C.N.S. CRISIS

Kernig's sign may signal a life-threatening CNS disorder: meningitis or subarachnoid hemorrhage. If you elicit a positive Kernig's sign in a patient suspected of having either disorder, immediately inform the doctor. Take the patient's vital signs to obtain baseline information. Then test for Brudzinski's sign to obtain further evidence of meningeal irritation. (See *Testing for Brudzinski's Sign,* page 135.) Next, ask the patient or his family to describe the onset of illness. Typically, progressive onset of headache, fever, nuchal rigidity, and confusion suggests meningitis. Conversely, sudden onset of severe headache, nuchal rigidity, photophobia, and possibly loss of consciousness usually indicates subarachnoid hemorrhage.

MENINGITIS	SUBARACHNOID HEMORRHAGE
If you suspect meningitis, ask about recent infections—especially tooth abscesses. Usually, meningitis is a complication of another bacterial infection. As ordered, draw blood for culture to determine the causative organism. Also find out if the patient has a history of I.V. drug abuse, open head injury, or endocarditis. Insert an I.V. line and administer antibiotics immediately.	*If you suspect subarachnoid hemorrhage,* ask about a history of hypertension, cerebral aneurysm, head trauma, or arteriovenous malformations. Also ask about sudden withdrawal of antihypertensive drugs. Check the patient's pupils for dilation, and assess for signs of increasing intracranial pressure, such as bradycardia, increased systolic blood pressure, and widened pulse pressure. Insert an I.V. line and administer supplemental oxygen.

leg pain • level of consciousness—decreased • lid lag • light flashes • low bir[
lymphadenopathy • masklike facies • McBurney's sign • McMurray's sign • m[
metrorrhagia • miosis • moon face • mouth lesions • murmurs • muscle atrop[
muscle spasms • muscle spasticity • muscle weakness • mydriasis • myoclon[
nausea • neck pain • night blindness • nipple discharge • nipple retraction •
rigidity • nystagmus • ocular deviation • oligomenorrhea • oliguria • opisthot[
dyskinesia • orthopnea • orthostatic hypotension • Ortolani's sign • Osler's nc
palpitations • papular rash • paralysis • paresthesias • paroxysmal nocturnal
d'orange • pericardial friction rub • peristaltic waves—visible • photophobia
rub • polydipsia • polyphagia • polyuria • postnasal drip • priapism • prurit[
psychotic behavior • ptosis • pulse—absent or weak • pulse—bounding • pul[
pulse pressure—widened • pulse rhythm abnormality • pulsus alternans • pu[
paradoxus • pupils—nonreactive • pupils—sluggish • purple striae • purpur[
pyrosis • raccoon's eyes • rebound tenderness • rectal pain • retractions—cos[
rhinorrhea • rhonchi • Romberg's sign • salivation—decreased • salivation—
scotoma • scrotal swelling • seizure—absence • seizure—focal • seizure—ge[
seizure—psychomotor • setting-sun sign • shallow respirations • skin—bron[
skin—mottled • skin—scaly • skin turgor—decreased • spider angioma • sp[
respirations • stool—clay-colored • stridor • syncope • tachycardia • tachypn[
tearing—increased • throat pain • tic • tinnitus • tracheal deviation • trache[
trismus • tunnel vision • uremic frost • urethral discharge • urinary frequen[
urinary incontinence • urinary urgency • urine cloudiness • urticaria • vagi[
postmenopausal • vaginal discharge • venous hum • vertigo • vesicular rash
loss • visual blurring • visual floaters • vomiting • vulvar lesions • weight ga[
loss—excessive • wheezing • wristdrop• abdominal distention • abdominal [
abdominal rigidity • accessory muscle use • agitation • alopecia • amenorrh[
analgesia • anhidrosis • anorexia • anosmia • anuria • anxiety • aphasia • a[
respirations • apraxia • arm pain • asterixis • ataxia • athetosis • aura • Ba[
pain • barrel chest • Battle's sign • Biot's respirations • bladder distention •
blood pressure increase • bowel sounds—absent • bowel sounds—hyperacti[
hypoactive • bradycardia • bradypnea • breast dimpling • breast nodule • b[
breath with ammonia odor • breath with fecal odor • breath with fruity od[
bruits • buffalo hump • butterfly rash • café-au-lait spots • capillary refill ti[
carpopedal spasm • cat cry • chest expansion—asymmetrical • chest pain •
respirations • chills • chorea • Chvostek's sign • clubbing • cogwheel rigidit[
confusion • conjunctival injection • constipation • corneal reflex—absent • c[
tenderness • cough—barking • cough—nonproductive • cough—productive
bony • crepitation—subcutaneous • cry—high-pitched • cyanosis • decerebr[
posture • deep tendon reflexes—hyperactive • deep tendon reflexes—hypoac[
diaphoresis • diarrhea • diplopia • dizziness • doll's eye sign—absent • dro[
dysmenorrhea • dyspareunia • dyspepsia • dysphagia • dyspnea • dystonia [
edema—generalized • edema of the arms • edema of the face • edema of th[
enuresis • epistaxis • eructation • erythema • exophthalmos • eye discharge
fasciculations • fatigue • fecal incontinence • fetor hepaticus • fever • flank
fontanelle bulging • fontanelle depression • footdrop • gag reflex abnormalit[
propulsive • gait—scissors • gait—spastic • gait—steppage • gait—waddlin[
gallop—ventricular • genital lesions in the male • grunting respirations • g[
swelling • gynecomastia • halitosis • halo vision • headache • hearing loss
Heberden's nodes • hematemesis • hematochezia • hematuria • hemianopia
hepatomegaly • hiccups • hirsutism • hoarseness • Homans' sign • hyperpi-

Leg Pain

Although leg pain often signifies a musculoskeletal disorder, this symptom can also result from more serious vascular or neurologic disorders. The pain may arise suddenly or gradually, and may be localized or affect the entire leg. Constant or intermittent, it may feel dull, burning, sharp, shooting, or tingling. Leg pain often affects locomotion, limiting weight bearing. Severe leg pain that follows cast application for a fracture may signal limb-threatening compartment syndrome. Sudden onset of severe leg pain in a patient with underlying vascular insufficiency may signal acute deterioration, possibly requiring an arterial graft or amputation.

Assessment

If the patient has acute leg pain and a history of trauma, quickly take his vital signs and assess the leg's neurovascular status. Observe leg position and check for swelling, gross deformities, or abnormal rotation. Check distal pulses, and note skin color and temperature. Immediately inform the doctor if the affected leg is pale, cool, and pulseless. These findings may indicate impaired circulation, which could require emergency surgery.

When the patient's condition permits, ask him when the pain began and have him describe its intensity, character, and pattern. Is the pain worse in the morning, at night, or with movement? If it doesn't prevent him from walking, must he rely on a crutch or other assistive device? Also ask him about the presence of other signs and symptoms.

Find out if the patient has a history of leg injury or surgery and if he or a family member has a history of joint, vascular, or back problems. Also ask what medications the patient is taking and whether they've helped to relieve his leg pain.

Begin the physical examination by watching the patient walk, if his condition permits. Observe how he holds his leg while standing and sitting. Palpate the legs, buttocks, and lower back to determine the extent of pain and tenderness. If the doctor has ruled out fracture, test range of motion in the hip and knee. Also check reflexes with the patient's leg straightened and raised, noting any action that causes pain. Then compare both legs for symmetry, movement, and active range of motion. If the patient wears a leg cast, splint, or restrictive dressing, carefully check distal circulation, sensation, and mobility, and stretch his toes to elicit any associated pain.

HIGHLIGHTING CAUSES OF LOCAL LEG PAIN

Various disorders cause hip, knee, ankle, or foot pain, which may radiate to surrounding tissues and be reported as leg pain. Local pain is often accompanied by tenderness, swelling, and deformity in the affected area.

Hip pain
Arthritis
Avascular necrosis
Bursitis
Dislocation
Fracture
Sepsis
Tumor

Knee pain
Arthritis
Bursitis
Chondromalacia
Contusion
Cruciate ligament
  injury
Dislocation
Fracture
Meniscal injury
Osteochondritis dissecans
Phlebitis
Popliteal cyst
Radiculopathy
Ruptured extensor
  mechanism
Sprain

Ankle pain
Achilles tendon contracture
Arthritis
Dislocation
Fracture
Sprain
Tenosynovitis

Foot pain
Arthritis
Bunion
Callus or corn
Dislocation
Flat foot
Fracture
Gout
Hallux rigidus
Hammer toe
Ingrown toenail
Köhler's disease
Morton's neuroma
Occlusive vascular
  disease
Plantar fasciitis
Plantar wart
Radiculopathy
Tabes dorsalis
Tarsal tunnel syndrome

Medical causes

- **Bone neoplasm.** Continuous deep or boring pain, often worse at night, may be the first symptom. Later, skin breakdown and impaired circulation may occur, along with cachexia, fever, and impaired mobility.
- **Compartment syndrome.** Progressive, intense, lower leg pain that increases with passive muscle stretching is a cardinal sign of this limb-threatening disorder. Restrictive dressings or traction may aggravate the pain, which typically worsens despite analgesia. Other findings may include muscle weakness and paresthesias, but apparently normal distal circulation. With irreversible muscle ischemia, you'll also find paralysis and absent pulse.
- **Fracture.** Severe, acute pain accompanies swelling and ecchymosis in the affected leg. Movement produces extreme pain, and the leg may be unable to bear weight. Neurovascular status distal to the fracture may be impaired, causing paresthesias, absent pulse, mottled cyanosis, and cool skin. Deformity, muscle spasms, and bony crepitation may occur.
- **Infection.** Local leg pain, erythema, swelling, and warmth characterize both soft tissue and bone infections. Fever and tachycardia may be present with other systemic signs.
- **Occlusive vascular disease.** Continuous cramping pain in the legs and feet may worsen with walking, inducing claudication. The patient may report increased pain at night and complain of cold feet and cold intolerance. Examination may reveal ankle and lower leg edema, decreased or absent pulses, and decreased capillary refill time.
- **Sciatica.** Pain radiates down the back of the leg along the sciatic nerve. Pain may be described as shooting, aching, or tingling. Typically, activity exacerbates the pain and rest relieves it. The patient may limp to avoid aggravating the leg pain and may have difficulty moving from a sitting to a standing position.
- **Strain or sprain.** Acute strain causes

sharp, transient pain and rapid swelling, followed by leg tenderness and ecchymosis. Chronic strain produces stiffness, soreness, and generalized leg tenderness several hours after the injury; active and passive motion may be painful or impossible. A sprain causes local pain, especially during joint movement; ecchymosis and possibly local swelling and loss of mobility develop.

• **Thrombophlebitis.** Discomfort may range from calf tenderness to severe pain accompanied by swelling, warmth, and a feeling of heaviness in the affected leg. The patient may also have fever, chills, malaise, muscle cramps, and a positive Homans' sign. Assessment may reveal visibly engorged, palpable superficial veins.

• **Varicose veins.** Mild-to-severe leg symptoms may develop, including nocturnal cramping; a feeling of heaviness; diffuse, dull aching after prolonged standing or walking; and aching during menses. Assessment may reveal palpable nodules, orthostatic edema, and stasis pigmentation of the calves and ankles.

• **Venous stasis ulcers.** Localized pain and bleeding arise from infected ulcerations on the calves. Mottled, bluish pigmentation is characteristic, and local edema may also occur.

Special considerations

If the patient has acute leg pain, closely monitor his neurovascular status by frequently checking distal pulses and assessing the temperature and color of both legs. Also monitor thigh and calf circumference to assess bleeding into tissues from a possible fracture site. Prepare him for X-rays. Use sandbags to immobilize the leg; apply ice and possibly skeletal traction, as ordered. If a fracture isn't suspected, prepare the patient for laboratory tests to detect an infectious agent or for such tests as venography, Doppler ultrasonography, or plethysmography to determine vascular competency. Withhold food and fluids until the need for surgery has

been eliminated, and withhold analgesics until the doctor makes a preliminary diagnosis.

If the patient has chronic leg pain, instruct him in using anti-inflammatory drugs and performing range-of-motion exercises. If necessary, teach him how to use a cane, walker, or other assistive device. Discuss with the patient and his family any life-style changes that may be necessary until leg pain resolves. If physical therapy is ordered, stress the importance of establishing a daily exercise regime.

Pediatric pointers

Common pediatric causes of leg pain include fracture, osteomyelitis, and bone neoplasms. If parents fail to give an adequate explanation for a leg fracture, consider the possibility of child abuse.

Level of Consciousness— Decreased

A decrease in level of consciousness (LOC)—from lethargy to stupor to coma—usually results from neurologic disorders and often signals life-threatening complications of hemorrhage, trauma, or cerebral edema. However, this sign can also result from metabolic, gastrointestinal, musculoskeletal, urologic, and cardiopulmonary disorders; severe nutritional deficiency; the effects of toxins; and drug use. LOC can deteriorate suddenly or gradually and can remain altered temporarily or permanently.

Consciousness is controlled by the reticular activating system (RAS), an intricate network of neurons whose axons extend from the brain stem, thalamus, and hypothalamus to the cerebral cortex. Disturbance in any part of this integrated system prevents the intercommunication that makes consciousness possible. Cerebral dysfunction characteristically produces the least dramatic decrease in a patient's level of consciousness. In contrast, dysfunction of the reticular activating system produces the most dramatic decrease in a patient's level of consciousness—coma.

The most sensitive indicator of decreased level of consciousness is a change in the patient's mental status. However, the Glasgow Coma Scale can also be used to quickly evaluate a patient's level of consciousness, based on his ability to respond to verbal, sensory, and motor stimulation.

Assessment

Use the Glasgow Coma Scale to quickly determine the severity of decreased LOC and to obtain baseline data. (See *Glasgow Coma Scale: Grading Level of Consciousness,* page 454.) If the patient's score is 13 or less, immediately notify the doctor. Insert an artificial airway, elevate the head of the bed 30° and, if spinal cord injury's been ruled out, turn the patient's head to the side. Prepare to suction the patient, if necessary. Remember to hyperventilate him first to reduce carbon dioxide levels. Then, assess the rate, rhythm, and depth of spontaneous respirations. Support breathing with an Ambu bag, if necessary. If the patient's Glasgow Coma Scale score is 7 or less, be prepared to assist with intubation and emergency resuscitation as necessary.

Next, assess the patient's circulation by checking carotid pulse, heart rate and rhythm, and blood pressure. Continue to monitor his vital signs, being alert for signs of increasing ICP, such as bradycardia and widening pulse pressure.

When you're confident the patient's airway, breathing, and circulation are stabilized, perform a neurologic examination.

Try to obtain history information from the patient, if he's lucid, and from his family. Did the patient complain of headache, dizziness, nausea, visual or hearing disturbances, weakness, fatigue, or any other problems before his LOC decreased? Has his family noticed any changes in the patient's behavior, personality, memory, or temperament? Also ask about a history of neurologic disease, cancer, or recent trauma; drug and alcohol use; and the development of other signs and symptoms.

Because decreased LOC can result from disorders that affect virtually every body system, tailor the remainder of your assessment according to the patient's associated symptoms.

Medical causes

● *Adrenal crisis.* Decreased LOC, ranging from lethargy to coma, may develop within 8 to 12 hours of onset. Early associated findings include progressive weakness; irritability; anorexia; headache; nausea and vomiting; diarrhea; abdominal pain; and fever. Later signs include hypotension; rapid, thready pulse; oliguria; cool, clammy skin; and flaccid extremities. The patient with chronic adrenocortical hypofunction may have hyperpigmented skin and mucous membranes.

● *Brain abscess.* Decreased LOC varies from drowsiness to deep stupor, depending on abscess size and site. Early signs reflect increasing ICP: constant intractable headache, nausea, vomiting, and seizures. Typical later features include ocular disturbances, such as nystagmus, vision loss, pupillary inequality, and signs of infection, such as fever. Other findings may include personality changes, confusion, abnormal behavior, dizziness, facial weakness, aphasia, ataxia, tremor, and hemiparesis.

● *Brain tumor.* LOC decreases slowly, from lethargy to coma. The patient may also experience apathy, behavior changes, memory loss, and decreased attention span; he may complain of morning headache, dizziness, vision loss, ataxia, or sensorimotor disturbances. Aphasia and seizures are possible, along with signs of hormonal imbalance, such as fluid retention or amenorrhea. In later stages, papilledema, vomiting, bradycardia, and widening pulse pressure also appear. The patient may exhibit a decorticate or decerebrate posture.

• *Cerebral aneurysm (ruptured).* Somnolence, confusion and, at times, stupor characterize a moderate bleed; deep coma occurs in often-fatal severe bleeding. Usually, onset is abrupt, with sudden, severe headache, nausea, and vomiting. Nuchal rigidity, back and leg pain, fever, restlessness, irritability, occasional seizures, and blurred vision reflect meningeal irritation. The type and severity of other findings depend on the site and severity of the hemorrhage, and may include hemiparesis, hemisensory defects, dysphagia, and visual defects.

• *Cerebral contusion.* Usually unconscious for a prolonged period, the patient may develop dilated, nonreactive pupils and decorticate or decerebrate posture. If he's conscious or recovers consciousness, he may be drowsy, confused, disoriented, agitated, or even violent. Associated findings may include blurred or double vision, fever, headache, pallor, diaphoresis, tachycardia, altered respirations, aphasia, and hemiparesis. Residual effects may include seizures, impaired mental status, slight hemiparesis, and vertigo.

• *Cerebrovascular accident (CVA).* LOC changes vary in degree and onset but aren't a CVA hallmark. *Thrombotic CVA* is typically preceded by multiple transient ischemic attacks, and may occur abruptly or evolve over several minutes, hours, or days. *Embolic CVA* occurs without warning, and deficits reach their peak almost at once. *Hemorrhagic CVA* deficits usually develop progressively over minutes or hours.

Associated findings vary with CVA type and severity and may include disorientation; intellectual deficits, such as memory loss and poor judgment; personality changes; and emotional lability. Other possible findings include dysarthria, dysphagia, ataxia, aphasia,

apraxia, agnosia, unilateral sensorimotor loss, and visual disturbances. In addition, urinary retention or incontinence, constipation, headache, vomiting, and seizures may occur.

• *Diabetic ketoacidosis.* This potentially life-threatening disorder produces a fairly rapid decrease in LOC, ranging from lethargy to coma. This is often preceded by polydipsia, polyphagia, and polyuria. The patient may complain of weakness, anorexia, abdominal pain, nausea, and vomiting. He may also exhibit orthostatic hypotension; fruity breath odor; Kussmaul's respirations; warm, dry skin; and a rapid, thready pulse.

• *Encephalitis.* Within 24 to 48 hours after onset, the patient may develop LOC changes ranging from lethargy to coma. He may also have abrupt onset of fever, headache, nuchal rigidity, vomiting, irritability, seizures, aphasia, ataxia, hemiparesis, nystagmus, photophobia, myoclonus, and cranial nerve palsies.

• *Encephalomyelitis (postvaccinal).* This life-threatening disorder produces rapid LOC deterioration from drowsiness to coma. The patient also experiences rapid onset of nuchal rigidity, vomiting, and seizures.

• *Encephalopathy.* In *hepatic encephalopathy,* signs and symptoms develop in four stages. *Prodromal stage:* slight personality changes (disorientation, forgetfulness, slurred speech) and slight tremor. *Impending stage:* tremor progressing to asterixis (the hallmark of hepatic encephalopathy), lethargy, aberrant behavior, and apraxia. *Stuporous stage:* stupor and hyperventilation, with the patient noisy and abusive when aroused. *Comatose stage:* coma with decerebrate posture, hyperactive reflexes, positive Babinski's reflex, and fetor hepaticus.

In life-threatening *hypertensive encephalopathy,* LOC progressively decreases from lethargy to stupor to coma. In addition to markedly elevated blood pressure, the patient may experience severe headache, vomiting, sei-

GLASGOW COMA SCALE: GRADING LEVEL OF CONSCIOUSNESS

You've probably heard terms such as *lethargic, obtunded,* or *stuporous* used to describe progressive decrease in a patient's level of consciousness. However, the Glasgow Coma Scale provides a more accurate, less subjective method of recording such changes, grading consciousness in relation to eye opening and motor and verbal responses.

To use the Glasgow Coma Scale, test the patient's ability to respond to verbal,

motor, and sensory stimulation. The scoring system doesn't determine exact level of consciousness, but it does provide an easy way to describe the patient's basic status and helps to detect and interpret changes from baseline. A decreased reaction score in one or more categories may signal impending neurologic crisis. A patient scoring 7 or less is comatose and probably has severe neurologic damage.

TEST		REACTION	SCORE
Eyes		Open spontaneously	4
		Open to verbal command	3
		Open to pain	2
		No response	1
Best motor response		Obeys verbal command	6
		Localizes painful stimulus	5
		Flexion—withdrawal	4
		Flexion—abnormal (decorticate rigidity)	3
		Extension (decerebrate rigidity)	2
		No response	1
Best verbal response		Oriented and converses	5
		Disoriented and converses	4
		Inappropriate words	3
		Incomprehensible sounds	2
		No response	1
Total			3 to 15

zures, visual disturbances, transient paralysis, and eventually Cheyne-Stokes respirations.

In *hypoglycemic encephalopathy,* LOC rapidly deteriorates from lethargy to coma. Early signs and symptoms include nervousness, restlessness, and confusion; hunger; alternate flushing and cold sweats; and headache, trembling, and palpitations. Blurred vision progresses to motor weakness, hemiplegia, dilated pupils, pallor, decreased pulse, shallow respirations, and seizures. Flaccidity and decerebrate posture appear late.

Depending on its severity, *hypoxic encephalopathy* produces a sudden or gradual decrease in LOC, leading to coma and brain death. Early, the pa-

tient appears confused and restless, with cyanosis and increased heart and respiratory rates and blood pressure. Later, his respiratory pattern becomes abnormal, and assessment reveals decreased pulse, blood pressure, and deep tendon reflexes (DTRs); Babinski's reflex; absent doll's eye sign; and fixed pupils.

In *uremic encephalopathy,* LOC decreases gradually from lethargy to coma. Early, the patient may appear apathetic, inattentive, confused, and irritable and may complain of headache, nausea, fatigue, and anorexia. Other findings may include vomiting, tremors, edema, papilledema, hypertension, cardiac dysrhythmias, dyspnea, rales, Kussmaul's and Cheyne-

Stokes respirations, and oliguria.

• *Epidural hemorrhage (acute).* This life-threatening posttraumatic disorder produces momentary loss of consciousness followed by a lucid interval. While lucid, the patient has severe headache, nausea, vomiting, and bladder distention. Rapid deterioration in consciousness follows, possibly leading to coma. Other findings: irregular respirations, seizures, decreased and bounding pulse, increased pulse pressure, hypertension, unilateral or bilateral fixed and dilated pupils, unilateral hemiparesis or hemiplegia, decerebrate posture, and Babinski's reflex.

• *Heatstroke.* As body temperature increases, LOC gradually decreases from lethargy to coma. Early signs and symptoms include malaise, tachycardia, tachypnea, orthostatic hypotension, muscle cramps, and syncope. The patient may be irritable, anxious, and dizzy and may report severe headache. His skin will be hot, flushed, and diaphoretic; later, when fever exceeds 105° F. (40.5° C.), the skin becomes hot, flushed, and anhidrotic. Pulse and respiratory rate increase markedly, while blood pressure drops precipitously. Other findings may include vomiting, diarrhea, dilated pupils, and Cheyne-Stokes respirations.

• *Hypercapnia with pulmonary disease.* LOC decreases gradually from lethargy to coma, but prolonged coma is rare. The patient becomes confused or drowsy and develops asterixis and muscle twitching. He may complain of headache and exhibit mental dullness, papilledema, and small, reactive pupils.

• *Hyperglycemic hyperosmolar nonketotic coma.* LOC decreases rapidly from lethargy to coma. Early findings may include polyuria, polydipsia, weight loss, and weakness. Later, the patient may develop hypotension, poor skin turgor, dry skin and mucous membranes, tachycardia, tachypnea, oliguria, and seizures.

• *Hypernatremia.* This disorder, life-threatening if acute, causes LOC to deteriorate from lethargy to coma. The patient will be irritable and exhibit twitches progressing to seizures. Other associated signs and symptoms may include a weak, thready pulse; nausea; malaise; fever; thirst; flushed skin; and dry mucous membranes.

• *Hyperventilation syndrome.* Brief episodes of unconsciousness follow stress-induced deep, rapid breathing associated with anxiety and agitation. Accompanying findings include dizziness, circumoral and peripheral paresthesias, twitching, carpopedal spasm, and dysrhythmias.

• *Hypokalemia.* LOC gradually decreases to lethargy; coma is rare. Other findings include confusion, nausea, vomiting, diarrhea, and polyuria; weakness, decreased reflexes, and malaise; and dizziness, hypotension, and dysrhythmias.

• *Hyponatremia.* This disorder, life-threatening if acute, produces decreased LOC in late stages. Early nausea and malaise may progress to behavior changes, incoordination, and eventually seizures and coma.

• *Hypothermia.* In *severe hypothermia* (temperature below 90° F., or 32.2° C.), LOC decreases rapidly from lethargy to coma. DTRs disappear, and ventricular fibrillation occurs—possibly followed by cardiopulmonary arrest. In *mild-to-moderate hypothermia,* the patient may experience memory loss and slurred speech in addition to shivering, weakness, fatigue, and apathy. Other early signs include ataxia, muscle stiffness, and hyperactive DTRs; diuresis; tachycardia and decreased respiratory rate and blood pressure; and cold, pale skin. Later, muscle rigidity and decreased reflexes may develop, along with peripheral cyanosis, bradycardia, dysrhythmias, severe hypotension, decreased respirations, and oliguria.

• *Intracerebral hemorrhage.* This life-threatening disorder produces rapid, steady loss of consciousness within hours, often accompanied by severe headache, dizziness, nausea, and vomiting. Associated signs and symptoms vary and may include increased blood pressure, irregular respirations, Babinski's reflex, seizures, aphasia, decreased sensations, hemiplegia, decorticate or decerebrate posture, and dilated pupils.

• *Meningitis.* Confusion and irritability are expected, although stupor, coma, and seizures may occur in severe meningitis. Fever develops early, possibly accompanied by chills. Associated findings include severe headache, nuchal rigidity, hyperreflexia, and possibly opisthotonos. The patient exhibits Kernig's and Brudzinski's signs and possibly ocular palsies, photophobia, facial weakness, and hearing loss.

• *Myxedema crisis.* The patient may show swift LOC decrease to stupor or just slow mentation and confusion. Associated findings include severe hypothermia, hypoventilation, hypotension and bradycardia, hypoactive reflexes, periorbital and peripheral edema, and seizures.

• *Poisoning.* Toxins such as lead, carbon monoxide, and snake and spider venoms can cause varying degrees of decreased LOC. Confusion is common, as are headache, nausea, and vomiting. Other general features include hypotension, cardiac dysrhythmias, dyspnea, sensorimotor loss, and seizures.

• *Pontine hemorrhage.* A sudden, rapid decrease in LOC to the point of coma occurs within minutes, and death within hours. The patient may also exhibit total paralysis; decerebrate posture; Babinski's reflex; absent doll's eye sign; and bilateral miosis, although pupils remain reactive to light.

• *Seizure disorders. Complex partial seizure* produces decreased LOC, manifested as a blank stare, purposeless behavior (picking at clothing, wandering, lip-smacking or chewing motions), and unintelligible speech. The seizure may be heralded by an aura and followed by several minutes of mental confusion.

Absence seizure usually involves a brief change in LOC, indicated by blinking or eye rolling, blank stare, and slight mouth movements.

Generalized tonic-clonic seizure typically begins with a loud cry and sudden loss of consciousness. Muscle spasm alternates with relaxation. Tongue-biting, incontinence, labored breathing, apnea, and cyanosis may also occur. Consciousness returns after the seizure, but the patient remains confused and may have difficulty talking. He may complain of drowsiness, fatigue, headache, muscle aching, and weakness and may fall into deep sleep.

Atonic seizure produces sudden unconsciousness for a few seconds.

Status epilepticus, rapidly recurring seizures without intervening periods of physiologic recovery and return of consciousness, can be life-threatening.

• *Shock.* Decreased LOC—lethargy progressing to stupor and coma—occurs late. Associated findings include confusion, anxiety, and restlessness; hypotension; tachycardia; weak pulse with narrowing pulse pressure; dyspnea; oliguria; and cool, clammy skin. *Hypovolemic shock* also produces massive or insidious bleeding, either internally or externally. *Cardiogenic shock* may produce chest pain or dysrhythmias and signs of congestive heart failure, such as dyspnea, cough, edema, distended neck veins, or weight gain. *Septic shock* may be accompanied by high fever and chills. *Anaphylactic shock* usually involves stridor.

• *Subdural hematoma (chronic).* LOC deteriorates slowly. Signs and symptoms include confusion, decreased ability to concentrate, and personality changes accompanied by headache, giddiness, seizures, and a dilated ipsilateral pupil with ptosis.

• *Subdural hemorrhage (acute).* In this potentially life-threatening disorder, consciousness progressively decreases from somnolence to coma, preceded by agitation and confusion. The patient may also experience headache, fever, unilateral pupil dilation, decreased pulse and respirations, widening pulse pressure, seizures, hemiparesis, and Babinski's reflex.

• **Thyroid storm.** LOC decreases suddenly and can progress to coma. Irritability, restlessness, confusion, and psychotic behavior precede the deterioration. Associated signs and symptoms include tremors and weakness; visual disturbances; tachycardia, dysrhythmias, and angina; warm, moist, flushed skin; and vomiting, diarrhea, and fever to 105° F. (40.5° C.).

• **Transient ischemic attack.** Abrupt decrease in LOC varies in severity and disappears gradually within 24 hours. Site-specific findings may include vision loss, nystagmus, aphasia, dizziness, dysarthria, unilateral hemiparesis or hemiplegia, tinnitus, paresthesias, dysphagia, or staggering or incoordinated gait.

Other causes
• **Alcohol.** Use of alcohol causes varying degrees of sedation, irritability, and incoordination; intoxication frequently causes stupor.
• **Drugs.** Sedation and other degrees of decreased LOC can result from overdose of barbiturates, other central nervous system depressants, and aspirin.

Special considerations
Reassess the patient's LOC and neurologic status at least hourly. Carefully monitor ICP, intake, and output. Ensure airway patency and proper nutrition. Take necessary precautions to help ensure the patient's safety. Keep him on bed rest with the side rails up. Apply restraints only if absolutely necessary, since their use may increase his agitation and confusion. Talk to the patient even if he's comatose; your voice may help reorient him to reality.

Pediatric pointers
The primary cause of decreased LOC in children is head trauma, which most often results from physical abuse or motor vehicle accident. Other causes include accidental poisoning, hydrocephalus, and meningitis or brain abscess following ear or respiratory infection. To reduce the parents' anxiety,

include them in the child's care. Offer them support and realistic explanations of their child's condition.

Lid Lag
[Graefe's sign]

A cardinal sign of thyrotoxicosis, lid lag is the inability of the upper eyelid to follow the eye's downward movements. Testing for lid lag involves holding a finger, penlight, or other target above the patient's eye level, then moving it downward and observing eyelid movement as his eyes follow the target. This sign is demonstrated when a rim of sclera appears between the upper lid margin and the iris when the patient lowers his eyes, when one lid closes more slowly than the other, or when both lids close slowly and incompletely with jerky movements. Lid lag results from chronic contraction of Müller's muscle in the upper eyelid.

Assessment
Ask the patient when he first noticed lid lag or its possible manifestation, incomplete closure of the eyelid. Explore other signs and symptoms, and ask about a history of thyroid disease. Next, perform a physical examination, focusing on the effects of thyrotoxicosis, such as an enlarged thyroid, diaphoresis, tremors, and exophthalmos.

Medical cause
• **Thyrotoxicosis.** This disorder may produce bilateral lid lag and other ocular effects, including exophthalmos, decreased blinking, eye dryness and discomfort, and conjunctival injection. Restricted eye movement may produce diplopia. Assessment also reveals the classic effects of thyrotoxicosis: enlarged thyroid, nervousness, heat intolerance, weight loss despite increased appetite, diaphoresis, diarrhea, tremors, and palpitations.

DIFFERENTIATING LID LAG AND BILATERAL PTOSIS

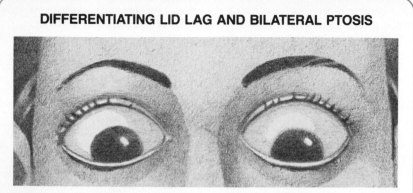

In lid lag (above), the upper eyelid is retracted—it *lags behind* the downward movement of the eye and exposes a rim of sclera above the iris.

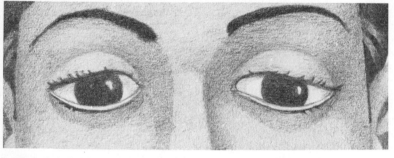

In bilateral ptosis (above), the upper eyelid *sags* and covers the sclera. Sometimes, ptosis is incorrectly called *lid lag*—a term that conveys an image of weakening and drooping.

Because thyrotoxicosis affects virtually every body system, it can produce many additional findings. For example, central nervous system effects include clumsiness, shaky handwriting, and emotional lability. Integumentary effects may include smooth, warm, flushed, and thickened skin with itchy patches; fine, soft hair with premature graying and increased loss; friable nails; and onycholysis.

Cardiopulmonary involvement causes constant dyspnea; tachycardia; full, bounding pulse; widened pulse pressure; visible point of maximal impulse; and, occasionally, systolic murmur.

Besides nausea and vomiting, gastrointestinal findings may include anorexia, diarrhea, and hepatomegaly. Musculoskeletal findings may include weakness, fatigue, and atrophy, along with paralysis and occasionally acropachy.

Women may report oligomenorrhea or amenorrhea; men may show gynecomastia; and both sexes may experience decreased libido.

Special considerations
If lid lag is accompanied by exophthalmos, provide privacy to ease the patient's self-consciousness. Do not cover the affected eye with a gauze pad or other object, since removal could destroy the corneal epithelium.

Pediatric pointers
Children may have lid lag associated with aberrant regeneration of cranial nerve III or, rarely, thyrotoxicosis.

Light Flashes

A cardinal symptom of vision-threatening retinal detachment, light flashes can occur locally or throughout the visual field. Usually, the patient reports seeing spots, stars, or lightning streaks. Light flashes can arise suddenly or gradually, and can indicate temporary or permanent vision impairment. Most often, light flashes signal the splitting of the posterior vitreous membrane into two layers; the inner layer detaches from the retina while the outer layer remains fixed to it. The sensation of light flashes may result from vitreous traction on the retina, hemorrhage caused by a tear in the retinal capillary, or strands of solid vitreous floating in a local pool of liquid vitreous.

Assessment

Until retinal detachment is ruled out, restrict the patient's eye and body movement. Have another nurse immediately call an ophthalmologist; he'll perform a funduscopic examination to rule out retinal detachment or gauge its extent.

Ask the patient when the light flashes began. Can he pinpoint their location or do they occur throughout the visual field? Find out if he's experiencing any eye pain or headache, and have him describe it. Also ask if he wears or has ever worn corrective lenses, and if he or a family member has a history of eye or vision problems. Also ask if he has any other medical problems—especially hypertension or diabetes mellitus, which can cause retinopathy and possibly retinal detachment. Be sure to obtain an occupational history, too, since the patient's light flashes may be related to job stress or to eye strain.

Perform a complete eye and vision examination, especially if trauma is apparent or suspected. First, inspect the external eye, lids, lashes, and tear puncta for any abnormalities and the iris and sclera for signs of bleeding. Observe pupil size and shape, and check for reaction to light, for accommodation, and for the consensual light response. Next, test visual acuity in each eye. Then test visual fields; be sure to document any light flashes the patient reports during this test.

Medical causes

• **Head trauma.** A patient who has sustained minor head trauma may report "seeing stars" when the injury occurs. He may also complain of localized pain at the injury site, along with generalized headache and dizziness. Later, he may develop nausea, vomiting, and decreased level of consciousness.

• **Migraine headache.** Light flashes—possibly accompanied by an aura—may herald a classic migraine headache. As these symptoms subside, the patient typically experiences a severe, throbbing, unilateral headache that usually lasts 1 to 12 hours and may be accompanied by numbness and tingling of the lips, face, or hands; slight confusion; dizziness; photophobia; nausea; and vomiting.

• **Retinal detachment.** Light flashes described as floaters or spots are localized in the portion of the visual field where the retina is detaching. With macular involvement, the patient may experience painless visual impairment resembling a curtain covering the visual field.

• **Vitreous detachment.** Sudden onset of light flashes may be accompanied by visual floaters. Often both eyes are affected, but usually one at a time.

Special considerations

If the patient has retinal detachment, prepare him for reattachment surgery. Explain that after surgery, he may need to continue wearing bilateral eye patches and may have activity and position restrictions until the retina heals completely.

If the patient doesn't have retinal detachment, reassure him that his light flashes are temporary and don't indicate eye damage. For the patient with migraine headache, maintain a quiet, darkened environment, encourage sleep, and administer analgesics as ordered.

Pediatric pointers
Children most often experience light flashes after minor head trauma.

Low Birth Weight

Two groups of infants are born weighing less than the normal minimum birth weight of 5½ lb (2,500 g)—those who are born prematurely (before the 37th week of gestation) and those who are small for gestational age (SGA). The premature infant weighs an appropriate amount for his gestational age and probably would have matured normally if carried to term. Conversely, the SGA infant weighs less than the normal amount for his age, even if carried to term. Differentiating the two helps direct the search for a cause. In the premature infant, low birth weight usually results from a disorder that prevents the uterus from retaining the fetus, interferes with the normal course of pregnancy, causes premature separation of the placenta, or stimulates uterine contractions before term. In the SGA infant, intrauterine growth may be retarded by a disorder that interferes with the placental circulation, fetal development, or maternal health. Regardless of the cause, low birth weight is linked with higher infant morbidity and mortality and can signal a life-threatening emergency.

Assessment
Because low birth weight is associated with poorly developed body systems, particularly the respiratory, your first priority is to monitor the infant's respiratory status. Be alert for signs of distress, such as apnea, grunting respirations, intercos-

tal or xiphoid retractions, or a respiratory rate exceeding 60 breaths/minute after the first hour of life. If you detect any of these signs, immediately notify the doctor and prepare to resuscitate the infant. Assist with endotracheal intubation or provide supplemental oxygen with an oxygen hood.

Monitor the infant's axillary temperature. Decreased fat reserves may keep him from maintaining normal body temperature, and a drop below 97.8° F. (36.5° C.) will exacerbate respiratory distress by increasing oxygen consumption. To maintain normal body temperature, use an overbed warmer or an isolette. (If these are unavailable, use a wrapped rubber bottle filled with warm water, but be careful to avoid hyperthermia.) Cover the infant's head to prevent heat loss.

When the infant's condition permits, assess neuromuscular and physical maturity to determine gestational age. (See *Ballard Scale: Calculating Gestational Age,* pages 462 and 463.) Then continue with a routine neonatal examination.

Medical causes
This section lists the fetal and placental causes of low birth weight, as well as the associated signs and symptoms present in the infant at birth. See *Maternal Causes of Low Birth Weight* for other causes of low birth weight.
• *Chromosomal aberrations.* Abnormalities in chromosomal number, size, or configuration cause low birth weight and possibly multiple congenital anomalies in a premature or SGA infant. For example, the infant with trisomy 21 (Down's syndrome) may be SGA and have prominent epicanthal folds, flat-bridged nose, protruding tongue, palmar simian creases, muscular hypotonia, and an umbilical hernia.
• *Cytomegalovirus infection.* Although low birth weight in this disorder is usually associated with premature birth, some infants may be SGA. Assessment at birth reveals these classic signs: petechiae and ecchymoses; jaun-

dice; and hepatosplenomegaly, which increases for several days. The infant also has high fever, lymphadenopathy, tachypnea, and dyspnea, along with prolonged bleeding at puncture sites.

• *Placental dysfunction.* Low birth weight and a wasted appearance occur in an infant who's SGA. The infant may be symmetrically short or may appear relatively long for his low weight. Additional findings reflect the underlying cause. For example, if maternal hyperparathyroidism caused placental dysfunction, the infant may have muscle jerking and twitching, carpopedal spasm, ankle clonus, vomiting, tachycardia, and tachypnea.

• *Rubella (congenital).* Usually, the low-birth-weight infant with this disease is born at term but is SGA. A characteristic "blueberry muffin" rash accompanies cataracts, purpuric lesions, hepatosplenomegaly, and a large anterior fontanelle. Abnormal heart sounds, if present, vary with the type of associated congenital heart defect.

• *Toxoplasmosis (congenital).* The low-birth-weight infant may be either premature or SGA and may have hydrocephalus or microcephalus. Associated findings include fever, convulsions, lymphadenopathy, hepatosplenomegaly, jaundice, and rash. Other defects, which may occur months or years later, include strabismus, blindness, epilepsy, and mental retardation.

• *Varicella (congenital).* Low birth weight is accompanied by cataracts and skin vesicles.

Special considerations

To make up for low fat and glycogen stores in the low-birth-weight infant, initiate feedings as soon as assessment reveals that peristalsis and the suck, swallow, and gag reflexes are present, and continue to feed every 2 to 3 hours. Provide gavage or I.V. feeding for the sick or very premature infant. Check abdominal girth with each feeding, and check stools for blood, since increasing girth and bloody stools may indicate necrotizing enterocolitis. Per-

---

MATERNAL CAUSES OF LOW BIRTH WEIGHT

Various maternal factors can predispose an infant to low birth weight.

If the infant is small for his gestational age, consider these possible maternal causes:

• Alcohol and narcotics abuse
• Chronic maternal illness
• Cigarette smoking
• Hypertension
• Hypoxemia
• Malnutrition
• Toxemia

If the infant is born prematurely, consider these common maternal causes:

• Abruptio placentae
• Amnionitis
• Incompetent cervix
• Placenta previa
• Polyhydramnios
• Preeclampsia
• Premature rupture of membranes
• Severe maternal illness
• Urinary tract infection

---

form or assist with a sepsis workup to determine if low birth weight results from infection.

Check the infant's vital signs every 15 minutes for the first hour and at least once every hour thereafter until his condition stabilizes. Be alert for changes in temperature or behavior, feeding problems, or periods of apnea—possible indications of infection. Also monitor blood glucose levels and watch for signs of hypoglycemia, such as irritability, jitteriness, tremors, seizures, irregular respirations, lethargy, and a high-pitched or weak cry. And if the infant is receiving supplemental oxygen, carefully monitor arterial blood gas values and the oxygen concentration of inspired air to prevent retinopathy.

Monitor the infant's urine output by weighing diapers before and after voiding. Check urine color, measure specific gravity, and test for the presence of glucose, blood, or protein. Also watch for changes in the infant's skin color, since increasing jaundice may

BALLARD SCALE: CALCULATING GESTATIONAL AGE

For quick calculation of gestational age, use this expanded version of the Ballard Scale, which grades gestational age in relation to neuromuscular and physical maturity. To use this scale, test the infant in each neuromuscular and physical category, assign the appropriate score, and, at the end of the test, total the scores. Then check the grading table at the bottom of page 463 for the corresponding gestational age.

NEUROMUSCULAR MATURITY	0	1	2	3	4	5
Posture. Place infant in supine position and observe degree of flexion in arms and legs.						
Square window. Flex infant's wrist against forearm until you meet resistance, and measure angle.	90°	60°	45°	30°	0°	
Arm recoil. Extend infant's forearm and release; after arm recoils, measure angle at elbow.	180°		100°-180°	90°-100°	< 90°	
Popliteal angle. With infant's pelvis flat on a hard surface, flex his thigh at hip until knee is close to chest. Extend his lower leg until you meet resistance, and measure popliteal angle.	180°	160	130°	110°	90°	< 90°
Scarf sign. Draw infant's hand across his chest as far over the opposite shoulder as it will go. Note relationship of elbow to chest midline.						
Heel to ear. Draw infant's foot toward his ear until you meet resistance. Note distance between foot and ear.						

PHYSICAL MATURITY	0	1	2	3	4	5
Skin. Examine skin over entire body. Observe for cracking at wrist and ankle.	Gelatinous, red, transparent	Smooth, pink, visible veins	Superficial peeling and/or rash, few veins	Superficial cracking, pale area, rare veins	Parchment-like cracking, no vessels	Leathery, cracked, wrinkled
Lanugo. Examine the infant's back for extent of body hair.	None	Abundant	Thinning	Bald areas	Mostly bald	
Plantar creases. Examine skin on soles of the infant's feet and note location of any creases.	No crease	Faint red marks	Anterior transverse crease	Creases over anterior two thirds	Creases over entire sole	
Breast. Inspect, palpate, and measure breast tissue diameter to evaluate breast development and nipple formation.	Barely perceptible	Flat areola, no bud	Stippled areola, 1- to 2-mm bud	Raised areola, 3- to 4-mm bud	Full areola, 5-to 10-mm bud	
Ear. Palpate infant's ear to determine extent of cartilage formation. Gently fold upper pinna toward infant's face, release it, and observe response.	Pinna flat, stays folded	Slightly curved pinna, soft, with slow recoil	Well-curved pinna, soft with ready recoil	Formed and firm, with instant recoil	Thick cartilage, ear stiff	
Male genitalia. Place infant in supine position and inspect and palpate scrotum.	Scrotum empty, no rugae		Testes descended, few rugae	Testes down, good rugae	Testes pendulous, deep rugae	
Female genitalia. Place infant in supine position and inspect genitalia.	Prominent clitoris and labia minora		Labia majora and minora equally prominent	Labia majora large; minora small	Clitoris and labia minora completely covered	

GRADING GESTATIONAL AGE

TOTAL SCORE	5	10	15	20	25	30	35	40	45	50
AGE (Weeks)	26	28	30	32	34	36	38	40	42	44

indicate hyperbilirubinemia.

Encourage the parents to participate in their infant's care to strengthen bonding, and allow ample time for their questions.

Lymphadenopathy

Lymphadenopathy—enlargement of one or more lymph nodes—may result from increased production of lymphocytes or reticuloendothelial cells, or from infiltration of cells not normally present. This sign may be generalized (involving three or more node groups) or localized. Generalized lymphadenopathy may be caused by an inflammatory process, such as bacterial or viral infection; connective tissue disease; endocrine disorder; or neoplasm. Localized lymphadenopathy most commonly results from infection or trauma affecting the drained area.

Normally, lymph nodes range from 0.5 to 2.5 cm and are discrete, mobile, nontender, and nonpalpable. Nodes that exceed 3 cm are cause for concern. They may be tender and erythematous—suggesting a draining lesion. Or they may be hard and fixed, tender or nontender—suggesting malignancy.

Assessment

Ask the patient when he first noticed the swelling and if it's on one side of his body or both. Are the swollen areas sore, hard, or red? Ask if he has recently had a cold or virus, or any other health problems. Also ask if a biopsy has ever been done on any nodes, as this may indicate a previously diagnosed malignancy. Find out if the patient has a family history of cancer.

Palpate the entire lymph node system to determine the extent of lymphadenopathy and detect any other areas of local enlargement. Use the pads of your index and middle fingers to move the skin over underlying tissues at the nodal area. If you detect enlarged nodes, note their size in centimeters and whether they're fixed or mobile, tender or nontender. Also note texture: Is the node discrete or does the area feel matted? If you detect tender, erythematous lymphadenopathy, check the area drained by that part of the lymph system for signs of infection, such as erythema and swelling.

Medical causes

• *Brucellosis.* Generalized lymphadenopathy most often affects cervical and axillary lymph nodes, making them tender. The disease usually begins insidiously with easy fatigability, headache, backache, anorexia, and arthralgias; it may also begin abruptly with chills, fever, and diaphoresis. Other effects include weight loss, pain or pressure over the vertebrae or down the peripheral nerve pathways, and possibly hepatosplenomegaly. Chronic brucellosis may also produce recurrent depression, sleep disturbances, and impotence. Abscesses may form in the testes, ovaries, kidneys, and brain.

• *Cytomegalovirus infection.* Generalized lymphadenopathy occurs in the immunocompromised patient. It's accompanied by fever, malaise, rash, and hepatosplenomegaly.

• *Hodgkin's lymphoma.* The extent of lymphadenopathy determines the stage of malignancy—from stage-one involvement of a single lymph node region to stage-four generalized lymphadenopathy. Usually, nodes in the neck enlarge first and become hard, swollen, movable, nontender, and discrete. Other common early findings include pruritus and, in older patients, fatigue, weakness, night sweats, malaise, weight loss, and unexplained fever (usually to 101° F., or 38.3° C.). Occasionally, relapsing fever occurs, accompanied at times by chills. If mediastinal lymph nodes enlarge, tracheal and esophageal pressure produces dyspnea and dysphagia. Dry cough, hyperpigmentation, pallor, and hepatosplenomegaly may also occur. Later, jaundice and nerve pain develop.

• *Infectious mononucleosis.* Characteristic, painful lymphadenopathy involves cervical, axillary, and inguinal nodes. Typically, prodromal symptoms, such as headache, malaise, and fatigue, occur 3 to 5 days before the appearance of the classic triad of lymphadenopathy, sore throat, and temperature fluctuations with an evening peak of about 102° F. (38.9° C.). Hepatosplenomegaly may also develop, along with signs and symptoms of stomatitis, exudative tonsillitis, or pharyngitis.

• *Leptospirosis.* Lymphadenopathy occurs infrequently in this rare disease. More common findings include sudden onset of fever and chills, malaise, myalgia, headache, nausea and vomiting, and abdominal pain.

• *Leukemia (acute lymphocytic).* Generalized lymphadenopathy is accompanied by fatigue, malaise, pallor, and low fever. The patient also experiences prolonged bleeding time, swollen gums, weight loss, bone or joint pain, and hepatosplenomegaly. Occasionally, dyspnea, tachycardia, palpitations, and abdominal pain may occur. Later findings may include confusion, headaches, vomiting, seizures, papilledema, and nuchal rigidity.

• *Leukemia (chronic lymphocytic).* Generalized lymphadenopathy appears early, along with fatigue, malaise, and fever. As the disease progresses, hepatosplenomegaly, severe fatigue, and weight loss occur. Other late findings include bone tenderness, edema, pallor, dyspnea, tachycardia, palpitations, bleeding, and often macular or nodular lesions.

• *Mycosis fungoides.* Lymphadenopathy occurs in stage three of this rare, chronic malignant lymphoma. It's accompanied by ulcerated brownish red tumors that are painful and itchy.

• *Non-Hodgkin's lymphoma.* Painless enlargement of one or more peripheral lymph nodes is the most common sign of this malignancy, with generalized lymphadenopathy characterizing stage four. Dyspnea, cough, and hepato-splenomegaly occur, along with systemic complaints of fever to 101° F. (38.3° C.), night sweats, fatigue, malaise, and weight loss.

• *Rheumatoid arthritis.* Lymphadenopathy is an early, nonspecific finding associated with fatigue, malaise, continuous low fever, weight loss, and vague arthralgias and myalgias. Later, the patient develops joint tenderness, swelling, and warmth; joint stiffness after inactivity; and subcutaneous nodules on the elbows. Eventually, joint deformity, muscle weakness, and atrophy may occur.

• *Sarcoidosis.* Generalized, bilateral hilar, and right paratracheal lymphadenopathy with splenomegaly are common. Initial findings are arthralgia, fatigue, malaise, and weight loss. Other findings vary with the site and extent of fibrosis. Typical cardiopulmonary findings include breathlessness, cough, substernal chest pain, and dysrhythmias. Musculoskeletal and cutaneous features may include muscle weakness and pain, phalangeal and nasal mucosal lesions, and subcutaneous skin nodules. Common ophthalmic signs and symptoms include eye pain, photophobia, and nonreactive pupils. CNS involvement may produce cranial or peripheral nerve palsies and convulsions.

• *Sjögren's syndrome.* Lymphadenopathy of the parotid and submaxillary nodes may occur in this rare disorder. Assessment reveals cardinal signs—dry eyes and mouth—with possible photosensitivity, poor vision, eye fatigue, nasal crusting, and epistaxis.

• *Syphilis (secondary).* Generalized lymphadenopathy occurs in stage two and may be accompanied by macular, papular, pustular, or nodular rash on the arms, trunk, palms, soles, face, and scalp. Headache, malaise, anorexia, weight loss, nausea, vomiting, sore throat, and low fever may occur.

• *Systemic lupus erythematosus.* Generalized lymphadenopathy often accompanies the hallmark butterfly rash, photosensitivity, Raynaud's phenome-

REVIEWING CAUSES AND AREAS OF LOCALIZED LYMPHADENOPATHY

When you detect an enlarged lymph node, palpate the entire lymph node system to determine the extent of lymphadenopathy. Include the lymph nodes indicated below in your assessment.

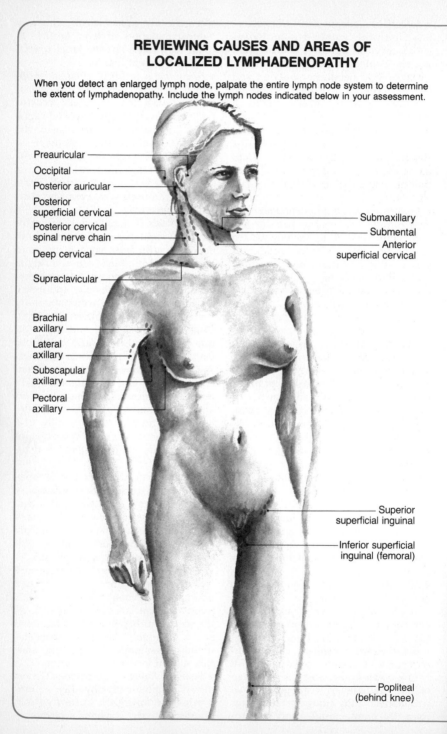

Preauricular

Occipital

Posterior auricular

Posterior superficial cervical

Posterior cervical spinal nerve chain

Deep cervical

Supraclavicular

Brachial axillary

Lateral axillary

Subscapular axillary

Pectoral axillary

Submaxillary

Submental

Anterior superficial cervical

Superior superficial inguinal

Inferior superficial inguinal (femoral)

Popliteal (behind knee)

non, and joint pain and stiffness. Pleuritic chest pain and cough may appear with systemic findings such as fever, anorexia, and weight loss.
- **Tuberculous lymphadenitis.** Lymphadenopathy may be restricted to superficial lymph nodes, or it may be generalized. Affected lymph nodes may become fluctuant and drain to surrounding tissue, and may be accompanied by fever, chills, weakness, and fatigue.
- **Waldenström's macroglobulinemia.** Lymphadenopathy may appear with hepatosplenomegaly. Associated signs and symptoms include retinal hemorrhage, pallor, and signs of congestive heart failure, such as neck vein distention and crackles. The patient shows decreased level of consciousness, abnormal reflexes, and signs of peripheral neuritis. Weakness, fatigue, weight loss, epistaxis, and gastrointestinal bleeding may also occur.

Other causes
- **Drugs.** Phenytoin may cause generalized lymphadenopathy.
- **Immunizations.** Typhoid vaccination may also cause generalized lymphadenopathy.

Special considerations
If the patient has fever above 101° F. (38.3° C.), provide antipyretics, tepid sponge baths, or a hypothermia blanket, as ordered.

Expect to obtain blood for routine blood work, a platelet count, and liver and renal function studies. Prepare the patient for other scheduled diagnostic tests, such as chest X-ray, liver and spleen scan, lymph node biopsy, or lymphography to visualize the lymphatic system. If tests reveal infection, check institutional policy regarding isolation requirements. Also observe isolation precautions if the patient has any draining wounds or lesions.

Pediatric pointers
Infection is the most common cause of lymphadenopathy in children.

A variety of disorders can cause localized lymphadenopathy. Most often, this sign results from infection or trauma affecting the drained area. The list below matches some common causes of lymphadenopathy with the areas they affect.

OCCIPITAL
Roseola
Scalp infection
Seborrheic dermatitis
Tick bite
Tinea capitis

AURICULAR
Erysipelas
Herpes zoster ophthalmicus
Infection
Rubella
Squamous cell carcinoma
Styes or chalazion
Tularemia

CERVICAL
Cat-scratch fever
Facial or oral cancer
Infection
Mucocutaneous lymph node syndrome
Rubella
Rubeola
Thyrotoxicosis
Tonsillitis
Tuberculosis
Varicella

SUBMAXILLARY AND SUBMENTAL
Cystic fibrosis
Dental infection
Gingivitis
Glossitis

SUPRACLAVICULAR
Neoplastic disease

AXILLARY
Breast cancer
Lymphoma

INGUINAL AND FEMORAL
Carcinoma
Chancroid
Lymphogranuloma venereum
Syphilis

POPLITEAL
Infection

masklike facies • McBurney's sign • McMurray's sign • melena • menorrhagia
miosis • moon face • mouth lesions • murmurs • muscle atrophy • muscle flac
spasms • muscle spasticity • muscle weakness • mydriasis • myoclonus • nas
pain • night blindness • nipple discharge • nipple retraction • nocturia • nucl
nystagmus • ocular deviation • oligomenorrhea • oliguria • opisthotonos • orc
orthopnea • orthostatic hypotension • Ortolani's sign • Osler's nodes • otorrh
palpitations • papular rash • paralysis • paresthesias • paroxysmal nocturnal
d'orange • pericardial friction rub • peristaltic waves—visible • photophobia
rub • polydipsia • polyphagia • polyuria • postnasal drip • priapism • prurit
psychotic behavior • ptosis • pulse—absent or weak • pulse—bounding • pul
pulse pressure—widened • pulse rhythm abnormality • pulsus alternans • pt
paradoxus • pupils—nonreactive • pupils—sluggish • purple striae • purpur
pyrosis • raccoon's eyes • rebound tenderness • rectal pain • retractions—cos
rhinorrhea • rhonchi • Romberg's sign • salivation—decreased • salivation—
scotoma • scrotal swelling • seizure—absence • seizure—focal • seizure—ger
seizure—psychomotor • setting-sun sign • shallow respirations • skin—bron
skin—mottled • skin—scaly • skin turgor—decreased • spider angioma • spl
respirations • stool—clay-colored • stridor • syncope • tachycardia • tachypn
tearing—increased • throat pain • tic • tinnitus • tracheal deviation • trache
trismus • tunnel vision • uremic frost • urethral discharge • urinary frequen
urinary incontinence • urinary urgency • urine cloudiness • urticaria • vagin
postmenopausal • vaginal discharge • venous hum • vertigo • vesicular rash
loss • visual blurring • visual floaters • vomiting • vulvar lesions • weight ga
loss—excessive • wheezing • wristdrop• abdominal distention • abdominal
abdominal rigidity • accessory muscle use • agitation • alopecia • amenorrh
analgesia • anhidrosis • anorexia • anosmia • anuria • anxiety • aphasia • a
respirations • apraxia • arm pain • asterixis • ataxia • athetosis • aura • Ba
pain • barrel chest • Battle's sign • Biot's respirations • bladder distention •
blood pressure increase • bowel sounds—absent • bowel sounds—hyperacti
hypoactive • bradycardia • bradypnea • breast dimpling • breast nodule • b
breath with ammonia odor • breath with fecal odor • breath with fruity odc
bruits • buffalo hump • butterfly rash • café-au-lait spots • capillary refill tir
carpopedal spasm • cat cry • chest expansion—asymmetrical • chest pain •
respirations • chills • chorea • Chvostek's sign • clubbing • cogwheel rigidit
confusion • conjunctival injection • constipation • corneal reflex—absent •
tenderness • cough—barking • cough—nonproductive • cough—productive
bony • crepitation—subcutaneous • cry—high-pitched • cyanosis • decerebr
posture • deep tendon reflexes—hyperactive • deep tendon reflexes—hypoac
diaphoresis • diarrhea • diplopia • dizziness • doll's eye sign—absent • dro
dysmenorrhea • dyspareunia • dyspepsia • dysphagia • dyspnea • dystonia
edema—generalized • edema of the arms • edema of the face • edema of th
enuresis • epistaxis • eructation • erythema • exophthalmos • eye discharge
fasciculations • fatigue • fecal incontinence • fetor hepaticus • fever • flank
fontanelle bulging • fontanelle depression • footdrop • gag reflex abnormali
propulsive • gait—scissors • gait—spastic • gait—steppage • gait—waddlin
gallop—ventricular • genital lesions in the male • grunting respirations • g
swelling • gynecomastia • halitosis • halo vision • headache • hearing loss
Heberden's nodes • hematemesis • hematochezia • hematuria • hemianopia
hepatomegaly • hiccups • hirsutism • hoarseness • Homans' sign • hyperpi
hypopigmentation • impotence • insomnia • intermittent claudication • Jane

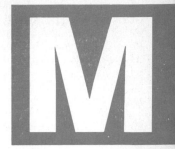

Masklike Facies

A total loss of facial expression, masklike facies results from bradykinesia—usually due to extrapyramidal damage. Even the rate of eye blinking is reduced—to 1 to 4 blinks per minute—producing a characteristic "reptillian" stare. Although a neurologic disorder is the most common cause, masklike facies can also result from certain systemic diseases and the effects of drugs and toxins. The sign often develops insidiously, at first mistaken by the observer for depression or apathy.

Assessment

Ask the patient and his family or friends when they first noticed the masklike facial expression and any other signs or symptoms. Find out what medications the patient's taking, if any, and ask about any changes in dosage or schedule. Determine the degree of facial muscle weakness by asking the patient to smile and to wrinkle his forehead. Typically, the patient's responses are slowed.

Medical causes

• **Carbon monoxide poisoning.** Masklike facies usually develops several weeks after acute poisoning. The patient may also have rigidity, dementia, impaired sensory function, choreoathetosis, generalized seizures, and myoclonus.

• **Dermatomyositis.** Masklike facies reflects muscle soreness and weakness extending from the face and neck to the shoulder and pelvic girdle. Dysphagia and dysphonia develop. Characteristic cutaneous signs involve edema and dusky lilac suffusion of the eyelid margin or periorbital tissue; an erythematous rash on the face, neck, upper back, chest, arms, and nail beds; and violet (Gottron's) papules dorsal to the interphalangeal joint.

• **Manganese poisoning (chronic).** Masklike facies develops gradually, along with a resting tremor and personality changes. The patient also experiences chorea, propulsive gait, dystonia, and rigidity. Later, extreme muscle weakness and fatigue occur.

• **Parkinson's disease.** Masklike facies occurs early but is often overlooked. More noticeable signs include muscle rigidity, which may be uniform (lead-pipe rigidity) or jerky (cogwheel rigidity), and an insidious tremor, which usually begins in the fingers (unilateral pill-roll tremor), increases during stress or anxiety, and decreases during purposeful movement or sleep. Typically, the patient exhibits stooped posture and propulsive gait, speaks in a high-pitched monotone, and may have drooling, dysphagia, and dysarthria.

• **Scleroderma.** A late sign, masklike facies develops along with a smooth, wrinkle-free appearance, "pinching" of the mouth, and possibly contractures, as facial skin becomes tight and inelastic. Other later features include pain, stiffness, and swelling of joints and foreshortened fingers. Skin on the fingers and then on the hands and forearms thickens and becomes taut and shiny. Gastrointestinal dysfunction produces frequent reflux and heartburn; weight loss; diarrhea or constipation; and malodorous floating stools.

Other causes
● *Drugs.* Phenothiazines (particularly piperazine derivatives) and other antipsychotics frequently cause masklike facies as well as other extrapyramidal effects. In addition, metoclopramide and metyrosine infrequently cause masklike facies. This sign usually improves when the drug is reduced or discontinued.

Special considerations
If the patient's masklike facies results from Parkinson's disease, explain to his family that the sign may hide facial clues to depression—a common symptom of Parkinson's disease.

Pediatric pointers
Masklike facies occurs in the juvenile form of Parkinson's disease.

McBurney's Sign

A telltale indicator of localized peritoneal inflammation in appendicitis, McBurney's sign is tenderness elicited

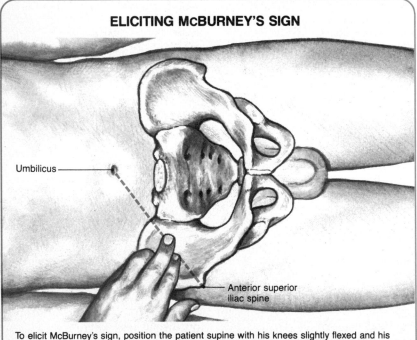

ELICITING McBURNEY'S SIGN

Umbilicus

Anterior superior iliac spine

To elicit McBurney's sign, position the patient supine with his knees slightly flexed and his abdominal muscles relaxed. Then, palpate deeply and slowly in the right lower quadrant over McBurney's point—located one-third of the distance from the anterior superior iliac spine to the umbilicus. Point tenderness, a positive McBurney's sign, indicates appendicitis.

by palpating the right lower quadrant over McBurney's point. Before McBurney's sign is elicited, the abdomen is inspected for distention and auscultated for hypoactive or absent bowel sounds.

Assessment

Ask the patient about abdominal pain. When did it begin? Does coughing, movement, eating, or elimination worsen or help relieve it? Also ask about the development of any other signs and symptoms.

Continue light palpation of the patient's abdomen to detect additional tenderness, rigidity, guarding, or pain. Observe the patient's facial expression for signs of pain, such as grimacing or wincing.

Medical cause

• *Appendicitis.* McBurney's sign appears within the first 2 to 12 hours, after initial pain in the epigastric and periumbilical area shifts to the right lower quadrant (McBurney's point). This persistent point pain increases with walking or coughing. Nausea and vomiting are present from the start. Boardlike abdominal rigidity and rebound tenderness accompany cutaneous hyperalgia, fever, constipation or diarrhea, tachycardia, retractive respirations, anorexia, and moderate malaise.

Rupture of the appendix causes a sudden cessation of pain. Then, signs of peritonitis develop, such as severe abdominal pain, pallor, hypoactive or absent bowel sounds, diaphoresis, and high fever.

Special considerations

As ordered, draw blood for laboratory tests and prepare the patient for abdominal X-rays to confirm appendicitis. Expect to prepare the patient for appendectomy.

Pediatric pointers

McBurney's sign is also elicited in children with appendicitis.

McMurray's Sign

Frequently an indicator of meniscal injury, McMurray's sign is a palpable, audible click or pop elicited by manipulating the leg. It results when gentle manipulation of the leg traps torn cartilage and then lets it snap free. Because eliciting this sign forces the surface of the tibial plateau against the femoral condyles, it's contraindicated in patients with suspected fractures of the tibial plateau or femoral condyles.

A positive McMurray's sign augments other findings commonly associated with meniscal injury, such as severe knee pain and decreased range of motion.

Assessment

After McMurray's sign has been elicited, find out if the patient is experiencing acute knee pain. Then ask him to describe any recent knee injury. For example, did his injury place twisting external or internal force on the knee, or did he experience blunt knee trauma from a fall? Also ask about previous knee injury, surgery, or prosthetic replacement, or other joint problems, such as arthritis, which could have weakened the knee. Ask if anything aggravates or relieves the pain and if he needs assistance to walk.

Have the patient point to the exact area of pain. Assess the leg's range of motion, both passive and with resistance. Next check for cruciate ligament stability by noting anterior or posterior movement of the tibia on the femur (drawer sign). Finally, measure the quadriceps muscles in both legs for symmetry.

Medical cause

• *Meniscal tear.* In this injury, McMurray's sign can frequently be elicited. Associated signs and symptoms may include acute knee pain at the medial or lateral joint line (depending on

ELICITING McMURRAY'S SIGN

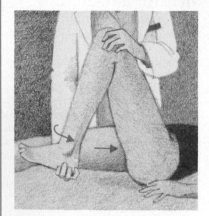
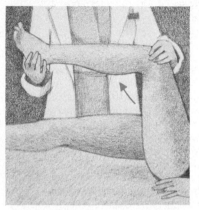

Eliciting this sign requires special training and gentle manipulation of the patient's leg to avoid extending a meniscal tear or locking the knee. If you've been trained to elicit McMurray's sign, place the patient in a supine position and flex his affected knee until his heel nearly touches his buttock. Place your thumb and index finger on either side of the knee joint space and grasp his heel with your other hand. Then rotate the foot and lower leg laterally to test the posterior meniscus. Keeping his foot in a lateral position, extend the knee to a 90° angle to test the anterior meniscus. A palpable or audible click—a positive McMurray's sign—indicates a meniscal tear.

injury site) and decreased range of motion or locking of the knee joint. Quadriceps weakening and atrophy frequently occur.

Special considerations
Prepare the patient for knee X-rays, arthroscopy, and arthrography, as ordered, and obtain any previous X-rays for comparison. If trauma precipitated the knee pain and McMurray's sign, an effusion or hemarthrosis may occur. Prepare the patient for aspiration of the joint. Immobilize and apply ice to the knee, and assist with application of a cast or a knee immobilizer.

Instruct the patient to elevate the affected leg and to perform straight leg–raising exercises up to 200 times a day. As appropriate, teach him how to use crutches. Also tell him the prescribed dosage and schedule of analgesics and anti-inflammatory drugs. Help him adjust to lifestyle changes by providing support and including significant others in teaching.

Pediatric pointers
McMurray's sign in adolescents is most commonly elicited in meniscal tear from sports injury. It may also be elicited in children with congenital discoid lateral meniscus.

Melena

A common sign of upper GI bleeding, melena is the passage of black, tarry stools. Characteristic color results from hydrochloric acid acting on the blood as it travels through the GI tract. At least 60 ml of blood is needed to produce this sign.

Severe melena can signal acute bleeding and life-threatening hypovolemic shock. Usually, melena indicates bleeding from the esophagus, stomach, or duodenum, although it can also indicate bleeding from the jejunum, ileum, or ascending colon. In addition, this sign can result from swallowing blood, as in epistaxis; from certain drugs; and from alcohol. Because false melena may occur from ingestion of lead, bismuth, or licorice (which produces black stools without the presence of blood), all black stools should be tested for the presence of occult blood.

Assessment

If the patient is experiencing severe melena, quickly take orthostatic vital signs to detect hypovolemic shock, while another nurse immediately notifies the doctor. A decrease of 10 mm Hg or more in systolic pressure, or an increase of 10 beats or more in pulse rate indicates volume depletion. Quickly look for other signs of shock, such as tachycardia, tachypnea, and cool, clammy skin. Insert a large-bore I.V. to administer replacement fluids and allow blood transfusion. Place the patient flat with his head turned to the side and his feet elevated. Administer supplemental oxygen as needed.

If the patient's condition permits, ask when he first noticed that his stools had become black and tarry. Has this happened before? Ask about the development of other signs and symptoms, particularly hematemesis or hematochezia; and about use of anti-inflammatory drugs, alcohol, or other GI irritants. Find out if the patient has a history of GI lesions, such as hemorrhoids.

Next, inspect the patient's mouth and nasopharynx for evidence of bleeding. Perform an abdominal examination that includes auscultation, palpation, and percussion.

Medical causes

● *Colon cancer.* On the right side of the colon, early tumor growth may cause melena accompanied by abdominal aching, pressure, or dull cramps. As the disease progresses, the patient develops weakness, fatigue, exertional dyspnea, and vertigo. Eventually, he also develops diarrhea or obstipation, anorexia, weight loss, vomiting, and other signs of intestinal obstruction, such as abdominal distention and abnormal bowel sounds.

On the left side, melena is a later sign. Early tumor growth commonly causes rectal bleeding accompanied by intermittent abdominal fullness or cramping and rectal pressure. As the disease progresses, the patient may develop obstipation, diarrhea, or pencil-shaped stools. At this stage, bleeding from the colon becomes obvious, with melena or hematochezia and mucus in or on the stools.

● *Diverticulitis.* Melena may occur as occult blood in the stool or as acute hemorrhage. Other findings may include episodic left lower quadrant pain and tenderness, constipation, and, possibly, a palpable abdominal mass.

● *Esophageal carcinoma.* Melena is a late sign. Increasing obstruction first produces painless dysphagia, then rapid weight loss. The patient may experience steady chest pain and a feeling of substernal fullness, nausea, vomiting, and hematemesis. Other related findings may include hoarseness, cough (possibly hemoptysis), hiccups, sore throat, and halitosis.

● *Esophageal varices (ruptured).* This life-threatening disorder can produce melena, possibly alternating with hematochezia, and hematemesis. Usually, melena is preceded by signs of shock, such as tachycardia, tachypnea, hypotension, and cool, clammy skin. Agitation or confusion signal developing hepatic encephalopathy.

● *Gastric carcinoma.* Melena and altered bowel habits may occur late in this uncommon cancer. More common findings include insidious onset of upper abdominal discomfort and chronic dyspepsia. Anorexia and slight nausea often occur, along with hematemesis, pallor, fatigue, weight loss, and a feeling of abdominal fullness.

● *Gastritis.* Melena and hematemesis are common. The patient may also experience mild epigastric or abdominal discomfort, belching, nausea, vomiting, fever, and malaise.

● *Malaria.* Melena may accompany persistent high fever and orthostatic hypotension in severe malaria. Other possible features include hemoptysis, vomiting, abdominal pain, diarrhea, oliguria, and convulsions, delirium, or coma. These findings are interspersed throughout the malarial paroxysm—chills, then high fever, and then profuse diaphoresis.

● *Mallory-Weiss syndrome.* Melena and hematemesis follow vomiting. Severe upper abdominal bleeding leads to signs and symptoms of shock, such as tachycardia, tachypnea, hypotension, and cool, clammy skin. The patient may also have epigastric or back pain.

● *Mesenteric vascular occlusion.* This life-threatening disorder produces slight melena with 2 to 3 days of persistent, mild abdominal pain. Later, abdominal pain becomes severe and may be accompanied by tenderness, distention, guarding, and rigidity. The patient may also experience anorexia, vomiting, fever, and profound shock.

● *Peptic ulcer.* Melena may signal life-threatening hemorrhage from vascular penetration. The patient may also have nausea, vomiting, hematemesis, hematochezia, and diffuse epigastric pain that's gnawing, burning, or sharp. With hypovolemic shock come tachycardia, tachypnea, hypotension, and cool, clammy skin. Assessment may reveal abdominal rigidity and guarding.

● *Thrombocytopenia.* Melena or hematochezia may accompany other manifestations of bleeding tendency: hematemesis, epistaxis, petechiae, ecchymoses, hematuria, vaginal bleeding, and characteristic blood-filled oral bullae. Typically, the patient experiences malaise, fatigue, weakness, and lethargy.

● *Typhoid fever.* Melena or hematochezia occurs late in this disorder and may be accompanied by hypotension and

COMPARING MELENA TO HEMATOCHEZIA

With GI bleeding, it's the site, amount, and rate of blood flow through the GI tract that determine if a patient will develop melena (black, tarry stools) or hematochezia (bright red, bloody stools). Usually, melena indicates *upper* GI bleeding, and hematochezia indicates *lower* GI bleeding. However, in some disorders, melena may alternate with hematochezia. This chart helps differentiate these two often-related signs.

SIGN	SITES	CHARACTERISTICS
Melena	Esophagus, stomach, duodenum; rarely, jejunum, ileum, ascending colon	Black, loose, tarry stools. Delayed or minimal passage of blood through GI tract.
Hematochezia	Usually distal to or affecting the colon; rapid hemorrhage of 1 liter or more is associated with esophageal, stomach, or duodenal bleeding	Bright red or dark mahogany-colored stools; pure blood; blood mixed with formed stool; or bloody diarrhea. Reflects lower GI bleeding or rapid blood loss and passage of undigested blood through GI tract.

hypothermia. Other late findings may include mental dullness or delirium, marked abdominal distention and diarrhea, marked weight loss, and profound fatigue.

• *Yellow fever.* Melena, hematochezia, and hematemesis are ominous signs of hemorrhage, a classic feature, along with jaundice. Other findings may include fever, headache, nausea, epistaxis, and dizziness.

Other causes

• *Drugs and alcohol.* Aspirin, other nonsteroidal anti-inflammatories, and alcohol can all cause melena as a result of gastric irritation.

Special considerations

Continue to monitor the patient's vital signs, and observe him closely for signs of hypovolemic shock. As a general comfort measure, encourage bed rest, and keep the patient's perianal area clean and dry to prevent skin irritation and breakdown. As ordered, prepare the patient for diagnostic tests, including blood studies, gastroscopy or other endoscopic studies, barium swallow, and upper GI series.

Pediatric pointers

Newborns may experience melena neonatorum due to extravasation of blood into the alimentary canal. In older children, melena most commonly results from peptic ulcer, gastritis, and Meckel's diverticulum.

Menorrhagia

Profuse or extended menstrual bleeding, menorrhagia may occur as a single episode or a chronic sign. Normal menstrual flow lasts about 5 days and produces a total blood loss of 60 to 250 ml. In menorrhagia, the menstrual period may be extended and total blood loss can range from 80 ml to overt hemorrhage. Usually a result of gynecologic disorders, this relatively common sign can also result from endocrine and hematologic disorders, stress, and certain drugs and procedures.

Assessment

Evaluate hemodynamic status by taking orthostatic vital signs. Immediately call the doctor if the patient shows an increase of 10 beats/minute in pulse rate, a decrease of 10 mm Hg in systolic blood pressure, or any other signs of hypovolemic shock, such as pallor, tachycardia, tachypnea, and cool, clammy skin. Insert a large-gauge I.V. to begin fluid replacement. Place the patient in a supine position with her feet elevated, and administer supplemental oxygen as needed. Prepare her for a pelvic examination to help determine the cause of bleeding.

When the patient's condition permits, obtain a history. Determine her age at menarche, the duration of menstrual periods, and the interval between them. Establish the date of her last menses and ask about any recent changes in her normal menstrual pattern. Have her describe the character and amount of bleeding. For example, how many pads or tampons does she use? Has she noted clots or tissue in the blood? Ask, too, about the development of other signs and symptoms prior to and during the menstrual period.

Next, ask if the patient is sexually active. Does she use a method of birth control? If so, what kind? Could she be pregnant? Ask about any past pregnancies, since endometriosis most often occurs in multiparous women over age 40. Note the number of pregnancies, the outcome of each, and any pregnancy-related complications. Find out the dates of her most recent pelvic examination and Pap smear and the details of any previous gynecologic infections or neoplasms. Also ask about any previous episodes of abnormal bleeding and the outcome of any treatment.

If possible, obtain a pregnancy history of the patient's mother, and determine if the patient was exposed to diethylstilbestrol in utero.

Ask the patient about her general health and past medical history. Note particularly if the patient or her family has a history of thyroid, adrenal, or hepatic disease, blood dyscrasias, or tuberculosis, since these may predispose to menorrhagia. Also ask about past surgical procedures and any recent emotional stress. Find out, too, about any X-ray or other radiation therapy, as this may indicate prior treatment for menorrhagia.

Medical causes

● *Blood dyscrasias.* Menorrhagia is one of a number of possible signs of bleeding, such as epistaxis, bleeding gums, purpura, hematemesis, hematuria, or melena.

● *Congestive heart failure.* Chronic passive venous congestion occasionally produces persistent menorrhagia. Other findings include dyspnea, edema of the ankles and feet, fatigue, crackles, abnormal heart sounds, and jugular vein distention.

● *Dysfunctional uterine bleeding.* Menorrhagia is a less common sign than metrorrhagia. The bleeding can be constant or intermittent.

● *Endometriosis.* Menorrhagia is the most common sign of this disorder. Typically, the patient also reports pain in the lower abdomen, vagina, posterior pelvis, and back.

● *Hypothyroidism.* Menorrhagia is a frequent early sign, along with such nonspecific findings as fatigue, cold intolerance, constipation, and weight gain despite anorexia. As hypothyroidism progresses, intellectual and motor activity decrease; the skin becomes dry, pale, cool, and doughy; the hair becomes dry and sparse; and the nails become thick and brittle. Myalgia, hoarseness, decreased libido, and infertility commonly occur. Eventually, the patient develops a characteristic dull, expressionless face and edema of the face, hands, and feet. Deep tendon reflexes are delayed, and bradycardia and abdominal distention may occur.

● *Uterine fibroids.* Menorrhagia is the most common sign, but other forms of abnormal uterine bleeding, as well as dysmenorrhea or leukorrhea, can also occur. Possible related findings include abdominal pain, a feeling of abdominal heaviness, backache, constipation, urinary urgency or frequency, and an enlarged uterus.

Other causes

● *Drugs.* Use of oral contraceptives may cause sudden onset of profuse, prolonged menorrhagia. Anticoagulants can also produce menorrhagia.

● *Intrauterine devices.* Menorrhagia can result from the use of intrauterine contraceptive devices.

● *Surgery and procedures.* Cervical conization or cauterization can cause menorrhagia.

Special considerations

Continue to monitor the patient closely for signs of hypovolemia. Monitor intake and output and estimate uterine blood loss by recording the number of sanitary napkins or tampons used. To help decrease blood flow, encourage the patient to rest and to avoid strenuous activities.

Prepare the patient for a pelvic examination if one hasn't already been performed, and obtain blood and urine samples for pregnancy testing.

Pediatric pointers

Irregular menstrual function in young girls may be accompanied by hemorrhage and resulting anemia.

Metrorrhagia

Metrorrhagia—uterine bleeding that occurs irregularly between menstrual periods—is usually light, although it can range from staining to hemorrhage. Most often, this common sign reflects slight physiologic bleeding from the endometrium during ovulation. However, metrorrhagia may be the only indication of an underlying gynecologic disorder and can also result from stress, drugs, and treatments.

Assessment

Begin your assessment by obtaining a thorough menstrual history. Ask the patient when she began menstruating and about the duration of her menstrual periods, the interval between them, and the average number of tampons or pads she uses. When does metrorrhagia usually occur in relation to her period? Does she experience any other signs and symptoms? Find out the date of her last menses, and ask about any other recent changes in her normal menstrual pattern. Get details of any previous gynecologic problems. If applicable, obtain a contraceptive and obstetric history. Record the dates of her last Pap smear and pelvic examination. Next, ask the patient about her general health and any recent changes. Is she under emotional stress? If possible, obtain a pregnancy history of the patient's mother. Was the patient exposed to diethylstilbestrol in utero? (This drug has been linked to vaginal adenosis.)

Medical causes

• *Cervicitis.* This nonspecific infection may cause spontaneous bleeding, spotting, or posttraumatic bleeding. Assessment reveals red, granular, irregular lesions on the external cervix. Purulent vaginal discharge, lower abdominal pain, and fever may occur.
• *Dysfunctional uterine bleeding.* Abnormal uterine bleeding not caused by pregnancy or major gynecologic disorders usually occurs as metrorrhagia, although menorrhagia is possible. Bleeding may be profuse or scant, intermittent or constant.
• *Endometrial polyps.* This disorder may produce metrorrhagia, but most patients are asymptomatic.

• *Endometriosis.* Metrorrhagia may be the only indication of this disorder, or it may accompany pelvic discomfort and dyspareunia.
• *Endometritis.* Infection of the endometrium results in metrorrhagia and purulent vaginal discharge. It also produces fever, lower abdominal pain, and abdominal muscle spasm.
• *Gynecologic carcinoma.* Metrorrhagia often occurs as an early sign of these carcinomas. Later, the patient may experience weight loss, pelvic pain, fatigue, and possibly an abdominal mass.
• *Syphilis.* Primary- or secondary-stage syphilis may cause metrorrhagia and postcoital bleeding. In primary syphilis, one or more usually painless chancres erupt on the genitalia and possibly other areas. In secondary syphilis, generalized lymphadenopathy may appear, along with a rash on the arms, trunk, palms, soles, face, and scalp. Other features of this stage include headache, malaise, anorexia, weight loss, nausea, vomiting, sore throat, and possibly low fever.
• *Vaginal adenosis.* This disorder commonly produces metrorrhagia. Palpation reveals roughening or nodules in affected vaginal areas.

Other causes

• *Drugs.* Anticoagulants and oral contraceptives may cause metrorrhagia.
• *Surgery and procedures.* Cervical conization and cauterization may cause metrorrhagia.

Special considerations

As ordered, obtain blood and urine samples for pregnancy testing and assist with pelvic examination. Encourage bed rest to reduce bleeding, and administer analgesics if metrorrhagia is accompanied by discomfort. Monitor the amount of bleeding by recording the number of pads or tampons used.

Pediatric pointers

Girls who have recently begun menstruating may mistake irregular periods for metrorrhagia.

Miosis

Miosis—pupillary constriction caused by contraction of the sphincter muscle in the iris—occurs normally as a response to fatigue, increased light, and administration of miotic drugs; as part of the eye's accommodation reflex; and as part of the aging process (pupil size steadily decreases from adolescence to about age 60). However, it can also stem from ocular and neurologic disorders, trauma, systemic drugs, and contact lens overuse. A rare form of miosis—Argyll Robertson pupils—can stem from tabes dorsalis and diverse neurologic disorders. Occurring bilaterally, these miotic (often pinpoint), unequal, and irregularly shaped pupils don't dilate properly with mydriatic drug use and fail to react to light, although they do constrict on accommodation.

Assessment

Begin by asking the patient if he's experiencing other ocular symptoms, and have him describe their onset, duration, and intensity. Does he wear contact lenses? During your history, be sure to ask about trauma, serious systemic disease, and use of topical and systemic medications.

Now, perform a thorough eye assessment. Examine and compare both pupils for size (many persons have a normal discrepancy), color, shape, reaction to light, accommodation, and consensual light response. Examine both eyes for additional signs, and then evaluate extraocular muscle function by assessing the six cardinal fields of gaze. Finally, test visual acuity in each eye, with and without correction, paying particular attention to blurred or decreased vision in the miotic eye.

Medical causes

• **Cerebrovascular arteriosclerosis.** Miosis is usually unilateral, depending on the site and extent of vascular damage. Other findings may include visual blurring, slurred speech or possibly aphasia, loss of muscle tone, memory loss, vertigo, and headache.

• **Chemical burns.** An opaque cornea may make miosis hard to detect. However, chemical burns may also cause moderate-to-severe pain, diffuse conjunctival injection, inability to keep the eye open, visual blurring, and blistering.

• **Cluster headache.** Ipsilateral miosis, tearing, conjunctival injection, and ptosis often accompany a severe cluster headache, along with facial flushing and sweating, bradycardia, restlessness, and nasal stuffiness or rhinorrhea.

• **Corneal foreign body.** Miosis in the affected eye occurs with pain, a foreign body sensation, slight vision loss, conjunctival injection, photophobia, and profuse tearing.

• **Corneal ulcer.** Miosis in the affected eye appears with moderate pain, visual blurring and possibly some vision loss, and diffuse conjunctival injection.

• **Horner's syndrome.** Moderate miosis is common in this syndrome and occurs ipsilaterally to the lesion. Related ipsilateral findings include a sluggish pupillary reflex, slight enophthalmos, moderate ptosis, facial anhidrosis, transient conjunctival injection, and vascular headache. When the syndrome is congenital, the iris on the affected side may appear lighter.

• **Hyphema.** Usually the result of blunt trauma, hyphema can cause miosis with moderate pain, visual blurring, diffuse conjunctival injection, and slight eyelid swelling. The eyeball may feel harder than normal.

• **Iritis (acute).** Miosis typically occurs in the affected eye along with decreased pupillary reflex, severe eye pain, photophobia, visual blurring, conjunctival injection, and possibly pus accumulation in the anterior chamber.

• **Neuropathy.** Two forms of neuropathy occasionally produce Argyll Robertson pupils. In *diabetic neuropathy*, related effects may include paresthesias and other sensory disturbances, extremity pain, postural hypotension, impotence, incontinence, and leg muscle weakness and atrophy. In *alcoholic neuropathy*, related effects are progressive, variable muscle weakness and wasting, various sensory disturbances, and hypoactive deep tendon reflexes.

• *Parry-Romberg syndrome.* This facial hemiatrophy typically produces miosis, sluggish pupillary reflexes, enophthalmos, nystagmus, ptosis, and different-colored irises.

• *Pontine hemorrhage.* Bilateral miosis is characteristic, along with rapid onset of coma, total paralysis, decerebrate posture, absent doll's eye sign, and a positive Babinski's sign.

• *Tabes dorsalis.* This tertiary form of syphilis is marked by Argyll Robertson pupils, ataxic gait, paresthesias, loss of proprioception, analgesia, thermanesthesia, Charcot's joints, and possibly impotence.

• *Uveitis.* Anterior *uveitis* commonly produces miosis in the affected eye, moderate-to-severe eye pain, severe conjunctival injection, and photophobia. In *posterior uveitis*, miosis is accompanied by gradual onset of eye pain, photophobia, visual floaters, visual blurring, conjunctival injection, and, often, distorted pupil shape.

Other causes

• *Drugs.* Such topical drugs as acetylcholine, carbachol, demecarium bromide, echothiophate iodide, and pilocarpine are used to treat eye disorders specifically for their miotic effect. Such systemic drugs as barbiturates, cholinergics, cholinesterase inhibitors, clonidine (overdose), guanethidine, opiates, and reserpine also cause miosis, as does deep anesthesia.

Special considerations

Since any ocular abnormality can be a source of fear and anxiety, be sure to reassure and support the patient. Clearly explain any diagnostic tests ordered, which may include a complete

ophthalmologic examination or a neurologic workup.

Pediatric pointers

Miosis occurs frequently in the neonate, simply because he's asleep or sleepy most of the time. Bilateral miosis occurs in congenital microcoria.

Moon Face

Moon face, a distinctive facial adiposity, usually indicates hypercortisolism resulting from ectopic or excessive pituitary production of adrenocorticotropic hormone (ACTH), adrenal adenoma or carcinoma, or long-term glucocorticoid therapy. Its typical characteristics include marked facial roundness, a double chin, prominent upper lip, and full supraclavicular fossae. Although the presence of moon face doesn't help differentiate causes of hypercortisolism, it indicates a need for diagnostic testing.

Assessment

Ask the patient when he first noticed his facial adiposity, and try to obtain a preonset photograph to help evaluate the extent of the change.

Ask about weight gain and any personal or family history of endocrine disorders, obesity, or cancer. Has the patient noticed any fatigue, irritability, depression, or confusion? If the patient's a female of childbearing age, determine the date of her last menses and whether she's experienced any menstrual irregularities.

If the patient's receiving glucocorticoids, ask the name of the medication, dosage and schedule, route of administration, and reason for therapy. Also ask if the dosage has ever been modified and, if so, when and why.

Take the patient's vital signs, weight, and height. Also assess the patient's overall appearance for other characteristic signs of hypercortisolism, including virilism in a female or gynecomastia in a male.

Medical cause

• *Hypercortisolism.* Moon face varies in severity, depending on the degree of cortisol excess and weight gain. The patient typically exhibits buffalo hump, truncal obesity with slender arms and legs, and thin, transparent skin with purple striae and ecchymoses. Other cushingoid features include acne, diaphoresis, fatigue, muscle wasting and weakness, poor wound healing, elevated blood pressure, and personality changes.

In addition to these findings, a woman may experience hirsutism and amenorrhea or oligomenorrhea; a man may experience gynecomastia and impotence.

Other causes

• *Drugs.* Moon face may result from prolonged use of glucocorticoids, such as cortisone, dexamethasone, hydrocortisone, and prednisone.

Special considerations

Relieve the patient's concern about his body image by explaining that moon face and other disconcerting cushingoid effects can usually be corrected by treating the underlying disorder or by discontinuing or modifying glucocorticoid therapy.

Clearly explain to the patient any diagnostic tests the doctor orders. These may include serum and urine 17-hydroxycorticosteroid studies, and a 2-day, low-dose dexamethasone test followed by a 2-day, high-dose dexamethasone test.

Pediatric pointers

Moon face is rare in children. In an infant or a young child, it usually indicates adrenal adenoma or carcinoma, or, rarely, cri du chat syndrome. After age 7, it usually indicates abnormal pituitary secretion of ACTH in bilateral adrenal hyperplasia.

Mouth Lesions

Mouth lesions include ulcers (the most common type), cysts, firm nodules, hemorrhagic lesions, papules, vesicles, bullae, and erythematous lesions. They may occur anywhere on the lips, cheeks, hard and soft palate, salivary glands, tongue, gingivae, or mucous membranes. Many are painful and readily detected. Some, however, are asymptomatic; when these occur deep in the mouth, they may be discovered only through a complete oral examination.

Mouth lesions can result from trauma, infection, systemic diseases, drugs, and radiation therapy.

Assessment

Begin your assessment with a thorough history. Ask the patient when the lesions appeared and whether he's noticed any pain, odor, or drainage. Also ask about associated complaints, particularly skin lesions. Obtain a complete medication history, including drug allergies, and a complete medical history. Note especially any malignancy, sexually transmitted disease, recent infection, or trauma. Ask about his dental history, including oral hygiene habits, frequency of dental examinations, and the date of his most recent dental visit.

Next, perform a complete oral examination, noting lesion sites and character. Examine the patient's lips for color and texture. Inspect and palpate the buccal mucosa and tongue for color, texture, and contour; note especially any painless ulcers on the sides or base of the tongue. Hold the tongue with a piece of gauze, lift it, and examine its underside and the floor of the mouth. Depress the tongue with a tongue blade and examine the oropharynx. Inspect teeth and gums, noting missing, broken, or discolored teeth; dental caries; excessive debris;

COMMON MOUTH LESIONS

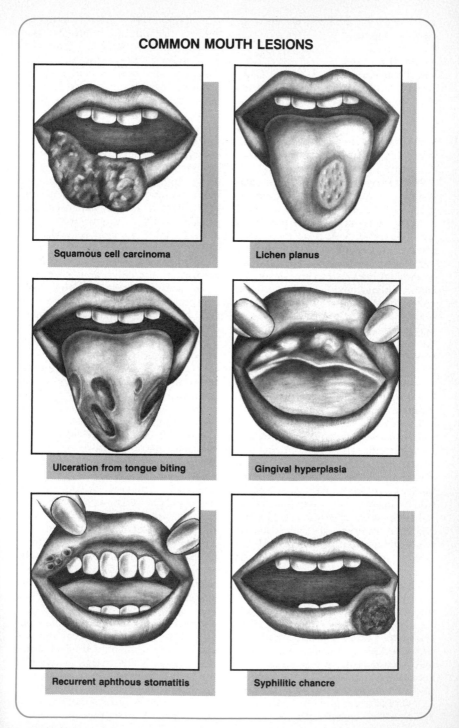

Squamous cell carcinoma

Lichen planus

Ulceration from tongue biting

Gingival hyperplasia

Recurrent aphthous stomatitis

Syphilitic chancre

and bleeding, inflamed, swollen, or discolored gums.

Medical causes

• *Actinomycosis (cervicofacial).* This chronic fungal infection typically produces small, firm, flat, painful or painless swellings on the oral mucosa and under the skin of the jaw and neck. Swellings may indurate and abscess, producing fistulas with a characteristic purulent yellow discharge.

• *Behçet's syndrome.* This chronic, progressive syndrome produces small, painful ulcers on the lips, gums, buccal mucosa, and tongue. In severe cases, the ulcers also develop on the palate, pharynx, and esophagus. Typically, the ulcers have a reddened border and are covered with a gray or yellow exudate. Similar lesions appear on the scrotum and penis or labia majora; small pustules or papules on the trunk and limbs; and painful erythematous nodules on the shins. Ocular lesions may also be present. Other findings include dysphagia, halitosis, and systemic effects, such as fever, malaise, and arthralgia. The patient may have gastrointestinal complaints.

• *Candidiasis.* This common fungal infection characteristically produces soft, elevated plaques on the buccal mucosa, tongue, and sometimes the palate, gingivae, and floor of the mouth; the plaques may be wiped away. The lesions of *acute atrophic candidiasis* are red and painful. In contrast, the lesions of *chronic hyperplastic candidiasis* are white and firm. Localized areas of redness, pruritus, and foul odor may be present.

• *Discoid lupus erythematosus.* Oral lesions are common, typically appearing on the tongue, buccal mucosa, and palate as erythematous areas with white spots and radiating white striae. Associated findings include skin lesions on the face, possibly extending to the neck, ears, and scalp; if the scalp is involved, alopecia may result. Hair follicles are enlarged and filled with scale. Telangiectasia may be present.

• *Epulis (giant cell).* This rare lesion occurs on the gingival or alveolar process, anterior to the molars. Dark red, pedunculated or sessile, and 0.5 to 1.5 cm in diameter, it commonly ulcerates to produce a concave defect in the underlying bone. Gingivae bleed easily with slight trauma.

• *Erythema multiforme.* This acute inflammatory skin disease produces sudden onset of vesicles and bullae on the lips and buccal mucosa. In addition, erythematous macules and papules form symmetrically on the hands, arms, feet, legs, face, and neck, and possibly in the eyes and on the genitalia. Lymphadenopathy may also occur. With visceral involvement (Stevens-Johnson syndrome), additional findings include fever, malaise, cough, throat and chest pain, vomiting, diarrhea, myalgias, arthralgias, fingernail loss, blindness, hematuria, and signs of renal failure.

• *Gingivitis (acute necrotizing ulcerative).* This condition causes a sudden onset of gingival ulcers covered with a grayish white pseudomembrane. Other findings may include tender or painful gingivae, intermittent gingival bleeding, and halitosis. A severe condition may induce fever, cervical adenopathy, headache, and malaise.

• *Gonorrhea.* Painful lip ulcerations may occur, along with rough, reddened, bleeding gingivae (possibly necrotic and covered by a yellowish pseudomembrane), and a swollen, ulcerated tongue. Related effects vary. Most men develop dysuria, purulent urethral discharge, and a reddened, edematous urinary meatus. Most women remain asymptomatic, but others may develop inflammation and a greenish yellow cervical discharge.

• *Herpes simplex.* In primary infection, a brief period of prodromal tingling and itching, accompanied by fever and pharyngitis, is followed by eruption of vesicles on any part of the oral mucosa, especially the tongue, gums, and cheeks. Vesicles form on an erythematous base, then rupture and leave a painful ulcer, followed by a yellowish crust. Other findings include submaxillary lymphadenopathy, increased salivation, halitosis, anorexia, and keratoconjunctivitis. Recurrence causes characteristic vesicular eruptions on the lips or buccal mucosa.

• *Herpes zoster.* This common viral infection may produce painful vesicles on the buccal mucosa, tongue, uvula, pharynx, and larynx. Small red nodules often erupt unilaterally around the thorax or vertically on the arms and legs, and rapidly become vesicles filled with clear fluid or pus; vesicles dry and form scabs about 10 days after eruption. Fever and general malaise accompany pruritus, paresthesia or hyperesthesia, and tenderness (usually unilateral) along the course of the involved sensory nerve.

• *Inflammatory fibrous hyperplasia.* This painless nodular swelling of the buccal mucosa typically results from cheek trauma or irritation. It's characterized by pink, smooth, pedunculated areas of soft tissue.

• *Lichen planus.* Oral lesions develop on the buccal mucosa or, less often, on the tongue as painless, white or gray, velvety, threadlike papules. These precede the eruption of violet papules with white lines or spots, most often on the genitalia, lower back, ankles, and anterior lower legs; pruritus; nail distortion; and alopecia.

• *Mucous duct obstruction.* Obstruction produces a ranula—a painless, slow-growing mucocele on the floor of the mouth near the ducts of the submandibular and sublingual glands.

• *Pemphigoid (benign mucosal).* This autoimmune disease is characterized by vesicles on the oral mucous membranes, conjunctiva, and, less often, the skin. Mouth lesions typically develop months or even years before other manifestations and may occur as desquamative patchy gingivitis or as a vesicobullous eruption. Secondary fibrous bands may lead to dysphagia, hoarseness, and blindness. Recurrent skin lesions include vesicobullous eruptions,

usually on the inguinal area and extremities, and an erythematous, vesicobullous plaque on the scalp and face near the affected mucous membranes.

• *Pemphigus.* This chronic skin disease is characterized by vesicles and bullae that appear in cycles. On the oral mucosa, bullae rupture, leaving painful lesions that bleed easily. Associated signs and symptoms include bullae anywhere on the body, denudation of the skin, and pruritus.

• *Pyogenic granuloma.* Often the result of trauma or irritation, this soft, painless nodule, papule, or polypoid mass most commonly appears on the gingivae but can also erupt on the lips, tongue, or buccal mucosa. The affected area may be smooth or have a warty surface; erythema develops in the surrounding mucosa. The lesions may ulcerate, producing a purulent exudate.

• *Squamous cell carcinoma.* In this disease, a painless ulcer with an elevated, indurated border usually erupts in areas of leukoplakia. It's most common on the lower lip but may also occur on the lateral border of the tongue and on the floor of the mouth.

• *Stomatitis (aphthous).* This common disease is characterized by recurrent, painful ulcerations of the oral mucosa, most often on the dorsum of the tongue, gingiva, and hard palate. In *recurrent aphthous stomatitis minor*, the ulcer begins as a single or multiple erosion covered by a gray membrane and surrounded by a red halo. It is commonly found on the buccal and lip mucosa and junction, tongue, soft palate, pharynx, gingivae, and all places not bound to the periosteum. In *recurrent aphthous stomatitis major*, large, painful ulcers are commonly found on the lips, cheek, tongue, and soft palate; they may last for up to 6 weeks and may leave a scar. Similar lesions may appear on the vagina, penis, rectum, or larynx, with associated rheumatoid arthritis or conjunctivitis.

• *Syphilis.* *Primary* syphilis typically produces a solitary painful ulcer (chancre) on the lip, tongue, palate, tonsil, or gingiva. The ulcer appears as a crater with undulated, raised edges and a shiny center; lip chancres may develop a crust. Similar lesions may appear on the fingers, breasts, or genitals, and regional lymph nodes may become enlarged and tender. During the *secondary* stage, multiple painless ulcers covered by a grayish white plaque may erupt on the tongue, gingivae, or buccal mucosa. A macular, papular, pustular, or nodular rash appears, usually on the arms, trunk, palms, soles, face, and scalp; genital lesions usually subside. Other findings may include generalized lymphadenopathy, headache, malaise, anorexia, weight loss, nausea, vomiting, sore throat, low fever, metrorrhagia, and postcoital bleeding. At the *tertiary* stage, lesions (often gummas—chronic, painless, superficial nodules or deep granulomatous lesions) develop on the skin and mucous membranes, especially the tongue and palate. Hepatic, respiratory, cardiovascular, or neurologic dysfunction may also occur.

• *Systemic lupus erythematosus.* Oral lesions are common and appear as erythematous areas associated with edema, petechiae, a tendency to bleed, and a superficial ulcer with a red halo. Primary effects include nondeforming arthritis, butterfly rash across the nose and cheeks, and photosensitivity.

• *Trauma.* The most common cause of oral lesions, trauma can produce ulcers anywhere in the mouth.

• *Tuberculosis (oral mucosal).* This rare disorder produces a painless ulcer (most often on the tongue) and, sometimes, caseation. Other findings include lymphadenopathy, fatigue, weakness, anorexia, gradual weight loss, persistent cough, low fever, and night sweats.

Other causes

• *Drugs.* Various chemotherapeutic agents can directly produce stomatitis. In addition, allergic reactions to penicillin, sulfonamides, gold, quinine, streptomycin, phenytoin, aspirin, and barbiturates often cause lesions to erupt.

• *Radiation therapy.* This treatment may produce oral lesions.

Special considerations

If the patient's mouth ulcers are painful, provide a topical anesthetic such as lidocaine, as ordered. Instruct him to avoid irritants, such as highly seasoned foods, citrus fruits, alcohol, and tobacco. For mouth care, avoid using lemon-glycerin swabs, since they can dry and irritate the lesions.

As appropriate, teach the patient proper oral hygiene. If toothbrushing is contraindicated, instruct him to use a mouth rinse, such as normal saline solution or half-strength hydrogen peroxide, and to avoid commercial mouthwashes that contain alcohol. Tell him to notify his doctor if any mouth lesions don't heal within 2 weeks.

Pediatric pointers

Causes of mouth ulcers in children include chicken pox, measles, scarlet fever, diphtheria, and hand-foot-and-mouth disease. In neonates, mouth ulcers can result from candidiasis or congenital syphilis.

Murmurs

Murmurs are auscultatory sounds heard within the heart chambers or major arteries. They're classified by their timing and duration in the cardiac cycle, auscultatory location, loudness, configuration, pitch, and quality. *Timing* can be characterized as systolic, holosystolic (continuous throughout systole), diastolic, or continuous throughout systole and diastole; systolic and diastolic murmurs can be further characterized as early, middle, or late. *Location* refers to the area of maximum loudness, such as the apex, the lower left sternal border, or an intercostal space. *Loudness* is graded on a scale of I to VI, with I signifying the faintest audible murmur. *Configuration,* or shape, refers to the nature of loudness—crescendo, decrescendo, crescendo-decrescendo, decrescendo-crescendo, plateau (even), or variable (uneven). The murmur's *pitch* may be high or low. Its *quality* may be described as harsh, rumbling, blowing, scratching, buzzing, musical, or squeaking.

Murmurs can reflect accelerated blood flow through normal or abnormal valves; forward blood flow through a narrowed or irregular valve or into a dilated vessel; blood backflow through an incompetent valve, septal defect, or patent ductus arteriosus; or decreased blood viscosity. Often the result of organic heart disease, murmurs occasionally may signal an emergency situation—for example, a loud holosystolic murmur after acute myocardial infarction (MI) may signal papillary muscle rupture. Murmurs may also result from surgical implantation of a prosthetic valve.

Some murmurs are innocent or functional. An *innocent systolic murmur* is generally soft, medium-pitched, and loudest along the left sternal border at the second or third intercostal space. It's exacerbated by physical activity, excitement, fever, pregnancy, anemia, or thyrotoxicosis. Examples include *Still's murmur* in children and *mammary souffle,* often heard over either breast during late pregnancy and early postpartum.

Assessment

If you discover a murmur, try to determine its type through careful auscultation. (See *Identifying Common Murmurs.*) Use the bell of your stethoscope for low-pitched murmurs; the diaphragm for high-pitched murmurs.

Next, obtain a patient history. Ask if the murmur is a new discovery or has been known since birth or childhood. Find out if the patient has experienced any associated symptoms, particularly palpitations, dizziness, syncope, chest

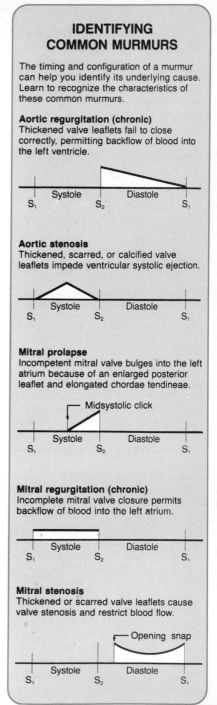

IDENTIFYING COMMON MURMURS

The timing and configuration of a murmur can help you identify its underlying cause. Learn to recognize the characteristics of these common murmurs.

Aortic regurgitation (chronic)
Thickened valve leaflets fail to close correctly, permitting backflow of blood into the left ventricle.

S_1 Systole S_2 Diastole S_1

Aortic stenosis
Thickened, scarred, or calcified valve leaflets impede ventricular systolic ejection.

S_1 Systole S_2 Diastole S_1

Mitral prolapse
Incompetent mitral valve bulges into the left atrium because of an enlarged posterior leaflet and elongated chordae tendineae.

Midsystolic click

S_1 Systole S_2 Diastole S_1

Mitral regurgitation (chronic)
Incomplete mitral valve closure permits backflow of blood into the left atrium.

S_1 Systole S_2 Diastole S_1

Mitral stenosis
Thickened or scarred valve leaflets cause valve stenosis and restrict blood flow.

Opening snap

S_1 Systole S_2 Diastole S_1

WHEN MURMURS MEAN EMERGENCY

Although not normally a sign of an emergency, murmurs—especially newly developed ones—may signal a serious complication in patients with bacterial endocarditis or recent acute myocardial infarction (MI).

When caring for a patient with known or suspected bacterial endocarditis, carefully auscultate for any new murmurs. Their development along with crackles, distended neck veins, orthopnea, and dyspnea may herald congestive heart failure.

Regular auscultation is also important in a patient who has experienced an acute MI. A loud decrescendo holosystolic murmur at the apex that radiates to the axilla and left sternal border or throughout the chest is significant, particularly in association with a widely split S₂ and an atrial gallop (S₄). This murmur, when accompanied by signs of acute pulmonary edema, usually indicates the development of acute mitral regurgitation due to rupture of the chordae tendineae—a medical emergency.

pain, dyspnea, and fatigue. Explore the patient's medical history, noting especially any incidence of rheumatic fever, heart disease, or heart surgery, particularly prosthetic valve replacement.

Now perform a systematic physical examination. Note especially the presence of cardiac dysrhythmias, jugular vein distention, and such pulmonary signs as dyspnea, orthopnea, and crackles. Is the patient's liver tender or palpable? Does he have peripheral edema?

Medical causes

• *Aortic regurgitation.* *Acute aortic regurgitation* typically produces a soft, short diastolic murmur over the left sternal border that's best heard when the patient sits and leans forward. S₂ may be soft or absent. Sometimes, a soft, short midsystolic murmur may also be heard over the second right intercostal space. Associated signs and symptoms may include tachycardia, dyspnea, distended neck veins, crackles, increased fatigue, and pale, cool extremities.

Chronic aortic regurgitation causes a high-pitched, blowing, decrescendo diastolic murmur that's best heard over the second or third right intercostal space or the left sternal border with the patient sitting, leaning forward, and holding his breath after deep expiration. An Austin Flint murmur—a rumbling, mid- to late diastolic murmur best heard at the apex—may also occur. Complications may not occur until age 40 to 50; then, typical findings include palpitations, tachycardia, anginal pain, increased fatigue, dyspnea, orthopnea, and crackles.

• *Aortic stenosis.* In this valvular disorder, the murmur is systolic, beginning after S₁ and ending at or before aortic valve closure. It's harsh and grating, medium-pitched, and crescendo-decrescendo. Loudest over the second right intercostal space, this murmur may also be heard at the apex, at the suprasternal notch (Erb's point), and over the carotid arteries. In advanced disease, S₂ may be heard as a single sound, with inaudible aortic closure. An early systolic ejection click at the apex is typical; it's absent when the valve is severely calcified. Associated signs and symptoms usually don't appear until age 30 in congenital aortic stenosis, age 30 to 65 in stenosis due to rheumatic disease, and after age 65 in calcific aortic stenosis. They may include dizziness, syncope, dyspnea, fatigue, and anginal pain.

• *Cardiomyopathy (hypertrophic obstructive).* This disorder generates a harsh late systolic murmur, ending at S₂. Best heard over the left sternal border and at the apex, the murmur is often accompanied by an audible S₃ or S₄. Major associated symptoms are dyspnea and chest pain; palpitations, dizziness, and syncope may also occur.

• *Complete heart block.* This disorder commonly produces a short, crescendo-decrescendo diastolic murmur following atrial contraction, best heard at the apex. S_1 may be paradoxical. Associated signs and symptoms may include fatigue, dizziness, or syncope.

• **Mitral prolapse.** This disorder generates a mid- to late systolic click with a high-pitched late systolic crescendo murmur, best heard at the apex. Occasionally, multiple clicks may be heard, with or without a systolic murmur. Accompanying signs and symptoms may include migraine headaches, dizziness, syncope, palpitations, chest pain, dyspnea, severe episodic fatigue, and mood swings.

• **Mitral regurgitation.** *Acute mitral regurgitation* is characterized by an early systolic or holosystolic decrescendo murmur at the apex, along with a widely split S_2 and often an S_4. Accompanying findings typically include tachycardia and signs of acute pulmonary edema.

Chronic mitral regurgitation produces a high-pitched, blowing, holosystolic plateau murmur that is loudest at the apex and usually radiates to the axilla or back. Fatigue, dyspnea, and palpitations may also occur.

• **Mitral stenosis.** In this valvular disorder, the murmur is soft, low-pitched, rumbling, decrescendo-crescendo, and diastolic, accompanied by a loud S_1 and an opening snap—a cardinal sign. It's best heard at the apex with the patient in the left lateral position. In severe stenosis, the murmur of mitral regurgitation may also be heard. Other findings may include hemoptysis, exertional dyspnea and fatigue, and signs of acute pulmonary edema.

• **Myxomas.** A *left atrial myxoma* (most common) usually produces a middiastolic murmur and a holosystolic murmur that's loudest at the apex, with an S_4, an early diastolic thudding sound (tumor plop), and a loud, widely split S_1. Related features may include dyspnea, orthopnea, chest pain, fatigue, weight loss, and syncope.

A *right atrial myxoma* causes a late diastolic rumbling murmur, a holosystolic crescendo murmur, and tumor plop, best heard at the lower left sternal border. Other findings include fatigue, peripheral edema, ascites, and hepatomegaly.

A *left ventricular myxoma* (very rare) produces a systolic murmur best heard at the lower left sternal border, dysrhythmias, dyspnea, and syncope.

A *right ventricular myxoma* commonly generates a systolic ejection murmur with delayed S_2 and a tumor plop, best heard at the left sternal border. It's accompanied by peripheral edema, hepatomegaly, ascites, dyspnea, and syncope.

• **Papillary muscle rupture.** In this life-threatening complication of acute MI, a loud holosystolic murmur can be auscultated at the apex. Related findings include severe dyspnea, chest pain, syncope, hemoptysis, tachycardia, and hypotension.

• **Tricuspid regurgitation.** This valvular abnormality is characterized by a soft, high-pitched, holosystolic blowing murmur that increases with inspiration (Carvallo's sign); it's best heard over the lower left sternal border and the xiphoid area. Following a lengthy asymptomatic period, exertional dyspnea and orthopnea may develop, along with neck vein distention, ascites, peripheral cyanosis and edema, and muscle wasting.

• **Tricuspid stenosis.** This valvular disorder produces a diastolic murmur similar to that of mitral stenosis, but louder with inspiration. S_1 may also be louder. Associated signs and symptoms may include fatigue, distended neck veins, ascites, hepatomegaly, and dyspnea.

Other causes

• **Treatments.** Prosthetic valve replacement may cause variable murmurs, depending on the location, valve composition, and method of operation.

Special considerations

Prepare the patient for diagnostic tests, such as electrocardiography and ech-

DETECTING CONGENITAL MURMURS

HEART DEFECT	TYPE OF MURMUR
Aorticopulmonary septal defect	*Small defect:* a continuous rough or crackling murmur best heard at the upper left sternal border and below the left clavicle, possibly accompanied by a systolic ejection click *Large defect:* a harsh systolic murmur heard at the left sternal border.
Atrial septal defect	A midsystolic, spindle-shaped murmur of grade II-III intensity heard at the upper left sternal border, with a fixed splitting of S_2. Large shunts may also produce a low- to medium-pitched early diastolic murmur over the lower left sternal border.
Bicuspid aortic valve	An early systolic, loud, high-pitched ejection sound or click that's best heard at the apex. It's frequently accompanied by a soft, early or midsystolic murmur at the upper right sternal border. The aortic component of S_2 is usually accentuated at the apex.
Coarctation of the aorta	Usually a systolic ejection click at the base of the heart, at the apex, and occasionally over the carotid arteries, often accompanied by a systolic ejection murmur at the base. This disorder may also produce a blowing diastolic murmur of aortic insufficiency or an apical pansystolic murmur of unknown origin.
Common atrioventricular canal defects (endocardial cushion defect)	*With a competent mitral valve:* a midsystolic, spindle-shaped murmur of grade II-III intensity heard at the upper left sternal border, with a fixed splitting of S_2; may be accompanied by a low- to medium-pitched early diastolic murmur over the lower left sternal border *With an incompetent mitral valve:* an early systolic or holosystolic decrescendo murmur at the apex, along with a widely split S_2 and often an S_4.
Ebstein's anomaly	A soft, high-pitched holosystolic blowing murmur that increases with inspiration (Carvallo's sign), best heard over the lower left sternal border and the xiphoid area; possibly accompanied by a low-pitched diastolic rumbling murmur at the apex. Fixed splitting of S_2 and a loud split S_4 also occur.
Left ventricular–right atrial communication	A holosystolic, grade II-IV decrescendo murmur heard along the lower left sternal border, accompanied by a normal S_2; large shunts also produce a diastolic rumbling murmur over the apex.
Mitral atresia	A nonspecific systolic murmur and a diastolic flow rumble at the lower left sternal border, with a loud and single S_2.

ocardiography. Since any cardiac abnormality will be frightening to the patient, provide emotional support.

Pediatric pointers

Innocent murmurs, such as Still's murmur, are frequently heard in young children and often disappear at puberty. Pathognomonic heart murmurs in infants and young children most commonly result from congenital heart disease, such as atrial and ventricular septal defects. (See *Detecting Congenital Murmurs.*) Other murmurs can be acquired, as with rheumatic heart disease.

HEART DEFECT	TYPE OF MURMUR
Partial anomalous pulmonary venous connection	A midsystolic, spindle-shaped, grade II-III murmur at the upper left sternal border, possibly accompanied by a low- to medium-pitched early diastolic murmur over the lower left sternal border.
Patent ductus arteriosus	A continuous rough or crackling murmur best heard at the upper left sternal border and below the left clavicle.
Pulmonic regurgitation	An early to middiastolic, soft, medium-pitched crescendo-decrescendo murmur best heard at the second or third right intercostal space.
Pulmonic stenosis	An early systolic, harsh, grade IV-VI crescendo-decrescendo murmur at the second left intercostal space, possibly radiating along the left sternal border.
Single atrium	A holosystolic regurgitant murmur at the apex, accompanied by a fixed splitting of S_2.
Supravalvular aortic stenosis	A systolic ejection murmur best heard over the second right intercostal space or higher in the episternal notch or over the right lower neck. The aortic closure sound is usually preserved, and no ejection clicks are heard.
Tetralogy of Fallot	A midsystolic murmur with a systolic thrill palpable at the left midsternal border; softer murmurs occurring earlier in systole generally indicate a more severe obstruction.
Tricuspid atresia	Variable, depending on associated defects.
Trilogy of Fallot	A systolic, harsh crescendo-decrescendo murmur, best heard at the upper left sternal border with radiation toward the left clavicle. The pulmonic component of S_2 becomes progressively softer with increasing degrees of obstruction.
Ventricular septal defect	*Small defect:* usually a holosystolic (but may be limited to early or midsystole), grade II-IV decrescendo murmur heard along the lower left sternal border, accompanied by a normal S_2 *Large defect:* a holosystolic murmur at the lower left sternal border and a midsystolic rumbling murmur at the apex, accompanied by an increased S_1 at the lower left sternal border and an increased pulmonic component of S_2.

Muscle Atrophy

[Muscle wasting]

Muscle atrophy results from prolonged muscle immobility or disuse. When deprived of regular exercise, muscle fibers lose both bulk and length, producing a visible loss of muscle size and contour and apparent emaciation or deformity in the affected area. Even slight atrophy usually causes some loss of motion or power.

Atrophy most commonly stems from

neuromuscular disease or injury. However, it may also stem from certain metabolic and endocrine disorders and prolonged immobility. Some muscle atrophy also occurs with aging.

Assessment
Ask the patient when and where he first noticed the muscle wasting and how it has progressed. Also ask about any associated symptoms, particularly weakness and recent weight loss. Review the patient's medical history for chronic illnesses; musculoskeletal or neurologic disorders, including trauma; and endocrine and metabolic disorders. Ask about his use of alcohol and drugs, particularly steroids.

Begin the physical examination by determining the extent of atrophy. Visually evaluate small and large muscles. Check all major muscle groups for size, tonicity, and contractility. Test motor strength (see *Testing Muscle Strength*, pages 500 and 501) and measure the circumference of all limbs, comparing sides. (See *Measuring Limb Circumference*, page 492.) Check for muscle contractures in all limbs by fully extending joints and noting any pain or resistance. Complete the examination by palpating peripheral pulses for quality and rate, assessing sensory function in and around the atrophied area, and testing deep tendon reflexes.

Medical causes
• *Amyotrophic lateral sclerosis.* Initial symptoms of this progressive disease include muscle weakness and atrophy that typically begin in one hand, spread to the arm, and then develop in the other hand and arm. Eventually, weakness and atrophy spread to the trunk, neck, tongue, larynx, pharynx, and legs; progressive respiratory muscle weakness leads to respiratory insufficiency. Other findings: muscle flaccidity, fasciculations, hyperactive deep tendon reflexes, slight leg muscle spasticity, dysphagia, impaired speech, excessive drooling, and depression.

• *Burns.* Fibrous scar tissue formation, pain, and loss of serum proteins from severe burns can limit muscle movement, resulting in atrophy.

• *Cerebrovascular accident.* CVA may produce contralateral or bilateral weakness, and eventually atrophy, of the arms, legs, face, and tongue. Associated signs and symptoms depend on the site and extent of vascular damage and may include dysarthria, aphasia, ataxia, apraxia, agnosia, and ipsilateral paresthesias or sensory losses. The patient may have visual disturbances, altered level of consciousness, amnesia and poor judgment, personality changes, and emotional lability. He may also have bowel and bladder dysfunction, vomiting, headache, and seizures.

• *Compartment syndrome and Volkmann's ischemic contracture.* In this acute disorder, muscle atrophy is a late sign of irreversible ischemia, along with contractures, paralysis, and loss of pulses. Earlier signs and symptoms include severe pain that's increased by passive muscle movement, along with weakness and paresthesias.

• *Herniated disk.* Here, pressure on nerve roots leads to muscle weakness, disuse, and ultimately atrophy. The primary symptom is severe lower back pain, possibly radiating to the buttocks, legs, and feet and often accompanied by muscle spasms. Diminished reflexes and sensory changes may also occur.

• *Hypercortisolism.* This disorder may cause limb weakness and eventually atrophy. Related cushingoid features include buffalo hump, moon face, truncal obesity, purple striae, thin skin, acne, easy bruising, poor wound healing, elevated blood pressure, fatigue, hyperpigmentation, and diaphoresis. The male patient may be impotent, while the female patient may have hirsutism and menstrual irregularities.

• *Hypothyroidism.* Reversible weakness and atrophy of proximal limb muscles may occur in hypothyroidism. Accompanying findings commonly include muscle cramps and stiffness; cold intolerance; weight gain despite anorexia; mental dullness; dry, pale, cool, doughy skin; puffy face, hands, and feet; and bradycardia.

• *Meniscal tear.* Quadriceps muscle atrophy, resulting from prolonged knee immobility and muscle weakness, is a classic sign of this traumatic disorder.

• *Multiple sclerosis.* This degenerative disease may produce arm and leg atrophy as a result of chronic progressive weakness; spasticity and contractures may also develop. Associated signs and symptoms often wax and wane and may include diplopia and blurred vision, nystagmus, hyperactive deep tendon reflexes, sensory loss or paresthesias, dysarthria, dysphagia, incoordination, ataxic gait, intention tremors, emotional lability, impotence, and urinary dysfunction.

• *Osteoarthritis.* This chronic disorder eventually causes atrophy proximal to involved joints as a result of progressive weakness and disuse. Other late signs and symptoms include bony joint deformities, such as Heberden's nodes on the distal interphalangeal joints, crepitus and fluid accumulation, and contractures.

• *Parkinson's disease.* In this disorder, muscle rigidity, weakness, and disuse may produce muscle atrophy. The patient may have insidious tremors that usually begin in the fingers (unilateral pill-rolling tremor), worsen with stress, and ease with purposeful movement and sleep. He may also have bradykinesia, a characteristic propulsive gait, a high-pitched, monotone voice, masklike facies, drooling, dysphagia, dysarthria, and occasionally oculogyric crisis or blepharospasm.

• *Peripheral nerve trauma.* Injury to or prolonged pressure on a peripheral nerve leads to muscle weakness and atrophy. Accompanying findings may include paresthesias or sensory loss, pain, and loss of reflexes supplied by the damaged nerve. Paralysis may also occur.

• *Peripheral neuropathy.* In this disorder, muscle weakness progresses slowly to flaccid paralysis and eventually atrophy. Distal extremity muscles are generally affected first. Associated findings may include loss of vibration sense; paresthesias, hyperesthesia, or anesthesia in the hands and feet; mild-to-sharp, burning pain; anhidrosis; glossy red skin; and diminished or absent deep tendon reflexes.

• *Protein deficiency.* Prolonged protein deficiency may lead to muscle weakness and atrophy. Other findings: chronic fatigue, apathy, anorexia, lethargy, dry skin, and dull, sparse, dry hair.

• *Rheumatoid arthritis.* Muscle atrophy occurs in the late stages of this disorder, as joint pain and stiffness decrease range of motion and discourage muscle use. Other late-stage findings may include flexion contractures, bony deformities, rheumatoid nodules, and crepitation upon joint rotation.

• *Spinal cord injury.* Trauma to the spinal cord can produce severe muscle weakness and flaccid, then spastic, paralysis, eventually leading to atrophy. Other signs and symptoms depend on the level of the injury but may include respiratory insufficiency or paralysis, sensory losses, bowel and bladder dysfunction, hyperactive deep tendon reflexes, positive Babinski's reflex, sexual dysfunction, priapism, hypotension, and anhidrosis (usually unilateral).

• *Thyrotoxicosis.* This disorder may produce insidious, generalized muscle weakness and atrophy. Related findings include extreme anxiety, fatigue, heat intolerance, diaphoresis, tremors, tachycardia, palpitations, ventricular or atrial gallop, dyspnea, weight loss, and an enlarged thyroid. Exophthalmos may be present.

Other causes

• *Drugs.* Prolonged steroid therapy interferes with muscle metabolism and leads to atrophy, most prominently in the limbs.

• *Immobility.* Prolonged immobilization from bed rest, casts, splints, or

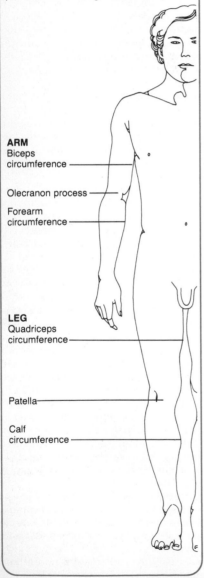

MEASURING LIMB CIRCUMFERENCE

To ensure accurate and consistent limb circumference measurements, use a consistent reference point each time and measure with the limb in full extension. The diagram below shows the correct reference points for arm and leg measurements.

ARM
Biceps circumference

Olecranon process

Forearm circumference

LEG
Quadriceps circumference

Patella

Calf circumference

traction may cause muscle weakness and atrophy.

Special considerations

Since contractures can occur as atrophied muscle fibers shorten, help the patient maintain muscle length by encouraging him to perform frequent active range-of-motion exercises. If he's unable to actively move a joint, provide active-assistive or passive exercises, and apply splints or braces to maintain muscle length. If you find resistance to full extension during exercises, use heat, pain medication, or relaxation techniques to relax the muscle. Then slowly stretch it to full extension. (*Caution*: don't pull or strain the muscle—you may tear muscle fibers and cause further contracture.) If these techniques fail to correct the contracture, use moist heat, a whirlpool bath, resistive exercises, or ultrasound therapy. If these techniques aren't effective, surgical release of contractures may be necessary.

As ordered, prepare the patient for electromyography, nerve conduction studies, muscle biopsy, and X-rays or computed tomography scans.

Pediatric pointers

In young children, profound muscle weakness and atrophy can result from muscular dystrophy (particularly Duchenne's type). Atrophy may also result from cerebral palsy and poliomyelitis, and from paralysis associated with meningocele and myelomeningocele.

Muscle Flaccidity

[Muscle hypotonicity]

Flaccid muscles are profoundly weak and soft, with decreased resistance to movement, increased mobility, and greater-than-normal range of motion. The result of disrupted muscle innervation, flaccidity can be localized to a limb or muscle group or generalized over the entire body. Its onset may be acute, as in trauma, or chronic, as in neurologic disease. Muscle flaccidity may be life-threatening if it affects the respiratory system.

Assessment

If the patient's flaccidity results from trauma, ensure that his cervical spine has been stabilized and notify the doctor. Quickly assess his respiratory status. If you note signs of respiratory insufficiency—dyspnea, shallow respirations, nasal flaring, and cyanosis—administer oxygen by nasal cannula or mask, and prepare to assist with intubation and mechanical ventilation.

If the patient isn't in distress, ask about the onset and duration of muscle flaccidity and any precipitating factors. Also ask about associated symptoms, particularly weakness, other muscle changes, and sensory losses or paresthesias.

Examine the affected muscles for atrophy, which indicates a chronic problem. Test muscle strength and check deep tendon reflexes in all limbs.

Medical causes

• *Amyotrophic lateral sclerosis.* In this disorder, progressive muscle weakness and paralysis are accompanied by generalized flaccidity. Typically, these effects begin in one hand, spread to the arm, and then develop in the other hand and arm. Eventually, they spread to the trunk, neck, tongue, larynx, pharynx, and legs; progressive respiratory muscle weakness leads to respiratory insufficiency. Other findings may include muscle cramps and coarse fasciculations, hyperactive deep tendon reflexes, slight leg muscle spasticity, dysphagia, dysarthria, excessive drooling, and depression.

• *Brain lesions.* Frontal and parietal lobe lesions may cause contralateral flaccidity, weakness or paralysis, and eventually spasticity. Other findings may include hyperactive deep tendon reflexes, positive Babinski's sign, loss of proprioception, analgesia, anesthesia, and thermanesthesia.

• *Cerebellar disease.* Here, generalized muscle flaccidity is accompanied by ataxia, dysmetria, intention tremor, slight muscle weakness, fatigue, and dysarthria.

• *Guillain-Barré syndrome.* This disorder causes muscle flaccidity from rapidly progressive muscle deterioration. Progression is typically symmetrical and ascending, moving from the feet to the arms and facial nerves within 24 to 72 hours of onset. Associated findings include sensory loss or paresthesias, absent deep tendon reflexes, tachycardia (or, less often, bradycardia), fluctuating hypertension and postural hypotension, diaphoresis, incontinence, dysphagia, dysarthria, hypernasality, and facial diplegia. Weakness may progress to total motor paralysis and respiratory failure.

• *Peripheral nerve trauma.* Peripheral nerve damage can produce flaccidity, paralysis, and loss of sensation and reflexes in the innervated area.

• *Peripheral neuropathy.* This disorder may produce muscle flaccidity, most commonly in the legs, as a result of chronic progressive muscle weakness and paralysis. It may also cause mild to sharp burning pain, glossy red skin, anhidrosis, and loss of vibration sensation. Paresthesia, hyperesthesia, or anesthesia may affect the hands and feet. Deep tendon reflexes may be hypoactive or absent.

• *Poliomyelitis.* Flaccidity develops late in this disorder from chronic muscle weakness that progresses to paralysis.

• *Seizure disorder.* Brief periods of syncope and generalized flaccidity commonly follow a grand mal seizure. Muscle tone returns rapidly once the patient regains consciousness.

• *Spinal cord injury.* Spinal shock can result in acute muscle flaccidity or spasticity below the level of injury. Associated signs and symptoms also occur below the level of injury and may include paralysis; absent deep tendon reflexes; analgesia; thermanesthesia; loss of proprioception and vibration, touch, and pressure sensation; and anhidrosis (usually unilateral). Hypotension, bowel and bladder dysfunction, and impotence or priapism may also occur. Injury in the C1 to C5 region can produce respiratory paralysis and bradycardia.

Special considerations
Provide regular, systematic, passive range-of-motion exercises to preserve joint mobility and to increase circulation. Reposition a patient with generalized flaccidity every 2 hours, as ordered, to protect him from skin breakdown. Pad bony prominences and other pressure points, and prevent thermal injury by testing bathwater yourself before the patient bathes. Treat isolated flaccidity by supporting the affected limb in a sling or with a splint.

Prepare the patient for diagnostic tests, such as cranial and spinal X-rays or computed tomography scans and electromyography.

Pediatric pointers
Pediatric causes of muscle flaccidity include myelomeningocele, Lowe's disease, Werdnig-Hoffmann disease, and muscular dystrophy. An infant or young child with generalized flaccidity may lie in a froglike position, with his hips and knees abducted.

Muscle Spasms
[Muscle cramps]

Muscle spasms are strong, painful contractions. They can occur in virtually any muscle but are most common in the calf and foot. Muscle spasms typically result from simple muscle fatigue, from exercise, and during pregnancy. However, they may also occur in electrolyte imbalances and neuromuscular disorders, or as the result of certain drugs. They're often precipitated by movement and can usually be relieved by slow stretching.

Assessment
If the patient complains of frequent or unrelieved spasms in many muscles, accompanied by paresthesias in his hands and feet, quickly attempt to elicit Chvostek's and Trousseau's signs. If these signs are present, suspect hypocalcemia and notify the doctor immediately. Assess respiratory function, watching for the development of laryngospasm; provide supplemental oxygen as necessary, and prepare to assist with intubation and mechanical ventilation. Draw blood for calcium levels and arterial blood gas analysis, and insert an I.V. for administration of a calcium supplement, as ordered. Monitor cardiac status, and prepare to begin resuscitation if necessary.

If the patient isn't in distress, ask when the spasms began. How long did they last? How painful were they? Did anything worsen or abate the pain? Ask about other symptoms, such as weakness, sensory loss, or paresthesias.

Evaluate muscle strength and tone. Then, check all major muscle groups, and note whether any movements precipitate spasms. Test the presence and quality of all peripheral pulses, and examine the limbs for color and temperature changes. Test capillary refill time and inspect for edema, especially in the involved area. Finally, test reflexes and sensory function in all extremities.

Medical causes
• *Amyotrophic lateral sclerosis.* In this disorder, muscle spasms may accompany progressive muscle weakness and atrophy that typically begin in one hand, spread to the arm, and then spread to the other hand and arm. Eventually, muscle weakness and atrophy affect the trunk, neck, tongue, larynx, pharynx, and legs; progressive respiratory muscle weakness leads to

respiratory insufficiency. Other findings may include muscle flaccidity progressing to spasticity, coarse fasciculations, hyperactive deep tendon reflexes, dysphagia, impaired speech, excessive drooling, and depression.

• *Arterial occlusive disease.* Arterial occlusion typically produces spasms and intermittent claudication in the leg, with residual pain. Associated findings are usually localized to the legs and feet and include loss of peripheral pulses, pallor or cyanosis, decreased sensation, hair loss, dry or scaling skin, edema, and ulcerations.

• *Dehydration.* Sodium loss may produce limb and abdominal cramps. Other findings may include a slight fever, decreased skin turgor, dry mucous membranes, tachycardia, postural hypotension, muscle twitching, seizures, nausea, vomiting, and oliguria.

• *Fracture.* Localized spasms and pain are mild if the fracture's nondisplaced, intense if it's severely displaced. Other findings: swelling, limited mobility, and possibly bony crepitation.

• *Hypocalcemia.* The classic feature is tetany—a syndrome of muscle cramps and twitching, carpopedal and facial muscle spasms, and convulsions, possibly with stridor. Both Chvostek's and Trousseau's signs may be elicited. Related findings include paresthesias of the lips, fingers, and toes; choreiform movements; hyperactive deep tendon reflexes; fatigue; palpitations; and cardiac dysrhythmias.

• *Hypothyroidism.* Muscle involvement may produce spasms and stiffness, along with leg muscle hypertrophy or proximal limb weakness and atrophy. Other findings: forgetfulness and mental instability; fatigue; cold intolerance; dry, pale, cool, doughy skin; puffy face, hands, and feet; periorbital edema; dry, sparse, brittle hair; bradycardia; and weight gain despite anorexia.

• *Muscle trauma.* Excessive muscle strain may cause mild to severe spasms. The injured area may be painful, swollen, reddened, and warm.

• *Respiratory alkalosis.* Acute onset of muscle spasms may be accompanied by twitching and weakness, carpopedal spasms, circumoral and peripheral paresthesias, vertigo, syncope, pallor, and extreme anxiety. In severe alkalosis, cardiac dysrhythmias may occur.

• *Spinal injury or disease.* Muscle spasms can result from spinal injury, such as cervical extension injury or spinous process fracture, or from spinal disease, such as infection.

Other causes

• *Drugs.* Common spasm-producing drugs include diuretics, corticosteroids, and estrogens.

Special considerations

Depending on the cause, help alleviate your patient's spasms by slowly stretching the affected muscle in the direction opposite the contraction. Or have the patient stand, preferably on a cold surface, such as tile or marble. If necessary, administer a mild analgesic.

Diagnostic studies may include serum calcium and sodium levels, thyroid function tests, and blood flow studies or arteriography.

Pediatric pointers

Muscle spasms rarely occur in children. However, their presence may indicate hypoparathyroidism, osteomalacia, rickets or, rarely, congenital torticollis.

Muscle Spasticity

[Muscle hypertonicity]

Spasticity is a state of excessive muscle tone with increased resistance to stretching and heightened reflexes. It's detected by evaluating a muscle's response to passive movement; a spastic muscle offers an initial resistance that suddenly gives way—a phenomenon known as the clasp-knife reflex. Caused by an upper motor neuron lesion, spasticity most commonly occurs in the arm and leg muscles. Long-term spasticity results in muscle fibrosis and contractures.

Assessment

Once you detect spasticity, ask the patient about its onset, duration, and progression. What, if any, events precipitated onset? Has he experienced other muscular changes or related symptoms? Does his medical history reveal any incidence of trauma or degenerative or vascular disease?

Take the patient's vital signs and perform a complete neurologic examination. Test reflexes and assess motor and sensory function in all limbs. Evaluate muscles for wasting and contractures.

During your assessment, keep in mind that generalized spasticity and trismus in a patient with a recent skin puncture or laceration indicates tetanus. If you suspect this rare disorder, assess for signs of respiratory distress and notify the doctor. If necessary, provide ventilatory support and monitor the patient closely.

Medical causes

● *Amyotrophic lateral sclerosis.* This disorder commonly produces spasticity, spasms, coarse fasciculations, hyperactive deep tendon reflexes, and a positive Babinski's sign. Earlier effects include progressive muscle weakness and flaccidity that typically begin in the hands and arms and eventually spread to the trunk, neck, larynx, pharynx, and legs; progressive respiratory muscle weakness leads to respiratory insufficiency. Other findings may include dysphagia, dysarthria, excessive drooling, and depression.

● *Cerebrovascular accident.* Spastic paralysis may develop on the affected side following the acute stage of CVA. Associated findings vary with the site and extent of vascular damage and may include dysarthria, aphasia, ataxia, apraxia, agnosia, ipsilateral paresthesias or sensory losses, visual disturbances, altered level of consciousness,

amnesia and poor judgment, personality changes, emotional lability, bowel and bladder dysfunction, headache, vomiting, and seizures.

● *Epidural hemorrhage.* In this disorder, bilateral limb spasticity is a late and ominous sign. Other findings may include a momentary loss of consciousness after head trauma, followed by a lucid interval and then a rapid deterioration in consciousness. The patient may also have unilateral hemiparesis or hemiplegia; seizures; fixed, dilated pupils; high fever; decreased and bounding pulse; widened pulse pressure; elevated blood pressure; irregular respiratory pattern; and decerebrate posture. A positive Babinski's sign can be elicited.

● *Multiple sclerosis.* Muscle spasticity, hyperreflexia, and contractures may eventually develop in this disorder; earlier muscle changes include progressive weakness and atrophy. Associated signs and symptoms often wax and wane and may include diplopia, blurred vision, nystagmus, sensory loss or paresthesias, dysarthria, dysphagia, incoordination, ataxic gait, intention tremors, emotional lability, impotence, and urinary dysfunction.

● *Spinal cord injury.* Spasticity commonly results from cervical and high thoracic spinal cord injury, especially from incomplete lesions. Spastic paralysis in the affected limbs follows initial flaccid paralysis; typically, spasticity and muscle atrophy increase for up to 1½ to 2 years after the injury, then gradually regress to flaccidity. Associated signs and symptoms vary with the level of the injury but may include respiratory insufficiency or paralysis, sensory losses, bowel and bladder dysfunction, hyperactive deep tendon reflexes, positive Babinski's sign, sexual dysfunction, priapism, hypotension, anhidrosis, and bradycardia.

● *Tetanus.* This rare, life-threatening disease produces varying degrees of spasticity. In generalized tetanus, the most common form, early signs and symptoms include jaw and neck stiff-

HOW SPASTICITY DEVELOPS

Motor activity is controlled by pyramidal and extrapyramidal tracts that originate in the motor cortex and extend down the spinal cord. The pyramidal tract stimulates muscle action, while the extrapyramidal tract inhibits it. Nerve fibers from the two tracts converge and synapse at the anterior horn in the spinal cord. Together, they maintain segmental muscle tone through a mechanism known as the *stretch reflex arc*. This arc, shown in simplified form below, is basically a negative feedback loop in which muscle stretch (stimulation) causes reflexive contraction (inhibition), thus maintaining muscle length and tone.

Damage to the extrapyramidal tract (or to the originating area of the motor cortex) results in loss of inhibition and disruption of the stretch reflex arc. Uninhibited muscle stretch produces exaggerated, uncontrolled muscle activity, eventually resulting in spasticity.

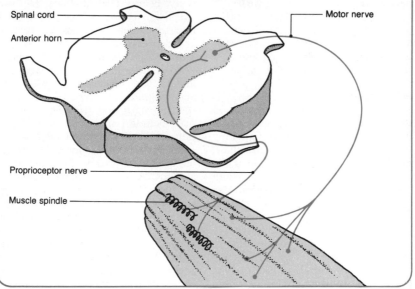

Spinal cord

Anterior horn

Motor nerve

Proprioceptor nerve

Muscle spindle

ness, trismus, headache, irritability, restlessness, low-grade fever with chills, tachycardia, diaphoresis, and hyperactive deep tendon reflexes. As the disease progresses, painful involuntary spasms may spread and cause boardlike abdominal rigidity, opisthotonos, and a characteristic grotesque grin known as risus sardonicus. Reflex spasms may occur in any muscle group with the slightest stimulus. Glottal, pharyngeal, or respiratory muscle involvement can cause death by asphyxia or cardiac failure.

Special considerations
Prepare the patient for diagnostic tests, which may include electromyography, muscle biopsy, or intracranial or spinal computed tomography. Administer pain medications and antispasmodics as ordered. Passive range-of-motion exercises, splinting, traction, and application of heat may help relieve spasms and prevent contractures. Keep the patient in a calm, quiet environment to help relieve spasms and prevent recurrence; encourage bed rest as appropriate. In cases of prolonged, uncontrollable spasticity, as in spastic paralysis, nerve blocks or surgical transection may be necessary for permanent relief.

Pediatric pointers
In children, muscle spasticity may be a sign of cerebral palsy.

Muscle Weakness

Muscle weakness is detected by measuring the strength of an individual muscle or a muscle group. Demonstrable muscle weakness can result from nerve degeneration or injury, or from altered chemical regulation at the neuromuscular junction or within the muscle itself. It occurs in a variety of neurologic and musculoskeletal disorders; in certain metabolic, endocrine, and cardiovascular disorders; as a response to certain drugs; and as a result of prolonged immobilization.

Assessment

Begin by determining the location of the patient's muscle weakness. Ask if he has difficulty with any specific movements, such as rising from a chair. Find out when he first noticed the weakness and whether it worsens with exercise or as the day progresses. Also ask about any associated symptoms, particularly muscle or joint pain, altered sensory function, and fatigue.

Obtain a medical history, noting especially chronic disease, such as hyperthyroidism; musculoskeletal or neurologic problems, including recent trauma; family history of chronic muscle weakness, especially in males; and alcohol and drug use.

Focus your physical assessment on evaluating muscle strength. Test all major muscles bilaterally. (See *Testing Muscle Strength,* pages 500 and 501.) Do *not* attempt to elicit pain during the tests; if the patient complains of pain, ease or discontinue resistance and have him try the movements again. Remember that the patient's dominant arm, hand, and leg tend to be somewhat stronger than their nondominant counterparts.

Now, test sensory function in the involved areas and in corresponding contralateral areas. Also test deep tendon reflexes bilaterally.

Medical causes

● *Amyotrophic lateral sclerosis.* This progressive disease typically begins with muscle weakness and atrophy in one hand that rapidly spreads to the arm, and then to the other hand and arm. Eventually, these effects spread to the trunk, neck, tongue, larynx, pharynx, and legs; progressive respiratory muscle weakness leads to respiratory insufficiency. Other signs and symptoms may include muscle flaccidity or spasticity; coarse fasciculations; hyperactive deep tendon reflexes; dysphagia; impaired speech; excessive drooling; and depression.

● *Anemia.* This disorder can cause varying degrees of muscle weakness and fatigue, exacerbated by exertion and temporarily relieved by rest. Associated signs and symptoms vary but may include pallor, tachycardia, paresthesias, and bleeding tendencies.

● *Cerebrovascular accident.* Depending on the site and extent of vascular damage, a CVA may produce contralateral or bilateral weakness of the arms, legs, face, and tongue, possibly progressing to hemiplegia and atrophy. Associated effects may include dysarthria, aphasia, ataxia, apraxia, agnosia, ipsilateral paresthesias or sensory losses, visual disturbances, altered level of consciousness, amnesia and poor judgment, personality changes, bowel and bladder dysfunction, headache, vomiting, and seizures.

● *Guillain-Barré syndrome.* In this disorder, rapidly progressive, symmetrical weakness ascends from the feet to the arms and facial nerves and may progress to total motor paralysis and respiratory failure. Associated findings include sensory loss or paresthesias, muscle flaccidity, loss of deep tendon reflexes, tachycardia (or, less often, bradycardia), fluctuating hypertension and postural hypotension, diaphoresis, bowel and bladder incontinence, facial diplegia, dysphagia, dysarthria, and hypernasality.

● *Head trauma.* Severe head injury can cause varying degrees of muscle weakness. Other findings may include decreased level of consciousness, otorrhea or rhinorrhea, raccoon's eyes and Battle's sign, sensory disturbances, and signs of increased intracranial pressure.

• *Herniated disk.* Here, pressure on nerve roots leads to muscle weakness, disuse, and ultimately atrophy. The primary symptom is severe low back pain, possibly radiating to the buttocks, legs, and feet—usually on one side. Diminished reflexes and sensory changes may also occur.

• *Hodgkin's lymphoma.* Here, muscle weakness may accompany the classic sign of lymphadenopathy. Other findings: paresthesias, fatigue, and weight loss.

• *Hypercortisolism.* This disorder may cause limb weakness and eventually atrophy. Related cushingoid features include buffalo hump, moon face, truncal obesity, purple striae, thin skin, acne, elevated blood pressure, fatigue, hyperpigmentation, easy bruising, poor wound healing, and diaphoresis. The male patient may be impotent; the female patient may have hirsutism and menstrual irregularities.

• *Hypothyroidism.* Reversible weakness and atrophy of proximal limb muscles may occur in hypothyroidism. Accompanying findings commonly include muscle cramps; cold intolerance; weight gain despite anorexia; mental dullness; dry, pale, doughy skin; puffy face, hands, and feet; and bradycardia.

• *Multiple sclerosis.* Muscle weakness in one or more limbs may progress to atrophy, spasticity, and contractures. Other findings typically wax and wane and may include diplopia and blurred vision, nystagmus, hyperactive deep tendon reflexes, sensory loss or paresthesias, dysarthria, dysphagia, incoordination, ataxic gait, intention tremors, emotional lability, impotence, and urinary dysfunction.

• *Myasthenia gravis.* Gradually progressive skeletal muscle weakness and fatigue are the cardinal symptoms of this disorder. Typically, weakness is mild upon awakening but worsens during the day. Early signs may include weak eye closure, ptosis, and diplopia; a blank, masklike facies; difficulty chewing and swallowing; nasal regurgitation of fluid with hypernasality; and a hanging jaw and bobbing head. Respiratory muscle involvement may eventually lead to respiratory failure.

• *Osteoarthritis.* This chronic disorder causes progressive muscle disuse and weakness that leads to atrophy.

• *Paget's disease.* As this disease progresses, muscle weakness or paralysis may develop, along with paresthesias and pain.

• *Parkinson's disease.* Muscle weakness accompanies rigidity in this degenerative disorder. Related findings include a unilateral pill-rolling tremor, propulsive gait, dysarthria, bradykinesia, drooling, dysphagia, masklike facies, and a high-pitched, monotonic voice.

• *Peripheral nerve trauma.* Prolonged pressure on or injury to a peripheral nerve causes muscle weakness and atrophy. Other findings: paresthesias or sensory loss, pain, and loss of reflexes supplied by the damaged nerve.

• *Peripheral neuropathy.* In this disorder, muscle weakness progresses slowly to flaccid paralysis, generally affecting distal extremities first. It may be accompanied by loss of vibration sense; paresthesias, hyperesthesia, or anesthesia in the hands and feet; hypoactive or absent deep tendon reflexes; mild to sharp and burning pain; anhidrosis; and glossy red skin.

• *Poliomyelitis.* Rapidly developing asymmetrical muscle weakness, progressing to flaccid paralysis, occurs in *paralytic poliomyelitis.* Associated signs and symptoms include moderate fever, headache, vomiting, lethargy, irritability, and widespread pain. As the disorder progresses, it may produce loss of superficial and deep reflexes, paresthesias, hyperalgesia, urine retention, constipation, abdominal distention, nuchal rigidity, and Hoyne's, Kernig's, and Brudzinski's signs. *Bulbar paralytic poliomyelitis* produces

TESTING MUSCLE STRENGTH

Obtain an overall picture of your patient's motor function by testing strength in ten selected muscle groups. Ask the patient to attempt normal range-of-motion movements against your resistance. If the muscle group is weak, vary the amount of resistance as necessary to permit accurate assessment. If necessary, position the patient so his limbs don't have to resist gravity, and repeat the test.

ARM MUSCLES

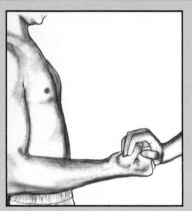

Biceps. With your hand on the patient's hand, have him flex his forearm against your resistance; observe for biceps contraction.

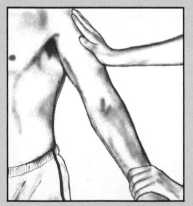

Deltoid muscle. With the patient's arm fully extended, place one hand over his deltoid muscle and the other on his wrist. Ask him to abduct his arm to a horizontal position against your resistance; as he does so, palpate for deltoid contraction.

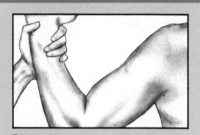

Triceps. Have the patient abduct and hold his arm midway between flexion and extension. Hold and support his arm at the wrist, and ask him to extend it against your resistance. Observe for triceps contraction.

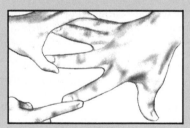

Dorsal interossei. Have the patient extend and spread his fingers, and tell him to try and resist your attempt to squeeze them together.

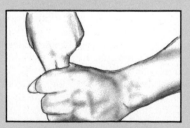

Forearm and hand (grip). Have the patient grasp your middle and index fingers and squeeze as hard as he can.

Rate muscle strength on a scale from 0 to 5:
0 = Total paralysis
1 = Visible or palpable contraction, but no movement
2 = Full muscle movement with force of gravity eliminated
3 = Full muscle movement against gravity, but no movement against resistance
4 = Full muscle movement against gravity; partial movement against resistance
5 = Full muscle movement against both gravity and resistance—normal strength.

LEG MUSCLES

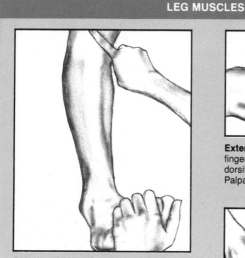

Anterior tibial. With the patient's leg extended, place your hand on his foot and ask him to dorsiflex his ankle against your resistance.

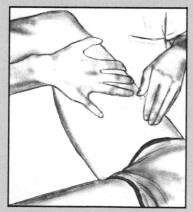

Psoas. While you support his leg, have the patient raise his knee and then flex his hip against your resistance. Observe for psoas muscle contraction.

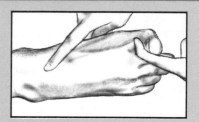

Extensor hallucis longus. With your finger on the patient's great toe, have him dorsiflex the toe against your resistance. Palpate for extensor hallucis contraction.

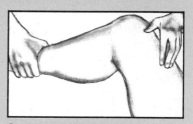

Quadriceps. Have the patient bend his knee slightly while you support his lower leg. Then ask him to extend the knee against your resistance; as he's doing so, palpate for quadriceps contraction.

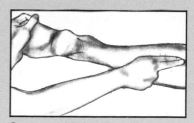

Gastrocnemius. With the patient on his side, support his foot and ask him to plantar-flex his ankle against your resistance. Palpate for gastrocnemius contraction.

symptoms of encephalitis along with facial weakness, dysphasia, dysphagia, and respiratory abnormalities.

• *Polymyositis.* This disorder produces insidious or acute onset of symmetrical limb and trunk muscle weakness and tenderness. Weakness may progress to facial, neck, pharyngeal, and laryngeal muscles. Associated findings: hypoactive deep tendon reflexes, dysphagia, and dysphonia.

• *Potassium imbalance.* In *hypokalemia,* temporary generalized muscle weakness may be accompanied by nausea, vomiting, diarrhea, decreased mentation, leg cramps, diminished reflexes, malaise, polyuria, dizziness, hypotension, and dysrhythmias. In *hyperkalemia,* weakness may progress to flaccid paralysis accompanied by irritability and confusion, hyperreflexia, paresthesias or anesthesia, oliguria, anorexia, nausea, diarrhea, abdominal cramps, tachycardia or bradycardia, and dysrhythmias.

• *Protein deficiency.* Prolonged protein deficiency may lead to muscle weakness and wasting, chronic fatigue, apathy, anorexia, lethargy, dry skin, and dull, sparse, dry hair.

• *Rheumatoid arthritis.* Here, muscle weakness may accompany increased warmth, swelling, and tenderness in involved joints; pain; and stiffness restricting motion.

• *Seizure disorder.* Temporary generalized muscle weakness may occur after a grand mal seizure; other postictal findings include headache, muscle soreness, and profound fatigue.

• *Spinal trauma and disease.* Trauma can cause severe muscle weakness, leading to flaccidity or spasticity and, eventually, paralysis. Infection, tumor, and cervical spondylosis or stenosis can also cause muscle weakness.

• *Thyrotoxicosis.* This disorder may produce insidious, generalized muscle weakness and atrophy. Its other effects include anxiety, fatigue, heat intolerance, diaphoresis, tremors, tachycardia, palpitations, ventricular or atrial gallop, dyspnea, weight loss, an enlarged thyroid, and warm, flushed skin. Exophthalmos may be present.

Other causes

• *Drugs.* Generalized muscle weakness can result from prolonged corticosteroid use, digitalis toxicity, and excessive doses of dantrolene. Aminoglycoside antibiotics may worsen weakness in patients with myasthenia gravis.

• *Immobility.* Immobilization in a cast, a splint, or traction can lead to muscle weakness in the involved extremity; prolonged bed rest or inactivity results in generalized muscle weakness.

Special considerations

Provide assistive devices as necessary, and protect the patient from injury. If he has concomitant sensory loss, guard against decubitus ulcer formation and thermal injury. With chronic weakness, provide range-of-motion exercises or splint limbs as necessary. Arrange therapy sessions to allow for adequate rest periods, and administer pain medications as ordered.

Prepare the patient for blood tests, muscle biopsy, electromyography, nerve conduction studies, and X-rays or computed tomography scans.

Pediatric pointers

Muscular dystrophy, usually the Duchenne type, is a major cause of muscle weakness in children.

Mydriasis

Mydriasis—pupillary dilation caused by contraction of the dilator of the iris—is a normal response to decreased light, strong emotional stimuli, and topical administration of mydriatic and cycloplegic drugs. It can also result from ocular and neurologic disorders, eye trauma, and disorders that decrease level of consciousness. Mydriasis may be a side effect of antihistamines or other drugs.

Assessment

Begin by asking the patient about any other eye problems, such as pain, blurring, diplopia, or visual field defects. Obtain a health history, focusing on eye or head trauma, glaucoma and other ocular problems, and neurologic and vascular disorders. Also obtain a complete medication history. Next, perform a thorough eye and pupil examination. Inspect and compare the pupils' size, color, and shape (many people normally have unequal pupils). Also test each pupil for light reflex, consensual response, and accommodation. Check the eyes for ptosis, swelling, and ecchymosis. Test visual acuity in both eyes with and without correction. Evaluate extraocular muscle function by checking the six cardinal fields of gaze.

Keep in mind that mydriasis appears in two ocular emergencies: acute closed-angle glaucoma and traumatic iridoplegia. If a report of acute pain or trauma makes you suspect either disorder, call the doctor immediately.

Medical causes

● *Adie's syndrome.* This disorder is characterized by abrupt unilateral mydriasis, poor or absent pupillary reflexes, visual blurring, and cramplike eye pain. Deep tendon reflexes may be hyperactive or absent.

● *Aortic arch syndrome.* Bilateral pupillary mydriasis commonly occurs late in this syndrome. Other ocular findings may include visual blurring, transient vision loss, and diplopia. Related findings may include dizziness and syncope; neck, shoulder, and chest pain; bruits; loss of radial and carotid pulses; paresthesias; and intermittent claudication. Blood pressure may be decreased in the arms.

● *Botulism.* Botulinum toxin causes bilateral mydriasis, usually 12 to 36 hours after ingestion. Other early findings are loss of pupillary reflexes, visual blurring, diplopia, ptosis, strabismus and extraocular muscle palsies, anorexia, nausea, vomiting, diarrhea, and dry mouth. Vertigo, hearing loss, hoarse- ness, hypernasality, dysarthria, dysphagia, progressive muscle weakness, and loss of deep tendon reflexes soon follow.

● *Brain stem infarction.* This rare disorder may cause bilateral mydriatic, fixed pupils. Associated signs and symptoms vary but may include paralysis of all extremities, sudden coma, decerebrate posturing, dysconjugate gaze, and respiratory pattern changes.

● *Carotid artery aneurysm.* Here, unilateral mydriasis may be accompanied by bitemporal hemianopia, decreased visual acuity, hemiplegia, decreased level of consciousness, headache, aphasia, behavioral changes, and hypoesthesia.

● *Glaucoma (acute closed-angle).* This ocular emergency is characterized by moderate mydriasis and loss of pupillary reflex in the affected eye, accompanied by abrupt onset of excruciating pain, decreased visual acuity, visual blurring, halo vision, conjunctival injection, and a cloudy cornea.

● *Oculomotor nerve palsy.* Unilateral mydriasis is often the first sign of this disorder. It's soon followed by ptosis, diplopia, decreased pupillary reflexes, exotropia, and complete loss of accommodation. Focal neurologic signs may accompany signs of increased intracranial pressure.

● *Traumatic iridoplegia.* Eye trauma often paralyzes the sphincter of the iris, causing mydriasis and loss of pupillary reflex; usually, this is transient. Associated findings may include a quivering iris (iridodonesis), ecchymosis, pain, and swelling.

Other causes

● *Drugs.* Mydriasis can be caused by anticholinergics, antihistamines, sympathomimetics, barbiturates (in overdose), estrogens, and tricyclic antidepressants; it also occurs commonly early in anesthesia induction. Topical mydriatics and cycloplegics, such as phenylephrine, atropine, homatropine, scopolamine, cyclopentolate, and tropicamide, are administered specifically for their mydriatic effects.

GRADING PUPIL SIZE

To ensure accurate evaluation of pupillary size, compare your patient's pupils to the scale below. Keep in mind that maximum constriction may be less than 1 mm and maximum dilation greater than 9 mm.

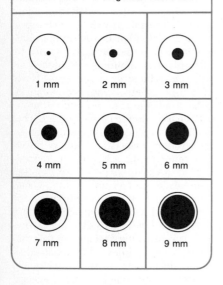

1 mm	2 mm	3 mm
4 mm	5 mm	6 mm
7 mm	8 mm	9 mm

● **Surgery.** Traumatic mydriasis commonly results from ocular surgery.

Special considerations

If the patient's mydriasis is the result of mydriatic drugs received during an eye examination, explain that he'll likely experience some photophobia and loss of accommodation. Instruct him to wear dark glasses and to avoid bright light, and reassure him that the condition is only temporary.

Diagnostic tests will depend on assessment findings and may include a complete ophthalmologic examination and a thorough neurologic workup. Explain any diagnostic tests to the patient.

Pediatric pointers

Mydriasis occurs in children as a result of ocular trauma, drugs, Adie's syndrome, and, most frequently, increased intracranial pressure.

Myoclonus

Myoclonus—sudden, shocklike contractions of a single muscle or muscle group—occurs in various neurologic disorders and often heralds onset of a seizure. These contractions may be isolated or repetitive, rhythmic or arrhythmic, symmetrical or asymmetrical, synchronous or asynchronous, and generalized or focal. Often, they're precipitated by a sensory stimulus, such as bright flickering light, a loud sound, or unexpected physical contact. One type, *intention myoclonus*, is evoked by intentional muscle movement, probably by a proprioceptive mechanism.

Myoclonus occurs normally just before falling asleep and as a part of the natural startle reaction. It also occurs with some poisonings and, rarely, as a complication of hemodialysis.

Assessment

If you observe myoclonus, notify the doctor immediately, and assess the patient for seizure activity. If he has a seizure, gently help him lie down. (If he's on a hard surface, place a pillow or a rolled-up towel under his head to prevent concussion.) Loosen any constrictive clothing, especially around the neck, and turn his head to one side to prevent airway occlusion or aspiration of secretions. Insert an oral airway or a suction catheter to maintain airway patency; if necessary, provide manual ventilation using an Ambu bag.

If the patient is stable, assess his level of consciousness and mental status. Then ask him about the frequency, severity, location, and circumstances of the myoclonus. Has he ever had a seizure? If so, did myoclonus precede it? Is the myoclonus ever precipitated by a sensory stimulus?

During the physical examination, check for muscle rigidity and wasting, and test deep tendon reflexes.

Medical causes

- **Alzheimer's disease.** Generalized myoclonus may occur in advanced stages of this slowly progressive dementia. Other late findings may include mild choreoathetoid movements, muscle rigidity, bowel and bladder incontinence, delusions, and hallucinations.
- **Creutzfeldt-Jakob disease.** Diffuse myoclonic jerks appear early in this rapidly progressive dementia. Initially random, they gradually become more rhythmic and symmetrical, often occurring in response to sensory stimuli. Associated effects may include ataxia, aphasia, hearing loss, muscle rigidity and wasting, fasciculations, hemiplegia, and visual disturbances or, possibly, blindness.
- **Encephalitis (viral).** In this disease, myoclonus is usually intermittent and either localized or generalized. Associated findings vary but may include rapidly decreasing level of consciousness, fever, headache, irritability, nuchal rigidity, vomiting, seizures, aphasia, ataxia, hemiparesis, facial muscle weakness, nystagmus, ocular palsies, and dysphagia.
- **Encephalopathy.** Hepatic encephalopathy occasionally produces myoclonic jerks in association with asterixis and focal or generalized seizures.

  Hypoxic encephalopathy may produce generalized myoclonus or convulsions almost immediately after restoration of cardiopulmonary function. The patient may also have a residual intention myoclonus.

  Uremic encephalopathy often produces myoclonic jerks and seizures. Other signs and symptoms include apathy, fatigue, irritability, headache, confusion, gradually decreasing level of consciousness, nausea, vomiting, oliguria, edema, and papilledema. The patient may also have elevated blood pressure, dyspnea, dysrhythmias, and abnormal respirations.
- **Epilepsy.** In idiopathic epilepsy, localized myoclonus is usually confined to an arm or leg and occurs singly or in short bursts, often upon awakening.

It's often more frequent and severe during the prodromal stage of a major generalized seizure, after which it diminishes in frequency and intensity.

Myoclonic jerks are usually the first signs of myoclonic epilepsy, the most common cause of progressive myoclonus. At first, myoclonus is infrequent and localized; but over a period of months it becomes more frequent and involves the entire body, disrupting voluntary movement (intention myoclonus). As the disease progresses, myoclonus is accompanied by generalized seizures and dementia.
- **Poisoning.** Acute intoxication with methyl bromide, bismuth, or strychnine may produce an acute onset of myoclonus and confusion.

Other causes

- **Treatments.** Facial or generalized myoclonus is an unusual complication of long-term hemodialysis.

Special considerations

If your patient's myoclonus is progressive, take seizure precautions. Keep an oral airway, suction equipment, and padded tongue blade at his bedside, and pad the side rails. Because myoclonus may cause falls, remove potentially harmful objects from the patient's environment, and remain with him while he walks. Be sure to instruct the patient and his family about the need for safety precautions.

As ordered, administer drugs that suppress myoclonus: ethosuximide, 5-hydroxytryptophan, phenobarbital, clonazepam, or carbidopa. An EEG may be ordered to evaluate myoclonus and related brain activity.

Pediatric pointers

Although myoclonus is relatively uncommon in infants and children, it can result from subacute sclerosing panencephalitis, severe meningitis, progressive poliodystrophy, West's disease, childhood myoclonic epilepsy, and encephalopathies, such as Reye's syndrome.

nasal flaring • nausea • neck pain • night blindness • nipple discharge • nipp
nuchal rigidity • nystagmus • ocular deviation • oligomenorrhea • oliguria • o
dyskinesia • orthopnea • orthostatic hypotension • Ortolani's sign • Osler's no
palpitations • papular rash • paralysis • paresthesias • paroxysmal nocturnal
d'orange • pericardial friction rub • peristaltic waves—visible • photophobia •
rub • polydipsia • polyphagia • polyuria • postnasal drip • priapism • prurit
psychotic behavior • ptosis • pulse—absent or weak • pulse—bounding • puls
pulse pressure—widened • pulse rhythm abnormality • pulsus alternans • pu
paradoxus • pupils—nonreactive • pupils—sluggish • purple striae • purpura
pyrosis • raccoon's eyes • rebound tenderness • rectal pain • retractions—cost
rhinorrhea • rhonchi • Romberg's sign • salivation—decreased • salivation—i
scotoma • scrotal swelling • seizure—absence • seizure—focal • seizure—gen
seizure—psychomotor • setting-sun sign • shallow respirations • skin—bronz
skin—mottled • skin—scaly • skin turgor—decreased • spider angioma • sple
respirations • stool—clay-colored • stridor • syncope • tachycardia • tachypne
earing—increased • throat pain • tic • tinnitus • tracheal deviation • trachea
rismus • tunnel vision • uremic frost • urethral discharge • urinary frequenc
urinary incontinence • urinary urgency • urine cloudiness • urticaria • vagina
postmenopausal • vaginal discharge • venous hum • vertigo • vesicular rash •
oss • visual blurring • visual floaters • vomiting • vulvar lesions • weight gai
oss—excessive • wheezing • wristdrop • abdominal distention • abdominal m
abdominal rigidity • accessory muscle use • agitation • alopecia • amenorrhe
nalgesia • anhidrosis • anorexia • anosmia • anuria • anxiety • aphasia • ap
respirations • apraxia • arm pain • asterixis • ataxia • athetosis • aura • Bab
ain • barrel chest • Battle's sign • Biot's respirations • bladder distention • b
blood pressure increase • bowel sounds—absent • bowel sounds—hyperactiv
ypoactive • bradycardia • bradypnea • breast dimpling • breast nodule • br
reath with ammonia odor • breath with fecal odor • breath with fruity odo
ruits • buffalo hump • butterfly rash • café-au-lait spots • capillary refill tim
arpopedal spasm • cat cry • chest expansion—asymmetrical • chest pain • C
espirations • chills • chorea • Chvostek's sign • clubbing • cogwheel rigidity
onfusion • conjunctival injection • constipation • corneal reflex—absent • co
enderness • cough—barking • cough—nonproductive • cough—productive •
ony • crepitation—subcutaneous • cry—high-pitched • cyanosis • decerebra
osture • deep tendon reflexes—hyperactive • deep tendon reflexes—hypoact
iaphoresis • diarrhea • diplopia • dizziness • doll's eye sign—absent • droo
ysmenorrhea • dyspareunia • dyspepsia • dysphagia • dyspnea • dystonia •
dema—generalized • edema of the arms • edema of the face • edema of the
nuresis • epistaxis • eructation • erythema • exophthalmos • eye discharge •
asciculations • fatigue • fecal incontinence • fetor hepaticus • fever • flank p
ontanelle bulging • fontanelle depression • footdrop • gag reflex abnormaliti
ropulsive • gait—scissors • gait—spastic • gait—steppage • gait—waddling
allop—ventricular • genital lesions in the male • grunting respirations • gu
velling • gynecomastia • halitosis • halo vision • headache • hearing loss •
eberden's nodes • hematemesis • hematochezia • hematuria • hemianopia •
epatomegaly • hiccups • hirsutism • hoarseness • Homans' sign • hyperpig
ypopigmentation • impotence • insomnia • intermittent claudication • Janev
w pain • jugular vein distention • Kehr's sign • Kernig's sign • leg pain • l
ecreased • lid lag • light flashes • low birth weight • lymphadenopathy • m
cBurney's sign • McMurray's sign • melena • menorrhagia • metrorrhagia

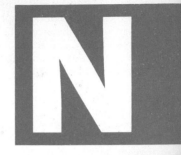

Nasal Flaring

Nasal flaring is the abnormal dilatation of the nostrils. Usually occurring during inspiration, nasal flaring may occasionally occur during expiration or throughout the respiratory cycle. It indicates respiratory dysfunction, ranging from mild difficulty to potentially life-threatening respiratory distress.

Assessment

If you note nasal flaring in your patient, quickly assess his respiratory status and notify the doctor. Inspiratory chest movement, absent breath sounds, cyanosis, diaphoresis, and tachycardia point to complete airway obstruction. As necessary, deliver back blows or abdominal thrusts (Heimlich maneuver) to relieve the obstruction. If these don't clear the airway, be prepared to assist with emergency intubation or tracheostomy and mechanical ventilation.

If the patient's airway isn't obstructed but he displays breathing difficulty, administer oxygen by nasal cannula or face mask, and be prepared to assist with intubation and mechanical ventilation as needed. Insert an I.V. for fluid and medication access. Begin cardiac monitoring, and obtain a chest X-ray and samples for arterial blood gas and electrolyte studies.

Once the patient is stabilized, obtain a pertinent history. Ask about cardiac and pulmonary disorders, such as asthma. Does the patient have allergies? Has he had a recent illness, such as a respiratory infection, or trauma?

Medical causes

● *Adult respiratory distress syndrome (ARDS).* ARDS causes increased respiratory difficulty, with nasal flaring, dyspnea, tachypnea, diaphoresis, cyanosis, scattered crackles, and rhonchi. It also causes tachycardia, anxiety, and decreased level of consciousness.

● *Airway obstruction. Complete obstruction* above the tracheal bifurcation causes sudden nasal flaring, absent breath sounds despite intercostal retractions and marked accessory muscle use, tachycardia, diaphoresis, cyanosis, decreasing level of consciousness, and eventually respiratory arrest.

Partial obstruction causes nasal flaring with inspiratory stridor, gagging, wheezing, violent cough, marked accessory muscle use, agitation, cyanosis, and hoarseness.

● *Anaphylaxis.* Severe reactions can produce respiratory distress with nasal flaring, stridor, wheezing, accessory muscle use, intercostal retractions, and dyspnea. Associated signs and symptoms may include nasal congestion, sneezing, pruritus, urticaria, erythema, diaphoresis, angioedema, weakness, hoarseness, dysphagia, and, rarely, vomiting, nausea, diarrhea, urinary urgency, and incontinence. Cardiac dysrhythmias and signs of shock may occur late.

• *Asthma (acute).* An asthmatic attack can cause nasal flaring, dyspnea, tachypnea, prolonged expiratory wheezing, accessory muscle use, cyanosis, and a dry or productive cough. Auscultation may reveal rhonchi, crackles, and decreased or absent breath sounds. Other findings: anxiety, tachycardia, and increased blood pressure.

• *Chronic obstructive pulmonary disease.* This disorder can lead to acute respiratory failure secondary to pulmonary infection or edema. Nasal flaring is accompanied by prolonged pursed-lip expiration; accessory muscle use; loose, rattling, productive cough; cyanosis; reduced chest expansion; crackles; rhonchi; wheezing; and dyspnea.

• *Pneumonia (bacterial).* Here, nasal flaring occurs with dyspnea, tachypnea, high fever, and sudden shaking chills. An initially dry and hacking cough later becomes productive. Stabbing chest pain worsens with movement and respirations. Auscultation reveals decreased or absent breath sounds, fine crackles, and pleural friction rub. Percussion reveals dullness.

• *Pneumothorax.* This acute disorder can result in respiratory distress with nasal flaring, dyspnea, tachypnea, shallow respirations, hyperresonance or tympany on percussion, agitation, distended neck veins, tracheal deviation, and cyanosis. Other findings typically include sharp chest pain, tachycardia, hypotension, cold and clammy skin, diaphoresis, and subcutaneous crepitation. Breath sounds may be decreased or absent on the affected side; similarly, chest wall motion may be decreased on the affected side.

Similar findings can occur with hydrothorax, chylothorax, or hemothorax, depending on the amount of fluid accumulation.

• *Pulmonary edema.* This disorder typically produces nasal flaring, severe dyspnea, wheezing, and a cough that produces frothy, pink sputum. Increased accessory muscle use may occur with tachycardia, cyanosis, hypotension, crackles, distended neck veins, peripheral edema, and decreased level of consciousness.

• *Pulmonary embolus.* Signs of this potentially life-threatening disorder may include nasal flaring, dyspnea, tachypnea, wheezing, cyanosis, pleural friction rub, and productive cough (possibly hemoptysis). Its other effects include sudden chest tightness or pleuritic pain, tachycardia, hypotension, low-grade fever, syncope, marked anxiety, and restlessness.

Other causes

• *Diagnostic tests.* Pulmonary function tests, such as vital capacity testing, can produce nasal flaring with forced inspiration or expiration.

• *Treatments.* Certain respiratory treatments, such as deep breathing, can cause nasal flaring.

Special considerations

To help ease breathing, place the patient in a high Fowler's position. If he's at risk for aspirating secretions, place him in a modified Trendelenburg's or side-lying position. If necessary, suction frequently to remove oropharyngeal secretions. Administer humidified oxygen to thin secretions and decrease airway drying and irritation. Provide adequate hydration to liquefy secretions. Reposition the patient every hour and encourage coughing and deep breathing. Avoid administering sedatives or opiates, which can depress the cough reflex or respirations. Continually assess the patient's respiratory status, and check his vital signs every 30 minutes or as necessary.

Prepare the patient for diagnostic tests, such as chest X-rays, lung scan, pulmonary arteriography, sputum culture, complete blood count, arterial blood gas analysis, and 12-lead EKG.

Pediatric pointers
Nasal flaring is an important sign of respiratory distress in infants and very young children, who can't verbalize their discomfort. Common causes include airway obstruction, hyaline membrane disease, croup, and acute epiglottitis.

Nausea

Nausea is a sensation of profound revulsion to food or of impending vomiting. Often accompanied by autonomic signs, such as hypersalivation, diaphoresis, tachycardia, pallor, and tachypnea, it's closely associated with both anorexia and vomiting.

Nausea, a common symptom of GI disorders, also occurs with fluid and electrolyte imbalances; infections; and metabolic, endocrine, labyrinthine, and cardiac disorders; and as a result of drug therapy, surgery, and radiation. Often present during the first trimester of pregnancy, nausea may also arise from severe pain, anxiety, alcohol intoxication, overeating, or ingestion of distasteful food or liquids.

Assessment
Begin by obtaining a complete medical history. Focus on GI, endocrine, and metabolic disorders; recent infections; and cancer and its treatment. Ask about medication use and alcohol consumption. If the patient's a female of child-bearing age, ask if she is or could be pregnant. Have the patient characterize the onset, duration, and intensity of the nausea, and its precipitating or alleviating factors. Ask about any associated complaints, particularly vomiting, abdominal pain, anorexia and weight loss, changes in bowel habits or stool character, excessive belching or flatus, and a sensation of bloating.

Now, inspect the skin for jaundice, bruises, and spider angiomas, and assess skin turgor. Next, inspect the abdomen for distention, auscultate for bowel sounds and bruits, palpate for rigidity and tenderness, and test for rebound tenderness. Palpate and percuss the liver for enlargement. Assess other body systems as appropriate.

Medical causes
● *Adrenal insufficiency.* Common GI findings in this endocrine disorder include nausea, vomiting, anorexia, and diarrhea. Other findings may include weakness, fatigue, weight loss, bronze skin, hypotension, and a weak, irregular pulse.
● *Appendicitis.* With acute appendicitis, a brief period of nausea may accompany onset of abdominal pain. Pain typically begins as vague epigastric or periumbilical discomfort and rapidly progresses to severe stabbing pain localized in the right lower quadrant (McBurney's sign). Associated findings usually include abdominal rigidity and tenderness, cutaneous hyperalgesia, fever, constipation or diarrhea, tachycardia, anorexia, and moderate malaise.
● *Cholecystitis (acute).* Here, nausea often follows severe right upper quadrant pain that may radiate to the back or shoulders. Associated findings include mild vomiting, abdominal tenderness and, possibly, rigidity and distention, fever with chills, and diaphoresis.
● *Cholelithiasis.* In this disorder, nausea accompanies attacks of severe right upper quadrant or epigastric pain after ingestion of fatty foods. Other findings include vomiting, abdominal tenderness and guarding, flatulence, belching, epigastric burning, pyrosis, tachycardia, and restlessness. Occlusion of the common bile duct may cause jaundice, clay-colored stools, fever, and chills.
● *Cirrhosis.* Insidious early symptoms of cirrhosis typically include nausea and vomiting, anorexia, abdominal pain, and constipation or diarrhea. As the disease progresses, jaundice and hepatomegaly may occur with abdominal distention, spider angiomas, palmar

erythema, severe pruritus, dry skin, fetor hepaticus, enlarged superficial abdominal veins, mental changes, and bilateral gynecomastia and testicular atrophy or menstrual irregularities.

• *Congestive heart failure.* This disorder may produce nausea and vomiting, particularly with right heart failure. Associated findings include tachycardia, ventricular gallop, profound fatigue, dyspnea, crackles, peripheral edema, and jugular vein distention.

• *Diverticulitis.* Besides nausea, diverticulitis causes intermittent abdominal pain, constipation, low-grade fever, and frequently a palpable mass.

• *Ectopic pregnancy.* Nausea, vomiting, vaginal bleeding, and lower abdominal pain occur in this potentially life-threatening disorder.

• *Electrolyte imbalances.* Such disturbances as hyponatremia or hypernatremia, hypokalemia, and hypercalcemia frequently cause nausea and vomiting. Other effects: cardiac dysrhythmias, tremors or seizures, anorexia, malaise, and weakness.

• *Gastric cancer.* This rare cancer may produce vague GI symptoms—mild nausea, anorexia, upper abdominal discomfort, and chronic dyspepsia. Fatigue, weight loss, weakness, hematemesis, melena, and altered bowel habits are also common.

• *Gastritis.* Nausea is common in this disorder, especially after ingestion of alcohol, aspirin, spicy foods, or caffeine. Vomiting of mucus or blood, epigastric pain, belching, fever, and malaise may also occur.

• *Gastroenteritis.* This disorder causes nausea, vomiting, diarrhea, and abdominal cramping. Fever, malaise, hyperactive bowel sounds, abdominal pain and tenderness, and possibly signs of dehydration may also develop.

• *Hepatitis.* Nausea is an insidious early symptom of viral hepatitis. Vomiting, fatigue, myalgia and arthralgia, headache, anorexia, photophobia, pharyngitis, cough, and fever also occur early in the preicteric phase.

• *Hyperemesis gravidarum.* Unremitting nausea and vomiting that persist beyond the first trimester are characteristic of this disorder of pregnancy. Vomitus ranges from undigested food, mucus, and bile early in the disorder to a "coffee-ground" appearance in later stages. Associated findings include weight loss, signs of dehydration, headache, and delirium.

• *Infection.* Acute localized or systemic infection often produces nausea. Other findings commonly include fever, headache, fatigue, and malaise.

• *Intestinal obstruction.* Nausea occurs frequently, especially with high small intestinal obstruction. Vomiting may be bilious or fecal; abdominal pain is usually episodic and colicky but can become severe and steady with strangulation. Constipation occurs early in large intestinal and later in small intestinal obstruction; obstipation may signal complete obstruction. Bowel sounds are typically hyperactive in partial obstruction, and hypoactive or absent in complete obstruction. Abdominal distention and tenderness occur, possibly with visible peristaltic waves and a palpable abdominal mass.

• *Irritable bowel syndrome.* Nausea, dyspepsia, and abdominal distention may occur in this syndrome. Other findings: lower abdominal pain, abdominal tenderness, diurnal diarrhea alternating with constipation or normal bowel function, and small stools with visible mucus.

• *Labyrinthitis.* Nausea and vomiting commonly occur with this acute inner ear inflammation. More significant findings include severe vertigo, progressive hearing loss, nystagmus, and possibly otorrhea.

• *Ménière's disease.* This disease causes sudden, brief, recurrent attacks of nausea, vomiting, vertigo, tinnitus, diaphoresis, and nystagmus. It also causes hearing loss.

• *Mesenteric artery ischemia.* Here, nausea and vomiting may accompany severe cramping abdominal pain, especially after meals. Other findings: diarrhea or constipation, abdominal tenderness and bloating, anorexia, weight loss, and abdominal bruits.

• *Mesenteric venous thrombosis.* Insidious or acute onset of nausea, vomiting, and abdominal pain occur here, with diarrhea or constipation, abdominal distention, hematemesis, and melena.

• *Metabolic acidosis.* This acid-base imbalance may produce nausea and vomiting, anorexia, diarrhea, Kussmaul's respirations, and decreased level of consciousness.

• *Migraine headache.* Nausea and vomiting may occur in the prodromal stage, along with photophobia, light flashes, increased sensitivity to noise, and possibly partial vision loss and paresthesias of the lips, face, and hands.

• *Motion sickness.* In this disorder, nausea and vomiting are brought on by motion or rhythmic movement. Headache, dizziness, fatigue, diaphoresis, and dyspnea may also occur.

• *Myocardial infarction.* Nausea and vomiting may occur, but the cardinal symptom is severe substernal chest pain that may radiate to the left arm, jaw, or neck. Dyspnea, pallor, clammy skin, diaphoresis, and altered blood pressure also occur.

• *Pancreatitis (acute).* Nausea, usually followed by vomiting, is an early symptom of pancreatitis. Common associated findings include steady, severe pain in the epigastrium or left upper quadrant that may radiate to the back; abdominal tenderness and rigidity; diminished bowel sounds; and fever. Tachycardia, restlessness, hypotension, skin mottling, and cold, sweaty extremities may occur in severe cases.

• *Peptic ulcer.* In this disorder, nausea and vomiting may follow attacks of sharp or burning epigastric pain. Attacks typically occur when the stomach is empty or after ingestion of alcohol, caffeine, or aspirin; they're relieved by eating or antacids. Hematemesis or melena may also occur.

• *Peritonitis.* Nausea and vomiting usually accompany acute abdominal pain localized to the area of inflammation. Other findings may include high fever with chills; tachycardia; hypoactive or absent bowel sounds; abdominal distention and tenderness (including rebound tenderness); weakness; pale, cold skin; diaphoresis; hypotension; shallow respirations; and hiccups.

• *Preeclampsia.* Nausea and vomiting commonly occur in this disorder of pregnancy, along with rapid weight gain, epigastric pain, generalized edema, elevated blood pressure, oliguria, severe frontal headache, and blurred or double vision.

• *Renal and urologic disorders.* Cystitis, pyelonephritis, calculi, uremia, and other disorders of this system can cause nausea. Related findings reflect the specific disorder.

• *Thyrotoxicosis.* In this disorder, nausea and vomiting may accompany the classic findings of severe anxiety, heat intolerance, weight loss despite increased appetite, diaphoresis, diarrhea, tremor, tachycardia, and palpitations. Other signs may include exophthalmos, ventricular or atrial gallop, and an enlarged thyroid gland.

• *Ulcerative colitis.* Nausea, vomiting, and anorexia may occur here, but the most common symptom is recurrent diarrhea with blood, pus, and mucus.

Other causes

• *Drugs.* Common nausea-producing drugs include antineoplastic agents, opiates, ferrous sulfate, levodopa, oral potassium chloride replacements, estrogens, sulfasalazine, antibiotics, quinidine, anesthetic agents, and digitalis and theophylline (overdose).

• *Radiation and surgery.* Radiation therapy may cause nausea and vomiting. Postoperative nausea and vomiting are common, especially after abdominal surgery.

Special considerations

If your patient's experiencing severe nausea, prepare him for blood tests to determine fluid, electrolyte, and acid-base balance. Have him breathe deeply to ease his nausea; keep his room air fresh and clean-smelling by removing bedpans and emesis basins promptly after use and by providing adequate ventilation. Since he could easily aspirate vomitus when supine, elevate his head or position him on his side.

Because pain can precipitate or intensify nausea, administer pain medications promptly, as ordered. If possible, give medications by injection or suppository to prevent exacerbating nausea. Be alert for abdominal distention and hypoactive bowel sounds when you administer antiemetics: these signs may indicate gastric retention. If you detect these, immediately insert a nasogastric tube, as ordered.

Pediatric pointers

Nausea, frequently described as stomachache, is one of the most common childhood complaints. Often the result of overeating, it can also occur with diverse disorders, ranging from acute infections to a conversion reaction caused by fear.

Neck Pain

Neck pain may originate from any neck structure, ranging from the meninges and cervical vertebrae to its blood vessels, muscles, and lymphatic tissue. This symptom can also be referred from other areas of the body. Its location, onset, and pattern help determine its origin and underlying causes. Neck pain most commonly results from trauma and degenerative, congenital, inflammatory, metabolic, and neoplastic disorders.

Assessment

If the patient's neck pain is due to trauma, your first priority is to ensure proper cervical spine immobilization, preferably with a long backboard and a Philadelphia collar. Then take his vital signs, and perform a quick neurologic assessment. If he shows signs of respiratory distress (a result of phrenic nerve involvement), administer oxygen and assist with intubation and mechanical ventilation as necessary. Ask the patient (or his companion, if the patient can't answer) how the injury occurred. Then examine the neck for abrasions, swelling, lacerations, erythema, and ecchymoses.

If the patient hasn't sustained trauma, find out the severity and onset of his neck pain. Where in the neck does he feel pain? Does anything relieve or worsen the pain? Also ask about the development of other symptoms. Next, focus on the patient's current and past illnesses and injuries, diet, medication use, and family health history.

Thoroughly inspect the patient's neck, shoulders, and cervical spine for swelling, masses, erythema, and ecchymoses. Assess range of motion in his neck by having him turn his head from side to side; note the degree of pain produced by these movements. Check the sensation in his arms and assess his hand grasp and arm reflexes. Attempt to elicit Brudzinski's and Kernig's signs, and palpate the cervical lymph nodes for enlargement.

Medical causes

● *Ankylosing spondylitis.* Intermittent, moderate to severe neck pain and stiffness with severely restricted range of motion is a classic finding in this disorder. Associated signs and symptoms also occur intermittently and may include low back pain and stiffness, low-grade fever, malaise, anorexia, fatigue, and occasionally iritis.

● *Cervical extension injury.* Anterior or posterior neck pain may develop within hours or days following a whiplash injury. Anterior pain usually diminishes within several days, but posterior pain persists and may even intensify. Associated findings may include tenderness, swelling and nuchal rigidity, occipital headache, muscle spasms, visual blurring, and unilateral miosis on the affected side.

● *Cervical fibrositis.* This disorder may

produce anterior neck pain that radiates to one or both shoulders. Pain is intermittent and variable, often changing with weather patterns. Other findings are nonspecific but frequently include point tenderness over involved muscles.

● *Cervical spine fracture.* Fracture at C1 to C4 often results in sudden death; survivors may experience severe neck pain that restricts all movement, intense occipital headache, quadriplegia, and respiratory paralysis.

● *Cervical spine infection.* Acute infection can cause moderate neck pain that restricts motion. Other findings may include fever, muscle spasms, local tenderness, dysphagia, paresthesias, and muscle weakness.

● *Cervical spine tumor.* Metastatic tumors typically produce persistent neck pain that increases with movement and isn't relieved by rest; *primary tumors* cause mild to severe pain along a specific nerve root. Other findings depend on the lesions and may include paresthesias, arm and leg weakness that progresses to atrophy and paralysis, and bladder and bowel incontinence.

● *Cervical spondylosis.* This degenerative process produces posterior neck pain that restricts movement and is aggravated by it. Pain may radiate down either arm and may accompany paresthesias and weakness.

● *Cervical stenosis.* This slowly progressive disorder, frequently asymptomatic, may produce nonspecific neck pain, paresthesias, and muscle weakness or paralysis.

● *Esophageal trauma.* An esophageal mucosal tear or a pulsion diverticulum may produce mild neck pain, chest pain, edema, hemoptysis, and dysphagia.

● *Hemorrhage (subarachnoid).* This life-threatening condition may cause moderate to severe neck pain and rigidity, headache, and a decreased level of consciousness (LOC). Kernig's and Brudzinski's signs are present.

● *Herniated cervical disk.* This disorder characteristically causes variable neck pain that restricts movement and is aggravated by it. It also causes referred pain, paresthesias and other sensory disturbances, and arm weakness.

● *Hodgkin's lymphoma.* This disorder eventually may result in generalized pain that may affect the neck. Lymphadenopathy, the classic sign, may ac-

APPLYING A PHILADELPHIA COLLAR

A lightweight molded polyethylene collar designed to hold the neck straight with the chin slightly elevated and tucked in, the Philadelphia cervical collar immobilizes the cervical spine, decreases muscle spasms, and relieves some pain. It also prevents further injury and promotes healing. When applying the collar, fit it snugly around the patient's neck and attach the Velcro fasteners or buckles at the back. Be sure to check the patient's airway and his neurovascular status to ensure that the collar isn't too tight. Also make sure that the collar isn't placed too high in front, which can hyperextend the neck. In a patient with a neck sprain, hyperextension may cause the ligaments to heal in a shortened position; in a patient with a cervical spine fracture, it could cause serious neurologic damage.

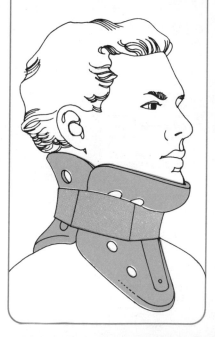

NECK PAIN: CAUSES AND ASSOCIATED FINDINGS

S&S CAUSES	MAJOR ASSOCIATED SIGNS AND SYMPTOMS													
	Arm pain	Back pain	Brudzinski's sign	Decreased LOC	Decreased range of motion	Deformity	Dysphagia	Dyspnea	Ecchymoses	Fatigue	Fever	Headache	Hemoptysis	Hoarseness
Ankylosing spondylitis		●								●	●			
Cervical extension injury												●		
Cervical fibrositis														
Cervical spine fracture					●							●		
Cervical spine infection					●		●				●			
Cervical spine tumor														
Cervical spondylosis	●													
Cervical stenosis														
Esophageal trauma							●						●	
Hemorrhage (subarachnoid)			●	●								●		
Herniated cervical disk	●	●												
Hodgkin's lymphoma										●	●			
Laryngeal cancer							●	●					●	●
Lymphadenitis											●			

Kernig's sign	Lymphadenopathy	Malaise	Muscle spasms	Nuchal rigidity	Paralysis	Paresthesias	Swelling	Tenderness	Weakness
		●		●					
			●	●			●		
									●
					●				
			●			●		●	●
						●	●		●
							●		●
						●	●		●
							●		
●			●						
						●			●
	●	●				●			●
	●								
	●	●						●	

(continued)

company paresthesias, muscle weakness, fever, fatigue, weight loss, malaise, and hepatomegaly.

• *Laryngeal cancer.* Neck pain that radiates to the ear develops late in this disorder. The patient may also have dysphagia, dyspnea, hemoptysis, stridor, hoarseness, and cervical lymphadenopathy.

• *Lymphadenitis.* In this disorder, enlarged and inflamed cervical lymph nodes cause acute pain and tenderness. Fever, chills, and malaise may also occur.

• *Meningitis.* Neck pain may accompany characteristic nuchal rigidity. Related findings include fever, headache, photophobia, positive Brudzinski's and Kernig's signs, and decreased level of consciousness.

• *Neck sprain.* Minor sprains typically produce pain, slight swelling, stiffness, and restricted range of motion. Ligament rupture causes pain, marked swelling, ecchymosis, muscle spasms, and nuchal rigidity with head tilt.

• *Osteoporosis.* Neck pain occurs rarely in this disorder, which usually affects the thoracic or lumbar vertebrae. Cervical vertebrae involvement produces tenderness and deformity.

• *Paget's disease.* This slowly developing disease is often asymptomatic in its early stages. As it progresses, cervical vertebrae deformity may produce severe, persistent neck pain, along with paresthesias and arm weakness or paralysis.

• *Rheumatoid arthritis.* This disorder most often affects peripheral joints, but it can also involve the cervical vertebrae. Acute inflammation may cause moderate to severe pain that radiates along a specific nerve root; increased warmth, swelling, and tenderness in involved joints; stiffness restricting range of motion; paresthesias and muscle weakness; low-grade fever; anorexia; malaise; and fatigue. Some pain and stiffness remain after the acute phase.

• *Spinous process fracture.* Fracture near the cervicothoracic junction produces

NECK PAIN: CAUSES AND ASSOCIATED FINDINGS (continued)

CAUSES	Arm pain	Back pain	Brudzinski's sign	Decreased LOC	Decreased range of motion	Deformity	Dysphagia	Dyspnea	Ecchymoses	Fatigue	Fever	Headache	Hemoptysis	Hoarseness
Meningitis			•	•							•	•		
Neck sprain					•					•				
Osteoporosis		•				•								
Paget's disease						•								
Rheumatoid arthritis					•						•	•		
Spinous process fracture					•	•								
Thyroid trauma								•	•					
Torticollis														
Tracheal trauma							•	•					•	•

acute pain radiating to the shoulders. Associated findings include swelling, exquisite tenderness, restricted range of motion, muscle spasms, and deformity.

• *Thyroid trauma.* Besides mild to moderate neck pain, thyroid trauma may cause local swelling and ecchymosis. If a hematoma forms, it can cause dyspnea.

• *Torticollis.* In this neck deformity, severe neck pain accompanies recurrent unilateral stiffness and muscle spasms that produce a characteristic head tilt.

• *Tracheal trauma. Fracture of the tracheal cartilage,* a life-threatening condition, produces moderate to severe neck pain and respiratory difficulty. *Torn tracheal mucosa* produces mild to moderate pain and may result in airway occlusion, hemoptysis, hoarseness, and dysphagia.

Special considerations
Promote patient comfort by giving anti-inflammatory drugs and analgesics, as ordered. Prepare him for diagnostic tests, such as X-rays, computed tomography scan, blood tests, and cerebrospinal fluid analysis.

Pediatric pointers
The most common causes of neck pain in children are meningitis and trauma. A rare cause of neck pain is congenital torticollis.

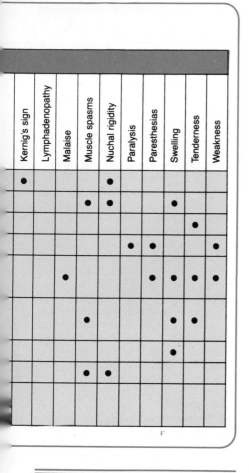

Night Blindness
[Nyctalopia]

Often difficult to identify, this symptom refers to impaired vision in the dark, especially after entering a darkened room or while driving at night. A symptom of choroidal and retinal degeneration, night blindness occurs in various ocular disorders and as an early indicator of vitamin A deficiency. In some patients, though, night blindness occurs without underlying pathology, simply reflecting poor adaptation to the dark. In these patients, it's often accompanied by myopia.

Assessment
If the patient complains of difficulty seeing at night, ask when he first noticed the problem. Is it intermittent or steadily worsening? Is it worse at certain times or in certain conditions? Also ask about other ocular symptoms, such as eye pain, blurred or halo vision, floaters or spots, and photophobia.

Explore any history of glaucoma, cataracts, and familial degeneration of vision. If no ocular problems are apparent, briefly evaluate the patient's nutritional status for possible vitamin A deficiency.

Examine the eyes for ptosis, abnormal tearing, discharge, and conjunctival injection. Test visual acuity and visual fields in both eyes and, if trained and equipped, measure intraocular pressure. Check pupillary response, and evaluate extraocular muscle function by testing the six cardinal fields of gaze.

Medical causes
• *Cataracts.* Night blindness and halo vision occur early in senile-type cataract formation. As the cataract matures, it causes gradual, painless visual blurring and vision loss, sometimes with visible lens opacity.

• *Choroidal dystrophies.* Night blindness and decreased peripheral vision may occur early in choroidal dystrophies. Disease progression causes loss of central vision.

• *Fundus albipunctatus.* Night blindness is the chief complaint in this retinal and choroidal disease. Multiple small, round, yellow-white dots are present on the retina.

• *Fundus flavimaculatus.* In this disease, night blindness may be pronounced or may be an incidental finding. Irregular yellow or white lesions appear deep in the retina.

• *Glaucoma.* Night blindness occurs late in chronic open-angle glaucoma, with halo vision, gradually impaired bilateral visual acuity, loss of peripheral vision, and possibly slight eye pain.

• *Goldman-Favre dystrophy.* In this disorder, night blindness is usually the chief complaint. The retina resembles that seen in retinitis pigmentosa.

• *Oguchi's disease.* This rare, hereditary retinal and choroidal degeneration produces night blindness and a retina with a yellowish metallic sheen.

• *Optic nerve atrophy.* This disorder may cause night blindness, visual field and color vision defects, and decreased visual acuity. Pupillary reactions are sluggish, and optic disk pallor is evident.

• *Retinitis pigmentosa.* In this hereditary retinal degeneration, night blindness is characteristically the first symptom, usually arising in adolescence. Scattered black pigmentary bodies form in a characteristic "bone-spicule" arrangement on the retina. As the disease progresses, the visual field gradually constricts, causing tunnel or "gun barrel" vision and eventually total blindness.

• *Vitamin A deficiency.* Night blindness is typically the first symptom of vitamin A deficiency. Associated findings may include xerophthalmia (conjunctival dryness) and Bitot's spots (gray-white conjunctival plaques). The patient may complain of visual blurring or vision loss. His skin may be dry and scaly. His mucous membranes may be shrunken and hardened.

Special considerations

Since any visual impairment is frightening to the patient, you'll need to provide emotional support. Help decrease his anxiety and enhance cooperation by explaining scheduled diagnostic tests, such as electroretinography, in simple terms.

Pediatric pointers

Since children generally don't have adequate body reserves of vitamin A, they're especially prone to deficiency and resulting night blindness.

Nipple Discharge

Nipple discharge can occur spontaneously or can be elicited by nipple stimulation. It's characterized as intermittent or constant, unilateral or bilateral, and by color, consistency, and composition. Its incidence increases with age and parity. This sign rarely occurs (but is more likely to be pathologic) in men and in nulligravid, regularly menstruating women. It's relatively common and often normal in parous women. A thick, grayish discharge—benign epithelial debris from inactive ducts—can often be elicited in middle-aged parous women. Colostrum, a thin, yellowish or milky discharge, often occurs in the last weeks of pregnancy.

Nipple discharge can signal serious underlying disease, particularly when accompanied by other breast changes. Significant causes include endocrine disorders, cancer, certain drugs, and blocked lactiferous ducts.

Assessment

Ask the patient when she first noticed the discharge, and determine its duration, extent, quantity, color, and consistency. Has she had other nipple and breast changes, such as pain, tenderness, itching, warmth, changes in contour, and lumps? If she reports a lump, question her about its onset, location, size, and consistency.

Obtain a complete gynecologic and obstetric history, and determine her normal menstrual cycle and the date of her last menses. Ask if she experiences breast swelling and tenderness, bloating, irritability, headaches, abdominal cramping, nausea, or diarrhea before or during menses. Note the number, date, and outcome of her pregnancies and, if she breastfed, the approximate time of her last lactation. Also check for any risk factors of breast cancer—family history, previous or current malignancies, nulliparity or first pregnancy after age 30, early menarche, or late menopause.

Start your physical examination by characterizing the discharge. If the discharge isn't frank, try to elicit it. (See *Eliciting Nipple Discharge*.) Then examine the nipples and breasts with the patient in four different positions: sitting with her arms at her sides, with her arms overhead, and with her hands pressing on her hips; and leaning forward so her breasts hang. Check for nipple deviation, flattening, retraction, redness, asymmetry, thickening, excoriation, erosion, or cracking. Inspect her breasts for asymmetry, irregular contours, dimpling, erythema, and peau d'orange. With the patient supine, palpate the breasts and axilla for lumps, giving special attention to the areolae. Note the size, location, delineation, consistency, and mobility of any lump you find.

Medical causes

• **Breast abscess.** This disorder, most common in lactating women, may produce a thick, purulent discharge from a cracked nipple or infected duct. Associated findings include abrupt onset of high fever with chills; breast pain, tenderness, and erythema; a palpable soft nodule or generalized induration; and possibly nipple retraction.

• **Breast cancer.** This may cause bloody, watery, or purulent discharge from a normal appearing nipple. More characteristic findings include a hard, irregular, fixed lump; erythema; dimpling; peau d'orange; changes in contour; nipple deviation, flattening, or retraction; axillary lymphadenopathy; and possibly breast pain.

• **Choriocarcinoma.** Galactorrhea (a white or grayish milky discharge) may result from this highly malignant neoplasm, which can follow pregnancy. Other characteristics include persistent uterine bleeding and bogginess after delivery or curettage.

• **Herpes zoster.** This virus can stimulate the thoracic nerves, causing bilateral, spontaneous, intermittent galactorrhea. Other characteristics: shooting or burning pain, eruption of small red nodules or vesicles on the thorax and possibly the arms and legs, pruritus and paresthesias or hyperesthesia in affected areas, and fever and malaise.

• **Hypothyroidism.** This disorder occasionally causes galactorrhea. Related findings include bradycardia; weight gain despite anorexia; decreased mentation; periorbital edema; puffy face, hands, and feet; brittle, sparse hair;

ELICITING NIPPLE DISCHARGE

If your patient has a history or evidence of nipple discharge, you can attempt to elicit it during your examination. Position the patient supine, and gently squeeze her nipple between your thumb and index finger; note any discharge through the nipple. Then place your fingers on the areola, as shown, and palpate the entire areolar surface, watching for any discharge through areolar ducts.

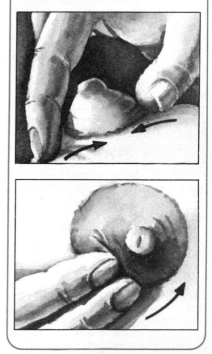

and dry, doughy, pale, cool skin.

● **Intraductal papilloma.** Unilateral serous, serosanguineous, or bloody nipple discharge is the predominant sign of this disorder. Discharge may be intermittent or profuse and constant, and can often be stimulated by gentle pressure around the areola. Subareolar nodules, breast pain, and tenderness may occur.

● **Mammary duct ectasia.** A thick, sticky, grayish discharge may be the first sign of this disorder; it may be bilateral and is usually spontaneous. Other findings include a rubbery, poorly delineated lump beneath the areola, with a blue-green discoloration of the overlying skin; nipple retraction and redness, swelling, tenderness, and burning pain in the areola and nipple.

● **Paget's disease.** Serous or bloody discharge emits from denuded skin on the nipple, which is red, intensely itchy, and possibly eroded or excoriated.

● **Prolactin-secreting pituitary tumor.** Bilateral galactorrhea may occur with this tumor. Other findings: amenorrhea, infertility, and decreased libido and vaginal secretions.

● **Proliferative (fibrocystic) breast disease.** This benign disorder occasionally causes bilateral clear, purulent, or bloody discharge. Multiple round, soft, tender nodules are usually palpable in both breasts, although they may occur singly. Usually, nodules are mobile. Nodule size, tenderness, and discharge increase during the luteal phase of the menstrual cycle.

● **Trauma.** Bilateral galactorrhea can result from trauma to the breasts.

Other causes

● **Drugs.** Galactorrhea can be caused by psychotropic agents, particularly phenothiazines and tricyclic antidepressants; some antihypertensives (reserpine and methyldopa); oral contraceptives; cimetidine; metoclopramide; and verapamil.

● **Surgery.** Chest wall surgery may stimulate the thoracic nerves, causing intermittent bilateral galactorrhea.

Special considerations

Although nipple discharge is usually insignificant, it can be very frightening to the patient. Help relieve her anxieties by clearly explaining the nature and origin of her discharge. Apply a breast binder, if ordered, which may reduce discharge by eliminating nipple stimulation.

Diagnostic tests may include tissue biopsy (if a breast lump is found), cytologic study of discharge, mammography, ultrasonography, transillumination, and serum prolactin.

Pediatric pointers

Nipple discharge in children and adolescents is rare. When it does occur, it's almost always nonpathologic, as in the bloody discharge that sometimes accompanies onset of menarche. Infants of both sexes may experience a milky breast discharge beginning 3 days after birth and lasting up to 2 weeks.

Nipple Retraction

Nipple retraction, the inward displacement of the nipple below the level of surrounding breast tissue, may indicate an inflammatory breast lesion or cancer. It results from scar tissue formation within a lesion or large mammary duct. As the scar tissue shortens, it pulls adjacent tissue in, causing nipple deviation, flattening, and finally retraction.

Assessment

Ask the patient when she first noticed retraction of the nipple. Has she experienced other nipple changes, such as itching, discoloration, discharge, or excoriation? Has she had breast pain, lumps, redness, swelling, or warmth? Obtain a history, noting risk factors of breast cancer, such as a family history or previous malignancy.

Carefully examine both nipples and breasts with the patient sitting upright

DIFFERENTIATING NIPPLE RETRACTION FROM INVERSION

Nipple retraction is often confused with nipple inversion, a common abnormality that's often congenital and doesn't usually signal underlying disease. A *retracted* nipple appears flat and broad, whereas an *inverted* nipple can be pulled out from the sulcus where it hides.

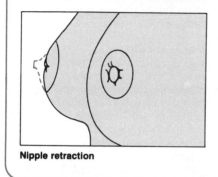

Nipple retraction

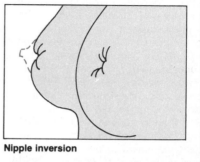

Nipple inversion

with her arms at her sides, with her hands pressing on her hips, and with her arms overhead; and with the patient leaning forward so her breasts hang. Look for redness, excoriation, and discharge; nipple flattening and deviation; and breast asymmetry, dimpling, or contour differences.

Try to evert the nipple by gently squeezing the areola. With the patient supine, palpate both breasts for lumps, especially beneath the areola. Mold breast skin over the lump or gently pull it up toward the clavicle, looking for accentuated nipple retraction. Also palpate axillary lymph nodes.

Medical causes
• *Breast abscess.* This disorder, most common in lactating women, occasionally produces unilateral nipple retraction. More frequent findings include high fever with chills; breast pain, erythema, and tenderness; breast induration or soft mass; and cracked, sore nipples, possibly with purulent discharge.
• *Breast cancer.* Unilateral nipple retraction is often accompanied by a hard, fixed nodule beneath the areola, as well as other breast nodules. Other nipple changes include itching, burning, erosion, and watery or bloody discharge. Breast changes commonly include dimpling, altered contour, peau d'orange, ulceration, tenderness (possibly pain), redness, and warmth. Axillary lymph nodes may be enlarged.
• *Fat necrosis.* This unlikely cause of nipple retraction closely mimics breast cancer, producing a firm, painless, irregular, fixed, benign nodule. Other findings: skin dimpling, tenderness, and ecchymoses.
• *Mammary duct ectasia.* Nipple retraction commonly occurs along with a poorly defined, rubbery nodule beneath the areola, with a blue-green skin discoloration; areolar burning, itching, swelling, tenderness, and erythema; and nipple pain with a thick, sticky, grayish discharge.
• *Mastitis.* Nipple retraction, deviation, cracking, or flattening may occur with a breast nodule, warmth, erythema, tenderness, and edema. Fatigue, high fevers, and chills may be present.

Special considerations
Prepare the patient for diagnostic tests, including mammography, cytology of nipple discharge, and biopsy.

Pediatric pointers
Nipple retraction doesn't occur in prepubescent females.

Nocturia

Nocturia—excessive urination at night—may result from disruption of the normal diurnal pattern of urine concentration or from overstimulation of the nerves and muscles that control urination. Normally, more urine is concentrated during the night than during the day. As a result, most persons excrete three to four times more urine during the day, and can sleep for 6 to 8 hours during the night without being awakened. In nocturia, the patient may awaken one or more times during the night to empty his bladder and excrete 700 ml or more of urine.

Although nocturia usually results from renal and lower urinary tract disorders, it may result from certain cardiovascular, endocrine, and metabolic disorders. This common sign may also result from drugs that induce diuresis, particularly when they're taken at night, and from the ingestion of large quantities of fluids, especially caffeinated beverages or alcohol, at bedtime.

Assessment

Begin your assessment by exploring the history of the patient's nocturia. When did it begin? How often does it occur? Can the patient identify a specific pattern? Precipitating factors? Also note the volume of urine voided. Ask the patient about any change in the color, odor, or consistency of his urine. Has he changed his usual pattern or volume of fluid intake? Next, explore associated symptoms. Ask about pain or burning on urination, difficulty initiating a urinary stream, costovertebral angle tenderness, and flank, upper abdominal, or suprapubic pain.

Determine if the patient or his family has a history of renal or urinary tract disorders or endocrine and metabolic diseases, particularly diabetes. Is the patient taking drugs that increase urinary output, such as diuretics, cardiac output, such as diuretics, cardiac glycosides, and antihypertensives?

Focus your physical examination on palpating and percussing the kidneys, the costovertebral angle, and the bladder. Carefully inspect the urinary meatus. Inspect a urine specimen for color, odor, and the presence of sediment.

Medical causes

• *Benign prostatic hypertrophy.* Common in men older than age 50, this disorder produces nocturia when significant urethral obstruction develops. Typically, it causes frequency, hesitancy, incontinence, reduced force and caliber of the urinary stream, and possibly hematuria. Oliguria may also occur. Palpation reveals a distended bladder and an enlarged prostate. The patient may also complain of lower abdominal fullness, perineal pain, and constipation.

• *Bladder neoplasm.* A late sign of this neoplasm, nocturia involves frequent voiding of small to moderate amounts of urine. Besides hematuria, the most common sign, associated characteristics include bladder distention; urinary frequency and urgency; dysuria; pyuria; bladder, rectal, flank, back, or leg pain; vomiting; diarrhea; and insomnia. Signs and symptoms of urinary tract infection, such as tenesmus, low-grade fever, and perineal pain, may also occur.

• *Congestive heart failure.* Nocturia may develop early here—the result of increased glomerular filtration associated with movement of edematous fluid from dependent areas during recumbency. Other early effects include fatigue, jugular vein distention, dyspnea, orthopnea, tachycardia, and a dry cough with wheezing. Later, the patient may develop tachypnea, weight gain, hypotension, oliguria, and cyanosis. He may also display marked hepatomegaly.

• *Cystitis.* All three forms of cystitis may cause nocturia marked by frequent, small voidings and accompanied by dysuria and tenesmus. *Bacterial cystitis* may also cause urinary urgency;

hematuria; fatigue; suprapubic, perineal, flank, and low back pain; and occasionally low-grade fever. Most common in women between the ages of 25 and 60, *chronic interstitial cystitis* is characterized by Hunner's ulcers— small, punctate, bleeding lesions in the bladder; it also causes gross hematuria. *Viral cystitis* also causes urinary urgency, hematuria, and fever.

• *Diabetes insipidus.* The result of antidiuretic hormone deficiency, this disorder usually produces nocturia early in its course. It's characterized by periodic voiding of moderate to large amounts of urine. Diabetes insipidus can also produce polydipsia.

• *Diabetes mellitus.* An early sign of diabetes mellitus, nocturia involves frequent, large voidings. Associated features include daytime polyuria, polydipsia, polyphagia, weakness, fatigue, weight loss, and, possibly, signs of dehydration, such as dry mucous membranes and poor skin turgor.

• *Hypercalcemic nephropathy.* In this disorder, nocturia involves the periodic voiding of moderate to large amounts of urine. Related findings: daytime polyuria, polydipsia, and occasionally hematuria and pyuria.

• *Hypokalemic nephropathy.* Again, nocturia involves the periodic voiding of moderate to large amounts of urine. Associated findings typically include polydipsia, daytime polyuria, muscle weakness or paralysis, and hypoactive bowel sounds.

• *Prostatic neoplasm.* The second leading cause of cancer deaths in men, this disorder is usually asymptomatic in early stages. Later, it produces nocturia characterized by infrequent voiding of moderate amounts of urine. Other characteristic effects include dysuria (most common symptom), difficulty initiating a urinary stream, bladder distention, urinary frequency, weight loss, pallor, weakness, perineal pain, and constipation. Palpation reveals a hard, irregularly shaped prostate.

• *Pyelonephritis (acute).* Nocturia occurs frequently in this inflammatory disorder; it's usually characterized by infrequent voiding of moderate amounts of urine. The urine may appear cloudy. Associated signs and symptoms include a high, sustained fever with chills, fatigue, flank pain, costovertebral angle tenderness, weakness, dysuria, hematuria, urinary frequency and urgency, and tenesmus. Occasionally, anorexia, nausea, vomiting, and hypoactive bowel sounds may also occur.

• *Renal failure (chronic).* Nocturia occurs relatively early in this disorder and is usually characterized by infrequent voiding of moderate amounts of urine. As the disorder progresses, oliguria or even anuria develops. Other widespread effects of chronic renal failure include fatigue, ammonia breath odor, Kussmaul's respirations, peripheral edema, elevated blood pressure, decreased level of consciousness, muscle twitching, anorexia, constipation or diarrhea, petechiae, ecchymoses, pruritus, yellow- or bronze-tinged skin, nausea, and vomiting.

Other causes

• *Drugs.* Any drug that mobilizes edematous fluid or produces diuresis (for example, diuretics and cardiac glycosides) may cause nocturia; obviously, this effect depends on when the drug is administered.

Special considerations

Nursing care includes maintaining fluid balance, ensuring adequate rest, and providing patient education. Monitor vital signs, intake and output, and daily weight; continue to document the frequency of nocturia, amount, and specific gravity. Plan administration of diuretics for daytime hours, if possible. Also plan rest periods to compensate for sleep lost because of nocturia.

Prepare the patient for diagnostic tests, which may include routine urinalysis, urine concentration and dilution studies, and serum blood urea nitrogen, creatinine, and electrolyte levels.

Pediatric pointers

In children, nocturia may be voluntary or involuntary. The latter is commonly known as enuresis, or bedwetting. With the exception of prostate disorders, causes of nocturia are generally the same for children and adults.

Nuchal Rigidity

Frequently an early sign of meningeal irritation, nuchal rigidity refers to profound stiffness of the neck that prevents flexion. To elicit this sign, attempt to passively flex the patient's neck and touch his chin to his chest. In nuchal rigidity, this maneuver triggers pain and muscle spasms. The patient may also notice nuchal rigidity when he attempts to flex his neck during daily activities.

This sign may herald life-threatening subarachnoid hemorrhage or meningitis. It may also be a late sign of cervical arthritis, in which joint mobility is gradually lost. Transient, mild neck stiffness may accompany muscle tension, muscle spasms, or myalgia, and must be differentiated from true nuchal rigidity.

Assessment

After eliciting nuchal rigidity, notify the doctor immediately, and attempt to elicit Kernig's and Brudzinski's signs. Quickly assess the patient's level of consciousness and take his vital signs. Note signs of increased intracranial pressure, such as increased systolic pressure, bradycardia, and widened pulse pressure. If these signs are present, start an I.V. for drug administration and deliver oxygen, as necessary. Draw a specimen for routine blood studies, as ordered.

Next, obtain a patient history, relying on family members if altered consciousness prevents the patient from responding. Ask about the onset and duration of neck stiffness. Were there any precipitating factors? Also ask about associated symptoms, such as headache, fever, nausea and vomiting, and motor and sensory changes. Check for a history of hypertension, head trauma, cerebral aneurysm or arteriovenous malformation, endocarditis, recent infection (especially tooth abscess), or recent dental work. Then, obtain a complete drug history.

If the patient has no other signs of meningeal irritation, ask about a history of arthritis or neck trauma. Can the patient recall pulling a muscle in his neck? Inspect the patient's hands for swollen, tender joints, and palpate the neck for pain or tenderness.

Medical causes

● *Cervical arthritis.* In this disorder, nuchal rigidity develops gradually. Initially, the patient may complain of neck stiffness in the early morning or after a period of inactivity. Stiffness then becomes increasingly severe and frequent. Pain on movement, especially with lateral motion or head turning, is common. Typically, arthritis also affects other joints, especially in the hands.

● *Encephalitis.* This viral infection may cause nuchal rigidity accompanied by other signs of meningeal irritation, such as positive Kernig's and Brudzinski's signs. Usually, nuchal rigidity appears abruptly and is preceded by headache, vomiting, and fever. The patient may display a rapidly decreasing level of consciousness, progressing from lethargy to coma within 24 to 48 hours of onset. Associated features include seizures, ataxia, hemiparesis, nystagmus, and cranial nerve palsies, such as dysphagia and ptosis.

● *Meningitis.* Nuchal rigidity is an early sign in this disorder. It's accompanied by other signs of meningeal irritation—positive Kernig's and Brudzinski's signs, hyperreflexia, and possibly opisthotonos. Other early features include fever with chills, headache, photophobia, and vomiting. Initially, the patient is confused and irritable; later, he may become stuporous and seizure-prone or may slip into coma. Cranial nerve involvement may cause ocular palsies, facial weakness, and hearing loss. An erythematous papular rash occurs in some forms of viral meningitis, while a purpuric rash may occur in meningococcal meningitis.

• *Subarachnoid hemorrhage.* In this acute disorder, nuchal rigidity develops immediately after bleeding into the subarachnoid space. Examination may detect positive Kernig's and Brudzinski's signs. Typically, the patient experiences abrupt onset of severe headache, photophobia, fever, nausea and vomiting, dizziness, cranial nerve palsies, and focal neurologic signs, such as hemiparesis or hemiplegia. His level of consciousness deteriorates rapidly, possibly progressing to coma. Signs of increased intracranial pressure, such as bradycardia and altered respiratory pattern, may also occur.

Special considerations
Prepare the patient for diagnostic tests, such as computed tomography scans and cervical spinal X-rays.

Monitor the patient's vital signs, intake and output, and neurologic status closely. Avoid routine administration of narcotic analgesics, since they may mask signs of increasing intracranial pressure. Enforce strict bed rest; keep the head of the patient's bed elevated at least 30° to help reduce intracranial pressure.

Pediatric pointers
Nuchal rigidity is a reliable sign of meningeal irritation in children.

Nystagmus

Nystagmus refers to the involuntary oscillations of one or—more commonly—both eyeballs. These oscillations are usually rhythmical and may be horizontal, vertical, or rotary. They may be transient or sustained and may occur spontaneously or on deviation or fixation of the eyes. Although nystagmus is fairly easy to identify, the patient may be unaware of it unless it affects his vision.

Nystagmus may be classified as pendular or jerk. *Pendular nystagmus* consists of horizontal (pendular) or vertical (seesaw) oscillations that are equal in both directions and resemble the movements of a clock's pendulum. *Jerk nystagmus* (convergence-retraction, downbeat, and vestibular) has a fast component and then a slow—perhaps unequal—corrective component in the opposite direction (see *Classifying Nystagmus,* page 526).

Nystagmus is considered a *supranuclear* ocular palsy. That is, it results from pathology in the visual perceptual area, vestibular system, cerebellum, or brain stem rather than in the extraocular muscles or cranial nerves III, IV, and VI. Its causes are varied and include brain stem or cerebellar lesions, multiple sclerosis, encephalitis, labyrinthine disease, and drug toxicity. Occasionally, nystagmus is entirely normal; it's also considered a normal response in the unconscious patient during the doll's eye test (oculocephalic stimulation) or the cold caloric water test (oculovestibular stimulation).

Assessment
Begin by asking the patient how long he's had nystagmus. Does it occur intermittently? Does it affect his vision? Ask about recent infection, especially of the ear or respiratory tract, and about head trauma and cancer. Does the patient or anyone in his family have a history of cerebrovascular accident (CVA)? Then explore associated signs and symptoms. Ask about vertigo, dizziness, tinnitus, nausea or vomiting, numbness, weakness, bladder dysfunction, and fever.

Begin the physical examination by assessing the patient's level of consciousness and vital signs. Be alert for signs of increased intracranial pres-

CLASSIFYING NYSTAGMUS

JERK NYSTAGMUS

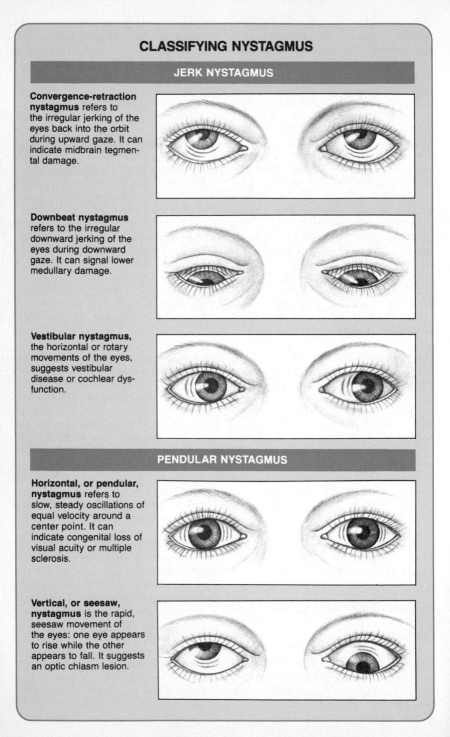

Convergence-retraction nystagmus refers to the irregular jerking of the eyes back into the orbit during upward gaze. It can indicate midbrain tegmental damage.

Downbeat nystagmus refers to the irregular downward jerking of the eyes during downward gaze. It can signal lower medullary damage.

Vestibular nystagmus, the horizontal or rotary movements of the eyes, suggests vestibular disease or cochlear dysfunction.

PENDULAR NYSTAGMUS

Horizontal, or pendular, nystagmus refers to slow, steady oscillations of equal velocity around a center point. It can indicate congenital loss of visual acuity or multiple sclerosis.

Vertical, or seesaw, nystagmus is the rapid, seesaw movement of the eyes: one eye appears to rise while the other appears to fall. It suggests an optic chiasm lesion.

sure, such as pupillary changes, drowsiness, elevated systolic pressure, and altered respiratory pattern. Next, assess nystagmus fully by testing extraocular muscle function: ask the patient to focus straight ahead and then to follow your finger up, down, and in an "X" across his face. Note when nystagmus occurs, as well as its velocity and direction. Finally, test reflexes, motor and sensory function, and the cranial nerves.

Medical causes

● *Brain tumor.* Insidious onset of jerk nystagmus may occur with tumors of the brain stem and cerebellum. Associated characteristics include deafness, dysphagia, nausea and vomiting, vertigo, and ataxia. Brain stem compression by the tumor may cause signs of increased intracranial pressure, such as altered level of consciousness, bradycardia, widening pulse pressure, and elevated systolic blood pressure.

● *Cerebrovascular accident.* A CVA involving the posterior inferior cerebellar artery may cause sudden horizontal or vertical jerk nystagmus that may be gaze-dependent. Other findings include dysphagia, dysarthria, loss of pain and temperature sensation on the ipsilateral face and contralateral trunk and limbs, ipsilateral Horner's syndrome (unilateral ptosis, pupillary constriction, and facial anhidrosis), and cerebellar signs, such as ataxia and vertigo. Signs of increased intracranial pressure, such as altered level of consciousness, bradycardia, widening pulse pressure, and elevated systolic pressure, may also occur.

● *Encephalitis.* In this disorder, jerk nystagmus is typically accompanied by altered level of consciousness, ranging from lethargy to coma. Usually, it's preceded by sudden onset of fever, headache, and vomiting. Among other features are nuchal rigidity, seizures, aphasia, ataxia, photophobia, and cranial nerve palsies, such as dysphagia and ptosis.

● *Head trauma.* Brain stem injury may cause jerk nystagmus, which is usually horizontal. The patient may also display pupillary changes, altered respiratory pattern, coma, and decerebrate posture.

● *Labyrinthitis (acute).* This inner ear inflammation causes sudden onset of jerk nystagmus, accompanied by dizziness, vertigo, tinnitus, nausea, and vomiting. The fast component of the nystagmus is toward the unaffected ear. Gradual sensorineural hearing loss may also occur.

● *Ménière's disease.* This inner ear disorder is characterized by acute attacks of jerk nystagmus, severe nausea and vomiting, dizziness, vertigo, progressive hearing loss, tinnitus, and diaphoresis. Typically, the direction of jerk nystagmus varies from one attack to the next. Attacks may last from 10 minutes to several hours.

● *Multiple sclerosis.* In this disorder, jerk or pendular nystagmus may occur intermittently. Usually, it's preceded by diplopia, blurred vision, and paresthesias. Related signs and symptoms may include muscle weakness or paralysis, spasticity, hyperreflexia, intention tremor, gait ataxia, dysphagia, dysarthria, impotence, and emotional instability. The patient may also have constipation, and urinary frequency, urgency, and incontinence.

Other causes

● *Drugs and alcohol.* Jerk nystagmus may result from barbiturate, phenytoin, or carbamazepine toxicity or from alcohol intoxication.

Special considerations

Prepare the patient for diagnostic tests, such as electronystagmography and a cerebral computed tomography scan.

Pediatric pointers

In children, pendular nystagmus may be idiopathic, or it may sometimes result from early impaired vision associated with such disorders as optic atrophy, albinism, congenital cataracts, and severe astigmatism.

ocular deviation • oligomenorrhea • oliguria • opisthotonos • orofacial dyskin
orthostatic hypotension • Ortolani's sign • Osler's nodes • otorrhea • pallor • p
rash • paralysis • paresthesias • paroxysmal nocturnal dyspnea • peau d'oran
rub • peristaltic waves—visible • photophobia • pica • pleural friction rub • p
polyuria • postnasal drip • priapism • pruritus • psoas sign • psychotic beha
absent or weak • pulse—bounding • pulse pressure—narrowed • pulse press
rhythm abnormality • pulsus alternans • pulsus bisferiens • pulsus paradoxu
pupils—sluggish • purple striae • purpura • pustular rash • pyrosis • raccoo
tenderness • rectal pain • retractions—costal and sternal • rhinorrhea • rhon
salivation—decreased • salivation—increased • salt craving • scotoma • scrot
absence • seizure—focal • seizure—generalized tonic-clonic • seizure—psych
sign • shallow respirations • skin—bronze • skin—clammy • skin—mottled •
turgor—decreased • spider angioma • splenomegaly • stertorous respirations
stridor • syncope • tachycardia • tachypnea • taste abnormalities • tearing—i
tic • tinnitus • tracheal deviation • tracheal tugging • tremors • trismus • tu
frost • urethral discharge • urinary frequency • urinary hesitancy • urinary i
urgency • urine cloudiness • urticaria • vaginal bleeding—postmenopausal •
venous hum • vertigo • vesicular rash • violent behavior • vision loss • visual
floaters • vomiting • vulvar lesions • weight gain—excessive • weight loss—e
wristdrop • abdominal distention • abdominal mass • abdominal pain • abd
accessory muscle use • agitation • alopecia • amenorrhea • amnesia • analge
anorexia • anosmia • anuria • anxiety • aphasia • apnea • apneustic respira
pain • asterixis • ataxia • athetosis • aura • Babinski's reflex • back pain • b
sign • Biot's respirations • bladder distention • blood pressure decrease • blo
bowel sounds—absent • bowel sounds—hyperactive • bowel sounds—hypoa
bradypnea • breast dimpling • breast nodule • breast pain • breast ulcer • b
odor • breath with fecal odor • breath with fruity odor • Brudzinski's sign •
butterfly rash • café-au-lait spots • capillary refill time—prolonged • carpope
chest expansion—asymmetrical • chest pain • Cheyne-Stokes respirations • c
sign • clubbing • cogwheel rigidity • cold intolerance • confusion • conjunct
constipation • corneal reflex—absent • costovertebral angle tenderness • cou
nonproductive • cough—productive • crackles • crepitation—bony • crepitat
cry—high-pitched • cyanosis • decerebrate posture • decorticate posture • d
hyperactive ^ deep tendon reflexes—hypoactive • depression • diaphoresis •
dizziness • doll's eye sign—absent • drooling • dysarthria • dysmenorrhea •
dyspepsia • dysphagia • dyspnea • dystonia • dysuria • earache • edema—g
arms • edema of the face • edema of the legs • enophthalmos • enuresis • e
erythema • exophthalmos • eye discharge • eye pain • facial pain • fascicul
incontinence • fetor hepaticus • fever • flank pain • flatulence • fontanelle b
depression • footdrop • gag reflex abnormalities • gait—bizarre • gait—pro
gait—spastic • gait—steppage • gait—waddling • gallop—atrial • gallop—v
n the male • grunting respirations • gum bleeding • gum swelling • gyneco
vision • headache • hearing loss • heat intolerance • Heberden's nodes • hen
hematochezia • hematuria • hemianopia • hemoptysis • hepatomegaly • hic
hoarseness • Homans' sign • hyperpigmentation • hyperpnea • hypopigmen
insomnia • intermittent claudication • Janeway's spots • jaundice • jaw pai
distention • Kehr's sign • Kernig's sign • leg pain • level of consciousness—
lashes • low birth weight • lymphadenopathy • masklike facies • McBurney
sign • melena • menorrhagia • metrorrhagia • miosis • moon face • mouth
muscle atrophy • muscle flaccidity • muscle spasms • muscle spasticity • m

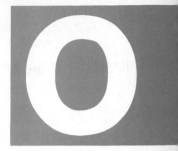

Ocular Deviation

Ocular deviation refers to abnormal eye movement that may be *conjugate* (both eyes move together) or *dysconjugate* (one eye moves differently from the other). This common sign may result from ocular, neurologic, endocrine, and systemic disorders that interfere with the muscles, nerves, or brain centers governing eye movement. Occasionally, it signals a life-threatening disorder, such as ruptured cerebral aneurysm (see *Ocular Deviation: Its Characteristics and Causes in Cranial Nerve Damage*, page 530).

Normally, eye movement is directly controlled by the extraocular muscles innervated by the oculomotor, trochlear, and abducens nerves (cranial nerves III, IV, and VI). Together, these muscles and nerves direct a visual stimulus to fall on corresponding parts of the retina. Dysconjugate ocular deviation may result from unequal muscle tone (nonparalytic strabismus) or from muscle paralysis associated with cranial nerve damage (paralytic strabismus). Conjugate ocular deviation may result from disorders that affect the centers in the cerebral cortex and brain stem responsible for conjugate eye movement. Typically, such disorders cause *gaze palsy*—difficulty moving the eyes in one or more directions.

Assessment

If the patient displays ocular deviation, quickly take his vital signs and assess for altered level of consciousness, pupil changes, motor or sensory dysfunction, and severe headache. If possible, ask the patient's family about behavioral changes. Is there a history of recent head trauma? Notify the doctor at once if you suspect an acute neurologic disorder. Prepare to assist with respiratory support, if necessary. Also prepare the patient for emergency neurologic tests, such as a computed tomography scan.

If the patient isn't in distress, find out how long he's had the ocular deviation. Is it accompanied by double vision, eye pain, or headache? Also ask if he's noticed any associated motor or sensory changes, or fever.

Check for a history of hypertension, diabetes, allergies, and thyroid, neurologic, or muscular disorders. Then obtain a thorough ocular history. Has the patient ever had extraocular muscle imbalance, eye or head trauma, or eye surgery?

During the physical examination, observe the patient for partial or complete ptosis. Does he spontaneously tilt his head or turn his face to compensate for ocular deviation? Check for eye redness or periorbital edema. Assess visual acuity, then evaluate extraocular

OCULAR DEVIATION: ITS CHARACTERISTICS AND CAUSES IN CRANIAL NERVE DAMAGE

CHARACTERISTICS	CRANIAL NERVE AND EXTRAOCULAR MUSCLES INVOLVED	PROBABLE CAUSES
Inability to focus the eye upward, downward, inward, and outward; drooping eyelid; and, except in diabetes, a dilated pupil in the affected eye	Oculomotor nerve (III); medial rectus, superior rectus, inferior rectus, and inferior oblique muscles	Cerebral aneurysm, diabetes, temporal lobe herniation from increased intracranial pressure, brain tumor
Loss of downward and outward movement in the affected eye	Trochlear nerve (IV), superior oblique muscle	Head trauma
Loss of outward movement in the affected eye	Abducens nerve (VI), lateral rectus muscle	Brain tumor

muscle function by testing the six cardinal fields of gaze.

Medical causes

• *Brain tumor.* Ocular deviation varies, depending upon the site and extent of the tumor. Associated signs and symptoms may include headache that's most severe in the morning, behavioral changes, memory loss, dizziness, confusion, vision loss, motor and sensory dysfunction, aphasia, and possibly signs of hormonal imbalance. The patient's level of consciousness may slowly deteriorate from lethargy to coma. Late signs include papilledema, vomiting, increased systolic blood pressure, widening pulse pressure, and decorticate posture.

• *Cavernous sinus thrombosis.* In this disorder, ocular deviation may be accompanied by diplopia, photophobia, exophthalmos, orbital and eyelid edema, corneal haziness, diminished or absent pupillary reflexes, and impaired visual acuity. Other features may include high fever, headache, malaise, nausea and vomiting, convulsions, and tachycardia. Retinal hemorrhages and papilledema are late signs.

• *Cerebral aneurysm.* When an aneurysm near the internal carotid artery compresses the oculomotor nerve, it may produce features that resemble third cranial nerve palsy. Typically, ocular deviation and diplopia are the presenting signs. Other cardinal findings include ptosis, a dilated pupil on the affected side, and a severe, unilateral headache, usually in the frontal area. Rupture of the aneurysm abruptly intensifies the pain, which may be accompanied by nausea and vomiting. Bleeding from the site causes meningeal irritation, resulting in nuchal rigidity, back and leg pain, fever, irritability, occasional seizures, and blurred vision. There may also be hemiparesis, dysphagia, visual defects, and other signs and symptoms associated with intracranial bleeding.

• *Cerebrovascular accident.* This life-threatening disorder may cause ocular deviation, depending on the site and extent of the stroke. Accompanying features are also variable and may include altered level of consciousness, contralateral hemiplegia and sensory loss, dysarthria, dysphagia, homonymous hemianopia, blurred vision, and diplopia. There may also be urinary retention and/or incontinence, constipation, behavioral changes, headache, vomiting, and seizures.

• *Diabetes mellitus.* A leading cause of isolated third cranial nerve palsy, especially in the middle-aged patient with longstanding mild diabetes, this disorder may cause ocular deviation and ptosis. Typically, the patient also complains of sudden onset of diplopia and pain.

• *Encephalitis.* This infection causes ocular deviation and diplopia in some patients. Typically, it begins abruptly with fever, headache, and vomiting, followed by signs of meningeal irritation, such as nuchal rigidity, and of neuronal damage, such as seizures, aphasia, ataxia, hemiparesis, cranial nerve palsies, and photophobia. The patient's level of consciousness may rapidly deteriorate from lethargy to coma within 24 to 48 hours after onset.

• *Head trauma.* Ocular deviation varies with the site and extent of head trauma. The patient may have visible soft tissue injury, bony deformity, facial edema, and clear or bloody otorrhea or rhinorrhea. Besides these obvious signs of trauma, he may also have blurred vision, diplopia, nystagmus, behavioral changes, headache, motor and sensory dysfunction, and a decreased level of consciousness that may progress to coma. Signs of increased intracranial pressure—such as bradycardia, increased systolic pressure, and widening pulse pressure—may also occur.

• *Multiple sclerosis.* Ocular deviation may be an early sign of this disorder. Accompanying it are diplopia, blurred vision, and sensory dysfunction, such as paresthesias. Other signs and symptoms may include nystagmus, constipation, muscle weakness, paralysis, spasticity, hyperreflexia, intention tremor, gait ataxia, dysphagia, dysarthria, impotence, and emotional instability. There may also be urinary frequency, urgency, and incontinence.

• *Myasthenia gravis.* In this disorder, ocular deviation may accompany the more common presenting signs of diplopia and ptosis. This disorder may affect only the eye muscles or may progress to other muscle groups, causing altered facial expression, difficulty chewing, dysphagia, weakened voice, and impaired fine hand movements. Signs of respiratory distress reflect weakness of the diaphragm and other respiratory muscles.

• *Ophthalmoplegic migraine.* Most common in young adults, this disorder produces ocular deviation and diplopia that persist for days after the pain subsides. Associated signs and symptoms include unilateral headache, possibly with ptosis on the same side; temporary hemiplegia; and sensory deficits. Irritability, depression, or slight confusion may also occur.

• *Orbital blow-out fracture.* In this fracture, the inferior rectus muscle may become entrapped, resulting in limited extraocular movements and ocular deviation. Typically, the patient's upward gaze is absent; other directions of gaze may be affected if edema is dramatic. The globe may also be displaced downward and inward. Associated signs and symptoms include pain, diplopia, nausea, periorbital edema, and ecchymosis.

• *Orbital cellulitis.* This disorder may cause sudden onset of ocular deviation and diplopia. Other signs and symptoms include unilateral eyelid edema and erythema, hyperemia, chemosis, and extreme orbital pain. Purulent discharge makes eyelashes matted and sticky. Proptosis is a late sign.

• *Orbital tumor.* Ocular deviation occurs as the tumor gradually enlarges. Associated findings include proptosis, diplopia, and possibly blurred vision.

• *Thyrotoxicosis.* This disorder may produce exophthalmos—proptotic or protruding eyes—which, in turn, causes limited extraocular movements and ocular deviation. Usually, the patient's upward gaze weakens first, followed by diplopia. Other features are lid retraction, a wide-eyed staring gaze, excessive tearing, edematous eyelids, and, sometimes, inability to close the eyes. Cardinal features of thyrotoxicosis include tachycardia, palpitations, weight loss despite increased appetite, diarrhea, tremors, an enlarged thyroid, dyspnea, nervousness, diaphoresis, heat intolerance, and an atrial or ventricular gallop.

Special considerations

Continue to monitor the patient's vital signs and neurologic status if you suspect an acute neurologic disorder. Take seizure precautions, if necessary. Also prepare the patient for diagnostic tests, such as blood studies, orbital and skull X-rays, and computed tomography scan.

Pediatric pointers

In children, the most common cause of ocular deviation is nonparalytic strabismus. Normally, children achieve binocular vision by age 3 to 4 months. Although severe strabismus is readily apparent, mild strabismus must be confirmed by tests for misalignment, such as the corneal light reflex test and the cover test. Testing is crucial—early corrective measures help preserve binocular vision and cosmetic appearance. Also, mild strabismus may indicate retinoblastoma, a tumor that may be asymptomatic before age 2, except for a characteristic whitish reflex in the pupil.

Oligomenorrhea

In most women, menstrual bleeding occurs every 28 days plus or minus 4 days. Although some variation is normal, menstrual bleeding at intervals of greater than 36 days may indicate oligomenorrhea—abnormally infrequent menstrual bleeding characterized by three to six menstrual cycles per year. When menstrual bleeding does occur, it's usually profuse (greater than 70 ml), prolonged (up to 10 days), and laden with clots and tissue. Occasionally, scant bleeding or spotting occurs between these heavy menses. Oligomenorrhea may develop suddenly or after a period of gradually lengthening cycles. Although this sign may alternate with normal menstrual bleeding, it can progress to secondary amenorrhea.

Because oligomenorrhea is frequently associated with anovulation, it's common in infertile, early postmenarchal, and perimenopausal women. Usually, this sign reflects abnormalities of the hormones that govern normal proliferation and shedding of the endometrium. It may result from ovarian, pituitary, and other metabolic disorders and from the effects of certain drugs. It may also result from emotional or physical stress—such as sudden weight change, debilitating illness, or rigorous physical training.

Assessment

After asking the patient how old she is, find out when menarche occurred. Has the patient ever experienced normal menstrual cycles? When did she begin having abnormal cycles? Ask her to describe the pattern of bleeding. How many days does the bleeding last, and how frequently does it occur? Are there clots and tissue fragments in her menstrual flow? Note when she last had menstrual bleeding.

Next, determine if she's having symptoms of ovulatory bleeding. Does she experience mild, cramping abdominal pain 14 days before she bleeds? Is the bleeding accompanied by premenstrual symptoms, such as breast tenderness, irritability, bloating, weight gain, nausea, and diarrhea? Does she have cramping or pain with bleeding? Also check for a history of infertility. Does the patient have any children? Is she trying to conceive? Ask if she's currently using oral contraceptives or if she's ever used them in the past. If she has, find out when she stopped taking them.

Then ask about previous gynecologic disorders, such as ovarian cysts. If the patient's breastfeeding, has she experienced any problems with milk production? If she hasn't been breastfeeding recently, has she noticed milk leaking from her breasts? Ask about recent weight gain or loss. Is the patient less than 80% of her ideal weight? If so, does she claim that she's overweight? Ask if she's exercising more vigorously than usual.

Screen for metabolic disorders by asking about excessive thirst, frequent urination, or fatigue. Has the patient been jittery or had palpitations? Ask about headache, dizziness, and impaired peripheral vision. Complete the history by finding out what drugs the patient is taking.

Begin the physical examination by taking the patient's vital signs and weighing her. Inspect for increased facial hair growth, sparse body hair, male distribution of fat and muscle, acne, and clitoral enlargement. Note if the skin is abnormally dry or moist, and check hair texture. Also be alert for signs of psychological or physical stress.

Medical causes

• *Adrenal hyperplasia.* In this disorder, oligomenorrhea may be accompanied by signs of androgen excess, such as clitoral enlargement and male distribution of hair, fat, and muscle mass. If this disorder is congenital, the patient may have never had normal menses.

• *Anorexia nervosa.* Anorexia nervosa may cause sporadic oligomenorrhea or amenorrhea. Its cardinal symptom, though, is a morbid fear of being fat associated with weight loss of more than 20% of ideal body weight. Typically, the patient displays dramatic skeletal muscle atrophy and loss of fatty tissue; dry or sparse scalp hair; lanugo on the face and body; and blotchy or sallow, dry skin. Other features may include constipation, sleep disturbances, hypotension, bradycardia, and cold intolerance.

• *Diabetes mellitus.* Oligomenorrhea

may be an early sign in this disorder. In juvenile-onset diabetes, the patient may have never had normal menses. Associated signs and symptoms include excessive hunger, polydipsia, polyuria, weakness, fatigue, dry mucous membranes, poor skin turgor, and weight loss.

• *Polycystic ovary disease.* Close to one quarter of women with polycystic ovary disease have oligomenorrhea; however, some may have amenorrhea, menometrorrhagia, or irregular menses. Infertility and enlarged, palpable ovaries are also common. Other features vary but may include signs of androgen excess—male distribution of body hair and muscle mass, facial hair growth, acne, and, occasionally, obesity.

• *Prolactin-secreting pituitary tumor.* Oligomenorrhea or amenorrhea may be the first sign of a prolactin-secreting pituitary tumor. Accompanying signs and symptoms include bilateral galactorrhea, infertility, loss of libido, and sparse pubic hair. Headache and visual field disturbances—such as diminished peripheral vision, blurred vision, diplopia, and hemianopia—signal tumor expansion.

• *Sheehan's syndrome.* This pituitary disorder usually follows severe obstetrical hemorrhage. Oligomenorrhea or amenorrhea may be accompanied by failure to lactate, sparse pubic and axillary hair, decreased libido, and fatigue.

• *Thyrotoxicosis.* This disorder may produce oligomenorrhea accompanied by reduced fertility. Its cardinal signs and symptoms include nervousness, irritability, weight loss despite increased appetite, dyspnea, tachycardia, palpitations, diarrhea, tremors, diaphoresis, heat intolerance, an enlarged thyroid, and possibly exophthalmos. An S_3 or S_4 gallop may also occur.

Other causes

• *Drugs.* Drugs that increase androgen levels—such as corticosteroids, ACTH, anabolic steroids, and danocrine—may cause oligomenorrhea. Oral contraceptives may be associated with delayed resumption of normal menses when their use is discontinued; however, 95% of women resume normal menses within 3 months. Other drugs that may cause oligomenorrhea include phenothiazine derivatives and amphetamines.

Special considerations

Prepare the patient for diagnostic tests, such as blood hormone levels, thyroid studies, and computed tomography scan. The patient also may be asked to record her basal body temperature to determine if she's having ovulatory cycles. Provide her with blank charts, and teach her how to keep them accurately.

Remind the patient that she can still become pregnant even though she isn't menstruating normally. Discuss contraceptive measures, as appropriate.

Pediatric pointers

Teenage girls may experience oligomenorrhea associated with immature hormonal function. However, prolonged oligomenorrhea or the development of amenorrhea may signal congenital adrenal hyperplasia or Turner's syndrome.

Oliguria

A cardinal sign of renal and urinary tract disorders, oliguria is clinically defined as urinary output of less than 400 ml per 24 hours. Typically, this sign occurs abruptly and may herald serious—possibly life-threatening—hemodynamic instability. Its causes can be classified as prerenal (decreased renal blood flow), intrarenal (intrinsic renal damage), or postrenal (urinary tract obstruction); the pathophysiology differs for each classification (see *How Oliguria Develops,* pages 536 and 537). Oliguria associated with a prerenal or postrenal cause is usually promptly reversible with treatment, although it may lead to intrarenal damage if untreated. However, oliguria associated with an intrarenal cause is usually more persistent and may be irreversible.

Assessment

Begin by asking the patient about his usual daily voiding pattern, including frequency and amount. When did he first notice changes in this pattern and in the color, odor, or consistency of his urine? Ask about pain or burning on urination. Note his normal daily fluid intake. Has he recently been drinking more or less? Has he had recent episodes of diarrhea or vomiting that might cause fluid loss? Next, explore associated complaints, especially fatigue, loss of appetite, thirst, dyspnea, chest pain, or recent weight gain.

Check for a history of renal, urinary tract, or cardiovascular disorders. Note recent traumatic injury or surgery associated with significant blood loss, as well as recent blood transfusions. Was the patient exposed to nephrotoxic agents, such as heavy metals, organic solvents, anesthetics, or radiographic contrast media? Next, obtain a drug history.

Begin the physical examination by taking the patient's vital signs and weighing him. Assess his overall appearance for edema. Palpate both kidneys for tenderness and enlargement, and percuss for costovertebral angle (CVA) tenderness. Also inspect the flank area for edema or erythema. Auscultate the heart and lungs for abnormal sounds, and over the periumbilical area for renal artery bruits.

As ordered, obtain a urine sample and inspect it for abnormal color, odor, or sediment. Use reagent strips to test for glucose, protein, and blood. Also, use a urinometer to measure specific gravity.

Medical causes

• *Acute tubular necrosis (ATN).* An early sign of ATN, oliguria may occur abruptly (in shock) or gradually (in nephrotoxicity). Usually, it persists for about 2 weeks, followed by polyuria. Related features may include signs of hyperkalemia (muscle weakness and cardiac dysrhythmias); uremia (anorexia, confusion, lethargy, twitching, convulsions, pruritus, and Kussmaul's respirations); and congestive heart failure (edema, jugular vein distention, crackles, and dyspnea).

• *Benign prostatic hypertrophy.* Common in men over age 50, this disorder commonly causes oliguria from urethral obstruction. It also causes urinary frequency and incontinence, nocturia, and possibly hematuria along with a distended bladder, an enlarged prostate, a sensation of lower abdominal fullness, perineal pain, and constipation.

• *Bladder neoplasm.* This disorder also produces oliguria due to urethral obstruction. Its cardinal sign, hematuria, may be accompanied by bladder, rectal, flank, back, or leg pain. Other findings include bladder distention, nocturia, dysuria, pyuria, vomiting, diarrhea, insomnia, and signs and symptoms of urinary tract infection—tenesmus, low-grade fever, and urinary frequency and urgency.

• *Calculi.* Oliguria or anuria may result from stones lodging in the kidneys, ureters, or the bladder outlet. Associated effects include urinary urgency and frequency, dysuria, and hematuria or pyuria. Usually, the patient experiences renal colic—excruciating pain that travels from the CVA to the flank, suprapubic region, and external genitalia. This pain may be accompanied by nausea, vomiting, hypoactive bowel sounds, abdominal distention, and occasionally fever and chills.

• *Cirrhosis.* In severe cirrhosis, hepatorenal syndrome may develop with oliguria, ascites, edema, fatigue, weakness, jaundice, hypotension, tachycardia, and signs of gastrointestinal bleeding, such as hematemesis.

• *Congestive heart failure (CHF).* Oliguria may occur in left ventricular failure as a result of low cardiac output and decreased renal perfusion. Accompanying signs and symptoms include dyspnea, fatigue, weakness, peripheral edema, distended jugular veins, tachycardia, tachypnea, crackles, and a dry or productive cough. In advanced CHF, the patient may also have orthopnea, cyanosis, clubbing, ventricular gallop, and hemoptysis.

• *Glomerulonephritis (acute).* This disorder produces oliguria or anuria. Other features are mild fever, fatigue, hematuria, generalized edema, elevated blood pressure, headache, nausea and vomiting, flank and abdominal pain, and signs of pulmonary congestion (dyspnea and productive cough).

• *Hypovolemia.* Any disorder that decreases circulating fluid volume can produce oliguria. Associated findings may include orthostatic hypotension, apathy, fatigue, muscle weakness, anorexia, nausea, profound thirst, dizziness, sunken eyeballs, poor skin turgor, and dry mucous membranes.

• *Pyelonephritis (acute).* Accompanying the sudden onset of oliguria in this disorder are high fever with chills, fatigue, flank pain, CVA tenderness, weakness, nocturia, dysuria, hematuria, urinary frequency and urgency, and tenesmus. The urine may appear cloudy. Occasionally, the patient also has anorexia, nausea, and vomiting.

• *Renal artery occlusion (bilateral).* This disorder may produce oliguria, or, more commonly, anuria. Other features include severe, constant upper abdominal and flank pain, nausea and vomiting, and hypoactive bowel sounds. The patient also develops a fever 1 to 2 days after the occlusion.

• *Renal failure (chronic).* Oliguria is a major sign of end-stage chronic renal failure. Associated findings reflect progressive uremia and may include fatigue, weakness, irritability, uremic fetor, ecchymoses and petechiae, peripheral edema, elevated blood pressure, confusion, drowsiness, coarse muscle twitching, muscle cramps, peripheral neuropathies, anorexia, nausea and vomiting, constipation or diar-

HOW OLIGURIA DEVELOPS

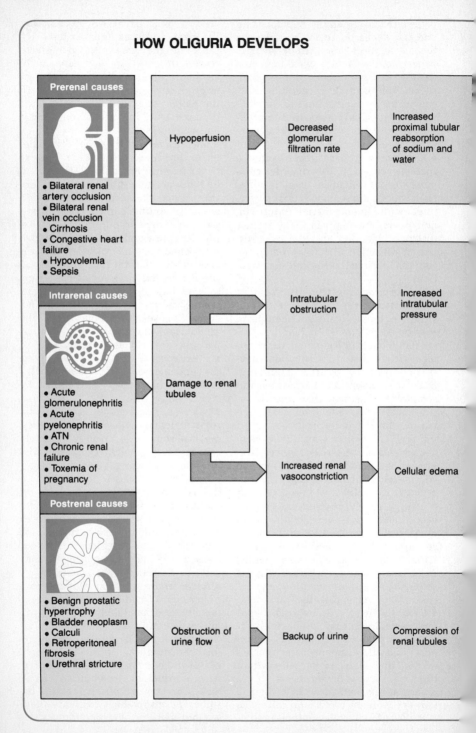

Prerenal causes

- Bilateral renal artery occlusion
- Bilateral renal vein occlusion
- Cirrhosis
- Congestive heart failure
- Hypovolemia
- Sepsis

Hypoperfusion → Decreased glomerular filtration rate → Increased proximal tubular reabsorption of sodium and water

Intrarenal causes

- Acute glomerulonephritis
- Acute pyelonephritis
- ATN
- Chronic renal failure
- Toxemia of pregnancy

Damage to renal tubules → Intratubular obstruction → Increased intratubular pressure

Damage to renal tubules → Increased renal vasoconstriction → Cellular edema

Postrenal causes

- Benign prostatic hypertrophy
- Bladder neoplasm
- Calculi
- Retroperitoneal fibrosis
- Urethral stricture

Obstruction of urine flow → Backup of urine → Compression of renal tubules

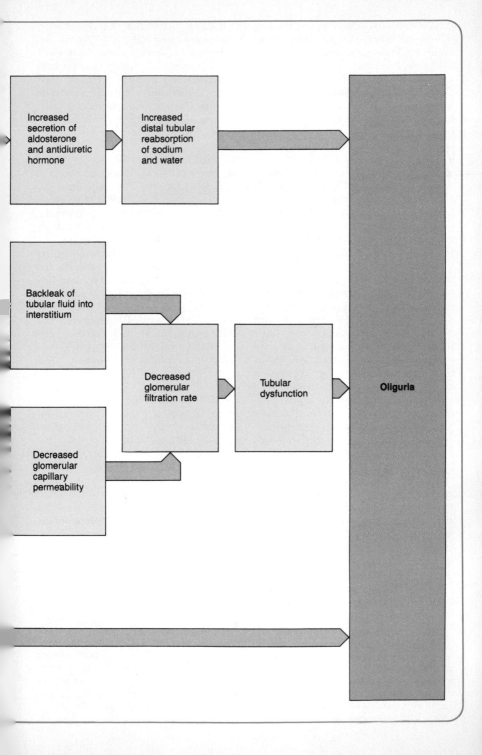

rhea, stomatitis, pruritus, pallor, and yellow- or bronze-tinged skin. Eventually, convulsions, coma, and uremic frost may develop.

• **Renal vein occlusion (bilateral).** This disorder occasionally causes oliguria accompanied by acute low back and flank pain, CVA tenderness, fever, pallor, hematuria, enlarged, palpable kidneys, and possibly signs of uremia.

• **Retroperitoneal fibrosis.** Oliguria may result from bilateral ureteral obstruction by dense fibrous tissue. Other effects may include urinary frequency, hematuria, diffuse low back pain, anorexia, weight loss, nausea and vomiting, fatigue, malaise, low-grade fever, and elevated blood pressure.

• **Sepsis.** Any condition that results in sepsis may produce oliguria, along with fever, chills, restlessness, confusion, diaphoresis, anorexia, vomiting, diarrhea, pallor, hypotension, and tachycardia. The patient may have signs of local infection, such as dysuria and wound drainage. In severe infection, he may develop lactic acidosis marked by Kussmaul's respirations.

• **Toxemia of pregnancy.** In severe preeclampsia, oliguria may be accompanied by elevated blood pressure, dizziness, diplopia, blurred vision, epigastric pain, nausea and vomiting, irritability, and severe frontal headache. Typically, the oliguria is preceded by generalized edema and sudden weight gain of more than 3 lb/week during the second trimester or more than 1 lb/week during the third trimester. If preeclampsia progresses to eclampsia, the patient has seizures and may slip into coma.

• **Urethral stricture.** This disorder produces oliguria accompanied by chronic urethral discharge, urinary frequency and urgency, dysuria, pyuria, and diminished urinary stream.

Other causes

• **Diagnostic studies.** Radiographic studies that use contrast media may cause nephrotoxicity and oliguria.

• **Drugs.** Oliguria may result from drugs that cause decreased renal perfusion (diuretics), nephrotoxicity (most notably, aminoglycosides and chemotherapeutic agents, such as cisplatin and methotrexate), urinary retention (adrenergic and anticholinergic agents) or urinary obstruction associated with precipitation of urinary crystals (sulfonamides).

Special considerations

Monitor vital signs, intake and output, and daily weight. Maintain fluid restrictions (usually 600 ml to 1 liter more than the patient's urine output for the previous day). Provide a diet low in sodium, potassium, and protein.

The doctor may order laboratory tests to determine whether the patient's oliguria is reversible; such tests may include serum blood urea nitrogen and creatinine levels, urea and creatinine clearance, urine sodium levels, and urine osmolality. He may also order abdominal X-rays, ultrasonography, computed tomography scan, and a renal scan.

Pediatric pointers

In the neonate, oliguria may result from edema or dehydration. Major causes include congenital heart disease, respiratory distress syndrome, sepsis, congenital hydronephrosis, acute tubular necrosis, and renal vein thrombosis. Common causes of oliguria in children between ages 1 and 5 are acute poststreptococcal glomerulonephritis and hemolytic uremic syndrome. After age 5, causes of oliguria are similar to those in adults.

Opisthotonos

A cardinal sign of meningeal irritation, opisthotonos is characterized by a severely arched, rigid back; hyperextended neck; the heels bent back; and the arms and hands flexed at the joints. Usually, this posture occurs spontaneously and continuously; however, it may be aggravated by movement. Presumably, opisthotonos represents a protective reflex since it immobilizes the spine, alleviating the pain associated with meningeal irritation.

Most commonly caused by meningitis, opisthotonos may also result from subarachnoid hemorrhage, Arnold-Chiari syndrome, and tetanus. Occasionally, it occurs in achondroplastic dwarfism, although not necessarily as an indicator of meningeal irritation.

Opisthotonos is far more common in children—especially infants—than in adults. It's also more exaggerated in children—the result of nervous system immaturity.

Assessment

Report opisthotonos to the doctor at once. If the patient is stuporous or comatose, quickly assess his vital signs, and employ resuscitative measures as appropriate. Place the patient in a bed, with side rails raised and padded, or in a crib.

When the patient's condition permits, obtain a history. Consult a family member of the young child or infant. Ask about a history of cerebral aneurysm or arteriovenous malformation and about hypertension. Also note any recent infection that may have spread to the nervous system. Explore associated signs and symptoms, such as headache, chills, and vomiting.

Focus the physical examination on the patient's neurologic status. Assess level of consciousness and test sensorimotor and cranial nerve function. Then check for Brudzinski's and Kernig's signs and for nuchal rigidity.

Medical causes

● *Arnold-Chiari syndrome.* In this syndrome, opisthotonos is typically accompanied by hydrocephalus with its characteristic, enlarged head; thin, shiny scalp with distended veins; and underdeveloped neck muscles. The infant usually also has a high-pitched, shrill cry, abnormal leg muscle tone, anorexia, vomiting, nuchal rigidity, irritability, noisy respirations, and a weak sucking reflex.

OPISTHOTONOS: A SIGN OF MENINGEAL IRRITATION

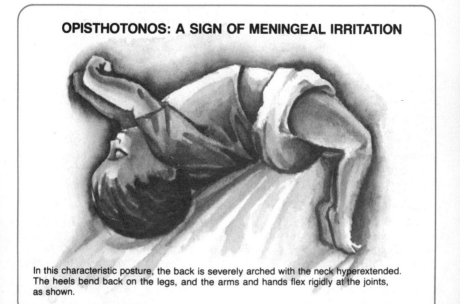

In this characteristic posture, the back is severely arched with the neck hyperextended. The heels bend back on the legs, and the arms and hands flex rigidly at the joints, as shown.

• **Meningitis.** In this infection, opisthotonos accompanies other signs of meningeal irritation, including nuchal rigidity, positive Brudzinski's and Kernig's signs, and hyperreflexia. Meningitis also causes cardinal signs of infection—moderate to high fever with chills and malaise—and of increased intracranial pressure—headache, vomiting, and, rarely, papilledema. Associated features include irritability; photophobia; diplopia, deafness, and other cranial nerve palsies; and decreased level of consciousness that may progress to seizures and coma.

• **Subarachnoid hemorrhage.** This disorder may also produce opisthotonos along with other signs of meningeal irritation, such as nuchal rigidity and positive Kernig's and Brudzinski's signs. Focal signs of hemorrhage—severe headache, hemiplegia or hemiparesis, aphasia, and photophobia—and other vision problems may also occur. With increasing intracranial pressure, the patient may develop bradycardia, elevated blood pressure, altered respiratory pattern, seizures, and vomiting. His level of consciousness may rapidly deteriorate, resulting in coma; then, decerebrate posture may alternate with opisthotonos.

• **Tetanus.** This life-threatening infection can cause opisthotonos. Initially, trismus occurs. Eventually, muscle spasms may affect the abdomen, producing boardlike rigidity; the back, resulting in opisthotonos; or the face, producing risus sardonicus. Spasms may affect the respiratory muscles, causing distress. Tachycardia, diaphoresis, hyperactive deep tendon reflexes, and convulsions may develop.

Other causes
• **Antipsychotics.** Phenothiazines and other antipsychotic drugs may cause opisthotonos, usually as part of an acute dystonic reaction.

Special considerations
Assess neurologic status and vital signs frequently. Make the patient as comfortable as possible; place him in a side-lying position with pillows for support. If meningitis is suspected, institute respiratory isolation. A lumbar puncture may be ordered to identify the causative microorganism and to analyze cerebrospinal fluid. If subarachnoid hemorrhage is suspected, prepare the patient for a computed tomography scan.

Orofacial Dyskinesia

Orofacial dyskinesia—abnormal movements involving muscles of the face, mouth, eyes, and occasionally neck—may be unilateral or bilateral, and constant or intermittent. Sometimes described as a facial tic, this sign is more common in women than in men, especially after age 50.

The pathophysiology of orofacial dyskinesia isn't clearly understood. Although the dyskinesia may result from hemifacial spasm disease and the effects of certain drugs, it's frequently idiopathic. Presumably, it results from pressure on the facial nerves associated with an extrapyramidal lesion or from a chemical imbalance. Psychogenic factors may also play a role—a theory supported by the fact that emotional upset aggravates the dyskinesia.

Assessment
If the patient abruptly displays orofacial dyskinesia, notify the doctor and review the patient's current medication regimen. If he's taking a phenothiazine or other antipsychotic, withhold the drug, if ordered, and prepare to give 50 mg of diphenhydramine to reverse the drug's effects. If the patient has difficulty swallowing, take necessary precautions to prevent choking and have suction equipment on hand.

If the patient's dyskinesia is chronic, begin by asking him when it began. Then obtain a complete drug history. Also note a history of seizures. Next, closely examine the patient's dyskinesia. Is it unilateral or bilateral? Does it involve the entire face or only part of it? Are neck muscles involved? Does the patient have any voluntary control over the movements? Characterize the abnormal movements. Are they constant or repetitive and intermittent? Listen to the patient's speech—does it sound abnormal? Is he able to swallow?

Medical cause
• **Hemifacial spasm.** This disorder is characterized by unilateral, intermittent spasms of muscles of the face, eye, and mouth. The patient may have some voluntary control over the spasms. Typically, the spasms are aggravated by emotional upset and disappear during sleep. Spasms may interfere with swallowing and speech.

Other causes
• **Metoclopramide and metyrosine.** Rarely, these drugs cause orofacial dyskinesia.
• **Phenothiazines and other antipsychotics.** These drugs may cause orofacial dyskinesia and other extrapyramidal effects. Typically, the movements are sustained and involve the eyes, mouth, face, and neck. Lip retraction and difficulty swallowing are common. Among the *phenothiazines,* the piperazine derivatives—acetophenazine, perphenazine, prochlorperazine, fluphenazine, and trifluoperazine—most frequently cause this sign. The aliphatic phenothiazines—chlorpromazine, promazine, and trifluopromazine—occasionally cause it. The piperidine phenothiazines—thioridazine, piperacetazine, and mesoridazine—rarely cause orofacial dyskinesia. *Other antipsychotics—*haloperidol, thiothixene, and loxapine—commonly cause orofacial dyskinesia.

Special considerations
Prepare the patient for diagnostic studies, such as blood screening for drugs and computed tomography scan.

If orofacial dyskinesia is drug-induced, assure the patient and his family that movements typically disappear 24 to 72 hours after stopping the drug. If orofacial dyskinesia is uncontrollable, advise the patient and his family that drug therapy—including phenobarbital, L-dopa, or carbamazepine—or psychotherapy may be beneficial.

Pediatric pointers
In children, orofacial dyskinesia is usually drug-induced. It may also result from Gilles de la Tourette's syndrome, seizure disorders, and dystonia musculorum deformans.

Orthopnea

Orthopnea—difficulty breathing in the supine position—is a common symptom of cardiopulmonary disorders that produce dyspnea. It's often a subtle symptom; the patient may complain that he can't catch his breath when lying down or mention that he sleeps most comfortably in a reclining chair or propped up by pillows. Derived from this complaint is the common classification as two- or three-pillow orthopnea.

Orthopnea presumably results from increased hydrostatic pressure in the pulmonary vasculature associated with increased venous return in the supine position. It may be aggravated by obesity, which restricts diaphragmatic excursion. Assuming the upright position relieves orthopnea by impairing venous return, which reduces hydrostatic pressure, and by enhancing diaphragmatic excursion, which increases inspiratory volume.

Assessment
Begin your assessment by asking the patient if he has a history of cardiopulmonary disorders, such as myocardial infarction, rheumatic heart disease, valvular disease, emphysema, or chronic bronchitis. Does the patient smoke? If so, how much? Explore as-

sociated symptoms, noting especially any complaints of cough, nocturnal or exertional dyspnea, fatigue, weakness, loss of appetite, or chest pain.

When examining the patient, check for other signs of increased respiratory effort, such as accessory muscle use, shallow respirations, and tachypnea. Also note barrel chest. Inspect the patient's skin for pallor or cyanosis, and the fingers for clubbing. Observe and palpate for edema, and check for jugular vein distention. Auscultate the lungs and heart.

Medical causes

• *Chronic obstructive pulmonary disease.* This disorder typically produces orthopnea and other dyspneic complaints, accompanied by accessory muscle use, tachypnea, tachycardia, and paradoxical pulse. Auscultation may reveal diminished breath sounds, rhonchi, crackles, and wheezing. The patient may also have a dry or productive cough with copious sputum. Other features include anorexia, weight loss, and edema. Barrel chest, cyanosis, and clubbing are usually late signs.

• *Left ventricular failure.* Orthopnea occurs late in this disorder. If heart failure is acute, orthopnea may begin suddenly; if chronic, it may be constant. The earliest symptom of this disorder is progressively severe dyspnea. Other common early symptoms include Cheyne-Stokes respirations, paroxysmal nocturnal dyspnea, fatigue, weakness, and a cough that may occasionally produce clear or blood-tinged sputum. Tachycardia, tachypnea, and crackles may also occur.

Other late findings may include cyanosis, clubbing, ventricular gallop, and hemoptysis. Left ventricular failure may also lead to signs of shock— hypotension, thready pulse, and cold, clammy skin.

• *Mediastinal tumor.* Orthopnea is an early sign of this disorder, resulting from pressure of the tumor against the trachea, bronchus, or lung when the patient lies down. However, many patients are asymptomatic until the tumor enlarges. Then, it produces retrosternal chest pain, dry cough, hoarseness, dysphagia, stertorous respirations, palpitations, and cyanosis. Examination reveals suprasternal retractions on inspiration, bulging of the chest wall, tracheal deviation, dilated jugular and superficial chest veins, and edema of the face, neck, and arms.

Special considerations

To relieve orthopnea, place the patient in semi-Fowler's or high Fowler's position; if this doesn't help, have him lean over a bedside table with his chest forward. If necessary, administer oxygen via nasal cannula. (Remember that patients with COPD require a low flow rate of 1 to 3 liters/minute.) If dyspnea persists when the patient's in the upright position, notify the doctor. He may order an EKG, chest X-ray, and pulmonary function tests for further evaluation.

Pediatric pointers

Common causes of orthopnea in children include congestive heart failure, croup syndrome, cystic fibrosis, and asthma.

Orthostatic Hypotension

[Postural hypotension]

In orthostatic hypotension, the patient's blood pressure drops 10 mm Hg or more when he rises from a supine to a sitting or standing position. This common sign indicates failure of compensatory vasomotor responses to adjust to position changes. It's typically associated with dizziness, syncope, or blurred vision, and may occur in a hypotensive, normotensive, or hypertensive patient. Although frequently a nonpathologic sign in the elderly, orthostatic hypotension may result from prolonged bed rest, fluid and electrolyte imbalance, endocrine or systemic disorders, and the effects of drugs.

To detect orthostatic hypotension, take and compare blood pressure readings with the patient supine, sitting, and then standing.

Assessment

If you detect orthostatic hypotension, quickly check for tachycardia, altered level of consciousness, and pale, clammy skin. If these signs are present, suspect hypovolemic shock and have another nurse notify the doctor immediately. Insert a large-bore I.V. for fluid or blood replacement. Take the patient's vital signs every 15 minutes, and monitor his intake and output.

If the patient's in no danger, obtain a history. Ask the patient if he frequently experiences dizziness, weakness, or fainting when he stands. Also ask him about associated symptoms, particularly fatigue, orthopnea, impotence, nausea, headache, and abdominal or chest discomfort. Then obtain a complete drug history.

Begin the physical examination by checking the patient's skin turgor. Palpate peripheral pulses and auscultate the heart and lungs. Finally, test muscle strength and observe his gait for unsteadiness.

Medical causes

• *Adrenal insufficiency.* This disorder typically begins insidiously, with progressively severe signs and symptoms. Orthostatic hypotension may be accompanied by fatigue, muscle weakness, anorexia, nausea and vomiting, weight loss, abdominal pain, irritability, and a weak, irregular pulse. Another common feature is hyperpigmentation—bronze coloring of the skin—which is especially prominent on the face, lips, gums, tongue, buccal mucosa, elbows, palms, knuckles, waist, and knees. Diarrhea, constipation, decreased libido, amenorrhea, and syncope may also occur along with enhanced taste, smell, and hearing.

• *Amyloidosis.* Orthostatic hypotension is commonly associated with amyloid infiltration of the autonomic nerves. Associated signs and symptoms vary widely and may include anginal chest pain, tachycardia, dyspnea, orthopnea, fatigue, and cough.

• *Diabetic autonomic neuropathy.* Here, orthostatic hypotension may be accompanied by syncope, dysphagia, constipation or diarrhea, painless bladder distention with overflow incontinence, impotence, and retrograde ejaculation.

• *Hyperaldosteronism.* This disorder typically produces orthostatic hypotension with sustained elevated blood pressure. Most other clinical effects of hyperaldosteronism result from hypokalemia, which increases neuromuscular irritability and produces muscle weakness, intermittent flaccid paralysis, fatigue, headache, paresthesias, and possibly tetany with positive Trousseau's and Chvostek's signs. The patient may also have visual disturbances, nocturia, polydipsia, and personality changes.

• *Hyponatremia.* In this disorder, orthostatic hypotension is typically accompanied by headache, profound thirst, tachycardia, nausea and vomiting, abdominal cramps, muscle twitching and weakness, fatigue, oliguria or anuria, cold clammy skin, poor skin turgor, irritability, seizures, and decreased level of consciousness. Cyanosis, thready pulse, and eventually vasomotor collapse may occur in severe sodium deficit.

• *Hypovolemia.* Mild to moderate hypovolemia may cause orthostatic hypotension associated with apathy, fatigue, muscle weakness, anorexia, nausea, and profound thirst. The patient may also develop dizziness, oliguria, sunken eyeballs, poor skin turgor, and dry mucous membranes.

• *Pheochromocytoma.* Although this disorder may produce orthostatic hypotension, its cardinal sign is paroxysmal or sustained hypertension. Typ-

PATIENT-TEACHING AID

PERFORMING PREAMBULATION EXERCISES

Dear Patient:

To help minimize the effects of orthostatic hypotension, such as dizziness and blurred vision when you stand up, perform these leg exercises before getting out of bed.

Lie flat on your back, and flex one knee slightly, keeping your heel on the bed.

Lift your heel off the bed and try to straighten your leg.

Flex your knee again, and lower your heel to the bed.

Straighten your leg.

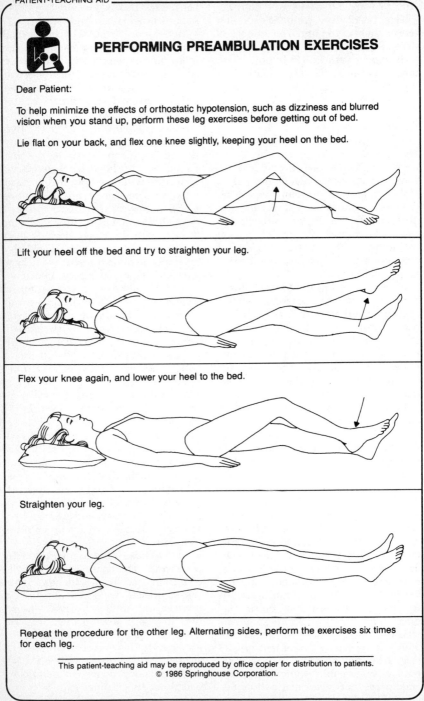

Repeat the procedure for the other leg. Alternating sides, perform the exercises six times for each leg.

ically, the patient is pale or flushed and diaphoretic, and his extreme anxiety makes him appear panicky. Associated signs and symptoms include tachycardia, palpitations, chest and abdominal pain, paresthesias, tremors, nausea and vomiting, low-grade fever, insomnia, and headache.

Other causes
• *Drugs.* Certain drugs may cause orthostatic hypotension by reducing circulating blood volume, causing blood vessel dilatation, or depressing the sympathetic nervous system. These drugs include antihypertensives (especially guanethidine and the initial dosage of prazosin), tricyclic antidepressants, phenothiazines, L-dopa, nitrates, monoamine oxidase inhibitors, morphine, bretylium, and spinal anesthesia. Large doses of diuretics can also cause orthostatic hypotension.
• *Treatments.* Orthostatic hypotension is commonly associated with prolonged bed rest (24 hours or longer). It may also result from sympathectomy, which disrupts normal vasoconstrictive mechanisms.

Special considerations
Monitor the patient's fluid balance by carefully recording his intake and output and weighing him daily. To help minimize orthostatic hypotension, advise the patient to change his position *gradually*. Elevate the head of the patient's bed, and help him to a sitting position with his feet dangling over the side of the bed. If he can tolerate this position, have him sit in a chair for brief periods. Immediately return him to bed if he becomes dizzy or pale or displays other signs of hypotension.

Always keep the patient's safety in mind. Never leave him unattended while he's sitting or walking; evaluate his need for assistive devices, such as a cane or walker.

Prepare the patient for diagnostic tests, such as serum electrolyte and drug levels, urinalysis, 12-lead EKG, and chest X-ray.

Pediatric pointers
Because normal blood pressure is lower in children than in adults, you must be familiar with normal age-specific values to detect orthostatic hypotension. From birth to age 3 months, normal systolic pressure is 40 to 80 mm Hg; from age 3 months to 1 year, 80 to 100 mm Hg; and from age 1 to 12, 100 mm Hg plus 2 mm Hg for every year over age 1. Diastolic blood pressure is first heard at about age 4; it's normally 60 mm Hg at this age and gradually increases to 70 mm Hg by age 12.

The causes of orthostatic hypotension in children may be the same as those in adults.

Ortolani's Sign

Ortolani's sign—a click or popping sensation that's felt and often heard on abduction of the newborn's thighs—indicates congenital dislocation of the hip (congenital hip dysplasia). Screening for this sign is an important part of newborn care, because early detection and treatment of congenital hip dysplasia improve the infant's chances of developing a healthy, functional joint.

Assessment
After eliciting Ortolani's sign, assess the infant for asymmetrical gluteal folds, limited hip abduction, and unequal leg length. Report your assessment data to the doctor for further orthopedic evaluation.

Medical cause
• *Congenital hip dysplasia.* Most common in females and in American Indians, this disorder produces Ortolani's sign, possibly accompanied by limited hip abduction and unequal gluteal folds. Usually, though, the infant has no gross deformity or pain. In complete dysplasia, his affected leg may

DETECTING CONGENITAL HIP DYSPLASIA

When assessing the newborn, attempt to elicit
Ortolani's sign to detect congenital hip dysplasia.
Begin by placing the infant supine with his
knees and hips flexed. Observe for symmetry.

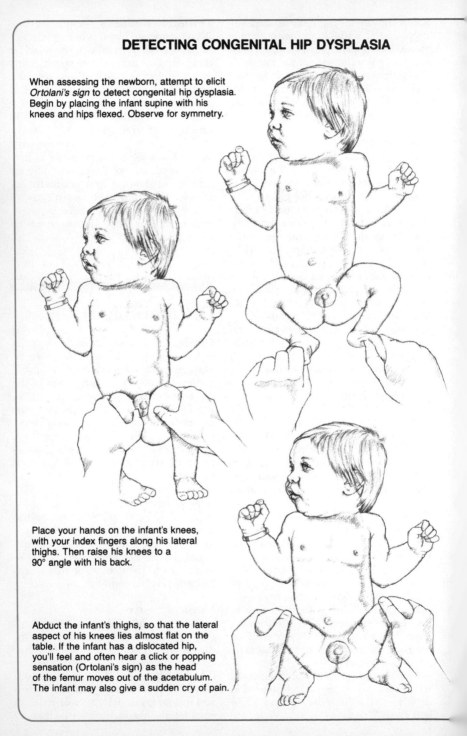

Place your hands on the infant's knees,
with your index fingers along his lateral
thighs. Then raise his knees to a
90° angle with his back.

Abduct the infant's thighs, so that the lateral
aspect of his knees lies almost flat on the
table. If the infant has a dislocated hip,
you'll feel and often hear a click or popping
sensation (Ortolani's sign) as the head
of the femur moves out of the acetabulum.
The infant may also give a sudden cry of pain.

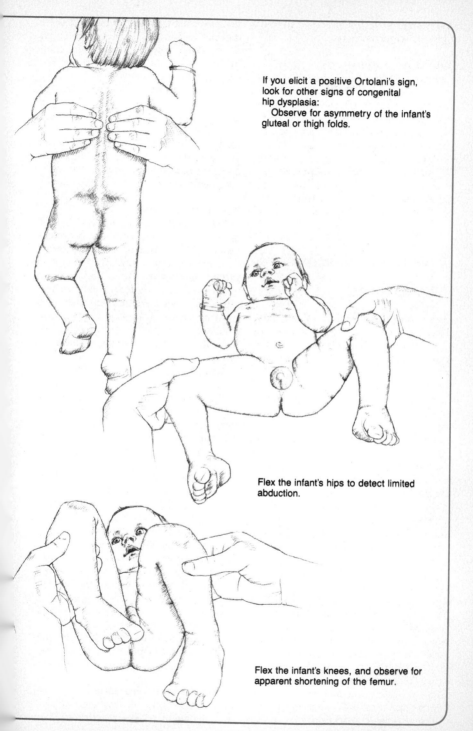

If you elicit a positive Ortolani's sign, look for other signs of congenital hip dysplasia:

Observe for asymmetry of the infant's gluteal or thigh folds.

Flex the infant's hips to detect limited abduction.

Flex the infant's knees, and observe for apparent shortening of the femur.

appear shorter, or his affected hip may appear more prominent.

Special considerations

Ortolani's sign can be elicited only during the first 4 to 6 weeks of life—the optimum time for effective corrective treatment. If treatment is delayed, congenital hip dysplasia may cause degenerative hip changes, lordosis, joint malformation, and soft-tissue damage. Various methods of abduction are used to produce a stable joint, including double-diapering, soft splinting devices, and a plaster hip spica cast.

Osler's Nodes

Osler's nodes are tender, raised, pea-sized, red or purple lesions that erupt on the palms, soles, and especially the pads of the fingers and toes. They're a rare, but reliable, sign of infective endocarditis, and are pathognomonic of the subacute form. However, the nodes usually develop after other telling signs and symptoms and disappear spontaneously within several days. How and why they develop is uncertain; they may result from emboli caught in peripheral capillaries, or may reflect an immunologic reaction to the causative organism. Osler's nodes must be distinguished from the even less common Janeway's lesions—small, painless, erythematous lesions that erupt on the palms and soles.

Assessment

If you discover Osler's nodes, explore the patient's history for clues to the cause of infective endocarditis. Has the patient had recent surgery or dental work? Invasive procedures of the urinary or gynecologic tract? Does he have a prosthetic valve or an arteriovenous fistula for hemodialysis? Note any history of cardiac disorders and murmurs, or recent upper respiratory, skin, or urinary tract infection. Also find out if the patient's been using intravenous drugs. Then explore associated complaints, such as chills, fatigue, anorexia, and night sweats.

After taking the patient's vital signs, auscultate the heart for murmurs and gallops and the lungs for crackles. Inspect the skin and mucous membranes for petechiae and other lesions. If you suspect intravenous drug abuse, inspect the patient's arms and other areas for needle tracks.

Medical causes

• *Acute infective endocarditis.* This type of endocarditis occasionally produces Osler's nodes. Among its more classic features are acute onset of high, intermittent fever with chills and signs of congestive heart failure, such as dyspnea, peripheral edema, and distended jugular veins. Janeway's spots and Roth's spots are more common in this form than in the subacute form; petechiae may also occur.

Embolization may abruptly occur, causing organ infarction or peripheral vascular occlusion with hematuria, chest or limb pain, paralysis, blindness, and other diverse effects.

• *Subacute infective endocarditis.* Osler's nodes are pathognomonic of this form of endocarditis. A suddenly changing murmur or the discovery of a new murmur is another cardinal sign. Associated signs and symptoms may include intermittent fever, pallor, weakness, fatigue, arthralgia, night sweats, tachycardia, anorexia and weight loss, splenomegaly, clubbing, and petechiae. Occasionally, Janeway's spots, subungual splinter hemorrhages, and Roth's spots also appear. Signs of congestive heart failure may occur with extensive valvular damage.

Embolization may develop, producing signs and symptoms that vary depending on the location of the emboli.

Special considerations

Monitor the patient's vital signs to evaluate the effectiveness of antibiotic therapy against infective endocarditis. Later, discuss measures to prevent reinfection, such as prophylactic antibiotic administration before dental or invasive procedures.

Pediatric pointers

In children, Osler's nodes may result from infective endocarditis associated with congenital heart defects or rheumatic fever.

Otorrhea

Otorrhea—drainage from the ear—may be bloody (otorrhagia), purulent, clear, or serosanguineous. Its onset, duration, and severity provide clues to the underlying cause. This sign may result from disorders that affect the external ear canal or the middle ear, including allergy, infection, neoplasms, trauma, and collagen diseases. Otorrhea may occur alone or with other symptoms, such as ear pain.

Assessment

Begin your assessment by asking the patient when the otorrhea began, noting how he recognized it. Did he clean the drainage from deep within the ear canal, or did he wipe it from the auricle? Have him describe the color, consistency, and odor of the drainage. Is it clear, purulent, or bloody? Does it occur in one or both ears? Is it continuous or intermittent? If the patient wears cotton in his ear to absorb the drainage, ask how often he changes it.

Then explore associated otologic symptoms, especially pain. Is there tenderness on movement of the pinna or tragus? Ask about vertigo, which is absent in disorders of the external ear canal. Also ask about tinnitus.

Next, check the patient's medical history for recent upper respiratory infection or head trauma. Also ask how he cleans his ears and if he's an avid swimmer. Note a history of cancer, der-

matitis, or immunosuppressive therapy.

Focus the physical examination on the patient's external ear, middle ear, and tympanic membrane. (If his symptoms are unilateral, examine the uninvolved ear first.) Inspect the external ear, and apply pressure on the tragus and mastoid area to elicit tenderness. Then insert an otoscope, using the largest speculum that will comfortably fit into the ear canal. If necessary, clean cerumen, pus, or other debris from the canal. Observe for edema, erythema, crusts, or polyps. Inspect the tympanic membrane, which should look like a shiny, pearl-gray cone. Note color changes, perforation, absence of the normal light reflex (a cone of light appearing toward the bottom of the drum), or a bulging membrane.

Next, test hearing acuity. Have the patient occlude one ear while you whisper some common two-syllable words toward the unoccluded ear. Stand behind him so he doesn't read your lips, and ask him to repeat what he heard. Perform the test on the other ear using different words. Then use a tuning fork to perform the Weber and Rinne tests. (See *Differentiating Conductive and Sensorineural Hearing Loss*, page 374.)

Complete your assessment by palpating the patient's neck and his preauricular, parotid, and postauricular (mastoid) areas for lymphadenopathy. Also test the function of cranial nerves VII, IX, X, and XI.

Medical causes

• *Allergy.* An allergy associated with tympanic membrane perforation may cause clear or cloudy otorrhea, rhinorrhea, and itchy, watery eyes.

• *Aural polyps.* These polyps may produce foul, purulent, and perhaps blood-streaked discharge. If they occlude the external ear canal, the polyps may cause partial hearing loss.

• *Basilar skull fracture.* In this disorder, otorrhea may be clear and watery, representing cerebrospinal fluid (CSF) leakage, or bloody, representing hemorrhage. Occasionally, inspection reveals blood behind the eardrum. The otorrhea may be accompanied by hearing loss, CSF or bloody rhinorrhea, periorbital ecchymosis (raccoon's eyes), and mastoid ecchymosis (Battle's sign). Cranial nerve palsies, decreased level of consciousness, and headache are other common findings.

• *Dermatitis of the external ear canal.* In *contact dermatitis,* vesicles produce clear, watery otorrhea with edema and erythema of the external ear canal.

Infectious eczematoid dermatitis causes purulent otorrhea with erythema and crusting of the external ear canal.

In *seborrheic dermatitis,* otorrhea consists of greasy scales and flakes. The scalp, forehead, and cheeks are also marked by pruritic, scaly lesions.

• *Epidural abscess.* In this disorder, profuse, creamy otorrhea is accompanied by steady, throbbing ear pain; fever; and temporal or temporoparietal headache on the ipsilateral side.

• *Mastoiditis.* This disorder causes thick, purulent, yellow otorrhea that becomes increasingly profuse. Its cardinal features include low-grade fever and dull aching and tenderness in the mastoid area. Postauricular erythema and edema may push the auricle out from the head; pressure within the edematous mastoid antrum may produce swelling and obstruction of the external ear canal, causing conductive hearing loss.

• *Myringitis (infectious).* In *acute infectious myringitis,* small, reddened, blood-filled blebs erupt in the external ear canal, the tympanic membrane, and, occasionally, the middle ear. Spontaneous rupture of these blebs causes serosanguineous otorrhea. Other features are severe ear pain, tenderness over the mastoid process, and, rarely, fever and hearing loss.

Chronic infectious myringitis causes purulent otorrhea, pruritus, and gradual hearing loss.

• *Otitis externa.* Acute otitis externa, commonly known as swimmer's ear, usually causes purulent, yellow, sticky, foul-smelling otorrhea. Inspection may reveal white-green debris in the external ear canal. Associated findings include edema, erythema, pain, and itching of the auricle and external ear canal; severe tenderness with movement of the mastoid, tragus, mouth, or jaw; tenderness and swelling of surrounding nodes; and partial conductive hearing loss. The patient may also have a low-grade fever and a headache ipsilateral to the affected ear.

Chronic otitis externa usually causes scanty, intermittent otorrhea that may be serous or purulent and possibly foul-smelling. Its primary symptom, though, is itching. Related findings include edema and slight erythema.

Life-threatening *malignant otitis externa* produces debris in the ear canal, which may build up against the tympanic membrane, causing severe pain that's especially acute during manipulation of the tragus or auricle. Most common in diabetics and immunosuppressed patients, this fulminant bacterial infection may also cause pruritus, tinnitus, and, possibly, unilateral hearing loss.

• *Otitis media.* In *acute otitis media,* rupture of the tympanic membrane produces bloody, purulent otorrhea and relieves continuous or intermittent ear pain. Typically, a conductive hearing loss worsens over several hours.

In *acute suppurative otitis media,* the patient may also have signs and symptoms of upper respiratory infection—sore throat, cough, nasal discharge, headache. Other features may include dizziness, fever, nausea, and vomiting.

Chronic otitis media causes intermittent, purulent, foul-smelling otorrhea associated with frequent perforation of the tympanic membrane. Conductive hearing loss occurs gradually and may be accompanied by pain, nausea, and vertigo.

• *Perichondritis.* In this disorder, multiple fistulas may open on the auricle or external ear canal, causing purulent otorrhea. Typically, the auricle is edematous and erythematous, with thickened skin.

• **Trauma.** Bloody otorrhea may result from trauma, such as a blow to the external ear, a foreign body in the ear, or barotrauma. Usually, the bleeding is minimal or moderate; it may be accompanied by partial hearing loss.

• **Tuberculosis.** Pulmonary tuberculosis may spread through the upper airway to the middle ear, causing chronic ear infection. The tympanic membrane thickens, ruptures, and produces a watery otorrhea and mild hearing loss. Cervical adenopathy may also occur.

• **Tumor (benign).** A benign tumor of the glomus jugulare (jugular bulb) may cause bloody otorrhea. Initially, the patient may complain of throbbing discomfort and tinnitus that resembles the sound of his heartbeat. Associated signs and symptoms include gradually progressive stuffiness in the affected ear, vertigo, conductive hearing loss, and possibly a reddened mass behind the tympanic membrane.

• **Tumor (malignant).** *Squamous cell carcinoma of the external ear* causes purulent otorrhea with itching; deep, boring ear pain; hearing loss; and, in late stages, facial paralysis.

In *squamous cell carcinoma of the middle ear,* blood-tinged otorrhea occurs early, typically accompanied by hearing loss on the affected side. Pain and facial paralysis are late features.

• **Wegener's granulomatosis.** This rare, necrotizing granulomatous vasculitis causes frequent perforation of the tympanic membrane and serosanguineous otorrhea. The patient may have a slowly progressive hearing loss, a cough (possibly hemoptysis), wheezing, shortness of breath, pleuritic chest pain, hemorrhagic skin lesions, epistaxis, and signs of severe sinusitis.

Special considerations

As ordered, apply warm, moist compresses, heating pads, or hot water bottles to the patient's ears to relieve inflammation and pain. Use cotton wicks to gently clean the draining ear or to apply topical drugs. Keep ear drops at room temperature; instillation of cold ear drops may cause vertigo.

Advise the patient with chronic ear problems to avoid forceful nose blowing when he has an upper respiratory infection, to avoid channeling infected secretions into the middle ear. Instruct him to blow his nose with his mouth open. Also remind him to cleanse his ears with a washcloth *only,* and not to stick anything in his ear (such as a hairpin or a cotton-tipped applicator) that might cause injury. If the patient is a swimmer, instruct him to wear earplugs and to wash and dry his ears thoroughly after swimming. Have him report recurring ear pain and drainage, especially in the absence of upper respiratory infection, as this may be a sign of cancer.

A ruptured tympanic membrane usually heals spontaneously. However, tell the patient to avoid water while it heals; instruct him to insert lubricated cotton balls into his ear canal before he showers or shampoos.

Pediatric pointers

When you examine or clean a child's ear, remember that the auditory canal lies horizontally and that the pinna must be pulled *downward* and *backward.* Restrain a child during an ear procedure by having him sit on a parent's or another nurse's lap with the ear to be examined facing you. Have him put one arm around the helper's waist and the other down at his own side, and then ask the helper to hold the child in place. Or, if you are alone with the child, have him lie on his abdomen with his arms at his sides and his head turned so the affected ear faces the ceiling. Bend over him, restraining his upper body with your elbows and upper arms.

Otitis media is the most common cause of otorrhea in infants and young children. Children are also likely to insert foreign bodies into their ears, resulting in infection, pain, and purulent discharge.

pallor • palpitations • papular rash • paralysis • paresthesias • paroxysmal n
d'orange • pericardial friction rub • peristaltic waves—visible • photophobia
rub • polydipsia • polyphagia • polyuria • postnasal drip • priapism • pruriti
psychotic behavior • ptosis • pulse—absent or weak • pulse—bounding • pul
pulse pressure—widened • pulse rhythm abnormality • pulsus alternans • pu
paradoxus • pupils—nonreactive • pupils—sluggish • purple striae • purpura
pyrosis • raccoon's eyes • rebound tenderness • rectal pain • retractions—cos
rhinorrhea • rhonchi • Romberg's sign • salivation—decreased • salivation—i
scotoma • scrotal swelling • seizure—absence • seizure—focal • seizure—gen
seizure—psychomotor • setting-sun sign • shallow respirations • skin—bronz
skin—mottled • skin—scaly • skin turgor—decreased • spider angioma • sple
respirations • stool—clay-colored • stridor • syncope • tachycardia • tachypne
tearing—increased • throat pain • tic • tinnitus • tracheal deviation • trachea
trismus • tunnel vision • uremic frost • urethral discharge • urinary frequen
urinary incontinence • urinary urgency • urine cloudiness • urticaria • vagin
postmenopausal • vaginal discharge • venous hum • vertigo • vesicular rash
loss • visual blurring • visual floaters • vomiting • vulvar lesions • weight ga
loss—excessive • wheezing • wristdrop• abdominal distention • abdominal
abdominal rigidity • accessory muscle use • agitation • alopecia • amenorrh
analgesia • anhidrosis • anorexia • anosmia • anuria • anxiety • aphasia • a
respirations • apraxia • arm pain • asterixis • ataxia • athetosis • aura • Bal
pain • barrel chest • Battle's sign • Biot's respirations • bladder distention •
blood pressure increase • bowel sounds—absent • bowel sounds—hyperacti
hypoactive • bradycardia • bradypnea • breast dimpling • breast nodule • b
breath with ammonia odor • breath with fecal odor • breath with fruity odo
bruits • buffalo hump • butterfly rash • café-au-lait spots • capillary refill ti
carpopedal spasm • cat cry • chest expansion—asymmetrical • chest pain •
respirations • chills • chorea • Chvostek's sign • clubbing • cogwheel rigidit
confusion • conjunctival injection • constipation • corneal reflex—absent • o
tenderness • cough—barking • cough—nonproductive • cough—productive
bony • crepitation—subcutaneous • cry—high-pitched • cyanosis • decerebr
posture • deep tendon reflexes—hyperactive • deep tendon reflexes—hypoac
diaphoresis • diarrhea • diplopia • dizziness • doll's eye sign—absent • dro
dysmenorrhea • dyspareunia • dyspepsia • dysphagia • dyspnea • dystonia •
edema—generalized • edema of the arms • edema of the face • edema of th
enuresis • epistaxis • eructation • erythema • exophthalmos • eye discharge
fasciculations • fatigue • fecal incontinence • fetor hepaticus • fever • flank
fontanelle bulging • fontanelle depression • footdrop • gag reflex abnormalit
propulsive • gait—scissors • gait—spastic • gait—steppage • gait—waddlin
gallop—ventricular • genital lesions in the male • grunting respirations • g
swelling • gynecomastia • halitosis • halo vision • headache • hearing loss
Heberden's nodes • hematemesis • hematochezia • hematuria • hemianopia
hepatomegaly • hiccups • hirsutism • hoarseness • Homans' sign • hyperpi
hypopigmentation • impotence • insomnia • intermittent claudication • Jane
jaw pain • jugular vein distention • Kehr's sign • Kernig's sign • leg pain •
decreased • lid lag • light flashes • low birth weight • lymphadenopathy •
McBurney's sign • McMurray's sign • melena • menorrhagia • metrorrhagia
mouth lesions • murmurs • muscle atrophy • muscle flaccidity • muscle spa
muscle weakness • mydriasis • myoclonus • nasal flaring • nausea • neck
nipple discharge • nipple retraction • nocturia • nuchal rigidity • nystagm

Pallor

Pallor is abnormal paleness or loss of skin color, which may develop suddenly or gradually. Although generalized pallor affects the entire body, it's most apparent on the face, conjunctiva, oral mucosa, and nail beds. Localized pallor commonly affects a single limb.

How easily pallor is detected varies with skin color and the thickness and vascularity of underlying subcutaneous tissue. At times, it's merely a subtle lightening of skin color. It may be difficult to detect in dark-skinned persons; sometimes it's only evident on their conjunctiva and oral mucosa.

Pallor may result from decreased peripheral oxyhemoglobin *or* decreased total oxyhemoglobin. The former reflects diminished peripheral blood flow associated with peripheral vasoconstriction or arterial occlusion or with low cardiac output. (Transient peripheral vasoconstriction may occur with exposure to cold, causing nonpathologic pallor.) The latter most commonly results from anemia, the chief cause of pallor.

Assessment

 If the patient suddenly develops generalized pallor, quickly assess for signs of shock, such as tachycardia, hypotension, and de-creased level of consciousness. Notify the doctor immediately, and prepare to infuse fluids or blood rapidly. Keep emergency resuscitation equipment nearby.

If the patient's condition permits, take a complete history. Does the patient or anyone in his family have a history of anemia? What about chronic disorders, such as renal failure, congestive heart failure, or diabetes, which might lead to anemia? Ask about the patient's diet, particularly his intake of green vegetables. Then explore the pallor more fully. Find out when the patient first noticed it. Is pallor constant or intermittent? Does it occur when he's exposed to the cold? Try to determine if the patient is under emotional stress. Explore associated signs and symptoms, such as dizziness, fainting, weakness and fatigue on exertion, chest pain, palpitations, menstrual irregularities, or loss of libido. If the pallor is confined to one or both legs, ask the patient if walking is painful. Do his legs feel cold or numb? If the pallor is confined to his fingers, ask about tingling and numbness.

Start the physical exam by taking the patient's vital signs. Be sure to check for orthostatic hypotension. Auscultate the heart for gallops and murmurs and the lungs for crackles. Check the patient's skin temperature—cold extrem-

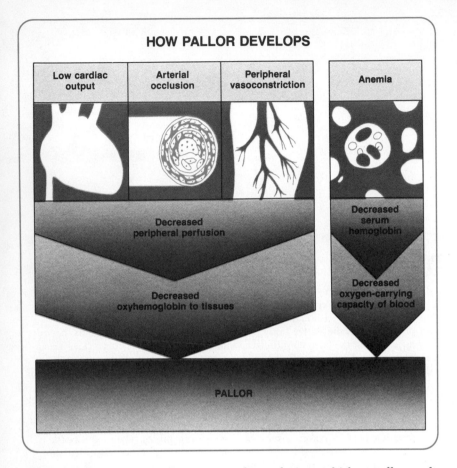

HOW PALLOR DEVELOPS

Low cardiac output	Arterial occlusion	Peripheral vasoconstriction	Anemia

Decreased peripheral perfusion

Decreased serum hemoglobin

Decreased oxyhemoglobin to tissues

Decreased oxygen-carrying capacity of blood

PALLOR

ities commonly occur with vasoconstriction or arterial occlusion. Also note skin ulceration. Finally, palpate peripheral pulses. An absent pulse in a pale extremity may indicate arterial occlusion, whereas a weak pulse may indicate low cardiac output.

Medical causes
• *Anemia.* Typically, pallor develops gradually in this disorder. The patient's skin color may also appear sallow or grayish. Other effects may include fatigue, dyspnea, tachycardia, bounding pulse, atrial gallop, systolic bruit over the carotid arteries, and possibly crackles and bleeding tendencies.
• *Arterial occlusion (acute).* Pallor develops abruptly in the extremity with

the occlusion, which usually results from an embolus. A line of demarcation develops, separating the cool, pale, cyanotic, and mottled skin below the occlusion from the normal skin above it. Accompanying the pallor may be severe pain, intense intermittent claudication, paresthesias, and paresis in the affected extremity. Absent pulses and diminished capillary refill below the occlusion are also characteristic.
• *Arterial occlusive disease (chronic).* Here, pallor is also specific to an extremity—usually one leg, but occasionally both legs or an arm. It develops gradually from obstructive arteriosclerosis or thrombus formation and is aggravated by elevating the extremity. Associated findings include intermit-

tent claudication, weakness, cool skin, diminished pulses in the extremity, and possibly ulceration and gangrene.

• **Cardiac dysrhythmias.** Cardiac dysrhythmias that seriously reduce cardiac output, such as complete heart block and attacks of tachyarrhythmia, may cause acute onset of pallor. Other features include irregular, rapid, or slow pulse; dizziness; weakness and fatigue; hypotension; confusion; palpitations; diaphoresis; oliguria; and, possibly, loss of consciousness.

• **Frostbite.** Pallor is localized to the frostbitten area, such as the feet, hands, or ears. Typically, the area feels cold, waxy, and, perhaps, hard in deep frostbite. The skin doesn't blanch and sensation may be absent. As the area thaws, the skin turns purplish blue. Blistering and gangrene may then follow if the frostbite was severe.

• **Orthostatic hypotension.** In this condition, pallor occurs abruptly on rising from a recumbent position to a sitting or standing position. A precipitous drop in blood pressure and dizziness are also characteristic. Occasionally, the patient loses consciousness for several minutes.

• **Raynaud's disease.** Pallor of the fingers upon exposure to cold or stress is a hallmark of this disease. Typically, the fingers abruptly turn pale, then cyanotic; with rewarming, they become red and paresthetic. In chronic disease, ulceration may occur.

• **Shock.** Two forms of shock initially cause acute onset of pallor and cool, clammy skin. In *hypovolemic shock,* other early signs include restlessness, thirst, slight tachycardia, and tachypnea. As shock progresses, the skin becomes increasingly clammy, pulse becomes more rapid and thready, and hypotension develops with narrowing pulse pressure. Other signs may include oliguria, subnormal body temperature, and decreased level of consciousness. In *cardiogenic shock,* the signs and symptoms are similar, but usually more profound.

• **Vasopressor syncope.** Sudden onset of pallor immediately precedes or accompanies loss of consciousness during syncopal attacks. These common fainting spells may be triggered by emotional stress or pain and usually last only a few seconds or minutes. Before loss of consciousness, the patient may have diaphoresis, nausea, yawning, hyperpnea, weakness, confusion, tachycardia, and dim vision. He then develops bradycardia, hypotension, a few clonic jerks, and dilated pupils with loss of consciousness.

Special considerations

If the patient has chronic *generalized* pallor, prepare him for blood studies and, possibly, bone marrow biopsy. If the patient has *localized* pallor, he may require arteriography to accurately determine the cause.

When pallor results from low cardiac output, administer blood and fluid replacements or such drugs as diuretics, cardiotonics, and antiarrhythmics, as ordered. Frequently monitor the patient's vital signs, intake and output, EKG, and hemodynamic status.

Pediatric pointers

In children, pallor stems from the same causes as it does in adults. It can also stem from congenital heart defects and chronic lung disease.

Palpitations

Defined as a conscious awareness of one's heart beat, palpitations are usually felt over the precordium or in the throat or neck. The patient may describe them as pounding, jumping, turning, fluttering, flopping, or as missing or skipping beats. They may be regular or irregular, fast or slow, paroxysmal or sustained.

Although frequently insignificant, this common symptom may result from cardiac and metabolic disorders and from the effects of certain drugs. Nonpathologic palpitations may occur with a newly implanted prosthetic valve because its clicking sound heightens the patient's awareness of his heartbeat. Transient palpitations may accompany emotional stress, such as fright, anger, and anxiety, or physical stress, such as exercise and fever. They can also accompany use of stimulants, such as tobacco and caffeine.

To help characterize the palpitations, ask the patient to simulate their rhythm by tapping his finger on a hard surface. An irregular "skipped beat" rhythm points to premature ventricular contractions, whereas an episodic racing rhythm that ends abruptly suggests paroxysmal atrial tachycardia.

Assessment

If the patient complains of palpitations, ask about dizziness and shortness of breath, then inspect for pale, cool, clammy skin. Take his vital signs, noting hypotension and irregular or abnormal pulse. If these signs are present, suspect cardiac dysrhythmias and notify the doctor immediately. Prepare to begin cardiac monitoring, and start an I.V. to administer antiarrhythmic drugs.

If the patient isn't in distress, perform a more complete cardiac history and physical examination. Ask about cardiovascular or pulmonary disorders, which may produce dysrhythmias. Does he have a history of hypertension or hypoglycemia? Obtain a drug history. Has the patient recently started digitalis therapy? Also ask about caffeine, tobacco, and alcohol consumption. Then explore associated symptoms, such as weakness, fatigue, and anginal pain. Finally, auscultate for gallops, murmurs, and abnormal breath sounds.

Medical causes

• *Acute anxiety attack.* In this disorder, palpitations may be accompanied by diaphoresis, facial flushing, and trembling. Almost invariably, the patient hyperventilates, which may lead to diz-

ziness, weakness, and syncope. Other typical findings include tachycardia, precordial pain, shortness of breath, restlessness, and insomnia.

• *Anemia.* Palpitations may occur in anemia, especially on exertion. Pallor, fatigue, and dyspnea are also common. Associated signs may include a systolic ejection murmur, bounding pulse, tachycardia, crackles, an atrial gallop, and a systolic bruit over the carotid arteries.

• *Aortic insufficiency.* This disorder may produce sustained or paroxysmal palpitations accompanied by anginal pain, pallor, and dyspnea. Strong, abrupt carotid pulsations may also occur. Auscultatory findings may include Duroziez's sign (a murmur heard over the femoral artery during both systole and diastole); a large, diffuse apical heave; a decrescendo, high-pitched, and blowing diastolic murmur along the lower left sternal border; possibly an early systolic murmur; and a ventricular gallop. In severe aortic insufficiency, there may be widened pulse pressure, an atrial gallop, and an Austin Flint murmur.

• *Cardiac dysrhythmias.* Paroxysmal or sustained palpitations may occur here, with dizziness, weakness, and fatigue. Other features may include irregular, rapid, or slow pulse; decreased blood pressure; confusion; pallor; oliguria; and diaphoresis.

• *Hypertension.* In this disorder, the patient may be asymptomatic or may complain of sustained palpitations alone or with headache, dizziness, tinnitus, and fatigue. Typically, his blood pressure exceeds 140/90 mm Hg. Nausea and vomiting, seizures, and decreased level of consciousness may also occur.

• *Hypocalcemia.* Typically, this disorder produces palpitations, weakness, and fatigue. It progresses from paresthesias to muscle tension and carpopedal spasms. Assessment may also reveal muscle twitching, hyperactive deep tendon reflexes, chorea, and positive Chvostek's and Trousseau's signs.

• *Hypoglycemia.* When blood glucose levels drop significantly, the sympathetic nervous system triggers adrenalin production, which may cause sustained palpitations accompanied by fatigue, irritability, hunger, cold sweats, tremors, tachycardia, anxiety, and headache. Eventually, central nervous system effects—blurred or double vision, muscle weakness, hemiplegia, and altered level of consciousness—may also develop.

• *Mitral prolapse.* This valvular disorder may cause paroxysmal palpitations accompanied by sharp, stabbing, or aching precordial pain. Its hallmark, though, is a midsystolic click followed by an apical systolic murmur. Associated signs and symptoms may include dyspnea, dizziness, severe fatigue, migraine headache, anxiety, paroxysmal tachycardia, crackles, and peripheral edema.

• *Mitral stenosis.* Early features of this disorder typically include sustained palpitations with dyspnea and fatigue on exertion. Auscultation also reveals a loud S_1 or opening snap and a rumbling diastolic murmur at the apex. Related effects may include an atrial gallop and, in advanced mitral stenosis, orthopnea, dyspnea at rest, and paroxysmal nocturnal dyspnea.

• *Pheochromocytoma.* This rare adrenal medulla tumor causes episodic hypermetabolism, commonly associated with paroxysmal palpitations. Its cardinal sign is dramatically elevated blood pressure, which may be sustained or paroxysmal. Associated features may include tachycardia, headache, chest or abdominal pain, diaphoresis, warm and pale or flushed skin, paresthesias, tremors, insomnia, nausea and vomiting, and anxiety.

• *Thyrotoxicosis.* A characteristic symptom in this disorder, sustained palpitations may be accompanied by tachycardia, dyspnea, weight loss despite increased appetite, diarrhea, tremors, nervousness, diaphoresis, heat intolerance, and, possibly, exophthalmos and an enlarged thyroid. An atrial or ventricular gallop may also occur.

Other causes

• *Drugs.* Palpitations may result from drugs that precipitate cardiac dysrhythmias or increase cardiac output, such as cardiac glycosides, sympathomimetics, ganglionic blockers, and atropine.

Special considerations

Prepare the patient for diagnostic tests, such as an EKG and chest X-ray. Remember that even mild palpitations may cause your patient much concern. Maintain a quiet, comfortable environment to minimize anxiety and perhaps decrease palpitations.

Pediatric pointers

Palpitations in children commonly result from fever and congenital heart defects, such as patent ductus arteriosus and septal defects. Because children are often unable to describe this complaint, you'll have to focus your assessment on objective measurements—cardiac monitoring, physical examination, and laboratory tests.

Papular Rash

This rash consists of small, raised, circumscribed—and perhaps discolored—lesions known as papules. It may erupt anywhere on the body in various configurations and may be acute or chronic. Papular rashes characterize many cutaneous disorders; they may also result from allergy and from infectious, neoplastic, and systemic disorders.

Assessment

Your first step is to assess the papular rash fully: note its color, configuration, and location on the patient's body. Find out when it erupted. Has the patient noticed any changes in the rash since then? Is it itchy or burning? Painful or

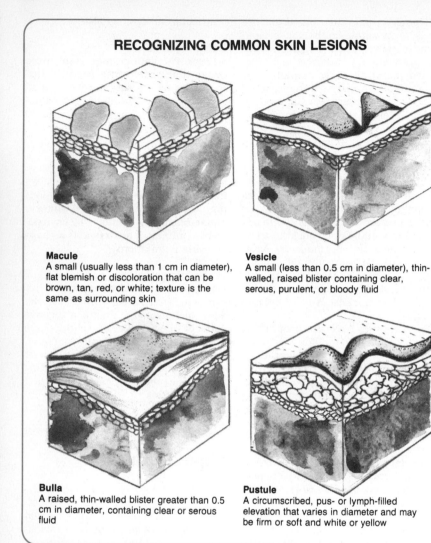

RECOGNIZING COMMON SKIN LESIONS

Macule
A small (usually less than 1 cm in diameter), flat blemish or discoloration that can be brown, tan, red, or white; texture is the same as surrounding skin

Vesicle
A small (less than 0.5 cm in diameter), thin-walled, raised blister containing clear, serous, purulent, or bloody fluid

Bulla
A raised, thin-walled blister greater than 0.5 cm in diameter, containing clear or serous fluid

Pustule
A circumscribed, pus- or lymph-filled elevation that varies in diameter and may be firm or soft and white or yellow

tender? Also have him describe associated signs and symptoms, such as fever, headache, and GI distress.

Next, obtain a medical history, including allergies, previous rashes or skin disorders, infections, childhood diseases, sexually transmitted diseases, and neoplasms. Has the patient recently been bitten by an insect or rodent, or been exposed to anyone with an infectious disease? Finally, obtain a complete drug history.

Medical causes

• *Acne vulgaris.* In this disorder, rupture of enlarged comedones produces inflamed—and perhaps, painful and pruritic—papules, pustules, nodules, or cysts on the face and sometimes the shoulders, chest, and back.

• *Dermatomyositis.* Grotton's papules—flat, violet lesions on the dorsum of the finger joints—are pathognomonic of this disorder, as is the dusky lilac discoloration of periorbital tissue and lid

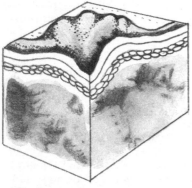

Wheal
A slightly raised, firm lesion of variable size and shape, surrounded by edema; skin may be red or pale

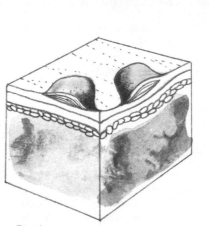

Papule
A small, solid, raised lesion less than 1 cm in diameter, with red-to-purple skin discoloration

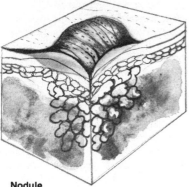

Nodule
A small, firm, circumscribed elevation approximately 1 to 2 cm in diameter; skin discoloration may be present

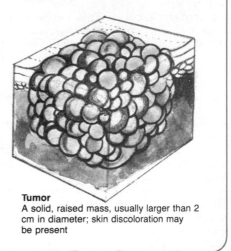

Tumor
A solid, raised mass, usually larger than 2 cm in diameter; skin discoloration may be present

margins. These signs may be accompanied by a transient, erythematous, macular rash in a malar distribution on the face and sometimes on the scalp, forehead, neck, upper torso, and arms. This rash may be preceded by symmetrical muscle soreness and weakness in the pelvis, upper extremities, shoulders, neck, and possibly the face.

• *Erythema chronicum migrans.* Transmitted through a tick bite, this rare systemic disorder is characterized by a papular or macular rash that starts from a single lesion (usually on the leg) that spreads at the margins while clearing centrally. The rash commonly appears on the thighs, trunk, or upper arms, and may exceed 50 cm in diameter. It may be accompanied by fever, chills, headache, malaise, nausea and vomiting, fatigue, backache, knee pain, and stiff neck.

• *Follicular mucinosis.* In this cutaneous disorder, perifollicular papules or plaques are accompanied by prominent alopecia.

• *Fox-Fordyce disease.* This chronic disorder is marked by pruritic papules on the axillae, pubic area, and areolae associated with apocrine sweat gland inflammation. Sparse hair growth in these areas is also common.

• *Gonococcemia.* In this chronic infection, sporadic eruption of an erythematous macular rash is characteristic, although fistulas and petechiae may appear. Typically, the rash affects the distal extremities and rapidly becomes maculopapular, vesiculopustular, and frequently hemorrhagic. Bullae may form. The mature lesion is raised, has a gray, necrotic center, and is surrounded by erythema; it heals in 3 to 4 days. Eruptions are often accompanied by fever and joint pain.

• *Granuloma annulare.* This benign, chronic disorder produces papules that usually coalesce to form plaques. The papules spread peripherally to form a ring with a normal or slightly depressed center. They usually appear on the feet, legs, hands, or fingers, and may be pruritic or asymptomatic.

• *Infectious mononucleosis.* A maculopapular rash that resembles rubella is an early sign of this infection in 10% of patients. Typically, it's preceded by headache, malaise, and fatigue. The rash may be accompanied by sore throat, cervical lymphadenopathy, and fluctuating temperature with an evening peak of 101° to 102 °F. (38.3° to 38.9° C.). Splenomegaly and hepatomegaly may also develop.

• *Insect bites.* Venom from insect bites—especially ticks, lice, flies, and mosquitoes—may produce an allergic reaction associated with a papular, macular, or petechial rash. The rash is usually accompanied by nonspecific signs and symptoms, such as fever, myalgia, headache, lymphadenopathy, nausea, and vomiting.

• *Kaposi's sarcoma.* This neoplastic disorder is characterized by purple or blue papules or macules on the extremities, ears, and nose. These lesions decrease in size upon firm pressure and then return to their original size within 10 to 15 seconds. They may become scaly and ulcerate with bleeding. Two variants—classic and acute generalized—affect the elderly and AIDS patients. Fever, weight loss, hepatomegaly, and splenomegaly may occur.

• *Leprosy.* This chronic infectious disorder produces a variety of skin lesions. Early papular or macular lesions are symmetrical, erythematous, or hypopigmented and may spread over the entire skin surface. Later, plaques and nodules form, especially on the ear lobes, nose, eyebrows, and forehead. Associated signs and symptoms include hypoesthesia or anesthesia, anhidrosis, and dry, scaly skin in affected areas; enlarged, palpable peripheral nerves with severe neuralgia; and muscle atrophy and contractures.

• *Lichen amyloidosus.* This idiopathic cutaneous disorder produces discrete, firm, hemispherical, pruritic papules on the anterior tibiae. Papules may be brown or yellow, smooth or scaly.

• *Lichen planus.* Characteristic lesions of this disorder are discrete, flat, angular or polygonal, violet papules, often marked with white lines or spots. They may be linear or coalesce into plaques and most commonly appear on the lumbar region, genitalia, ankles, anterior tibiae, and the wrists. Lesions usually develop first on the buccal mucosa as a lacy network of white or gray threadlike papules or plaques. Pruritus, distorted fingernails, and atrophic alopecia commonly occur.

• *Mycosis fungoides.* Stage I (premycotic stage) of this rare malignant lymphoma is marked by the eruption of erythematous, pruritic macules on the trunk and extremities. In Stage II, these lesions coalesce into papules and plaques, and nodes become irregular. Stage III is characterized by large, irregular, brown-to-red tumors that ulcerate and are painful and itchy.

• *Necrotizing vasculitis.* In this systemic disorder, crops of purpuric, but otherwise asymptomatic, papules are typical. Some patients also have low-grade fever, headache, myalgia, arthralgia, and abdominal pain.

● *Parapsoriasis (chronic).* This disorder mimics psoriasis, producing small-to-moderate sized, asymptomatic papules with a thin, adherent scale, primarily on the trunk, hands, and feet.

● *Perioral dermatitis.* This inflammatory disorder causes an erythematous eruption of discrete, tiny papules and pustules on the nasolabial fold, chin, and upper lip area. This eruption may be pruritic and painful.

● *Pityriasis rosea.* This disorder begins with an erythematous "herald patch"—a slightly raised, oval lesion about 2 to 6 cm in diameter that may appear anywhere on the body. A few days to weeks later, yellow-to-tan or erythematous patches with scaly edges appear on the trunk, arms, and legs, often erupting along body cleavage lines in a characteristic "pine tree" pattern. These pruritic patches are about 0.5 to 1 cm in diameter.

● *Pityriasis rubra pilaris.* This rare, chronic disorder initially produces scaling seborrhea on the scalp that spreads to the face and ears. Scaly red patches then develop on the palms and soles; these patches thicken, become keratotic, and may develop painful fissures. Later, follicular papules erupt on the hands and forearms, then spread over wide areas of the trunk, neck, and extremities. These papules coalesce into large, scaly, erythematous plaques. Striated fingernails may appear.

● *Polymorphic light eruption.* Abnormal reactions to light may produce papular, vesicular, or nodular rashes on sun-exposed areas. Other symptoms may include pruritus, headache, and malaise.

● *Psoriasis.* Typically, this disorder begins with small, erythematous papules on the scalp, chest, elbows, knees, back, buttocks, and genitalia. These papules are pruritic and sometimes painful. Eventually they enlarge and coalesce, forming elevated, red, scaly plaques covered by characteristic silver scales, except in moist areas such as the genitalia. These scales may flake off easily or thicken, covering the plaque. Associated features include pitted fingernails and arthralgia.

● *Rat-bite fever.* A maculopapular or petechial rash develops on the palms and soles several weeks after a bite from an infected rodent. Other findings typically include pain, redness, and swelling at the bite site; tender regional lymph nodes; fever with chills; malaise; headache; and myalgia.

● *Rosacea.* This hyperemic disorder is characterized by persistent erythema, telangiectasia, and recurrent eruption of papules and pustules on the forehead, malar areas, nose, and chin. Eventually, eruptions recur more frequently and erythema deepens. Rhinophyma may occur in severe cases.

● *Sarcoidosis.* This multisystem granulomatous disorder may produce crops of small, erythematous or yellow-brown papules around the eyes and mouth and on the nose, nasal mucosa, and upper back. Associated findings may include dyspnea with a nonproductive cough, fatigue, arthralgia, weight loss, lymphadenopathy, vision loss, and dysphagia.

● *Seborrheic keratosis.* In this cutaneous disorder, benign skin tumors begin as small, yellow-brown papules on the chest, back, or abdomen; they eventually enlarge and become deeply pigmented. However, in blacks, these papules may remain small and affect only the malar part of the face (dermatosis papulosa nigra).

● *Syphilis.* A discrete, reddish brown, mucocutaneous rash and general lymphadenopathy herald the onset of secondary syphilis. The rash may be papular, macular, pustular, or nodular. Typically, it erupts between rolls of fat on the trunk and proximally on the arms, palms, soles, face, and scalp. Lesions in warm, moist areas enlarge and erode, producing highly contagious, pink or grayish white condylomata lata. In addition, the patient may have mild headache, malaise, anorexia, weight loss, nausea and vomiting, sore throat, low-grade fever, temporary alopecia, and brittle, pitted nails.

• *Syringoma.* In this disorder, adenoma of the sweat glands produces a yellowish or erythematous papular rash on the face (especially the eyelids), neck, and upper chest.

• *Systemic lupus erythematosus (SLE).* This disorder is characterized by a "butterfly rash" of erythematous maculopapules or discoid plaques that appears in a malar distribution across the nose and cheeks. Similar rashes may appear elsewhere, especially on exposed body areas. Other cardinal features include photosensitivity and nondeforming arthritis, especially in the hands, feet, and large joints. Among widespread effects are patchy alopecia, mucous membrane ulceration, low-grade or spiking fever, chills, lymphadenopathy, anorexia, weight loss, abdominal pain, diarrhea or constipation, dyspnea, tachycardia, hematuria, headache, and irritability.

Other causes
• *Drugs.* Transient maculopapular rashes, usually on the trunk, may accompany reactions to many drugs, including antibiotics, such as tetracycline, ampicillin, cephalosporins, and sulfonamides; benzodiazepines, such as diazepam; lithium; phenylbutazone; gold salts; allopurinol; isoniazid; and salicylates.

Special considerations
Advise the patient to keep his skin clean and dry, to wear loose-fitting, nonirritating clothing, and to avoid scratching his rash. Instruct him to promptly report any change in its color, size, or configuration and the onset of itching or bleeding. Also have him avoid excessive exposure to direct sunlight and apply a protective sunscreen before going outdoors.

Apply cool compresses or an antipruritic lotion, such as Sarna lotion, as ordered. Administer antihistamines for allergic reactions and antibiotics for infections, as ordered.

Pediatric pointers
Common causes of papular rashes in children include infectious diseases, such as molluscum contagiosum; scarlet fever; scabies; insect bites; allergies or drug reactions; and congenital cutaneous disorders, such as miliaria profunda.

Paralysis

Paralysis, the total loss of voluntary motor function, results from severe cortical or pyramidal tract damage. It occurs in cerebrovascular disorders, degenerative neuromuscular disease, trauma, tumors, or central nervous system infection. Acute paralysis may be an early indicator of a life-threatening disorder, such as Guillain-Barré syndrome. Paralysis can be local or widespread, symmetrical or asymmetrical, transient or permanent, and spastic or flaccid. It's often classified according to location and severity as paraplegia (sometimes transient paralysis of the legs), quadriplegia (permanent paralysis of the arms, legs, and body below the level of the spinal lesion), or hemiplegia (unilateral paralysis of varying severity and permanence). Incomplete paralysis with profound weakness (paresis) may precede total paralysis in some patients.

Assessment
If the patient's paralysis has developed suddenly, suspect trauma or an acute vascular insult. After ensuring that the patient's spine is properly immobilized, quickly assess his level of consciousness and take his vital signs. Elevated systolic blood pressure, widening pulse pressure, and bradycardia may signal increasing intracranial pressure; notify the doctor immediately, and, if possi-

ble, elevate the patient's head 30° to decrease intracranial pressure. Assess his respiratory status, and be prepared to administer oxygen, insert an artificial airway, or assist with intubation and mechanical ventilation, as needed. To help determine the nature of his injury, attempt to elicit an account of the precipitating events. If the patient's unable to respond, try to find an eyewitness.

If the patient's in no immediate danger, perform a complete neurologic assessment. Start with the history, relying on family members for information, as necessary. Ask about the onset, duration, intensity, and progression of paralysis and about the events preceding its development. Focus medical history questions on the incidence of degenerative neurologic or neuromuscular disease, recent infectious illness, sexually transmitted disease, cancer, or recent injury. Explore related symptoms, noting fever, headache, visual disturbances, dysphagia, nausea and vomiting, bowel or bladder dysfunction, muscle pain or weakness, and fatigue.

Next, perform a complete neurologic examination, testing cranial nerve, motor, and sensory function and deep tendon reflexes. Assess strength in all major muscle groups (see *Testing Muscle Strength*, pages 500 and 501), and note any muscle atrophy. Document all findings to serve as a baseline.

Medical causes

● *Amyotrophic lateral sclerosis.* This invariably fatal disorder produces spastic or flaccid paralysis in the body's major muscle groups, eventually progressing to total paralysis. Earlier findings include progressive muscle weakness, fasciculations, and muscle atrophy, often beginning in the arms and hands. Cramping and hyperreflexia are also common. Respiratory muscle and brain stem involvement produces dyspnea and possibly respiratory distress. Developing cranial nerve paralysis causes dysarthria, dysphagia, drooling, chok-

ing, and difficulty chewing.

● *Bell's palsy.* Bell's palsy, a disease of cranial nerve VII, causes transient, unilateral facial muscle paralysis. The affected muscles sag and eyelid closure is impossible. Other signs include increased tearing, drooling, and a diminished or absent corneal reflex.

● *Botulism.* This bacterial toxin infection can cause rapidly descending muscle weakness that progresses to paralysis within 2 to 4 days after the ingestion of contaminated food. Respiratory muscle paralysis leads to dyspnea and respiratory arrest. Nausea, vomiting, diarrhea, blurred or double vision, bilateral mydriasis, dysarthria, and dysphagia are some early findings.

● *Brain abscess.* Advanced abscess in the frontal or temporal lobe can cause hemiplegia accompanied by other late findings, such as ocular disturbances, unequal pupils, decreased level of consciousness, ataxia, tremors, and signs of infection.

● *Brain tumor.* A tumor affecting the motor cortex of the frontal lobe may cause contralateral hemiparesis that progresses to hemiplegia. Onset is gradual, but paralysis is permanent without treatment. In early stages, frontal headache and behavioral changes may be the only indicators. Eventually, seizures, aphasia, and signs of increased intracranial pressure (decreased level of consciousness and vomiting) develop.

● *Cerebrovascular accident (CVA).* A CVA involving the motor cortex can produce contralateral paresis or paralysis. Onset may be sudden or gradual, and paralysis may be transient or permanent. Associated signs and symptoms vary widely and may include headache, vomiting, seizures, decreased level of consciousness and mental acuity, dysarthria, dysphagia, ataxia, contralateral paresthesias or sensory loss, apraxia, agnosia, aphasia, visual disturbances, emotional lability, and bowel and bladder dysfunction.

● *Conversion disorder.* Hysterical paralysis, a classic conversion symptom, is characterized by the loss of voluntary movement with no obvious physical cause. It can affect any muscle group, appears and disappears unpredictably, and may occur with histrionic behavior (manipulative, dramatic, vain, irrational) or a strange indifference.

• *Encephalitis.* Variable paralysis develops in the late stages of this disorder. Earlier signs and symptoms include rapidly decreasing level of consciousness (possibly coma), fever, headache, photophobia, vomiting, signs of meningeal irritation (nuchal rigidity, positive Kernig's and Brudzinski's signs), aphasia, ataxia, nystagmus, ocular palsies, myoclonus, and seizures.

• *Guillain-Barré syndrome.* This syndrome is characterized by a rapidly developing, but reversible, ascending paralysis. It commonly begins as leg muscle weakness and progresses symmetrically, sometimes affecting even the cranial nerves, producing dysphagia, nasal speech, and dysarthria. Respiratory muscle paralysis may be life-threatening. Other effects may include transient paresthesias, orthostatic hypotension, tachycardia, diaphoresis, and bowel and bladder incontinence.

• *Head trauma.* Cerebral injury can cause paralysis due to cerebral edema and increased intracranial pressure. Onset is usually sudden. Location and extent vary, depending on the injury. Associated findings also vary but may include decreased level of consciousness; sensory disturbances, such as paresthesias and loss of sensation; headache; blurred or double vision; nausea and vomiting; and focal neurologic disturbances.

• *Migraine headache.* Hemiparesis, scotomas, paresthesias, confusion, dizziness, photophobia, or other transient symptoms may precede the onset of a throbbing unilateral headache and may persist after it subsides.

• *Multiple sclerosis.* In this disorder, paralysis commonly waxes and wanes until the later stages, when it may become permanent. Its extent can range from monoplegia to quadriplegia. In most patients, visual and sensory disturbances (paresthesias) are the earliest symptoms. Later findings are widely variable and may include muscle weakness and spasticity, nystagmus, hyperreflexia, intention tremor, gait ataxia, dysphagia, dysarthria, impotence, and constipation. Urinary frequency, urgency, and incontinence may also occur.

• *Myasthenia gravis.* In this neuromuscular disease, profound muscle weakness and abnormal fatigability may produce paralysis of certain muscle groups. Paralysis is usually transient in early stages but becomes more persistent as the disease progresses. Associated findings depend on the areas of neuromuscular involvement; they may include weak eye closure, ptosis, diplopia, lack of facial mobility, dysphagia, nasal speech, and frequent nasal regurgitation of fluids. Neck muscle weakness may cause the patient's jaw to drop and his head to bob. Respiratory muscle involvement can lead to respiratory distress—dyspnea, shallow respirations, and cyanosis.

• *Neurosyphilis.* Irreversible hemiplegia may occur in the late stages of neurosyphilis. Dementia, cranial nerve palsies, tremors, and abnormal reflexes are other late findings.

• *Parkinson's disease.* Tremor, bradykinesia, and lead-pipe or cogwheel rigidity are the classic signs of Parkinson's disease. Extreme rigidity can progress to paralysis, particularly in the extremities. In most cases, paralysis resolves with prompt treatment of the disease.

• *Peripheral nerve trauma.* Severe injury to a peripheral nerve or group of nerves results in the loss of motor and sensory function in the innervated area. Muscles become flaccid and atrophied, and reflexes are lost. If transection isn't complete, paralysis may be temporary.

• *Peripheral neuropathy.* Typically, this syndrome produces muscle weakness that may lead to flaccid paralysis and atrophy. Related effects may include

UNDERSTANDING SPINAL CORD SYNDROMES

When the patient's spinal cord is incompletely severed, he will have partial motor and sensory loss. Most incomplete cord lesions fit into one of the syndromes described below.

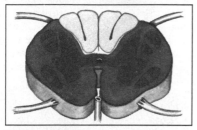

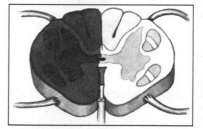

Anterior cord syndrome, most commonly resulting from a flexion injury, causes motor paralysis and loss of pain and temperature sensation below the level of injury. Touch, proprioception, and vibration sensation are usually preserved.

Brown-Séquard syndrome can result from flexion, rotation, or penetration injuries. It's characterized by unilateral motor paralysis ipsilateral to the injury and loss of pain and temperature sensation contralateral to the injury.

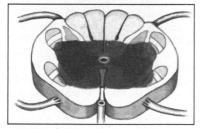

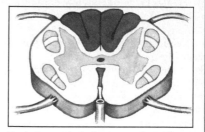

Central cord syndrome is caused by hyperextension or flexion injuries. Motor loss is variable and greater in the arms than in the legs; sensory loss is usually slight.

Posterior cord syndrome, produced by a cervical hyperextension injury, causes only a loss of proprioception and loss of light touch sensation. Motor function remains intact.

paresthesias, loss of vibration sensation, hypoactive or absent deep tendon reflexes, neuralgia, and skin changes, such as anhidrosis.

• *Poliomyelitis.* This disorder can produce insidious, permanent flaccid paralysis and hyporeflexia. Sensory function remains intact, but the patient loses voluntary muscle control.

• *Rabies.* This acute disorder produces progressive flaccid paralysis, vascular collapse, coma, and death within 2 weeks of contact with an infected animal. Prodromal signs and symptoms—fever; headache; hyperesthesia; paresthesias, coldness, and itching at the bite site; photophobia; tachycardia; shallow respirations; and excessive salivation, lacrimation, and perspiration—develop almost immediately. Within 2 to 10 days, a phase of excitement begins with agitation, cranial nerve dysfunction (pupil changes, hoarseness, facial weakness, ocular palsies), tachycardia or bradycardia, cyclic respirations, high fever, urinary retention, drooling, and hydrophobia.

• *Seizure disorders.* Seizures, particularly focal seizures, can cause transient local paralysis (Todd's paralysis). Any part of the body may be affected, although paralysis tends to occur contralateral to the side of the irritable focus.

• **Spinal cord injury.** Complete spinal cord transection results in permanent spastic paralysis below the level of injury. Reflexes may return after resolution of spinal shock. Partial transection causes variable paralysis and paresthesias, depending on the location and extent of injury (see *Understanding Spinal Cord Syndromes*, page 565).

• **Spinal cord tumors.** Paresis, pain, paresthesias, and variable sensory loss may occur along the nerve distribution pathway served by the affected cord segment. Eventually, this may progress to spastic paralysis with hyperactive deep tendon reflexes (unless the tumor is in the cauda equina, which produces hyporeflexia) and, perhaps, bladder and bowel incontinence. Paralysis is permanent without treatment.

• **Subarachnoid hemorrhage.** This potentially life-threatening disorder can produce sudden paralysis. Duration may be temporary, resolving with decreasing edema, or permanent, if tissue destruction has occurred. Other acute effects are severe headache, mydriasis, photophobia, aphasia, sharply decreased level of consciousness, nuchal rigidity, vomiting, and seizures.

• **Syringomyelia.** This degenerative spinal cord disease produces segmental paresis, leading to flaccid paralysis of the hands and arms. Reflexes are absent, and loss of pain and temperature sensation is distributed over the neck, shoulders, and arms in a capelike pattern.

• **Thoracic aortic aneurysm.** Occlusion of spinal arteries by a ruptured thoracic aortic aneurysm may cause sudden onset of transient bilateral paralysis. Severe chest pain radiating to the neck, shoulders, back, and abdomen and a sensation of tearing in the thorax are prominent symptoms. Related findings include syncope, pallor, diaphoresis, dyspnea, tachycardia, cyanosis, diastolic heart murmur, and abrupt loss of radial and femoral pulses or wide variations in pulses and blood pressure between arms and legs. Paradoxically, though the patient appears to be in shock, his systolic blood pressure is often normal or elevated.

• **Transient ischemic attack (TIA).** Episodic TIAs may cause transient unilateral paresis or paralysis accompanied by paresthesias, blurred or double vision, dizziness, aphasia, dysarthria, decreased level of consciousness, and other site-dependent effects.

Other causes
• **Drugs.** Therapeutic use of neuromuscular blocking agents, such as pancuronium or curare, produces paralysis.
• **Electroconvulsive therapy.** This therapy can produce acute, but transient, paralysis.

Special considerations
Because a paralyzed patient is particularly susceptible to the complications of prolonged immobility, provide frequent position changes, meticulous skin care, and frequent chest physiotherapy. He may benefit from passive range-of-motion exercises to maintain muscle tone, application of splints to prevent contractures, and the use of footboards or other devices to prevent footdrop. If his cranial nerves are affected, the patient will have difficulty chewing and swallowing. Provide a liquid or soft diet, and keep suction equipment on hand in case aspiration occurs. Feeding tubes or I.V. hyperalimentation may be necessary in severe paralysis. Paralysis and accompanying visual disturbances may make ambulation hazardous; provide a call light and show the patient how to call for help. As appropriate, arrange for physical, speech, or occupational therapy.

Pediatric pointers
Besides the obvious causes—trauma, infection, or tumors—children may contract paralysis from hereditary and congenital disorders, such as Tay-Sachs disease, Werdnig-Hoffmann disease, spina bifida, and cerebral palsy.

Paresthesias

Paresthesias are abnormal sensations—often described as numbness, prickling, or tingling—felt along peripheral nerve pathways. These sensations are generally not painful; unpleasant or painful sensations are termed *dysesthesias*. Paresthesias may develop suddenly or gradually and may be transient or permanent.

A common symptom of many neurologic disorders, paresthesias may also result from certain systemic disorders and the effects of drugs. They reflect damage or irritation of the parietal lobe, thalamus, spinothalamic tract, or spinal or peripheral nerves—the circuit responsible for transmission and interpretation of sensory stimuli.

Assessment

First explore the paresthesias. When did they begin? Have the patient describe their character and distribution. Also ask about associated signs and symptoms, such as sensory loss and paresis or paralysis. Next, take a medical history, including neurologic, cardiovascular, metabolic, renal, and chronic inflammatory disorders, such as arthritis or lupus. Has the patient sustained trauma or had recent surgery or invasive procedures that may have injured peripheral nerves?

Focus the physical examination on the patient's neurologic status. Assess his level of consciousness and cranial nerve function. Test muscle strength and deep tendon reflexes in limbs affected by paresthesias. Systematically evaluate light touch, pain, temperature, vibration, and position sensation (see *Testing for Analgesia*, pages 44 and 45). Also note skin color and temperature, and palpate pulses.

Medical causes

● *Arterial occlusion (acute).* In this disorder, sudden paresthesias and cold-ness may develop in one or both legs with a saddle embolus. Paresis, intermittent claudication, and aching pain at rest are also characteristic. The extremity becomes mottled with a line of temperature and color demarcation at the level of occlusion. Pulses are absent below the occlusion, and capillary refill is diminished.

● *Arteriosclerosis obliterans.* This disorder produces paresthesias, intermittent claudication (most common symptom), diminished or absent popliteal and pedal pulses, pallor, paresis, and coldness in the affected leg.

● *Arthritis.* Rheumatoid or osteoarthritic changes in the cervical spine may cause paresthesias in the neck, shoulders, and arms. Less frequently the lumbar spine is affected, causing paresthesias in one or both legs and feet. Painful or stiff back and neck and hypoactive deep tendon reflexes may also occur.

● *Brain tumor.* Tumors affecting the sensory cortex in the parietal lobe may cause progressive contralateral paresthesias accompanied by agnosia, apraxia, agraphia, homonymous hemianopia, and loss of proprioception.

● *Buerger's disease.* In this inflammatory occlusive disorder, exposure to cold makes the feet cold, cyanotic, and numb; later, they redden, become hot, and tingle. Intermittent claudication, which is aggravated by exercise and relieved by rest, is also common. Occasionally, Buerger's disease affects the hands, possibly resulting in painful fingertip ulcerations. Other findings include weak peripheral pulses, migratory superficial thrombophlebitis, and, in later stages, ulceration, muscle atrophy, and gangrene.

● *Cerebrovascular accident (CVA).* Although contralateral paresthesias may occur in CVA, sensory loss is more common. Associated features vary with the artery affected. There may be contralateral hemiplegia, decreased level of consciousness, homonymous hemianopia, and others.

● *Guillain-Barré syndrome.* In this syndrome, transient paresthesias may precede muscle weakness, which usually begins in the legs and ascends to the arms and facial nerves. Eventually, weakness may progress to paralysis. Other clinical features may be dysarthria, dysphagia, nasal speech, orthostatic hypotension, bladder and bowel incontinence, diaphoresis, tachycardia, and possibly signs of life-threatening respiratory muscle paralysis.

• **Head trauma.** Unilateral or bilateral paresthesias may occur when head trauma causes concussion or contusion; however, sensory loss is more common. Other findings may include variable paresis or paralysis, decreased level of consciousness, headache, blurred or double vision, nausea and vomiting, dizziness, and seizures.

• **Heavy metal or solvent poisoning.** Exposure to industrial or household products containing lead, mercury, thallium, or organophosphates may cause paresthesias of acute or gradual onset. Mental status changes, tremors, weakness, seizures, and gastrointestinal distress also occur commonly.

• **Herniated disk.** Herniation of a lumbar or cervical disk may cause acute or gradual onset of paresthesias along the distribution pathways of affected spinal nerves. Other neuromuscular effects include severe pain, muscle spasms, and weakness that may progress to atrophy unless herniation is relieved.

• **Herpes zoster.** An early symptom of this disorder, paresthesias occur in the dermatome supplied by the affected spinal nerve. Within several days, this dermatome is marked by a pruritic, erythematous, vesicular rash associated with sharp, shooting, or burning pain.

• **Hyperventilation syndrome.** Usually triggered by acute anxiety, this syndrome may produce transient paresthesias in the hands, feet, and perioral area, accompanied by agitation, vertigo, syncope, pallor, muscle twitching and weakness, carpopedal spasm, and cardiac dysrhythmias.

• **Hypocalcemia.** An early symptom of hypocalcemia, asymmetrical paresthesias usually occur in the fingers, toes, and circumoral area. Among other manifestations are muscle weakness, twitching, or cramps; palpitations; hyperactive deep tendon reflexes; carpopedal spasm; and positive Chvostek's and Trousseau's signs.

• **Migraine headache.** Paresthesias in the hands, face, and perioral area may herald an impending migraine headache. Other prodromal symptoms may include scotomas, hemiparesis, confusion, dizziness, and photophobia. These effects may persist during the characteristic throbbing headache and continue after it subsides.

• **Multiple sclerosis (MS).** In this disorder, demyelination of the sensory cortex or spinothalamic tract may produce paresthesias—often one of the earliest symptoms of MS. Like other effects of MS, paresthesias commonly wax and wane until the later stages, when they may become permanent. Associated findings may include muscle weakness, spasticity, hyperreflexia, and others.

• **Peripheral nerve trauma.** Injury to any of the major peripheral nerves may cause paresthesias—often dysesthesias—in the area supplied by that nerve. Paresthesias begin shortly after trauma and may be permanent. Other effects may be flaccid paralysis or paresis, hyporeflexia, and variable sensory loss.

• **Peripheral neuropathy.** This syndrome may cause progressive paresthesias in all extremities. The patient also commonly displays muscle weakness, which may lead to flaccid paralysis and atrophy; loss of vibration sensation; diminished or absent deep tendon reflexes; neuralgia; and cutaneous changes, such as glossy, red skin and anhidrosis.

• **Rabies.** Paresthesias, coldness, and itching at the site of an animal bite herald the prodromal stage of rabies. Other prodromal effects are fever, headache, photophobia, hyperesthesia, tachycardia, shallow respirations, and excessive salivation, lacrimation, and perspiration.

• *Raynaud's disease.* Exposure to cold or stress makes the fingers turn pale, cold, and cyanotic; with rewarming, they become red and paresthetic. Ulceration may occur in chronic cases.

• *Seizure disorders.* Seizures originating in the parietal lobe usually cause paresthesias of the lips, fingers, and toes. Paresthesias may also be an aura that warns of tonic-clonic seizures.

• *Spinal cord injury.* Paresthesias may occur in partial spinal cord transection, after spinal shock resolves. They may be unilateral or bilateral, occurring at or below the level of the lesion. Associated sensory and motor loss is variable (see *Understanding Spinal Cord Syndromes,* page 565).

• *Spinal cord tumors.* Typically, these tumors produce paresthesias, paresis, pain, and variable sensory loss along the nerve distribution pathway served by the affected cord segment. Eventually, paresis may progress to spastic paralysis with hyperactive deep tendon reflexes (unless the tumor is in the cauda equina, which produces hyporeflexia) and, possibly, bladder and bowel incontinence.

• *Systemic lupus erythematosus.* This disorder infrequently causes paresthesias. Its primary clinical features include nondeforming arthritis, usually involving the hands, feet, and large joints; photosensitivity; and a characteristic "butterfly" rash that appears across the nose and cheeks.

• *Tabes dorsalis.* In this form of neurosyphilis, paresthesias—especially of the legs—are a common, but late, symptom. Other effects may include ataxia, loss of proprioception and pain and temperature sensation, absent deep tendon reflexes, Charcot's joints, Argyll Robertson pupils, incontinence, and impotence.

• *Thoracic outlet syndrome.* Paresthesias occur suddenly in this syndrome when the affected arm is raised and abducted. The arm also becomes pale and cool with diminished pulses. Unequal blood pressure between arms may be noted.

• *Transient ischemic attack.* Typically, paresthesias occur abruptly in an attack and are limited to one arm or another isolated part of the body. They usually last about 10 minutes and are accompanied by paralysis or paresis. Associated findings may include decreased level of consciousness, dizziness, unilateral vision loss, nystagmus, aphasia, dysarthria, tinnitus, facial weakness, dysphagia, and ataxic gait.

• *Vitamin B deficiency.* Chronic thiamine or vitamin B_{12} deficiency may cause paresthesias and weakness in the arms and legs. Burning leg pain, hypoactive deep tendon reflexes, and variable sensory loss are common in thiamine deficiency; vitamin B_{12} deficiency also produces mental status changes and impaired vision.

Other causes

• *Drugs.* Phenytoin, chemotherapeutic agents (such as vincristine, vinblastine, and procarbazine), D-penicillamine, isoniazid, nitrofurantoin, chloroquine, and parenteral gold therapy may produce transient paresthesias that disappear when the drug is discontinued.

• *Radiation therapy.* Long-term radiation therapy may eventually cause peripheral nerve damage, producing paresthesias.

Special considerations

Since paresthesias are often accompanied by patchy sensory loss, teach the patient safety measures. For example, have him test bathwater with a thermometer and smoke cigarettes carefully to avoid burning his fingers.

Pediatric pointers

Although children may experience paresthesias associated with the same causes as adults, they're frequently unable to describe this symptom. Nevertheless, hereditary polyneuropathies are usually first recognized in childhood.

Paroxysmal Nocturnal Dyspnea

Typically dramatic and terrifying to the patient, this sign refers to an attack of dyspnea that abruptly awakens the patient. An attack often causes diaphoresis, coughing, and wheezing. It abates after the patient sits up or stands for several minutes, but may recur every 2 to 3 hours.

Paroxysmal nocturnal dyspnea is an early sign of left ventricular failure. It can reflect decreased respiratory drive, impaired left ventricular function, enhanced reabsorption of interstitial fluid, and increased thoracic blood volume. All of these pathophysiologic mechanisms cause dyspnea to worsen when the patient lies down.

Assessment

Begin by exploring the patient's complaint of dyspnea. Does he have a dyspneic attack at other times, such as after exertion or while sitting down? If so, what type of activity triggers the attack? Does he have coughing, wheezing, fatigue, or weakness during an attack? Find out if the patient sleeps with his head elevated and, if so, on how many pillows. Obtain a cardiopulmonary history. Does the patient or a family member have a history of myocardial infarction, coronary artery disease, or hypertension? Chronic bronchitis, emphysema, or asthma? Has the patient had cardiac surgery?

Now perform a physical examination. Begin by taking the patient's vital signs and forming an overall impression of his appearance. Is he noticeably cyanotic or edematous? Auscultate the lungs for crackles and wheezing, and the heart for gallops and dysrhythmias.

Medical cause

● *Left ventricular failure.* Dyspnea—on exertion, during sleep, and eventually even at rest—is an early sign of left ventricular failure. It's characteristically accompanied by Cheyne-Stokes respirations, diaphoresis, weakness, wheezing, and a persistent, nonproductive cough or a cough that produces clear or blood-tinged sputum.

As the patient's condition worsens, he develops tachycardia, tachypnea, pulsus alternans (often initiated by a premature beat), a ventricular gallop, and crackles.

In advanced left ventricular failure, the patient may also have severe orthopnea, cyanosis, clubbing, hemoptysis, and cardiac dysrhythmias. In addition, the patient may develop signs and symptoms of shock, such as hypotension, weak pulse, and cold, clammy skin.

Special considerations

Prepare the patient for diagnostic tests, such as chest X-ray, echocardiography, exercise electrocardiography, and cardiac blood pool imaging.

If the hospitalized patient experiences paroxysmal nocturnal dyspnea, assist him to a sitting position, or help him walk around the room. If necessary, provide low-flow supplemental oxygen. Try to calm him, since anxiety can exacerbate dyspnea.

Pediatric pointers

In a child, paroxysmal nocturnal dyspnea usually stems from congenital heart defects that precipitate ventricular failure. Help relieve the child's dyspnea by elevating his head and calming him.

Peau d'Orange

["Orange-peel" skin]

Usually a late sign of breast cancer, peau d'orange is the edematous thickening and pitting of breast skin. This slowly developing sign can also occur with breast or axillary lymph node infection. Its striking orange-peel appearance stems from lymphatic edema around deepened hair follicles.

Assessment
Ask the patient when she first detected peau d'orange. Has she noticed any lumps, pain, or other breast changes? Does she have related symptoms, such as malaise and achiness? Is she lactating or has she recently weaned her infant?

In a well-lit examining room, observe the patient's breasts. Estimate the extent of the peau d'orange and check for erythema. Assess the nipples for discharge, deviation, retraction, dimpling, and cracking. Now gently palpate the area of peau d'orange, noting warmth or induration. Then palpate the entire breast, noting any fixed or mobile lumps, and the axillary lymph nodes, noting enlargement. Finally, take the patient's temperature.

Medical causes
● *Breast abscess.* Usually affecting lactating women with milk stasis, this infection causes peau d'orange, malaise, breast tenderness and erythema, and a sudden fever possibly accompanied by shaking chills. A cracked nipple may exude pus, and an indurated or palpable soft mass may be present.

● *Breast cancer.* Advanced breast cancer is the most likely cause of peau d'orange, which usually begins in the dependent part of the breast or the areola. Palpation typically reveals a firm, immobile mass that adheres to the skin above the area of peau d'orange. Inspection of the breasts may reveal changes in contour, size, or symmetry. Inspection of the nipples may reveal deviation, erosion, retraction, and a thin and watery, bloody, or purulent discharge. The patient may report a burning and itching sensation in the nipples as well as a sensation of warmth or heat in the breast. Breast pain may occur, but it's not a reliable indicator of malignancy.

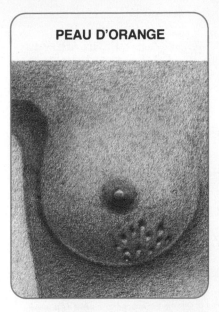

PEAU D'ORANGE

● *Tuberculosis of the axillary lymph nodes.* Rarely, peau d'orange occurs as one or more axillary lymph nodes enlarge. Nodal enlargement is usually painless but may be accompanied by mild fever, fatigue, and weight loss.

Special considerations
Because peau d'orange usually signals advanced breast cancer, you'll need to provide emotional support for the patient. Encourage her to express her fears and concerns. Clearly explain expected diagnostic tests, such as mammography and breast biopsy.

Pediatric pointers
None.

Pericardial Friction Rub

Often transient, a pericardial friction rub is a scratching, grating, or crunching sound that occurs when two inflamed layers of the pericardium slide

PERICARDIAL FRICTION RUB OR MURMUR?

Is the sound you hear a pericardial friction rub or a murmur? Here's how to tell.

The classic pericardial friction rub has three sound components, which are related to the phases of the cardiac cycle. In some patients, however, the rub's presystolic and/or early diastolic sounds may be inaudible, causing it to resemble the murmur of mitral insufficiency or aortic stenosis and regurgitation.

If you don't detect the classic three-component sound, you can distinguish a pericardial friction rub from a murmur by auscultating again and asking yourself these questions:

How deep is the sound?

A pericardial friction rub usually sounds superficial; a murmur sounds deeper in the chest.

Does the sound radiate?

A pericardial friction rub usually doesn't radiate; a murmur may radiate widely.

Does the sound vary with inspiration or changes in patient position?

A pericardial friction rub is usually loudest during inspiration and is best heard when the patient leans forward. A murmur varies in timing and duration with both factors.

---

over one another. Ranging from faint to loud, this abnormal sound is best heard along the lower left sternal border during deep inspiration. It indicates pericarditis, which can result from acute infection, cardiac and renal disorders, postpericardiotomy syndrome, and certain drugs, such as procainamide and antineoplastic agents.

Occasionally, a pericardial friction rub can resemble a murmur (see *Pericardial Friction Rub or Murmur?*) or a pleural friction rub (see *Comparing Auscultation Findings,* pages 580 and 581). However, the classic pericardial friction rub has three components. (See *Understanding Pericardial Friction Rubs.*)

Assessment

Obtain a complete medical history, noting especially cardiac dysfunction. Has the patient recently had a myocardial infarction or cardiac surgery? Has he ever had pericarditis or rheumatic disorders, such as rheumatoid arthritis or systemic lupus erythematosus? Does he have chronic renal failure or an infection? If the patient complains of chest pain, ask him to describe its character and location. What relieves the pain? What worsens it?

Take the patient's vital signs, noting especially hypotension, tachycardia, irregular pulse, tachypnea, and fever. Inspect for jugular vein distention, edema, ascites, and hepatomegaly. Auscultate the lungs for crackles.

Medical cause

• *Pericarditis.* A pericardial friction rub is the hallmark of *acute pericarditis.* This disorder also causes sharp precordial or retrosternal pain that usually radiates to the left shoulder and neck. The pain worsens when the patient breathes deeply, coughs, or lies flat and, possibly, when he swallows. It abates when he sits up and leans forward. He may also have fever, dyspnea, tachycardia, and dysrhythmias.

In *chronic constrictive pericarditis,* a pericardial friction rub develops gradually. It's accompanied by signs of decreased cardiac filling and output, such as peripheral edema, ascites, jugular vein distention on inspiration (Kussmaul's sign), and hepatomegaly. Dyspnea, orthopnea, pulsus paradoxus, and chest pain may also occur.

Special considerations

Continue to monitor the patient's cardiovascular status. If the pericardial friction rub disappears, be alert for signs of cardiac tamponade: pallor; cool, clammy skin; hypotension; tachycardia; tachypnea; pulsus paradoxus;

and increased jugular vein distention. If these signs occur, prepare the patient for pericardiocentesis to prevent cardiovascular collapse.

Ensure that the patient gets adequate rest. As ordered, give anti-inflammatory drugs, antiarrhythmics, diuretics, or antimicrobials to treat the underlying cause. If necessary, prepare him for a pericardiectomy to promote adequate cardiac filling and contraction.

Pediatric pointers

Bacterial pericarditis may develop during the first two decades of life, most commonly before age 6. Although a pericardial friction rub may occur, other signs and symptoms—fever, tachycardia, dyspnea, chest pain, jugular vein distention, and hepatomegaly—more reliably indicate this life-threatening disorder.

A pericardial friction rub may occur after surgery to correct congenital cardiac anomalies. However, it usually vanishes without development of pericarditis.

Peristaltic Waves— Visible

In intestinal obstruction, peristalsis temporarily increases in strength and frequency as the intestine tries to force its contents past the obstruction. As a result, visible peristaltic waves may roll across the abdomen. Typically, these waves appear suddenly and vanish quickly, because increased peristalsis overcomes the obstruction or the gastrointestinal tract becomes atonic. Peristaltic waves are best detected by stooping at the supine patient's side and inspecting the abdominal contour.

Visible peristaltic waves may also reflect normal stomach and intestinal contractions in thin patients or in malnourished patients with abdominal muscle atrophy.

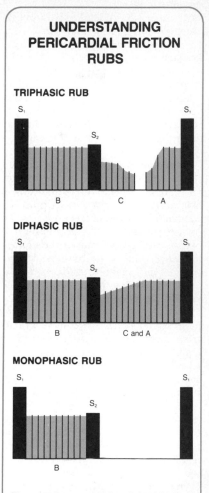

UNDERSTANDING PERICARDIAL FRICTION RUBS

The complete, or classic, rub is triphasic. Its three sound components are linked to phases of the cardiac cycle: the *presystolic* component (A) reflects atrial systole and precedes the first heart sound (S_1). The *systolic* component (B)—usually the loudest—reflects ventricular systole and occurs between the first and second heart sounds (S_2). The *early diastolic* component (C) reflects ventricular diastole and follows the second heart sound.

Sometimes, the early diastolic component merges with the presystolic component, producing a diphasic to-and-fro sound on auscultation. In other patients, auscultation may detect only one component—a monophasic rub, typically during ventricular systole.

Assessment

After observing peristaltic waves, collect pertinent history data. For example, ask about a history of pyloric ulcer, stomach cancer, or chronic gastritis, which can lead to pyloric obstruction. Also ask about conditions leading to intestinal obstruction, such as intestinal tumors or polyps, gallstones, chronic constipation, and a hernia. Has the patient recently had abdominal surgery?

Determine if the patient has related symptoms. Spasmodic abdominal pain, for example, accompanies small-bowel obstruction, whereas colicky pain accompanies pyloric obstruction. Is the patient nauseated? Has he vomited? If he has vomited, ask about the consistency and color of the vomitus. Lumpy vomitus may contain undigested food particles. Green or brown vomitus may contain bile or fecal matter.

Now, with the patient supine, inspect the abdomen for distention, surgical scars and adhesions, or visible loops of bowel. Auscultate for bowel sounds, noting high-pitched, tinkling sounds. Next, jar the patient's bed (or roll the patient from side to side) and auscultate for a succussion splash—a splashing sound in the stomach that indicates pyloric obstruction. Palpate the abdomen for rigidity and tenderness, and percuss for tympany. Check the skin and mucous membranes for dryness and poor skin turgor, indicating dehydration. Take the patient's vital signs, noting especially tachycardia and hypotension, which indicate hypovolemia.

Medical causes

• *Large-bowel obstruction.* Visible peristaltic waves in the upper abdomen are an early sign of this obstruction. Obstipation, however, may be the earliest finding. Other characteristic signs and symptoms develop more slowly than in small-bowel obstruction. They may include nausea, colicky abdominal pain (milder than in small-bowel obstruction), gradual and eventually marked abdominal distention, and hyperactive bowel sounds.

• *Pyloric obstruction.* Peristaltic waves may be detected in a swollen epigastrium or in the left upper quadrant, usually beginning near the left rib margin and rolling from left to right. Related findings include vague epigastric discomfort or colicky pain after eating, nausea, vomiting, anorexia, and weight loss. Auscultation reveals a loud succussion splash.

• *Small-bowel obstruction.* Early signs of mechanical obstruction of the small bowel include peristaltic waves rolling across the upper abdomen and intermittent, cramping periumbilical pain. Associated signs and symptoms include nausea, vomiting of bilious or, later, fecal material, and constipation; in partial obstruction, diarrhea may be present. Hyperactive bowel sounds and slight abdominal distention also occur early.

Special considerations

Because visible peristaltic waves are often an early sign of intestinal obstruction, you'll need to monitor the patient's status and prepare him for diagnostic evaluation and treatment. Be sure to withhold food and fluids, and explain the purpose and procedure of abdominal X-rays and barium studies, which can confirm obstruction.

If tests confirm obstruction, nasogastric suctioning may be used to decompress the stomach and small bowel. Provide frequent oral hygiene, and watch for a thick, swollen tongue and dry mucous membranes, indicating dehydration. Monitor vital signs and intake and output frequently.

Pediatric pointers

In infants, visible peristaltic waves may indicate pyloric stenosis. In small children, peristaltic waves may normally be visible because of their protuberant abdomens. Or visible waves may indicate bowel obstruction stemming from congenital anomalies, volvulus, or swallowing a foreign body.

Photophobia

A common symptom, photophobia is an abnormal sensitivity to light. In many patients, photophobia simply indicates increased eye sensitivity without an underlying pathology. In some patients, it can indicate excessive wearing of contact lenses or poorly fitted lenses. But, in others, this symptom can indicate systemic disorders, ocular disorders or trauma, or use of certain drugs.

Assessment

If your patient reports photophobia, find out when it began and how severe it is. Did it follow eye trauma? A chemical splash or exposure to the rays of a sun lamp? If photophobia results from trauma, avoid eye manipulation. Ask the patient about eye pain and have him describe its location, duration, and intensity. Does he have a sensation of a foreign body in his eye? Does he have any other signs and symptoms, such as increased tearing and vision changes?

Next, take the patient's vital signs and assess his neurologic status. Follow this with a careful eye examination, inspecting the eyes' external structures for any abnormalities. Examine the conjunctiva and sclera, noting especially their color. Characterize the amount and consistency of any discharge. Then check pupillary reaction to light. Evaluate extraocular muscle function by testing the six cardinal fields of gaze, and test visual acuity in both eyes.

During your assessment, keep in mind that photophobia can accompany life-threatening meningitis, although it's not a cardinal sign of meningeal irritation.

Medical causes

● *Burns.* In *chemical burns*, photophobia and eye pain may be accompanied by erythema and blistering on the face and lids, miosis, diffuse conjunctival injection, and corneal changes. The patient may be unable to keep the eye(s) open, and his vision is blurred.

In *ultraviolet radiation burns*, photophobia occurs with moderate to severe eye pain. These symptoms develop about 12 hours after exposure to the rays of a welding arc or sun lamp.

● *Conjunctivitis.* When conjunctivitis affects the cornea, it causes photophobia. Other common findings include conjunctival injection, increased tearing, a foreign body sensation, a feeling of fullness around the eyes, and eye pain, burning, and itching. *Allergic conjunctivitis* is distinguished by a stringy eye discharge and milky red injection. *Bacterial conjunctivitis* tends to cause a copious, mucopurulent, flaky eye discharge that may make the eyelids stick together, as well as brilliant red conjunctiva. *Fungal conjunctivitis* produces a thick, purulent discharge, extreme redness, and crusting, sticky eyelids. *Viral conjunctivitis* causes copious tearing with little discharge as well as enlargement of the preauricular lymph nodes.

● *Corneal abrasion.* A common finding with corneal abrasion, photophobia is usually accompanied by excessive tearing, conjunctival injection, visible corneal damage, and a foreign body sensation in the eye. Blurred vision and eye pain may occur.

● *Corneal foreign body.* Photophobia may occur with miosis, intense eye pain, a foreign body sensation, slightly impaired vision, conjunctival injection, and profuse tearing. A dark speck may be visible on the cornea.

● *Corneal ulcer.* This vision-threatening disorder causes severe photophobia and eye pain that's aggravated by blinking. Impaired visual acuity may accompany blurring, eye discharge, and sticky eyelids. Conjunctival injection may occur even though the cornea appears white and opaque. A *bacterial ulcer* may also cause an irregularly shaped corneal ulcer and unilateral pupillary constriction. A *fungal ulcer* may be surrounded by progressively clearer rings.

• *Dry eye syndrome.* This disorder may produce photophobia but more characteristically causes eye pain, conjunctival injection, a foreign body sensation, itching, excessive mucus secretion, and possibly decreased tearing and difficulty moving the eyelids.

• *Iritis (acute).* Severe photophobia may result from this disorder, along with marked conjunctival injection, moderate to severe eye pain, and blurred vision. The pupil may be constricted and may respond poorly to light.

• *Keratitis (interstitial).* This corneal inflammation causes photophobia, eye pain, blurred vision, dramatic con-

PHOTOPHOBIA: CAUSES AND ASSOCIATED FINDINGS

CAUSES	Conjunctival injection	Corneal changes	Eye discharge	Eyelid edema	Eye pain	Foreign body sensation	Nuchal rigidity	Pupillary changes	Tearing—increased	Vision changes	Visual floaters	Vomiting
Burns (chemical)	●	●			●			●		●		
Burns (ultraviolet)					●							
Conjunctivitis	●		●		●	●			●			
Corneal abrasion	●	●			●	●			●	●		
Corneal foreign body	●	●			●	●		●	●	●		
Corneal ulcer	●	●	●		●			●		●		
Dry eye syndrome	●		●		●	●						
Interstitial keratitis	●	●			●					●		
Iritis (acute)	●				●			●		●		
Meningitis (acute bacterial)							●	●				●
Migraine headache										●		●
Scleritis	●				●				●			
Sclerokeratitis		●			●							
Trachoma		●	●	●	●				●	●		
Uveitis (anterior)	●				●			●				
Uveitis (posterior)	●				●			●		●	●	

junctival injection, and grayish pink corneas.

• **Meningitis (acute bacterial).** A common symptom of this disorder, photophobia may occur with other signs of meningeal irritation, such as nuchal rigidity, hyperreflexia, and opisthotonos. Brudzinski's and Kernig's signs can be elicited. Fever, an early finding, may be accompanied by chills. Related effects may include headache, vomiting, ocular palsies, facial weakness, pupillary abnormalities, and hearing loss. In severe meningitis, seizures may occur along with stupor progressing to coma.

• **Migraine headache.** Photophobia and noise sensitivity are prominent features of a common migraine. Typically severe, this aching or throbbing headache may also cause fatigue, blurred vision, nausea, and vomiting.

• **Scleritis.** This disorder may cause photophobia, severe eye pain, conjunctival injection, and a bluish purple sclera. The eye may tear profusely.

• **Sclerokeratitis.** Inflammation of the sclera and cornea causes photophobia, eye pain, burning, and irritation.

• **Trachoma.** At first, trachoma resembles bacterial conjunctivitis, producing photophobia, visible conjunctival follicles, red and edematous eyelids, pain, increased tearing, and discharge. Without treatment, conjunctival follicles enlarge into inflamed papillae that later become yellow or gray; small blood vessels invade the cornea under the upper lid. Eventually, entropion may occur with corneal scarring, visual distortion, and possibly dry eyes.

• **Uveitis.** Both anterior and posterior uveitis can cause photophobia. Typically, *anterior uveitis* also produces moderate to severe eye pain, severe conjunctival injection, and a small, nonreactive pupil. *Posterior uveitis* develops slowly, causing visual floaters, eye pain, pupil distortion, conjunctival injection, and blurred vision.

Other causes

• **Drugs.** Mydriatics—such as phenylephrine, atropine, scopolamine, cyclo-pentolate, and tropicamide—can cause photophobia due to ocular dilation. Amphetamines, cocaine, and ophthalmic antifungal drugs—such as trifluridine, vidarabine, and idoxuridine—can also cause photophobia.

Special considerations

Promote patient comfort by darkening the room and telling him to close both eyes. If photophobia persists at home, suggest that he wear dark glasses.

As ordered, prepare the patient for diagnostic tests, such as corneal scraping and slit-lamp examination.

Pediatric pointers

Suspect photophobia in any child who squints, rubs his eyes frequently, or wears sunglasses indoors and outside.

Congenital disorders, such as syphilis and albinism, and childhood diseases, such as measles and rubella, can cause photophobia.

Pica

Pica refers to the craving and ingestion of normally inedible substances, such as plaster, charcoal, clay, wool, ashes, paint, or dirt. In children, the most commonly affected group, pica typically results from nutritional deficiencies. However, in adults, pica may reflect a psychological disturbance.

Depending on the substance eaten, pica can lead to poisoning and gastrointestinal disorders.

Assessment

Begin your assessment by determining what substances the patient has been eating. If he has eaten toxic substances, such as lead, notify the doctor and the poison control center.

Ask the parents to describe their child's eating habits and nutritional history. When did he first display pica? Does he always crave the same substance? Is he listless or irritable?

Check the patient's vital signs, noting especially bradycardia, tachycardia, or hypotension. Then inspect the abdomen for visible peristaltic waves or other abnormalities. Also observe the hair, skin, and mucous membranes for changes, such as dryness or pallor.

Medical causes

• *Anemia (iron deficiency).* Chronic, severe iron deficiency anemia may cause pica for dirt, paint, cornstarch, nails, or clay. It may also cause fatigue, irritability, listlessness, and anorexia. The patient may complain of light-headedness, headache, an inability to concentrate, dysphagia, and dyspnea on exertion. His muscle tone is poor and his extremities may have paresthesias. His nails are brittle and spoon-shaped, his tongue is smooth, and his skin and mucous membranes are pale.

• *Malnutrition.* Severe malnutrition and starvation may cause pica for any substance, including dirt. Besides marked weight loss, the patient may have muscle wasting and paresthesias in the extremities. He appears lethargic and apathetic. His skin is dry, thin, and flaky. His sparse, dull hair falls out easily. His nails are brittle, his cheeks are dark and swollen, and his lips are red and swollen. The patient may also have nausea, vomiting, hepatomegaly, bradycardia, hypotension, slow and shallow respirations, and amenorrhea or gonadal atrophy.

• *Psychological disorders.* Profound psychological impairments, such as schizophrenia and autism, can lead to pica.

Special considerations

Teach the child's parents the effects of poisoning and give them the telephone number of the local poison control center. Refer them to a dietitian for nutritional counseling.

As ordered, prepare the patient for blood tests, a toxicology screen, and stool examination for ova and parasites. If tests fail to reveal an organic disorder, refer the patient for psychological evaluation.

Pleural Friction Rub

Commonly resulting from pulmonary disorders or trauma, this loud, coarse, grating, creaking, or squeaking sound may be auscultated over one or both lungs during late inspiration or early expiration. It's heard best over the low axilla or the anterior, lateral, or posterior bases of the lung fields with the patient upright. Sometimes intermittent, it may resemble crackles or a pericardial friction rub (see *Comparing Auscultation Findings*, pages 580 and 581).

A pleural friction rub indicates inflammation of the visceral and parietal pleural lining, which causes congestion and edema. The resultant fibrinous exudate covers both pleural surfaces, displacing the fluid that's normally between them and causing the surfaces to rub together.

Assessment

When you detect a pleural friction rub, quickly assess for signs of respiratory distress: shallow or decreased respirations; crowing, wheezing, or stridor; dyspnea; increased accessory muscle use; intercostal or suprasternal retractions; cyanosis; and nasal flaring. Also check for hypotension, tachycardia, and a decreased level of consciousness. If you detect signs of distress, have another nurse notify the doctor while you open and maintain an airway. Then assist with endotracheal intubation and give supplemental oxygen. Insert a large-bore I.V. to deliver drugs and fluids, as ordered. Elevate the patient's head 30°. Monitor cardiac status constantly and check vital signs frequently.

If the patient isn't in severe distress, explore related symptoms. Find out if he has had chest pain. If so, ask him to describe its location and severity. How long does his chest pain last? Does it radiate to his shoulder, neck, or upper abdomen? Does the pain worsen with breathing, movement, coughing, or sneezing? Does it abate if he splints his chest, holds his breath, or exerts pressure or lies on the affected side?

Ask the patient about a history of rheumatoid arthritis, respiratory or cardiovascular disorders, recent trauma, asbestos exposure, or radiation therapy. If he smokes, obtain a history in pack years.

Characterize the pleural friction rub by auscultating the lungs with the patient sitting upright and breathing deeply and slowly through his mouth. Is the friction rub unilateral or bilateral? Also listen for absent or diminished breath sounds, noting their location and timing in the respiratory cycle. Do abnormal breath sounds clear with coughing? Observe for clubbing and pedal edema, which may indicate a chronic disorder. Then palpate for decreased chest motion and percuss for flatness or dullness.

Medical causes

● *Asbestosis.* Besides a pleural friction rub, this disorder may cause dyspnea on exertion, a cough, chest pain, and crackles. Clubbing is a late sign.

● *Lung cancer.* A pleural friction rub may be heard in the affected area of the lung. Other effects may include a cough (with possible hemoptysis), dyspnea, chest pain, weight loss, anorexia, fatigue, clubbing, fever, and wheezing.

● *Pleurisy.* A pleural friction rub occurs early in this disorder. However, the cardinal symptom is sudden, intense chest pain that's usually unilateral and located in the lower and lateral parts of the chest. Deep breathing, coughing, or thoracic movement aggravates the pain. Decreased breath sounds and inspiratory crackles may be heard over the painful area. Other findings: dyspnea, tachypnea, tachycardia, cyanosis, fever, and fatigue.

● *Pneumonia (bacterial).* A pleural fric-

tion rub occurs in this disorder, which usually starts with a dry, painful, hacking cough that rapidly becomes productive. Related effects develop suddenly: shaking chills, high fever, headache, dyspnea, pleuritic chest pain, tachypnea, tachycardia, grunting respirations, nasal flaring, dullness to percussion, and cyanosis. Auscultation reveals decreased breath sounds and fine crackles.

● *Pulmonary embolism.* An embolism can cause a pleural friction rub over the affected area of the lung. Usually, the first symptom is sudden dyspnea that may be accompanied by anginal or pleuritic chest pain. Other clinical features include a nonproductive cough or a cough that produces blood-tinged sputum, tachycardia, tachypnea, low-grade fever, restlessness, and diaphoresis. Less common findings include massive hemoptysis, chest splinting, leg edema, and, with a large embolus, cyanosis, syncope, and jugular vein distention. Crackles, diffuse wheezing, decreased breath sounds, and signs of circulatory collapse may also occur.

● *Rheumatoid arthritis.* This disorder infrequently causes a unilateral pleural friction rub. More typical early findings include fatigue, persistent low-grade fever, weight loss, and vague arthralgias and myalgias. Later findings include warm, swollen, painful joints; joint stiffness after inactivity; subcutaneous nodules on the elbows; joint deformity; and muscle weakness and atrophy.

● *Systemic lupus erythematosus.* Pulmonary involvement can cause a pleural friction rub, hemoptysis, dyspnea, pleuritic chest pain, and crackles. More characteristic effects include a butterfly rash, nondeforming joint pain and stiffness, and photosensitivity. Fever, anorexia, weight loss, and lymphadenopathy may also occur.

● *Tuberculosis (pulmonary).* In this disorder, a pleural friction rub may occur over the affected part of the lung. Early signs and symptoms include weight loss, night sweats, low-grade fever in

COMPARING AUSCULTATION FINDINGS

During auscultation, you may detect a pleural friction rub, a pericardial friction rub, or crackles—three abnormal sounds that are often confused. Use this chart to help identify auscultation findings.

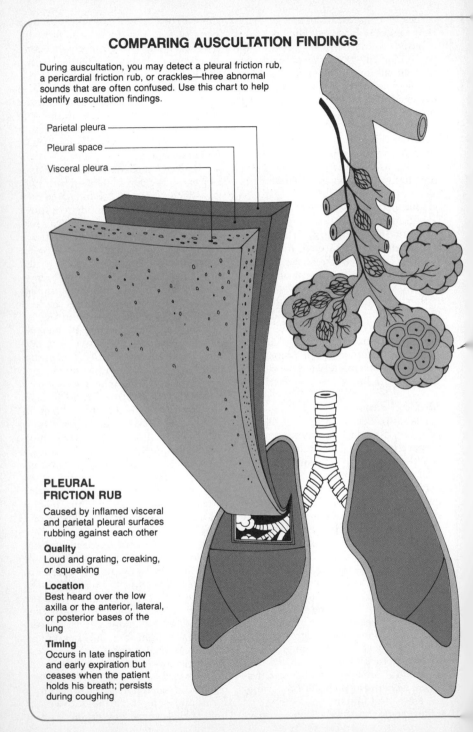

Parietal pleura

Pleural space

Visceral pleura

PLEURAL FRICTION RUB

Caused by inflamed visceral and parietal pleural surfaces rubbing against each other

Quality
Loud and grating, creaking, or squeaking

Location
Best heard over the low axilla or the anterior, lateral, or posterior bases of the lung

Timing
Occurs in late inspiration and early expiration but ceases when the patient holds his breath; persists during coughing

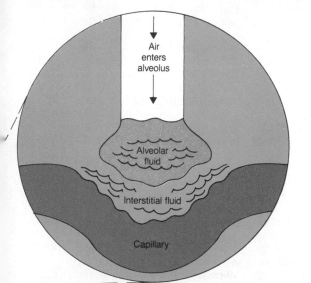

CRACKLES

Caused by air suddenly
entering fluid-filled airways

Quality
Nonmusical clicking or
rattling

Location
Best heard at less distended
and more dependent
areas of the lungs, usually
at the bases

Timing
Occurs chiefly during
inspiration

Endocardium

Myocardium

Visceral
pericardium

Pericardial space

Parietal
pericardium

Fibrous
pericardium

PERICARDIAL FRICTION RUB

Caused by inflamed layers
of the pericardium rubbing
against each other

Quality
Hard and grating, scratching,
or crunching

Location
Best heard along the lower
left sternal border

Timing
Occurs in relation to heartbeat. Most noticeable
during deep inspiration and
continues even when the
patient holds his breath

the afternoon, malaise, dyspnea, anorexia, and easy fatigability. Progression of the disorder usually produces pleuritic pain, fine crackles over the upper lobes, and a productive cough with blood-streaked sputum. Advanced tuberculosis can cause chest wall retraction, tracheal deviation, and dullness to percussion.

Other causes
• *Treatments.* Thoracic surgery and radiation therapy can cause a pleural friction rub.

Special considerations
Continue to monitor the patient's respiratory status and vital signs.

Because pleuritic pain often accompanies a pleural friction rub, teach your patient splinting maneuvers to increase his comfort. Also apply a heating pad over the affected area and, as ordered, administer analgesics for pain relief.

Although coughing may be painful, instruct the patient not to suppress it because coughing and deep breathing help prevent respiratory complications. However, if the patient's persistent dry, hacking cough tires him, administer antitussives. (Avoid giving narcotics, which can further depress respirations.) As ordered, administer oxygen and antibiotics.

Prepare the patient for diagnostic tests, such as chest X-rays.

Pediatric pointers
Auscultate for a pleural friction rub in any child who has grunting respirations, reports chest pain, or protects his chest by holding it or lying on one side. Usually, a pleural friction rub in a child is an early sign of pleurisy.

Polydipsia

Polydipsia refers to excessive thirst—a common symptom associated with endocrine disorders and certain drugs. It may reflect reduced fluid intake, increased urinary output (as in diabetes mellitus), or excessive loss of water and salt (as in profuse sweating).

Assessment
If your patient has polydipsia, take his blood pressure and pulse in the supine and standing positions. A decrease of 10 mm Hg in systolic pressure and a pulse rate increase of 10 beats/minute from the supine to the standing position may indicate hypovolemia. If you detect these changes, notify the doctor and ask the patient about recent weight loss. If ordered, infuse I.V. replacement fluids.

Next, obtain a history. Find out how much fluid the patient drinks each day. How often does he urinate? How much does he typically urinate? Does the need to urinate awaken him at night? Ask about any recent weight loss or change in appetite. Determine if he or anyone in his family has diabetes or kidney disease. What medications does he use? Has his life-style changed recently? If so, have these changes upset him?

Finally, check for signs of dehydration, such as dry mucous membranes and decreased skin turgor.

Medical causes
• *Diabetes insipidus.* This disorder characteristically produces polydipsia. It may also cause excessive voiding of dilute urine and mild to moderate nocturia. In severe cases, it causes fatigue and signs of dehydration.
• *Diabetes mellitus.* Polydipsia is a classic finding in this disorder. Other characteristic effects include polyuria, polyphagia, nocturia, weakness, fatigue, and weight loss. Signs of dehydration may occur.
• *Hypercalcemia.* As this disorder progresses, the patient develops polydipsia, polyuria, nocturia, constipation, paresthesias and, occasionally, hematuria and pyuria. Severe hypercalcemia can progress quickly to vomiting, decreased level of consciousness, and renal failure.

• *Hypokalemia.* This electrolyte imbalance can cause nephropathy, resulting in polydipsia, polyuria, and nocturia. Related hypokalemic effects include muscle weakness or paralysis, fatigue, decreased bowel sounds, hypoactive deep tendon reflexes, and dysrhythmias.

• *Psychogenic polydipsia.* This uncommon disorder causes polydipsia and polyuria, usually without nocturnal awakening. Signs of psychiatric disturbances, such as anxiety or depression, typically occur. Other findings may include headache, blurred vision, weight gain, edema, elevated blood pressure and, occasionally, stupor and coma. Signs of heart failure may develop with overhydration.

• *Renal disorders (chronic).* Chronic renal disorders, such as glomerulonephritis and pyelonephritis, damage the kidneys, causing polydipsia and polyuria. Associated signs and symptoms may include nocturia, weakness, elevated blood pressure, pallor and, in later stages, oliguria.

• *Sheehan's syndrome.* Polydipsia, polyuria, and nocturia occur in this syndrome of postpartum pituitary necrosis. Other features include fatigue, failure to lactate, amenorrhea, decreased pubic and axillary hair growth, and reduced libido.

• *Sickle cell anemia.* As nephropathy develops, polydipsia and polyuria occur. They may be accompanied by abdominal pain and cramps, arthralgia and, occasionally, lower extremity skin ulcers and bone deformities, such as kyphosis and scoliosis.

• *Thyrotoxicosis.* This disorder infrequently causes polydipsia. Characteristic findings include tachycardia, palpitations, weight loss despite increased appetite, diarrhea, tremors, an enlarged thyroid, dyspnea, nervousness, diaphoresis, and heat intolerance. Exophthalmos may occur.

Other causes

• *Drugs.* Diuretics and demeclocycline may produce polydipsia. Phenothiazines and anticholinergics can cause dry mouth, making the patient so thirsty that he drinks compulsively.

Special considerations

Carefully monitor the patient's fluid balance by recording his total intake and output. Weigh the patient at the same time each day, in the same clothing, and using the same scale. Regularly check blood pressure and pulse in the supine and standing positions to detect orthostatic hypotension, which may indicate hypovolemia. Because thirst is usually the body's way of compensating for water loss, give the patient ample liquids.

Pediatric pointers

In children, polydipsia usually stems from diabetes insipidus or diabetes mellitus. Rare causes include pheochromocytoma, neuroblastoma, and medullary cystic disease. However, some children have habitual polydipsia that's unrelated to any disease.

Polyphagia
[Hyperphagia]

Polyphagia refers to voracious or excessive eating before satiety. This common symptom can be persistent or intermittent, resulting primarily from endocrine and psychological disorders, as well as from certain drugs. Depending on the underlying cause, polyphagia may or may not cause weight gain.

Assessment

Begin your assessment by asking the patient what he has eaten and drunk within the last 24 hours. (If the patient easily recalls this information, ask about the 2 previous days' intake for a broader view of his dietary habits.) Note the frequency of meals and the amount and types of food eaten. Find out if the patient's eating habits have changed recently. Has he always had a large appetite? Does his overeating alternate with periods of anorexia? Ask about conditions that may trigger overeating, such as stress, depression, or menstruation. Does the patient actually feel hungry, or does he eat simply because food is available? Does he ever vomit or have a headache after overeating?

Explore related signs and symptoms. Has the patient recently gained or lost weight? Does he feel tired, nervous, or excitable? Has he experienced heat intolerance, dizziness, or palpitations? Diarrhea or increased thirst or urination? Obtain a complete drug history, including use of laxatives or enemas.

During the physical examination, weigh the patient. Tell him his current weight, and watch for any expression of disbelief or anger. Inspect the skin to detect dryness or poor turgor. Palpate the thyroid for enlargement.

Medical causes

● *Anxiety.* Polyphagia may result from mild to moderate anxiety or emotional stress. Typically, *mild anxiety* produces restlessness, sleeplessness, irritability, repetitive questioning, and constant seeking of attention and reassurance. With *moderate anxiety,* selective inattention and difficulty concentrating may also occur. Other effects of anxiety may include muscle tension, diaphoresis, gastrointestinal distress, palpitations, tachycardia, and urinary and sexual dysfunction.

● *Bulimia.* Most common in women aged 18 to 29, bulimia causes polyphagia that alternates with self-induced vomiting, fasting, or diarrhea. The patient typically weighs less than normal but has a morbid fear of obesity. She appears depressed, has low self-esteem, and conceals her overeating.

● *Diabetes mellitus.* In this disorder, polyphagia occurs with weight loss, polydipsia, and polyuria. It's accompanied by nocturia, weakness, fatigue, and signs of dehydration, such as dry mucous membranes and poor skin turgor.

● *Migraine headache.* Polyphagia sometimes precedes a migraine headache. Other prodromal signs and symptoms may include fatigue, nausea, vomiting, and a visual aura. Light and noise sensitivity may also occur.

● *Premenstrual syndrome.* Appetite changes, typified by food cravings and binges, are common in this syndrome. Abdominal bloating, the most common associated finding, may occur with behavioral changes, such as depression and insomnia. Headache, paresthesias, and other neurologic symptoms may also occur. Related findings include diarrhea or constipation, edema and temporary weight gain, palpitations, back pain, breast swelling and tenderness, oliguria, and easy bruising.

● *Thyrotoxicosis.* This disorder can produce weight loss despite constant polyphagia. Other characteristics include weakness, nervousness, diarrhea, tremors, diaphoresis, and dyspnea. The patient's hair and nails are thin and brittle, and his thyroid is enlarged. He may also have palpitations, tachycardia, heat intolerance, and possibly exophthalmos and an atrial or ventricular gallop.

Other causes

● *Drugs.* Corticosteroids and cyproheptadine may increase appetite, causing weight gain.

Special considerations

Offer the patient with polyphagia emotional support, and help him understand its underlying cause. As needed, refer the patient and his family for psychological counseling.

Pediatric pointers

In children, polyphagia commonly results from juvenile diabetes. In infants 6 to 18 months old, it can result from a malabsorptive disorder, such as celiac disease. However, polyphagia may occur normally in a child who's experiencing a sudden growth spurt.

Polyuria

A relatively common sign, polyuria is the daily production and excretion of more than 2,500 ml (2.5 liters) of urine. It's usually reported by the patient as increased voidings, especially when it occurs at night. Polyuria is aggravated by overhydration, consumption of caffeine or alcohol, and excessive ingestion of salt, glucose, or other hyperosmolar substances.

Polyuria most commonly results from drugs, such as diuretics, and from psychological, neurologic, and renal disorders. It can reflect central nervous system dysfunction that diminishes or suppresses secretion of antidiuretic hormone (ADH), which regulates fluid balance. Or, when ADH levels are normal, it can reflect renal impairment. In both of these pathophysiologic mechanisms, the renal tubules fail to reabsorb sufficient water, causing polyuria.

Assessment

Because the patient with polyuria is at risk for developing hypovolemia, evaluate fluid status first. Take vital signs, noting especially increased body temperature, tachycardia, and orthostatic hypotension. Inspect for dry skin and mucous membranes, decreased skin turgor and elasticity, and reduced perspiration. Is the patient unusually tired or thirsty? Has he recently lost more than 5% of his body weight? If you detect these effects of hypovolemia, notify the doctor and infuse replacement fluids, as ordered.

If the patient doesn't display signs of hypovolemia, explore the frequency and pattern of the polyuria. When did it begin? How long has it lasted? Was it precipitated by a certain event? Ask the patient to describe the pattern and amount of his daily fluid intake. Find out about any current or past psychiatric disorders and chronic hypokalemia or hypercalcemia. Check for a history of visual deficits, headaches, or head trauma, which may precede diabetes insipidus. Also check for a history of urinary tract obstruction, diabetes mellitus, and renal disorders. Find out the schedule and dosage of any drugs the patient is currently taking.

Perform a neurologic examination, noting especially any change in the patient's level of consciousness (LOC). Then palpate the bladder and inspect the urethral meatus. Obtain a urine specimen and check its specific gravity.

Medical causes

● *Acute tubular necrosis.* During the diuretic phase of this disorder, polyuria of less than 8 liters/day gradually subsides after 8 to 10 days. Urine specific gravity (1.010 or less) increases as the polyuria subsides. Related findings include weight loss, decreasing edema, and nocturia.

● *Diabetes insipidus.* Extreme polyuria—up to 30 liters/day—can occur in this disorder. However, polyuria of about 5 liters/day with a specific gravity of 1.005 or less is a more common finding. Polyuria is often accompanied by polydipsia, nocturia, fatigue, and signs of dehydration, such as poor skin turgor and dry mucous membranes.

● *Diabetes mellitus.* In this disorder, polyuria seldom exceeds 5 liters/day, while urine specific gravity typically exceeds 1.020. The patient usually has polydipsia, polyphagia, weight loss, weakness, fatigue, and nocturia. He may also display signs of dehydration.

● *Glomerulonephritis (chronic).* Polyuria gradually progresses to oliguria in this disorder. Urine output is usually less than 4 liters/day; specific gravity is about 1.010. Related gastrointestinal effects include anorexia, nausea, and vomiting. Other findings: drowsiness, fatigue, edema, headache, elevated blood pressure, and dyspnea. Nocturia, hematuria, and mild to severe proteinuria may occur.

● *Hypercalcemia.* Elevated plasma calcium levels may lead to nephropathy, usually producing polyuria of less than

5 liters/day with a specific gravity of about 1.010. Accompanying signs and symptoms include polydipsia, nocturia, constipation, paresthesias and, occasionally, hematuria and pyuria. In severe hypercalcemia, the patient's condition worsens rapidly and he experiences anorexia, vomiting, stupor progressing to coma, and renal failure.

• **Hypokalemia.** Prolonged potassium depletion may lead to nephropathy, producing polyuria—usually less than 5 liters/day with a specific gravity of about 1.010. Associated findings in-

POLYURIA: CAUSES AND ASSOCIATED FINDINGS

CAUSES	Anorexia	Blood pressure increase	Constipation	Dyspnea	Dysuria	Edema	Fatigue	Fever	Flank pain	Headache	Hematuria	LOC—altered	Mucous membrane dryness
Acute tubular necrosis						•							
Diabetes insipidus							•						•
Diabetes mellitus							•						•
Glomerulonephritis (chronic)	•	•		•		•	•			•	•		
Hypercalcemia	•		•							•	•		
Hypokalemia							•						
Postobstructive uropathy						•							•
Psychogenic polydipsia		•				•				•		•	
Pyelonephritis (acute)	•				•			•	•		•		
Pyelonephritis (chronic)	•	•					•						
Sheehan's syndrome							•						
Sickle cell anemia							•						

clude polydipsia, muscle weakness or paralysis, hypoactive deep tendon reflexes, fatigue, hypoactive bowel sounds, nocturia, and dysrhythmias.

• **Postobstructive uropathy.** After resolution of a urinary tract obstruction, polyuria—usually more than 5 liters/day with a specific gravity of less than 1.010—occurs for several days before gradually subsiding. Resolving bladder distention and edema may occur with nocturia and weight loss. Occasionally, signs of dehydration appear.

• **Psychogenic polydipsia.** Most common in women over age 30, this disorder usually produces dilute polyuria of 3 to 15 liters/day, depending on fluid intake. The patient may appear depressed and have a headache and blurred vision. She may have weight gain, edema, elevated blood pressure and, occasionally, stupor or coma. In severe overhydration, she may display signs of heart failure.

• **Pyelonephritis.** Acute pyelonephritis usually results in polyuria of less than 5 liters/day with a low but variable specific gravity. Other findings may include persistent high fever, flank pain, hematuria, costovertebral angle tenderness, chills, weakness, dysuria, urinary frequency and urgency, tenesmus, and nocturia. Occasionally, nausea, anorexia, vomiting, and hypoactive bowel sounds may occur.

Chronic pyelonephritis produces polyuria of less than 5 liters/day that declines as renal function worsens. Usually, urine specific gravity is about 1.010, but it may be higher if proteinuria is present. Other effects include irritability, paresthesias, fatigue, nausea, vomiting, drowsiness, anorexia, pyuria and, in late stages, elevated blood pressure.

• **Sheehan's syndrome.** This syndrome of postpartum pituitary necrosis may cause polyuria of over 5 liters/day with a specific gravity of 1.001 to 1.005. Associated findings include polydipsia, nocturia, and fatigue. Reproductive effects include failure to lactate, amenorrhea, decreased pubic and axillary hair growth, and reduced libido.

• **Sickle cell anemia.** This disorder may cause nephropathy, typically producing polyuria that amounts to less than 5 liters/day with a specific gravity of about 1.020. Additional findings include polydipsia, fatigue, abdominal

Nocturia	Paresthesias	Personality changes	Polydipsia	Polyphagia	Pyuria	Vomiting	Weakness	Weight gain	Weight loss
•									•
•			•						
•			•	•			•		•
•						•			
•	•		•			•	•		
•			•				•		
•									•
		•						•	
•							•	•	
	•					•	•		
•			•						
			•						

cramps, arthralgia and, occasionally, leg ulcers and bony deformities.

Other causes
- **Diagnostic tests.** Transient polyuria can result from radiographic tests that use contrast media.
- **Drugs.** Diuretics characteristically produce polyuria. Cardiotonics, vitamin D, demeclocycline, phenytoin, lithium, methoxyflurane, and propoxyphene can also produce polyuria.

Special considerations
Maintaining an adequate fluid balance is your primary concern when the patient has polyuria. Record intake and output accurately, and weigh him daily. Closely monitor the patient's vital signs to detect fluid imbalance, and encourage him to drink adequate fluids.

Prepare the patient for serum electrolyte, osmolality, blood urea nitrogen, and creatinine studies to monitor fluid and electrolyte status. If ordered, prepare him for a fluid deprivation test to determine the cause of polyuria.

Pediatric pointers
The major causes of polyuria in children are congenital nephrogenic diabetes insipidus, medullary cystic disease, polycystic renal disease, and distal renal tubular acidosis.

Because a child's fluid balance is more delicate than an adult's, check his urine specific gravity at each voiding, and be alert for signs of dehydration.

Postnasal Drip

Postnasal drip is a sinus or nasal discharge that flows behind the nose and into the throat. This symptom typically results from infection or allergies—a thick, tenacious, and purulent discharge suggests infection, whereas a watery discharge usually suggests an allergy. Postnasal drip may also result from environmental irritants.

Assessment
Ask the patient when his postnasal drip began and if it's continuous or intermittent. Does it occur during a certain season? What relieves the postnasal drip? What aggravates it? Ask about related signs and symptoms, such as a cough, sinus pain, headache, and nasal congestion. Next, take an allergy history and find out about occupational exposure to environmental irritants, such as chemical fumes or dust.

If the patient has mucosal swelling, use a vasoconstricting nasal spray before beginning the nasal examination. Then use a nasal speculum to assess the mucous membranes, which are normally pink to dull red. Observe the size and shape of the turbinates and septum, noting any abnormal structures and characterizing the secretions. If the patient wears dentures, ask him to remove them before you examine his throat. Use a warmed, size 0 postnasal mirror and a tongue depressor to examine the oropharynx and nasopharynx for drainage. Finally, palpate the sinus areas for swelling and tenderness. (See *Palpating the Sinuses.*)

Medical causes
- **Environmental irritants.** Exposure to environmental irritants, such as fumes, smoke, or dust, may cause postnasal drip. Other findings depend on the type of irritant and the duration of exposure but may include a cough and itching or burning eyes, nose, and throat.
- **Rhinitis.** Two types of rhinitis—allergic and vasomotor—can produce postnasal drip. In *allergic rhinitis,* symptoms can occur seasonally, as with hay fever, or year-round, as with chronic rhinitis. Nasal obstruction and edematous, pale nasal mucosa may be apparent. The mucosal surface appears smooth and shiny, and the turbinates fill the air space and press against the nasal septum. The patient has swollen, red eyelids and conjunctivae and excessive tearing. He also has paroxysmal sneezing, a thin nasal discharge, a diminished sense of smell, frontal or tem-

PALPATING THE SINUSES

When your patient reports postnasal drip, assess his sinuses for swelling and tenderness—telltale signs of sinusitis. To do this, carefully press up with your thumb on the areas illustrated below. Avoid placing pressure on the eyes.

Tenderness and swelling beneath the middle of his eyebrows may indicate frontal sinusitis; over his cheeks, maxillary sinusitis.

Frontal sinuses

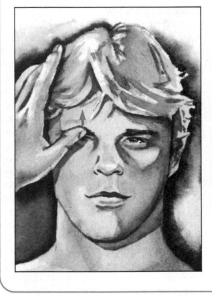

Maxillary sinuses

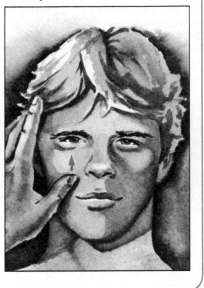

poral headache, and eye, nose, and possibly throat itching.

A recurrent postnasal drip occurs with *vasomotor rhinitis,* which can be aggravated by dry air. Related effects may include engorged inferior turbinates, nasal obstruction, sneezing, watery or sticky rhinorrhea, a pink nasal septum, and bluish mucosa.

• *Sinusitis.* This disorder commonly produces postnasal drip. It may also cause headache, sinus pain, purulent rhinorrhea, halitosis, red, swollen nasal mucosa and turbinates, fever, sore throat, cough, and malaise.

Special considerations

Teach the patient with postnasal drip how to use medications safely. Remind him not to use decongestants for more than a month at a time. If he has hy-pertension, instruct him to avoid systemic decongestants. Caution against overuse of nose drops, which can produce rebound rhinitis. If he has allergic rhinitis, recommend antihistamines.

If sinus pain accompanies postnasal drip, apply wet hot packs to the sinuses. Instruct the patient to avoid nasal irritants, such as tobacco smoke.

As ordered, prepare the patient for diagnostic tests, such as sinus X-rays and culture and sensitivity studies.

Pediatric pointers

If a child has postnasal drip (less common in children than a runny nose), inspect his nose by pushing its tip upward to visualize the anterior nares. If the child's under age 5, use a small postnasal mirror to examine his nasopharynx.

Priapism

A urologic emergency, priapism is a persistent, painful erection that's unrelated to sexual excitation. This relatively rare sign may begin during sleep and appear to be a normal erection, but it may last for several hours or days. It's usually accompanied by a severe, constant, dull aching in the penis. Despite this, the patient may be too embarrassed to seek medical help and may try to achieve detumescence through continued sexual activity.

Priapism occurs when the veins of the corpora cavernosa fail to drain correctly, resulting in persistent engorgement of the tissues. Without prompt treatment, penile ischemia and thrombosis occur. In about half of all cases, priapism is idiopathic and develops without apparent predisposing factors. Secondary priapism results from blood disorders, neoplasms, trauma, and certain drugs.

Assessment

 If your patient has priapism, notify the doctor immediately. Apply an ice pack to the patient's penis, administer analgesics, and insert an indwelling catheter to relieve urinary retention, as ordered. If ordered, assist with procedures to remove blood from the corpora cavernosa, such as irrigation and surgery.

When the patient's condition permits, ask him when the priapism began. Is it continuous or intermittent? Has he had a prolonged erection before? If so, what did he do to relieve it? How long did he remain detumescent? Does he have pain or tenderness when he urinates? Has he noticed any changes in sexual function?

Explore the patient's medical history. If he reports sickle cell anemia, find out about any factors that could precipitate a crisis, such as dehydration and infections. Ask if he's recently suffered genital trauma, and obtain a thorough drug history.

Examine the patient's penis, noting its color and temperature. Check for any loss of sensation, and look for signs of infection, such as redness or drainage. Finally, take his vital signs, particularly noting fever.

Medical causes

• **Cerebrovascular accident (CVA).** A CVA may cause priapism, but sensory loss and aphasia may prevent the patient from noticing or describing it. Other findings depend on the CVA's location and extent but may include contralateral hemiplegia, seizures, headache, dysarthria, dysphagia, ataxia, apraxia, and agnosia. Visual deficits include homonymous hemianopia, blurring, decreased acuity, and diplopia. Urinary retention or incontinence, constipation, and vomiting may also occur.

• **Genitourinary infection.** Priapism occurs rarely with infection. Typical effects include fever, chills, urethral discharge, dysuria, urinary urgency and frequency, and nocturia.

• **Granulocytic leukemia (chronic).** Priapism is an uncommon sign of this disorder. More characteristic effects include fatigue, weakness, malaise, lymphadenopathy, pallor, dyspnea, tachycardia, and bleeding tendencies. Hepatosplenomegaly, bone tenderness, low-grade fever, weight loss, and anorexia may also occur.

• **Penile carcinoma.** Carcinoma that exerts pressure on the corpora cavernosa can cause priapism. Usually, the first sign is a painless ulcerative lesion or an enlarging warty growth on the glans or foreskin, which may be accompanied by localized pain, a foul-smelling discharge from the prepuce, a firm lump near the glans, and lymphadenopathy. Later findings may include bleeding, dysuria, urinary retention, and bladder distention.

• **Penile trauma.** Priapism can occur with bruising, abrasions, swelling, pain, and hematuria.

• **Sickle cell anemia.** In this disorder,

painful priapism can occur without warning, usually on awakening. A history of priapism, impaired growth and development, and increased susceptibility to infection may be present. Related findings include tachycardia, pallor, weakness, hepatomegaly, dyspnea, joint swelling, joint or bone aching, chest pain, persistent fatigue, murmurs, leg ulcers and, possibly, jaundice and gross hematuria.

In sickle cell crisis, signs and symptoms of sickle cell anemia may worsen and others, such as abdominal pain and low-grade fever, may appear.

• *Spinal cord injury.* In this condition, the patient may be unaware of the onset of priapism. Related effects depend on the extent and level of the injury and may include autonomic signs, such as bradycardia.

• *Thrombocytopenia.* This disorder uncommonly produces priapism. More typical characteristics include blood-filled bullae in the mouth and local bleeding, such as epistaxis, ecchymosis, and hematuria. Central nervous system bleeding may cause decreased level of consciousness. Fatigue, weakness, and lethargy may occur.

Other causes
• *Drugs.* Priapism can result from phenothiazines, thioridazine, trazodone, androgenic steroids, and some antihypertensives.

Special considerations
As ordered, prepare the patient for blood tests to help determine the cause of his priapism. If he requires surgery, keep his penis flaccid postoperatively by applying a pressure dressing. At least once every 30 minutes, inspect the glans for signs of vascular compromise, such as coolness or pallor.

Pediatric pointers
In neonates, priapism can result from hypoxia but usually resolves with oxygen therapy. Priapism is more likely to develop in children with sickle cell disease than in adults with the disease.

Pruritus
[Itching]

Often provoking scratching in an attempt to gain relief, this unpleasant sensation affects the skin, certain mucous membranes, and the eyes. Most severe at night, pruritus may also worsen with increased skin temperature, poor skin turgor, local vasodilation, dermatoses, and stress.

The most common symptom of dermatologic disease, pruritus may also result from local and systemic disorders and from drug use. Physiologic pruritus, such as pruritic urticarial papules and plaques of pregnancy, may occur in primigravidas late in the third trimester. It can also stem from emotional upsets or contact with skin irritants.

Assessment
If the patient reports pruritus, have him describe its onset, frequency, and intensity. If pruritus occurs at night, ask him whether it prevents him from falling asleep or awakens him after he falls asleep. (Generally, pruritus related to dermatoses prevents—but doesn't disturb—sleep.) Does exercise, stress, fear, depression, or illness seem to aggravate the itching? Ask about contact with skin irritants, previous skin disorders, and related symptoms. Then obtain a complete drug history.

Examine the patient for signs of scratching, such as excoriation, purpura, scabs, scars, or lichenification. Look for primary lesions to help confirm dermatoses.

Medical causes
• *Anemia (iron deficiency).* This disorder occasionally produces pruritus. Initially asymptomatic, anemia can later cause dyspnea on exertion, fatigue, listlessness, pallor, irritability, headache, tachycardia, poor muscle tone,

and possibly murmurs. Chronic anemia causes spoon-shaped and brittle nails, cracked mouth corners, a smooth tongue, and dysphagia.

• *Cimex lectularius (bedbugs)*. Typically, bedbug bites produce itching and burning over the ankles and lower legs, along with clusters of purpuric spots.

• *Conjunctivitis*. Regardless of the type, conjunctivitis causes eye itching, burning, and pain along with photophobia, conjunctival injection, a foreign body sensation, excessive tearing, and a feeling of fullness around the eye.

Allergic conjunctivitis may also cause milky redness and a stringy eye discharge. *Bacterial conjunctivitis* typically causes brilliant redness and a mucopurulent, flaky discharge that may make the eyelids stick together. *Fungal conjunctivitis* produces a thick, purulent discharge and crusting and sticking of the eyelid. *Viral conjunctivitis* may cause copious tearing—but little discharge—and preauricular lymph node enlargement.

• *Dermatitis*. Several types of dermatitis can cause pruritus accompanied by a skin lesion. *Atopic dermatitis* begins with intense, severe pruritus and an erythematous rash on dry skin at flexion points (antecubital fossa, popliteal area, and neck). During a flare-up, scratching may produce edema, scaling, and pustules. In chronic atopic dermatitis, lesions may progress to dry, scaly skin with white dermatographia, blanching, and lichenification.

Mild irritants and allergies can cause *contact dermatitis,* with itchy small vesicles that may ooze and scale and are surrounded by redness. Severe reaction can produce marked localized edema.

Dermatitis herpetiformis, most common in men between the ages of 20 and 50, initially causes intense pruritus and stinging. Eight to twelve hours later, symmetrically distributed lesions form on the buttocks, shoulders, elbows, and knees. Sometimes, they also form on the neck, face, and scalp. These lesions are erythematous and papular, bullous, or pustular.

• *Hemorrhoids*. Anal pruritus may occur here, along with rectal pain and constipation. External hemorrhoids may be seen outside the external anal sphincter; internal hemorrhoids are less obvious and less painful but are more likely to cause rectal bleeding.

• *Hepatobiliary disease*. An important diagnostic clue to liver and gallbladder disease, pruritus is often accompanied by jaundice and may be generalized or localized to the palms and soles. Other characteristics may include right upper quadrant pain, clay-colored stools, chills and fever, flatus, belching and a bloated feeling, epigastric burning, and bitter fluid regurgitation. Later, liver disease may produce mental changes, ascites, bleeding tendencies, spider angiomas, palmar erythema, dry skin, fetor hepaticus, enlarged superficial abdominal veins, bilateral gynecomastia, testicular atrophy or menstrual irregularities, and hepatomegaly.

• *Herpes zoster*. In this disorder, pruritus may precede eruption of lesions and may be accompanied by malaise, fever, erythema, and sharp, shooting, or burning pain. Macular lesions erupt later, usually spreading over the thorax or over the arms and legs. If nodules appear, they rapidly evolve into fluid- or pus-filled vesicles that later dry and form scabs. Localized paresthesia or hyperesthesia may occur.

• *Hodgkin's lymphoma*. This disorder, which is most common in young adults, initially causes mild pruritus on the lower part of the body. As the disorder progresses, the pruritus may become severe and unresponsive to treatment. Early nonspecific findings include persistent fever (occasionally cyclic fever and chills), night sweats, fatigue, weight loss, malaise, and painless swelling of a cervical lymph node. Other lymph nodes may enlarge rapidly and cause pain, or they may enlarge slowly and be painless. Later findings may include retroperitoneal node enlargement, hepatomegaly, splenomegaly, dyspnea, dysphagia, dry cough, hyperpigmentation, jaundice, and pallor.

● *Leukemia (chronic lymphocytic).* Pruritus occurs uncommonly in this disorder. More characteristic effects include fatigue, malaise, generalized lymphadenopathy, fever, hepatomegaly, splenomegaly, weight loss, pallor, bleeding, and palpitations.

● *Lichen planus.* This common skin disease can cause moderate to severe pruritus that's aggravated by stress. Characteristic oral lesions (white or gray, velvety, threadlike papules that look like lace) develop on the buccal mucosa and may cause pain. Violet papules with white lines or spots develop later, usually on the genitalia, lower back, ankles, and shins. Nail distortion and atrophic alopecia may also occur.

● *Lichen simplex chronicus.* Persistent rubbing and scratching cause localized pruritus and a circumscribed scaling patch with sharp margins. Later, the skin thickens and papules form.

● *Multiple myeloma.* Infrequently, this disorder produces pruritus near the xanthomas. Other findings: severe, constant back pain that increases with exercise; achiness; joint swelling and tenderness; fever; malaise; and slight peripheral neuropathy.

● *Mycosis fungoides.* Pruritus may precede other symptoms of this neoplastic disease by 10 years. It may persist into the first, or premycotic, stage, accompanied by erythematous lesions.

● *Myringitis (chronic).* This disorder produces pruritus in the affected ear, along with a purulent discharge and gradual hearing loss.

● *Pediculosis (lice).* A prominent symptom, pruritus occurs in the area of infestation. *Pediculosis capitis* (head lice) may also cause scalp excoriation from scratching, along with matted, foul-smelling, lusterless hair; occipital and cervical lymphadenopathy; and oval, gray-white nits on hair shafts.

Pediculosis corporis (body lice) initially causes small red papules (usually on the shoulders, trunk, or buttocks), which become urticarial from scratch-

---

PATIENT-TEACHING AID

CONTROLLING ITCHING

Dear Patient:

To reduce your itching and increase your comfort, follow these simple steps:
● Avoid scratching or rubbing the itchy areas. Ask your family to let you know if you're scratching, because you may be unaware of it. Keep your fingernails short to avoid skin damage from any unconscious scratching.
● Wear cool, light, loose bedclothes. Avoid wearing rough clothing—particularly wool—over the itchy area.
● Take tepid baths, using little soap and rinsing thoroughly. Try a skin-soothing oatmeal or cornstarch bath for a change.
● Apply an emollient lotion after bathing to soften and cool the skin.
● Apply cold compresses to the itchy area.
● Use topical ointments and take prescribed medications, as directed.
● Avoid prolonged exposure to excessive heat and humidity. For maximum comfort, keep room temperatures at 68° to 70° F. (20° to 21.1° C.) and humidity at 30% to 40%.
● Take up an enjoyable hobby that distracts you from the itching during the day and leaves you tired enough to sleep at night.

---

ing. Later, rashes or wheals may develop. Untreated, *pediculosis corporis* produces dry, discolored, thickly encrusted, scaly skin with bacterial infection and scarring. In severe cases, it produces headache, fever, and malaise.

With *pediculosis pubis* (pubic lice), scratching commonly produces skin irritation. Nits or adult lice and erythematous, itching papules may appear in pubic hair or hair around the anus, abdomen, or thighs.

● *Pityriasis rosea.* Typically, this disorder produces mild to severe pruritus that's aggravated by a hot bath or shower. Usually, it begins with an erythematous herald patch—a slightly raised, oval lesion about 2 to 6 cm in diameter. After a few days or weeks, scaly yellow-tan or erythematous patches erupt on the trunk and extremities and persist for 2 to 6 weeks. Occasionally, these patches are macular, vesicular, or urticarial.

• *Polycythemia vera.* This hematologic disorder can produce pruritus that's generalized or localized to the head, neck, face, and extremities. Typically, the pruritus is aggravated by a hot bath or shower and can last from a few minutes to an hour. The patient's oral mucosa may be deep purplish red, especially on the gingivae and tongue. His engorged gingivae ooze blood with even slight trauma. Related findings include headache, dizziness, fatigue, dyspnea, paresthesias, impaired mentation, tinnitus, double or blurred vision, scotoma, hypotension, intermittent claudication, urticaria, ruddy cyanosis, and ecchymosis. Gastrointestinal effects include epigastric distress, weight loss, and hepatosplenomegaly.

• *Psoriasis.* Here, pruritus and pain are common. Typically, psoriasis begins with small erythematous papules that enlarge or coalesce to form red elevated plaques with silver scales on the scalp, chest, elbows, knees, back, buttocks, and genitals. Nail pitting and joint stiffness may occur.

• *Psychogenic pruritus.* Localized or generalized pruritus occurs without symptoms of dermatologic or systemic disease. Anxiety or emotional lability may be evident.

• *Renal failure (chronic).* Pruritus may develop gradually or suddenly in this disorder. It may be accompanied by ammonia breath odor, oliguria or anuria, lassitude, fatigue, irritability, decreased mental acuity, convulsions, coarse muscular twitching, muscle cramps, peripheral neuropathies, and coma. Renal failure also causes diverse GI effects, such as anorexia, constipation or diarrhea, nausea, and vomiting.

• *Scabies.* Typically, scabies causes localized pruritus that intensifies at night. The pruritus may become generalized and persist up to 2 weeks after treatment. Threadlike lesions from 1 to 10 cm long appear with a swollen nodule or red papule. In males, crusty lesions may form on the glans penis, penile shaft, and scrotum. In females, lesions may form on the wrists, elbows, axilla, waistline, and nipples. Excoriation from scratching is common.

• *Thyrotoxicosis.* Generalized pruritus may precede or accompany this disorder's characteristic effects: tachycardia, palpitations, weight loss despite increased appetite, diarrhea, tremors, an enlarged thyroid, dyspnea, nervousness, diaphoresis, heat intolerance, and possibly exophthalmos.

• *Tinea pedis.* This fungal infection causes severe foot pruritus, pain with walking, scales and blisters between the toes, and a dry, scaly squamous inflammation on the entire sole.

• *Urticaria.* Extreme pruritus and stinging occur as transient erythematous or whitish wheals form on the skin or mucous membranes. Commonly, prickly sensations precede the wheals, which may affect any part of the body and may range from pinpoint to palm-sized or larger.

Pruritus may also occur with *urticaria pigmentosa.* In this disorder, reddish brown macules or papules or, less commonly, nodules or plaques occur. Other signs and symptoms may include flushing, tachycardia, hypotension, and nausea.

• *Vaginitis.* This disorder frequently causes localized pruritus and a foul-smelling vaginal discharge that may be purulent, white or gray, and curdlike. Perineal pain and urinary dysfunction may also occur.

Other cause

• *Drug hypersensitivity.* When mild and localized, an allergic reaction to such drugs as penicillin and sulfonamides can cause pruritus, erythema, an urticarial rash, and edema. However, in a severe drug reaction, anaphylaxis may occur.

Special considerations

Administer topical corticosteroids, antihistamines, or tranquilizers, as ordered. Suggest ways to control pruritus. (See *Controlling Itching,* page 593.)

If the patient doesn't have a localized infection or skin lesions, suspect a systemic disease and prepare him for a CBC and differential, erythrocyte sedimentation rate, protein electrophoresis, and radiologic studies.

Pediatric pointers

Many adult disorders also cause pruritus in children. However, they may affect different parts of the body. For instance, scabies may affect the head in infants, but not in adults. Pityriasis rosea may affect the face, hands, and feet of adolescents.

Some childhood diseases, such as measles and chicken pox, can cause pruritus. Hepatic diseases can also produce pruritus in children as bile salts accumulate on the skin.

Psoas Sign

A positive psoas sign—increased abdominal pain when the patient moves his leg against resistance—indicates direct or reflexive irritation of the psoas muscles. This sign, which can be elicited on the right or left side, usually indicates appendicitis but may also occur with localized abscesses. It's elicited in a patient with abdominal or lower back pain *after* completion of the abdominal examination to prevent spurious assessment findings. (See *Eliciting Psoas Sign,* pages 596 and 597.)

Assessment

If you elicit a positive psoas sign in a patient with abdominal pain, suspect appendicitis. Quickly check the patient's vital signs and have another nurse notify the doctor. Prepare the patient for surgery: explain the procedure, restrict food and fluids, and withhold analgesics, which can mask symptoms. Administer I.V. fluids to prevent dehydration, but do *not* give cathartics or enemas, which can cause a ruptured appendix and lead to peritonitis.

Check for Rovsing's sign by deeply palpating the patient's *left* lower quadrant. If he reports *right* lower quadrant pain, the sign is positive, indicating peritoneal irritation.

Medical causes

• *Appendicitis.* An inflamed retrocecal appendix can cause a positive right psoas sign. Early epigastric and periumbilical pain disappear only to worsen and localize in the right lower quadrant. This pain also worsens with walking or coughing. Related findings include nausea and vomiting, abdominal rigidity and rebound tenderness, and constipation or diarrhea. Fever, tachycardia, retractive respirations, anorexia, and malaise may also occur. If the appendix ruptures, additional findings may include sudden, severe pain, followed by signs of peritonitis, such as hypoactive or absent bowel sounds, high fever, and boardlike abdominal rigidity.

• *Retroperitoneal abscess.* After a lower retroperitoneal infection, an iliac or lumbar abscess can produce a positive right or left psoas sign and fever. An *iliac abscess* causes iliac or inguinal pain that may radiate to the hip, thigh, or knee; a tender mass in the lower abdomen or groin may be palpable. A *lumbar abscess* usually produces back tenderness and spasms on the affected side with a palpable lumbar mass; a tender abdominal mass without back pain may occur instead.

Special considerations

Monitor vital signs to detect complications, such as peritonitis. Promote patient comfort by position changes. For example, have the patient lie down and flex his right leg. Then have him sit upright.

Prepare the patient for diagnostic

ELICITING PSOAS SIGN

You can use two techniques to elicit a psoas sign in an adult with abdominal pain. With either technique, increased abdominal pain is a positive result, indicating psoas muscle irritation from an inflamed appendix or a localized abscess.

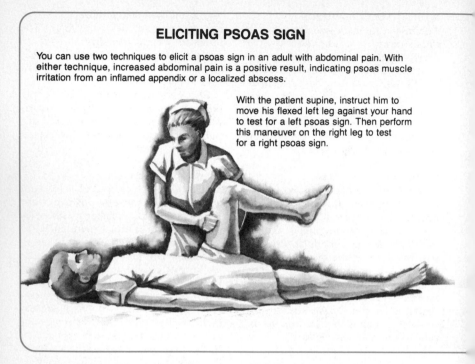

With the patient supine, instruct him to move his flexed left leg against your hand to test for a left psoas sign. Then perform this maneuver on the right leg to test for a right psoas sign.

tests, such as electrolyte studies and abdominal X-rays.

Pediatric pointers

Elicit psoas sign by asking the child to raise his head while you exert pressure on his forehead. Resulting right lower quadrant pain usually indicates appendicitis.

Psychotic Behavior

Psychotic behavior reflects an inability or unwillingness to recognize and acknowledge reality and to relate with others. It may begin suddenly or insidiously, progressing from vague complaints of fatigue, insomnia, or headache to withdrawal, social isolation, and preoccupation with certain issues.

Various behaviors together or separately can constitute psychotic behavior. These include delusions, illusions, hallucinations, bizarre language, and perseveration. *Delusions* are persistent beliefs that have no basis in reality or in the patient's knowledge or experience, such as delusions of grandeur. *Illusions* are misinterpretations of external sensory stimuli, such as a mirage in the desert. In contrast, *hallucinations* are sensory perceptions that do not result from external stimuli. *Bizarre language* reflects a communication disruption. It can range from echolalia (purposeless repetition of a word or phrase) and clang association (repetition of words or phrases that sound similar) to neologisms (creation and use of words whose meaning only the patient knows). *Perseveration,* a persistent verbal or motor response, may indicate organic brain disease. Motor changes include inactivity, excessive activity, and repetitive movements.

Assessment

Because the patient's behavior can make it difficult—or potentially dan-

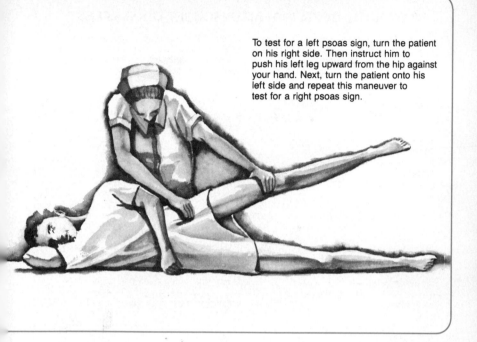

To test for a left psoas sign, turn the patient on his right side. Then instruct him to push his left leg upward from the hip against your hand. Next, turn the patient onto his left side and repeat this maneuver to test for a right psoas sign.

gerous—to obtain pertinent information, conduct the interview in a calm, safe, and well-lit room. Be sure to provide enough personal space to avoid threatening or agitating the patient. Ask him to describe his problem and any circumstances that may have precipitated it. Explore his use of alcohol or drugs, noting duration of use and amount. Ask the patient if he has had any illnesses or accidents in the last year.

As the patient talks, watch for cognitive, linguistic, or perceptual abnormalities, such as delusions. Do his thoughts and actions seem to match? Look for unusual gestures, posture, gait, tone of voice, or mannerisms.

Next, interview the patient's family. Which family members does the patient seem closest to? How does the family describe the patient's relationships, communication patterns, and role? Find out if anyone in his family has been previously hospitalized for psychiatric or emotional illness.

Finally, evaluate the patient's environment. Ask about his educational and employment history. What is his (or his family's) socioeconomic status? Are community services available to them? How does the patient spend his leisure time? Does he have friends? Has he ever had a close emotional relationship?

Medical causes

● *Organic disorders.* Various disorders may produce psychotic behavior. These include alcohol withdrawal syndrome, cerebral hypoxia, and nutritional disorders. Endocrine disorders, such as adrenal dysfunction, and severe infections, such as encephalitis, can also cause psychotic behavior. Neurologic causes include Alzheimer's disease and other dementias.

● *Psychiatric disorders.* Psychotic behavior usually occurs with bipolar disorders, personality disorders, schizophrenia, and traumatic stress disorders.

PSYCHOTIC BEHAVIOR: AN UNSOUGHT DRUG EFFECT

Certain drugs can cause psychotic behavior and other psychiatric signs and symptoms, ranging from depression to violent behavior. Usually, these effects occur during therapy and resolve when the drug is discontinued. If your patient is receiving one of these common drugs and exhibits the behavior described below, notify the doctor immediately. He may want to change the dosage or substitute another drug.

DRUG	PSYCHIATRIC SIGNS AND SYMPTOMS
albuterol	Hallucinations, paranoia
alprazolam	Anger, hostility
amantadine	Visual hallucinations, nightmares
asparaginase	Confusion, depression, paranoia
atropine and anticholinergics	Auditory, visual, and tactile hallucinations; memory loss; delirium; fear; paranoia
bromocriptine	Mania, delusions, sudden relapse of schizophrenia, paranoia, aggressive behavior
cardiac glycosides	Paranoia, euphoria, amnesia, visual hallucinations
cimetidine	Hallucinations, paranoia, confusion, depression, delirium
clonidine	Delirium, hallucinations, depression
corticosteroids (prednisone, ACTH, cortisone)	Mania, catatonia, depression, confusion, paranoia, hallucinations
cycloserine	Anxiety, depression, confusion, paranoia, hallucinations
dapsone	Insomnia, agitation, hallucinations
diazepam	Suicidal thoughts, rage, hallucinations, depression
disopyramide	Agitation, paranoia, auditory and visual hallucinations, panic
disulfiram	Delirium, auditory hallucinations, paranoia, depression
indomethacin	Hostility, depression, paranoia, hallucinations
lidocaine	Disorientation, hallucinations, paranoia
methyldopa	Severe depression, amnesia, paranoia, hallucinations
methysergide	Depersonalization, hallucinations
propranolol	Severe depression, hallucinations, paranoia, confusion
thyroid hormones	Mania, hallucinations, paranoia
vincristine	Hallucinations

Other causes

● **Drugs.** Certain drugs can cause psychotic behavior. (See *Psychotic Behavior: An Unsought Drug Effect*). However, almost any drug can provoke psychotic behavior as a rare, severe adverse or idiosyncratic reaction.

● **Surgery.** Postoperative delirium and depression may produce psychotic behavior.

Special considerations

Continuously evaluate the patient's orientation to reality. Help him build a conception of reality by calling him by his preferred name, telling him your name, describing where he is, and using clocks and calendars.

Encourage the patient's involvement in structured activities. However, if he's nonverbal or incoherent, be sure to spend time with him—simply sitting or walking with him, or talking about the day, the season, the weather, or other concrete topics. Avoid making time commitments that you can't keep: this will only upset the patient and may make him withdraw further.

Refer the patient for psychological evaluation. Administer antipsychotics or other drugs, as ordered, and prepare him for transfer to a mental health center, if necessary.

Don't overlook the patient's physiologic needs. Check his eating habits to avoid dehydration and malnutrition, and monitor his elimination patterns, especially if he's receiving psychotropic drugs, which can cause constipation.

Pediatric pointers

In children, psychotic behavior may result from early infantile autism, symbiotic infantile psychosis, and childhood schizophrenia—all of which can retard development of language, abstract thinking, and socialization.

The adolescent patient with psychotic behavior may have a history of several days' drug use or lack of sleep or food, which must be corrected before therapy can begin.

CONTROLLING PSYCHOTIC BEHAVIOR

A patient who displays psychotic behavior may be terrified and unable to differentiate between himself and his environment. To control this patient's behavior and to prevent injury to the patient, staff, and others, you'll need to act calmly and quickly, following these guidelines.

● Remove potentially dangerous objects, such as belts or metal utensils, from the patient's environment.

● Help the patient discern what is real and unreal in an honest and genuine way.

● Be straightforward, concise, and non-threatening when speaking to the patient. Discuss simple, concrete subjects and avoid theories or philosophical issues.

● Positively reinforce the patient's perceptions of reality, and correct his misperceptions in a matter-of-fact way.

● *Never* argue with the patient. However, don't support his misperceptions.

● If the patient is frightened, stay with him.

● Touch the patient to provide reassurance *only* if you've tested this before and know that it's safe.

● Move the patient to a safer, less stimulating environment.

● Provide one-on-one nursing care if the patient's behavior is extremely bizarre, disturbing to other patients, or dangerous to himself.

Ptosis

Ptosis is the excessive drooping of the upper eyelid. In severe ptosis, the patient may not be able to raise his eyelids voluntarily.

This sign can be constant, progressive, or intermittent, and unilateral or bilateral. When it's unilateral, it's easy to detect by comparing the eyelids' relative positions. When it's bilateral or mild, it's difficult to detect—the eyelids may be abnormally low, covering the upper part of the iris or even part of the pupil instead of overlapping the iris slightly. Other clues include a furrowed forehead or a tipped-back head—both of these help the patient see under his drooping lids. However, because ptosis can resemble enophthalmos, exophthalmometry may be required (see *Differentiating Enophthalmos from Ptosis,* page 284).

Ptosis can be classified as congenital or acquired. Congenital ptosis results from levator muscle underdevelopment or disorders of the third cranial (oculomotor) nerve. Acquired ptosis may result from trauma to or inflammation of these muscles and nerves, or from certain drugs, systemic diseases, intracranial lesions, and life-threatening aneurysms. But the most common cause is age, which reduces muscle elasticity and produces senile ptosis.

Assessment

Ask your patient when his ptosis began and if it has worsened or improved. Determine if he's had recent eye trauma. (If he has, avoid manipulating the eye to prevent further damage.) Ask about eye pain or headache and determine its location and severity. Has the patient experienced any vision changes? If so, have him describe them. Obtain a drug history, noting especially any chemotherapeutic agents.

Assess the degree of ptosis, and check for eyelid edema, exophthalmos, deviation, or conjunctival injection. Evaluate extraocular muscle function by testing the six cardinal fields of gaze. Carefully examine the pupils' size, color, shape, and reaction to light, and test visual acuity.

Keep in mind that ptosis infrequently indicates a life-threatening condition. For example, sudden unilateral ptosis can herald a cerebral aneurysm.

Medical causes

● *Alcoholism.* Long-term alcohol abuse can cause ptosis and such complications as severe weight loss, jaundice, ascites, and mental disturbances.

● *Botulism.* Acute cranial nerve dysfunction causes hallmark signs of ptosis, dysarthria, dysphagia, and diplopia. Other findings include dry mouth, sore throat, weakness, vomiting, diar-

rhea, hyporeflexia, and dyspnea.

● *Cerebral aneurysm.* An aneurysm that compresses the oculomotor nerve can cause sudden ptosis, along with diplopia, a dilated pupil, and inability to rotate the eye. These may be the first signs of this life-threatening disorder.

With rupture, an aneurysm typically produces sudden severe headache, nausea, vomiting, and decreased level of consciousness. Other findings may include nuchal rigidity, back and leg pain, fever, restlessness, irritability, occasional seizures, blurred vision, hemiparesis, sensory deficits, dysphagia, and visual defects.

● *Dacryoadenitis.* Ptosis may accompany unilateral exophthalmos, limited extraocular movements, eyelid edema and erythema, conjunctival injection, eye pain, and diplopia.

● *Hemangioma.* This orbital tumor can produce ptosis, exophthalmos, limited extraocular movements, and blurred vision.

● *Horner's syndrome.* This disorder causes moderate unilateral ptosis that almost disappears when the patient opens his eyes widely. Common accompanying findings include unilateral miosis and ipsilateral anhidrosis of the face and neck, which may spread to the entire body. Other signs and symptoms may include transient conjunctival injection, vascular headache on the affected side, and vertigo.

● *Lacrimal gland tumor.* This disorder frequently produces mild to severe ptosis, depending on the tumor's size and location. It may also cause brow elevation, exophthalmos, eye deviation, and possibly eye pain.

● *Lead poisoning.* Usually, ptosis develops over 3 to 6 months. Other effects: anorexia, nausea, vomiting, diarrhea, colicky abdominal pain, a lead line in the gums, decreased level of consciousness, tachycardia, hypotension and, possibly, irritability and peripheral nerve weakness.

● *Myasthenia gravis.* Gradual bilateral ptosis is often the first sign of this disorder. It may be mild to severe and

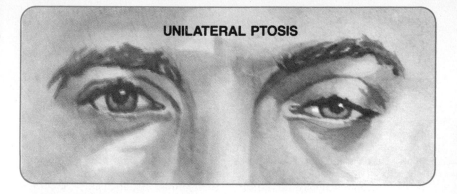

UNILATERAL PTOSIS

accompanied by weak eye closure and diplopia. Other characteristics include muscle weakness and fatigue that eventually may lead to paralysis. Depending on the muscles affected, other findings may include masklike facies, difficulty chewing or swallowing, dyspnea, cyanosis, and others.

• *Myotonic dystrophy.* This disorder may cause mild to severe bilateral ptosis. Distinctive cataracts with iridescent dots in the cortex, miosis, diplopia, decreased tearing, and muscular and testicular atrophy may also occur.

• *Ocular muscle dystrophy.* In this disorder, bilateral ptosis progresses slowly to complete eyelid closure. Related signs and symptoms include progressive external ophthalmoplegia and muscle weakness and atrophy of the upper face, neck, trunk, and limbs.

• *Ocular trauma.* Trauma to the nerve or muscles that control the eyelids can cause mild to severe ptosis. Depending on the damage, eye pain, lid swelling, ecchymosis, and decreased visual acuity may also occur.

• *Parinaud's syndrome.* This form of ophthalmoplegia can cause ptosis, enophthalmos, nystagmus, lid retraction, dilated pupils with absent or poor light response, and papilledema. The patient's ocular muscles fail to move voluntarily.

• *Parry-Romberg syndrome.* Unilateral ptosis and facial hemiatrophy occur with this disorder. Other signs may include miosis, sluggish pupil reaction to light, enophthalmos, irises that don't match in color, ocular muscle paralysis, nystagmus, and neck, shoulder, trunk, and extremity atrophy.

• *Subdural hematoma (chronic).* Ptosis may be a late sign, along with unilateral pupillary dilation and sluggishness. Headache, behavioral changes, and decreased level of consciousness often occur.

Other causes

• *Drugs.* Vinca alkaloids can produce ptosis.

Special considerations

Prepare the patient for diagnostic studies, such as the tensilon test and slit-lamp examination. If he needs surgery to correct levator muscle dysfunction, explain the procedure to him.

If the patient has decreased visual acuity, orient him to his surroundings. As ordered, provide special spectacle frames that suspend the eyelid by traction with a wire crutch. Most often, these frames are used to help patients with temporary paresis or those who aren't good candidates for surgery.

Pediatric pointers

Parents typically discover congenital ptosis when their child is an infant. Usually, the ptosis is unilateral, constant, and accompanied by lagophthalmos, which causes the infant to sleep with his eyes open. If this occurs, teach proper eye care to prevent drying.

Pulse—Absent or Weak

An absent or weak pulse may be generalized or affect only one extremity. (See *Evaluating Peripheral Pulses*, page 607.) When generalized, this sign is an important indicator of such life-threatening conditions as shock. Localized loss or weakness of a pulse that's normally present and strong may indicate arterial occlusion, which could require emergency surgery. However, the pressure of palpation may temporarily diminish or obliterate superficial pulses, such as the posterior tibial or the dorsal pedal. Thus, bilateral weakness or absence of these pulses doesn't necessarily indicate underlying pathology.

Assessment

After detecting an absent or weak pulse, quickly palpate the remaining arterial pulses to distinguish between localized or generalized loss or weakness. Next, quickly check other vital signs, assess cardiopulmonary status, and obtain a brief history. Based on your findings, proceed with emergency interventions. (See *Managing Absent or Weak Pulse*, pages 604 and 605.)

Medical causes

• *Aortic aneurysm (dissecting).* When the dissecting aneurysm affects circulation to the innominate, left common carotid, subclavian, or femoral arteries, it causes weak or absent arterial pulses distal to the affected area. However, 25% of patients with this life-threatening condition may have normal peripheral pulses. Tearing pain usually develops suddenly in the chest and neck and may radiate to the upper and lower back and abdomen. Blood pressure may be lower in the patient's legs than in his arms. Other findings may include syncope, weakness or transient paralysis of the legs, the diastolic murmur of aortic insufficiency, systemic hypotension, and mottled skin below the waist. The patient may be diaphoretic and have prolonged capillary refill time in his feet.

• *Aortic arch syndrome.* This syndrome produces weak or abruptly absent carotid pulses and unequal or absent radial pulses. Usually, this is preceded by night sweats, pallor, nausea, anorexia, weight loss, arthralgia, and Raynaud's phenomenon. Other findings may include hypotension in the arms; neck, shoulder, and chest pain; paresthesias; intermittent claudication; bruits; visual disturbances; and dizziness and syncope.

• *Aortic bifurcation occlusion (acute).* This rare disorder produces abrupt absence of all leg pulses. The patient reports moderate to severe pain in the legs and, less often, in the abdomen, lumbosacral area, or perineum. His legs are cold, pale, numb, and flaccid.

• *Aortic stenosis.* In this disorder, the carotid pulse is sustained, but weak. Dyspnea, chest pain, and syncope dominate the clinical picture. The patient commonly has an atrial (S_4) or ventricular (S_3) gallop and may have a harsh systolic ejection murmur. Other findings may include crackles, palpitations, fatigue, and narrowed pulse pressure.

• *Arterial occlusion.* In *acute occlusion,* arterial pulses distal to the obstruction are unilaterally weak and then absent. The affected limb is cool, pale, and cyanotic, with prolonged capillary refill time, and the patient complains of moderate to severe pain and paresthesias. A line of color and temperature demarcation develops at the level of obstruction. Varying degrees of limb paralysis may also occur, along with intense intermittent claudication. In *chronic occlusion,* occurring in disorders such as arteriosclerosis or Buerger's disease, pulses in the affected limb weaken gradually.

• *Cardiac tamponade.* Life-threatening cardiac tamponade causes a weak, rapid pulse accompanied by these classic findings: pulsus paradoxus, jugular vein distention, hypotension, and muffled heart sounds. Narrowed pulse pressure, pericardial friction rub, and hepatomegaly may also occur. The patient may appear anxious, restless, and cyanotic. He may have chest pain, clammy skin, dyspnea, and tachypnea.

• *Dysrhythmias.* Cardiac dysrhythmias may produce generalized weak pulses accompanied by cool, clammy skin. Other findings reflect the dysrhythmia's severity and may include hypotension, chest pain, dizziness, and decreased level of consciousness.

• *Peripheral vascular disease.* This disorder causes a gradual weakening and loss of peripheral pulses. The patient complains of aching pain distal to the occlusion that worsens with exercise and abates with rest. The skin feels cool and shows decreased hair growth. With occlusion in the descending aorta or femoral areas, the male patient may experience impotence.

• *Pulmonary embolism.* This disorder causes generalized weak, rapid pulse. It also may cause abrupt onset of chest pain, tachycardia, apprehension, syncope, diaphoresis, and cyanosis. Acute respiratory effects may include tachypnea, dyspnea, decreased breath sounds, crackles, and a cough—possibly with blood-tinged sputum.

• *Shock.* In *anaphylactic shock*, pulses become rapid and weak and then uniformly absent within seconds or minutes after exposure to an allergen. Before this, the patient experiences hypotension, anxiety, restlessness, feelings of doom, intense itching, a pounding headache, and possibly urticaria. Other findings: dyspnea, stridor, and hoarseness; chest or throat tightness; skin flushing; nausea, abdominal cramps, and urinary incontinence; seizures; and narrowed pulse pressure.

In *cardiogenic shock*, peripheral pulses are absent and central pulses are weak, depending on the degree of vascular collapse. A drop in systolic blood pressure to 30 mm Hg below baseline, or a sustained reading below 80 mm Hg produces poor tissue perfusion. Resulting signs include cold, pale,

clammy skin; tachycardia; rapid, shallow respirations; oliguria; and restlessness, confusion, and obtundation.

In *hypovolemic shock*, all pulses in the extremities become weak and then uniformly absent, depending on the severity of hypovolemia. As shock progresses, remaining pulses become thready and more rapid. Early signs of cardiogenic shock include cool, pale skin, restlessness, thirst, and tachypnea. Late signs include hypotension with narrowing pulse pressure, clammy skin, a drop in urine output to less than 25 ml/hour, confusion, decreased level of consciousness, and possibly hypothermia.

In *septic shock*, all pulses in the extremities first become weak. Depending on the degree of vascular collapse, pulses may then become uniformly absent. Shock is heralded by chills, sudden fever, and possibly nausea, vomiting, and diarrhea. Typically, the skin is flushed, warm, and dry, and tachycardia and tachypnea occur. As shock progresses, thirst, hypotension, anxiety, restlessness, and confusion develop. Pulse pressure narrows and the skin becomes cold, clammy, and cyanotic. The patient experiences severe hypotension, oliguria or anuria, respiratory failure, and coma.

• *Thoracic outlet syndrome.* A patient with this syndrome may have a gradual or abrupt weakness or loss of the pulses in the arms, depending on how quickly vessels in the neck compress. These pulse changes commonly occur after the patient works with his hands above his shoulders, lifts a weight, or abducts his arm. Paresthesias and pain occur along the ulnar distribution of the arm and disappear immediately when the patient returns his arm to a neutral position. In addition, the patient may have asymmetrical blood pressure and cool, pale skin.

Other causes
• *Treatments.* Localized pulse absence may occur distal to arteriovenous fistulas or shunts for dialysis.

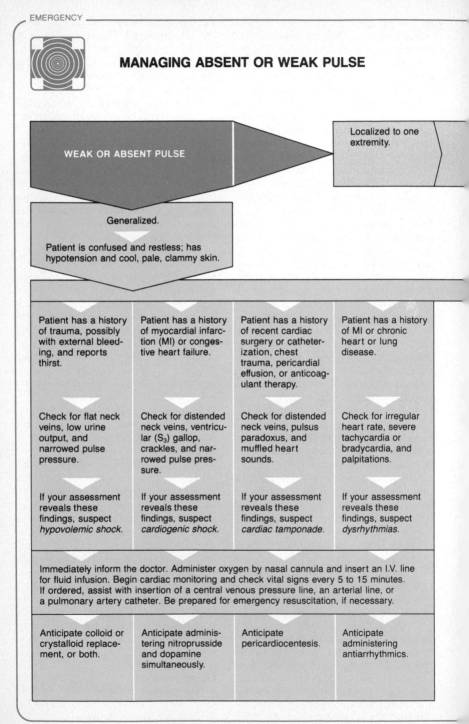

MANAGING ABSENT OR WEAK PULSE

WEAK OR ABSENT PULSE

Localized to one extremity.

Generalized.

Patient is confused and restless; has hypotension and cool, pale, clammy skin.

Patient has a history of trauma, possibly with external bleeding, and reports thirst.	Patient has a history of myocardial infarction (MI) or congestive heart failure.	Patient has a history of recent cardiac surgery or catheterization, chest trauma, pericardial effusion, or anticoagulant therapy.	Patient has a history of MI or chronic heart or lung disease.
Check for flat neck veins, low urine output, and narrowed pulse pressure.	Check for distended neck veins, ventricular (S₃) gallop, crackles, and narrowed pulse pressure.	Check for distended neck veins, pulsus paradoxus, and muffled heart sounds.	Check for irregular heart rate, severe tachycardia or bradycardia, and palpitations.
If your assessment reveals these findings, suspect *hypovolemic shock.*	If your assessment reveals these findings, suspect *cardiogenic shock.*	If your assessment reveals these findings, suspect *cardiac tamponade.*	If your assessment reveals these findings, suspect *dysrhythmias.*

Immediately inform the doctor. Administer oxygen by nasal cannula and insert an I.V. line for fluid infusion. Begin cardiac monitoring and check vital signs every 5 to 15 minutes. If ordered, assist with insertion of a central venous pressure line, an arterial line, or a pulmonary artery catheter. Be prepared for emergency resuscitation, if necessary.

Anticipate colloid or crystalloid replacement, or both.	Anticipate administering nitroprusside and dopamine simultaneously.	Anticipate pericardiocentesis.	Anticipate administering antiarrhythmics.

An absent or weak pulse can result from several life-threatening disorders. Your assessment and interventions will vary depending on whether the weak or absent pulse is generalized or affects one extremity. They'll also depend on associated signs and symptoms. Use the flowchart below to help you establish priorities for managing this emergency successfully.

Assess affected extremity for cool, mottled skin and pain.

If your assessment reveals these findings, suspect *arterial occlusive disease.*

Immediately inform the doctor. Prepare the patient for diagnostic tests, such as arteriography, aortography, or Doppler ultrasonography, to confirm or rule out arterial occlusion. Do not elevate the affected extremity. Start an I.V. line in an unaffected arm or leg, and administer heparin or streptokinase, as ordered. Anticipate preparing the patient for emergency embolectomy or peripheral angioplasty.

Patient has a history of trauma, congenital heart disease, or hypertension and reports severe, tearing chest pain.	Patient has a history of severe infection— frequently gram-negative, urinary, or respiratory infection.	Patient has a history of an insect sting, drug ingestion, or exposure to other possible allergen.	Patient has a history of venous stasis or deep vein thrombosis and reports sharp, substernal chest pain.
Check for pulse quality and blood pressure variation between extremities.	Check for fever, chills, and widened pulse pressure.	Check for urticaria, wheezing or stridor, and dyspnea.	Check for dyspnea, crackles, pleural friction rub, and hemoptysis.
If your assessment reveals these findings, suspect *dissecting aortic aneurysm.*	If your assessment reveals these findings, suspect *septic shock.*	If your assessment reveals these findings, suspect *anaphylactic shock.*	If your assessment reveals these findings, suspect *pulmonary embolism.*

Immediately inform the doctor. Administer oxygen by nasal cannula and insert an I.V. line for fluid infusion. Begin cardiac monitoring and check vital signs every 5 to 15 minutes. If ordered, assist with insertion of a central venous pressure line, an arterial line, or a pulmonary artery catheter. Be prepared for emergency resuscitation, if necessary.

Anticipate preparing the patient for surgery and administering an antihypertensive or nitroprusside.	Anticipate administering antibiotics and vasopressors.	Anticipate emergency intubation or cricothyrotomy and administration of epinephrine.	Anticipate possible intubation and anticoagulant or thrombolytic therapy.

Special considerations

Continue to monitor the patient's vital signs to detect untoward changes in his condition. Monitor hemodynamic status by measuring daily weight and hourly or daily intake and output and by assessing central venous pressure.

Pediatric pointers

Radial, dorsal pedal, and posterior tibial pulses aren't easily palpable in infants and small children, so be careful not to mistake these normally hard-to-find pulses for weak or absent pulses. Instead, palpate the brachial, popliteal, or femoral pulses to evaluate arterial circulation to the extremities. In children and young adults, weak or absent femoral and more distal pulses may indicate coarctation of the aorta.

Pulse—Bounding

Produced by large waves of pressure as blood ejects from the left ventricle with each contraction, a bounding pulse is strong and easily palpable and may be visible over superficial peripheral arteries. It's characterized by regular, recurrent expansion and contraction of the arterial walls and isn't obliterated by the pressure of palpation. A healthy person develops a bounding pulse during exercise, pregnancy, or periods of anxiety. However, this sign also results from fever and certain endocrine, hematologic, and cardiovascular disorders that increase the basal metabolic rate.

Assessment

After you detect a bounding pulse, check other vital signs, then auscultate the heart and lungs for any abnormal sounds, rates, or rhythms. Ask the patient if he's noticed any weakness, fatigue, shortness of breath, or other health changes. Review his medical history for hyperthyroidism, anemia, or cardiovascular disorders, and ask about his use of alcohol.

Medical causes

● *Alcoholism (acute).* Vasodilation of acute alcoholism produces a rapid, bounding pulse and flushed face. An odor of alcohol on the patient's breath and an ataxic gait are common. Other findings may include hypothermia, bradypnea, stertorous respirations, nausea, vomiting, diuresis, decreased level of consciousness, and seizures.

● *Anemia.* In this disorder, bounding pulse may be accompanied by capillary pulsations, a systolic ejection murmur, tachycardia, an atrial gallop (S_4), and a systolic bruit over the carotid artery. Associated findings include fatigue, pallor, dyspnea, and possibly bleeding tendencies.

● *Aortic insufficiency.* Sometimes called a water-hammer pulse, the bounding pulse associated with this condition is characterized by a rapid, forceful expansion of the arterial pulse followed by rapid contraction. Widened pulse pressure also occurs. *Acute aortic insufficiency* may produce signs and symptoms of left ventricular failure and cardiovascular collapse, such as weakness, severe dyspnea, hypotension, a ventricular gallop (S_3), and tachycardia. Additional findings may include pallor, chest pain, palpitations, or strong, abrupt carotid pulsations. The patient may also have pulsus bisferiens, an early systolic murmur, a murmur heard over the femoral artery during systole and diastole (Duroziez's sign), and a high-pitched diastolic murmur that starts with the second heart sound. An apical diastolic rumble (Austin Flint murmur) may also occur, especially with heart failure. Most patients with *chronic aortic insufficiency* remain asymptomatic until the age of 40 or 50, when exertional dyspnea, increased fatigue, orthopnea and, eventually, paroxysmal nocturnal dyspnea may develop.

● *Febrile disorder.* Fever can cause a bounding pulse. Accompanying find-

EVALUATING PERIPHERAL PULSES

The rate, amplitude, and symmetry of peripheral pulses provide important clues to cardiac function and the quality of peripheral perfusion. To gather these clues, palpate peripheral pulses lightly with the pads of your index, middle, and ring fingers—as space permits.

Rate. Count all pulses for at least 30 seconds (60 seconds when recording vital signs). The normal rate is between 60 and 100 beats/minute.

Amplitude. Palpate the blood vessel during ventricular systole. Describe pulse amplitude by using a scale like the one below:

4+	bounding
3+	normal
2+	difficult to palpate
1+	weak, thready
0	absent

Use a stick figure to easily document the location and amplitude of all pulses.

Symmetry. Simultaneously palpate pulses (except for the carotid pulse) on both sides of the patient's body, and note any inequality. Always assess peripheral pulses methodically, moving from the arms to the legs.

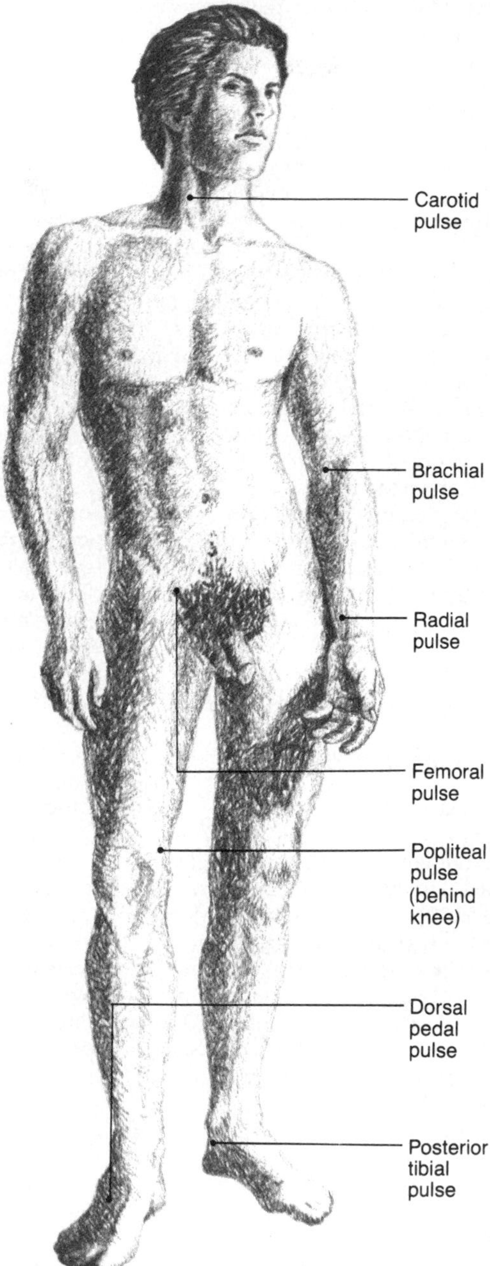

Carotid pulse

Brachial pulse

Radial pulse

Femoral pulse

Popliteal pulse (behind knee)

Dorsal pedal pulse

Posterior tibial pulse

ings reflect the specific disorder.

• *Thyrotoxicosis.* This disorder produces a rapid, full, bounding pulse. Associated findings may include tachycardia, palpitations, an S_3 or S_4 gallop, and weight loss despite increased appetite. In addition, the patient may have diarrhea, an enlarged thyroid, dyspnea, tremors, nervousness, and exophthalmos. His skin will be warm, moist, and diaphoretic, and he may be hypersensitive to heat.

Special considerations

Prepare the patient for diagnostic laboratory and radiographic studies. If bounding pulse is accompanied by rapid or irregular heartbeat, you may need to connect the patient to a cardiac monitor for further evaluation.

Pediatric pointers

Bounding pulse can be normal in infants or children, because arteries lie close to the skin surface. It can also result from patent ductus arteriosus if the left-to-right shunt is large.

Pulse Pressure— Narrowed

Pulse pressure, the difference between systolic and diastolic blood pressures, is measured by sphygmomanometry or intraarterial monitoring. Normally, systolic pressure exceeds diastolic by about 40 mm Hg. Narrowed pressure—a difference of less than 30 mm Hg—occurs when peripheral vascular resistance increases, cardiac output declines, or intravascular volume markedly decreases (see *Understanding Pulse Pressure Changes,* page 610). In conditions that cause mechanical obstruction, such as aortic stenosis, pulse pressure is directly related to the severity of the underlying condition. Usually a late sign, narrowed pulse pressure alone doesn't signal an emergency,

even though it commonly occurs in shock and other life-threatening disorders.

Assessment

After you detect a narrowed pulse pressure, check for other signs of heart failure, such as hypotension, tachycardia, dyspnea, distended neck veins, and decreased urinary output. Also check for changes in skin temperature or color, strength of peripheral pulses, and level of consciousness. Auscultate the heart for murmurs, and ask about a history of chest pain, dizziness, or syncope. Inform the doctor of your findings.

Medical causes

• *Aortic stenosis.* Narrowed pulse pressure occurs late in significant stenosis. This disorder also produces an atrial or ventricular gallop; chest pain; a harsh, systolic ejection murmur; dyspnea; and syncope. Additional findings may include crackles, palpitations, fatigue, and diminished carotid pulses.

• *Cardiac tamponade.* In this life-threatening disorder, pulse pressure narrows approximately 10 to 20 mm Hg. Pulsus paradoxus, neck vein distention, hypotension, and muffled heart sounds are classic. The patient may be anxious, restless, and cyanotic, with clammy skin and chest pain. He may exhibit dyspnea, tachypnea, decreased level of consciousness, and a weak, rapid pulse. Pericardial friction rub and hepatomegaly may also occur.

• *Congestive heart failure.* Narrowed pulse pressure occurs relatively late. It may accompany tachypnea; palpitations; dependent edema; steady weight gain despite nausea and anorexia; chest tightness; slowed mental response; hypotension; diaphoresis; pallor; and oliguria. Assessment reveals a ventricular gallop, inspiratory crackles, and possibly a tender, palpable liver. Later, dullness develops over the lung bases, and hemoptysis, cyanosis, marked hepatomegaly, and marked pitting edema may occur.

• *Shock.* In *anaphylactic shock,* narrowed pulse pressure occurs late, preceded by a rapid, weak pulse that soon becomes uniformly absent. Within seconds or minutes after exposure to an allergen, the patient experiences hypotension, anxiety, restlessness, and feelings of doom, along with intense itching, a pounding headache, and possibly urticaria. Other possible findings: dyspnea, stridor, and hoarseness; chest or throat tightness; skin flushing; nausea, abdominal cramps, and urinary incontinence; and seizures.

In *cardiogenic shock*, narrowed pulse pressure occurs relatively late. Typically, peripheral pulses are absent and central pulses are weak. A drop in systolic pressure to 30 mm Hg below baseline, or a sustained reading below 80 mm Hg not attributable to medication produces poor tissue perfusion. Poor perfusion produces tachycardia; tachypnea; cold, pale, clammy skin; cyanosis; oliguria; restlessness; confusion; and obtundation.

In *hypovolemic shock*, narrowed pulse pressure occurs as a late sign. All peripheral pulses become first weak and then uniformly absent. Deepening shock leads to hypotension, urine output of less than 25 ml/hour, confusion, decreased level of consciousness, and possibly hypothermia.

In *septic shock*, narrowed pulse pressure is a relatively late sign. All of the patient's peripheral pulses become first weak and then uniformly absent. As shock progresses, the patient has oliguria, thirst, anxiety, restlessness, confusion, and hypotension. His extremities become cool and cyanotic, and eventually his skin becomes cold and clammy. The patient also eventually develops severe hypotension, persistent oliguria or anuria, respiratory failure, and coma.

Special considerations

Monitor the patient closely for changes in pulse rate or quality and for hypotension. Prepare him for diagnostic studies, such as echocardiography, to detect valvular heart disease.

Pediatric pointers

In children, narrowed pulse pressure can result from congenital aortic stenosis, as well as from disorders that affect adults.

Pulse Pressure— Widened

Pulse pressure is the difference between systolic and diastolic blood pressures. Normally, systolic pressure is about 40 mm Hg higher than diastolic. Widened pulse pressure—a difference greater than 50 mm Hg—commonly occurs as a physiologic response to fever, hot weather, or exercise. However, it can also result from certain neurologic and cardiovascular disorders that reduce arterial compliance or cause backflow of blood into the heart with each contraction; chief among these is a life-threatening increase in intracranial pressure (ICP). Widened pulse pressure can easily be identified by monitoring arterial blood pressure and is commonly detected during routine sphygmomanometric recordings.

Assessment

If the patient's level of consciousness is decreased, and you suspect that his widened pulse pressure results from increased ICP, check his vital signs while another nurse immediately notifies the doctor. Maintain a patent airway, and prepare to hyperventilate the patient with an Ambu bag to help reduce PCO_2 levels and, thus, ICP. Perform a thorough neurologic examination to serve as a baseline for assessing subsequent changes. Use the Glasgow Coma Scale to evaluate the patient's level of consciousness. (See *Glasgow Coma Scale: Grading Level of Consciousness*, page 454.) Also check cranial nerve function—especially in cranial nerves III, IV, and VI—and assess pupillary re-

UNDERSTANDING PULSE PRESSURE CHANGES

Two major factors affect pulse pressure—the amount of blood, or *stroke volume,* that the ventricles eject into the arteries with each beat, and the arteries' *peripheral resistance* to blood flow. These two factors affect systolic and diastolic blood pressures and, as a result, pulse pressure. For example, pulse pressure narrows when systolic pressure falls (lower right),

diastolic pressure rises (upper left), or both. These changes reflect decreased stroke volume, increased peripheral resistance, or both.

Pulse pressure widens when systolic pressure rises (upper right), diastolic pressure falls (lower left), or both. These changes reflect increased stroke volume, decreased peripheral resistance, or both.

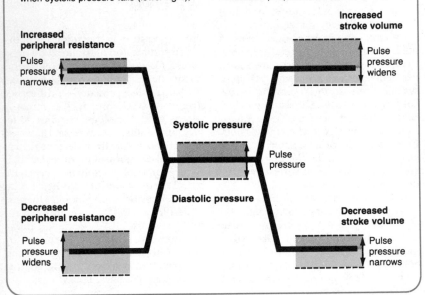

actions, reflexes, and muscle tone. If ordered, assist with insertion of an ICP monitor and begin monitoring ICP.

If you don't suspect increased ICP, ask about associated symptoms, such as chest pain, shortness of breath, weakness, fatigue, or syncope. Check for edema and auscultate for murmurs.

Medical causes

• *Aortic insufficiency.* In acute aortic insufficiency, pulse pressure widens progressively as the valve deteriorates, and a bounding pulse and an atrial gallop (S₄) develop. These signs may be accompanied by chest pain; palpitations; pallor; strong, abrupt carotid pulsations; pulsus bisferiens; and signs of congestive heart failure, such as crack-

les, dyspnea, and distended neck veins. Auscultation may reveal several murmurs, such as an early systolic murmur (common) and an apical diastolic rumble (Austin Flint murmur).

• *Arteriosclerosis.* In this disorder, reduced arterial compliance causes progressive widening of pulse pressure, which becomes permanent without treatment of the underlying disorder. It's preceded by moderate hypertension and accompanied by signs of vascular insufficiency, such as claudication and speech disturbances.

• *Febrile disorders.* Fever can cause widened pulse pressure. Accompanying symptoms vary depending on the specific disorder.

• *Increased intracranial pressure.* Widening pulse pressure is an intermediate to late sign of increased ICP. Although decreased level of consciousness is the earliest and most sensitive indicator of this life-threatening condition, the onset and progression of widening pulse pressure also parallel rising ICP. (Even a gap of only 50 mm Hg can signal a rapid deterioration in the patient's condition.) Assessment reveals Cushing's triad: bradycardia, hypertension, and respiratory pattern changes. Other findings may include headache, vomiting, and impaired or unequal motor movement. The patient may also have visual disturbances, such as blurring or photophobia, and pupillary changes.

Special considerations

If the patient has increased ICP, continually reassess his neurologic status, and compare your findings carefully with those of previous assessments. Immediately notify the doctor if you detect any change. Be alert for restlessness, confusion, unresponsiveness, or decreased level of consciousness, but remember that *subtle changes* in the patient's condition, rather than the abrupt development of any one sign or symptom, often signal increasing ICP.

Pediatric pointers

Increased ICP causes widened pulse pressure in children. Patent ductus arteriosus (PDA) can also cause it but this sign may not be evident at birth. The older child with PDA experiences exertional dyspnea, with pulse pressure that widens even further on exertion.

Pulse Rhythm Abnormality

An abnormal pulse rhythm is an irregular expansion and contraction of the peripheral arterial walls. It may be persistent or sporadic, and rhythmic or arrhythmic. Detected by palpating the radial or carotid pulse, an abnormal rhythm is typically reported first by the patient, who complains instead of palpitations. This important finding reflects an underlying cardiac dysrhythmia, which may range from benign to life-threatening. Dysrhythmias are commonly associated with cardiovascular, renal, respiratory, metabolic, and neurologic disorders, as well as the effects of drugs, diagnostic tests, and treatments.

Assessment

Quickly assess the patient for signs of reduced cardiac output, such as decreased level of consciousness, hypotension, or dizziness. If you detect these signs, immediately notify the doctor. Promptly obtain an EKG and possibly a chest X-ray, and begin cardiac monitoring. Insert an I.V. line for emergency cardiac drugs and give oxygen by nasal cannula or mask. Closely monitor the patient's vital signs, pulse quality, and cardiac rhythm: accompanying bradycardia or tachycardia may result in poor tolerance of the abnormal rhythm and cause further decline in cardiac output. Keep emergency intubation and suction equipment handy.

If the patient's condition permits, ask if he's experiencing any pain. If so, find out when the pain started and where it's located. Does it radiate? Ask about a history of heart disease and treatments for dysrhythmias. Find out what medications the patient is currently taking and if he's complying with the prescribed dosage and schedule. Digitalis toxicity, cessation of antiarrhythmic drugs, and use of quinidine and sympathomimetics (such as epinephrine) may cause dysrhythmias.

Now check the patient's apical and peripheral arterial pulses. An apical rate exceeding a peripheral arterial rate indicates a pulse deficit, which may also cause associated signs and symptoms of low cardiac output. Next, evaluate heart sounds: a long pause between S_1 ("lub") and S_2 ("dub") may

ABNORMAL PULSE RHYTHM:
CLUE TO CARDIAC DYSRHYTHMIAS

An abnormal pulse rhythm may be your only clue that the patient has a cardiac dysrhythmia. But this sign doesn't help you pinpoint the specific type of dysrhythmia. For that, you need a cardiac monitor or an electrocardiogram (EKG) machine. These devices record the electrical current generated by the heart's conduction system and display this information

DYSRHYTHMIA

Sinus arrhythmia

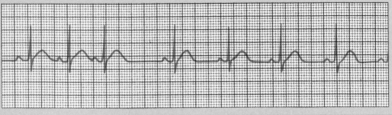

Premature atrial contractions (PACs)

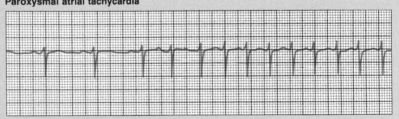

Paroxysmal atrial tachycardia

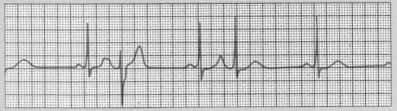

Atrial fibrillation

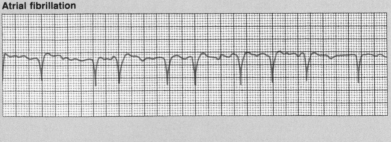

on an oscilloscope screen or a strip-chart recorder. Besides rhythm disturbances, they can identify conduction defects and electrolyte imbalances.

The EKG strips below show some common cardiac dysrhythmias that can cause abnormal pulse rhythms.

PULSE RHYTHM AND RATE	CLINICAL IMPLICATIONS
Irregular rhythm; fast, slow, or normal rate.	• Vagal effect of respiration on heart rate increases with inspiration and decreases with expiration. • May result from drugs, as in digitalis toxicity. • Occurs most often in children and young adults.
Irregular rhythm during PACs; fast, slow, or normal rate.	• Occasional PAC may be normal. • Isolated PACs indicate atrial irritation—for example, from anxiety or excessive caffeine intake. Increasing PACs may herald other atrial dysrhythmias. • May result from congestive heart failure, ischemic heart disease, acute respiratory failure, chronic obstructive pulmonary disease (COPD), or use of digitalis, aminophylline, or adrenergic drugs.
Irregular rhythm at abrupt onset or end of dysrhythmia; heart rate exceeds 140 beats/minute.	• May occur in otherwise normal, healthy persons with physical or psychological stress, hypoxia, or hypokalemia; may be associated with excessive use of caffeine or other stimulants, with use of marijuana, and with digitalis toxicity. • Indicates intrinsic abnormality of atrioventricular (AV) conduction system; may herald more serious ventricular dysrhythmia or precipitate angina or congestive heart failure.
Irregular rhythm; atrial rate exceeds 400 beats/minute; fast, slow, or normal ventricular rate.	• May result from congestive heart failure, COPD, hyperthyroidism, sepsis, pulmonary embolus, mitral valve disease, digitalis toxicity (rarely), atrial irritation, postcoronary bypass, or valve replacement surgery. • Because atria don't contract, preload isn't consistent, so cardiac output changes with each beat. Emboli may also result.

(continued)

ABNORMAL PULSE RHYTHM:
CLUE TO CARDIAC DYSRHYTHMIAS *(continued)*

DYSRHYTHMIA

Premature junctional contractions (PJCs)

Second-degree AV heart block, Mobitz Type I (Wenckebach)

Second-degree AV heart block, Mobitz Type II

Premature ventricular contractions (multifocal)

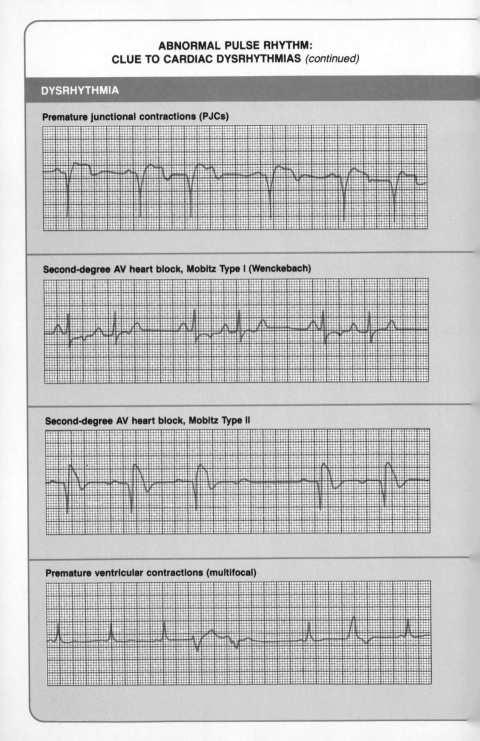

PULSE RHYTHM AND RATE	CLINICAL IMPLICATIONS
Irregular rhythm during PJCs; fast, slow, or normal rate.	• May result from myocardial infarction (MI) or ischemia, excessive caffeine intake, and most commonly digitalis toxicity (from enhanced automaticity). • Increasing PJCs may herald other dysrhythmias.
Irregular rhythm; fast, slow, or normal rate.	• Often transient; may progress to complete heart block. • May result from inferior wall MI, digitalis or quinidine toxicity, vagal stimulation, and arteriosclerotic heart disease.
Irregular rhythm; slow or normal rate.	• May progress to complete heart block. • May result from degenerative disease of conduction system, ischemia of AV node in anterior MI, anteroseptal infarction, or digitalis or quinidine toxicity.
Usually irregular rhythm with a long pause after the premature beat; fast, slow, or normal rate.	• Indicates ventricular irritability; may initiate ventricular tachycardia or ventricular fibrillation. • May result from heart failure, old or acute MI, contusion with trauma, myocardial irritation by a ventricular catheter, hypoxia, drug toxicity, electrolyte imbalance, or stress.

indicate a conduction defect. A faint or absent S_1 and an easily audible S_2 may indicate atrial fibrillation or flutter. You may hear the two heart sounds close together on certain beats—possibly indicating premature atrial contractions—or other variations in heart rate or rhythm. Take the patient's apical and radial pulses while you listen for heart sounds. In some dysrhythmias, such as premature ventricular contractions, you may hear the beat with your stethoscope but not feel it over the radial artery. This indicates an ineffective contraction that failed to produce a peripheral pulse. Now count the apical pulse for 60 seconds, noting the frequency of skipped peripheral beats. Report your findings to the doctor.

Medical causes

• *Dysrhythmias.* An abnormal pulse rhythm may be the only sign of a cardiac dysrhythmia. (See *Abnormal Pulse Rhythm: Clue to Cardiac Dysrhythmias,* pages 612 to 615.) The patient may complain of palpitations, a fluttering heartbeat, or weak and skipped beats. Pulses may be weak and rapid or slow. Depending on the specific dysrhythmia, dull chest pain or discomfort and hypotension may occur. Associated findings, if any, reflect decreased cardiac output. Neurologic findings, for example, include confusion, dizziness, light-headedness, decreased level of consciousness, and, sometimes, seizures. Other findings include decreased urine output, dyspnea, tachypnea, pallor, and diaphoresis.

Special considerations

If ordered, prepare the patient for transfer to a cardiac or intensive care unit. If the patient remains in your care, he may require bed rest or help with ambulation, depending on the severity of his symptoms. To prevent falls and injury, raise the side rails of the patient's bed and don't leave him unattended while he's sitting or walking. Check his vital signs frequently to detect associated bradycardia, tachycar-

dia, hypertension or hypotension, tachypnea, and dyspnea. Also monitor intake and output and the patient's daily weight.

If ordered, collect blood samples for serum electrolyte, cardiac enzyme, and drug level studies. Prepare the patient for a chest X-ray and a 12-lead EKG. If possible, obtain a previous EKG to compare with current findings. If ordered, prepare the patient for 24-hour Holter monitoring. Stress to the patient the importance of keeping a diary of his activities and any symptoms that develop, to correlate with the incidence of dysrhythmias.

Instruct the patient to avoid smoking and caffeine, which increase dysrhythmias. If he has a history of failing to comply with prescribed antiarrhythmic therapy, help him develop strategies to overcome this.

Pediatric pointers

Dysrhythmias also produce pulse rhythm abnormalities in children.

Pulsus Alternans

A sign of severe left ventricular failure, pulsus alternans is a beat-to-beat change in the size and intensity of a peripheral pulse. Although pulse rhythm remains regular, strong and weak contractions alternate. (See *Comparing Arterial Pressure Waves,* pages 618 and 619.) An alternation in the intensity of heart sounds and of existing heart murmurs may accompany this sign.

Pulsus alternans is thought to result from the change in stroke volume that occurs with beat-to-beat alteration in the left ventricle's contractility. Recumbency or exercise increases venous return and reduces the abnormal pulse, which often disappears with treatment for heart failure. Rarely, a patient with normal left ventricular function has pulsus alternans, but the abnormal pulse seldom persists for more than 10 to 12 beats.

Although most easily detected by sphygmomanometry, pulsus alternans can be detected by palpating the brachial, radial, or femoral artery when systolic pressure varies from beat to beat by more than 20 mm Hg. Because the small changes in arterial pressure that occur during normal respirations may obscure this abnormal pulse, you'll need to have the patient hold his breath during palpation. Apply *light* pressure to avoid obliterating the weaker pulse.

When using a sphygmomanometer to detect pulsus alternans, inflate the cuff 10 to 20 mm Hg above the systolic pressure as determined by palpation, then slowly deflate it. At first, you'll hear only the strong beats. With further deflation, all beats will become audible and palpable, and then equally intense. (The difference between this point and the peak systolic level is often used to determine the degree of pulsus alternans.) When the cuff is removed, pulsus alternans returns.

Occasionally, the weak beat is so small that no palpable pulse is detected at the periphery. This produces total pulsus alternans, an apparent halving of the pulse rate.

Assessment

Pulsus alternans indicates a critical change in the patient's status. After you detect it, quickly check other vital signs and have another nurse immediately notify the doctor. Closely assess the patient's heart rate, respiratory pattern, and blood pressure. Auscultate for a ventricular gallop (S₃) and increased crackles.

Medical cause

• *Left ventricular failure.* In this disorder, pulsus alternans is often initiated by a premature beat. It's almost always associated with a ventricular gallop. Other findings may include hypotension and cyanosis. Possible respiratory findings include exertional and paroxysmal nocturnal dyspnea, orthop-

nea, tachypnea, Cheyne-Stokes respirations, hemoptysis, and crackles. Fatigue and weakness are common.

Special considerations

If left ventricular failure develops suddenly, prepare the patient for transfer to an intensive or cardiac care unit. Meanwhile, elevate the head of his bed to promote respiratory excursion and increase oxygenation. The doctor may adjust the patient's current treatment plan to improve cardiac output, reduce the heart's workload, and promote diuresis.

Pediatric pointers

Pulsus alternans, which also occurs in a child with heart failure, may be difficult to assess if the child's crying or restless. Try to quiet the child by holding him, if his condition permits.

Pulsus Bisferiens

A bisferiens pulse is a hyperdynamic, double-beating pulse characterized by two systolic peaks separated by a midsystolic dip. Both peaks may be equal or either may be larger; most often, though, the first peak is taller or more forceful than the second. The first peak (percussion wave) is believed to be the pulse pressure and the second (tidal wave), reverberation from the periphery. (See *Comparing Arterial Pressure Waves,* pages 618 and 619.) Pulsus bisferiens occurs in conditions, such as aortic insufficiency, in which a large volume of blood is rapidly ejected from the left ventricle. The pulse can be palpated in peripheral arteries or observed on an arterial pressure wave recording.

To detect pulsus bisferiens, *lightly* palpate the carotid, brachial, radial, or femoral artery. (The pulse is easiest to palpate in the carotid artery.) At the same time, listen to the patient's heart sounds to determine if the two palpable peaks occur during systole. If they do, you'll feel the double pulse between the first and second heart sounds.

Assessment

After you detect a bisferiens pulse, review the patient's history for cardiac disorders. Next, find out what medication he's taking, if any, and ask if he has any other illnesses. Also ask about the development of any associated signs and symptoms, such as dyspnea, chest pain, or fatigue. Find out how long he's had these symptoms and if they change with activity or rest. Now, take his vital signs and auscultate for abnormal heart or lung sounds.

Medical causes.

● *Aortic insufficiency.* This heart defect is the most common organic cause of bisferiens pulse. Most patients with *chronic aortic insufficiency* are asymptomatic until age 40 or 50. However, exertional dyspnea, worsening fatigue, orthopnea, and, eventually, paroxysmal nocturnal dyspnea may develop.

Acute aortic insufficiency may produce signs and symptoms of left ventricular failure and cardiovascular collapse, such as weakness, severe dyspnea, hypotension, ventricular gallop (S_3), and tachycardia. Additional findings may include chest pain, palpitations, pallor, and strong, abrupt carotid pulsations. The patient may also have widened pulse pressure and one or more murmurs, especially an apical diastolic rumble (Austin Flint murmur).

● *Aortic stenosis with aortic insufficiency.* A bisferiens pulse is commonly seen in aortic stenosis when moderately severe aortic insufficiency also occurs. In aortic stenosis, the pulse rises slowly and the second wave of the double beat is the more forceful one. Frequently, this is accompanied by dyspnea and fatigue. Chest pain and syncope are not specific in the combined lesion, although they suggest predominant aortic stenosis.

● *High cardiac output states.* Pulsus bis-

COMPARING ARTERIAL PRESSURE WAVES

The percussion wave in the **normal arterial pulse** reflects ejection of blood into the aorta (early systole). The tidal wave is the peak of the pulse wave (later systole). And the dicrotic notch marks the beginning of diastole.

Pulsus alternans is a beat-to-beat alternation in pulse size and intensity. Although the rhythm of pulsus alternans is regular, the volume varies. If you take the blood pressure of a patient with this abnormality, you'll first hear a loud Korotkoff sound and then a soft sound, continually alternating. Pulsus alternans frequently accompanies states of poor contractility that occur with left ventricular failure.

Pulsus bisferiens is a double-beating pulse with two systolic peaks. The first beat reflects pulse pressure and the second beat reflects reverberation from the periphery. Pulsus bisferiens commonly occurs in aortic insufficiency or high cardiac output states.

Pulsus paradoxus is an exaggerated decline in blood pressure during inspiration, resulting from an increase in negative intrathoracic pressure. A pulsus paradoxus that exceeds 10 mm Hg is considered abnormal and may result from cardiac tamponade, constrictive pericarditis, or severe lung disease.

Inspiration

Expiration

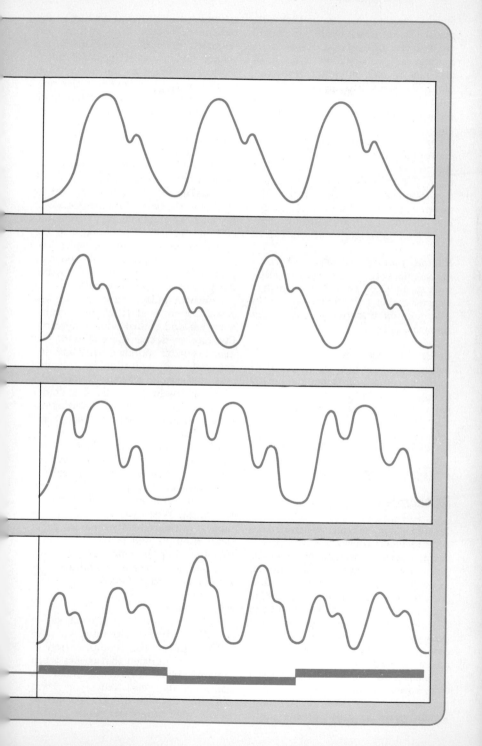

feriens commonly occurs in high-output states, such as anemia, thyrotoxicosis, fever, or exercise. Associated findings vary with the underlying cause and may include moderate tachycardia, a cervical venous hum, and widened pulse pressure.

• **Hypertrophic obstructive cardiomyopathy.** About 40% of patients with this disorder have pulsus bisferiens because of a pressure gradient in the left ventricular outflow tract. Recorded more often than it's palpated, the pulse rises rapidly, and the first wave is the more forceful one. Associated findings may include a systolic murmur, dyspnea, angina, fatigue, and syncope.

Special considerations
Prepare the patient for diagnostic tests, such as an EKG, chest X-ray, cardiac catheterization, or angiography, to help determine the underlying cause of the abnormal pulse.

Pediatric pointers
Pulsus bisferiens may be palpated in children with a large patent ductus arteriosus, as well as those with congenital aortic stenosis and insufficiency.

Pulsus Paradoxus

[Paradoxical pulse]

Paradoxical pulse is an exaggerated decline in blood pressure during inspiration. Normally, systolic pressure falls less than 10 mm Hg during inspiration. In pulsus paradoxus, however, it falls more than 10 mm Hg. (See *Comparing Arterial Pressure Waves*, pages 618 and 619.) When systolic pressure falls more than 20 mm Hg, the peripheral pulses may be barely palpable or may disappear during inspiration.

Pulsus paradoxus is thought to result from an inspirational increase in negative intrathoracic pressure. Normally, systolic pressure drops during inspiration because of blood pooling in the pulmonary system. This, in turn, reduces left ventricular filling and stroke volume and transmits negative intrathoracic pressure to the aorta. Such conditions as chronic obstructive pulmonary disease or cardiac tamponade further impede blood flow from the left ventricle during inspiration and produce paradoxical pulse.

To accurately detect and measure paradoxical pulse, use a sphygmomanometer or intraarterial monitoring device. Inflate the blood pressure cuff 10 to 20 mm Hg beyond the peak systolic pressure. Then deflate the cuff at a rate of 2 mm Hg/second until you hear the first Korotkoff sound during expiration. Note the systolic pressure. As you continue to slowly deflate the cuff, observe the patient's respiratory pattern. If a paradoxical pulse is present, the Korotkoff sounds will disappear with inspiration and return with expiration. Continue to deflate the cuff until you hear Korotkoff sounds during both inspiration and expiration, and, again, note the systolic pressure. Now subtract this reading from the first one to determine the degree of paradoxical pulse. A difference of more than 10 mm Hg is abnormal.

You can also detect paradoxical pulse by palpating the radial pulse over several cycles of slow inspiration and expiration. Marked pulse diminution during inspiration indicates paradoxical pulse. When you check for paradoxical pulse, remember that irregular heart rhythms and tachycardia cause variations in pulse amplitude and must be ruled out before a true paradoxical pulse can be identified.

Assessment

A paradoxical pulse may signal cardiac tamponade—a life-threatening complication of pericardial effusion that occurs when sufficient blood or fluid accumulates to compress the heart. After you detect paradoxical pulse, quickly take the patient's other vital signs, while another nurse immediately informs the doctor. Check for additional signs and symptoms of cardiac tamponade, such as dyspnea, tachypnea, diaphoresis, distended neck veins, tachycardia, narrowed pulse pressure, and hypotension. If necessary, assist with emergency pericardiocentesis to aspirate blood or fluid from the pericardial sac. Then evaluate the effectiveness of pericardiocentesis by measuring the degree of pulsus paradoxus; it should decrease after aspiration.

If the patient doesn't have cardiac tamponade, find out if he has a history of chronic cardiac or pulmonary disease. Ask about the development of associated signs and symptoms, such as a cough or chest pain. Then auscultate for abnormal breath sounds.

Medical causes

• *Cardiac tamponade.* Pulsus paradoxus commonly occurs in this disorder. However, if intrapericardial pressure rises abruptly and profound hypotension occurs, paradoxical pulse may be difficult to detect. In severe tamponade, assessment also reveals these classic findings: hypotension, diminished or muffled heart sounds, and jugular vein distention. Related findings include chest pain, pericardial friction rub, narrowed pulse pressure, anxiety, restlessness, clammy skin, and hepatomegaly. Characteristic respiratory signs and symptoms include dyspnea, tachypnea, and cyanosis; the patient typically sits up and leans forward to facilitate breathing.

If cardiac tamponade develops gradually, paradoxical pulse may be accompanied by weakness, anorexia, and weight loss. The patient may also have chest pain, but he won't have muffled heart sounds or severe hypotension.

• *Chronic obstructive pulmonary disease (COPD).* The wide fluctuations in intrathoracic pressure that are characteristic of this disorder produce pulsus paradoxus and possibly tachycardia. Other findings vary but may include dyspnea, tachypnea, wheezing, productive or nonproductive cough, accessory muscle use, barrel chest, and clubbing. The patient may show labored, pursed-lip breathing after exertion or even at rest. Typically, he'll sit leaning forward to facilitate breathing. Auscultation reveals decreased breath sounds, rhonchi, and crackles. Weight loss, cyanosis, and edema may occur.

• *Pericarditis (chronic constrictive).* Paradoxical pulse can occur in up to 50% of patients with this disorder. Other findings include pericardial friction rub, chest pain, exertional dyspnea, orthopnea, hepatomegaly, and ascites. The patient also exhibits peripheral edema and Kussmaul's sign—distended neck veins that become more prominent on inspiration.

• *Pulmonary embolism (massive).* Decreased left ventricular filling and stroke volume in massive pulmonary embolism produces pulsus paradoxus. It also produces syncope and severe apprehension, dyspnea, tachypnea, and pleuritic chest pain. The patient appears cyanotic, with distended neck veins. He may succumb to circulatory collapse, with hypotension and a weak, rapid pulse. Infarction may produce hemoptysis, along with decreased breath sounds and a pleural friction rub over the affected area.

• *Right ventricular infarction.* This infarction may produce pulsus paradoxus and elevated jugular venous or central venous pressure. Other findings are similar to those of myocardial infarction.

Special considerations

Prepare the patient for an echocardiogram to visualize cardiac motion and to help determine the causative disorder. Monitor the patient's vital signs and frequently check the degree of paradox. Inform the doctor immediately if you note a steady increase in the degree of paradox. Such an increase may indicate recurring or worsening cardiac tamponade or impending respiratory arrest in severe COPD. Vigorous respiratory treatment—such as chest physiotherapy—may avoid the need for endotracheal intubation.

Pediatric pointers

Paradoxical pulse often occurs in children with chronic pulmonary disease, especially during an acute asthmatic attack. Children with pericarditis may also develop pulsus paradoxus due to cardiac tamponade, although this disorder more commonly affects adults. A paradoxical pulse above 20 mm Hg is a reliable indicator of cardiac tamponade in these patients; a change of 10 to 20 mm Hg is equivocal.

Pupils—Nonreactive

Nonreactive (fixed) pupils fail to constrict in response to light or dilate when the light is removed. The development of a unilateral or bilateral nonreactive response indicates an important change in the patient's condition and could signal a life-threatening emergency and possibly brain death. It also occurs with use of certain optic drugs.

To assess pupillary reaction to light, first test the patient's *direct light reflex*. Darken the room, and cover one of the patient's eyes while you hold open the opposite eyelid. Using a bright penlight, bring the light toward the patient from the side and shine it directly into his opened eye. If normal, the pupil will promptly constrict. Now test the *consensual light reflex*. Hold the patient's eyelids open and shine the light into one eye while watching the pupil of the opposite eye. If normal, both pupils will promptly constrict. Repeat both procedures in the opposite eye. A unilateral or bilateral nonreactive response indicates dysfunction of cranial nerves II and III, which mediate the pupillary light reflex. (See *Innervation of Direct and Consensual Light Reflexes*, page 624.)

Assessment

If the patient is unconscious and develops unilateral or bilateral nonreactive pupil(s), quickly take his vital signs while another nurse immediately informs the doctor. Be alert for decerebrate or decorticate posture, bradycardia, elevated systolic blood pressure, widened pulse pressure, and the development of other untoward changes in the patient's condition. Remember, a unilateral dilated, nonreactive pupil may be an early sign of uncal brain herniation. The doctor may adjust the patient's current treatment or order emergency surgery to try to decrease intracranial pressure (ICP). If the patient isn't already being treated for increased ICP, insert an I.V. line to administer diuretics, osmotics, and corticosteroids. You may also need to start the patient on controlled hyperventilation.

If the patient isn't unconscious, obtain a brief history. Ask him what type of eye drops he's using, if any, and when they were last instilled. Also ask if he's experiencing any pain, and, if so, try to determine its location, intensity, and duration. Assess the patient's visual acuity in both eyes. Then test the pupillary reaction to accommodation: normally, both pupils constrict equally as the patient shifts his glance from a distant to a near object. Next, hold a penlight at the side of each eye and examine the cornea and iris for any abnormalities. As ordered, assist in measuring intraocular pressure with a tonometer. Or estimate intraocular pressure by placing your second and third fingers over the patient's closed eyelid. If the eyeball feels rock hard, suspect elevated intraocular pressure. Assist the doctor in performing an ophthalmoscopic examination. He may also use a slit lamp to examine the eye. If the patient has experienced ocular trauma, don't manipulate the affected eye. After the examination, cover the affected eye with a protective metal shield, but don't let the shield rest on the globe.

Medical causes

• **Adie's syndrome.** This syndrome produces abrupt onset of unilateral mydriasis, along with sluggish or nonreactive pupillary response. It also may produce blurred vision and cramplike eye pain. Eventually, both eyes may be affected. Musculoskeletal assessment reveals hypoactive or absent deep tendon reflexes in the arms and legs.

• **Botulism.** Bilateral mydriasis and nonreactive pupils usually appear 12 to 36 hours after ingestion of tainted food. Other early findings are blurred vision, diplopia, ptosis, strabismus, and extraocular muscle palsies, along with anorexia, nausea, vomiting, diarrhea, and dry mouth. Vertigo, deafness, hoarseness, nasal voice, dysarthria, and dysphagia follow. Progressive muscle weakness and absent deep tendon reflexes usually evolve over 2 to 4 days. This results in severe constipation and paralysis of respiratory muscles with respiratory distress.

• **Encephalitis.** As this disease progresses, initially sluggish pupils become dilated and nonreactive. Decreased accommodation and other symptoms of cranial nerve palsies, such as dysphagia, develop. Within 48 hours after onset, encephalitis causes a decreased level of consciousness, high fever, headache, vomiting, and nuchal rigidity. Aphasia, ataxia, nystagmus, hemiparesis, and photophobia may occur with seizures.

• **Familial amyloid polyneuropathy.** This disorder produces sluggish or nonreactive pupils and miosis. Corneal opacities may affect visual acuity. The patient may also have anhidrosis, orthostatic hypotension, alternating diarrhea and constipation, and impotence. Initially, he'll experience paresthesias and possibly pain in the feet and lower legs; later, absent deep tendon reflexes and thinning legs.

• **Glaucoma (acute closed-angle.)** In this ophthalmic emergency, examination reveals a moderately dilated, nonreactive pupil in the affected eye. Conjunctival injection, corneal clouding, and decreased visual acuity also occur. The patient experiences sudden onset of blurred vision, followed by excrutiating pain in and around the affected eye. Commonly, he reports seeing halos around white lights at night. Severely elevated intraocular pressure frequently induces nausea and vomiting.

• **Iris disease (degenerative or inflammatory).** This disease causes pupillary nonreactivity in the affected eye(s). Visual acuity also may decrease.

• **Midbrain lesions.** Although rare, these lesions produce bilateral midposition nonreactive pupils. Other findings include loss of upward gaze, coma, central neurogenic hyperventilation, bradycardia, hemiparesis or hemiplegia, and decorticate or decerebrate posture.

• **Ocular trauma.** Severe damage to the iris or optic nerve may produce a nonreactive, dilated pupil in the affected eye (traumatic iridoplegia). It's usually transitory but can be permanent. Slit lamp examination frequently reveals a V-shaped notch in the pupillary rim, indicating a tear in the iris sphincter muscle. Usually, the patient experiences eye pain. Other findings may include eye edema and ecchymoses.

• **Oculomotor nerve palsy.** Often, the first signs of this oculomotor ophthalmoplegia are a dilated, nonreactive pupil and loss of the accommodation reaction. These findings may occur in one eye or both, depending on whether the palsy is unilateral or bilateral. Among the causes of total third cranial nerve paralysis is life-threatening brain herniation. *Central herniation* causes bilateral midposition nonreactive pupils, whereas *uncal herniation* initially causes a unilateral dilated, nonreactive pupil. Other common findings include diplopia, ptosis, outward deviation of the eye, and inability to elevate or adduct the eye. Additional findings depend on the palsy's underlying cause.

• **Uveitis.** A small, nonreactive pupil typifies *anterior uveitis*, appearing suddenly with severe eye pain, conjunctival injection, and photophobia. In *posterior uveitis*, similar features

INNERVATION OF DIRECT AND CONSENSUAL LIGHT REFLEXES

Two reactions—direct and consensual—constitute the pupillary light reflex. Normally, when a light is shined directly onto the retina of one eye, the parasympathetic nerves are stimulated to cause brisk constriction of that pupil—the *direct light reflex*. The pupil of the opposite eye also constricts—the *consensual light reflex*.

The optic nerve (CN II) mediates the afferent arc of this reflex from each eye, while the oculomotor nerve (CN III) mediates the efferent arc to both eyes. A nonreactive or sluggish response in one or both pupils indicates dysfunction of these cranial nerves—usually due to degenerative disease of the central nervous system.

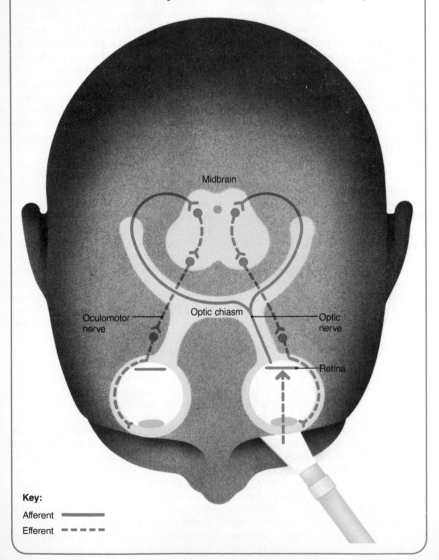

Midbrain

Oculomotor nerve

Optic chiasm

Optic nerve

Retina

Key:

Afferent ——————

Efferent - - - - - -

develop insidiously, along with blurred vision and distorted pupil shape.

• *Wernicke's disease.* Nonreactive pupils are a late sign in this disease, which initially produces intention tremor accompanied by sluggish pupillary reaction. Other ocular findings include diplopia, gaze paralysis, nystagmus, ptosis, decreased visual acuity, and conjunctival injection. The patient may also exhibit postural hypotension, tachycardia, ataxia, apathy, and confusion.

Other causes

• *Drugs.* Instillation of topical mydriatics and cycloplegics may induce a temporarily nonreactive pupil in the affected eye. Use of glutethimide and deep ether anesthesia produces medium-sized or slightly enlarged pupils, which remain nonreactive for several hours. Opiates, such as heroin and morphine, cause pinpoint pupils with a minimal light response that can be seen only with a magnifying glass. And atropine poisoning produces widely dilated, nonreactive pupils.

Special considerations

If the patient is conscious, monitor his pupillary light reflex to detect changes. If he's unconscious, close his eyes to prevent corneal exposure. (Use tape to secure the eyelids, if needed.)

Pediatric pointers

Children have nonreactive pupils for the same reasons as adults. The most common cause is oculomotor nerve palsy from increased ICP.

Pupils—Sluggish

Sluggish pupillary reaction is an abnormally slow pupil response to light. It can occur in one pupil or both, unlike the normal reaction, which is always bilateral. A sluggish reaction accompanies degenerative disease of the central nervous system and diabetic neuropathy. It can occur normally in the elderly, whose pupils become smaller and less responsive with age.

To assess pupillary reaction to light, first test the patient's *direct light reflex.* Darken the room, and cover one of the patient's eyes while you hold open the opposite eyelid. Using a bright penlight, bring the light toward the patient from the side and shine it directly into his opened eye. If normal, the pupil will promptly constrict. Now test the *consensual light reflex.* Hold both of the patient's eyelids open, and shine the light into one eye while watching the pupil of the opposite eye. If normal, both pupils will promptly constrict. Repeat both procedures to test light reflexes in the opposite eye. A sluggish reaction in one or both pupils indicates dysfunction of cranial nerves II and III, which mediate the pupillary light reflex. (See *Innervation of Direct and Consensual Light Reflexes.*)

Assessment

After you detect a sluggish pupillary reaction, assess the patient's visual function. Start by testing visual acuity in both eyes. Then test the pupillary reaction to accommodation: the pupils should constrict equally as the patient shifts his glance from a distant to a near object. Next, hold a penlight at the side of each eye and examine the cornea and iris for irregularities, scars, and foreign bodies. As ordered, assist the doctor in measuring intraocular pressure with a tonometer. Or you can estimate intraocular pressure without a tonometer by placing your fingers over the patient's closed eyelid. If the eyeball feels rock hard, suspect elevated intraocular pressure. Assist the doctor with an ophthalmoscopic examination. The doctor may also use a slit lamp to examine the eye.

Medical causes

• *Adie's syndrome.* This syndrome produces abrupt onset of unilateral mydriasis and sluggish pupillary response, possibly progressing to a nonreactive response. The patient may complain of blurred vision and cramplike eye pain. Eventually, both eyes may be affected. Musculoskeletal assessment also reveals hypoactive or absent deep tendon reflexes in the arms and legs.

● *Diabetic neuropathy.* A patient with long-standing diabetes mellitus may have a sluggish pupillary response. He may also have orthostatic hypotension and syncope. Additional findings may include dysphagia, episodic constipation or diarrhea, painless bladder distention with overflow incontinence, retrograde ejaculation, and impotence.

● *Encephalitis.* This disorder initially produces a bilateral sluggish pupillary response. Later, pupils become dilated and nonreactive, and decreased accommodation may occur, along with other cranial nerve palsies, such as dysphagia and facial weakness. Within 24 to 48 hours after onset, encephalitis causes a decreased level of consciousness, headache, high fever, vomiting, and nuchal rigidity. In addition, aphasia, ataxia, nystagmus, hemiparesis, and photophobia may occur. The patient may exhibit seizure activity and myoclonic jerks.

● *Familial amyloid polyneuropathy.* A patient with this disorder will have sluggish or nonreactive pupils, accompanied by miosis and corneal opacities that may affect visual acuity. The patient may also have anhidrosis, orthostatic hypotension, alternating diarrhea and constipation, and impotence. Initially, he'll experience paresthesias and possibly pain in the feet and lower legs. Later, absent deep tendon reflexes and thinning legs may hamper walking.

● *Herpes zoster.* The patient with herpes zoster affecting the nasociliary nerve may have a sluggish pupillary response. Examination of the conjunctiva will reveal follicles. Additional ocular findings include a serous discharge, absence of tears, ptosis, and extraocular muscle palsy.

● *Iritis (acute).* In this disorder, the affected eye exhibits a sluggish pupillary response and conjunctival injection. The pupil may remain constricted; if posterior synechiae have formed, the pupil will also be irregularly shaped. The patient will report sudden onset of eye pain and photophobia and may also have blurred vision.

● *Multiple sclerosis.* This disorder may produce small, irregularly shaped pupils that react better to accommodation than to light. Additional ocular findings may include ptosis, nystagmus, diplopia, and blurred vision. In most patients, visual problems and sensory impairment, such as paresthesias, are the earliest indications. Later, a variety of features may develop, including muscle weakness and paralysis; intention tremor, spasticity, hyperreflexia, and gait ataxia; dysphagia and dysarthria; constipation; urinary urgency, frequency, and incontinence; impotence; and emotional instability.

● *Myotonic dystrophy.* In this disorder, sluggish pupillary reaction may be accompanied by lid lag, ptosis, miosis, and possibly diplopia. The patient may have decreased visual acuity from cataract formation. Muscular weakness and atrophy and testicular atrophy may occur.

● *Tertiary syphilis.* Sluggish pupillary reaction (especially in Argyll Robertson pupils) occurs in the late stage of neurosyphilis, along with marked weakness of the extraocular muscles, visual field defects, and possibly cataractous changes in the lens. The patient may complain of orbital rim pain, which worsens at night. Lid edema, decreased visual acuity, and exophthalmos may also occur. Tertiary lesions appear on the skin and mucous membranes. Liver, respiratory, cardiovascular, and additional neurologic dysfunction may also occur.

● *Wernicke's disease.* Initially, this disorder produces intention tremor accompanied by sluggish pupillary reaction. Later, pupils may become nonreactive. Additional ocular findings include diplopia, gaze paralysis, nystagmus, ptosis, decreased visual acuity, and conjunctival injection. The patient may also exhibit postural hypotension, tachycardia, ataxia, apathy, and confusion.

Special considerations
Sluggish pupillary reaction isn't diagnostically significant, although it occurs in a variety of disorders.

Pediatric pointers
Children experience sluggish pupillary reactions for the same reasons as adults.

Purple Striae

Purple striae—thin, purple streaks on the skin—characteristically occur in hypercortisolism along with other cushingoid signs, such as a buffalo hump and moon face. Although hypercortisolism can result from adrenocortical carcinoma, adrenal adenoma, and pituitary adenoma, it most commonly results from excessive use of glucocorticoid drugs.

The catabolic action of excess glucocorticoids on skin, fat, and muscle produces purple striae by inhibiting fibroblast activity, resulting in loss of collagen and connective tissue. This causes extreme thinning of the skin, which, along with erythrocytosis, is responsible for the striae's purple color. Although purple striae are most common over the abdominal area, they may also occur over the breasts, hips, buttocks, thighs, and axillae. They develop gradually and, with treatment, may gradually fade or decrease in size.

Assessment
Ask the patient when—and on what part of his body—he first noticed purple striae. To help determine the rate of progression, find out if he has photographs of himself before and over the course of striae development. Next, obtain a complete medication history. If the patient is receiving glucocorticoid therapy, find out the drug's name, the daily dosage and schedule, and the reason for treatment. Also, ask if the dosage has been altered recently and if the drug is given intramuscularly. Find out if the patient uses topical corticosteroid preparations, especially fluorinated products, and ask about concomitant use of occlusive dressings and, with large skin surface areas, the amount of corticosteroid applied.

Then examine the patient, and note all areas where purple striae appear. When checking for striae, remember that the patient's skin is extremely thin and susceptible to bruising.

Medical cause
● *Hypercortisolism.* In this disorder, purple striae—usually more than 1 cm wide—develop gradually over the abdomen and possibly the breasts, hips, buttocks, thighs, and axillae. Inspection also reveals moon face, buffalo hump, and truncal obesity—the cardinal signs of hypercortisolism. Other findings may include acne, ecchymoses, petechiae, muscle weakness and wasting, poor wound healing, excessive perspiration, hypertension, fatigue, and personality changes. Women may develop hirsutism, menstrual irregularities, and loss of ability to achieve orgasm. Men may have impotence.

Other causes
● *Drugs.* Excessive use of glucocorticoids can cause purple striae and other cushingoid effects.

Special considerations
Prepare the patient for diagnostic tests to confirm hypercortisolism and determine its cause. Expect to collect 24-hour urine samples before and during the 2-day low-dose and 2-day high-dose dexamethasone tests. Explain that follow-up tests may be performed.

Help the patient cope with changes

in his body image by clearly explaining the disease process and allowing him to openly express his concerns.

Pediatric pointers

Although relatively rare in childhood, hypercortisolism may occur at any age. In infancy and early years, it usually results from adrenal tumor, systemic absorption of topical corticosteroids applied excessively, or oral administration of glucocorticoids. After age 7, it usually stems from inappropriate pituitary secretion of adrenocorticotropic hormone, with bilateral adrenal hyperplasia.

Purpura

Purpura is the extravasation of red blood cells from the blood vessels into the skin, subcutaneous tissue, or mucous membranes. It's characterized by discoloration—usually purplish or brownish red—that's easily visible through the epidermis. Purpuric lesions include petechiae, ecchymoses, and hematomas. (See *Identifying Purpuric Lesions.*) Purpura differs from erythema in that it doesn't blanch with pressure because it involves blood in the tissues, not just dilated vessels.

Purpura results from damage to the endothelium of small blood vessels, coagulation defects, ineffective perivascular support, capillary fragility and permeability, or a combination of these factors. In turn, these faulty hemostatic factors can result from thrombocytopenia or other hematologic disorders, invasive procedures, and, of course, anticoagulant drugs.

Additional causes are nonpathologic. Purpura can be a consequence of aging, when loss of collagen decreases connective tissue support of upper skin blood vessels. In the elderly or cachectic person, skin atrophy and inelasticity and loss of subcutaneous fat increase susceptibility to minor trauma,

causing purpura to appear along the veins of the forearms, hands, legs, and feet. Prolonged coughing or vomiting can produce crops of petechiae in loose face and neck tissue. Violent muscle contraction, as occurs in seizures or weight lifting, sometimes results in localized ecchymoses from increased intraluminal pressure and rupture. High fever, which increases capillary fragility, can also produce purpura.

Assessment

After you detect purpura, ask the patient when he first noticed the lesion and if he has also noticed other lesions on his body. Does he or his family have a history of bleeding disorders or easy bruising? Find out what medications the patient is taking, if any, and ask him to describe his diet. Ask about recent trauma or transfusions and the development of associated signs, such as epistaxis, bleeding gums, hematuria, and hematochezia. Also ask about systemic complaints, such as fever, which may suggest infection. And if the patient's female, ask about heavy menstrual flow.

Inspect the patient's entire skin surface to determine the type, size, location, distribution, and severity of purpuric lesions. Also inspect the mucous membranes. Remember that the same mechanisms that cause purpura can also cause internal hemorrhage, although purpura isn't a cardinal indicator of this condition.

Medical causes

● *Autoerythrocyte sensitivity.* In this syndrome, painful ecchymoses appear either singly or in groups, usually preceded by local itching, burning, or pain. Frequently associated findings include epistaxis, hematuria, hematemesis, and menometrorrhagia. Abdominal pain, diarrhea, nausea, vomiting, syncope, headache, and chest pain also commonly occur. This syndrome can be linked to a psychiatric disorder, with associated anxiety, depression, hysteria, and masochism.

IDENTIFYING PURPURIC LESIONS

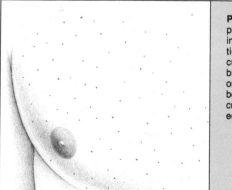

Petechiae are painless, round, pinpoint lesions, 1 to 3 mm in diameter. Caused by extravasation of red blood cells into cutaneous tissue, these red or brown lesions usually arise on dependent portions of the body. They appear and fade in crops and can group to form ecchymoses.

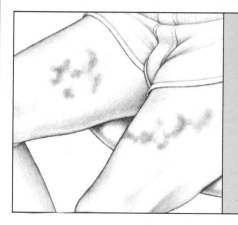

Ecchymoses, another form of blood extravasation, are larger than petechiae. These purple, blue, or yellow-green bruises vary in size and shape and can arise anywhere on the body as a result of trauma. Ecchymoses usually appear on the arms and legs of patients with bleeding disorders.

Hematomas are palpable ecchymoses that are painful and swollen. Usually the result of trauma, superficial hematomas are red, whereas deep hematomas are blue. Hematomas often exceed 1 cm in diameter, but their size varies widely.

● **Disseminated intravascular coagulation.** This syndrome can cause varying degrees of purpura, depending on its severity and underlying cause. Rarely, the patient develops life-threatening purpura fulminans, with symmetrical cutaneous and subcutaneous lesions on the arms and legs. Or he may have cutaneous oozing, hematemesis, or bleeding from incision or needle insertion sites. Other findings may include acrocyanosis; nausea; dyspnea; convulsions; severe muscle, back, and abdominal pain; and signs of acute tubular necrosis, such as oliguria.

● **Dysproteinemias.** In *multiple myeloma,* petechiae and ecchymoses accompany other bleeding tendencies: hematemesis, epistaxis, gum bleeding, and excessive bleeding after surgery. Similar findings occur in *cryoglobulinemia,* which may also produce a malignant maculopapular purpura. *Hyperglobulinemia* typically begins insidiously with occasional attacks of purpura over the lower legs and feet. Attacks eventually become more frequent and extensive, involving the entire lower leg and possibly the trunk. The purpura usually occurs after prolonged standing or exercise and may be heralded by skin burning or stinging. Leg edema, knee or ankle pain, and low-grade fever may precede or accompany the purpura, which gradually fades over 1 or 2 weeks. Persistent pigmentation develops after repeated attacks.

● **Easy bruising syndrome.** This syndrome is characterized by recurrent bruising on the legs, arms, and trunk, either spontaneously or following minor trauma. Bruising may be preceded by pain and is more common in women than in men, especially during menses.

● **Ehlers-Danlos syndrome (EDS).** Besides petechiae, this syndrome features easy bruising, epistaxis, gum bleeding, hematuria, melena, menorrhagia, and excessive bleeding after surgery. EDS characteristically produces soft, velvety, hyperelastic skin; hyperextensible joints; increased skin and blood vessel fragility; and repeated dislocations of the temporomandibular joint.

● **Idiopathic thrombocytopenic purpura (ITP).** Chronic ITP typically begins insidiously, with scattered petechiae that are most common on the distal arms and legs. Deep-lying ecchymoses may also occur. Other findings include epistaxis, easy bruising, hematuria, hematemesis, and menorrhagia.

● **Leukemia.** This disorder produces widespread petechiae on the skin, mucous membranes, retina, and serosal surfaces that persist throughout the course of the disease. Confluent ecchymoses are uncommon but may occur. The patient may also have swollen and bleeding gums, epistaxis, and other bleeding tendencies. Lymphadenopathy and splenomegaly are common.

Acute leukemias also produce severe prostration and high fever and may cause dyspnea, tachycardia, palpitations, and abdominal or bone pain. Confusion, headache, seizures, vomiting, papilledema, and nuchal rigidity may occur late in the disease.

Chronic leukemias begin insidiously with minor bleeding tendencies, malaise, fatigue, pallor, low-grade fever, anorexia, and weight loss.

● **Liver disease.** Hepatic disease may cause purpura, particularly ecchymoses, and other bleeding tendencies. Associated findings may include hepatomegaly, ascites, right upper quadrant pain, jaundice, nausea, vomiting, and anorexia.

● **Lymphomas.** T-cell (Hodgkin's) *lymphomas* initially may produce erythematous patches with some scaling. These lesions—which may be psoriasiform or parapsoriasiform—then become interspersed with nodules. Pruritus and discomfort are common. Later, tumors and ulcerations form, and nontender lymphadenopathy develops. *B-cell (non-Hodgkin's) lymphomas* may produce a scaling dermatitis with pruritus, which usually begins on the legs and then affects the entire body. Small pink-to-brown nodules and diffuse pigmentation also occur. In addition,

B-cell lymphomas typically produce painless peripheral lymphadenopathy, usually affecting the cervical nodes first. Other findings in both types of lymphoma include fever, fatigue, malaise, weight loss, and hepatosplenomegaly.

• *Myeloproliferative disorders.* These disorders, which include polycythemia vera, paradoxically can cause hemorrhage accompanied by ecchymoses and ruddy cyanosis. The oral mucosa takes on a deep purplish red hue, and slight trauma causes swollen gums to bleed. Other findings include pruritus, urticaria, and such nonspecific symptoms as lethargy, weakness, fatigue, and weight loss. The patient typically complains of headache, a sensation of fullness in the head, and rushing in the ears; dizziness and vertigo; dyspnea; paresthesias of the fingers; double or blurred vision and scotoma; and epigastric distress. He may also experience intermittent claudication, hypertension, hepatosplenomegaly, and impaired mentation.

• *Nutritional deficiencies.* In *vitamin C deficiency,* the characteristic pattern of purpura is perifollicular petechiae, which coalesce to form ecchymoses, in the "saddle area" of the thighs and buttocks. Additional hemorrhage occurs in arm and leg muscles (with phlebothrombosis), viscera, joints (with limb and joint pain), and nail beds. Related findings include scaly dermatitis; pallor; tender, swollen, bleeding gums and loosened teeth; dry mouth; and poor wound healing. Nonspecific symptoms include weakness, lethargy, and anorexia. Irritability, depression, insomnia, and hysteria may also develop.

Vitamin K deficiency produces abnormal bleeding tendencies, such as ecchymosis, gum bleeding, epistaxis, and hematuria. It also causes GI and intracranial bleeding.

Vitamin B_{12} deficiency can cause varying degrees of purpura. Its GI effects include anorexia, nausea, vomiting, weight loss, abdominal discomfort, and jaundice. Dyspnea, peripheral

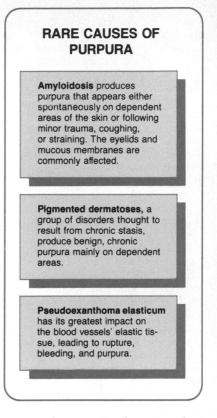

RARE CAUSES OF PURPURA

Amyloidosis produces purpura that appears either spontaneously on dependent areas of the skin or following minor trauma, coughing, or straining. The eyelids and mucous membranes are commonly affected.

Pigmented dermatoses, a group of disorders thought to result from chronic stasis, produce benign, chronic purpura mainly on dependent areas.

Pseudoexanthoma elasticum has its greatest impact on the blood vessels' elastic tissue, leading to rupture, bleeding, and purpura.

neuropathies, ataxia, glossitis, and occasional depression also occur.

Folic acid deficiency also can cause varying degrees of purpura. The patient may complain of fatigue, weakness, dyspnea, palpitations, nausea, and anorexia. He may be irritable and forgetful and report headaches and fainting spells. Additional findings include pallor, slight jaundice, and glossitis.

• *Septicemia.* Thrombocytopenia or the effects of toxins in acute infection can lead to purpura, especially in the form of petechiae. Associated findings may include fever, chills, headache, tachycardia, lethargy, diaphoresis, and anorexia. Signs and symptoms specific to the area of infection—for example, cough, wound drainage, or urinary burning— also occur.

• *Stasis.* Chronic stasis usually affects

the elderly, producing dusky reddish purpura on the legs after prolonged standing.

• *Systemic lupus erythematosus.* This chronic inflammatory disorder may produce purpura accompanied by other cutaneous findings, such as scaly patches on the scalp, face, neck, and arms; diffuse alopecia; telangiectasis; urticaria; and ulceration. The characteristic butterfly rash appears in the disorder's acute phase. Commonly associated signs and symptoms include nondeforming joint pain and stiffness, Raynaud's phenomenon, seizures, psychotic behavior, photosensitivity, fever, anorexia, weight loss, and lymphadenopathy.

• *Thrombotic thrombocytopenic purpura.* Generalized purpura is usually a presenting sign in this disorder. Other presenting signs and symptoms vary but may include hematuria, vaginal bleeding, jaundice, and pallor. Most patients have fever, and some may also experience fatigue, weakness, headache, nausea, abdominal pain, and arthralgias. Hepatosplenomegaly may occur. Finally, neurologic changes—including seizures, paresthesias, cranial nerve palsies, vertigo, and altered level of consciousness—may develop along with renal failure.

• *Trauma.* Traumatic injury can cause local or widespread purpura.

Other causes

• *Diagnostic tests.* Invasive procedures, such as venipuncture and arterial catheterization, may produce local ecchymoses and hematomas due to extravasated blood.

• *Drugs.* The anticoagulants heparin and coumadin can produce purpura.

• *Surgery and other procedures.* Any procedures that disrupt circulation, coagulation, or platelet activity or production may cause purpura. These include pulmonary and cardiac surgery, radiation therapy, chemotherapy, hemodialysis, multiple blood transfusions with platelet-poor blood, and use of plasma expanders, such as dextran.

Special considerations

Prepare the patient for diagnostic tests, as ordered. These may include a peripheral blood smear, bone marrow examination, and blood tests to determine platelet count, bleeding and coagulation times, capillary fragility, clot retraction, one-stage prothrombin time, activated partial thromboplastin time, and fibrinogen levels.

Reassure the patient that purpuric lesions are not permanent and will fade if the underlying cause can be successfully treated. Warn the patient not to use cosmetic fade creams or other products in an attempt to reduce pigmentation. If the patient has a hematoma, apply pressure and cold compresses initially to help reduce bleeding and swelling. After the first 24 hours, apply hot compresses to help speed absorption of blood.

Pediatric pointers

Newborns commonly have petechiae, particularly on the head, neck, and shoulders, after vertex deliveries. Thought to result from the trauma of birth, these petechiae disappear within a few days. Other causes in infants include thrombocytopenia, vitamin K deficiency, and infantile scurvy.

The most common type of purpura in children is allergic purpura. Other causes in children include trauma, hemophilia, autoimmune hemolytic anemia, Gaucher's disease, thrombasthenia, congenital factor deficiencies, Wiskott-Aldrich syndrome, acute ITP, von Willebrand's disease, and the rare but life-threatening purpura fulminans, which most often follows bacterial or viral infection. As a child grows and tests his motor skills, the risk of accidents multiplies, and ecchymoses and hematomas commonly occur. However, when you assess a child with purpura, be alert for signs of possible child abuse: bruises in different stages of resolution, from repeated beatings; bruise patterns resembling a familiar object, such as a belt, hand, or thumb and finger; and bruises on the face, buttocks, or genitals, areas unlikely to be injured accidentally.

Pustular Rash

A pustular rash is made up of crops of pustules—vesicles and bullae that fill with purulent exudate. These lesions vary greatly in size and shape and can be generalized or localized to the hair follicles or sweat glands. Pustules appear in skin and systemic disorders, with use of certain drugs, and with exposure to skin irritants. For example, people who've been swimming in salt water commonly develop a papulopustular rash under the bathing suit or elsewhere on the body from irritation by sea organisms (see *Recognizing Common Skin Lesions*, pages 558 and 559). Although many pustular lesions are sterile, pustular rash usually indicates infection. Any vesicular eruption, or even acute contact dermatitis, can become pustular if secondary infection occurs.

Assessment
Have the patient describe the appearance, location, and onset of the first pustular lesion. Did another type of skin lesion precede the pustule? Find out how the lesions spread. Ask what medications the patient takes and if he has applied any topical medication to his rash. If so, what type and when was it last applied? Find out if he has a family history of skin disorders.

Examine the entire skin surface, noting if it's dry, oily, moist, or greasy. Record the exact location and distribution of the skin lesions and their color, shape, and size.

Medical causes
• *Acne vulgaris.* Pustules typify inflammatory lesions of this disorder, which is accompanied by papules, nodules, cysts, and open comedones (black-heads). Lesions commonly appear on the face, shoulders, back, and chest. Other findings may include pain on pressure, pruritus, or burning. Chronic recurrent lesions produce scars.

• *Blastomycosis.* This fungal infection produces small, painless, nonpruritic macules or papules that can enlarge to well-circumscribed, verrucous, crusted, or ulcerated lesions edged by pustules. Localized infection may cause only one lesion; systemic infection, many lesions on the hands, feet, face, and wrists. Blastomycosis also produces signs of pulmonary infection, such as pleuritic chest pain and a dry, hacking or productive cough with occasional hemoptysis. Other effects may include fever, chills, anorexia, weight loss, fatigue, night sweats, malaise, and prostration. The patient may also develop soft tissue swelling and tenderness and warmth over bony lesions; painful swelling of the testes, epididymis, or prostate; deep perineal pain, pyuria, and hematuria; decreased level of consciousness; and a change in mood or affect.

• *Folliculitis.* This bacterial infection of hair follicles produces individual pustules, each pierced by a hair and possibly attended by pruritus. *Hot-tub folliculitis* produces pustules on areas covered by a bathing suit.

• *Furunculosis.* Crops of furuncles (purulent skin lesions involving hair follicles and sebaceous glands) typify this disorder. Furuncles usually begin as small, tender red pustules at the base of hair follicles. They're likely to occur on the face, neck, forearm, groin, axillae, buttocks, and legs, and to produce local pain, swelling, and redness. The pustules usually remain tense for 2 to 4 days and then become fluctuant. Rupture discharges pus and necrotic material. Then pain subsides, but erythema and edema may persist.

• *Gonococcemia.* This disorder produces a rash of scanty, pinpoint erythematous macules that rapidly become vesiculopustular, maculopapular, and, frequently, hemorrhagic.

Bullae may form. Mature lesions are elevated, with dirty gray necrotic centers and surrounding erythema. The rash appears on the distal part of the arms and legs, usually during the first day that other findings, such as fever and joint pain, occur. The rash disappears after 3 or 4 days but may recur with each episode of fever.

● **Nummular or annular dermatitis.** In this disorder, pustular lesions appear that are coinlike (nummular) or ringed (annular). Often, they ooze a purulent exudate, itch severely, and rapidly become crusted and scaly. There may be two or three lesions on the hands, but most often numerous lesions appear on the extensor surfaces of the extremities, posterior trunk, buttocks, and lower legs. A few small, scaling patches may remain for some time.

● **Pompholyx.** This common recurrent disorder characteristically produces symmetrical vesicular lesions that can become pustular. The lesions appear on the palms and, less often, on the soles and may be accompanied by minimal erythema and recurrent pruritus.

● **Pustular miliaria.** This anhidrotic disorder causes pustular lesions that begin as tiny erythematous papulovesicles located at sweat pores. Diffuse erythema may radiate from the lesion. The rash and associated burning and pruritus worsen with sweating.

● **Pustular psoriasis.** Small vesicles form and eventually become pustules in this disorder. The patient may report pruritus, burning, and pain. Localized pustular psoriasis usually affects the hands and feet. Generalized pustular psoriasis erupts suddenly in patients with psoriasis, psoriatic arthritis, or exfoliative psoriasis. Although generalized pustular psoriasis rarely occurs, it can occasionally be fatal.

● **Rosacea.** This chronic hyperemic disorder often produces telangiectasia with acute episodes of pustules, papules, and edema. Characterized by persistent erythema, this disorder may begin as a flush covering the forehead, malar region, nose, and chin. Inter-mittent episodes gradually become more persistent, and the skin—instead of returning to its normal color—develops variations in the intensity of the erythema.

● **Scabies.** Threadlike channels or burrows under the skin characterize this disorder, which can also produce pustules, vesicles, and excoriations. The lesions are 1 to 10 cm long, with a swollen nodule or red papule that contains the itch mite. In men, crusted lesions often develop on the glans, shaft, and scrotum. In women, lesions may form on the nipples. Lesions also develop on wrists, elbows, axillae, and waist. Related pruritus worsens with inactivity and warmth.

Other causes
● **Drugs.** Bromides and iodides commonly cause pustular rash. Other drug causes include adrenocorticotropic hormone, corticosteroids, dactinomycin, trimethadione, lithium, phenytoin, phenobarbital, isoniazid, oral contraceptives, androgens, and anabolic steroids.

Special considerations
Observe wound and skin isolation procedures until infection is ruled out by a gram stain or culture and sensitivity test of the pustule's contents. If the organism is infectious, remember not to allow any drainage to touch unaffected skin. Instruct the patient to keep toilet articles and linen separate from those of other family members. Associated pain and itching, altered body image, or stress of isolation may result in loss of sleep, anxiety, and depression. Give medications as ordered to relieve pain and itching, and encourage the patient to express his feelings.

Pediatric pointers
Among the various disorders that produce pustular rash in children are varicella, erythema toxicum neonatorum, candidiasis, impetigo, infantile acropustulosis, and acrodermatitis enteropathica.

Pyrosis

[Heartburn]

Caused by reflux of gastric contents into the esophagus, pyrosis is a substernal burning sensation that rises in the chest and may radiate to the neck or throat. It's frequently accompanied by regurgitation, which also results from gastric reflux. Because increased intraabdominal pressure contributes to reflux, pyrosis often occurs with pregnancy, ascites, or obesity. It also accompanies various gastrointestinal disorders, connective tissue disease, and use of numerous drugs. (See *How Pyrosis Occurs,* page 636.) Usually, pyrosis develops after meals or when the patient lies down (especially on his right side), bends over, lifts heavy objects, or exercises vigorously. Typically, pyrosis worsens with swallowing and improves when the patient sits upright or takes antacids.

A patient experiencing a myocardial infarction (MI) may mistake chest pain for pyrosis. However, he'll probably have other signs and symptoms—such as dyspnea, tachycardia, palpitations, nausea, and vomiting—that will help distinguish MI from pyrosis. And, of course, his chest pain won't be relieved by antacids.

Assessment

Ask the patient if he's experienced heartburn before. Do certain foods or beverages trigger it? Does stress or fatigue aggravate his discomfort? Also ask if movement, certain body positions, or ingestion of very hot or cold liquids worsens or helps relieve his heartburn. Ask about the location of the pain and determine if it radiates to other areas. Also find out if the patient regurgitates sour or bitter-tasting fluids along with the pyrosis. Does the patient have any associated signs and symptoms?

Medical causes

● *Esophageal cancer.* Pyrosis may be a sign of this cancer, depending on tumor size and location. The first and most common symptom is painless dysphagia that progressively worsens. Eventually, partial obstruction and rapid weight loss occur, and the patient may complain of steady pain in the front and back of the chest. He may also experience hoarseness, sore throat, nausea, vomiting, and a feeling of substernal fullness. Hematemesis, hemoptysis, and melena may also occur.

● *Esophageal diverticula.* Although usually asymptomatic, this disorder may cause pyrosis, regurgitation, and dysphagia. Other findings include chronic cough, halitosis, and a gurgling in the esophagus when liquids are swallowed. The patient may also complain of a bad taste in the mouth.

● *Gastroesophageal reflux disease.* Pyrosis, frequently severe, is the most common symptom of this disorder. The pyrosis tends to be chronic, usually occurs 30 to 60 minutes after eating, and may be triggered by certain foods or beverages. It worsens when the patient lies down or bends and abates when he sits or stands upright or takes antacids. Other findings include postural regurgitation, dysphagia, flatulent dyspepsia, and dull retrosternal pain that may radiate. Cough, halitosis, and, less commonly, odynophagia (painful swallowing) may also occur. If GI bleeding occurs, the patient may have bright red or dark brown hematemesis. Rarely, bleeding leads to signs of shock.

● *Obesity.* Increased intraabdominal pressure can contribute to reflux and resulting pyrosis.

● *Peptic ulcer disease.* Pyrosis and indigestion usually signal the start of a peptic ulcer attack. Most patients experience gnawing, burning pain in the left epigastrium, although some may report sharp pain. Typically, the pain arises 2 to 3 hours after eating or when the stomach is empty (frequently at night), and is relieved by eating or taking antacids. The pain may also occur

HOW PYROSIS OCCURS

Barrier to reflux, the lower esophageal sphincter (LES) normally relaxes only to allow food to pass from the esophagus into the stomach. But hormonal fluctuations, mechanical stress, and the effects of certain foods and drugs can lower LES pressure. When LES pressure falls and intraabdominal or intragastric pressure rises, the normally contracted LES relaxes inappropriately and allows reflux of gastric acid or bile secretions into the lower esophagus. There, the reflux irritates and inflames the esophageal mucosa, producing pyrosis.

Persistent inflammation can cause LES pressure to decrease even more and may trigger a recurrent cycle of reflux and pyrosis.

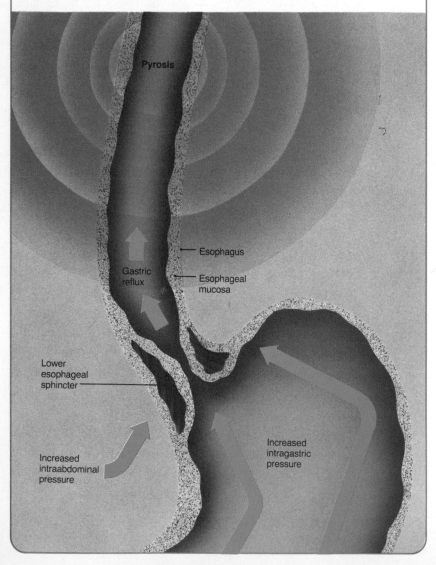

after ingestion of coffee, aspirin, alcohol, or possibly citrus juice. The patient may also have epigastric tenderness, nausea, vomiting, and GI bleeding.

• *Scleroderma.* This connective tissue disease may cause esophageal dysfunction resulting in reflux with pyrosis, the sensation of food sticking behind the breastbone, odynophagia, bloating after meals, and weight loss. Other GI effects include abdominal distention, constipation or diarrhea, and malodorous floating stools. Early signs of scleroderma include blanching, cyanosis, and stress- or cold-induced erythema of the fingers and toes. Later developments include finger and joint pain, stiffness, and swelling; skin thickening on the hands and forearms; masklike facies; and possibly contractures. In advanced disease, cardiac and renal involvement may produce dysrhythmias, dyspnea, cough, malignant hypertension, and signs of renal failure, such as oliguria.

Other causes
• *Drugs.* Various drugs may cause or aggravate pyrosis. Among these offenders are acetohexamide, tolbutamide, lypressin, aspirin, anticholinergic agents, and drugs that have anticholinergic effects.

Special considerations
Prepare the patient for diagnostic tests, such as barium swallow, upper GI series, esophagoscopy, and laboratory studies to test esophageal motility and acidity.

After the causative disorder is determined, teach the patient how to avoid a recurrence of pyrosis. Advise him to eat frequent small meals, to sit upright (especially after a meal), and to avoid lying down for at least 2 hours after a meal. Instruct him to avoid highly seasoned foods, caffeine, acidic juices, alcohol, bedtime snacks, and foods high in fat or carbohydrates, which reduce lower esophageal sphincter (LES) pressure. Also instruct

---

REGURGITATION: ITS MECHANISM AND CAUSES

When gastric reflux moves up the esophagus and passes through the upper esophageal sphincter, regurgitation occurs. Unlike vomiting, regurgitation is effortless and unaccompanied by nausea. It usually happens when the patient is lying down or bending over and often accompanies pyrosis. Aspiration of regurgitated gastric contents can lead to recurrent pulmonary infections.

In adults, regurgitation most often results from esophageal disorders, such as achalasia. However, it can also occur when the gag reflex is absent, as in bulbar palsy, or when the patient has an overfilled stomach or esophagus.

In infants, regurgitation can signal pyloric stenosis or dysphagia lusoria. Most often, though, infants "spit up" because their esophageal sphincters aren't fully developed during the first year of life. To help reduce regurgitation in the infant, teach parents to handle the infant gently during feeding and to burp him frequently. After feeding, place the infant on his right side or stomach with his head slightly elevated to avoid gravitational regurgitation and to help prevent aspiration.

---

the patient to avoid bending, coughing, engaging in vigorous exercise, wearing tight clothing, or gaining weight, thereby preventing increased intraabdominal pressure. Advise him to refrain from smoking and using drugs that reduce sphincter control.

If the patient's pyrosis is severe, instruct him to sleep with extra pillows or with 6″ wooden blocks under the head of the bed to reduce reflux by gravity. Tell him to take antacids, as ordered (usually 1 hour after meals and at bedtime). The doctor may also order medications that increase LES contraction, such as bethanechol.

Pediatric pointers
A child may have difficulty distinguishing esophageal pain from pyrosis. To gain information, help him describe the sensation.

raccoon's eyes • rebound tenderness • rectal pain • retractions—costal and st
rhonchi • Romberg's sign • salivation—decreased • salivation—increased • sa
scrotal swelling • seizure—absence • seizure—focal • seizure—generalized to
psychomotor • setting-sun sign • shallow respirations • skin—bronze • skin—
mottled • skin—scaly • skin turgor—decreased • spider angioma • splenome
respirations • stool—clay-colored • stridor • syncope • tachycardia • tachypn
tearing—increased • throat pain • tic • tinnitus • tracheal deviation • trache
trismus • tunnel vision • uremic frost • urethral discharge • urinary frequen
urinary incontinence • urinary urgency • urine cloudiness • urticaria • vagin
postmenopausal • vaginal discharge • venous hum • vertigo • vesicular rash
loss • visual blurring • visual floaters • vomiting • vulvar lesions • weight ga
loss—excessive • wheezing • wristdrop • abdominal distention • abdominal r
abdominal rigidity • accessory muscle use • agitation • alopecia • amenorrh
analgesia • anhidrosis • anorexia • anosmia • anuria • anxiety • aphasia • a
respirations • apraxia • arm pain • asterixis • ataxia • athetosis • aura • Bal
pain • barrel chest • Battle's sign • Biot's respirations • bladder distention • l
blood pressure increase • bowel sounds—absent • bowel sounds—hyperactiv
hypoactive • bradycardia • bradypnea • breast dimpling • breast nodule • br
breath with ammonia odor • breath with fecal odor • breath with fruity odo
bruits • buffalo hump • butterfly rash • café-au-lait spots • capillary refill tin
carpopedal spasm • cat cry • chest expansion—asymmetrical • chest pain •
respirations • chills • chorea • Chvostek's sign • clubbing • cogwheel rigidity
confusion • conjunctival injection • constipation • corneal reflex—absent • c
tenderness • cough—barking • cough—nonproductive • cough—productive •
bony • crepitation—subcutaneous • cry—high-pitched • cyanosis • decerebr
posture • deep tendon reflexes—hyperactive • deep tendon reflexes—hypoac
diaphoresis • diarrhea • diplopia • dizziness • doll's eye sign—absent • droc
dysmenorrhea • dyspareunia • dyspepsia • dysphagia • dyspnea • dystonia •
edema—generalized • edema of the arms • edema of the face • edema of the
enuresis • epistaxis • eructation • erythema • exophthalmos • eye discharge
fasciculations • fatigue • fecal incontinence • fetor hepaticus • fever • flank
fontanelle bulging • fontanelle depression • footdrop • gag reflex abnormalit
propulsive • gait—scissors • gait—spastic • gait—steppage • gait—waddling
gallop—ventricular • genital lesions in the male • grunting respirations • gu
swelling • gynecomastia • halitosis • halo vision • headache • hearing loss •
Heberden's nodes • hematemesis • hematochezia • hematuria • hemianopia
hepatomegaly • hiccups • hirsutism • hoarseness • Homans' sign • hyperpig
hypopigmentation • impotence • insomnia • intermittent claudication • Jane
jaw pain • jugular vein distention • Kehr's sign • Kernig's sign • leg pain •
decreased • lid lag • light flashes • low birth weight • lymphadenopathy • n
McBurney's sign • McMurray's sign • melena • menorrhagia • metrorrhagia
mouth lesions • murmurs • muscle atrophy • muscle flaccidity • muscle spa
muscle weakness • mydriasis • myoclonus • nasal flaring • nausea • neck p
nipple discharge • nipple retraction • nocturia • nuchal rigidity • nystagmu
oligomenorrhea • oliguria • opisthotonos • orofacial dyskinesia • orthopnea
Ortolani's sign • Osler's nodes • otorrhea • pallor • palpitations • papular r
paresthesias • paroxysmal nocturnal dyspnea • peau d'orange • pericardial
waves—visible • photophobia • pica • pleural friction rub • polydipsia • po
postnasal drip • priapism • pruritus • psoas sign • psychotic behavior • pto
weak • pulse—bounding • pulse pressure—narrowed • pulse pressure—wi

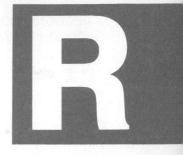

Raccoon's Eyes

Raccoon's eyes refer to bilateral periorbital ecchymoses that don't result from facial trauma. Usually an indicator of basilar skull fracture, this sign develops when damage at the time of fracture tears the meninges and causes the venous sinuses to bleed into the arachnoid villi and the cranial sinuses. Raccoon's eyes may be the only indicator of basilar skull fracture, which isn't always visible on skull X-rays. Their appearance signals the need for careful assessment to detect any underlying trauma, since a basilar skull fracture can injure cranial nerves, blood vessels, and the brain stem. Raccoon's eyes can also occur after a craniotomy if the surgery causes a meningeal tear.

Assessment

After you detect raccoon's eyes, check the patient's vital signs and try to find out when the head injury occurred. Then assess the extent of underlying trauma.

Start by evaluating the patient's level of consciousness with the Glasgow Coma Scale. (See *Glasgow Coma Scale: Grading Level of Consciousness*, page 454.) Next, assess function of the cranial nerves, especially the first (olfactory), third (oculomotor), fourth (trochlear), sixth (abducens), and seventh (facial). If the patient's condition permits, also test his visual acuity and gross hearing. Note any irregularities in the facial or skull bones, as well as any swelling, localized pain, or lacerations of the face and scalp. Check for ecchymoses over the mastoid bone. Inspect for hemorrhage or cerebrospinal fluid (CSF) leakage from the nose or ears. Test any drainage with a sterile 4″ x 4″ gauze pad, and note if you find a halo sign—a circle of clear fluid that surrounds the drainage, indicating CSF. Also, use a Dextrostix to test any clear drainage for glucose. A positive test indicates CSF since mucus doesn't contain glucose. Inform the doctor of your findings.

Medical cause

• *Basilar skull fracture.* This injury produces raccoon's eyes following head trauma that doesn't involve the orbital area. Associated signs and symptoms vary with the fracture site and may include pharyngeal hemorrhage, epistaxis, rhinorrhea, otorrhea, or a bulging tympanic membrane from blood or CSF. The patient may experience hearing difficulty, headache, nausea, vomiting, and altered level of consciousness. He may also have a positive Battle's sign. In addition, most patients experience cranial nerve palsies.

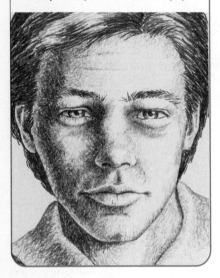
Other cause

• *Surgery.* Raccoon's eyes that occur after a craniotomy may indicate a meningeal tear and bleeding into the sinuses.

Special considerations

Keep the patient on complete bed rest, and position him as ordered. Perform a neurologic assessment every hour to reevaluate his level of consciousness. Also check vital signs hourly; be alert for such changes as bradypnea, bradycardia, hypertension, and fever. To avoid worsening a dural tear, instruct the patient not to blow his nose, cough vigorously, or strain. If otorrhea or rhinorrhea is present, don't attempt to stop the flow. Instead, place a sterile, loose gauze pad under the nose or ear to absorb the drainage. Monitor the amount and test it with a Dextrostix to confirm or rule out CSF leakage.

Never suction or pass a nasogastric tube through the patient's nose to prevent further tearing of the mucous membranes and infection. Observe the patient for signs and symptoms of meningitis, such as fever and nuchal rigidity, and expect to administer prophylactic antibiotics.

Prepare the patient for diagnostic tests, such as skull X-ray and possibly computed tomography. If the dural tear does not heal spontaneously, contrast cisternography may be performed to locate the tear, possibly followed by corrective surgery.

Pediatric pointers

Raccoon's eyes in children are most often caused by basilar skull fracture following a fall.

Rebound Tenderness

[Blumberg's sign]

A reliable indicator of peritonitis, rebound tenderness is intense, elicited abdominal pain caused by rebound of palpated tissue. The tenderness may be localized, as in an abscess, or generalized, as in perforation of an intraabdominal organ. Rebound tenderness usually occurs with abdominal pain, tenderness, and rigidity. When a patient has sudden, severe abdominal pain, this symptom is usually elicited to detect peritoneal inflammation.

Assessment

If you elicit rebound tenderness in a patient who's experiencing constant, severe abdominal pain, quickly take his vital signs and have another nurse immediately notify the doctor. Insert a large-bore I.V. catheter and begin administering I.V. fluids. Also insert an indwelling (Foley) catheter, and monitor intake and output. Give supplemental oxygen, as needed, and continue to monitor the patient for signs of shock, such as hypotension and tachycardia.

When the patient's condition permits, ask him to describe the events that led up to the tenderness. Does movement, exertion, or other activity relieve or aggravate the tenderness? Also ask about other signs and symptoms. Inspect the abdomen for distention, vis-ible peristaltic waves, or scars. Then auscultate for bowel sounds and characterize their motility. Finally, palpate for associated rigidity or guarding.

Medical cause

• *Peritonitis.* In this life-threatening disorder, rebound tenderness is accompanied by sudden and severe abdominal pain, which may be either diffuse or localized. Because movement worsens the patient's pain, he'll usually lie

ELICITING REBOUND TENDERNESS

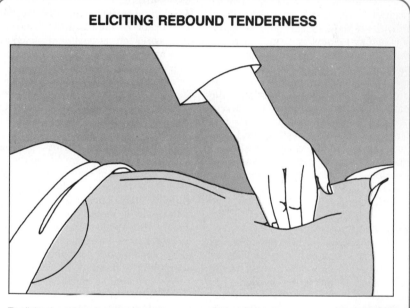

To elicit rebound tenderness, place the patient in a supine position, and push your fingers deeply and steadily into his abdomen, as shown above. Then quickly release the pressure. Pain that results from the rebound of palpated tissue—rebound tenderness—indicates peritoneal inflammation or peritonitis.

You can also elicit this symptom on a miniature scale by percussing the patient's abdomen lightly and indirectly (right). Better still, simply ask the patient to cough. This allows you to elicit rebound tenderness without having to touch the patient's abdomen and may also increase his cooperation, since he won't associate exacerbation of his pain with your actions.

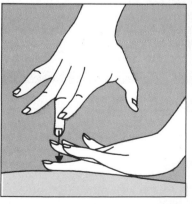

still. Typically, he'll display weakness, pallor, excessive sweating, and cold skin. He may also display hypoactive or absent bowel sounds; tachypnea; nausea; vomiting; abdominal distention, rigidity, and guarding; and a fever of 103° F. (39.4° C.) or higher. Inflammation of the diaphragmatic peritoneum may cause shoulder pain and hiccups.

Special considerations
Promote comfort by having the patient flex his knees or assume a semi-Fowler position. Administer analgesics carefully, since these drugs could mask associated symptoms. You may also administer antiemetics and antipyretics, as ordered. However, because of decreased intestinal motility and the probability of surgery, don't give the patient *oral* drugs or fluids. As ordered, obtain samples of blood, urine, and feces for laboratory testing, and prepare the patient for chest and abdominal X-rays, sonograms, and computed tomography scans. Finally, perform or assist the doctor with a rectal or pelvic examination.

Pediatric pointers
Eliciting rebound tenderness may be difficult in young children. Be alert for such clues as an anguished facial expression or intensified crying. When you elicit this symptom, use assessment techniques that produce minimal tenderness. For example, have the child hop or jump to allow tissue to rebound gently.

Rectal Pain

A common symptom of anorectal disorders, rectal pain is discomfort that arises in the anal-rectal area. Although the anal canal is separated from the rest of the rectum by the internal sphincter, the patient may refer to all local pain as rectal pain.

Because the mucocutaneous border of the anal canal and the perianal skin contains somatic nerve fibers, lesions in this area are especially painful. This pain may result from or be aggravated by diarrhea, constipation, or passage of hardened stools. It may also be aggravated by intense pruritus and continued scratching associated with drainage of mucus, blood, or fecal matter that irritates the skin and nerve endings.

Assessment
When your patient reports rectal pain, inspect for rectal bleeding; abnormal drainage, such as pus; or protrusions, such as skin tags or thrombosed hemorrhoids. Also observe the patient for inflammation and other lesions. Notify the doctor right away if you detect any of these findings, since he may want to perform an immediate rectal examination.

After your examination, proceed with your assessment by taking the patient's history. Ask him to describe the pain. Is it sharp or dull, burning or knifelike? How often does it occur? Ask if the pain is worse during or immediately after defecation. Does he avoid having bowel movements because of anticipated pain? Also find out what alleviates the pain.

Ask appropriate questions about the development of any associated signs and symptoms. Does the patient experience bleeding along with rectal pain? If so, find out how frequently this occurs and whether the blood is on the toilet tissue, on the surface of the stool, or in the toilet bowl. Is the blood bright or dark red? Also ask about other drainage, such as mucus or pus, and find out if the patient has constipation or diarrhea.

Medical causes
● *Anal carcinoma.* Rectal pain, bleeding, and tenesmus are typical findings in this rare disorder.
● *Anal fissure.* This longitudinal crack in the anal lining causes sharp rectal

pain on defecation. Typically, the patient experiences a burning sensation and gnawing pain that can continue up to 4 hours after defecation. Fear of provoking this pain may lead to acute constipation. The patient may also have anal pruritus and extreme tenderness and may report finding spots of blood on the toilet tissue after defecation.

• *Anorectal abscess.* This abscess can occur in various locations in the rectum and anus, causing pain in the perianal area. Typically, a superficial abscess produces constant, throbbing local pain that is exacerbated by sitting or walking. The local pain associated with a deeper abscess may begin insidiously, often occurring high in the rectum or even in the lower abdomen, and is accompanied by an indurated anal mass. The patient may also develop associated signs and symptoms, such as fever, malaise, anal swelling and inflammation, purulent drainage, and local tenderness.

• *Anorectal fistula.* Pain develops when a tract formed between the anal canal and skin temporarily seals. It persists until drainage resumes. Other chief complaints include pruritus and drainage of pus, blood, mucus, and occasionally stool.

• *Cryptitis.* This disorder results when particles of stool that are lodged in the anal folds decay and cause infection, which may produce dull anal pain or discomfort and anal pruritus.

• *Hemorrhoids.* Thrombosed or prolapsed hemorrhoids cause rectal pain that may worsen during defecation and abate after it. The patient's fear of provoking the pain may lead to constipation. Usually, rectal pain is accompanied by severe itching. Internal hemorrhoids may also produce mild, intermittent bleeding that characteristically occurs as spotting on the toilet tissue or on the stool surface. External hemorrhoids are visible outside the anal sphincter.

• *Proctalgia fugax.* In this disorder, muscle spasms of the rectum and pelvic floor produce sudden, severe episodes of rectal pain that last up to several minutes and then disappear. The patient may report being awakened by the pain.

• *Prostatic abscess.* This disorder occasionally produces rectal pain. Common associated findings include urinary retention and frequency, dysuria, and fever.

Special considerations

Apply analgesic ointment or suppositories, as ordered, and administer stool softeners, if needed. Be sure to stress to the patient the importance of proper diet to maintain soft stools and thus avoid aggravating pain during defecation.

Teach the patient how to apply hot, moist compresses. Also instruct him to give himself a sitz bath—this will ease his discomfort by helping to relieve the sphincter spasm associated with most anorectal disorders. However, if the patient's rectal pain results from prolapsed hemorrhoids, apply cold compresses to help shrink protruding hemorrhoids, avoid thrombosis, and reduce pain. If his condition permits, place him in Trendelenburg's position with his buttocks elevated to further relieve pain.

If ordered, prepare the patient for an anoscopic examination and proctosigmoidoscopy to determine the cause of rectal pain.

Because the patient may feel embarrassed by treatments and diagnostic tests involving the rectum, provide emotional support and as much privacy as possible.

Pediatric pointers

Observe any child with rectal pain for associated bleeding, drainage, and signs of infection (fever and irritability). Acute anal fissure is a common cause of rectal pain and bleeding in children, whose fear of provoking the pain may lead to constipation. Infants who seem to have pain on defecation should be evaluated for congenital anomalies of the rectum.

Retractions—Costal and Sternal

A cardinal sign of respiratory distress in infants and children, retractions are visible indentations of the soft tissue covering the chest wall. They may be suprasternal (directly above the sternum and clavicles), intercostal (between the ribs), subcostal (below the lower costal margin of the rib cage), or substernal (just below the xiphoid process). Retractions may be mild or severe, producing barely visible to deep indentations.

Normally, infants and young children use abdominal muscles for breathing, unlike older children and adults who use the diaphragm. When breathing requires extra effort, accessory muscles assist respiration, especially inspiration. Retractions typically accompany accessory muscle use.

Assessment

If the child displays retractions, quickly check for other signs of respiratory distress, such as cyanosis, tachypnea, and tachycardia. Have another nurse immediately notify the doctor while you monitor the child's respiratory status. Prepare for suctioning, insertion of an artificial airway, and administration of oxygen.

Observe the depth and location of retractions. Also note the rate, depth, and quality of respirations. Assess for accessory muscle use, nasal flaring during inspiration, or grunting during expiration. If the child has a cough, record the color, consistency, and odor of any sputum. Note if the child appears restless or lethargic. Finally, auscultate the child's lungs to detect abnormal breath sounds.

When the child's condition permits, ask his parents about his medical history. Was he born prematurely? Was the delivery complicated? Ask about recent signs of an upper respiratory infection, such as a runny nose, cough, or low-grade fever. How often has the child had respiratory problems in the past year? Has he been in contact with anyone who has had a cold, the flu, or other respiratory ailments? Did he aspirate any food, liquid, or foreign body? Inquire about any personal or family history of allergies or asthma.

Medical causes

• **Asthmatic attack.** Intercostal and suprasternal retractions may accompany an attack. They are preceded by dyspnea, wheezing, a hacking cough, and pallor. Related features may include cyanosis or flushing, crackles, rhonchi, diaphoresis, tachycardia, tachypnea, a frightened, anxious expression, and, in severe distress, nasal flaring.

• **Bronchiolitis.** Most common in children less than age 2, this acute lower respiratory tract infection may cause intercostal and subcostal retractions, nasal flaring, tachypnea, dyspnea, cough, restlessness, and possibly a slight fever. Periodic apnea may occur in infants less than 6 months old.

• **Congestive heart failure.** Usually linked to a congenital heart defect, this disorder may cause intercostal and substernal retractions along with nasal flaring, progressive tachypnea, and—in severe respiratory distress—grunting respirations, edema, and cyanosis. Other findings may include productive cough, crackles, jugular vein distention, tachycardia, right upper quadrant pain, anorexia, and fatigue.

• **Epiglottitis.** This life-threatening bacterial infection may precipitate severe respiratory distress with suprasternal, substernal, and intercostal retractions; stridor; nasal flaring; cyanosis; and tachycardia. Initially, it causes sudden onset of barking cough and high fever. Other early features include sore throat, hoarseness, dysphagia, drooling, dyspnea, and restlessness. The child becomes panicky as edema makes breathing difficult. Total airway occlusion may occur in 2 to 5 hours.

OBSERVING RETRACTIONS

When observing retractions in infants and children, be sure to note their exact location—an important clue to the cause and severity of respiratory distress. For example, subcostal and substernal retractions usually result from lower respiratory tract disorders, whereas suprasternal retractions usually result from upper respiratory tract disorders. Mild intercostal retractions alone may be normal. However, intercostal retractions accompanied by subcostal and substernal retractions may indicate moderate respiratory distress. Deep suprasternal retractions typically indicate severe distress.

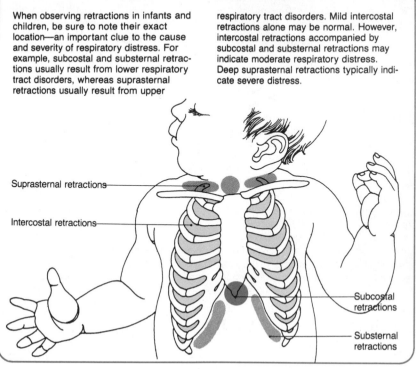

Suprasternal retractions

Intercostal retractions

Subcostal retractions

Substernal retractions

• *Laryngotracheobronchitis (acute).* In this viral infection, substernal and intercostal retractions typically follow low to moderate fever, runny nose, poor appetite, barking cough, hoarseness, and inspiratory stridor. Associated signs and symptoms may include tachycardia; shallow, rapid respirations; restlessness; irritability; and pale, cyanotic skin.

• *Pneumonia (bacterial).* This disorder begins with signs of acute infection—such as high fever and lethargy—followed by subcostal and intercostal retractions, nasal flaring, dyspnea, tachypnea, grunting respirations, cyanosis, and productive cough. Auscultation may reveal diminished breath sounds, scattered crackles, and sibilant rhonchi over the affected lung. GI effects may include vomiting, diarrhea, and abdominal distention.

• *Respiratory distress syndrome.* Substernal and subcostal retractions are an early sign of this life-threatening syndrome, which affects premature infants shortly after birth. Associated early signs include tachypnea, tachycardia, and expiratory grunting. As respiratory distress worsens, intercostal and suprasternal retractions typically occur, and apnea or irregular respirations replace grunting. Other effects are nasal flaring, cyanosis, lethargy, and eventual unresponsiveness, bradycardia, and hypotension. Auscultation may detect crackles over the lung bases on deep inspiration and harsh, diminished breath sounds. Oliguria and peripheral edema may occur.

• *Spasmodic croup.* This disorder causes attacks of barking cough, hoarseness, dyspnea, and restlessness. As distress worsens, the child may display suprasternal, substernal, and intercostal retractions; nasal flaring; tachycardia; cyanosis; and an anxious, frantic expression. These attacks usually subside within a few hours but tend to recur.

Special considerations
Continue to monitor the child's vital signs. Keep suction equipment and an appropriate-size airway at bedside.

If the infant weighs less than 15 lb, place him in an oxygen hood, as ordered. If he weighs more, place him in a cool mist tent instead. As ordered, perform chest physical therapy with postural drainage to help mobilize and drain excess lung secretions. (See *Positioning the Infant for Chest Physical Therapy*, pages 354 and 355.)

Prepare the child for chest X-rays, cultures, and arterial blood gas analysis. Explain the procedures to his parents, too, and have them calm and comfort the child.

Rhinorrhea
[Nasal discharge]

Common but rarely serious, rhinorrhea is the free discharge of thin nasal mucus. It can be self-limiting or chronic, resulting from nasal, sinus, or systemic disorders or from basilar skull fracture. This sign can also result from sinus or cranial surgery, excessive use of vasoconstricting nose drops or sprays, or an irritant, such as tobacco smoke, dust, and fumes. Depending on the cause, the discharge may be clear, purulent, bloody, or serosanguineous.

Assessment
Begin the history by asking the patient if the discharge runs from both nostrils. Is it intermittent or persistent? Did it begin suddenly or gradually? Does the position of his head affect it? Next, ask the patient to characterize the discharge. Is it watery, bloody, purulent, or foul-smelling? Is it copious or scanty? Does it worsen or improve with the time of day? Find out if the patient is taking any medications, especially nose drops or sprays. Has he been exposed to nasal irritants at home or at work? Has he had a recent head injury?

Examine the patient's nose, assessing airflow from each nostril. Evaluate the size, color, and condition of the turbinate mucosa (normally pale pink). Note if it's red, unusually pale, blue, or gray. Then examine the area beneath each turbinate and the sinus opening into each meatus, and trace purulent discharge to the involved sinus. Palpate over the frontal, ethmoid, and maxillary sinus for tenderness.

To detect secretions or thickened mucosa, perform transillumination of the maxillary and frontal sinuses. Finally, using a nonirritating substance, test for anosmia.

Medical causes
• *Basilar skull fracture.* A tear in the dura can lead to cerebrospinal rhinorrhea, which increases when the patient lowers his head. Associated findings may include epistaxis, otorrhea, and a bulging tympanic membrane from blood or fluid. A fracture may also cause headache, facial paralysis, nausea, vomiting, impaired eye movement, ocular deviation, vision and hearing loss, depressed level of consciousness, Battle's sign, and raccoon's eyes.
• *Cluster headache.* In this disorder, rhinorrhea can accompany severe unilateral headache. Related ocular effects include miosis, ipsilateral tearing, conjunctival injection, and ptosis. Other effects include flushing, facial diaphoresis, bradycardia, and restlessness.
• *Common cold.* An initial watery nasal discharge may become thicker and mucopurulent. Related findings include sneezing, nasal congestion, a dry and hacking cough, sore throat, mouth breathing, and transient loss of smell and taste. The patient may also have

PERFORMING TRANSILLUMINATION

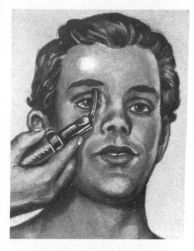

Transillumination of frontal sinuses
One way to determine the source of a nasal discharge is to transilluminate the patient's frontal and maxillary sinuses. First, darken the room. Then, gently press a penlight under the patient's right or left brow, close to the nose, and shield the light with your hand. You'll normally see a dim red glow through the air-filled frontal sinus; if you don't, suspect secretions or thickened mucosa. Repeat this procedure under the other brow.

Transillumination of maxillary sinuses
If the patient wears an upper denture, have him remove it. Then ask him to open his mouth wide. Tilt his head back slightly as you shine a penlight downward, on his right or left cheek, just below the inner aspect of the eye. Look through his open mouth at the hard palate. A red glow indicates his sinus is clear; its absence suggests secretions or thickened mucosa in the maxillary sinus. Repeat this procedure on the other cheek.

malaise, fatigue, myalgia, arthralgia, and a slight headache. His lips are dry, and his upper lip and nose are red.
• *Ethmoiditis.* In *acute bacterial ethmoiditis*, nasal discharge is yellow-gray or purulent; in *acute viral ethmoiditis*, it's mucoid. Other features include nasal congestion, frontal or orbital headache, fever, malaise, postnasal drip, and an impaired sense of smell and taste. Pain, erythema, and tenderness over bone in the upper lateral areas of the nose occur.

In *chronic ethmoiditis*, purulent discharge may be intermittent or persistent. Related findings include postnasal drip, headache, and impaired sense of smell and taste.
• *Mucormycosis.* Rhinocerebral mucormycosis causes a thin, serosanguineous nasal discharge and ulceration or perforation of the nasal septum. Other initial findings may include dull nasal pain; black, dusky red, or necrotic turbinates; low-grade fever; periorbital and facial edema; and erythema of the skin on the cheeks.
• *Nasal or sinus tumors.* Nasal tumors can produce intermittent, unilateral bloody or serosanguineous discharge, possibly purulent and foul-smelling. Nasal congestion, postnasal drip, and headache may also occur. In advanced stages, paranasal sinus tumors may cause a cheek mass or eye displacement, facial paresthesia, and nasal obstruction.
• *Rhinitis.* *Allergic rhinitis* produces an

episodic, profuse watery discharge. (Mucopurulent discharge indicates infection.) Typical associated findings include increased lacrimation; nasal congestion; itchy eyes, nose, and throat; postnasal drip; recurrent sneezing; mouth breathing; impaired sense of smell; and frontal or temporal headache. The turbinates are pale and engorged; the mucosa, pale and boggy.

In *atrophic rhinitis,* nasal discharge is scanty, purulent, and foul-smelling. Nasal obstruction is common, and the crusts may bleed on removal. The mucosa is pale pink and shiny.

In *vasomotor rhinitis,* a profuse and watery nasal discharge accompanies chronic nasal obstruction, sneezing, recurrent postnasal drip, and pale, swollen turbinates. The nasal septum is pink; the mucosa, blue.

• *Scleroma.* This rare, progressive condition produces watery nasal discharge that later becomes foul-smelling and encrusted. It also produces firm, bluish red nodules on the mucous membranes that can develop into scars and cause stenosis.

• *Sinusitis. Acute sphenoid sinusitis*— a disorder affecting immunosuppressed, diabetic, elderly, and debilitated patients—produces purulent nasal discharge that leads to obstruction. Its related effects include fever, malaise, and deep pain behind the eyes that's referred to the top or back of the head or to the mastoid area.

In *chronic frontal sinusitis,* intermittent and purulent discharge may lead to nasal obstruction. Other findings include postnasal drip and a constant headache associated with dull, localized tenderness over the sinus. Also, a purulent exudate covers the middle and superior turbinates.

In *chronic maxillary sinusitis,* mucopurulent discharge is intermittent and ipsilateral and may lead to unilateral nasal obstruction. Related features: facial aching, pain in the upper teeth, swelling and tenderness in the anterior maxilla, and postnasal drip.

• *Wegener's granulomatosis.* Besides a mucopurulent nasal discharge, this disorder causes conductive hearing loss, crusting and tissue necrosis of the nose, and epistaxis. Less common findings: sore throat, cough (possibly hemoptysis), wheezing, dyspnea, pleuritic chest pain, hemorrhagic skin lesions, and oliguria.

Other causes
• *Drugs.* Nasal sprays or drops containing vasoconstrictors may cause rebound rhinorrhea (rhinitis medicamentosa) if used longer than 3 weeks.
• *Surgery.* Following sinus or cranial surgery, cerebrospinal rhinorrhea may occur.

Special considerations
If ordered, prepare the patient for X-rays of the sinuses or the skull (in suspected skull fracture) and computed tomography scan.

As ordered, administer antihistamines, decongestants, analgesics, or antipyretics. Promote fluids to thin secretions. Warn the patient to avoid using over-the-counter nasal sprays for more than 5 days, unless ordered.

Pediatric pointers
Rhinorrhea may stem from choanal atresia, a foreign body in the nose, allergic or chronic rhinitis, acute ethmoiditis, or congenital syphilis.

Rhonchi

Rhonchi are continuous adventitious breath sounds detected by auscultation. They're usually louder and lower-pitched than crackles—more like a hoarse moan or a deep snore, though they may be described as rattling, sonorous, bubbling, rumbling, or musical. However, sibilant rhonchi, or wheezes, are high-pitched.

Rhonchi are heard over large airways, such as the trachea. They occur in pulmonary disorders when air flows through passages that have been narrowed by secretions, a tumor or foreign body, bronchospasm, or mucosal thickening. The resulting vibration of airway walls produces the rhonchi.

Assessment

If you auscultate rhonchi, take the patient's vital signs and be alert for signs of respiratory distress. Characterize the patient's respirations as rapid or slow, shallow or deep, and regular or irregular. Inspect the chest, noting use of accessory muscles. Is the patient audibly wheezing or gurgling? Auscultate for other abnormal breath sounds, such as crackles and a pleural friction rub. If detected, note the location. Are breath sounds diminished or absent? Next, percuss the chest.

If the patient has a cough, note its frequency and characterize its sound. If it's productive, examine the sputum for color, odor, consistency, and blood.

Ask related questions: Does the patient smoke? If so, obtain a history in pack years. Has he recently lost weight or felt tired or weak? Does he have asthma or other pulmonary disorders? Is he currently taking any prescribed or over-the-counter drugs?

During the assessment, keep in mind that thick or excessive secretions, bronchospasm, or inflammation of mucous membranes may lead to airway obstruction. If necessary, suction the patient and keep equipment available for inserting an airway. Keep bronchodilators available to treat bronchospasm.

Medical causes

• *Adult respiratory distress syndrome.* Fluid accumulation in this life-threatening disorder produces rhonchi and crackles. Initial features include rapid, shallow respirations and dyspnea, sometimes after the patient appears stable. Developing hypoxemia leads to intercostal and suprasternal retractions, diaphoresis, and fluid accumulation. As hypoxemia worsens, the patient displays increased breathing difficulty, restlessness, apprehension, decreased level of consciousness, cyanosis, motor dysfunction, and possibly tachycardia.

• *Aspiration of a foreign body.* A retained bronchial foreign body can cause inspiratory and expiratory rhonchi and wheezes due to increased secretions. Diminished breath sounds may be auscultated over the obstructed area. Fever, pain, and cough may also occur.

• *Asthma.* An asthmatic attack can cause rhonchi, crackles, and commonly wheezes. Other features include apprehension, a dry cough that later becomes productive, prolonged expirations, and intercostal and supraclavicular retractions on inspiration. There may also be increased accessory muscle use, nasal flaring, tachypnea, tachycardia, diaphoresis, and flushing or cyanosis.

• *Bronchiectasis.* This disorder causes lower-lobe rhonchi and crackles, which coughing may help relieve. Its classic sign is a cough that produces mucopurulent, foul-smelling, and possibly bloody sputum. Other findings include fever, weight loss, dyspnea on exertion, fatigue, malaise, halitosis, weakness, and late-stage clubbing.

• *Bronchitis.* Acute tracheobronchitis produces sonorous rhonchi and wheezes due to bronchospasm or increased mucus in the airways. Related findings include chills, sore throat, a low-grade fever (rising up to 102° F., or 38.9° C., in severe illness), muscle and back pain, and substernal tightness. A cough becomes productive as secretions increase.

In *chronic bronchitis*, auscultation may reveal scattered rhonchi, coarse crackles, wheezing, high-pitched piping sounds, and prolonged expirations. An early hacking cough later becomes productive. The patient also displays exertional dyspnea, increased accessory muscle use, barrel chest, cyanosis, tachypnea, and clubbing (a late sign).

• *Emphysema.* This disorder may cause sonorous rhonchi, but faint, high-pitched wheezes are more typical, together with weight loss; a mild, chronic, productive cough with scant sputum; exertional dyspnea; accessory muscle use on inspiration; tachypnea; and grunting expirations. Other features: anorexia, malaise, barrel chest, peripheral cyanosis, and late-stage clubbing.

• *Pneumonia. Bacterial pneumonias* can cause rhonchi and a dry cough that later becomes productive. Related signs and symptoms develop suddenly—with shaking chills, high fever, myalgias, headache, pleuritic chest pain, tachypnea, tachycardia, dyspnea, cyanosis, diaphoresis, decreased breath sounds, and fine crackles.

• *Pulmonary coccidioidomycosis.* This disorder causes rhonchi and wheezing. Other features include a cough with fever, occasional chills, pleuritic chest pain, sore throat, headache, backache, malaise, marked weakness, anorexia, hemoptysis, and an itchy macular rash.

Other causes
• *Diagnostic tests.* Pulmonary function tests or bronchoscopy can loosen secretions and mucus, causing rhonchi.
• *Respiratory therapy.* This may produce rhonchi from loosened secretions and mucus.

Special considerations
Prepare the patient for diagnostic tests, such as arterial blood gas analysis, pulmonary function studies, sputum analysis, and chest X-rays.

To ease the patient's breathing, place him in a semi-Fowler position, and reposition him every 2 hours. Or, if appropriate, encourage increased activity to promote drainage of secretions. Teach deep breathing and coughing techniques and splinting, if necessary.

If ordered, administer antibiotics, bronchodilators, and expectorants. Also, provide humidification to thin secretions, to relieve inflammation, and to prevent drying. Pulmonary physiotherapy with postural drainage and percussion can also help loosen secretions. Encourage fluids to help liquefy secretions and prevent dehydration.

Pediatric pointers
Because a respiratory tract disorder may begin abruptly and progress rapidly in an infant or child, observe carefully for signs of airway obstruction.

Rhonchi in children can result from bacterial pneumonia, cystic fibrosis, and croup syndrome.

Romberg's Sign

Relatively uncommon, a positive Romberg's sign refers to a patient's inability to maintain balance when standing erect with his feet together and his eyes closed. It indicates a proprioceptive disorder or a disorder of the spinal tracts (the posterior columns) that carry proprioceptive information—the perception of one's position in space and joint movements, and of pressure sensations—to the brain. Insufficient proprioceptive information causes an inability to execute precise movements and maintain balance without visual cues.

Assessment
Once you've detected a positive Romberg's sign, perform other neurologic screening tests. Why? Because a positive Romberg's sign only indicates the presence of a proprioceptive defect; it doesn't pinpoint its cause or location.

First, test proprioception. If the patient is able to maintain his balance with his eyes open, ask him to hop on one foot and then on the other. Next, ask him to do a knee bend, and to walk a straight line, placing heel to toe. Lastly, ask him to walk a short distance so you can evaluate his gait.

Test the patient's awareness of body-part position by changing the position of one of his fingers, or any other joint, while his eyes are closed. Ask him to describe the change you've made.

Now, test the patient's direction of movement. Ask him to close his eyes and to touch his nose with the index finger of one hand and then with the other. Ask him to repeat this movement several times, gradually increasing his speed. Then, test the accuracy of his movement by having him rapidly touch each finger of one hand to the thumb. Next, using a pin, test sensation in all dermatomes. Also test two-point discrimination by touching two pins (one in each hand) to his skin simultaneously. Does he feel one or two pinpricks? Finally, test and characterize the patient's deep tendon reflexes.

Test the patient's vibratory sense. Ask him to close his eyes; then apply a vibrating tuning fork to his clavicles, spinous processes, elbows, finger joints, knees, ankles, and toes. Hold it in each location until it stops vibrating. Tell the patient to report when he feels the vibrations start and stop.

Record all test results. Also, ask the patient if he's noticed sensory changes, such as numbness and tingling in his limbs. If so, when did they begin?

Medical causes

• *Multiple sclerosis.* Early features may include blurred vision, diplopia, and paresthesias. Besides a positive Romberg's sign, other findings may include nystagmus, constipation, muscle weakness and spasticity, and hyperreflexia. The patient may also have dysphagia, dysarthria, incontinence, urinary frequency and urgency, impotence, and emotional instability.

• *Peripheral nerve disease.* Besides a positive Romberg's sign, advanced disease may produce impotence, fatigue, and paresthesia, hyperesthesia, or anesthesia in the hands and feet. Related findings are incoordination, ataxia, burning pain in the affected area, progressive muscle weakness and atrophy, and loss of vibration sense. Deep tendon reflexes may be hypoactive.

• *Pernicious anemia.* A positive Romberg's sign and loss of proprioception in the lower limbs reflect peripheral nerve and spinal cord damage. Gait changes (usually ataxia), muscle weakness, impaired coordination,

paresthesias, and sensory loss may be present. Deep tendon reflexes may be hypoactive or hyperactive. Other findings include a sore tongue, a positive Babinski's reflex, fatigue, blurred vision, diplopia, and light-headedness.

• *Spinal cerebellar degeneration.* In this disorder, a positive Romberg's sign accompanies decreased visual acuity, fatigue, paresthesias, loss of vibration sense, incoordination, ataxic gait, and muscle weakness and atrophy. Deep tendon reflexes may be hypoactive.

• *Spinal cord disease.* A positive Romberg's sign may accompany fasciculations, muscle weakness and atrophy, and loss of proprioception, vibration, and other senses. Deep tendon reflexes may be hypoactive at the level of the lesion and hyperactive above it. Other features include loss of sphincter tone and pain.

• *Tabes dorsalis.* A positive Romberg's sign may occur, but burning extremity pain is this disorder's classic symptom. Other findings include ataxia, loss of proprioception in the lower limbs (common), and loss of pain and temperature sensation. As the disease progresses, deep tendon reflexes in the legs become hypoactive or absent, muscle tone decreases, and muscles atrophy. The patient may also have Charcot's joints and Argyll Robertson pupils.

• *Vestibular disorders.* Besides a positive Romberg's sign, these disorders commonly cause vertigo. They also cause nystagmus, nausea, and vomiting.

Special considerations

Help the patient with walking, especially in poorly lit areas. Also keep a night light on in his room, and raise the side rails of the bed. Encourage him to ask for assistance and to use visual cues to maintain his balance.

Pediatric pointers

Romberg's sign can't be tested in children until they can stand without support and follow commands. However, a positive sign in children commonly results from spinal cord disease.

salivation—decreased • salivation—increased • salt craving • scotoma • scrot
absence • seizure—focal • seizure—generalized tonic-clonic • seizure—psych
sign • shallow respirations • skin—bronze • skin—clammy • skin—mottled •
turgor—decreased • spider angioma • splenomegaly • stertorous respirations
stridor • syncope • tachycardia • tachypnea • taste abnormalities • tearing—i
tic • tinnitus • tracheal deviation • tracheal tugging • tremors • trismus • tu
frost • urethral discharge • urinary frequency • urinary hesitancy • urinary i
urgency • urine cloudiness • urticaria • vaginal bleeding—postmenopausal •
venous hum • vertigo • vesicular rash • violent behavior • vision loss • visual
floaters • vomiting • vulvar lesions • weight gain—excessive • weight loss—e
wristdrop• abdominal distention • abdominal mass • abdominal pain • abdo
accessory muscle use • agitation • alopecia • amenorrhea • amnesia • analge
anorexia • anosmia • anuria • anxiety • aphasia • apnea • apneustic respira
pain • asterixis • ataxia • athetosis • aura • Babinski's reflex • back pain • b
sign • Biot's respirations • bladder distention • blood pressure decrease • blo
bowel sounds—absent • bowel sounds—hyperactive • bowel sounds—hypoa
bradypnea • breast dimpling • breast nodule • breast pain • breast ulcer • b
odor • breath with fecal odor • breath with fruity odor • Brudzinski's sign •
butterfly rash • café-au-lait spots • capillary refill time—prolonged • carpope
chest expansion—asymmetrical • chest pain • Cheyne-Stokes respirations • c
sign • clubbing • cogwheel rigidity • cold intolerance • confusion • conjunct
constipation • corneal reflex—absent • costovertebral angle tenderness • cou
nonproductive • cough—productive • crackles • crepitation—bony • crepitat
cry—high-pitched • cyanosis • decerebrate posture • decorticate posture • d
hyperactive • deep tendon reflexes—hypoactive • depression • diaphoresis •
dizziness • doll's eye sign—absent • drooling • dysarthria • dysmenorrhea •
dyspepsia • dysphagia • dyspnea • dystonia • dysuria • earache • edema—g
arms • edema of the face • edema of the legs • enophthalmos • enuresis • ep
erythema • exophthalmos • eye discharge • eye pain • facial pain • fascicula
incontinence • fetor hepaticus • fever • flank pain • flatulence • fontanelle bu
depression • footdrop • gag reflex abnormalities • gait—bizarre • gait—prop
gait—spastic • gait—steppage • gait—waddling • gallop—atrial • gallop—v
in the male • grunting respirations • gum bleeding • gum swelling • gyneco
vision • headache • hearing loss • heat intolerance • Heberden's nodes • hen
hematochezia • hematuria • hemianopia • hemoptysis • hepatomegaly • hic
hoarseness • Homans' sign • hyperpigmentation • hyperpnea • hypopigment
insomnia • intermittent claudication • Janeway's spots • jaundice • jaw pair
distention • Kehr's sign • Kernig's sign • leg pain • level of consciousness—
flashes • low birth weight • lymphadenopathy • masklike facies • McBurney
sign • melena • menorrhagia • metrorrhagia • miosis • moon face • mouth
muscle atrophy • muscle flaccidity • muscle spasms • muscle spasticity • m
mydriasis • myoclonus • nasal flaring • nausea • neck pain • night blindnes
nipple retraction • nocturia • nuchal rigidity • nystagmus • ocular deviatio
oliguria • opisthotonos • orofacial dyskinesia • orthopnea • orthostatic hypo
Osler's nodes • otorrhea • pallor • palpitations • papular rash • paralysis •
nocturnal dyspnea • peau d'orange • pericardial friction rub • peristaltic w
photophobia • pica • pleural friction rub • polydipsia • polyphagia • polyur
priapism • pruritus • psoas sign • psychotic behavior • ptosis • pulse—abs
bounding • pulse pressure—narrowed • pulse pressure—widened • pulse r
pulsus alternans • pulsus bisferiens • pulsus paradoxus • pupils—nonreacti

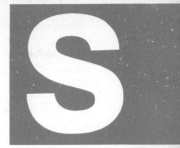

Salivation—Decreased
[Dry mouth, xerostomia]

Typically a common but minor complaint, diminished production or excretion of saliva most often results from mouth breathing. However, this symptom can also result from salivary duct obstruction, Sjögren's syndrome, the use of anticholinergics and other drugs, and the effects of radiation. It can even result from vigorous exercise or autonomic stimulation—for example, by fear.

Assessment
Evaluate the patient's complaint of dry mouth by asking pertinent history questions: When did he first notice the symptom? Was he exercising at the time? Is he currently taking any medication? Is his sensation of dry mouth intermittent or continuous? Is it related to or relieved by a particular activity? Ask about related symptoms, such as burning or itching eyes or changes in sense of smell or taste.

Now inspect the patient's mouth, including the mucous membranes, for any abnormalities. Observe his eyes for conjunctival irritation, matted lids, and corneal epithelial thickening. Perform simple tests of smell and taste to detect impairment of these senses. Next, check for enlarged parotid and submaxillary glands (see *Assessing Salivary Glands and Ductal Openings,* page 654). Palpate for tender or enlarged areas along the neck, too.

Medical causes
● *Salivary duct obstruction.* Usually associated with a salivary stone, this obstruction causes reduced salivation and local pain and swelling.
● *Sjögren's syndrome.* Diminished secretions from the lacrimal, parotid, and submaxillary glands produce the hallmarks of this disorder: decreased or absent salivation and dry eyes with a persistent burning, gritty sensation. The patient may also have dryness that involves the respiratory tract, vagina, and skin.

Related oral signs and symptoms include difficulty chewing, talking, and swallowing, as well as ulcers and soreness of the lips and mucosa. The parotid and submaxillary glands may be enlarged. Nasal crusting, epistaxis, fatigue, lethargy, nonproductive cough, abdominal discomfort, and polyuria may be present.

Other causes
● *Drugs.* Anticholinergics, antihistamines, tricyclic antidepressants, phenothiazines, clonidine hydrochloride, and narcotic analgesics may cause de-

ASSESSING SALIVARY GLANDS AND DUCTAL OPENINGS

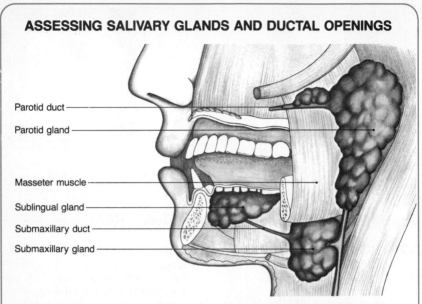

Parotid duct
Parotid gland
Masseter muscle
Sublingual gland
Submaxillary duct
Submaxillary gland

When a patient reports decreased saliva-tion, assess the parotid and submaxillary glands for enlargement and the ductal openings for salivary flow.

To detect an enlarged parotid gland, ask the patient to clench his teeth, thereby tensing the masseter muscle. Now, palpate the parotid duct (about 5 cm long); you should be able to feel it against the tensed muscle, on the cheek just below the zygomatic arch. Next, check the ductal orifice, opposite the second molar. Using a gloved finger, palpate the orifice for

enlargement, and observe for drainage.

Next, palpate the submaxillary gland. About the size of a walnut, it's located under the mandible, anterior to the angle of the jaw. Using a gloved finger, palpate the floor of the mouth for enlargement of the submaxillary ductal orifice.

Finally, test both ductal openings for salivary flow. Place cotton under the patient's tongue, have him sip pure lemon juice, and then remove the cotton and observe salivary flow from each opening. Document your findings.

---

creased salivation, which disappears after discontinuation of therapy.

• *Radiation.* Excessive irradiation of the mouth or face from antineoplastic treatments or dental X-rays may cause transient decreased salivation due to salivary gland atrophy.

Special considerations
If markedly reduced salivation inter-feres with speaking, eating, or swal-lowing, allow the patient extra time for these activities. Encourage him to in-crease his fluid intake during meals and to brush his teeth, floss, and use mouth-wash. Also encourage him to suck sour hard candies to relieve his dry mouth.

Pediatric pointers
Mouth breathing and anticholinergics are the primary causes of decreased salivation in children.

Salivation—Increased
[Polysialia, ptyalism]

This uncommon symptom may result from gastrointestinal disorders, espe-cially of the mouth. It also accompanies certain systemic disorders and may re-sult from the effects of drugs and toxins. Saliva may also accumulate because of difficulty swallowing. (See "Dysphagia.")

Assessment
A patient who complains of increased salivation may have overproductive salivary glands or difficulty swallowing. To distinguish these, first test for a gag reflex and observe the patient's ability to swallow and chew. Is he drooling? Is his chewing uncoordinated? An impaired gag reflex, drooling, and chewing incoordination suggest difficulty swallowing. Does he have related signs and symptoms, such as fatigue, fever, headache, or a sore throat? Ask about exposure to industrial toxins, such as mercury. Is the patient currently taking any medications? Note especially use of iodides, cholinergics, and miotics.

Now inspect the mouth and mucous membranes for lesions. If present, are they painful? Put on gloves and palpate the lesions, which may be suppurative or infectious. Describe them in your notes. Next, inspect the uvula, gingivae, and pharynx. Palpate the lymph nodes, and determine if the parotid glands are swollen or sore.

Medical causes
• *Arsenic poisoning.* Increased salivation infrequently occurs in this disorder. More common effects are diarrhea, diffuse skin hyperpigmentation, and edema of the eyelids, face, and ankles. The patient may have a garlicky breath odor, pruritus, alopecia, irritated mucous membranes, headache, drowsiness, and confusion. He may also have muscle aching, weakness, paresthesias, and seizures.
• *Mercury poisoning.* Stomatitis—involving increased salivation and a metallic taste—commonly occurs in mercury poisoning. The patient's teeth may be loose and his gums are painful, swollen, and prone to bleeding. A blue line appears on the gingivae. The patient may also have personality changes, abdominal cramps, diarrhea,

paresthesias, and tremors of the eyelids, lips, tongue, and fingers.
• *Stomatitis.* Mucosal ulcers may be accompanied by moderately increased salivation, mouth pain, fever, and erythema. Spontaneous healing usually occurs in 7 to 10 days, but scarring and recurrence are possible.
• *Syphilis.* In secondary syphilis, mucosal ulcers cause increased salivation that may persist up to a year. Related findings include fever, malaise, headache, anorexia, weight loss, nausea, vomiting, sore throat, and generalized lymphadenopathy. A rash appears on the arms, trunk, palms, soles, face, and scalp.
• *Tuberculosis.* Certain forms of tuberculosis may produce solitary, irregularly shaped mouth or tongue ulcers, covered with exudate, that cause increased salivation. Other findings: weight loss, anorexia, fever, fatigue, malaise, dyspnea, cough, night sweats (a common sign), and hemoptysis.

Other causes
• *Drugs.* Increased salivation may occur in iodide toxicity, but the earliest symptoms are a brassy taste and a burning sensation in the mouth and throat. Associated findings include sneezing, irritated eyelids, and (commonly) pain in the frontal sinus.

Pilocarpine and other miotics used to treat glaucoma may be absorbed systemically, increasing salivation. Cholinergics, such as bethanechol and neostigmine, may also cause this symptom.

Special considerations
Though annoying to the patient, increased salivation doesn't require treatments beyond those needed to correct the underlying disorder.

Pediatric pointers
Besides stemming from conditions that affect adults, increased salivation in children may also stem from congenital esophageal atresia. In this disorder, the infant is unable to swallow seemingly excessive saliva and frothy mucus.

Salt Craving

Craving salty foods is a compensatory response to the body's failure to adequately conserve sodium. Normally, the renal tubules reabsorb almost all sodium, allowing less than 1% of it to be excreted in the urine. This reabsorption is regulated by aldosterone, a hormone synthesized in the adrenal gland. However, adrenal dysfunction can reduce aldosterone levels, thereby impairing reabsorption and increasing excretion of sodium.

Assessment

Because normal salt intake varies widely, depending on dietary preferences and cultural differences, find out how much salt the patient typically uses. Has he increased this amount recently? Has he also experienced weakness, fatigue, anorexia, or weight loss? Has he felt dizzy or fainted? Check for a history of adrenal insufficiency or diabetes mellitus and for recent onset of polydipsia or polyuria. Inspect the patient's skin for hyperpigmentation or hypopigmentation. Take his vital signs, too, noting postural hypotension.

Remember that sudden or rapidly worsening salt craving may indicate adrenal crisis if it's accompanied by hypotension, tachycardia, oliguria, and cool, clammy skin.

Medical cause

• *Primary adrenal insufficiency.* Often called Addison's disease, this disorder reduces aldosterone secretion. As a result, the patient may exhibit an intense craving for salty food. He may display diffuse brown, tan, or bronze-to-black hyperpigmentation of exposed areas (such as the face, knees, and knuckles) and of nonexposed areas (such as palmar creases, the tongue, or buccal mucosa) and darkening of normally pigmented areas, moles, and scars. In about 15% of cases, the patient also displays hypopigmentation. Related findings include weakness, anorexia, nausea, irritability, vomiting, weight loss, abdominal pain, and slowly progressive fatigue.

Special considerations

Prepare the patient for laboratory tests, such as serum aldosterone and electrolytes, plasma cortisol and glucose, and urine 17-ketogenic steroids and 17-hydroxycorticosteroids. Special provocative studies may include the metyrapone test or the rapid ACTH test. Collect a urine specimen and use a reagent strip to test for glucose and acetone.

To check for volume depletion, monitor and record the patient's intake, output, and weight. Promote fluids and arrange for a diet that helps maintain adequate sodium and potassium levels. Be alert for signs of hyponatremia, such as hypotension, muscle twitching and weakness, and abdominal cramps. Also be alert for signs of hyperkalemia, such as muscle weakness, tachycardia, nausea, vomiting, and characteristic EKG changes—tented and elevated T waves, widened QRS complex, prolonged PR interval, flattened or absent P waves, and depressed ST segment.

If diagnostic tests confirm primary adrenal insufficiency, emphasize the importance of complying with lifelong steroid therapy, including glucocorticoids and mineralocorticoids. Teach the patient the signs and symptoms of steroid toxicity and underdosage. Also explain that his dosage may need to be increased during stress (infection, injury, even profuse sweating) to prevent adrenal crisis. Instruct him to carry a Medic Alert card at all times, stating that he takes a steroid and giving the drug's name and dosage. Teach him how to give himself a hydrocortisone injection, and tell him to keep hydrocortisone available in a prepared syringe for emergency use.

Pediatric pointers

Salt craving in children may stem from decompensated congenital adrenal hyperplasia, although this disorder usually responds adequately to steroid replacement. Adrenal insufficiency can also develop with surgery or acute illness. Salt craving may signal a change in condition requiring increased steroid dosage.

Scotoma

A scotoma is an area of partial or complete blindness within an otherwise normal or slightly impaired visual field. Usually located within the central 30° area, the defect ranges from absolute blindness to a barely detectable loss of visual acuity. Typically, the patient can pinpoint the scotoma's location in the visual field.

A scotoma can result from retinal, choroid, or optic nerve disorders. It can be classified as absolute, relative, or scintillating. An *absolute scotoma* refers to the total inability to see all sizes of test objects used in mapping the visual field. A *relative scotoma,* in contrast, refers to the ability to see only large test objects. A *scintillating scotoma* refers to the flashes or bursts of light commonly seen during a migraine headache.

Assessment
First, identify and characterize a scotoma, using such visual field tests as the tangent screen examination, the Goldmann perimeter test, and the automated perimetry test. (Two other visual field tests—confrontation testing and the Amsler grid—may also help identify a scotoma.)

Next, test the patient's visual acuity and inspect his pupils for size, equality, and reaction to light. If requested, assist with an ophthalmoscopic examination and measurement of intraocular pressure.

Explore the patient's history for eye disorders, vision problems, or chronic systemic disorders. Does the patient take medications or use eye drops?

Medical causes
● *Chorioretinitis.* Inflammation of the choroid produces a paracentral scotoma. Ophthalmoscopic examination reveals clouding and cells in the vitreous, subretinal hemorrhage, and neovascularization.
● *Glaucoma.* Prolonged elevation of intraocular pressure can cause an arcuate scotoma. Poorly controlled glaucoma can also cause cupping of the optic disk, loss of peripheral vision, and reduced visual acuity. The patient may also see rainbow-colored halos around lights.
● *Macular degeneration.* Any degenerative process or disorder affecting the fovea centralis results in a central scotoma. Ophthalmoscopic examination reveals changes in the macular area. The patient may notice subtle changes in visual acuity, in color perception, and in the size and shape of objects.
● *Migraine headache.* Transient scintillating scotomas, usually bilateral and often homonymous, can occur with a classic migraine aura. Besides pain, characteristic associated symptoms include paresthesias of the lips, face, or hands; slight confusion; dizziness; and photophobia.
● *Optic neuritis.* Inflammation, degeneration, or demyelination of the optic nerve produces central, circular, or centrocecal scotoma. The scotoma may be unilateral with involvement of one nerve or bilateral with involvement of both nerves. It can vary in size, density, and symmetry. The patient may have severe visual loss or blurring, lasting up to 3 weeks, and pain—especially with eye movement. Common ophthalmoscopic findings include hyperemia of the optic disk, retinal vein distention, blurred disk margins, and filling of the physiologic cup.
● *Retinal pigmentary degenerations.* These disorders cause premature retinal cell changes leading to cell death. One of these disorders, retinitis pig-

LOCATING SCOTOMAS

Scotomas, or "blind spots," are classified according to the affected area of the visual field. The normal scotoma—shown in the temporal region of the right eye—appears in black in all the illustrations.

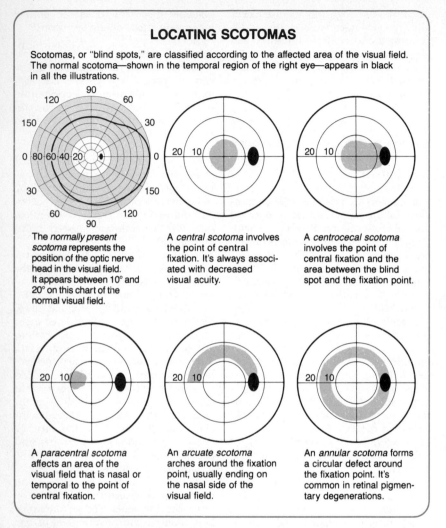

The *normally present scotoma* represents the position of the optic nerve head in the visual field. It appears between 10° and 20° on this chart of the normal visual field.

A *central scotoma* involves the point of central fixation. It's always associated with decreased visual acuity.

A *centrocecal scotoma* involves the point of central fixation and the area between the blind spot and the fixation point.

A *paracentral scotoma* affects an area of the visual field that is nasal or temporal to the point of central fixation.

An *arcuate scotoma* arches around the fixation point, usually ending on the nasal side of the visual field.

An *annular scotoma* forms a circular defect around the fixation point. It's common in retinal pigmentary degenerations.

mentosa, initially involves loss of peripheral rods: the resulting annular scotoma progresses concentrically until only a central field of vision (tunnel vision) remains. The earliest symptom—impaired night vision—appears during adolescence. Associated signs include narrowing of the retinal blood vessels and pallor of the optic disk. Eventually, with invasion of the macula, blindness may occur.

Special considerations
For the patient with an arcuate scotoma associated with glaucoma, emphasize regular testing of intraocular pressure and visual fields. In addition, teach the patient with a disorder involving the fovea centralis (or the area surrounding it) to periodically use the Amsler grid to detect progression of macular degeneration.

Pediatric pointers
In young children, visual field testing is difficult and requires patience. Confrontation testing is the method of choice.

Scrotal Swelling

Scrotal swelling occurs when a condition affecting the testicles, epididymis, or scrotal skin produces edema or a mass; the penis may or may not be involved. Scrotal swelling can be unilateral or bilateral and painful or painless. It can affect males of any age.

The sudden onset of painful scrotal swelling suggests torsion of a testicle or testicular appendages, especially in the prepubescent male. This emergency requires immediate surgery to untwist and stabilize the spermatic cord or to remove the appendage.

Assessment

If severe pain accompanies scrotal swelling, find out when the swelling began. If it began suddenly, notify a urologist immediately. Then, using a Doppler stethoscope, assess blood flow to the scrotum. If it's decreased or absent, suspect testicular torsion and prepare the patient for surgery. Withhold food and fluids, insert an I.V. line, as ordered, and apply an ice pack to the scrotum to reduce pain and swelling. The doctor may attempt to untwist the cord manually, but even if he's successful, the patient will still require surgery for stabilization.

If the patient isn't in distress, proceed with the history. Ask about injury to the scrotum, about urethral discharge, and about cloudy urine, increased urinary frequency, and dysuria. Is the patient sexually active? When was his last sexual contact? Find out about recent illnesses, particularly mumps. Does he have a history of prostate surgery or prolonged catheterization? Does changing his body position or level of activity affect the swelling?

Take the patient's vital signs, noting especially fever, and palpate his abdomen for tenderness. Then examine the entire genital area. Assess the scrotum with the patient supine and stand-ing. Note its size and color. Is the swelling unilateral or bilateral? Do you see signs of trauma or bruising? Gently palpate the scrotum for a cyst or a lump. Note especially tenderness or increased firmness. Check the testicles' position in the scrotum. Finally, transilluminate the scrotum to distinguish a fluid-filled cyst from a solid mass. (A solid mass can't be transilluminated.)

Medical causes

• *Elephantiasis of the scrotum.* In this disorder (common in some tropical countries), infection by a filaria worm obstructs lymphatic drainage, causing chronic gross scrotal edema and pain. Associated findings include other areas of pitting and, eventually, brawny edema, thickened subcutaneous tissue, hyperkeratosis, and skin fissures.

• *Epididymal cysts.* Located in the head of the epididymis, these cysts produce painless scrotal swelling.

• *Epididymal tuberculosis.* This disorder produces an enlarged scrotal mass separated from the testicle. Other findings may include palpable beading along the vas deferens, induration of the prostate or seminal vesicles, and pus or tubercle bacilli in the urine.

• *Epididymitis.* Key features of inflammation are pain, extreme tenderness, and swelling in the groin and scrotum. The patient waddles to avoid pressure on the groin and scrotum during walking. He may have high fever, malaise, urethral discharge and cloudy urine, and lower abdominal pain on the affected side. His scrotal skin may be hot, red, dry, flaky, and thin.

• *Gumma.* This rare, painless nodule can affect any bone or organ. If it affects the testicle, it causes edema.

• *Hernia.* Herniation of bowel into the scrotum can cause swelling and a soft or unusually firm scrotum. Occasionally, bowel sounds can be auscultated in the scrotum.

• *Hydrocele.* Fluid accumulation produces gradual scrotal swelling that's usually painless. The scrotum may be soft and cystic or firm and tense. Pal-

PATIENT-TEACHING AID

HOW TO EXAMINE YOUR TESTICLES

Dear Patient:

To help detect abnormalities early, you should examine your testicles once a month. (Schedule this exam for the same date every month.) The best time to examine your testicles is during or after a hot bath or shower. The heat causes the testicles to descend and relaxes the scrotum; this makes finding any abnormalities easier.

Now, follow these simple instructions, using the illustration (top right) to locate anatomic landmarks.

Check the scrotum
With one hand, lift your penis and check your scrotum (the pouch of skin containing the testicles and parts of the spermatic cords) for any change in shape or size and for reddened, distended veins. Expect the scrotum's left side to hang slightly lower than the right.

Check each testicle
Place your left thumb on the front of your left testicle and your index and middle fingers behind it, as shown (middle right). Gently but firmly roll the testicle between your thumb and fingers. Then, use your right hand to examine your right testicle in the same manner. Your testicles should feel smooth, rubbery, slightly tender, and movable within the scrotum.

If you notice any lumps, masses, or other changes, notify your doctor.

Check each spermatic cord
Locate the cordlike structure called the epididymis at the back of your testicles. Then locate the spermatic cord extending upward from it, as shown (bottom right).

Gently squeeze the spermatic cord above your left testicle between your thumb and the first two fingers of your left hand. Then repeat on the right side, using your right hand. Check for lumps and masses along the entire length of the cords.

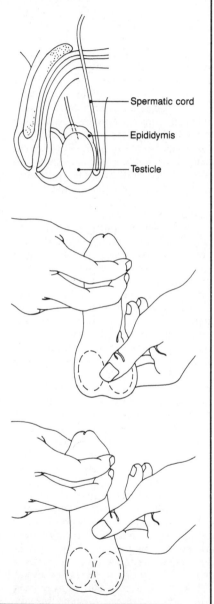

Spermatic cord

Epididymis

Testicle

pation reveals a round, nontender scrotal mass.

• *Idiopathic scrotal edema.* Swelling occurs quickly in this disorder and usually disappears within 24 hours. The affected testicle is pink.

• *Orchitis (acute).* Mumps may precipitate this disorder, which causes sudden painful swelling of one or, at times, both testicles. Related findings include a hot, reddened scrotum, fever of up to 104° F. (40° C.), chills, lower abdominal pain, nausea, vomiting, and extreme weakness. Urinary signs are usually absent.

• *Scrotal burns.* Burns cause swelling within 24 hours of injury. Depending on the burn's severity, associated findings may include severe pain, erythema, chafing, tissue sloughing, and maceration with a weeping exudate.

• *Scrotal trauma.* Blunt trauma causes scrotal swelling with bruising and severe pain. The scrotum may appear dark or bluish.

• *Spermatocele.* This painless or painful cystic mass lies above and behind the testicle and contains opaque fluid and sperm. Its onset may be acute or gradual. Less than 1 cm in diameter, it's movable and may be transilluminated.

• *Testicular torsion.* Most common before puberty, this urologic emergency causes scrotal swelling, sudden and severe pain, and possible elevation of the affected testicle within the scrotum. It may also cause nausea and vomiting.

• *Testicular tumor.* Typically painless, smooth, and firm, a testicular tumor produces swelling and a sensation of excessive weight in the scrotum.

• *Torsion of a hydatid of Morgagni.* Torsion of this small, pea-sized cyst severs its blood supply, causing a hard, painful swelling on the testicle's upper pole.

Other cause

• *Surgery.* An effusion of blood from surgery can produce a hematocele, leading to scrotal swelling.

Special considerations

As ordered, keep the patient on bed rest and give antibiotics. Provide adequate fluids, fiber, and stool softeners. Place a rolled towel between the patient's legs and under the scrotum to help reduce severe swelling. Or, if the patient has mild or moderate swelling, advise him to wear a loose-fitting athletic supporter lined with soft cotton dressings. Administer analgesics for several days, as ordered, to relieve his pain. Encourage sitz baths, and apply heat or ice packs to decrease inflammation.

Encourage the patient to perform testicular self-examination at home. (See *How to Examine Your Testicles.*) Prepare him for needle aspiration of fluid-filled cysts and other diagnostic tests, such as lung tomography and computed tomography of the abdomen, to rule out malignancies.

Pediatric pointers

Thorough physical assessment is especially important in children with scrotal swelling, who may be unable to give history data.

In children up to age 1, hernia or hydrocele of the cord may stem from abnormal fetal development. In infants, scrotal swelling may stem from ammonia-related dermatitis, if diapers aren't changed often enough. In prepubescent males, it most commonly results from torsion of the spermatic cord.

Other disorders producing scrotal swelling in children include epididymitis (rare before age 10), traumatic orchitis from contact sports, and mumps, which occurs most often after puberty.

Seizure—Absence

[Petit mal seizure]

Absence seizures are benign, generalized seizures thought to originate subcortically. These brief episodes of unconsciousness last 10 to 20 seconds and can occur 100 or more times a day, commonly causing periods of inattention. Absence seizures most often affect children between the ages of 4 and 12 and rarely persist beyond adolescence. Their first sign may be deteriorating school work and behavior. Their cause isn't known.

Absence seizures occur without warning. The patient suddenly stops all purposeful activity and stares blankly ahead—unable to see, hear, or feel. Absence seizures may produce automatisms, such as repetitive lip smacking, or mild clonic or myoclonic movements, including mild jerking of muscles in the eyelids. The patient may drop objects he's holding, and muscle relaxation may cause him to drop his head or arms or to slump. After the attack, the patient resumes activity, typically unaware of the episode.

Absence status, a rare form of absence seizure, occurs as a prolonged absence seizure or as repeated episodes of these seizures. Usually not life-threatening, it occurs most commonly in patients with preexisting absence seizures.

Assessment

If you suspect a patient is having an absence seizure, assess its occurrence and duration by reciting a series of numbers and then asking him to repeat them after the attack ends. The patient will be unable to do this. Or, if the seizures are occurring within minutes of each other, ask the patient to count for about 5 minutes. He'll stop counting during a seizure, then resume when it's over. Look for accompanying automatisms.

Find out if the family has noticed a change in behavior or deteriorating school work.

Medical cause

● *Idiopathic epilepsy.* Frequently, absence seizures are accompanied by automatisms and learning disability.

Special considerations

Explain the purpose of any diagnostic tests, such as computed tomography scans and electroencephalography. Teach the patient and his family about these seizures and how to recognize their onset, pattern, and duration. Include the child's teacher and school nurse in the teaching process, if possible. If the seizures are being controlled with drug therapy, emphasize the importance of strict compliance.

Seizure—Focal
[Simple partial seizure]

Resulting from an irritable focus in the cerebral cortex, a focal seizure typically lasts about 30 seconds and doesn't alter the patient's level of consciousness. Its type and pattern reflect the location of the irritable focus. A focal seizure may be classified as motor or somatosensory. A focal motor seizure, in turn, includes a jacksonian seizure and epilepsia partialis continua. A somatosensory seizure includes visual, olfactory, and auditory seizures.

A *focal motor seizure* is a series of unilateral clonic (muscle jerking) and tonic (muscle stiffening) movements of one part of the body. The patient's head and eyes characteristically turn away from the hemispheric focus—most commonly the frontal lobe near the motor strip. A tonic-clonic contraction of the trunk or extremities may follow.

A *jacksonian motor seizure* typically begins with a tonic contraction of a finger, the corner of the mouth, or one foot. Clonic movements follow, spreading to other muscles on the same side of the body, moving up the arm or leg, and eventually involving the whole side. Or clonic movements may spread to the opposite side, becoming generalized and leading to loss of consciousness. In the postictal phase, the patient may display paralysis (Todd's paralysis) in the affected limbs that usually resolves within 24 hours.

Epilepsia partialis continua causes clonic twitching of one muscle group, usually in the face, arm, or leg. Twitching occurs every few seconds and persists for hours, days, or months without spreading. Spasms affect the distal arm and leg muscles more frequently than the proximal ones; in the face, they affect the corner of the mouth, one or both eyelids and, occasionally, the neck or trunk muscles unilaterally.

A *focal somatosensory seizure* affects a localized body area on one side. Usually, this seizure initially causes numbness, tingling, or crawling or "electric" sensations; rarely, it may cause pain or burning sensations in the lips, fingers, or toes. A *visual seizure* involves sensations of darkness or of stationary or moving lights or spots—usually red at first, then blue, green, and yellow. It can affect both visual fields or the visual field on the side opposite the lesion. The irritable focus is in the occipital lobe. In contrast, the irritable focus in an *auditory* or *olfactory seizure* is in the temporal lobe.

Assessment

If you observe a patient during a focal seizure, notify the doctor immediately so he can witness the seizure, if possible. Record the patient's behavior in detail; your data may be critical in locating the lesion in the brain. Does the patient turn his head and eyes? If so, to what side? Where does movement first start? Does it spread? Because a partial seizure may become generalized, watch closely for loss of consciousness, bilateral tonicity and clonicity, cyanosis, tongue biting, and urinary incontinence. (See "Seizure—Generalized Tonic-Clonic.")

During the seizure, ask the patient to describe exactly what's happening. After the seizure, check his level of consciousness, and test for residual deficits (such as weakness in the involved extremity) and sensory disturbances.

Obtain a history: What happened before the seizure? Did the patient recognize its onset? If so, how did he recognize it—a smell, a visual disturbance, or a sound or visceral phenomenon, such as an unusual sensation in his stomach? How does this seizure compare with others the patient has had? Explore fully any history, recent or remote, of head trauma. Also check for a history of stroke or recent infection—especially with fever, headache, or a stiff neck.

Medical causes

• *Brain abscess.* Seizures can occur in the acute stage of abscess formation or after resolution of the abscess. Decreased level of consciousness varies from drowsiness to deep stupor. Early signs and symptoms reflect increased intracranial pressure and include constant, intractable headache, nausea, and vomiting. Later symptoms include ocular disturbances—such as nystagmus, decreased visual acuity, and unequal pupils. Other findings differ with the abscess site and may include aphasia, hemiparesis, and personality changes.

• *Brain tumor.* Focal seizures are commonly the earliest indicators of a brain tumor. The patient may report morning headache, dizziness, confusion, vision loss, and motor and sensory disturbances. He may also have aphasia, generalized seizures, ataxia, decreased level of consciousness, papilledema, vomiting, increased systolic blood pressure, and widening pulse pressure. Eventually, he may assume a decorticate posture.

• *Cerebrovascular accident (CVA).* A major cause of seizures in patients over age 50, a CVA may induce focal seizures within 6 months after its onset. Related effects depend on the type and extent of the CVA but may include decreased level of consciousness, contralateral hemiplegia, dysarthria, dysphagia, ataxia, unilateral sensory loss, apraxia, agnosia, and aphasia. A CVA may also cause visual deficits, memory loss, poor judgment, personality changes, emotional lability, headache, urinary retention or incontinence, and

BODY FUNCTIONS AFFECTED BY FOCAL SEIZURES

The body function normally governed at the site of the irritable focus determines a focal seizure's signs and symptoms.

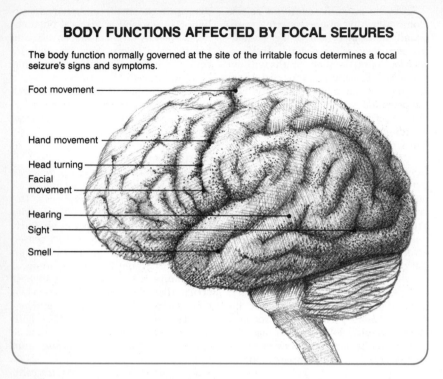

Foot movement

Hand movement

Head turning

Facial movement

Hearing

Sight

Smell

vomiting. It may cause generalized seizures.

• **Head trauma.** Any head injury can cause seizures, but penetrating wounds are characteristically associated with focal seizures. These seizures most commonly arise 3 to 15 months after injury, decrease in frequency after several years, and eventually stop. The patient may have generalized seizures and a decreased level of consciousness that may progress to coma.

• **Multiple sclerosis.** Rarely, this disorder begins with focal seizures; generalized seizures may also occur. Other findings may include visual deficits, paresthesias, constipation, muscle weakness, spasticity, paralysis, hyperreflexia, intention tremor, gait ataxia, dysphagia, and dysarthria. There may also be emotional lability, impotence, and urinary frequency, urgency, and incontinence.

• **Neurofibromatosis.** Multiple brain lesions cause focal seizures and, at times, generalized seizures. Inspection reveals café-au-lait spots, multiple skin tumors, scoliosis, and kyphoscoliosis. Related findings include dizziness, ataxia, progressive monocular blindness, nystagmus, and endocrine abnormalities.

• **Sarcoidosis.** Multiple lesions from this disorder affect the brain, producing focal and generalized seizures. Associated findings include a nonproductive cough with dyspnea, substernal pain, malaise, fatigue, arthralgia, myalgia, weight loss, tachypnea, dysphagia, skin lesions, and impaired vision.

Special considerations

No emergency care is necessary during a focal seizure, unless it progresses to a generalized seizure. (See "Seizure—Generalized Tonic-Clonic.") Remain with the patient during the seizure, and reassure him. After the seizure, instruct him to observe and record his seizures and to contact his doctor if their character or frequency changes. Also emphasize the importance of complying with prescribed drug therapy.

As ordered, prepare the patient for such diagnostic tests as a computed tomography scan and electroencephalography.

Pediatric pointers
In children more than in adults, focal seizures are likely to spread and become generalized. They typically cause the child's eyes, or his head and eyes, to turn to the side; in neonates, they cause mouth twitching, staring, or both.

Focal seizures in children can result from hemiplegic cerebral palsy, head trauma, child abuse, arteriovenous malformation, and Sturge-Weber syndrome. About 25% of febrile seizures may present as focal seizures.

Seizure—Generalized Tonic-Clonic

[Grand mal seizure]

Like other types of seizure, a generalized tonic-clonic seizure reflects the paroxysmal, uncontrolled discharge of central nervous system (CNS) neurons, leading to neurologic dysfunction. Unlike most other types of seizure, this cerebral hyperactivity isn't confined to the original focus or to a localized area but extends to the entire brain.

A generalized tonic-clonic seizure typically begins with a prodrome and may include an aura. As seizure activity spreads to the subcortical structures, the patient loses consciousness, falls to the ground, and may utter a loud cry that's precipitated by air rushing from the lungs through the vocal cords. His body stiffens (tonic phase), then undergoes rapid, synchronous muscle jerking and hyperventilation (clonic phase). Tongue biting, incon-

tinence, diaphoresis, profuse salivation, and signs of respiratory distress may also occur. The seizure usually stops after 2 to 5 minutes, when abnormal electrical conduction of neurons is completed. The patient then regains consciousness but displays confusion. He may complain of headache, fatigue, muscle soreness, and arm and leg weakness.

Generalized tonic-clonic seizures occur singly. The patient may be awake and active or sleeping. Possible complications include respiratory arrest due to airway obstruction from secretions, status epilepticus (occurring in 5% to 8% of patients), head or spinal injuries and bruises, Todd's paralysis and, rarely, cardiac arrest. Life-threatening status epilepticus is marked by prolonged seizure activity or by rapidly recurring seizures with no intervening periods of recovery. It's most commonly triggered by abrupt discontinuation of anticonvulsant drugs.

Generalized seizures may stem from brain tumors, vascular disorders, head trauma, infections, metabolic defects, drug and alcohol withdrawal syndromes, toxins, and genetic defects. These seizures may also stem from a focal seizure. In recurring seizures, or epilepsy, the cause may be unknown.

Assessment
If you witness the beginning of the seizure, stay with the patient and have another nurse notify the doctor immediately. Focus your care on observing the seizure and protecting the patient. Place a towel under his head to prevent injury, loosen his clothing, and move any sharp or hard objects out of his way. Never try to restrain him or force a hard object into his mouth; you may chip his teeth or fracture his jaw. Only at the start of the ictal phase can you safely insert a soft object into his mouth.

If possible during the seizure, turn the patient to one side to allow secretions to drain. Otherwise, do this at the end of the clonic phase when respirations return. (If they fail to return, check for airway obstruction and suction the patient, if necessary. Be prepared to assist with intubation and mechanical ventilation.) Protect the patient after the seizure by providing a safe area in which he can rest. As he awakens, reassure and reorient him. Check his vital signs and neurologic status. Carefully record these and your observations made during the seizure.

If the seizure lasts longer than 4 minutes or if a second seizure occurs before full recovery from the first, suspect status epilepticus. As ordered, establish an airway, start an I.V., give supplemental oxygen, and begin cardiac monitoring. Draw blood for appropriate studies. Turn the patient on his side, with his head in a semidependent position, to drain secretions and prevent aspiration. Periodically turn him to the opposite side, check his arterial blood gas results for hypoxemia, and give oxygen by mask, increasing the flow rate as ordered. If necessary, assist with intubation and mechanical ventilation (probably when seizure activity slows).

If ordered, give diazepam by slow I.V. push, repeated two or three times at 10- to 20-minute intervals, to stop the seizures. If the patient's not a known epileptic, the doctor may order an I.V. bolus of dextrose 50% (50 ml) or of thiamine (100 mg). Dextrose may stop the seizures if the patient's hypoglycemic; thiamine, if he's alcohol-dependent. If the patient's intubated, expect to insert a nasogastric tube to prevent vomiting and aspiration. However, if the patient hasn't been intubated, the doctor may forego this procedure, because the nasogastric tube itself can trigger the gag reflex and cause vomiting. Record your observations and the intervals between seizures.

If you didn't witness the seizure, obtain a description from the patient's companion. Ask when the seizure started and how long it lasted. Did the patient report any unusual sensations before the seizure began? Did the sei-

zure start in one area of the body and spread, or did it affect the entire body right away? Did the patient fall on a hard surface? Did his eyes or head turn? Did he turn blue? Did he lose bladder control? Did he have any other seizures before recovering?

If the patient may have a head injury, observe him closely for loss of consciousness, unequal or nonreactive pupils, and focal neurologic signs. Does he complain of headache and muscle soreness? Is he increasingly difficult to arouse when you check on him at 20-minute intervals? Examine his arms, legs, and face (including tongue) for injury, residual paralysis, or limb weakness.

Now obtain a history. Has the patient ever had generalized or focal seizures before? Are they frequent? Do other family members also have them? Is the patient receiving drug therapy? Does he take his medication regularly? Also ask about emotional or physical stress at the time the seizure occurred.

Medical causes

• *Alcohol withdrawal syndrome.* Sudden withdrawal from chronic alcohol dependence may cause seizures 7 to 48 hours later and status epilepticus. The patient may also be restless and have hallucinations, profuse diaphoresis, and tachycardia.

• *Arsenic poisoning.* Besides generalized seizures, arsenic poisoning may cause a garlicky breath odor, increased salivation, and generalized pruritus. Gastrointestinal effects include diarrhea, nausea, vomiting, and severe abdominal pain. Related effects include diffuse hyperpigmentation; sharply defined edema of the eyelids, face, and ankles; numbness or tingling of the extremities; alopecia; irritated mucous membranes; weakness; muscle aches; and peripheral neuropathy.

• *Barbiturate withdrawal.* In chronically intoxicated patients, barbiturate withdrawal may produce generalized seizures 2 to 4 days after the last dose. Status epilepticus is possible.

WHAT HAPPENS IN A GENERALIZED SEIZURE

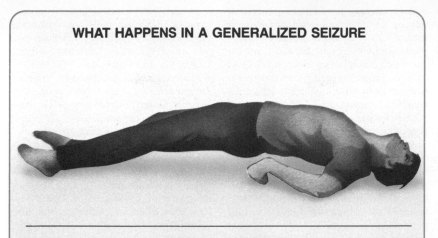

BEFORE THE SEIZURE

Prodromal signs and symptoms, such as myoclonic jerks, throbbing headache, and mood changes, may occur over several hours or days. Less common findings include abdominal pain or cramps, diarrhea or constipation, and facial pallor or redness. The patient may have premonitions of the seizure.

DURING THE SEIZURE

If a generalized seizure begins with an *aura,* this indicates that irritability in a specific area of the brain quickly became widespread. Common auras include palpitations, epigastric distress rapidly rising to the throat, head or eye turning, and sensory hallucinations.

Next, *loss of consciousness* occurs as a sudden discharge of intense electrical activity overwhelms the brain's subcortical center. The patient falls and experiences brief, bilateral myoclonic contractures. Air forced through spasmodic vocal cords may produce a birdlike, piercing cry.

During the *tonic phase,* skeletal muscles contract for about 10 to 20 seconds. The patient's eyelids are drawn up, his arms are flexed, and his legs are extended. His mouth opens wide, then snaps shut; he may bite his tongue. His respirations cease because of respiratory muscle spasm, and initial pallor of the skin and mucous membranes (the result of impaired venous return) changes to cyanosis secondary to apnea. The patient arches his back and slowly lowers his arms. Other effects include dilated, nonreactive pupils; greatly increased heart rate and blood pressure; increased salivation and tracheobronchial secretions; and profuse diaphoresis.

During the *clonic phase,* lasting about 60 seconds, mild trembling progresses to violent contractures or jerks. Other motor activity includes facial grimaces (with possible tongue biting) and violent expiration of bloody, foamy saliva from clonic contractures of thoracic cage muscles. Clonic jerks slowly decrease in intensity and frequency. The patient is still apneic.

AFTER THE SEIZURE

The patient's movements gradually cease and he becomes unresponsive to external stimuli. Other postseizure features include stertorous respirations from increased tracheobronchial secretions, equal or unequal pupils (but becoming reactive), and urinary incontinence due to brief muscle flaccidity. After about 5 minutes, the patient's level of consciousness increases, and he appears confused and disoriented. His muscle tone, heart rate, and blood pressure return to normal.

After several hours' sleep, the patient awakens exhausted and may have headache, sore muscles, and amnesia for the seizure.

• **Brain abscess.** Generalized seizures may occur in the acute stage of abscess formation or after the abscess disappears. Depending on the size and location of the abscess, decreased level of consciousness varies from drowsiness to deep stupor. Early signs and symptoms reflect increased intracranial pressure and include constant headache, nausea, vomiting, and focal seizures. Typical later features include ocular disturbances—such as nystagmus, impaired vision, and unequal pupils. Other findings differ with the abscess site but may include aphasia, hemiparesis, abnormal behavior, and personality changes.

• **Brain tumor.** Generalized seizures may occur, depending on the tumor's location and type. Other findings include a slowly decreasing level of consciousness, morning headache, dizziness, confusion, focal seizures, vision loss, motor and sensory disturbances, aphasia, and ataxia. Later findings: papilledema, vomiting, increased systolic blood pressure, widening pulse pressure, and (eventually) decorticate posture.

• **Cerebral aneurysm.** Occasionally, generalized seizures may occur with aneurysmal rupture. Premonitory signs and symptoms may last several days, but onset is typically abrupt with severe headache, nausea, vomiting, and decreased level of consciousness. Depending on the site and amount of bleeding, related signs and symptoms vary but may include nuchal rigidity, irritability, hemiparesis, hemisensory defects, dysphagia, photophobia, diplopia, ptosis, and a unilateral dilated pupil.

• **Cerebrovascular accident (CVA).** Seizures (focal more often than generalized) occur within 6 months of an ischemic CVA. Associated signs and symptoms vary with the location and extent of brain damage. They include decreased level of consciousness, contralateral hemiplegia, dysarthria, dysphagia, ataxia, unilateral sensory loss, apraxia, agnosia, and aphasia. There

may also be visual deficits, memory loss, poor judgment, personality changes, emotional lability, urinary retention or incontinence, constipation, headache, and vomiting.

• **Chronic renal failure.** End-stage renal failure produces rapid onset of twitching, trembling, myoclonic jerks, and generalized seizures. Related signs and symptoms include anuria or oliguria, fatigue, malaise, irritability, decreased mental acuity, muscle cramps, peripheral neuropathies, anorexia, and constipation or diarrhea. Integumentary effects include skin color changes (yellow, brown, or bronze), pruritus, and uremic frost. Other effects include ammonia breath odor, nausea and vomiting, ecchymoses, petechiae, gastrointestinal bleeding, mouth and gum ulcers, hypertension, and Kussmaul's respirations.

• **Eclampsia.** Generalized seizures are a hallmark of this disorder. Related findings include severe frontal headache, nausea and vomiting, vision disturbances, increased blood pressure, edema, and sudden weight gain. The patient may also have oliguria, irritability, hyperactive deep tendon reflexes, and a decreased level of consciousness.

• **Encephalitis.** Seizures are an early sign of this disorder, indicating a poor prognosis; they may also occur after recovery as a result of residual damage. Other findings include fever, headache, photophobia, nuchal rigidity, vomiting, aphasia, ataxia, hemiparesis, nystagmus, irritability, cranial nerve palsies (causing facial weakness, ptosis, dysphagia), and myoclonic jerks.

• **Head trauma.** In severe head trauma, generalized seizures occur at the time of injury. (Months later, focal seizures may occur.) Severe head trauma may also cause a decreased level of consciousness leading to coma; soft tissue injury of the face, head, or neck; clear or bloody drainage from the mouth, nose, or ears; facial edema; bony deformity of the face, head, or neck; Battle's sign; and lack of response to oculocephalic and oculovestibular stimulation. Motor and sensory deficits may occur along with altered respirations. Examination may reveal signs of increasing intracranial pressure, such as decreased response to painful stimuli, nonreactive pupils, bradycardia, increased systolic pressure, and widening pulse pressure. If the patient is conscious, he may have visual deficits, behavioral changes, and headache.

● *Hepatic encephalopathy.* Late in this disorder, generalized seizures may occur. Associated late-stage findings in the comatose patient include fetor hepaticus, asterixis, hyperactive deep tendon reflexes, and a positive Babinski's sign.

● *Hypertensive encephalopathy.* This life-threatening disorder may cause seizures, along with severely increased blood pressure, decreased level of consciousness, intense headache, vomiting, transient blindness, paralysis, and (eventually) Cheyne-Stokes respirations.

● *Hypoglycemia.* Generalized seizures usually occur in late stages of severe hypoglycemia. Accompanying findings include blurred or double vision, motor weakness, hemiplegia, trembling, excessive diaphoresis, tachycardia, myoclonic twitching, and decreased level of consciousness.

● *Hyponatremia.* Seizures develop when serum sodium levels fall below 125 mEq/liter. Hyponatremia also causes postural hypotension, headache, muscle twitching and weakness, fatigue, oliguria or anuria, cold and clammy skin, decreased skin turgor, irritability, lethargy, confusion, and stupor or coma. Excessive thirst, tachycardia, nausea, vomiting, and abdominal cramps may also occur. Severe hyponatremia may cause cyanosis and vasomotor collapse, with a thready pulse.

● *Hypoparathyroidism.* Worsening tetany causes generalized seizures. Chronic hypoparathyroidism produces neuromuscular irritability and hyperactive deep tendon reflexes.

● *Hypoxic encephalopathy.* Besides generalized seizures, this disorder may produce myoclonic jerks and coma. Later, if the patient has recovered, dementia, visual agnosia, choreoathetosis, and ataxia may occur.

● *Idiopathic epilepsy.* Frequently, the cause of recurrent seizures is unknown.

● *Intermittent acute porphyria.* Generalized seizures are a late sign of this disorder, indicating severe CNS involvement. This disorder also causes severe abdominal pain, tachycardia, psychotic behavior, muscle weakness, and sensory loss in the trunk.

● *Multiple sclerosis.* This disorder rarely produces generalized seizures. Characteristic findings include vision deficits, paresthesias, constipation, muscle weakness, paralysis, spasticity, hyperreflexia, intention tremor, ataxic gait, dysphagia, dysarthria, impotence, and emotional lability. There may be urinary frequency, urgency, and incontinence.

● *Neurofibromatosis.* Multiple brain lesions in this disorder cause focal and generalized seizures. Inspection reveals café-au-lait spots, multiple skin tumors, scoliosis, and kyphoscoliosis. Related findings: dizziness, ataxia, monocular blindness, and nystagmus.

● *Sarcoidosis.* Lesions may affect the brain, causing generalized and focal seizures. Associated findings include a nonproductive cough with dyspnea, substernal pain, malaise, fatigue, arthralgia, myalgia, weight loss, tachypnea, dysphagia, skin lesions, and impaired vision.

Other causes

● *Diagnostic tests.* Contrast agents used in radiologic tests may cause generalized seizures.

● *Drugs.* Toxic blood levels of aminophylline, theophylline, lidocaine, meperidine, penicillins, and cimetidine may cause generalized seizures. Phenothiazines, tricyclic antidepressants, alprostadil, amphetamines, isoniazid, and vincristine may cause seizures in patients with preexisting epilepsy.

Special considerations

Closely monitor the patient after the seizure, remaining alert for recurring seizure activity. Prepare him for a computed tomography scan and electroencephalography.

Emphasize strict compliance with drug therapy, and warn the patient about side effects. Stress the importance of regular follow-up appointments for blood studies and of having his family observe and record his seizure activity to ensure proper treatment.

Pediatric pointers

Generalized seizures are common in children. In fact, between 75% and 90% of epileptic patients experience their first seizure before age 20. Many children between the ages of 3 months and 3 years experience generalized seizures associated with fever; some of these children later develop seizures without fever. Generalized seizures may also stem from inborn errors of metabolism, perinatal injury, brain infections, Reye's syndrome, Sturge-Weber syndrome, arteriovenous malformation, lead poisoning, hypoglycemia, and idiopathic causes. Rarely, the pertussis component of the DPT vaccine causes seizures.

Seizure—Psychomotor

[Complex partial seizure, temporal lobe seizure]

A psychomotor seizure occurs when a focal seizure begins in the temporal lobe and causes an alteration in consciousness—usually confusion. A psychomotor seizure can occur at any age, but incidence usually increases during adolescence and adulthood. Two thirds of patients also have generalized seizures.

Typically, an aura—most often a complex hallucination or illusion—precedes a psychomotor seizure. The hallucination may be audiovisual (images with sounds), auditory (abnormal or normal sounds or voices from the patient's past), or olfactory (unpleasant smells, such as rotten eggs or burning materials). Other types of auras include feelings of déjà vu, unfamiliarity with surroundings, or depersonalization. Some patients become fearful or anxious or have an unpleasant feeling in the epigastric region that rises toward the chest and throat. The patient usually recognizes the aura and lies down before losing consciousness.

A period of unresponsiveness follows the aura. The patient may experience automatisms, appear dazed and wander aimlessly, perform inappropriate acts (such as undressing in public), be unresponsive, utter incoherent phrases, or, rarely, go into a rage or tantrum. After the seizure, he's confused, drowsy, and amnesic for the seizure. Behavioral automatisms rarely last longer than 5 minutes, but postseizure confusion and amnesia may persist.

Between attacks, the patient may exhibit slow and rigid thinking, outbursts of anger and aggressiveness, tedious conversation, a preoccupation with naive philosophical ideas, diminished libido, mood swings, and paranoid tendencies.

Assessment

If you witness a psychomotor seizure, notify the patient's doctor so he can observe it. Never attempt to restrain the patient. Instead, lead him gently to a safe area. (*Exception*: Don't approach him if he's angry or violent.) Calmly encourage him to sit down, and remain with him until he's fully alert. After the seizure, ask the patient if he experienced an aura. Remember to record all your observations and findings.

Medical causes

● *Brain abscess.* If the brain abscess is in the temporal lobe, psychomotor seizures commonly occur in the acute phase or after the abscess disappears.

Related effects may include headache, nausea, vomiting, generalized seizures, and a decreased level of consciousness. The patient may also have central facial weakness, auditory receptive aphasia, hemiparesis, and ocular disturbances.

• *Head trauma.* Severe trauma to the temporal lobe (especially from a penetrating injury) can produce psychomotor seizures months or years later. The seizures may decrease in frequency and eventually stop. Head trauma also causes generalized seizures and behavior and personality changes.

• *Herpes simplex encephalitis.* If the herpes simplex virus attacks the temporal lobe, psychomotor seizures can occur. Other features include fever, headache, coma, and generalized seizures.

• *Temporal lobe tumor.* Psychomotor seizures may be the first sign of this disorder. Other associated signs and symptoms include headache, pupillary changes, and mental dullness. Increased intracranial pressure may cause a decreased level of consciousness, vomiting, and possible papilledema.

Special considerations

After the seizure, remain with the patient to reorient him to his surroundings and to protect him from injury. Keep him in bed until he's fully alert, and remove harmful objects. Offer emotional support to the patient and his family, and teach them how to cope with seizures.

Prepare the patient for diagnostic tests, such as electroencephalography and computed tomography scans.

Pediatric pointers

Psychomotor seizures in children may resemble absence seizures. They can result from birth injury, abuse, infections, or neoplasms. In about one third of patients, their cause is unknown.

Repeated psychomotor seizures commonly lead to generalized seizures. Typically, the child wanders aimlessly (an automatism) during a seizure and may develop frightening hallucinations.

Setting-Sun Sign

[Sunset eyes]

Setting-sun sign describes the position of an infant's or young child's eyes as a result of pressure on cranial nerves III, IV, and VI. Both eyes are forced downward so that an area of sclera shows above the irises; in some patients, the irises appear to be forced outward.

Setting-sun sign reflects increased intracranial pressure (ICP). Typically, increased ICP results from space-occupying lesions—such as tumors—or from an accumulation of fluid in the brain's ventricular system, as occurs in hydrocephalus. It also results from intracranial bleeding or cerebral edema.

Setting-sun sign may be intermittent—for example, it may disappear when the infant is upright, because this position slightly reduces ICP. The sign may be elicited in a normal infant under age 4 weeks by suddenly changing his head position. It can also be elicited in a normal infant up to age 9 months by placing a bright light before his eyes and removing it quickly.

Assessment

If you observe the setting-sun sign in an infant, notify the doctor and assess the infant's neurologic status. Then obtain a brief history from the parents. Has the infant had a fall or even a minor trauma? When did this sign appear? Ask about early nonspecific signs of increasing ICP: has the infant's sucking reflex diminished? Is he irritable, restless, or unusually tired? Does he cry when moved? Is his cry high-pitched?

Now perform a physical examination, keeping in mind that neurologic responses are primarily reflexive during early infancy. Assess the infant's level of consciousness. Is he awake, irritable, or lethargic? Does he reach for a bright object or turn toward the sound of a music box? Observe his posture for normal flexion and extension or opisthotonos. Examine muscle tone, and observe for seizure automatisms.

Examine the infant's anterior fontanelle for bulging, measure his head circumference, and observe his breathing pattern. (Cheyne-Stokes respirations may accompany increased ICP.) Also check his pupillary response to light: unilateral or bilateral dilation occurs as ICP rises. Finally, elicit reflexes—diminished in increased ICP, especially Moro's reflex. Keep endotracheal intubation equipment available.

Medical cause

● *Increased ICP.* Transient or intermittent setting-sun sign often occurs late in increased ICP. The infant may have bulging, widened fontanelles, increased head circumference, and widened sutures. He may also exhibit a decreased level of consciousness, behavioral changes, high-pitched cry, pupillary abnormalities, and impaired motor movement. Other findings: increased systolic pressure, widened pulse pressure, bradycardia, changes in breathing pattern, vomiting, and seizures as ICP increases.

Special considerations

Nursing care of the infant with setting-sun sign includes monitoring of vital signs and neurologic status. Elevate the head of the crib, and monitor intake and output. If ordered, monitor ICP, restrict fluids, and insert an I.V. line to administer diuretics and corticosteroids. For severely increased ICP, the doctor may order endotracheal intubation and mechanical hyperventilation to reduce serum carbon dioxide levels and constrict cerebral vessels, or barbiturate coma or hypothermia therapy to lower metabolic rate.

Try to maintain a calm environment, and when the infant's crying, comfort him to help prevent stress-related ICP elevations. Encourage the parents' help, and offer emotional support.

IDENTIFYING SETTING-SUN SIGN

In this late sign of increased ICP in a young child, pressure on cranial nerves III, IV, and VI forces the eyes downward. As a result, a rim of sclera appears above the irises.

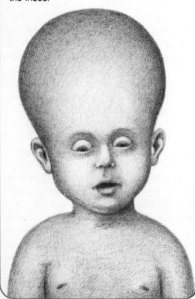

Shallow Respirations

Respirations are shallow when a diminished volume of air enters the lungs during inspiration. In an effort to obtain enough air, the patient with shallow respirations usually breathes at an accelerated rate. However, as he tires or as his muscles weaken, this compensatory increase in respirations diminishes, leading to inadequate gas exchange and such signs as dyspnea, cyanosis, confusion, agitation, loss of consciousness, and tachycardia.

Shallow respirations may develop suddenly or gradually and may last briefly or become chronic. They're a key sign of respiratory distress and neurologic deterioration. Causes include inadequate central respiratory control over breathing, neuromuscular disorders, increased resistance to airflow into the lungs, respiratory muscle fatigue or weakness, voluntary alterations in breathing, and decreased activity from prolonged bed rest.

Assessment

If you observe shallow respirations, be alert for impending respiratory failure or arrest. Is the patient severely dyspneic? Agitated or frightened? Look for signs of airway obstruction. If the patient's choking, perform a series of four back blows, then four abdominal thrusts, to try to expel the foreign object. Use suction if secretions occlude the patient's airway.

If the patient's also wheezing, check for stridor, nasal flaring, and use of accessory muscles. Administer oxygen with a face mask or an Ambu bag. Notify the doctor at once, and attempt to calm the patient. Administer epinephrine I.V., as ordered.

If the patient loses consciousness, insert an artificial airway and prepare for endotracheal intubation and ventilatory support. Measure his tidal volume and minute volume with a Wright respirometer to determine the need for mechanical ventilation. (See *Measuring Lung Volumes,* page 674.) Check arterial blood gas (ABG) levels, heart rate, and blood pressure. Tachycardia, increased or decreased blood pressure, poor minute volume, and deteriorating ABGs signal the need for intubation and mechanical ventilation.

If the patient isn't in severe respiratory distress, begin with the history. Ask about chronic illness and any surgery or trauma. Has the patient had a tetanus booster in the past 10 years? Does he have asthma, allergies, or a history of heart failure or vascular dis-

ease? Does he have chronic respiratory disorders or infections, or neurologic or neuromuscular disease? Does he smoke? Obtain a medication history, too, and explore the possibility of drug abuse.

Ask about the patient's shallow respirations: when did they begin? How long do they last? What makes them subside? What aggravates them? Ask about changes in appetite, weight, activity level, and behavior.

Begin the physical examination by assessing the patient's level of consciousness and his orientation to time, person, and place. Observe spontaneous movements, and test muscle strength and deep tendon reflexes. Next, inspect the chest for deformities or abnormal movements, such as intercostal retractions. Inspect the extremities for cyanosis and digital clubbing.

Now, palpate for expansion and diaphragmatic tactile fremitus, and percuss for hyperresonance or dullness. Auscultate for diminished, absent, or adventitious breath sounds and for abnormal or distant heart sounds. Do you note any peripheral edema? Finally, examine the abdomen for distention, tenderness, or masses.

Medical causes

● *Adult respiratory distress syndrome.* Initially, this life-threatening syndrome produces rapid, shallow respirations and dyspnea, at times after the patient appears stable. Hypoxemia leads to intercostal and suprasternal retractions, diaphoresis, and fluid accumulation, causing rhonchi and crackles. As hypoxemia worsens, the patient has increased breathing difficulty, restlessness, apprehension, decreased level of consciousness, cyanosis, and possibly tachycardia.

● *Amyotrophic lateral sclerosis (ALS).* Respiratory muscle weakness in this disorder causes progressive shallow respirations. Exertion may result in increased weakness and respiratory distress. ALS initially produces upper extremity muscle weakness and wast-

MEASURING LUNG VOLUMES

Use a Wright respirometer to measure tidal volume (the amount of air inspired with each breath) and minute volume (the volume of air inspired in a minute—or tidal volume multiplied by respiratory rate). You can connect the respirometer to an intubated patient's airway via an endotracheal tube (shown here) or a tracheostomy tube. If the patient isn't intubated, connect it to a face mask, making sure the seal over the patient's mouth and nose is airtight.

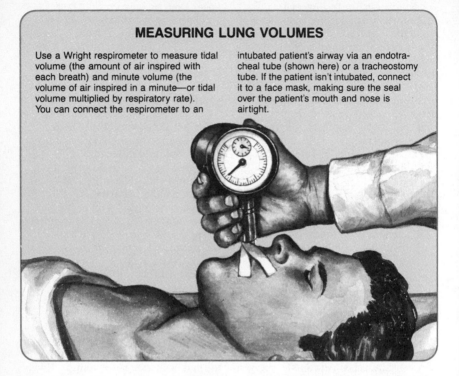

ing that, within several years, affect the trunk, neck, tongue, and muscles of the larynx, pharynx, and lower extremities. Associated signs and symptoms include muscle cramps and atrophy, hyperreflexia, slight spasticity of the legs, coarse fasciculations of the affected muscle, impaired speech, and difficulty chewing and swallowing.

● *Asthma.* In this disorder, bronchospasm and hyperinflation of the lungs cause rapid, shallow respirations. In adults, mild persistent signs and symptoms may worsen during severe attacks. Related respiratory effects include wheezing, rhonchi, a productive cough, dyspnea, prolonged expirations, intercostal and supraclavicular retractions on inspiration, nasal flaring, and use of accessory muscles. Chest tightness, tachycardia, diaphoresis, and flushing or cyanosis may occur.

● *Atelectasis.* Decreased lung expansion or pleuritic pain causes sudden onset of rapid, shallow respirations. Other signs and symptoms may include a dry cough, dyspnea, tachycardia, anxiety, cyanosis, and diaphoresis. Examination reveals dullness to percussion, decreased breath sounds and vocal fremitus, inspiratory lag, and substernal or intercostal retractions.

● *Botulism.* In this disorder, progressive muscle weakness and paralysis initially cause shallow respirations. Within 4 days, the patient develops respiratory distress from respiratory muscle paralysis. Early signs and symptoms include bilateral mydriasis and nonreactive pupils, anorexia, nausea, vomiting, diarrhea, dry mouth, blurred vision, diplopia, ptosis, strabismus, and extraocular muscle palsies. Others quickly follow: vertigo, deafness, hoarseness, constipation, nasal voice, dysarthria, and dysphagia.

● *Bronchiectasis.* Increased secretions obstruct airflow in the lungs, leading to shallow respirations and a productive cough with copious, foul-smelling, mucopurulent sputum (a classic finding). Other findings include hemoptysis, wheezes, rhonchi, coarse crackles during inspiration, and late-stage clubbing. The patient may complain of weight loss, fatigue, weakness and dyspnea on exertion, fever, malaise, and halitosis.

• *Chronic bronchitis.* Airway obstruction causes chronic shallow respirations. This disorder may begin with a nonproductive, hacking cough that later becomes productive. It may also cause prolonged expirations, wheezing, dyspnea, accessory muscle use, barrel chest, cyanosis, tachypnea, scattered rhonchi, coarse crackles, and clubbing (a late sign).

• *Coma.* Rapid, shallow respirations result from neurologic dysfunction or restricted chest movement.

• *Emphysema.* Increased breathing effort causes muscle fatigue, leading to chronic shallow respirations. The patient may also display dyspnea, anorexia, malaise, tachypnea, diminished breath sounds, cyanosis, pursed-lip breathing, accessory muscle use, barrel chest, chronic productive cough, and clubbing (a late sign).

• *Flail chest.* In this disorder, decreased air movement results in rapid, shallow respirations, paradoxical chest wall motion from rib instability, tachycardia, hypotension, ecchymoses, cyanosis, and pain over the affected area.

• *Guillain-Barré syndrome.* Progressive ascending paralysis causes rapid or progressive onset of shallow respirations. Muscle weakness begins in the lower limbs and extends finally to the face. Associated findings include paresthesias, dysarthria, diminished or absent corneal reflex, nasal speech, dysphagia, ipsilateral loss of facial muscle control, and flaccid paralysis.

• *Kyphoscoliosis.* Skeletal cage distortion can eventually cause rapid, shallow respirations from reduced lung capacity. It also causes back pain, fatigue, tracheal deviation, and dyspnea.

• *Multiple sclerosis.* Muscle weakness causes progressive shallow respirations. Early features may include diplopia, blurred vision, and paresthesias. Other possible findings are nystagmus, constipation, paralysis, spasticity, hyperreflexia, intention tremor, ataxic gait, dysphagia, dysarthria, urinary dysfunction, impotence, and emotional lability.

• *Muscular dystrophy.* With progressive thoracic deformity and muscle weakness, shallow respirations may occur along with waddling gait, contractures, scoliosis, lordosis, and muscle atrophy or hypertrophy.

• *Myasthenia gravis.* Progression of this disorder causes respiratory muscle weakness marked by shallow respirations, dyspnea, and cyanosis. Other effects: fatigue, weak eye closure, ptosis, diplopia, and difficulty chewing and swallowing.

• *Parkinson's disease.* Fatigue and weakness lead to progressive shallow respirations. Typically, this disorder slowly progresses to increased rigidity (lead-pipe or cogwheel), masklike facies, stooped posture, shuffling gait, dysphagia, drooling, dysarthria, and pill-rolling tremor.

• *Pleural effusion.* In this disorder, restricted lung expansion causes shallow respirations, beginning suddenly or gradually. Other findings: nonproductive cough, weight loss, dyspnea, and pleuritic chest pain. Examination reveals pleural friction rub, tachycardia, tachypnea, decreased chest motion, flatness to percussion, egophony, decreased or absent breath sounds, and decreased tactile fremitus.

• *Pneumonia.* Pulmonary consolidation results in rapid, shallow respirations. The patient may have dyspnea, fever, shaking chills, chest pain, cough, tachycardia, decreased breath sounds, crackles, and rhonchi. He may also have myalgias, fatigue, anorexia, headache, abdominal pain, cyanosis, and diaphoresis.

• *Pneumothorax.* This disorder causes sudden onset of shallow respirations and dyspnea. Related effects are tachycardia; tachypnea; sudden sharp, severe chest pain (often unilateral) worsening with movement; nonproductive cough; cyanosis; accessory muscle use; asymmetrical chest expansion; anxiety; restlessness; hyperresonance or tympany on the affected side; subcutaneous crepitation; decreased vocal fremitus; and diminished or absent breath sounds on the affected side.

● *Pulmonary edema.* Pulmonary vascular congestion causes rapid, shallow respirations. Early signs and symptoms include dyspnea on exertion, paroxysmal nocturnal dyspnea, and a nonproductive cough. Clinical features also include tachycardia, tachypnea, dependent crackles, and a ventricular gallop. Severe pulmonary edema produces more rapid and labored respirations; widespread crackles; a productive cough with frothy, bloody sputum; worsening tachycardia; dysrhythmias; cold, clammy skin; cyanosis; hypotension; and thready pulse.

● *Pulmonary embolism.* This disorder causes sudden rapid, shallow respirations and severe dyspnea with anginal or pleuritic chest pain. Other clinical features include tachycardia, tachypnea, a nonproductive cough or a productive cough with blood-tinged sputum, low-grade fever, restlessness, diaphoresis, pleural friction rub, crackles, diffuse wheezing, dullness to percussion, decreased breath sounds, and signs of circulatory collapse. Less common findings are massive hemoptysis, chest splinting, leg edema, and (with a large embolus) cyanosis, syncope, and distended neck veins.

● *Spinal cord injury.* Diaphragmatic breathing and shallow respirations may occur in injury to the C5 to C8 area. Other findings include quadriplegia with flaccidity followed by spastic paralysis, areflexia, hypotension, sensory loss below the level of injury, and bowel and bladder incontinence.

● *Tetanus.* In this now-rare disorder, spasm of the intercostal muscles and the diaphragm causes shallow respirations. Late findings typically include jaw pain and stiffening, difficulty opening the mouth, tachycardia, profuse diaphoresis, hyperactive deep tendon reflexes, and opisthotonos.

● *Upper airway obstruction.* Partial airway obstruction causes acute shallow respirations with sudden gagging and dry, paroxysmal coughing; hoarseness; stridor; and tachycardia. Other findings: dyspnea, decreased breath sounds, wheezing, and cyanosis.

Other causes

● *Drugs.* Narcotics, sedatives and hypnotics, tranquilizers, neuromuscular blockers, magnesium sulfate, and anesthetics can produce slow, shallow respirations.

● *Surgery.* After abdominal or thoracic surgery, pain associated with chest splinting and decreased chest wall motion may cause shallow respirations.

Special considerations

Prepare the patient for diagnostic tests: ABG analysis, pulmonary function tests, chest X-rays, or bronchoscopy.

Position the patient as nearly upright as possible to ease his breathing. (Help a postoperative patient splint his incision while coughing.) If he's taking a drug that depresses respirations, follow all precautions, and monitor him closely. Ensure adequate hydration, and use humidification as needed to thin secretions and to relieve inflamed, dry, or irritated airway mucosa. As ordered, administer humidified oxygen, bronchodilators, mucolytics, expectorants, or antibiotics.

Have the patient cough and deep-breathe every hour to clear secretions and to counteract possible hypoventilation. Turn him frequently. He may require chest physiotherapy, incentive spirometry, or intermittent positive-pressure breathing.

Pediatric pointers

In children, shallow respirations commonly indicate a life-threatening condition. Airway obstruction can occur rapidly; if it does, administer back blows or chest thrusts but *not* abdominal thrusts, which can damage internal organs.

Causes of shallow respirations in infants and children may include idiopathic (infant) respiratory distress syndrome, acute epiglottitis, diphtheria, aspiration of a foreign body, croup, acute bronchiolitis, cystic fibrosis, and bacterial pneumonia.

Observe the child to detect apnea. As needed, use humidification and suction, and administer supplemental oxygen. Give parenteral fluids to ensure adequate hydration. Chest physiotherapy may be required.

Skin—Bronze

The result of excess circulating melanin, a bronze skin tone tends to appear at pressure points—such as the knuckles, elbows, toes, and knees—and in creases on the palms and soles. Eventually, this hyperpigmentation may extend to the buccal mucosa and gums before covering the entire body. It may stem from endocrine disorders, malnutrition, biliary cirrhosis, and certain drugs.

Because bronzing develops gradually, it's sometimes mistaken for a suntan. However, the hyperpigmentation can affect the entire body, not just sun-exposed areas: sun exposure deepens the bronze color of exposed areas, but this effect gradually fades. In fair-skinned patients, the bronze tone can range from light to dark. It also varies with the disorder.

Assessment
Begin by asking the patient when the hyperpigmentation first appeared. Has its hue changed? When was he last exposed to the sun? Also ask about a history of infection, illness, surgery, or trauma. Does he have abdominal pain, weakness, fatigue, diarrhea, or constipation? Has he lost weight recently? If the patient's receiving maintenance

therapy for adrenal insufficiency, has his dosage been increased?

Examine the mucosa, gums, and scars for hyperpigmentation. Check for signs of dehydration and for abdominal distention, loss of body hair, and tissue and muscle wasting. Palpate for hepatosplenomegaly.

Medical causes
• *Adrenal hyperplasia.* In this disorder, the entire skin assumes a dark bronze tone within a few months. Other findings include visual field deficits and headache, resulting from an expanding pituitary lesion, and signs of androgen excess in females—clitoral enlargement and male distribution patterns of hair, fat, and muscle. Congenital adrenal hyperplasia causes irregular menses.

• *Adrenal insufficiency.* In this disorder, bronze skin is a classic sign that may precede other features of hypoadrenalism by many years. Other findings may include axillary and pubic hair loss, vitiligo, progressive fatigue, weakness, anorexia, nausea and vomiting, weight loss, orthostatic hypotension, weak and irregular pulse, abdominal pain, irritability, diarrhea or constipation, decreased libido, amenorrhea, and syncope. Enhanced taste, smell, and hearing may also occur.

• *Biliary cirrhosis.* This disorder causes bronze skin from melanosis of exposed areas of jaundiced skin: eyelids, palms, neck, and chest or back. Other findings: generalized pruritus, weakness, fatigue, jaundice, dark urine, pale stools with steatorrhea, decreased appetite with weight loss, and hepatomegaly.

• *Hemochromatosis.* An early sign is progressive, generalized bronzing accented by metallic gray-bronze skin on sun-exposed areas, genitals, and scars. Mucous membranes are affected less often. Early associated effects include weakness, lethargy, weight loss, abdominal pain, loss of libido, and polydipsia and polyuria. Later findings include hepatosplenomegaly, spider angiomas, joint swelling and tenderness, ascites, jaundice, edema, dysrhythmias, loss of body hair, and testicular atrophy.

• *Malnutrition.* As weight loss depletes body nutrients, bronzing develops along with apathy, lethargy, anorexia, weakness, and slow pulse and respirations. Other findings include paresthesias in the extremities; dull, sparse, dry hair; brittle nails; dark, swollen cheeks; dry, flaky skin; red, swollen lips; muscle wasting; and gonadal atrophy in males.

Other causes
• *Drugs.* Prolonged therapy with high doses of phenothiazines may cause gradual bronzing of the skin.

Special considerations
Prepare the patient for the ACTH stimulation test, thyroid function studies, CBC, electrolyte analysis, electrocardiography, and a computed tomography scan of the pituitary.

Pediatric pointers
Celiac disease can cause bronze skin in young children. Bronzing begins with the introduction of cereals and usually subsides later in childhood or adolescence. It also stems from adrenoleukodystrophy, a rare but life-threatening X-linked recessive disorder that affects boys and young men.

Skin—Clammy

Clammy skin—moist, cool, and often pale—is a sympathetic response to stress, which triggers release of the hormones epinephrine and norepinephrine. These hormones cause cutaneous vasoconstriction and secretion of cold sweat from eccrine glands, particularly on the palms, forehead, and soles.

Clammy skin typically accompanies shock, acute hypoglycemia, anxiety reactions, dysrhythmias, and heat exhaustion. It also occurs as a vasovagal reaction to severe pain associated with nausea, anorexia, epigastric distress, hyperpnea, tachypnea, weakness, confusion, tachycardia, and pupillary dilation or a combination of these findings. Marked bradycardia and syncope may follow.

Assessment
If you detect clammy skin, remember that rapid assessment and intervention are paramount. (See *Clammy Skin: A Key Finding.*) For example, ask about a history of insulin-dependent diabetes mellitus or cardiac disorders. Is the patient currently taking any medications, especially antiarrhythmics? Is he experiencing pain, nausea, or epigastric distress? Does he feel weak? Does he have a dry mouth? Diarrhea or increased urination?

Next, examine the pupils for dilation. Also check for abdominal distention and increased muscle tension.

Medical causes
• *Acute hypoglycemia.* Generalized cool, clammy skin or diaphoresis may accompany irritability, tremors, palpitations, hunger, headache, tachycardia, and anxiety. Central nervous system disturbances may include blurred vision, diplopia, confusion, motor weakness, hemiplegia, or coma.
• *Anxiety.* An acute anxiety attack often produces cold, clammy skin on the forehead, palms, and soles. Other features may include pallor, dry mouth, tachycardia or bradycardia, palpitations, and hypertension or hypotension. The patient may also have tremors, breathlessness, headache, muscle tension, nausea, vomiting, abdominal distention, diarrhea, increased urination, and sharp chest pain.
• *Cardiogenic shock.* Generalized cool, moist, pale skin accompanies confusion and restlessness, hypotension, tachycardia, tachypnea, narrowing pulse pressure, cyanosis, and oliguria.
• *Dysrhythmias.* Cardiac dysrhythmias may produce generalized cool, clammy

skin, mental status changes, dizziness, and hypotension.

• *Heat exhaustion.* In the acute stage, generalized cold, clammy skin accompanies an ashen-gray appearance, headache, confusion, syncope, giddiness, and a normal or subnormal temperature. The patient may have a rapid and thready pulse, nausea, vomiting, tachypnea, oliguria, thirst, muscle cramps, and hypotension.

• *Hypovolemic shock.* In this common form of shock, generalized pale, cold, clammy skin accompanies subnormal body temperature, hypotension with narrowing pulse pressure, tachycardia, tachypnea, and rapid, thready pulse. Other findings are flat neck veins, prolonged capillary refill time, decreased urine output, confusion, and decreased level of consciousness.

• *Septic shock.* The cold shock stage causes generalized cold, clammy skin. Associated findings include rapid and

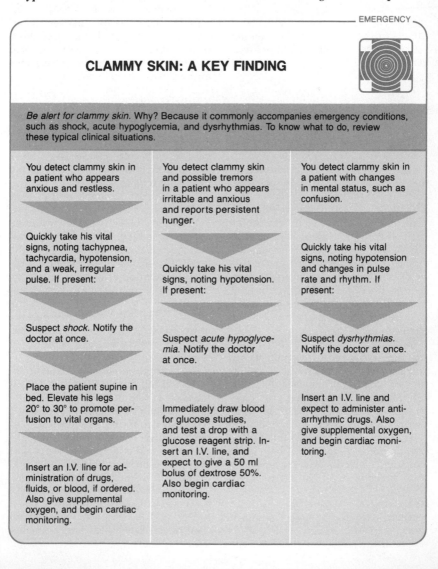

EMERGENCY

CLAMMY SKIN: A KEY FINDING

Be alert for clammy skin. Why? Because it commonly accompanies emergency conditions, such as shock, acute hypoglycemia, and dysrhythmias. To know what to do, review these typical clinical situations.

You detect clammy skin in a patient who appears anxious and restless.

Quickly take his vital signs, noting tachypnea, tachycardia, hypotension, and a weak, irregular pulse. If present:

Suspect *shock.* Notify the doctor at once.

Place the patient supine in bed. Elevate his legs 20° to 30° to promote perfusion to vital organs.

Insert an I.V. line for administration of drugs, fluids, or blood, if ordered. Also give supplemental oxygen, and begin cardiac monitoring.

You detect clammy skin and possible tremors in a patient who appears irritable and anxious and reports persistent hunger.

Quickly take his vital signs, noting hypotension. If present:

Suspect *acute hypoglycemia.* Notify the doctor at once.

Immediately draw blood for glucose studies, and test a drop with a glucose reagent strip. Insert an I.V. line, and expect to give a 50 ml bolus of dextrose 50%. Also begin cardiac monitoring.

You detect clammy skin in a patient with changes in mental status, such as confusion.

Quickly take his vital signs, noting hypotension and changes in pulse rate and rhythm. If present:

Suspect *dysrhythmias.* Notify the doctor at once.

Insert an I.V. line and expect to administer antiarrhythmic drugs. Also give supplemental oxygen, and begin cardiac monitoring.

thready pulse, severe hypotension, persistent oliguria or anuria, and respiratory failure.

Special considerations
Take the patient's vital signs frequently, and monitor urine output. If clammy skin occurs with an anxiety reaction or pain, offer the patient emotional support, administer pain medication as ordered, and provide a quiet environment.

Pediatric pointers
Infants in shock will not have clammy skin because of their immature sweat glands.

Skin—Mottled

Mottled skin is patchy discoloration indicating primary or secondary changes of the deep, middle, or superficial dermal blood vessels. It can result from hematologic, immune, or connective tissue disorders; chronic occlusive arterial disease; dysproteinemias; immobility; exposure to heat or cold; or shock. Or it can be a normal reaction, such as the diffuse mottling (cutis marmorata) that occurs when exposure to cold causes venous stasis in cutaneous blood vessels.

Mottling that occurs with other signs and symptoms most often affects the extremities, usually indicating restricted blood flow. For example, livedo reticularis, a characteristic network pattern of reddish blue discoloration, occurs when vasospasm of the mid-dermal blood vessels slows local blood flow in dilated superficial capillaries and small veins. Shock causes mottling from systemic vasoconstriction.

Assessment
Mottled skin may indicate an emergency condition requiring rapid assessment and intervention. (See *Mot-* *tled Skin: Know What to Do.*) However, if the patient isn't in distress, ask if the mottling began suddenly or gradually. What precipitated it? How long has he had it? Does anything make it go away? Does the patient have other symptoms, such as pain, numbness, or tingling in an extremity? If so, do they disappear with temperature changes?

Observe the patient's skin color, and palpate his arms and legs for skin texture, swelling, and temperature differences between extremities. Also palpate for the presence (or absence) of pulses and for their quality. Note breaks in the skin, muscle appearance, and hair distribution. Also assess motor and sensory function.

Medical causes
• *Acrocyanosis.* In this rare disorder, anxiety or exposure to cold can cause vasospasm in small cutaneous arterioles. This results in persistent symmetrical blue and red mottling of the affected hands and feet.

• *Acute arterial occlusion.* Initial signs include temperature and color changes. Pallor may change to blotchy cyanosis and livedo reticularis. Color and temperature demarcation develop at the level of obstruction. Other effects include sudden onset of pain in the extremity, and possibly paresthesias, paresis, and a sensation of cold in the affected area. Examination reveals diminished or absent pulses, prolonged capillary refill time, and diminished reflexes.

• *Arteriosclerosis obliterans.* Atherosclerotic buildup narrows intraarterial lumens, resulting in reduced blood flow through the affected artery. Obstructed blood flow to the extremities (most often the lower) produces such peripheral signs and symptoms as leg pallor, cyanosis, blotchy erythema, and livedo reticularis. Related findings include intermittent claudication (most common symptom), diminished or absent pedal pulses, and leg coolness. Other symptoms include coldness and paresthesias.

• *Buerger's disease.* This form of vasculitis produces unilateral or asymmetrical color changes and mottling, particularly livedo networking in the lower extremities. It also typically causes intermittent claudication and erythema along extremity blood vessels. During exposure to cold, the feet are cold, cyanotic, and numb; later they're hot, red, and tingling. Other findings: impaired peripheral pulses and peripheral neuropathy.

• *Cryoglobulinemia.* This necrotizing disorder causes patchy livedo reticularis, petechiae, and ecchymoses. Other findings include fever, chills, urticaria, melena, skin ulcers, epistaxis, Raynaud's phenomenon, eye hemorrhages, hematuria, and gangrene.

• *Hypovolemic shock.* Vasoconstriction from shock commonly produces skin mottling, initially in the knees and elbows. As shock worsens, mottling becomes generalized. Early signs: sudden onset of pallor, cool skin, restlessness, thirst, tachypnea, and slight tachycardia. As shock progresses, associated findings include cool, clammy skin; rapid, thready pulse; hypotension; narrowed pulse pressure; decreased urine output; subnormal temperature; confusion; and decreased level of consciousness.

• *Idiopathic or primary livedo reticularis.* Symmetrical, diffuse, initially asymptomatic mottling can involve the hands, feet, arms, legs, buttocks, and trunk. Initially, networking is intermittent and most pronounced on exposure to cold or stress; eventually, mottling persists even with warming.

• *Periarteritis nodosa.* Cutaneous findings may include asymmetrical, patchy livedo reticularis, palpable nodules along the distribution of medium-sized arteries, erythema, purpura, muscle wasting, ulcers, gangrene, and peripheral neuropathy.

• *Polycythemia vera.* This hematologic disorder produces livedo reticularis, hemangiomas, purpura, rubor, ulcerative nodules, and scleroderma-like lesions. Other symptoms include head-

ache, a vague feeling of fullness in the head, dizziness, vertigo, visual disturbances, dyspnea, and pruritus.

• *Rheumatoid arthritis.* This disorder may cause skin mottling. Early nonspecific signs and symptoms progress to joint pain and stiffness with subcutaneous nodules, most commonly on the elbows.

• *Systemic lupus erythematosus.* This connective tissue disorder can cause livedo reticularis, most commonly on the outer arms. Other signs and symptoms may include a butterfly rash, nondeforming joint pain and stiffness, photosensitivity, Raynaud's phenomenon, patchy alopecia, seizures, fever, anorexia, weight loss, lymphadenopathy, and emotional lability.

Other causes

• *Immobility.* Prolonged immobility may cause bluish, asymptomatic mottling, most noticeably in dependent extremities.

● *Thermal exposure.* Prolonged thermal exposure, as from a heating pad or hot water bottle, may cause erythema abigne—a localized, reticulated, brown-to-red mottling.

Special considerations
Typically, mottled skin results from chronic conditions. Teach patients to avoid tight clothing and overexposure to cold or to heating devices, such as hot water bottles and heating pads.

Pediatric pointers
Mottled skin in children stems from the same causes as in adults. A common cause in children is systemic vasoconstriction from shock.

Skin—Scaly

Scaly skin results when cells of the uppermost skin layer (stratum corneum) desiccate and shed, causing excessive accumulation of loosely adherent flakes of normal or abnormal keratin. Normally, skin cell loss is imperceptible; the appearance of scale indicates increased cell proliferation secondary to altered keratinization.

Scaly skin varies in texture from fine and delicate to branny, coarse, or stratified. Scales are typically dry, brittle, and shiny, but they can be greasy and dull. Their color ranges from whitish gray, yellow, or brown to a silvery sheen.

Usually benign, scaly skin occurs in fungal, bacterial, and viral infections (cutaneous or systemic), in lymphomas, and in lupus erythematosus; it's common in inflammatory skin diseases. A form of scaly skin—generalized fine desquamation—commonly follows prolonged febrile illness, sunburn, or thermal burn. Red patches of scaly skin that appear or worsen in the winter result from dry skin (or from actinic keratosis, common in the elderly). Drugs also cause scaly skin. Aggravating factors include cold, heat, immobility, and frequent bathing.

Assessment
Obtain a history: how long has the patient had scaly skin, and has he had it before? Where did it appear first? Did a lesion or skin eruption, such as erythema, precede it? Has the patient used a topical skin product recently? How often does he bathe? Has he had recent joint pain, illness, or malaise? Ask the patient about work exposure to chemicals, use of prescribed drugs, and a family history of skin disorders. Find out what kinds of soap, cosmetics, skin lotion, and hair preparations the patient uses.

Now examine the entire skin surface. Is it dry, oily, moist, or greasy? Observe the general pattern of skin lesions, and record their location. Note their color, shape, and size. Are they thick or fine? Do they itch? Does the patient have other lesions besides scaly skin? Examine the mucous membranes of his mouth, lips, and nose, and inspect his ears, hair, and nails.

Medical causes
● *Bowen's disease.* This common form of intraepidermal carcinoma causes painless, erythematous plaques that are widely distributed, raised, and indurated with a thick, hyperkeratotic scale and possibly ulcerated centers.

● *Dermatitis. Exfoliative dermatitis* begins with rapidly developing generalized erythema. Desquamation with fine scales or thick sheets of all or most of the skin surface may cause life-threatening hypothermia. Other possible complications include high cardiac output failure and septicemia. Systemic signs and symptoms may include low-grade fever, chills, malaise, lymphadenopathy, and gynecomastia.

In *nummular dermatitis*, round, pustular lesions often ooze purulent exudate, itch severely, and rapidly become encrusted and scaly. Lesions appear on the extensor surfaces of the limbs, posterior trunk, and buttocks.

Seborrheic dermatitis begins with erythematous, scaly papules that progress to larger scaly plaques, possibly involving the genitalia along with the scalp, chest, eyebrows, back, axillae, and umbilicus. Pruritus accompanies the scaling.

• *Dermatophytosis. Tinea capitis* produces lesions with reddened, slightly elevated borders and a central area of dense scaling; these lesions may become inflamed and pus-filled (kerions). Patchy alopecia and itching may also occur. *Tinea pedis* causes scaling and blisters between the toes. The squamous type produces diffuse, fine, branny scaling. Adherent and silvery white, it's most prominent in skin creases and may affect the entire dorsum of the foot. *Tinea corporis* produces crusty lesions. As they enlarge, their centers heal, causing the classic ringworm shape.

• *Discoid lupus erythematosus.* This cutaneous form of lupus may occur without systemic manifestations. Separate or coalescing lesions (macules, papules, or plaques), ranging from pink to purple, are covered with a yellow or brown crust. Enlarged hair follicles are filled with scale. Telangiectasia may be present. After this inflammatory stage, the lesions heal with hypopigmentation or hyperpigmentation and noncontractile scarring and atrophy. The disorder commonly involves the face or sun-exposed areas of the neck, ears, scalp, lips, and oral mucosa. Alopecia may also occur.

• *Lichen planus.* In this disorder, flat, violet lesions with a fine scale most commonly affect the lumbar region, genitalia, ankles, and anterior lower legs.

• *Lymphoma.* Hodgkin's disease and non-Hodgkin's lymphoma commonly cause scaly rashes. *Hodgkin's disease* may cause scaling dermatitis with pruritus that begins in the legs and spreads to the entire body. Remission and re-

currence are common. Small nodules and diffuse pigmentation are related signs. This disorder typically produces painless enlargement of the peripheral lymph nodes. Other signs and symptoms of lymphoma include fever, fatigue, weight loss, malaise, and hepatosplenomegaly.

Non-Hodgkin's lymphoma initially produces erythematous patches with some scaling that later become interspersed with nodules. Pruritus and discomfort are common; later, tumors and ulcers form. Progression produces nontender lymphadenopathy.

• *Parapsoriasis (chronic).* This disorder produces small or moderate-sized papules, with a thin, adherent scale, on the trunk, hands, and feet. Removal of the scale reveals a shiny brown surface.

• *Pityriasis. Pityriasis rosea*—an acute, benign, and self-limiting disorder—produces widespread scales. It begins with an erythematous, raised, oval herald patch anywhere on the body. A few days or weeks later, yellow-tan or erythematous patches with scaly edges erupt on the trunk and limbs and sometimes on the face, hands, and feet. Pruritus also occurs.

Pityriasis rubra pilaris, an uncommon disorder, initially produces seborrheic scaling on the scalp, progressing to the face and ears. Later, scaly red patches develop on the palms and soles, becoming diffuse, thick, fissured, hyperkeratotic, and painful. Lesions also appear on the hands, fingers, wrists, and forearms and then on wide areas of the trunk, neck, and limbs.

• *Psoriasis.* Silvery white, micaceous scales in this disorder cover erythematous plaques that have sharply defined borders. Psoriasis most commonly appears on the scalp, chest, elbows, knees, back, buttocks, and genitals. Associated signs and symptoms include nail pitting, pruritus, arthritis, and sometimes pain from dry, cracked, encrusted lesions.

• *Syphilis (secondary).* Papulosquamous, slightly scaly eruptions characterize this disorder. A ring-shaped pattern of copper-red papules usually forms on the face, arms, palms, soles, chest, back, and abdomen. Systemic signs and symptoms may include lymphadenopathy, malaise, weight loss, anorexia, nausea, vomiting, headache, sore throat, and low-grade fever.

• *Systemic lupus erythematosus.* This disorder produces a bright red maculopapular eruption with fine scales. Patches are sharply defined and involve the nose and malar regions of the face in a butterfly pattern—a primary sign. Similar characteristic rashes appear on other body surfaces; scaling occurs along the lower lip or anterior hair line. Other primary clinical features include photosensitivity, and joint pain and stiffness. Vasculitis can occur—leading to infarctive lesions, necrotic leg ulcers, or digital gangrene—as well as Raynaud's phenomenon, patchy alopecia, and mucous membrane ulcers. The disorder also produces nonspecific systemic effects.

• *Tinea versicolor.* This benign fungal skin infection typically produces macular hypopigmented, fawn-colored, or brown patches of varying sizes and shapes. All are slightly scaly. Lesions frequently affect the upper trunk, arms, and lower abdomen, sometimes the neck and, rarely, the face.

Other causes

• *Drugs.* Many drugs can produce scaling patches. Among them: penicillins, sulfonamides, barbiturates, quinidine, diazepam, phenytoin, and isoniazid.

Special considerations

Teach the patient proper skin care, and suggest lubricating baths and emollients. If scaling results from treatment with corticosteroids, withhold the drug, if ordered.

Prepare the patient for such diagnostic tests as a Wood's light examination, skin scraping, and skin biopsy.

Pediatric pointers

In children, scaly skin may stem from infantile eczema, pityriasis rosea, epi-

dermolytic hyperkeratosis, psoriasis, various forms of ichthyosis, atopic dermatitis, a viral infection (especially hepatitis B virus, which can cause Gianotti-Crosti syndrome), or an acute transient dermatitis. Desquamation may follow a febrile illness.

Skin Turgor— Decreased

Skin turgor—the skin's elasticity—is determined by observing the time required for the skin to return to its normal position after being stretched or pinched. With decreased turgor, pinched skin "holds" for up to 30 seconds, then slowly returns to its normal contour. Skin turgor is commonly assessed over the arm or the sternum, areas normally free of wrinkles and wide variations in tissue thickness.

Decreased skin turgor results from dehydration, or volume depletion, which moves interstitial fluid into the vascular bed to maintain circulating blood volume, leading to slackness in the skin's dermal layer. It's a normal finding in the elderly and in people with rapid weight loss; it also occurs in disorders affecting the gastrointestinal, renal, endocrine, and other systems.

Assessment

If your assessment reveals decreased skin turgor, ask the patient about food and fluid intake—and fluid loss. Has he had recent prolonged fluid loss from vomiting, diarrhea, draining wounds, or increased urination? Ask about a recent fever with sweating. Is he taking diuretics? If so, how often?

Now take the patient's vital signs, noting if his systolic blood pressure while supine is abnormally low (90 mm Hg or less), if it drops 10 mm Hg or more when he stands, or if his pulse increases 10 beats/minute on standing

ASSESSING SKIN TURGOR

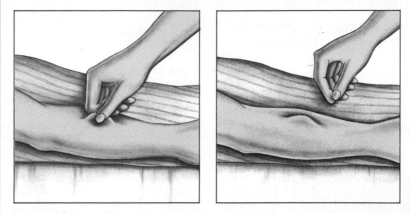

To assess skin turgor in an adult, pick up a fold of skin over the sternum or the arm, as shown at left. (In an infant, roll a fold of loosely adherent skin on the abdomen between your thumb and forefinger.) Then release it. Normal skin will immediately return to its previous contour. In decreased skin turgor, the fold of skin will "hold," as shown at right, for up to 30 seconds.

or sitting. If you detect these signs of orthostatic hypotension or resting tachycardia, call the doctor and start an I.V., as ordered, for fluid administration.

Assess the patient's level of consciousness for confusion and disorientation, signs of profound dehydration. Inspect his oral mucosa, the furrows of the tongue (especially under the tongue), and the axillae for dryness. Also check his neck veins for flatness, and monitor his urine output.

Medical cause
● *Dehydration.* Decreased skin turgor commonly occurs in moderate to severe dehydration. Associated findings include dry oral mucosa, decreased perspiration, resting tachycardia, orthostatic hypotension, dry and furrowed tongue, increased thirst, weight loss, oliguria, fever, and fatigue. As dehydration worsens, other findings include enophthalmos, lethargy, weakness, confusion, delirium or obtundation, anuria, and shock. Hypotension persists even when the patient lies down.

Special considerations
Even a small deficit in body fluid may be critical in patients with diminished total body fluid—young children, the elderly, the obese, or those patients who've rapidly lost a large amount of weight.

To prevent skin breakdown in the dehydrated patient with poor skin turgor, a decreased level of consciousness, and impaired peripheral circulation, turn him every 2 hours, and frequently massage his back and pressure points. Monitor his intake and output, administer I.V. fluid replacement, if ordered, and offer frequent oral fluids. Weigh the patient daily at the same time on the same scale. If his urine output falls below 30 ml/hour or his weight loss continues, notify the doctor. Also closely monitor the patient for signs of electrolyte imbalance.

Pediatric pointers
Diarrhea secondary to gastroenteritis is the most common cause of dehydration in children, especially from birth to age 2.

Spider Angioma

[Arterial spider, spider nevus, stellate angioma, vascular spider]

A spider angioma is a fiery red vascular lesion with an elevated central body, branching spiderlike legs, and a surrounding flush. A form of telangiectasia, this characteristic lesion ranges from a few millimeters to several centimeters in diameter and may be singular or multiple. Most commonly, it appears on the face and neck; less commonly, on the shoulders, thorax, arms, backs of the hands and fingers, and mucous membranes of the lips and nose. Rarely does it appear below the waist or on the lips, ears, nail beds, or palms. On palpation, the angioma may be slightly warmer than the surrounding skin and may have a pulsating central body.

Spider angiomas are most commonly associated with cirrhosis. They may also erupt in the second to third months of pregnancy, enlarge and multiply, then disappear about 6 weeks after delivery. Occasionally, a few lesions may persist. These lesions may also appear in normal patients—especially the elderly—but are smaller and fewer in number (nine or less). They may persist indefinitely or spontaneously disappear.

Assessment

Open your assessment by asking the patient how long he's had the spider angiomas and where they're located. Then carefully examine him yourself, noting the size and location of angiomas. Also check for other skin abnormalities, such as jaundice, dryness, and palmar erythema.

Medical cause

• *Cirrhosis.* Multiple spider angiomas are a hallmark of cirrhosis. Typically, they're a late sign, enlarging and multiplying as the disorder progresses. Associated signs and symptoms are widespread, varying with the degree of hepatic insufficiency and related portal hypertension. Splenomegaly and hematemesis, for example, point to portal hypertension.

Other skin effects in cirrhosis may include severe pruritus, extreme dryness, palmar erythema, and poor tissue turgor. Cardinal hepatic effects

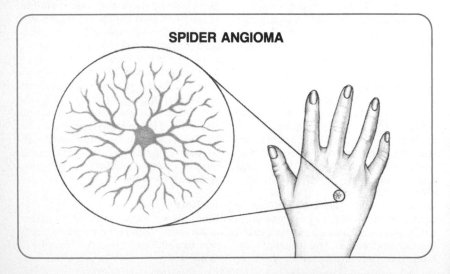

SPIDER ANGIOMA

may include jaundice, hepatomegaly, ascites, and leg edema. Right upper quadrant pain that worsens when the patient sits up or leans forward is common. The patient may also display hepatic encephalopathy with such key symptoms as slurred speech, asterixis, fetor hepaticus, and decreased level of consciousness that progresses to coma. The male patient may have testicular atrophy, gynecomastia, and loss of chest and axillary hair; the female patient, menstrual irregularities.

Special considerations
Treatment isn't indicated for spider angiomas during pregnancy. However, cautery, electrodesiccation, or freezing may be used to treat them in the patient with cirrhosis.

Pediatric pointers
Occasionally, spider angiomas occur in normal children. Typically, they're small and few, appearing on the back of the hands and forearms.

Splenomegaly

Because splenomegaly commonly occurs in many disorders, it isn't a diagnostic sign by itself. What's more, an enlarged spleen may occur in as many as 5% of normal adults. Usually, though, this sign points to infection, trauma, or hepatic, autoimmune, neoplastic, or hematologic disorders.

Because the spleen functions as the body's largest lymph node, splenomegaly can result from any process that triggers lymphadenopathy. For example, it may reflect reactive hyperplasia (a response to infection or inflammation), proliferation or infiltration of neoplastic cells, extramedullary hemopoiesis, phagocytic cell proliferation, increased blood cell destruction, or vascular congestion associated with portal hypertension.

Splenomegaly may be detected by light palpation under the left costal margin (see *How to Palpate for Splenomegaly,* page 688). Unfortunately, this technique isn't always advisable or effective. As a result, splenomegaly may need to be confirmed by a computed tomography or radionuclide scan.

Assessment
If the patient has a history of abdominal or thoracic trauma, do *not* palpate the abdomen, because this may aggravate internal bleeding. Instead, assess for left upper quadrant pain and signs of shock, such as tachycardia and tachypnea. If you detect these signs and symptoms, suspect splenic rupture and have another nurse notify the doctor immediately. Insert an I.V. for emergency fluid and blood replacement and administer oxygen. Also catheterize the patient to evaluate urine output, and begin cardiac monitoring. Prepare the patient for surgery, if ordered.

If you detect splenomegaly during a routine physical examination, begin by exploring associated signs and symptoms. Has the patient been unusually tired lately? Does he frequently have colds, sore throats, or other infections? Does he bruise easily? Ask about left upper quadrant pain, abdominal fullness, and early satiety. Finally, examine the patient's skin for pallor and ecchymoses. Palpate his axillae, groin, and neck for lymphadenopathy.

Medical causes
• *Amyloidosis.* Marked splenomegaly may occur here—the result of excessive protein deposits in the spleen. Associated signs and symptoms vary, depending on what other organs are involved. The patient may display signs of renal failure, such as oliguria and anuria, and signs of congestive heart failure, such as dyspnea, crackles, and tachycardia. Gastrointestinal effects may include a stiff, enlarged tongue, resulting in dysarthria, and constipation or diarrhea.

• *Brucellosis.* In severe cases of this rare

HOW TO PALPATE FOR SPLENOMEGALY

Detecting splenomegaly requires skillful and gentle palpation to avoid rupturing the enlarged organ. Follow these steps carefully:

• Position the patient supine and stand at her right side. Place your left hand under the left costovertebral angle and push lightly to move the spleen forward. Then press your right hand gently under the left front costal margin.

• Have the patient take a deep breath and then exhale. As she exhales, move your right hand along the tissue contours under the ribs' border, feeling for the spleen's edge. The enlarged spleen should feel like a firm mass that bumps against your fingers. Remember to begin palpation low enough in the abdomen to catch the edge of a massive spleen.

• Grade the splenomegaly as slight (1 to 4 cm below the costal margin), moderate (4 to 8 cm below the costal margin), or great (8 cm or more below the costal margin).

• Reposition the patient on her right side with her hips and knees flexed slightly to move the spleen forward. Then repeat the palpation procedure.

infection, splenomegaly is a major sign. Typically, brucellosis begins insidiously with fatigue, headache, backache, anorexia, and arthralgia. Later, it may cause hepatomegaly, lymphadenopathy, weight loss, and vertebral or peripheral nerve pain on pressure.

• *Cirrhosis.* About one third of patients with advanced cirrhosis develop moderate to marked splenomegaly. Among other late findings are jaundice, hepatomegaly, leg edema, hematemesis, and ascites. Signs of hepatic encephalopathy—such as asterixis, fetor hepaticus, slurred speech, and decreased level of consciousness that may progress to coma—are also common. Besides jaundice, skin effects may include severe pruritus, poor tissue turgor, spider angiomas, palmar erythema, pallor, and signs of bleeding tendencies. Endocrine effects may include menstrual irregularities or testicular atrophy, gynecomastia, and loss of chest and axillary hair. The patient may also have fever and right upper abdominal pain that's aggravated by sitting up or leaning forward.

• *Felty's syndrome.* Splenomegaly is characteristic in this syndrome that occurs in chronic rheumatoid arthritis. Associated findings are joint pain and deformity, sensory or motor loss, rheumatoid nodules, palmar erythema, lymphadenopathy, and leg ulcers.

• *Hepatitis.* Splenomegaly may occur in this disorder. More characteristic findings include hepatomegaly, vomiting, jaundice, and fatigue.

• *Histoplasmosis.* Acute disseminated histoplasmosis commonly produces splenomegaly and hepatomegaly. It may also cause lymphadenopathy, jaundice, fever, anorexia, emaciation, and signs of anemia, such as weakness, fatigue, pallor, and malaise. Occasionally, the patient's tongue, palate, epiglottis, and larynx become ulcerated, resulting in pain, hoarseness, and dysphagia.

• *Hypersplenism (primary).* In this syndrome, splenomegaly accompanies signs of pancytopenia—anemia, neutropenia, or thrombocytopenia. If the patient has anemia, findings may include weakness, fatigue, malaise, and pallor. If he has severe neutropenia, frequent bacterial infections are likely. If he has severe thrombocytopenia, easy bruising or spontaneous, widespread hemorrhage may occur.

• *Infectious mononucleosis.* A common sign of this disorder, splenomegaly is most pronounced during the second and third weeks of illness. Typically, it's accompanied by a triad of symptoms: sore throat, cervical lymphadenopathy, and fluctuating temperature with an evening peak of 101° to 102° F. (38.3° to 38.9° C.). Occasionally, hepatomegaly, jaundice, and a maculopapular rash may also occur.

• *Infective endocarditis (subacute).* This infection usually causes an enlarged, but nontender, spleen. Its classic sign, though, is a suddenly changing murmur or the discovery of a new murmur in the presence of fever. Other features include anorexia, pallor, weakness, night sweats, fatigue, tachycardia, weight loss, arthralgia, petechiae, and—in chronic cases—clubbing. If embolization occurs, there may be chest, abdominal, or limb pain; paralysis; hematuria; or blindness. Endocarditis may produce Osler's nodes (tender, raised, subcutaneous lesions on the fingers or toes), Roth's spots (hemorrhagic areas with white centers on the retina), and Janeway lesions (purplish macules on the palms or soles).

• *Leukemia.* Moderate to severe splenomegaly is an early sign of both acute and chronic leukemia. In chronic granulocytic leukemia, splenomegaly is sometimes painful. Accompanying it may be hepatomegaly, lymphadenopathy, fatigue, malaise, pallor, fever, gum swelling, bleeding tendencies, weight loss, anorexia, and abdominal, bone, and joint pain. At times, acute leukemia also causes dyspnea, tachycardia, and palpitations. In advanced disease, the patient may display confusion, headache, vomiting, seizures, papilledema, and nuchal rigidity.

• *Lymphoma.* Moderate to massive splenomegaly is a late sign here. It may be accompanied by hepatomegaly, painless lymphadenopathy, scaly dermatitis with pruritus, fever, fatigue, weight loss, and malaise.

• *Malaria.* Splenomegaly is common in malaria. Typically, it's preceded by the malarial paroxysm of chills, followed by high fever and then diaphoresis. Related effects may include headache, muscle pain, and hepatomegaly. In benign malaria, these paroxysms alternate with periods of well-being. In severe malaria, however, the patient may have persistent high fever, orthostatic hypotension, convulsions, delirium, coma, coughing (with possible hemoptysis), vomiting, abdominal pain, diarrhea, melena, oliguria or anuria, and possibly hemiplegia.

• *Pancreatic cancer.* This cancer may cause moderate to severe splenomegaly if tumor growth compresses the splenic vein. Its other characteristics include abdominal or back pain, anorexia, nausea and vomiting, weight loss, gastrointestinal bleeding, jaundice, pruritus, skin lesions, emotional lability, weakness, and fatigue. Palpation may reveal a tender abdominal mass and hepatomegaly, while auscultation reveals a bruit in the periumbilical area and left upper quadrant.

• *Polycythemia vera.* Late in this disorder, the spleen may become markedly enlarged, resulting in easy satiety, abdominal fullness, and left upper quadrant or pleuritic chest pain. Clinical features accompanying splenomegaly are widespread and numerous. The patient may have deep, purplish red oral mucous membranes, headache, dyspnea, dizziness, vertigo, weakness, and fatigue. He may also have finger and toe paresthesias, impaired mentation, tinnitus, blurred or double vision, scotoma, increased blood pressure, and intermittent claudication. Other signs and symptoms include pruritus, urticaria, ruddy cyanosis, epigastric distress, weight loss, hepatomegaly, and bleeding tendencies.

• *Sarcoidosis.* This granulomatous disorder may produce splenomegaly and hepatomegaly, possibly accompanied by vague abdominal discomfort. Its other signs and symptoms vary with the affected body system but may include nonproductive cough, dyspnea, malaise, fatigue, arthralgia, myalgia, weight loss, lymphadenopathy, skin lesions, irregular pulse, impaired vision, dysphagia, and seizures.

• *Splenic rupture.* Splenomegaly may result from massive hemorrhage in this disorder. The patient may also have left upper quadrant pain, abdominal rigidity, and Kehr's sign—pain referred to the left shoulder.

• *Thrombotic thrombocytopenic purpura.* This disorder may produce splenomegaly and hepatomegaly accompanied by fever, generalized purpura, jaundice, pallor, vaginal bleeding, and hematuria. Other effects may include fatigue, weakness, headache, pallor, abdominal pain, and arthralgias. Eventually, the patient develops signs of neurologic deterioration, such as seizures and decreased level of consciousness, and of renal failure, such as oliguria or anuria.

Special considerations

Prepare the patient for diagnostic studies, such as the complete blood count and radionuclide and computed tomography scans of the spleen.

Pediatric pointers

Besides the causes of splenomegaly described above, the pediatric patient may develop splenomegaly in congenital hemolytic anemia, Gaucher's disease, Niemann-Pick disease, hereditary spherocytosis, sickle cell disease, or beta-thalassemia (Cooley's anemia).

Stertorous Respirations

Characterized by a harsh, rattling, or snoring sound, stertorous respirations usually result from the vibration of relaxed oropharyngeal structures during sleep or coma, causing partial airway obstruction. Less often, these respirations result from retained mucus in the upper airway.

This common sign occurs in about 10% of normal individuals, especially middle-aged, obese men. It may be aggravated by use of alcohol or sedatives before bed, which increases oropharyngeal flaccidity, and by sleeping in the supine position, which allows the relaxed tongue to slip back into the airway. The major pathologic causes of stertorous respirations are obstructive sleep apnea and life-threatening upper airway obstruction associated with an oropharyngeal tumor or with uvular or palatal edema. This obstruction may also occur during the postictal phase of a generalized seizure when mucous secretions or a relaxed tongue blocks the airway.

Occasionally, stertorous respirations are mistaken for stridor, which is another sign of upper airway obstruction. However, stridor indicates laryngeal or tracheal obstruction, whereas stertorous respirations signal higher airway obstruction.

Assessment

If you detect stertorous respirations, check the patient's mouth and throat for edema, redness, and masses. If edema is marked, quickly take vital signs and notify the doctor immediately. Observe for signs and symptoms of respiratory distress, such as dyspnea, tachypnea, use of accessory muscles, intercostal muscle retractions, and cyanosis. Elevate the head of the bed 30° to help ease breathing and reduce the edema. Then administer supplemental oxygen by nasal cannula or face mask, and prepare to assist with intubation or tracheostomy and mechanical ventilation. Insert an I.V. for fluid and drug access, and begin cardiac monitoring.

If you detect stertorous respirations while the patient is sleeping, observe his breathing pattern for 3 to 4 minutes. Do noisy respirations cease when he turns on his side and recur when he assumes a supine position? Watch carefully for periods of apnea and note their length. When possible, question the patient's sleep partner about his snoring habits. Is she frequently awakened by the patient's snoring? Has she also observed the patient talk in his sleep or sleepwalk? Ask about characteristic signs of sleep deprivation, such as personality changes or decreased mental acuity.

Medical causes

• *Airway obstruction.* Regardless of its cause, partial airway obstruction may lead to stertorous respirations accompanied by wheezing, dyspnea, tachypnea and, later, intercostal retractions

and nasal flaring. If the obstruction becomes complete, the patient abruptly loses his ability to talk and displays diaphoresis, tachycardia, and inspiratory chest movement but absent breath sounds. Severe hypoxemia rapidly ensues, resulting in cyanosis, loss of consciousness, and cardiopulmonary collapse.

• *Obstructive sleep apnea.* Loud and disruptive snoring is a major characteristic of this syndrome, which commonly affects the obese. Typically, the snoring alternates with periods of sleep apnea, which usually end with loud, gasping sounds. Alternating tachycardia and bradycardia may occur.

Episodes of snoring and apnea recur in a cyclic pattern throughout the night. Sleep disturbances, such as somnambulism and talking during sleep, may also occur. Some patients display hypertension and ankle edema. Most awaken in the morning with a generalized headache, feeling tired and unrefreshed. The most common complaint is excessive daytime sleepiness. Lack of sleep may cause depression, hostility, and decreased mental acuity.

Other causes

• *Endotracheal surgery, intubation, or suction.* These procedures may cause significant palatal or uvular edema, resulting in stertorous respirations.

Special considerations

Continue to monitor the patient's respiratory status carefully. Administer corticosteroids or antibiotics and cool, humidified oxygen, as ordered, to reduce palatal or uvular inflammation and edema.

The doctor may order laryngoscopy and bronchoscopy to rule out airway obstruction.

Pediatric pointers

In children, the most common cause of stertorous respirations is nasal or pharyngeal obstruction secondary to tonsillar or adenoid hypertrophy or the presence of a foreign body.

Stool—Clay-Colored

Pale, putty-colored stools usually result from hepatic, gallbladder, or pancreatic disorders. Normally, bile pigments give the stool its characteristic brown color. However, hepatocellular degeneration or biliary obstruction may interfere with the formation or release of these pigments into the intestine, resulting in clay-colored stools. Commonly, these stools are associated with jaundice.

Assessment

After noting when the patient first noticed clay-colored stools, explore associated signs and symptoms, such as abdominal pain. Also ask about nausea and vomiting, fatigue, anorexia, weight loss, and dark urine. Does the patient have trouble digesting fatty foods or heavy meals? Does he bruise easily?

Next, review the patient's medical history for gallbladder, hepatic, or pancreatic disorders. Has he ever had biliary surgery? Has he recently undergone barium studies? (After barium studies, the patient has light-colored stools for several days; these may be mistaken for clay-colored stools.) Note a history of alcoholism or exposure to other hepatotoxins.

After assessing the patient's general appearance, take his vital signs and check his skin and eyes for jaundice. Then examine the abdomen; inspect for distention and auscultate for hypoactive bowel sounds. Percuss and palpate for masses and rebound tenderness. Finally, obtain urine and stool specimens for laboratory analysis.

Medical causes

• *Bile duct cancer.* Frequently a presenting sign of this cancer, clay-colored stools may be accompanied by jaundice, pruritus, and weight loss. Upper abdominal pain and bleeding tendencies may also occur.

• *Biliary cirrhosis.* Clay-colored stools typically follow unexplained pruritus that worsens at bedtime, weakness, fatigue, weight loss, and vague abdominal pain; these features may be present for years. Associated findings include jaundice, hyperpigmentation, and signs of malabsorption, such as nocturnal diarrhea; steatorrhea; purpura; and bone and back pain resulting from osteomalacia. The patient may also have hepatomegaly, hematemesis, ascites, edema, and xanthomas on his palms, soles, and elbows.

• *Cholangitis (sclerosing).* Characterized by fibrosis of the bile ducts, this chronic inflammatory disorder may cause clay-colored stools, chronic or intermittent jaundice, pruritus, and right upper abdominal pain.

• *Cholelithiasis.* Stones in the biliary tract may cause clay-colored stools, especially when they obstruct the common bile duct (choledocholithiasis). However, if the obstruction is intermittent, the stools may alternate between normal and clay color. Associated symptoms may include dyspepsia and—in sudden, severe obstruction—characteristic biliary colic. This right upper quadrant pain intensifies over several hours and may radiate to the epigastrium or shoulder blades. The pain is accompanied by tachycardia, restlessness, nausea, vomiting, upper abdominal tenderness, fever, chills, and jaundice.

• *Hepatic carcinoma.* Before clay-colored stools occur in this disorder, the patient usually has weight loss, weakness, and anorexia. Later, he may develop jaundice, right upper quadrant pain, hepatomegaly, ascites, dependent edema, and fever. A bruit, hum, or rubbing sound may be heard on auscultation if the carcinoma involves a large part of the liver.

• *Hepatitis.* In *viral hepatitis,* clay-colored stools signal the start of the icteric phase and are typically followed by jaundice within 1 to 5 days. Associated signs include mild weight loss and dark urine as well as continuation of some preicteric findings, such as anorexia and tender hepatomegaly. During the icteric phase, the patient may become irritable and develop right upper quadrant pain, splenomegaly, enlarged cervical lymph nodes, and severe pruritus. After jaundice disappears, the patient continues to experience fatigue, flatulence, abdominal pain or tenderness, and dyspepsia, although his appetite usually returns and hepatomegaly subsides. The posticteric phase generally lasts from 2 to 6 weeks, with full recovery in 6 months.

In cholestatic *nonviral hepatitis,* clay-colored stools occur with other signs of viral hepatitis.

• *Pancreatic cancer.* Common bile duct obstruction associated with this insidious cancer may cause clay-colored stools. Classic associated features include hepatomegaly, abdominal or back pain, jaundice, pruritus, nausea, vomiting, anorexia, weight loss, fatigue, weakness, and fever. Other possible effects are skin lesions, especially on the legs; emotional lability; splenomegaly; and signs of gastrointestinal bleeding. Auscultation may reveal a bruit in the periumbilical area and left upper quadrant.

• *Pancreatitis (acute).* This disorder may cause clay-colored stools, dark urine, and jaundice. Typically, it also causes severe epigastric pain that radiates to the back and is aggravated by lying down. Associated signs and symptoms may include nausea, vomiting, fever, abdominal rigidity and tenderness, hypoactive bowel sounds, and crackles at the lung bases. In severe pancreatitis, the patient is markedly restless and has tachycardia, mottled skin, and cold, sweaty extremities.

Other cause

• *Biliary surgery.* This surgery may cause bile duct stricture, resulting in clay-colored stools.

Special considerations
Prepare the patient for diagnostic tests, such as liver enzyme and serum bili-

rubin levels and stool analysis.

Pediatric pointers
Clay-colored stools may occur in infants with biliary atresia.

Stridor

A loud, harsh, musical respiratory sound, stridor results from obstruction in the trachea or larynx. Usually heard during inspiration, this sign may also occur during expiration in severe upper airway obstruction. It may begin as low-pitched "croaking" and progress to high-pitched "crowing" as respirations become more vigorous.

Life-threatening upper airway obstruction can stem from foreign body aspiration, increased secretions, intraluminal tumor, localized edema or muscle spasms, and external compression by a tumor or aneurysm.

Assessment
If you hear stridor, quickly check the patient's vital signs and assess for other signs of partial airway obstruction—choking or gagging, tachypnea, dyspnea, shallow respirations, intercostal retractions, nasal flaring, tachycardia, cyanosis, and diaphoresis. (Recognize that abrupt cessation of stridor signals complete obstruction in which the patient has inspiratory chest movement but absent breath sounds. Unable to talk, he quickly becomes lethargic and loses consciousness.) If you detect any signs of airway obstruction, have another nurse notify the doctor immediately while you try to clear the airway with back blows or abdominal thrusts (Heimlich maneuver). Next, administer oxygen by nasal cannula or face mask, or prepare for intubation or emergency tracheostomy and mechanical ventilation. Have equipment ready to suction any aspirated vomitus or blood through the endotracheal or tra-

cheostomy tube. Connect the patient to a cardiac monitor and position him upright to ease his breathing.

When the patient's condition permits, discuss his medical history with him or his family. First, find out when the stridor began. Has he had it before? Does he have an upper respiratory infection? If so, how long has he had it? Ask about a history of allergies, tu-mors, and respiratory and vascular disorders. Note recent exposure to smoke or noxious fumes or gases. Next, explore associated signs and symptoms. Is stridor accompanied by pain or cough?

Then examine the patient's mouth for excessive secretions, foreign matter, inflammation, and swelling. Assess his neck for swelling, masses, subcuta-

ASSISTING WITH
EMERGENCY ENDOTRACHEAL INTUBATION

For a patient with stridor, the doctor may order emergency endotracheal intubation to establish a patent airway and administer mechanical ventilation. Be prepared to assist with tube insertion or to insert the tube yourself, if your hospital's protocol allows. Just follow these essential steps:
• Gather the necessary equipment. If ordered, have a respiratory technician or another nurse set up the mechanical ventilator.
• Explain the procedure to your patient.
• Place the patient flat on his back with a small blanket or pillow under his head. This position aligns the axis of the oropharynx, posterior pharynx, and trachea.
• Check the cuff on the endotracheal tube for leaks.
• After intubation, inflate the cuff, using the minimal leak technique.

• Check tube placement by auscultating for bilateral breath sounds; observe the patient for chest expansion and feel for warm exhalations at the endotracheal tube's opening.
• Insert an oral airway or bite block.
• Secure the tube and airway with tape applied to skin treated with compound benzoin tincture.
• Suction secretions from the patient's mouth and endotracheal tube, as needed.
• Administer oxygen and/or initiate mechanical ventilation, as ordered.

After the patient's intubated, suction secretions at least every 2 hours and check cuff pressure once every shift (correcting any air leaks with the minimal leak technique). Prepare the patient for chest X-rays to check tube placement, and restrain and reassure him, as needed.

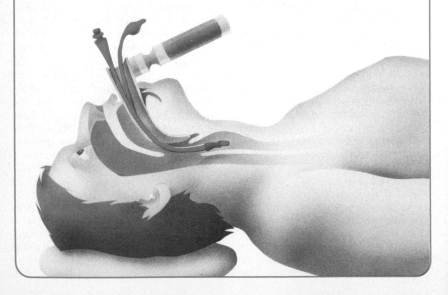

neous crepitation, or scars. Observe the patient's chest for delayed, decreased, or asymmetrical chest expansion. Auscultate for wheezes, rhonchi, crackles, rubs, and other abnormal breath sounds. Percuss for dullness, tympany, or flatness. Finally, note any burns or signs of trauma, such as ecchymoses and lacerations.

Medical causes

● *Airway trauma.* Local trauma to the upper airway commonly causes acute obstruction, resulting in the sudden onset of stridor. Accompanying this sign are dysphonia, dysphagia, hemoptysis, cyanosis, accessory muscle use, intercostal retractions, nasal flaring, tachypnea, progressive dyspnea, and shallow respirations. Palpation may reveal subcutaneous crepitation in the neck or upper chest.

● *Anaphylaxis.* In a severe allergic reaction, upper airway edema causes stridor and other signs of respiratory distress: nasal flaring, wheezing, accessory muscle use, intercostal retractions, and dyspnea. The patient may also have nasal congestion and profuse, watery rhinorrhea. Typically, these respiratory effects are preceded by a feeling of impending doom or fear, weakness, diaphoresis, sneezing, nasal pruritus, urticaria, erythema, and angioedema. Common associated findings include chest or throat tightness, dysphagia, and possibly signs of shock, such as hypotension, tachycardia, and cool, clammy skin.

● *Aspiration of a foreign body.* Sudden stridor is characteristic in life-threatening aspiration of a foreign body. Related findings are abrupt onset of dry, paroxysmal coughing, gagging or choking, hoarseness, tachycardia, wheezing, dyspnea, tachypnea, intercostal muscle retractions, diminished breath sounds, cyanosis, and shallow respirations. The patient's expression is typically anxious and distressed.

● *Hypocalcemia.* In this disorder, laryngospasm can cause stridor. Other findings: paresthesias, carpopedal spasm, and positive Chvostek's and Trousseau's signs.

● *Inhalation injury.* Within 48 hours after inhalation of smoke or noxious fumes, the patient may develop laryngeal edema and bronchospasms, resulting in stridor. Associated signs and symptoms may include singed nasal hairs, orofacial burns, coughing, hoarseness, sooty sputum, crackles, rhonchi, wheezes, and other signs of respiratory distress, such as dyspnea, accessory muscle use, intercostal retractions, and nasal flaring.

● *Laryngeal tumor.* Stridor is a late sign here and may be accompanied by dysphagia, dyspnea, enlarged cervical nodes, and pain that radiates to the ear. Typically, stridor is preceded by hoarseness, minor throat pain, and a mild, dry cough.

● *Laryngitis (acute).* This disorder may cause severe laryngeal edema, resulting in stridor and dyspnea. Its chief sign, though, is mild to severe hoarseness, perhaps with transient voice loss. Other findings: sore throat, dysphagia, dry cough, malaise, and fever.

● *Mediastinal tumor.* Often asymptomatic at first, this tumor may eventually compress the trachea and bronchi, resulting in stridor. Its other effects include hoarseness, brassy cough, tracheal shift or tug, dilated neck veins, swelling of the face and neck, stertorous respirations, and suprasternal retractions on inspiration. The patient may also report dyspnea, dysphagia, and pain in the chest, shoulder, or arm.

● *Retrosternal thyroid.* This anatomic abnormality causes stridor, dysphagia, cough, hoarseness, and tracheal deviation. It can also cause signs of thyrotoxicosis.

● *Thoracic aortic aneurysm.* If this aneurysm compresses the trachea, it may cause stridor accompanied by dyspnea, wheezing, and a brassy cough. Other characteristics may include hoarseness or complete voice loss, dysphagia, distended neck veins, prominent chest veins, tracheal tug, paresthesias or neuralgias, and edema of the face, neck, and arms. The patient may also complain of substernal, lower back, abdominal, or shoulder pain.

Other causes
● *Diagnostic tests.* Bronchoscopy or laryngoscopy may precipitate laryngospasm and stridor.
● *Treatments.* After prolonged intubation, the patient may have laryngeal edema and stridor when the tube is removed. Neck surgery, such as thyroidectomy, may cause laryngeal paralysis and stridor.

Special considerations
Continue to monitor the patient's vital signs closely. Prepare him for diagnostic tests, such as arterial blood gas analysis and chest X-rays, as ordered.

Pediatric pointers
Stridor is a major sign of airway obstruction in the pediatric patient. When you hear this sign, you must intervene quickly to prevent total airway obstruction. This emergency can happen more rapidly in a child because his airway is narrower than an adult's.

Causes of stridor include foreign body aspiration, croup syndrome, laryngeal diphtheria, pertussis, retropharyngeal abscess, and congenital abnormalities of the larynx.

Therapy for partial airway obstruction typically involves hot or cold steam in a mist tent or hood, parenteral fluids and electrolytes, and plenty of rest.

Syncope

A common neurologic sign, syncope (or faint) refers to transient loss of consciousness associated with impaired cerebral oxygenation. It usually occurs abruptly and lasts for seconds to minutes. Typically, the patient lies motionless with his skeletal muscles relaxed but sphincter muscles controlled. However, the depth of unconsciousness varies; some patients can hear voices or see blurred outlines, whereas others are unaware of their surroundings.

In many ways, syncope simulates death: the patient is strikingly pale with a slow, weak pulse, hypotension, and almost imperceptible breathing. If loss of consciousness lasts for 15 to 20 seconds, the patient may also develop convulsive, tonic-clonic movements. However, the common sequelae of a convulsive seizure—confusion, headache, and drowsiness—don't follow syncope.

Syncope may result from cardiac and cerebrovascular disorders, hypoxemia, and postural changes in the presence of autonomic dysfunction. It may also follow vigorous coughing (tussive syncope) and emotional stress, injury, shock, or pain (vasovagal syncope, or the common faint). Hysterical syncope may also follow emotional stress but isn't accompanied by other vasodepressor effects.

Assessment
If you witness syncope, place the patient in a supine position, elevate his legs, and loosen any tight clothing. Ensure a patent airway and take vital signs. If you detect tachycardia, bradycardia, or an irregular pulse, have another nurse notify the doctor. Meanwhile, place the patient on a cardiac monitor to detect dysrhythmias. Give oxygen and insert an I.V. for drug administration, if a dysrhythmia appears. Be prepared to begin cardiopulmonary resuscitation and to assist with cardioversion, defibrillation, or insertion of a temporary pacemaker, as needed.

If the patient reports syncope, collect information about the episode from the patient and his family. Did he feel weak, light-headed, nauseous, or sweaty just before he fainted? Did he get up quickly from a chair or from lying down? During the syncope, did he have muscle spasms or incontinence? How long was he unconscious? When he regained consciousness, was he alert or confused? Did he have a headache? Has he had syncope before? If so, how often does it occur?

Next, take the patient's vital signs and examine him for any injuries that may have occurred during his fall.

Medical causes

• *Aortic arch syndrome.* This syndrome produces syncope. The patient may have weak or abruptly absent carotid pulses and unequal or absent radial pulses. Early symptoms include night sweats, pallor, nausea, anorexia, weight loss, arthralgia, and Raynaud's phenomenon. He may also have hypotension in the arms; neck, shoulder, and chest pain; paresthesias; intermittent claudication; bruits; visual disturbances; and dizziness.

• *Aortic stenosis.* A cardinal late sign, syncope is accompanied by exertional dyspnea and anginal chest pain. Related findings include marked fatigue, orthopnea, paroxysmal nocturnal dyspnea, palpitations, and diminished carotid pulses. Typically, auscultation reveals atrial and ventricular gallops as well as a harsh, crescendo-decrescendo systolic ejection murmur that's loudest at the right sternal border of the second intercostal space.

• *Cardiac dysrhythmias.* Any dysrhythmia that decreases cardiac output and impairs cerebral circulation may cause syncope. Usually, other effects develop first, such as palpitations, pallor, confusion, diaphoresis, dyspnea, and hypotension. But in Adams-Stokes syndrome, syncope may occur several times daily without warning. During syncope, the patient has asystole, which may precipitate spasms and myoclonic jerks if prolonged. He also has an ashen-gray pallor that progresses to cyanosis, incontinence, bilateral Babinski's reflex, and fixed pupils.

• *Carotid sinus hypersensitivity.* Syncope is triggered here by compression of the carotid sinus, for example, by turning the head to one side or by wearing a tight collar. Usually, syncope lasts several minutes and is followed by mental clarity. Exertional dyspnea and anginal chest pain may also occur.

• *Hypoxemia.* Regardless of its cause, hypoxemia may produce syncope. Common related effects: confusion, tachycardia, restlessness, and incoordination.

• *Orthostatic hypotension.* Syncope occurs when the patient rises quickly from a recumbent position. It follows a drop of 10 to 20 mm Hg or more in systolic or diastolic blood pressure, tachycardia, pallor, dizziness, blurred vision, nausea, and diaphoresis.

• *Transient ischemic attack.* Marked by transient neurologic deficits, these attacks may produce syncope and decreased level of consciousness. Other findings vary with the affected artery but may include vision loss, nystagmus, aphasia, dysarthria, unilateral numbness, hemiparesis or hemiplegia, tinnitus, facial weakness, dysphagia, and staggering or uncoordinated gait.

• *Vagal glossopharyngeal neuralgia.* In this disorder, localized pressure may trigger pain in the base of the tongue, pharynx, larynx, tonsils, and ear, resulting in syncope that lasts for several minutes.

Other causes

• *Drugs.* Quinidine commonly causes syncope—and possibly sudden death—associated with ventricular fibrillation. Prazosin may cause severe orthostatic hypotension and syncope, usually after the first dose. Occasionally, griseofulvin, levodopa, and indomethacin produce syncope, too.

Special considerations

Continue to monitor the patient's vital signs closely. Advise him to pace his activities, to rise slowly from a recumbent position, to avoid standing still for a prolonged time, and to sit or lie down as soon as he feels faint.

Pediatric pointers

Syncope is much less common in children than in adults. It may result from cardiac or neurologic disorders, allergy, or emotional stress.

tachycardia • tachypnea • taste abnormalities • tearing—increased • throat p
tracheal deviation • tracheal tugging • tremors • trismus • tunnel vision • ur
discharge • urinary frequency • urinary hesitancy • urinary incontinence • u
cloudiness • urticaria • vaginal bleeding—postmenopausal • vaginal discharg
vertigo • vesicular rash • violent behavior • vision loss • visual blurring • vis
vulvar lesions • weight gain—excessive • weight loss—excessive • wheezing •
distention • abdominal mass • abdominal pain • abdominal rigidity • access
agitation • alopecia • amenorrhea • amnesia • analgesia • anhidrosis • anore
anxiety • aphasia • apnea • apneustic respirations • apraxia • arm pain • as
athetosis • aura • Babinski's reflex • back pain • barrel chest • Battle's sign •
bladder distention • blood pressure decrease • blood pressure increase • bow
bowel sounds—hyperactive • bowel sounds—hypoactive • bradycardia • bra
dimpling • breast nodule • breast pain • breast ulcer • breath with ammonia
odor • breath with fruity odor • Brudzinski's sign • bruits • buffalo hump •
lait spots • capillary refill time—prolonged • carpopedal spasm • cat cry • ch
asymmetrical • chest pain • Cheyne-Stokes respirations • chills • chorea • Ch
cogwheel rigidity • cold intolerance • confusion • conjunctival injection • co
reflex—absent • costovertebral angle tenderness • cough—barking • cough—
productive • crackles • crepitation—bony • crepitation—subcutaneous • cry—
cyanosis • decerebrate posture • decorticate posture • deep tendon reflexes—
reflexes—hypoactive • depression • diaphoresis • diarrhea • diplopia • dizzi
absent • drooling • dysarthria • dysmenorrhea • dyspareunia • dyspepsia • d
dystonia • dysuria • earache • edema—generalized • edema of the arms • ed
of the legs • enophthalmos • enuresis • epistaxis • eructation • erythema • e
discharge • eye pain • facial pain • fasciculations • fatigue • fecal incontinen
fever • flank pain • flatulence • fontanelle bulging • fontanelle depression • fo
abnormalities • gait—bizarre • gait—propulsive • gait—scissors • gait—spas
gait—waddling • gallop—atrial • gallop—ventricular • genital lesions in the
respirations • gum bleeding • gum swelling • gynecomastia • halitosis • hal
hearing loss • heat intolerance • Heberden's nodes • hematemesis • hematoch
hemianopia • hemoptysis • hepatomegaly • hiccups • hirsutism • hoarseness
hyperpigmentation • hyperpnea • hypopigmentation • impotence • insomnia
claudication • Janeway's spots • jaundice • jaw pain • jugular vein distention
sign • leg pain • level of consciousness—decreased • lid lag • light flashes •
lymphadenopathy • masklike facies • McBurney's sign • McMurray's sign • n
metrorrhagia • miosis • moon face • mouth lesions • murmurs • muscle atro
muscle spasms • muscle spasticity • muscle weakness • mydriasis • myoclon
nausea • neck pain • night blindness • nipple discharge • nipple retraction •
rigidity • nystagmus • ocular deviation • oligomenorrhea • oliguria • opistho
dyskinesia • orthopnea • orthostatic hypotension • Ortolani's sign • Osler's n
palpitations • papular rash • paralysis • paresthesias • paroxysmal nocturna
d'orange • pericardial friction rub • peristaltic waves—visible • photophobia
rub • polydipsia • polyphagia • polyuria • postnasal drip • priapism • pruri
psychotic behavior • ptosis • pulse—absent or weak • pulse—bounding • pu
pulse pressure—widened • pulse rhythm abnormality • pulsus alternans • p
paradoxus • pupils—nonreactive • pupils—sluggish • purple striae • purpu
pyrosis • raccoon's eyes • rebound tenderness • rectal pain • retractions—co
rhinorrhea • rhonchi • Romberg's sign • salivation—decreased • salivation—
scotoma • scrotal swelling • seizure—absence • seizure—focal • seizure—ge
seizure—psychomotor • setting-sun sign • shallow respirations • skin—bron

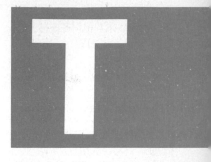

Tachycardia

Easily detected by counting the apical, carotid, or radial pulse, tachycardia is a heart rate greater than 100 beats/ minute. Usually, the patient also complains of palpitations or of his heart "racing." This common sign normally occurs in response to emotional or physical stress, such as excitement, exercise, pain, and fever. It may also result from use of stimulants, such as caffeine and tobacco. More importantly, though, tachycardia may be an early sign of a life-threatening disorder, such as cardiogenic or septic shock. It may also result from cardiovascular, respiratory, and metabolic disorders; electrolyte imbalance; and the effects of certain drugs, tests, and treatments (see *What Happens in Tachycardia*, page 700).

Assessment

After detecting tachycardia, your first priority is to assess for reduced cardiac output, which may initiate or result from tachycardia. Take the patient's other vital signs and assess his level of consciousness. If he has increased or decreased blood pressure and is drowsy or confused, have another nurse notify the doctor while you administer oxygen and begin cardiac monitoring. Insert an I.V. to allow fluid and drug administration, and gather emergency resuscitation equipment.

When the patient's condition permits, take a focused history. Find out if he has had palpitations before. If so, how were they treated? Explore associated symptoms. Is the patient dizzy or short of breath? Weak or fatigued? Is he experiencing chest pain? Next, ask about a history of trauma, diabetes, or cardiac, pulmonary, or thyroid disorders. Also obtain a drug history.

Now, inspect the patient's skin for pallor or cyanosis. Assess pulses, noting peripheral edema. Finally, auscultate the heart and lungs for abnormal sounds or rhythms.

Medical causes

• *Adrenocortical insufficiency.* In this disorder, tachycardia commonly occurs with a weak, irregular pulse. It's also accompanied by progressive weakness and fatigue, which may become so severe that the patient requires bed rest. Other features include abdominal pain, nausea and vomiting, altered bowel habits, weight loss, orthostatic hypotension, irritability, bronze skin, decreased libido, and syncope. Some patients report an enhanced sense of taste, smell, and hearing.

• *Adult respiratory distress syndrome*

WHAT HAPPENS IN TACHYCARDIA

Tachycardia represents the heart's effort to deliver more oxygen to body tissues by increasing the rate at which blood passes through the vessels. This sign can reflect overstimulation within the SA node, the atrium, the AV node, or the ventricles.

Because heart rate affects cardiac output (cardiac output = heart rate × stroke volume), tachycardia can lower cardiac output by reducing ventricular filling time and stroke volume (the output of each ventricle at every contraction). As cardiac output plummets, arterial pressure and peripheral perfusion decrease. Tachycardia further aggravates myocardial ischemia by increasing the heart's demand for oxygen while reducing the duration of diastole—the period of greatest coronary flow.

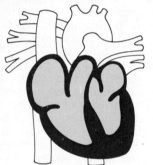

Normally, ventricular volume reaches 120 to 130 ml during diastolic filling.

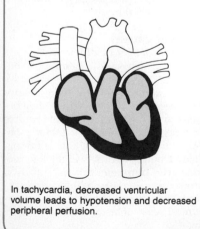

In tachycardia, decreased ventricular volume leads to hypotension and decreased peripheral perfusion.

(ARDS). Besides tachycardia, ARDS causes crackles, rhonchi, dyspnea, tachypnea, nasal flaring, and grunting respirations. Other findings: cyanosis, anxiety, and decreased level of consciousness.

• *Alcohol withdrawal syndrome.* Tachycardia can occur with tachypnea, profuse diaphoresis, fever, insomnia, and anorexia. The patient is characteristically anxious, irritable, and prone to visual and tactile hallucinations.

• *Anaphylactic shock.* In life-threatening anaphylactic shock, tachycardia and sudden hypotension develop within minutes after exposure to an allergen, such as penicillin or an insect sting. Typically, the patient is visibly anxious and has severe pruritus, perhaps with urticaria and a pounding headache. Other findings may include flushed and clammy skin, a cough, dyspnea, nausea, abdominal cramps, seizures, stridor, change or loss of voice associated with laryngeal edema, and urinary urgency and incontinence.

• *Anemia.* Tachycardia and bounding pulse are characteristic in anemia. Associated signs and symptoms include fatigue, pallor, dyspnea, and possibly bleeding tendencies. Auscultation may reveal an atrial gallop, a systolic bruit over the carotid arteries, and crackles.

• *Aortic insufficiency.* Accompanying tachycardia in this disorder are a "water-hammer" bounding pulse and a large, diffuse apical heave. In severe insufficiency, widened pulse pressure occurs. Auscultation may reveal an atrial or ventricular gallop, an early systolic murmur, an Austin Flint murmur (apical diastolic rumble), Duroziez's sign (a murmur over the femoral artery during systole and diastole), or a diastolic murmur that starts with the second heart sound, is decrescendo, high-pitched, and blowing, and is heard best at the left sternal border of the second and third intercostal space. Other findings may include anginal chest pain, dyspnea, palpitations, strong abrupt carotid pulsations, pallor, and signs of congestive heart failure, such as crackles and neck vein distention.

● *Aortic stenosis.* Typically, this valvular disorder causes tachycardia, a weak, thready pulse, and an atrial or ventricular gallop. Its chief features, though, are dyspnea, anginal chest pain, and syncope. Aortic stenosis also causes a harsh, crescendo-decrescendo systolic ejection murmur that's loudest at the right sternal border of the second intercostal space. Other findings may include palpitations, crackles, and fatigue.

● *Cardiac contusion.* The result of blunt chest trauma, this contusion may cause tachycardia, substernal pain, dyspnea and palpitations. Assessment may detect sternal ecchymoses and a pericardial friction rub.

● *Cardiac dysrhythmias.* Tachycardia may occur with a regular or irregular heart rhythm here. The patient may be hypotensive and report dizziness, palpitations, weakness, and fatigue. Depending on his heart rate, he may also have tachypnea, decreased level of consciousness, and pale, cool, clammy skin.

● *Cardiac tamponade.* In life-threatening cardiac tamponade, tachycardia commonly occurs with pulsus paradoxus, dyspnea, and tachypnea. The patient is visibly anxious and restless with cyanotic, clammy skin and distended neck veins. He may have muffled heart sounds, pericardial friction rub, chest pain, hypotension, narrowed pulse pressure, and hepatomegaly.

● *Cardiogenic shock.* Although many features of cardiogenic shock appear in other types of shock, they're usually more profound here. Accompanying tachycardia are weak, thready pulse; narrowing pulse pressure; hypotension; tachypnea; cold, pale, clammy, and cyanotic skin; oliguria; restlessness; and altered level of consciousness.

● *Chronic obstructive pulmonary disease (COPD).* Although the clinical picture varies widely in COPD, tachycardia is a common sign. Other characteristic findings include cough, tachypnea,

dyspnea, pursed-lip breathing, accessory muscle use, cyanosis, diminished breath sounds, rhonchi, crackles, and wheezing. Clubbing and barrel chest are usually late findings.

● *Congestive heart failure.* Especially common in left heart failure, tachycardia may be accompanied by a ventricular gallop, fatigue, dyspnea (exertional and paroxysmal nocturnal), and orthopnea. Eventually, the patient develops widespread effects, such as palpitations, narrowed pulse pressure, hypotension, tachycardia, crackles, dependent edema, weight gain, slowed mental response, diaphoresis, pallor, and possibly oliguria. Late signs include hemoptysis, cyanosis, and marked hepatomegaly and pitting edema.

● *Diabetic ketoacidosis.* This life-threatening disorder commonly produces tachycardia and a thready pulse. Its cardinal sign, though, is Kussmaul's respirations—abnormally rapid, deep breathing. Other signs and symptoms of acidosis may include fruity breath odor, orthostatic hypotension, generalized weakness, anorexia, nausea, vomiting, and abdominal pain. The patient's level of consciousness may vary from lethargy to coma.

● *Febrile illness.* Fever can cause tachycardia. Related findings reflect the specific disorder.

● *Hyperosmolar hyperglycemic nonketotic coma.* Rapidly deteriorating level of consciousness is typically accompanied by tachycardia, hypotension, tachypnea, seizures, oliguria, and severe dehydration with poor skin turgor and dry mucous membranes.

● *Hypertensive crisis.* Life-threatening hypertensive crisis is characterized by tachycardia, tachypnea, diastolic blood pressure that exceeds 120 mm Hg, and systolic blood pressure that may exceed 200 mm Hg. Typically, the patient develops pulmonary edema with neck vein distension, dyspnea, and pink, frothy sputum. Related findings may include chest pain, severe headache, drowsiness, confusion, anxiety, tinnitus, epistaxis, muscle twitching, seizures, nausea, and vomiting. Focal neurologic signs, such as paresthesias, may also occur.

• *Hypoglycemia.* A common sign of hypoglycemia, tachycardia is accompanied by hypothermia, nervousness, trembling, fatigue, malaise, weakness, headache, hunger, nausea, diaphoresis, and moist, clammy skin. Central nervous system effects may include blurred or double vision, motor weakness, hemiplegia, seizures, and decreased level of consciousness.

• *Hyponatremia.* Tachycardia is one effect of this electrolyte imbalance. Others include orthostatic hypotension, headache, muscle twitching and weakness, fatigue, oliguria or anuria, poor skin turgor, thirst, irritability, seizures, nausea, vomiting, and decreased level of consciousness that may progress to coma. Severe hyponatremia may cause cyanosis and signs of vasomotor collapse, such as thready pulse.

• *Hypovolemia.* Tachycardia can occur in this disorder. Associated findings include hypotension, decreased skin turgor, sunken eyeballs, thirst, syncope, and dry skin and tongue.

• *Hypovolemic shock.* Slight tachycardia is an early sign of life-threatening hypovolemic shock. It may be accompanied by tachypnea, restlessness, thirst, and pale, cool skin. As shock progresses, the patient's skin becomes clammy and his pulse increasingly rapid and thready. He may also develop hypotension, narrowed pulse pressure, oliguria, subnormal body temperature, and decreased level of consciousness.

• *Hypoxemia.* Tachycardia may accompany tachypnea, dyspnea, and cyanosis. Confusion, syncope, and incoordination may also occur.

• *Myocardial infarction.* This life-threatening disorder may cause tachycardia or bradycardia. Its classic symptom, however, is crushing substernal chest pain that may radiate to the left arm, jaw, neck, or shoulder. Auscultation may reveal an atrial gallop, a new mur-

mur, and crackles. Other signs and symptoms may include pallor, clammy skin, dyspnea, diaphoresis, nausea, vomiting, anxiety, restlessness, and increased or decreased blood pressure.

• *Neurogenic shock.* Tachycardia or bradycardia may occur. Related effects: tachypnea, apprehension, oliguria, variable body temperature, decreased level of consciousness, and warm, dry skin.

• *Orthostatic hypotension.* Tachycardia accompanies the characteristic signs in this condition: dizziness, syncope, pallor, blurred vision, diaphoresis, and nausea.

• *Pheochromocytoma.* Characterized by sustained or paroxysmal hypertension, this rare tumor may also cause tachycardia and palpitations. Other findings include headache, chest and abdominal pain, diaphoresis, pale or flushed, warm skin, paresthesias, tremors, nausea, vomiting, insomnia, and extreme anxiety—possibly even panic.

• *Pneumothorax.* Life-threatening pneumothorax causes tachycardia and other signs of distress, such as severe dyspnea and chest pain, tachypnea, and cyanosis. Related findings include dry cough, subcutaneous crepitation, absent or decreased breath sounds, and decreased vocal fremitus.

• *Pulmonary embolism.* In this disorder, tachycardia is usually preceded by sudden dyspnea and anginal or pleuritic chest pain. Common associated signs and symptoms include weak peripheral pulses, tachypnea, low-grade fever, restlessness, diaphoresis, and a dry cough or a cough with blood-tinged sputum.

• *Septic shock.* Initially, septic shock produces chills, sudden fever, tachycardia, tachypnea, and possibly nausea, vomiting, and diarrhea. The patient's skin is flushed, warm, and dry; his blood pressure, normal or slightly decreased. Eventually, he may display anxiety; restlessness; thirst; oliguria or anuria; cool, clammy, cyanotic skin; rapid, thready pulse; and severe hypotension. His level of consciousness may decrease progressively, culminating perhaps in a state of coma.

• **Thyrotoxicosis.** Tachycardia is a classic feature of this thyroid disorder, as are an enlarged thyroid, nervousness, heat intolerance, weight loss despite increased appetite, diaphoresis, diarrhea, tremors, and palpitations. Although also considered characteristic, exophthalmos is sometimes absent.

Because thyrotoxicosis affects virtually every body system, its associated signs and symptoms are diverse and numerous. Some examples include full and bounding pulse, widened pulse pressure, dyspnea, anorexia, nausea, vomiting, altered bowel habits, hepatomegaly, and muscle weakness, fatigue, and atrophy. The patient's skin is smooth, warm, and flushed, while the hair is fine and soft and may gray prematurely or fall out. The female patient may have reduced libido and oligomenorrhea or amenorrhea; the male patient, reduced libido and gynecomastia.

Other causes
• **Diagnostic tests.** Cardiac catheterization and electrophysiologic studies may induce transient tachycardia.
• **Drugs and alcohol.** Various drugs affect the nervous system, circulatory system, or heart muscle, resulting in tachycardia. Examples of these include sympathomimetics; phenothiazines; anticholinergics, such as atropine; thyroid drugs; vasodilators, such as hydralazine and nifedipine; nitrates, such as nitroglycerin; and alpha-adrenergic blockers, such as phentolamine. Alcohol intoxication may also cause tachycardia.
• **Surgery and pacemakers.** Cardiac surgery and pacemaker malfunction or wire irritation may cause tachycardia.

Special considerations
Continue to monitor the patient closely. If appropriate, prepare him for ambulatory electrocardiography. Also explain ordered diagnostic tests, such as blood work, pulmonary function studies, and 12-lead EKG.

Pediatric pointers
When assessing for tachycardia, recognize that normal rates for children are higher than for adults (see *Normal Pediatric Vital Signs*, pages 706 and 707.)

In children, tachycardia may result from patent ductus arteriosus as well as from many of the adult causes described above.

Tachypnea

A common sign of cardiopulmonary disorders, tachypnea is an abnormally fast respiratory rate—20 breaths or more per minute. It's easily detected by unobtrusively counting the patient's respirations. Generally, tachypnea indicates the need to increase minute volume—the amount of air breathed each minute. It may be accompanied by an increase in tidal volume—the volume of air inhaled or exhaled per breath—resulting in hyperventilation.

Tachypnea may result from reduced arterial oxygen tension or arterial oxygen content, decreased perfusion, or increased oxygen demand. Heightened oxygen demand, for example, may result from fever, exertion, anxiety, and pain. Tachypnea may also occur as a compensatory response to metabolic acidosis and may result from pulmonary irritation, stretch receptor stimulation, or neurologic disorders that upset medullary respiratory control. Generally, respirations increase by 4 breaths/minute for every 1 F. degree rise in body temperature.

Assessment
After detecting tachypnea, quickly assess cardiopulmonary status; check for cyanosis, chest pain, dyspnea, tachycardia, and hypotension. If you detect these signs, have another nurse notify the doctor immediately. If the patient has paradoxical chest movement, immediately

splint his chest with your hands or with sandbags. Then administer supplemental oxygen by nasal cannula or face mask and, if possible, place the patient in a semi-Fowler's position to help ease his breathing. Prepare to assist the doctor with intubation and mechanical ventilation if respiratory failure ensues. In addition, insert an I.V. for fluid and drug administration and begin cardiac monitoring.

When the patient's condition permits, obtain a medical history. Find out when the tachypnea began. Did it follow activity? Has the patient had it before? Then have him describe associated signs and symptoms, such as diaphoresis and recent weight loss. Is he anxious about anything or does he have a history of anxiety attacks? Be sure to note whether the patient is currently taking drugs for pain relief. How effective are they?

Begin the physical examination by taking the patient's other vital signs, if you haven't already done so, and observing his overall behavior. Does he seem restless? Next, auscultate the chest for abnormal heart and lung sounds. If the patient has a productive cough, record the color, amount, and consistency of sputum. Finally, assess the patient for jugular vein distention and check his skin for pallor, cyanosis, edema, and warmth or coolness.

Medical causes

● *Adult respiratory distress syndrome (ARDS).* In this life-threatening disorder, tachypnea and apprehension may be the earliest features. Tachypnea gradually worsens as fluid accumulates in the patient's lungs, causing them to stiffen. It's accompanied by accessory muscle use, grunting expirations, suprasternal and intercostal retractions, and crackles and rhonchi. Eventually, ARDS precipitates hypoxemia, resulting in tachycardia, dyspnea, cyanosis, extreme anxiety, mental sluggishnss, motor dysfunction, and transient hypertension.

● *Alcohol withdrawal syndrome.* A late

sign in the acute phase of this syndrome, tachypnea typically is accompanied by anorexia, insomnia, tachycardia, fever, and diaphoresis. The patient may also experience anxiety, irritability, and bizarre visual or tactile hallucinations.

● *Anaphylactic shock.* In this type of shock, tachypnea develops within minutes after exposure to an allergen, such as penicillin or insect venom. Accompanying features include anxiety, pounding headache, skin flushing and intense pruritus, and possibly diffuse urticaria. The patient may have widespread edema, affecting the eyelids, lips, tongue, hands, feet, and genitalia. Other findings in this life-threatening shock are cool, clammy skin; rapid, thready pulse; cough; dyspnea; stridor; and change or loss of voice associated with laryngeal edema.

● *Anemia.* Tachypnea may occur in this disorder, depending on the duration and severity of anemia. Associated signs and symptoms may include fatigue, pallor, dyspnea, tachycardia, postural hypotension, bounding pulse, an atrial gallop, and a systolic bruit over the carotid arteries.

● *Aspiration of a foreign body.* Life-threatening upper airway obstruction may result from aspiration of a foreign body. In *partial obstruction,* the patient abruptly develops a dry, paroxysmal cough with rapid, shallow respirations. Other signs and symptoms include dyspnea, gagging or choking, intercostal retractions, nasal flaring, cyanosis, decreased or absent breath sounds, hoarseness, and stridor or coarse wheezes. Typically, the patient appears frightened and distressed. *Complete obstruction* may rapidly cause asphyxia and death.

● *Asthma.* Tachypnea is common in life-threatening asthmatic attacks, which commonly occur at night. These attacks usually begin with mild wheezing and a dry cough that progresses to mucus expectoration. Eventually, the patient becomes apprehensive and develops prolonged expirations, intercostal and supraclavicular retractions on inspiration, accessory muscle use, severe audible wheezing, rhonchi, flaring nostrils, tachycardia, diaphoresis, and flushing or cyanosis.

● *Bronchiectasis.* Although this disorder may produce tachypnea, its classic sign is a chronic productive cough with copious, mucopurulent, foul-smelling sputum and, occasionally, hemoptysis. Related findings include coarse crackles on inspiration, dyspnea on exertion, rhonchi and halitosis. The patient may also have fever, malaise, weight loss, fatigue, and weakness. Clubbing is a common late sign.

● *Bronchitis (chronic).* Mild tachypnea may occur in this form of COPD, but it's not typically a predominant sign. Usually, chronic bronchitis begins with a dry, hacking cough that later produces copious sputum. Other characteristics include dyspnea, prolonged expirations, wheezing, scattered rhonchi, accessory muscle use, and cyanosis. Clubbing and barrel chest are late signs.

● *Cardiac dysrhythmias.* Depending on the patient's heart rate, tachypnea may occur along with hypotension, dizziness, palpitations, weakness, and fatigue. The patient's level of consciousness may be decreased.

● *Cardiac tamponade.* In life-threatening tamponade, tachypnea may accompany tachycardia, dyspnea, and pulsus paradoxus. Related findings include muffled heart sounds, pericardial friction rub, chest pain, hypotension, narrowed pulse pressure, and hepatomegaly. The patient is noticeably anxious and restless. His skin is clammy and cyanotic, and his neck veins are distended.

● *Cardiogenic shock.* Although signs of cardiogenic shock resemble signs of other types of shock, they're usually more severe. Besides tachypnea, the patient commonly has cold, pale, clammy, cyanotic skin; hypotension; tachycardia; narrowed pulse pressure; a ventricular gallop; oliguria; decreased level of consciousness; and

neck vein distention.

● *Emphysema.* This chronic pulmonary disorder commonly produces tachypnea accompanied by dyspnea on exertion. It may also cause anorexia, malaise, peripheral cyanosis, pursed-lip breathing, accessory muscle use, and chronic productive cough. Percussion yields a hyperresonant tone while auscultation reveals wheezes, crackles, and diminished breath sounds. Clubbing and barrel chest are late signs.

● *Febrile illness.* Fever can cause tachypnea, tachycardia, and other signs.

● *Flail chest.* Tachypnea usually appears early in this life-threatening disorder. Other findings include paradoxical chest wall movement, rib bruises and palpable fractures, localized chest pain, hypotension, and diminished breath sounds. The patient may also develop signs of respiratory distress, such as dyspnea and accessory muscle use.

● *Head trauma.* When trauma affects the brain stem, the patient may display central neurogenic hyperventilation, a form of tachypnea marked by rapid, even, and deep respirations. The tachypnea may be accompanied by other signs of life-threatening neurogenic dysfunction, such as coma, unequal and nonreactive pupils, seizures, hemiplegia, flaccidity, and hypoactive or absent deep tendon reflexes.

● *Hyperosmolar hyperglycemic nonketotic coma.* Rapidly deteriorating level of consciousness occurs with tachypnea, tachycardia, hypotension, seizures, oliguria, and signs of dehydration.

● *Hypovolemic shock.* An early sign of life-threatening hypovolemic shock, tachypnea is accompanied by cool, pale skin; restlessness; thirst; and mild tachycardia. As shock progresses, the patient's skin becomes clammy; his pulse, increasingly rapid and thready. Other findings include hypotension, narrowed pulse pressure, oliguria, subnormal body temperature, and decreased level of consciousness.

● *Interstitial fibrosis.* In this disorder, ta-

NORMAL PEDIATRIC VITAL SIGNS*

VITAL SIGNS	Newborn	2 years	4 years	6 years
Respiratory rate/minute				
Girls	28	26	25	24
Boys	30	28	25	24
Blood pressure (mm hg)				
Girls	—	98/60	98/60	98/64
Boys	—	96/60	96/60	98/62
Pulse rate/ minute				
Girls	130	110	100	100
Boys	130	110	100	100

*At rest

chypnea develops gradually and may become severe. Associated features may include dyspnea on exertion, pleuritic chest pain, a paroxysmal dry cough, crackles, late inspiratory wheezes, cyanosis, fatigue, and weight loss. Clubbing is a late sign.

• *Lung abscess.* In this abscess, tachypnea is usually paired with dyspnea and accentuated by fever. However, the chief sign is a productive cough with copious, purulent, foul-smelling, often bloody sputum. Other findings may include chest pain, halitosis, diaphoresis, chills, fatigue, weakness, anorexia, weight loss, and clubbing.

• *Lung, pleural, or mediastinal tumor.* This tumor may cause tachypnea along with dyspnea on exertion, cough, hemoptysis, and pleuritic chest pain. Other effects include weight loss, anorexia, and fatigue.

• *Mesothelioma (malignant).* Often related to asbestos exposure, this pleural mass initially produces tachypnea and dyspnea on mild exertion. Other classic symptoms are persistent, dull chest pain and aching shoulder pain that progresses to arm weakness and paresthesia. Later signs and symptoms include a cough, insomnia associated with pain, clubbing, and dullness over

	8 years	10 years	12 years	14 years	16 years
	24	22	20	18	16
	22	23	20	16	16
	104/68	110/72	114/74	118/76	120/78
	102/68	110/72	112/74	120/76	124/78
	90	90	90	85	80
	90	90	85	80	75

the malignant mesothelioma.

• *Neurogenic shock.* Tachypnea is characteristic in this life-threatening type of shock. It commonly occurs with apprehension, bradycardia or tachycardia, oliguria, fluctuating body temperature, and decreased level of consciousness that may progress to coma. The patient's skin is warm, dry, and perhaps flushed. He may experience nausea and vomiting.

• *Pneumonia (bacterial).* A common sign in this infection, tachypnea is usually preceded by a painful, hacking, dry cough that rapidly becomes productive. Other signs and symptoms quickly follow, including high fever, shaking chills, headache, dyspnea, pleuritic chest pain, tachycardia, grunting respirations, nasal flaring, and cyanosis. Auscultation reveals diminished breath sounds and fine crackles while percussion yields a dull tone.

• *Pneumothorax.* Tachypnea is a common sign of life-threatening pneumothorax. Typically, it's accompanied by severe, sharp, and commonly unilateral chest pain that's aggravated by chest movement. Associated signs and symptoms may include dyspnea, tachycardia, accessory muscle use, asymmetrical chest expansion, dry cough, cyanosis, anxiety, and restlessness. Examination of the affected lung reveals hyperresonance or tympany, subcutaneous crepitation, decreased vocal fremitus, and diminished or absent breath sounds. The patient with tension pneumothorax will also have a deviated trachea.

• *Pulmonary edema.* An early sign of this life-threatening disorder, tachypnea is accompanied by dyspnea on exertion, paroxysmal nocturnal dyspnea, and, later, orthopnea. Other features include a dry cough, crackles, tachycardia, and a ventricular gallop. In severe pulmonary edema, respirations become increasingly rapid and labored, tachycardia worsens, and crackles become more diffuse. The patient's cough also produces frothy, bloody sputum. Signs of shock—such as hypotension, thready pulse, and cold, clammy skin—may also occur.

• *Pulmonary embolism (acute).* Tachypnea occurs suddenly in life-threatening pulmonary embolism and is usually accompanied by dyspnea. The patient may complain of anginal or pleuritic chest pain. Other common characteristics include tachycardia, a dry or productive cough with blood-tinged sputum, low-grade fever, restlessness, and diaphoresis. Less common signs include massive hemoptysis, chest splinting, leg edema, and—with a large embolus—distended neck veins, cyanosis, and syncope. In addition, assessment may detect pleural friction rub, crackles, diffuse wheezing, dullness on percussion, diminished breath sounds, and signs of shock, such as hypotension and a weak, rapid pulse.

• *Pulmonary hypertension (primary).* In this rare disorder, tachypnea is usually a late sign accompanied by dyspnea on exertion, general fatigue, weakness, and syncopal episodes. The patient may complain of anginal chest pain on exertion that may radiate to the neck. Other effects may include a cough, hemoptysis, and hoarseness.

• *Septic shock.* Early in septic shock, the patient usually has tachypnea accompanied by sudden fever, chills, and possibly nausea, vomiting, and diarrhea. He may also have tachycardia and normal or slightly decreased blood pressure; his skin is flushed and warm, yet dry. As this life-threatening type of shock progresses, the patient may display anxiety; restlessness; decreased level of consciousness; hypotension; cool, clammy, and cyanotic skin; rapid, thready pulse; thirst; and oliguria that may progress to anuria.

Other causes

• *Salicylates.* Tachypnea may result from an overdose of these drugs.

Special considerations

Continue to monitor the patient's vital signs closely. Keep suction and emergency equipment nearby, and be prepared to assist with intubation and mechanical ventilation, if necessary.

As ordered, prepare the patient for diagnostic studies, such as arterial blood gas analysis, chest X-rays, and an EKG.

Pediatric pointers

When assessing for tachypnea, recognize that the normal respiratory rate varies with the child's age. (See *Normal Pediatric Vital Signs,* pages 706 and 707.) If you detect tachypnea, you'll need to rule out the causes listed above. Then consider these pediatric causes: congenital heart defects, meningitis, metabolic acidosis, and cystic fibrosis. Keep in mind, though, that hunger and anxiety may also cause tachypnea.

Taste Abnormalities

This symptom refers to several types of taste impairment. *Ageusia,* for example, refers to complete loss of taste; *hypogeusia,* partial loss of taste; and *dysgeusia,* distorted sense of taste. In *cacogeusia,* food may taste unpleasant or even revolting.

The sensory receptors for taste are the taste buds—concentrated over the tongue's surface and scattered over the palate, pharynx, and larynx. These buds can differentiate among sweet, salty, sour, and bitter stimuli. More complex flavors are perceived by taste and olfactory receptors together. In fact, much of what constitutes taste is actually smell; food odors typically stimulate the olfactory system more strongly than related food tastes stimulate the taste buds.

Any factor that interrupts transmission of taste stimuli to the brain may cause taste abnormalities (see *Tracing Taste Pathways to the Brain,* page 710). Taste abnormalities may result from trauma, infection, vitamin or mineral deficiency, neurologic or oral disorders, and the effects of drugs. Also, since tastes are most accurately perceived in a fluid medium, mouth dryness may interfere with taste.

Two major nonpathologic causes of impaired taste are aging, which normally reduces the number of taste buds, and heavy smoking (especially pipe smoking), which dries the tongue.

Assessment

After noting the patient's age, find out when his taste abnormality began. Then search for possible causes. Does the patient have a history of oral or other disorders? Has he recently had the flu? Any head trauma? Does he smoke? Is he receiving radiation treatments? Have the patient list drugs he's currently taking.

Now, thoroughly evaluate the patient's sense of taste. Gently withdraw his tongue slightly with a gauze sponge. Then use a moistened applicator to place a few crystals of salt or sugar on one side of the tongue. Wipe the tongue clean and ask the patient to identify the taste sensation. Repeat the test on the other side of the tongue. To test bitter taste sensation, apply a tiny amount of quinine to the base of the tongue. To test sour taste sensation, place electrodes on the surface of either side of

the tongue and use low-voltage direct current.

Finally, evaluate the patient's sense of smell. Pinch off one nostril and ask the patient to close his eyes and sniff through the open nostril to identify nonirritating odors, such as coffee, lime, and wintergreen. Repeat the test on the opposite nostril.

Medical causes

● *Basilar skull fracture.* When this fracture affects the cranial nerves, it may cause impaired taste. Usually, the patient is unable to taste aromatic flavors, although he can still correctly identify sweet, salty, sour, and bitter stimuli. He may have anosmia (usually permanent), epistaxis, rhinorrhea, otorrhea, Battle's sign, and raccoon's eyes. The patient may also experience headache, nausea and vomiting, hearing and vision loss, and decreased level of consciousness.

● *Bell's palsy.* Taste loss involving the anterior two thirds of the tongue is common in this disorder. Hemifacial muscle weakness or paralysis is also characteristic. The affected side of the patient's face sags and is masklike. Associated signs include drooling and tearing, diminished or absent corneal reflex, and difficulty blinking the affected eye.

● *Common cold.* Although impaired taste sense is a common complaint here, it's usually secondary to loss of smell. Other common features include rhinorrhea with nasal congestion; dry, hacking cough; sore throat; headache; fatigue; myalgia; arthralgia; and malaise.

● *Influenza.* After this viral infection, the patient may have hypogeusia and/or dysgeusia. Typically, he also reports an impaired sense of smell.

● *Oral cancer.* Approximately half of all oral tumors involve the tongue, especially the posterior portion and the lateral borders. These tumors may destroy or damage taste buds, resulting in impaired taste. The patient also has difficulty chewing and speaking, and

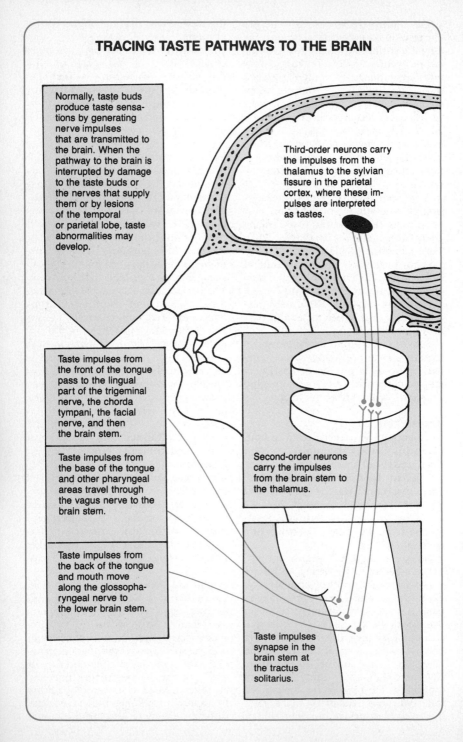

TRACING TASTE PATHWAYS TO THE BRAIN

Normally, taste buds produce taste sensations by generating nerve impulses that are transmitted to the brain. When the pathway to the brain is interrupted by damage to the taste buds or the nerves that supply them or by lesions of the temporal or parietal lobe, taste abnormalities may develop.

Third-order neurons carry the impulses from the thalamus to the sylvian fissure in the parietal cortex, where these impulses are interpreted as tastes.

Taste impulses from the front of the tongue pass to the lingual part of the trigeminal nerve, the chorda tympani, the facial nerve, and then the brain stem.

Taste impulses from the base of the tongue and other pharyngeal areas travel through the vagus nerve to the brain stem.

Taste impulses from the back of the tongue and mouth move along the glossopharyngeal nerve to the lower brain stem.

Second-order neurons carry the impulses from the brain stem to the thalamus.

Taste impulses synapse in the brain stem at the tractus solitarius.

he may demonstrate halitosis.

• *Sjögren's syndrome.* In this autosomal recessive disorder, impaired taste sense results from extreme mouth dryness associated with inadequate production of saliva. Ocular dryness is also characteristic; initially, it causes burning and pain around the eyes and under the lids. Later, the patient develops photosensitivity, impaired vision, and eye fatigue and redness. Other signs and symptoms may include mouth soreness; difficulty chewing, swallowing, and talking; dry cough; hoarseness; epistaxis; dry, scaly skin; decreased sweating; abdominal distress; and polyuria. Physical examination may reveal corneal ulceration, nasal crusting, and enlarged lacrimal, parotid, and submaxillary glands.

• *Thalamic syndromes.* Déjerine-Roussy syndrome, for example, may produce a distorted sense of taste. Typically, this symptom is preceded by contralateral sensory loss (both deep and cutaneous), transient hemiparesis, and homonymous hemianopia. Subsequently, the patient gradually regains sensation and may then experience pain or hyperpathia.

• *Viral hepatitis (acute).* Hypogeusia frequently precedes the jaundice of hepatitis by 1 to 2 weeks. Associated signs and symptoms in the preicteric phase include altered sense of smell, anorexia, nausea, vomiting, fatigue, malaise, headache, photophobia, sore throat, and a cough. The patient may also have muscle and joint aches.

• *Vitamin B_{12} deficiency.* In this vitamin deficiency, hypogeusia is accompanied by an impaired sense of smell, anorexia, weight loss, abdominal discomfort, and glossitis. The patient may also have yellow skin, peripheral neuropathy, dyspnea, ataxic gait, and occasional depression.

• *Zinc deficiency.* This mineral deficiency is common in patients with idiopathic hypogeusia, suggesting that zinc plays an important role in normal taste sensation. Common associated characteristics of zinc deficiency in-clude impaired or distorted sense of smell, cacogeusia, anorexia, soft and misshapen nails, and sparse hair growth. Palpation reveals an enlarged liver and spleen.

Other causes

• *Drugs.* Drugs that may distort taste include penicillamine, captopril, griseofulvin, lithium, rifampin, antithyroid preparations, procarbazine, vincristine, and vinblastine.

• *Radiation therapy.* Irradiation of the head or neck may cause excessive dryness of the mouth, resulting in impaired taste.

Special considerations

Modify the patient's diet, if necessary, so that he can distinguish and enjoy as many tastes as possible.

Pediatric pointers

Recognize that young children are frequently unable to differentiate between an abnormal taste sensation and a simple taste dislike.

Tearing Increase
[Epiphora]

Tears normally bathe the eyes, keeping the epithelium moist and flushing away foreign bodies. Excessive production of this clear fluid—or lacrimation—results from stimulation of the lacrimal glands.

Lacrimation may be classified as psychic and neurogenic. *Psychic lacrimation* normally occurs in response to emotional or physical stress, such as pain; it's the most common cause of increased tearing. *Neurogenic lacrimation* is triggered by reflex stimulation associated with ocular trauma or inflammation or with exposure to environmental irritants, such as strong light, dry or hot wind, or airborne allergens. This type of lacrimation may also accompany eyestrain, yawning, vomiting, and laughing.

Assessment

If the patient complains of increased tearing, begin by fully exploring this sign. When did it begin? Is it constant or intermittent? Minimal or excessive? Is increased tearing accompanied by pain? Next, ask about recent eye trauma and about ocular and systemic disorders. Then record what drugs the patient is currently taking. Note his occupation and the nature of his work. For example, does he read extensively or work with small or fine objects?

After taking vital signs, examine both eyes—unless the history suggests a perforating or penetrating injury. Carefully inspect the external structures. Do the eyelashes contain debris? Examine the eyelids for lesions and edema. Ask the patient to look straight ahead at a fixed object while you check for ptosis. Are the lid margins turned inward or outward? Examine the eyeballs. Do they appear sunken or bulging? Examine the conjunctiva for redness and abnormal drainage. Also note the color of the sclera. Hold a flashlight at the side of either eye and examine the cornea and iris for scars, irregularities, and foreign bodies. Evaluate extraocular muscle function by testing the six cardinal fields of gaze. (See *Testing Extraocular Muscles*, page 235.) Finally, test the patient's visual acuity.

Medical causes

● *Blepharophimosis.* Increased tearing and exposure keratitis—corneal inflammation with incomplete lid closure—are common signs. Examination also reveals ectropion; a small, expressionless face with deep-set eyes and pursed lips; and a high-arched palate.

● *Conjunctival foreign bodies and abrasions.* Increased tearing may accompany localized conjunctival injection, severe eye pain, and photophobia. A foreign body sensation may be present.

● *Conjunctivitis.* Typically, increased tearing is accompanied by conjunctival injection and itching in this disorder. *Allergic conjunctivitis* also causes ropy or stringy discharge. In *bacterial conjunctivitis,* other features include copious, purulent discharge; burning; a foreign body sensation; and possibly eye pain if the cornea is involved. Associated signs of *fungal conjunctivitis* include lid edema; burning; and copious, thick, purulent discharge that may form sticky crusts on the lids. The patient complains of photophobia and pain if the cornea is involved. Highly contagious *viral conjunctivitis* also causes a foreign body sensation, slight exudate, and lid edema. Other effects: fever, sore throat, diarrhea, and preauricular lymphadenopathy.

● *Corneal abrasion.* Marked by severe corneal pain that's aggravated by blinking, this injury also causes increased tearing. Associated features are a foreign body sensation, blurred vision, conjunctival injection, and photophobia, which makes opening the lids difficult.

● *Corneal foreign body.* When a foreign body lodges in the cornea, the patient will have increased tearing, blurred vision, a foreign body sensation, photophobia, eye pain, miosis, and conjunctival injection. A dark speck may also be visible in the cornea.

● *Corneal ulcers.* In this vision-threatening disorder, increased tearing is accompanied by severe photophobia and eye pain. Typically, the disorder begins with pain that's aggravated by blinking. Ulcers also cause blurred vision, conjunctival injection, and a white, opaque cornea. A bacterial ulcer also produces copious, purulent discharge that may form sticky crusts on the lids.

● *Dacryocystitis.* Increased tearing and purulent discharge are the chief complaints in this disorder, which is typically unilateral. Associated signs and symptoms include pain and tenderness around the tear sac with marked eyelid edema and redness near the lacrimal punctum. Pressure on the tear sac expresses a thick, purulent discharge or, in chronic cases, a mucoid discharge.

• **Episcleritis.** Commonly unilateral, this disorder causes increased tearing, photophobia, and—if the sclera is inflamed—eye pain and tenderness on palpation. Inspection reveals conjunctival injection and edema, a purplish pink sclera, and episcleral edema.

• **Herpes zoster.** Increased tearing usually occurs when herpes zoster affects the trigeminal nerve. It's accompanied by severe unilateral facial and eye pain that's followed by the eruption of vesicles within several days. The patient's eyelids are red and swollen with scanty serous discharge. Other common findings include a white, cloudy cornea and conjunctival injection.

• **Lid contractions.** Here, increased tearing usually results from stricture of the canaliculi. Because lid contractions are caused by burns or chemical or mechanical trauma, lid scars are also frequently visible.

• **Psoriasis vulgaris.** When these lesions affect the eyelids and extend into the conjunctiva, they may cause irritation with increased tearing and a foreign body sensation. Typically, the appearance of lesions follows signs of chronic conjunctivitis, such as copious mucoid discharge and conjunctival injection.

• **Punctum misplacement.** Increased tearing is characteristic when ectropion involves the punctum, causing misplacement. It may be accompanied by exposure keratitis.

• **Raeder's syndrome.** This syndrome is characterized by periodic symptomatic attacks for 5 minutes or longer. The patient may have increased tearing, ptosis, abnormal pupillary response, ipsilateral headache, and anhidrosis of the face and neck. Diplopia and enophthalmos may also occur.

• **Scleritis.** This rare, chronic disorder causes increased tearing, photophobia, and severe eye pain with tenderness on palpation. Examination reveals conjunctival injection and a bluish purple sclera.

• **Thyrotoxicosis.** This disorder may cause increased tearing, usually in both

CAUSES OF DECREASED TEARING

Decreased tearing, or hyposecretion, makes the patient's eyes uncomfortably dry. Usually, this symptom is associated with aging. However, it may also result from the following causes:

Anticholinergics. Decreased tearing commonly follows administration of anticholinergic (mydriatic) agents, such as atropine, scopolamine, cyclopentolate, and tropicamide.

Bonnevie-Ullrich syndrome. Characterized by congenital absence of the lacrimal gland, this syndrome also causes decreased tearing.

Keratoconjunctivitis sicca (dry eye syndrome). In this syndrome, atrophy of the lacrimal glands curtails tear production.

Ocular trauma. Decreased tearing may accompany healing and scar formation following acute ocular trauma.

Sarcoidosis. Decreased tearing results from inflammation of the lacrimal and salivary glands in this syndrome.

Stevens-Johnson syndrome. In this syndrome, decreased tearing is accompanied by purulent conjunctivitis and severe eye pain.

Vitamin A deficiency. Typically, this vitamin deficiency causes decreased tearing and poor night vision.

Treatment of nontraumatic decreased tearing usually involves a preparation of artificial tears in either drops or ointment.

eyes. Other ocular effects may include ptosis, lid edema, photophobia, a foreign body sensation, conjunctival injection, chemosis, diplopia and, at times, exophthalmos. Common associated features are heat intolerance, weight loss despite increased appetite, nervousness, sweating, diarrhea, tremors, tachycardia, palpitations, and an enlarged thyroid.

• *Trachoma.* An early sign of this disorder, increased tearing is accompanied by visible conjunctival follicles, red and edematous eyelids, pain, photophobia, and exudation. After about 1 month, if the infection is untreated, conjunctival follicles enlarge into inflamed papillae that later become yellow or gray. Also, small blood vessels invade the cornea under the upper lid.

Other causes

• *Cholinergics.* Miotics, such as pilocarpine, may increase tearing.

Special considerations

Obtain a tear specimen for culture, as ordered, and isolate the patient until a definite diagnosis is made. Also prepare him for Schirmer's test to measure tear production and secretion and for irrigation of the lacrimal drainage system, as ordered. Instruct him not to touch the unaffected eye to avoid possible cross-contamination.

Pediatric pointers

The most common pediatric causes of increased tearing include allergies, conjunctivitis, and the common cold.

Throat Pain

[Sore throat]

Throat pain refers to discomfort in any part of the pharynx: the nasopharynx, the oropharynx, or the hypopharynx. This common symptom ranges from a sensation of scratchiness to severe pain.

It's often accompanied by ear pain because cranial nerves IX and X innervate the pharynx as well as the middle and external ear.

Throat pain may result from infection, trauma, allergy, neoplasms, and certain systemic disorders. It may also follow surgery and endotracheal intubation. Nonpathologic causes include dry mucous membranes associated with mouth breathing and laryngeal irritation associated with alcohol consumption, inhaling smoke or chemicals like ammonia, and vocal strain.

Assessment

Ask the patient when he first noticed the pain and have him describe it. Has he had throat pain before? Is it accompanied by fever, ear pain, or dysphagia? Review the patient's medical history for throat problems, allergies, and systemic disorders.

Next, carefully examine the pharynx, noting redness, exudate, or swelling. Assess the oropharynx, using a warmed metal spatula or tongue blade, and the nasopharynx, using a warmed laryngeal mirror. Assist with laryngoscopic examination of the hypopharynx, as ordered. (If necessary, spray the soft palate and pharyngeal wall with a local anesthetic to prevent gagging.) Observe the tonsils for redness, swelling, or exudate, too. Also obtain an exudate specimen for culture. Then examine the patient's nose, using a nasal speculum. Also check his ears—especially if he reports ear pain. Finally, palpate the neck and oropharynx for nodules or lymph node enlargement.

Medical causes

• *Agranulocytosis.* In this disorder, sore throat may accompany other signs of infection, such as fever, chills, and headache. Typically, it follows progressive fatigue and weakness. Other findings may include nausea, vomiting, anorexia, and bleeding tendencies. Rough-edged ulcers with gray or black membranes may appear on the gums,

REVIEWING ANATOMY OF THE THROAT

The throat, or pharynx, is divided into three areas: the nasopharynx (the soft palate and posterior nasal cavity), the oropharynx (the area between the soft palate and upper edge of the epiglottis), and the hypopharynx (the area between the epiglottis and level of the cricoid cartilage). A disorder affecting any of these areas may cause sore throat, or throat pain. Pinpointing the causative disorder begins with accurate assessment of the throat structures illustrated here.

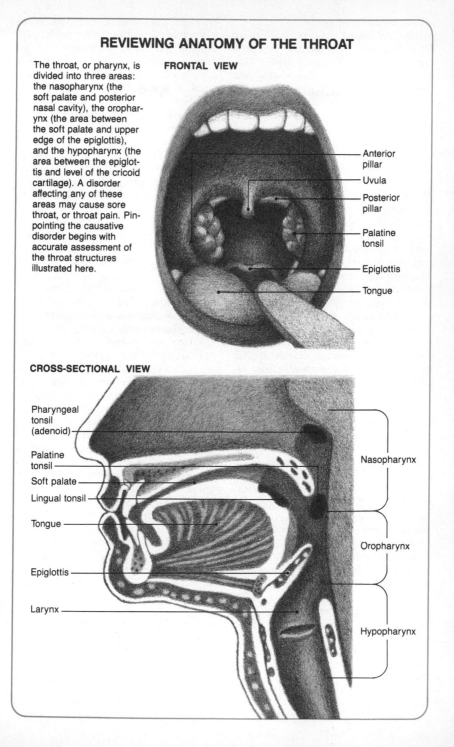

FRONTAL VIEW

- Anterior pillar
- Uvula
- Posterior pillar
- Palatine tonsil
- Epiglottis
- Tongue

CROSS-SECTIONAL VIEW

- Pharyngeal tonsil (adenoid)
- Palatine tonsil
- Soft palate
- Lingual tonsil
- Tongue
- Epiglottis
- Larynx

- Nasopharynx
- Oropharynx
- Hypopharynx

palate, or perianal area.

• *Allergic rhinitis.* Occurring seasonally or year-round, this disorder may produce sore throat. The patient will also complain of nasal congestion with thin nasal discharge, postnasal drip, paroxysmal sneezing, decreased sense of smell, frontal or temporal headache, and itchy eyes, nose, and possibly throat. Examination reveals pale and glistening nasal mucosa with edematous nasal turbinates, watery eyes, reddened conjunctiva and eyelids, and possibly swollen lids.

• *Bronchitis (acute).* This disorder may produce lower throat pain. Associated findings may include fever, chills, cough, and muscle and back pain. Auscultation reveals rhonchi, wheezing and, at times, crackles.

• *Common cold.* Sore throat may accompany cough, sneezing, nasal congestion, rhinorrhea, fatigue, headache, myalgia, and arthralgia.

• *Contact ulcers.* Common in men with stressful jobs, contact ulcers appear symmetrically on the vocal cords, resulting in sore throat. The pain is aggravated by talking and may be accompanied by referred ear pain and, occasionally, hemoptysis. Typically, the patient also has a history of chronic throat clearing.

• *Eagle's syndrome.* This syndrome results when an unusually long styloid process becomes trapped in a tonsillectomy scar. Palpation of this area will cause throat pain.

• *Foreign body.* A foreign body lodged in the palatine or lingual tonsil and pyriform sinus may produce localized throat pain. The pain may persist after the foreign body is dislodged until mucosal irritation resolves.

• *Glossopharyngeal neuralgia.* Triggered by a specific pharyngeal movement, such as yawning or swallowing, this condition causes unilateral, knifelike throat pain in the tonsillar fossa that may radiate to the ear.

• *Herpes simplex virus.* Sore throat may result from lesions on the oral mucosa, especially the tongue, gingivae, and cheeks. After causing brief prodromal discomfort (tingling and itching), lesions erupt into erythematous vesicles that eventually rupture and leave a painful ulcer, followed by a yellowish crust. In generalized infection, the vesicles are accompanied by submaxillary lymphadenopathy, halitosis, increased salivation, anorexia, and fever of up to 105° F. (40.5° C.).

• *Infectious mononucleosis.* Sore throat is one of the three classic findings in this infection. Other classic signs are cervical lymphadenopathy and fluctuating temperature with an evening peak of 101° to 102° F. (38.3° to 38.9° C.). Splenomegaly and hepatomegaly may also develop.

• *Influenza.* Patients with the flu commonly complain of sore throat, fever with chills, headache, weakness, malaise, muscle aches, cough, and occasionally hoarseness and rhinorrhea.

• *Laryngeal cancer.* In *extrinsic laryngeal cancer*, the chief symptom is pain or burning in the throat when drinking citrus juice or hot liquids, or a lump in the throat; in *intrinsic laryngeal cancer*, it's hoarseness that persists for more than 3 weeks. Later, clinical effects of metastases include dysphagia, dyspnea, a cough, enlarged cervical lymph nodes, and pain that radiates to the ear.

• *Laryngitis (acute).* This disorder produces sore throat. Its cardinal sign, though, is mild to severe hoarseness— perhaps with temporary loss of voice. Other findings are malaise, low-grade fever, dysphagia, dry cough, and tender, enlarged cervical lymph nodes.

• *Lymph follicular hypertrophy.* In this disorder, mild sore throat is accompanied by diffuse edema of the oropharynx.

• *Necrotizing ulcerative gingivitis (acute).* Also known as trench mouth, this disorder usually begins abruptly with sore throat and tender gums that ulcerate and bleed. A gray exudate may cover the gums and pharyngeal tonsils. Related signs and symptoms include a foul taste in the mouth, halitosis, cervical lymphadenopathy, headache, malaise, and fever.

• *Peritonsillar abscess.* A complication of bacterial tonsillitis, this abscess typically causes severe throat pain that radiates to the ear. Accompanying the pain may be dysphagia, drooling, dysarthria, halitosis, fever with chills, malaise, and nausea. Usually, the patient tilts his head to the side of the abscess. Examination may also reveal a deviated uvula, trismus, and tender cervical lymphadenopathy.

• *Pharyngeal burns.* First- or second-degree burns of the posterior pharynx may cause throat pain and dysphagia.

• *Pharyngitis.* Whether bacterial, fungal, or viral, pharyngitis may cause sore throat and localized erythema and edema. *Bacterial pharyngitis* begins abruptly with unilateral sore throat. Associated signs and symptoms include dysphagia, fever, malaise, headache, abdominal pain, myalgia, and arthralgia. Inspection reveals an exudate on the tonsil or tonsillar fossae, uvular edema, soft palate erythema, and tender cervical lymph nodes.

Also known as thrush, *fungal pharyngitis* causes diffuse sore throat—often described as a burning sensation—accompanied by pharyngeal erythema and edema. White plaques mark the pharynx, tonsil, tonsillar pillars, and base of the tongue; scraping these plaques uncovers a hemorrhagic base.

In *viral pharyngitis,* findings include diffuse sore throat, malaise, fever, and mild erythema and edema of the posterior oropharyngeal wall. The tonsils aren't inflamed, but the cervical lymph nodes may be enlarged.

• *Pharyngomaxillary space abscess.* A complication of untreated pharyngeal or tonsillar infection or tooth extraction, this abscess causes mild throat pain. Inspection reveals a bulge in the medial wall of the pharynx accompanied by swelling of the neck and at the jaw angle on the affected side. Other signs and symptoms may include fever, dysphagia, trismus, and possibly signs of respiratory distress.

• *Posterior tongue carcinoma.* In this carcinoma, localized throat pain may occur around a raised white lesion or ulcer. The pain may radiate to the ear and be accompanied by dysphagia.

• *Reflux laryngopharyngitis.* In this disorder, an incompetent gastroesophageal sphincter allows gastric juices to enter the hypopharynx and irritate the larynx, resulting in chronic sore throat and hoarseness. The adenoids may also appear red and swollen.

• *Sinusitis (acute).* This disorder may cause sore throat accompanied by purulent nasal discharge and postnasal drip, resulting in halitosis. Its other effects may include headache, malaise, cough, fever, and facial pain and swelling associated with nasal congestion.

• *Supraglottic cancer.* Early features include throat pain that radiates to the ear, dysphagia, and a muffled voice. Most common in smokers, the lesion appears as an exophytic wart on the epiglottis and causes hoarseness.

• *Tonsillar carcinoma.* Sore throat is the presenting symptom here. Unfortunately, the carcinoma is usually quite advanced before this symptom occurs. The pain radiates to the ear and is accompanied by a superficial ulcer on the tonsil or one that extends to the base of the tongue.

• *Tonsillitis.* In *acute tonsillitis,* mild to severe sore throat is usually the first symptom. The pain may radiate to the ears and be accompanied by dysphagia and headache. Related findings include malaise, fever with chills, halitosis, myalgia, arthralgia, and tender cervical lymphadenopathy. Examination reveals edematous, reddened tonsils with a purulent exudate.

Chronic tonsillitis causes mild sore throat, malaise, and tender cervical lymph nodes. The tonsils appear smooth, pink, and possibly enlarged, with a purulent debris in the crypts. Halitosis and a foul taste in the mouth are other common findings.

Unilateral throat pain just above the hyoid bone occurs in *lingual tonsillitis.* The lingual tonsils appear red and swollen and are covered with exudate. Other findings include a muffled voice, dysphagia, and tender cervical lymphadenopathy on the affected side.

- **Uvulitis.** This inflammation may cause throat pain or a sensation of something in the throat. Usually, the uvula is swollen and red; however, in allergic uvulitis, it's pale.

Other causes
- **Treatments.** Endotracheal intubation and local surgery, such as tonsillectomy and adenoidectomy, commonly cause sore throat.

Special considerations
Provide analgesic sprays or lozenges, as ordered, to relieve throat pain. Also prepare the patient for throat culture, complete blood count, and a Monospot test.

Pediatric pointers
In children, sore throat is a common complaint. It may result from many of the same disorders that affect adults. Other pediatric causes of sore throat include acute epiglottitis, herpangina, scarlet fever, acute follicular tonsillitis, and retropharyngeal abscess.

Tics

A tic is an involuntary, repetitive movement of a specific group of muscles—usually those of the face, neck, shoulders, trunk, and hands. Typically, this sign occurs suddenly and intermittently. It may involve a single isolated movement, such as lip smacking, grimacing, blinking, sniffing, tongue thrusting, throat clearing, hitching up one shoulder, or protruding the chin. Or it may involve a complex set of movements. Mild tics, such as twitching of an eyelid, are especially common.

Usually, tics are psychogenic and may be aggravated by stress or anxiety.

However, they're also associated with one rare affliction—Gilles de la Tourette's syndrome. Psychogenic tics, though, often begin between the ages of 5 and 10 as voluntary, coordinated, and purposeful actions that the child feels compelled to perform to decrease anxiety. Unless the tics are severe, the child may be unaware of them. The tics may subside as the child matures, or they may persist into adulthood.

To distinguish tics from minor seizures, remember that tics aren't associated with transient loss of consciousness or amnesia.

Assessment
Begin by asking the parents how long the child has had the tic. Can they identify any precipitating factors? Ask about stress in the child's life, such as difficult school work. Next, carefully observe the tic. Is it a purposeful or involuntary movement? Note whether it's localized or generalized and describe it in detail.

Medical cause
- **Gilles de la Tourette's syndrome.** Typically, this rare syndrome begins between the ages of 2 and 15 with a tic that involves the face or neck. Eventually, the tic spreads to the muscles of the shoulders, arms, trunk, and legs, and may be characterized by violent movement and outbursts of obscenities (coprolalia). The patient snorts, barks, and grunts and may emit explosive sounds, such as hissing, when he speaks. He may involuntarily repeat another person's words (echolalia) or movements (echopraxia). Occasionally, this syndrome subsides spontaneously or undergoes a prolonged remission; however, the syndrome may persist throughout life.

Special considerations
Psychotherapy and administration of tranquilizers may relieve the source of anxiety causing the tic. Many patients with Gilles de la Tourette's syndrome receive haloperidol or pimozide to control tics and reduce anxiety.

Tinnitus

Tinnitus literally means ringing in the ears, although many other abnormal sounds fall under this term. For example, tinnitus may be described as the sound of escaping air, running water, or the inside of a seashell or as a sizzling, buzzing, or humming noise. Occasionally, it's described as a roaring or musical sound. This common symptom may be unilateral or bilateral and constant or intermittent. Although the brain can adjust to or suppress constant tinnitus, intermittent tinnitus may be so disturbing that some patients contemplate suicide as their only source of relief.

Tinnitus can be classified in several ways. *Subjective tinnitus* (nonvibratory or nonpulsatile tinnitus) is heard only by the patient, while *objective tinnitus* (vibratory or pulsatile tinnitus) is also heard by the observer who places a stethoscope near the patient's affected ear. *Tinnitus aurium* refers to noise that the patient hears in his ears; *tinnitus cerebri,* to noise that he hears in his head.

No matter how tinnitus is classified, its pathophysiology remains the same. This symptom reflects stimulation of sensory auditory neurons, resulting in transmission of a sound impulse. Commonly resulting from ear disorders, tinnitus may also stem from cardiovascular and systemic disorders and from the effects of drugs. Nonpathologic causes of tinnitus include acute anxiety and presbycusis.

Assessment

Ask the patient to describe the tinnitus: its onset, pattern, pitch, location, and intensity. Is it accompanied by other symptoms, such as vertigo, headache, or hearing loss? Next, take a health history, including a complete drug history.

Using an otoscope, inspect the patient's ears and examine the tympanic membrane. To check for hearing loss, perform the Weber and Rinne tuning fork tests. (See *Differentiating Conductive and Sensorineural Hearing Loss,* page 374.) Auscultate for bruits in the neck; then compress the jugular or carotid artery to see if this affects the tinnitus. Finally, examine the nasopharynx for masses that might cause eustachian tube dysfunction and tinnitus.

Medical causes

● *Acoustic neuroma.* An early symptom of this eighth cranial nerve tumor, tinnitus precedes unilateral sensorineural hearing loss and vertigo. Facial paralysis, headache, nausea, vomiting, and papilledema may also occur.

● *Anemia.* Severe anemia may produce mild, reversible tinnitus accompanied by dim vision, syncope, and irritability. Other common effects of anemia include pallor, weakness, fatigue, exertional dyspnea, tachycardia, bounding pulse, atrial gallop, and a systolic bruit over the carotid arteries.

● *Atherosclerosis of the carotid artery.* In this disorder, the patient has constant tinnitus that can be stopped by applying pressure over the carotid artery. He also feels confused, weak, and unsteady when he rises in the morning or stands up quickly. Auscultation over the upper part of the neck, on the auricle, or near the ear on the affected side may detect a bruit. Palpation may reveal a weak carotid pulse.

● *Cervical spondylosis.* In this degenerative disorder, osteophytic growths may compress the vertebral arteries, resulting in tinnitus. Typically, a stiff neck and pain aggravated by activity produce tinnitus. Other features may include brief vertigo, nystagmus, hearing loss, and pain that radiates down the arms. Paresthesias or weakness may be present.

● *Ear canal obstruction.* When cerumen or a foreign body blocks the ear canal, tinnitus may occur with conductive hearing loss, itching, and a feeling of fullness or pain in the ear.

• *Eustachian tube patency.* Normally, the eustachian tube remains closed, except during swallowing. However, persistent patency of this tube can cause tinnitus, audible breath sounds, loud and distorted voice sounds, and a sense of fullness in the ear. Examination with a pneumatic otoscope reveals movement of the tympanic membrane with respirations. At times, breath sounds can be heard with a stethoscope placed over the auricle.

• *Glomus jugulare or tympanicum tumor.* Usually, vibratory tinnitus is the first symptom of this tumor. Other early features include a reddish blue mass behind the tympanic membrane and progressive conductive hearing loss. Later, total unilateral deafness is accompanied by ear pain and dizziness. Otorrhagia may also occur if the tumor breaks through the tympanic membrane.

• *Hypertension.* Bilateral, high-pitched tinnitus may occur in severe hypertension. Diastolic blood pressure exceeding 120 mm Hg may also cause severe, throbbing headache, restlessness, nausea, vomiting, blurred vision, seizures, and decreased level of consciousness.

• *Intracranial arteriovenous malformation.* A large malformation may cause pulsating tinnitus accompanied by a bruit over the mastoid process.

• *Labyrinthitis (suppurative).* In this disorder, tinnitus may accompany sudden, severe attacks of vertigo, unilateral or bilateral sensorineural hearing loss, nystagmus, dizziness, nausea, and vomiting.

• *Ménière's disease.* Most common in men between the ages of 55 and 65, this labyrinthine disease is characterized by attacks of low-pitched tinnitus, vertigo, and fluctuating sensorineural hearing loss. Usually, these attacks are unilateral and last from 10 minutes to several hours; they occur over a few days or weeks followed by a remission. Severe nausea, vomiting, diaphoresis, and nystagmus may also occur during attacks. The patient may report a feeling of fullness in the ear.

• *Noise.* Chronic exposure to noise, especially high-pitch sounds, may damage the ear's hair cells, causing tinnitus and a bilateral hearing loss. These symptoms may be temporary or permanent.

• *Ossicle dislocation.* Acoustic trauma—such as a slap on the ear—may cause ossicle dislocation, resulting in tinnitus, sensorineural hearing loss, and bleeding from the middle ear.

• *Otitis externa (acute).* Although not a major complaint here, tinnitus may result if debris in the external ear canal impinges on the tympanic membrane. More typical findings include pruritus, foul-smelling purulent discharge, and severe ear pain that's aggravated by manipulation of the tragus or auricle, teeth clenching, mouth opening, and chewing. Typically, the external ear canal appears red and edematous and may be occluded by debris, causing partial hearing loss.

• *Otitis media.* This infection may cause tinnitus and conductive hearing loss. However, its more characteristic features include ear pain, a red and bulging tympanic membrane, high fever, chills, and dizziness.

• *Otosclerosis.* In this disorder, the patient may describe ringing, roaring, or whistling tinnitus or a combination of these sounds. He may also report progressive hearing loss—which may lead to bilateral deafness—and vertigo. Audiologic evalution usually reveals that bone conduction is better than air conduction.

• *Palatal myoclonus.* In this disorder, muscles of the palate contract rhythmically—either intermittently or continuously—causing a clicking sound in the ear and vibratory tinnitus. The contractions are visible with a nasopharyngeal mirror.

• *Tympanic membrane perforation.* In this disorder, tinnitus and hearing loss go hand-in-hand. However, tinnitus is usually the chief complaint in a small perforation; hearing loss, in a larger one. Typically, these symptoms develop suddenly and may be accompanied by

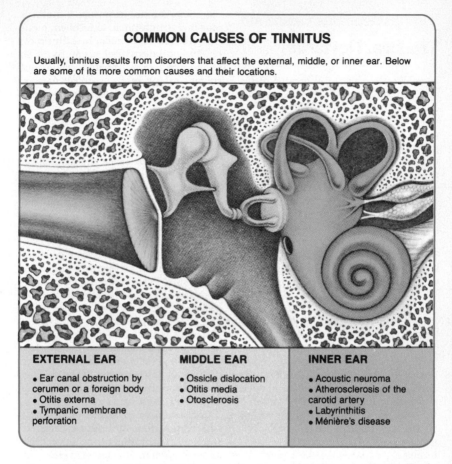

COMMON CAUSES OF TINNITUS

Usually, tinnitus results from disorders that affect the external, middle, or inner ear. Below are some of its more common causes and their locations.

EXTERNAL EAR
- Ear canal obstruction by cerumen or a foreign body
- Otitis externa
- Tympanic membrane perforation

MIDDLE EAR
- Ossicle dislocation
- Otitis media
- Otosclerosis

INNER EAR
- Acoustic neuroma
- Atherosclerosis of the carotid artery
- Labyrinthitis
- Ménière's disease

pain, vertigo, and a feeling of fullness in the ear.

Other causes
• *Drugs and alcohol.* An overdose of salicylates frequently causes reversible tinnitus. Quinine, alcohol, and indomethacin may also cause reversible tinnitus. Common drugs that may cause irreversible tinnitus include the aminoglycoside antibiotics (especially kanamycin, streptomycin, and gentamicin) and vancomycin.

Special considerations
Recognize that tinnitus usually can't be treated successfully. To help the patient tolerate this symptom, provide vasodilators, tranquilizers, and antiseizure drugs or encourage use of biofeedback and tinnitus maskers, as ordered. A tinnitus masker produces a band of noise about 1800 Hz, which helps block out tinnitus without hampering hearing. Also, a hearing aid may be prescribed to amplify environmental sounds, thereby obscuring tinnitus. At times, a device that combines features of a masker and hearing aid may be used to block out tinnitus.

Pediatric pointers
Maternal use of ototoxic drugs during the third trimester of pregnancy can cause labyrinthine damage in the fetus, resulting in tinnitus. This symptom may also occur in children with many of the disorders described above.

Tracheal Deviation

Normally, the trachea is located at the midline of the neck—except at the bifurcation, where it shifts slightly toward the right. Visible deviation from its normal position signals an underlying condition that can compromise pulmonary function and possibly cause respiratory distress. A hallmark of life-threatening tension pneumothorax, this sign occurs in disorders that produce mediastinal shift due to asymmetrical thoracic volume or pressure. In elderly persons, tracheal deviation to the right often stems from an elongated, atherosclerotic aortic arch, but this deviation isn't considered abnormal.

Assessment

If the patient exhibits signs of respiratory distress (tachypnea, dyspnea, stridor, nasal flaring, accessory muscle use, asymmetrical chest expansion, restlessness, and anxiety), notify the doctor at once. If possible, place the patient in semi-Fowler's position to aid respiratory excursion and improve oxygenation. Give supplemental oxygen, and prepare to intubate the patient, if necessary. As ordered, insert an I.V. line for fluid and drug administration. Palpate for subcutaneous crepitation in the neck and chest—a sign of tension pneumothorax. Prepare to assist with chest tube insertion to release trapped air or fluid and to restore normal intrapleural and intrathoracic pressure gradients.

If the patient doesn't display signs of distress, ask about a history of pulmonary or cardiac disorders, trauma, or infection. If he smokes, determine how much. Ask about associated symptoms, especially breathing difficulty, pain, and cough.

Medical causes

• *Atelectasis.* Extensive lung collapse can produce tracheal deviation toward the affected side. Respiratory findings may include dyspnea, tachypnea, pleuritic chest pain, dry cough, dullness on percussion, decreased vocal fremitus and breath sounds, inspiratory lag, and substernal or intercostal retraction. Tachycardia, cyanosis, anxiety, and diaphoresis may also occur.

• *Hiatal hernia.* Intrusion of abdominal viscera into the pleural space causes tracheal deviation toward the unaffected side. The degree of attendant respiratory distress depends on the extent of herniation. Other effects may include pyrosis, regurgitation or vomiting, and chest or abdominal pain.

• *Kyphoscoliosis.* This disorder can cause rib cage distortion and mediastinal shift, producing tracheal deviation toward the compressed lung. Respiratory effects include dry coughing, dyspnea, and asymmetrical chest expansion. Backache and fatigue commonly occur.

• *Mediastinal tumor.* Often asymptomatic in its early stages, this tumor, when large, can press against the trachea and nearby structures, causing tracheal deviation and dysphagia. Other late findings may include stridor, dyspnea, brassy cough, hoarseness, and stertorous respirations with suprasternal retraction. The patient may experience shoulder, arm, or chest pain, and edema of the neck, face, or arm. His neck and chest wall veins may be dilated.

• *Pleural effusion.* A large pleural effusion can shift the mediastinum to the contralateral side, producing tracheal deviation. Related effects may include dry cough, dyspnea, pleuritic pain, pleural friction rub, tachypnea, decreased chest motion, decreased or absent breath sounds, egophony, flatness on percussion, decreased tactile fremitus, fever, and weight loss.

• *Pulmonary fibrosis.* Asymmetrical fibrosis can cause tracheal deviation as the mediastinum shifts toward the affected side. Associated findings reflect the underlying condition and pattern of fibrosis. Dyspnea, cough, clubbing,

DETECTING SLIGHT TRACHEAL DEVIATION

Although gross tracheal deviation will be visible, detection of slight deviation requires palpation and perhaps even an X-ray. Try palpation first.

With the tip of your index finger, locate the patient's trachea by palpating between the sternocleidomastoid muscles. Then compare the trachea's position to an imaginary line drawn vertically through the suprasternal notch. Any deviation from midline is usually considered abnormal.

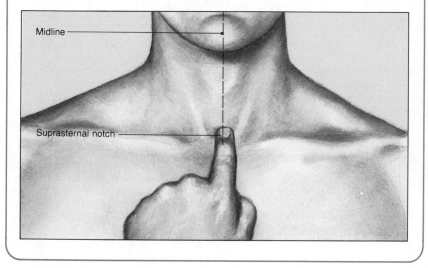

malaise, and fever are common.

• *Pulmonary tuberculosis.* With a large cavitation, tracheal deviation toward the affected side accompanies asymmetrical chest excursion, dullness on percussion, increased tactile fremitus, amphoric breath sounds, and inspiratory crackles. Insidious early effects include fatigue, anorexia, weight loss, fever, chills, and night sweats. Productive cough, hemoptysis, pleuritic chest pain, and dyspnea develop as the disease progresses.

• *Retrosternal thyroid.* This anatomic abnormality can displace the trachea. The gland is felt as a movable neck mass above the suprasternal notch. Dysphagia, cough, hoarseness, and stridor frequently occur. Signs of thyrotoxicosis may be present.

• *Tension pneumothorax.* This acute, life-threatening condition produces tracheal deviation toward the unaffected side. It's marked by a sudden onset of respiratory distress with sharp chest pain, dry cough, severe dyspnea, tachycardia, wheezing, cyanosis, accessory muscle use, nasal flaring, air hunger, and asymmetrical chest movement. Restless and anxious, the patient may also have subcutaneous crepitation in the neck and upper chest, decreased vocal fremitus, decreased or absent breath sounds on the affected side, distended neck veins, and hypotension.

• *Thoracic aortic aneurysm.* This disorder usually causes the trachea to deviate to the right. Highly variable associated findings may include stridor, dyspnea, wheezing, brassy cough, hoarseness, and dysphagia. Edema of the face, neck, or arm may occur with distended chest wall and neck veins. Substernal, neck, shoulder, or lower back pain may occur, possibly with paresthesias or neuralgia.

Special considerations
Because tracheal deviation usually signals a severe underlying disorder that can cause respiratory distress at any time, monitor the patient's respiratory and cardiac status constantly, and make sure that emergency equipment is readily available. Prepare the patient for diagnostic tests, such as chest X-ray, EKG, and arterial blood gas analysis.

Pediatric pointers
Keep in mind that respiratory distress often develops more rapidly in children than in adults.

Tracheal Tugging
[Cardarelli's sign, Castellino's sign, Oliver's sign]

A visible recession of the larynx and trachea that occurs in synchrony with cardiac systole, tracheal tugging commonly results from an aneurysm or a tumor near the aortic arch and may signal dangerous compression or obstruction of major airways. The tugging movement, best observed with the patient's neck hyperextended, reflects abnormal transmission of aortic pulsations because of compression and distortion of the heart, esophagus, great vessels, airways, and nerves.

Assessment
If you observe tracheal tugging, assess the patient for signs of respiratory distress, such as tachypnea, stridor, accessory muscle use, cyanosis, and agitation. If the patient's in distress, have another nurse call the doctor immediately while you check airway patency. Administer oxygen, and prepare to intubate the patient, if necessary. As ordered, insert an I.V. line for fluid and drug access, and institute cardiac monitoring.

If the patient isn't in distress, obtain a pertinent history. Ask about associated symptoms, especially pain, and about any history of cardiovascular disease, cancer, chest surgery, or trauma.

Now examine the patient's neck and chest for abnormalities. Palpate the neck for masses, enlarged lymph nodes, abnormal arterial pulsations, and tracheal deviation. Percuss and auscultate the lung fields for abnormal sounds, and auscultate the heart for murmurs.

Medical causes
• *Aortic arch aneurysm.* A large aneurysm can distort and compress surrounding tissues and structures, producing tracheal tugging. The cardinal sign of this aneurysm is severe pain in the substernal area, sometimes radiating to the back or side of the chest. A sudden increase in pain may herald impending rupture—a medical emergency. Depending on the aneurysm's site and size, associated findings may include a visible pulsatile mass in the first or second intercostal space or suprasternal notch, a diastolic murmur of aortic regurgitation, and an aortic systolic murmur and thrill in the absence of any peripheral signs of aortic stenosis. Dyspnea and stridor may occur with hoarseness, dysphagia, brassy cough, and hemoptysis. Distended jugular veins may also occur along with edema of the face, neck, or arm. Compression of the left main bronchus can cause atelectasis of the left lung.
• *Hodgkin's lymphoma.* Development of a tumor adjacent to the aortic arch can cause tracheal tugging. Initial signs and symptoms include usually painless cervical lymphadenopathy, sustained or remittent fever, fatigue, malaise, pruritus, night sweats, and weight loss. Swollen lymph nodes may become tender and painful. Later findings include dyspnea and stridor; dry cough; dys-

TRACHEAL TUGGING: CAUSES AND ASSOCIATED FINDINGS

S&S CAUSES	MAJOR ASSOCIATED SIGNS AND SYMPTOMS											
	Chest pain	Cough—brassy	Cough—crowing	Dyspnea	Edema of face, neck, or arm	Fever	Hemoptysis	Hoarseness	Lymphadenopathy	Murmur	Neck vein distention	Stridor
Aortic arch aneurysm	●	●		●	●		●	●		●	●	●
Hodgkin's lymphoma				●	●			●			●	●
Non-Hodgkin's lymphoma			●	●	●			●			●	●
Thymoma	●			●	●			●			●	

phagia; distended neck veins; edema of the face, neck, or arm; hepatosplenomegaly; hyperpigmentation, jaundice, or pallor; and neuralgia.

• *Non-Hodgkin's lymphoma.* Tracheal tugging may reflect anterior mediastinal lymphadenopathy or tumor development next to the aortic arch. The most common initial sign, though, is painless peripheral lymphadenopathy. Other early findings include fever, fatigue, malaise, night sweats, and weight loss. Later findings: a crowing cough, dyspnea, stridor, dysphagia, distended neck veins, neck edema, hepatomegaly, and splenomegaly.

• *Thymoma.* This rare tumor can cause tracheal tugging if it develops in the anterior mediastinum. Cough, chest pain, dysphagia, dyspnea, hoarseness, a palpable neck mass, distended neck veins, and edema of the face, neck, or upper arm are common findings.

Special considerations

Prepare the patient for diagnostic procedures, which may include chest X-ray, computed tomography scan, lymphangiography, aortography, bone marrow biopsy, liver biopsy, echocardiography, and a complete blood count.

Place the patient in semi-Fowler's position to ease respiration. Administer cough suppressants. Also give prescribed pain medications as ordered, but keep alert for signs of respiratory depression.

Pediatric pointers

In infants and children, tracheal tugging may indicate a mediastinal tumor, such as occurs in either Hodgkin's or non-Hodgkin's lymphoma. It may also be present in Marfan's syndrome.

Tremors

The most common involuntary muscle movement, tremors are regular rhythmic oscillations that result from alternate contraction and relaxation of opposing muscle groups. They're typical of extrapyramidal or cerebellar disorders and can also result from certain drugs.

Tremors can be characterized by their location, amplitude, and frequency. They're classified as resting, intention, or postural. *Resting tremors* occur only when an extremity is at rest and subside with movement. They include the classic pill-rolling tremor of Parkinson's disease. Conversely, *intention tremors* occur only with movement and subside with rest. *Postural (or action) tremors* appear when an extremity or the trunk is actively held in a particular posture or position. A slow postural tremor is known as an *essential tremor*. Tremors may also be elicited, such as asterixis—the characteristic flapping tremor in hepatic failure (see "Asterixis").

Stress or emotional upset tends to aggravate a tremor; alcohol use often diminishes it.

Assessment

Begin your assessment by asking the patient about the tremor's onset (sudden or gradual) and about its duration, progression, and any aggravating or alleviating factors. Does the tremor interfere with his normal activities? Does the patient have other symptoms? Has he noticed any behavioral changes or memory loss (the patient's family or friends may provide more accurate information on this)?

Explore the patient's personal and family medical history for neurologic (especially seizures), endocrine, or metabolic disorders. Obtain a complete drug history, noting especially the use of phenothiazines. Also ask about alcohol use.

Assess the patient's overall appearance and demeanor, noting mental status. Test range of motion and strength in all major muscle groups while observing for chorea, athetosis, dystonia, and other involuntary movements. Check deep tendon reflexes, and, if possible, observe the patient's gait.

Medical causes

• *Alcohol withdrawal syndrome.* Acute alcohol withdrawal following long-term dependence may first be manifested by resting and intention tremors that appear as soon as 7 hours after the last drink and progressively worsen. Other early signs and symptoms may include diaphoresis, tachycardia, elevated blood pressure, anxiety, restlessness, irritability, insomnia, headache, nausea, and vomiting. Severe withdrawal may produce delirium tremens marked by profound tremors, agitation, confusion, hallucinations, and possibly seizures.

• *Alkalosis.* Severe alkalosis may produce a severe intention tremor, along with twitching, carpopedal spasms, agitation, diaphoresis, and hyperventilation. The patient may complain of dizziness, tinnitus, palpitations, and peripheral and circumoral paresthesias.

• *Benign familial essential tremor.* This disorder of early adulthood produces a bilateral essential tremor that typically begins in the fingers and hands and may spread to the head, jaw, lips, and tongue. Laryngeal involvement may result in a quavering voice.

• *Cerebellar tumor.* Intention tremor may be an early sign of this disorder; related findings may include ataxia, nystagmus, incoordination, muscle weakness and atrophy, and hypoactive or absent deep tendon reflexes.

• *General paresis.* This effect of neurosyphilis may cause an intention tremor accompanied by clonus, a positive Babinski's reflex, ataxia, Argyll Robertson pupils, and a diffuse, dull headache.

• *Hypercapnia.* Elevated PCO_2 levels may result in a rapid, fine intention tremor. Other common findings include headache, fatigue, blurred vision, weakness, lethargy, and decreasing level of consciousness.

• *Hypoglycemia.* Acute hypoglycemia may produce a rapid, fine intention tremor accompanied by confusion, weakness, tachycardia, diaphoresis, and cold, clammy skin. Early patient complaints typically include mild generalized headache, profound hunger, nervousness, and blurred or double vision. The tremor may disappear as hypoglycemia worsens and hypotonia and decreased level of consciousness become evident.

• *Kwashiorkor.* Coarse intention and resting tremors may occur in the advanced stages of this rare disease. Examination reveals myoclonus, rigidity of all extremities, hyperreflexia, hepatomegaly, and pitting edema in the hands, feet, and sacral area. Other manifestations may include a flat affect, pronounced hair loss, and dry, peeling skin.

• *Manganese toxicity.* Early signs of manganese poisoning include resting tremor, chorea, propulsive gait, cogwheel rigidity, personality changes, amnesia, and masklike facies.

• *Multiple sclerosis (MS).* Intention tremor may be an early sign of MS. Like the disorder's other effects, it tends to wax and wane. Commonly, visual and sensory impairments are the earliest findings. Associated effects vary greatly and may include nystagmus, muscle weakness, paralysis, spasticity, hyperreflexia, ataxic gait, dysphagia, and dysarthria. Constipation, urinary frequency and urgency, incontinence, impotence, and emotional lability may also occur.

• *Parkinson's disease.* Tremors, a classic early sign of this degenerative disease, begin in the fingers and may eventually affect the foot, eyelids, jaw, lips, and tongue. The slow, regular, rhythmic resting (or occasionally intention) tremor takes the form of flexion-extension or abduction-adduction of the fingers or hand, or pronation-supination of the hand. Flexion-extension of the fingers combined with abduction-adduction of the thumb yields the characteristic pill-rolling tremor.

Leg involvement produces flexion-extension foot movement. Lightly closing the eyelids causes them to flutter. The jaw may move up and down, and

the lips may purse. The tongue, when protruded, may move in and out of the mouth in tempo with tremors elsewhere in the body. The rate of the tremor holds constant over time, but amplitude varies.

Other characteristic findings include cogwheel or lead-pipe rigidity, bradykinesia, propulsive gait with forward-leaning posture, monotone voice, masklike facies, drooling, dysphagia, dysarthria, and occasionally oculogyric crisis (eyes fix upward, with involuntary tonic movements) or blepharospasm (eyelids close completely).

• *Porphyria.* Involvement of the basal ganglia in porphyria can produce resting tremor with rigidity, accompanied by chorea and athetosis. As the disease progresses, generalized seizures may appear along with aphasia and hemiplegia.

• *Thalamic syndrome. Central midbrain syndromes* are heralded by contralateral ataxic tremors and other abnormal movements, along with Weber's syndrome (oculomotor palsy with contralateral hemiplegia), paralysis of vertical gaze, and stupor or coma. *Anteromedial-inferior thalamic syndrome* produces varying combinations of tremor, deep sensory loss, and hemiataxia. However, the main effect of this syndrome is an extrapyramidal dysfunction, such as hemiballismus or hemichoreoathetosis.

• *Thyrotoxicosis.* Neuromuscular effects of this disorder include a rapid, fine intention tremor of the hands and tongue, along with clonus, hyperreflexia, and Babinski's reflex. Other common signs and symptoms include tachycardia, cardiac dysrhythmias, palpitations, anxiety, dyspnea, diaphoresis, heat intolerance, weight loss despite increased appetite, diarrhea, an enlarged thyroid, and possibly exophthalmos.

• *Wernicke's disease.* Intention tremor is an early sign of this thiamine deficiency. Other characteristics include ocular abnormalities (such as gaze paralysis or nystagmus), ataxia, apathy, and confusion. Orthostatic hypotension and tachycardia may also develop in this disorder.

• *Wilson's disease.* This disorder of abnormal copper metabolism produces slow "wing-flapping" tremors in the arms and pill-rolling tremors in the hands; these appear early in the disease and progressively worsen. The most characteristic sign, however, is Kayser-Fleischer rings—rusty brown rings of pigment around the corneas. Other clinical features may include incoordination, dysarthria, chorea, ataxia, and muscle spasms and rigidity; abdominal distress; fatigue; personality changes; hypotension; syncope; and seizures. Liver and spleen enlargement may occur with ascites and jaundice. Hyperpigmentation may also occur.

Other causes
• *Drugs.* Phenothiazines (particularly piperazine derivatives, such as fluphenazine) and other antipsychotics may cause resting and pill-rolling tremors. Infrequently, metoclopramide and metyrosine also cause these tremors. Lithium toxicity, sympathomimetics (such as terbutaline and pseudoephedrine), amphetamines, and phenytoin can all cause essential tremors that disappear with dose reduction.

Special considerations
Severe intention tremors may interfere with the patient's ability to perform activities of daily living. Assist the patient with these activities as necessary, and take precautions against possible injury during such activities as walking or eating.

Pediatric pointers
The normal newborn may display coarse tremors with stiffening—an exaggerated hypocalcemic startle reflex—in response to noises and chills. Pediatric-specific causes of pathologic tremor include cerebral palsy, fetal alcohol syndrome, and maternal drug addiction.

Trismus
[Lockjaw]

A prolonged and painful tonic spasm of the masticatory jaw muscles, trismus is a characteristic early symptom of tetanus produced by the neuromuscular effects of tetanospasmin, a potentially lethal exotoxin. It can also result from drug therapy; occasionally, a milder form may be associated with neuromuscular involvement in other disorders, or with infection or disease of the jaw, teeth, parotid glands, or tonsils.

Assessment
Ask the patient about any recent injury (even a slight wound), infection, or animal bite. Does he have a history of epilepsy, neuromuscular disease, or endocrine or metabolic disorders? Obtain a complete drug history, including self-injected drugs, since the use of a contaminated needle may produce tetanus. Also ask about paresthesias or pain in the jaw, neck, or shoulders.

Perform a neurologic assessment, evaluating cranial nerve, motor, and sensory function and deep tendon reflexes. Try to elicit the jaw jerk reflex, since this test and a careful patient history usually establish the diagnosis.

Medical causes
• *Hypocalcemia.* Severe hypocalcemia can produce trismus and cramping spasms in virtually all muscle groups, except those of the eye. It also causes fatigue, weakness, chorea, and palpitations. Chvostek's and Trousseau's signs may be elicited.
• *Rabies.* Trismus often develops after a prodromal period of fever, headache, photophobia, hyperesthesia, and increasing restlessness and agitation. Other neuromuscular effects include excessive salivation, painful laryngeal and pharyngeal muscle spasms, and

PERFORMING THE JAW JERK TEST

If your patient reports difficulty in opening her mouth, perform the jaw jerk test because even slight trismus may indicate an otherwise asymptomatic mild localized tetanus. Here's how to elicit and interpret this important reflex: ask the patient to relax her jaw and slightly open her mouth. Then place your index finger over the middle of her chin and firmly tap it with a reflex hammer.

Normally, this tap produces sudden jaw closing. Then an inhibitory mechanism abruptly halts motor nerve activity, and the mouth remains closed. In trismus, however, this inhibitory mechanism fails and motor nerve activity increases, causing immediate spasm of jaw muscles.

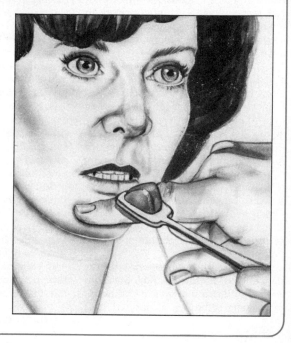

possibly respiratory distress.

• *Seizure disorders.* Trismus, along with spasms of other facial muscles, a limb, and the trunk, commonly occurs during a generalized tonic-clonic seizure.

• *Strychnine poisoning.* In this potentially fatal condition, tonic seizures characterized by trismus, leg muscle rigidity, and respiratory muscle spasm follow early symptoms of irritability and twitching.

• *Temporomandibular joint syndrome.* This syndrome causes trismus, facial pain, and mandibular dysfunction. The pain may be a severe dull ache or an intense spasm that radiates to the cheek, temple, lower jaw, ear, mastoid area, neck, or shoulders. Earache occurs without involvement of the tympanic membrane or external auditory canal.

• *Tetanus.* This acute, life-threatening infection is heralded by trismus, typically appearing within 14 days of initial infection. The painful spasms increase in frequency and intensity during the initial disease stage, then gradually subside. Although trismus is frequently the first manifestation of tetanus, it occasionally follows a short prodromal period of headache, restlessness, irritability, slight fever, chills, swelling at the wound site, and dysphagia. As the disease progresses, painful involuntary muscle spasms spread to other areas, such as the abdomen, producing boardlike rigidity; the back, resulting in opisthotonos; or the face, producing a characteristic grotesque grin (risus sardonicus). Tachycardia, diaphoresis, hyperactive deep tendon reflexes, and convulsions may develop. Spasms may affect the laryngeal or chest wall muscles.

Other causes

• *Drugs.* Phenothiazines (particularly the piperazine derivatives, such as fluphenazine) and other antipsychotics may produce an acute dystonic reaction marked by trismus, involuntary facial movements, and tonic spasms in the limbs. These complications usually occur early in drug therapy, sometimes after the initial dose.

Special considerations

Since inadequate ventilation from laryngeal or respiratory muscle spasm is a constant threat during the acute phase of tetanus, constantly assess the patient's respiratory status and make sure that oxygen and emergency airway equipment are readily available.

To treat tetanus, expect to administer human tetanus immune globulin, which neutralizes unbound toxin. Instruct the patient about the importance of annual booster injections to ensure immunization.

Maintain a quiet environment for the patient with trismus; darken his room and keep all stimulation to a minimum. Administer sedatives, as ordered.

Pediatric pointers

Trismus in a neonate can result from tetanus neonatorum, a disorder produced by introduction of the tetanus toxin through the umbilical cord. Trismus usually develops within 10 days of birth.

Tunnel Vision

[Gunbarrel vision, tubular vision]

Resulting from severe constriction of the visual field that leaves only a small central area of sight, tunnel vision is typically described as the sensation of looking through a tunnel or gun barrel. It may be unilateral or bilateral and usually develops gradually. This abnormality results from chronic open-angle glaucoma, advanced retinal degeneration, and laser photocoagulation therapy. Also a common complaint of malingerers, it can be verified or discounted by visual field examination performed by an ophthalmologist.

Assessment

Ask the patient when he first noticed a loss of peripheral vision. Then have him describe the progression of vision loss. Next, ask him to describe in detail exactly what and how far he can see peripherally. Explore the patient's personal and family history for ocular problems, especially progressive blindness that began at an early age.

To rule out malingering, observe the patient as he walks. A patient with severely limited peripheral vision may frequently bump into objects (and may even have bruises), whereas the malingerer will manage to avoid them.

If your assessment findings suggest tunnel vision, refer the patient to an ophthalmologist for further evaluation.

Medical causes

• *Chronic open-angle glaucoma.* In this insidious disorder, bilateral tunnel vision occurs late and slowly progresses to complete blindness. Other late findings include mild eye pain, halo vision, and reduced visual acuity (especially at night) that's uncorrectable with glasses.

• *Retinal pigmentary degeneration.* This group of hereditary disorders, such as retinitis pigmentosa, produces an annular scotoma that progresses concentrically, causing tunnel vision and eventually resulting in complete blindness, usually by age 50. Typically, impaired night vision, the earliest symptom, appears in the first or second decade of life. Ophthalmoscopic examination may reveal narrowed retinal blood vessels and a pale optic disk.

Other causes

• *Treatments.* Tunnel vision can result from laser photocoagulation therapy, which aims to correct retinal detachment.

Special considerations

To protect the patient from injury, be sure to remove all potentially dangerous objects and orient him to his surroundings.

If tunnel vision is permanent, teach the patient to move his eyes from side to side when he walks to avoid bumping into objects. Since any visual impairment is frightening, remember to reassure the patient and clearly explain diagnostic procedures, such as tonometry, perimeter examination, and visual field testing.

Pediatric pointers

In children with retinitis pigmentosa, night blindness foreshadows tunnel vision, which usually doesn't develop until later in the disease process.

COMPARING TUNNEL VISION AND NORMAL VISION

The patient with tunnel vision experiences drastic constriction of his peripheral visual field. The illustrations here convey the extent of this constriction, comparing test findings for normal and tunnel vision.

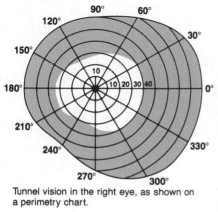
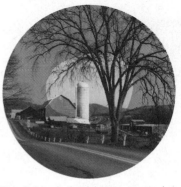
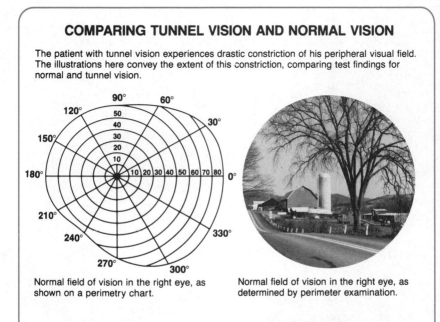

Normal field of vision in the right eye, as shown on a perimetry chart.

Normal field of vision in the right eye, as determined by perimeter examination.

Tunnel vision in the right eye, as shown on a perimetry chart.

Tunnel vision in the right eye, as seen in advanced glaucoma during perimeter examination.

uremic frost • urethral discharge • urinary frequency • urinary hesitancy • u
urinary urgency • urine cloudiness • urticaria • vaginal bleeding—postmeno
discharge • venous hum • vertigo • vesicular rash • violent behavior • vision
visual floaters • vomiting • vulvar lesions • weight gain—excessive • weight l
wheezing • wristdrop• abdominal distention • abdominal mass • abdominal
rigidity • accessory muscle use • agitation • alopecia • amenorrhea • amnesi
anhidrosis • anorexia • anosmia • anuria • anxiety • aphasia • apnea • apne
apraxia • arm pain • asterixis • ataxia • athetosis • aura • Babinski's reflex •
chest • Battle's sign • Biot's respirations • bladder distention • blood pressure
pressure increase • bowel sounds—absent • bowel sounds—hyperactive • bo
bradycardia • bradypnea • breast dimpling • breast nodule • breast pain • b
ammonia odor • breath with fecal odor • breath with fruity odor • Brudzins
hump • butterfly rash • café-au-lait spots • capillary refill time—prolonged •
cry • chest expansion—asymmetrical • chest pain • Cheyne-Stokes respiratior
Chvostek's sign • clubbing • cogwheel rigidity • cold intolerance • confusion
constipation • corneal reflex—absent • costovertebral angle tenderness • coug
nonproductive • cough—productive • crackles • crepitation—bony • crepitati
cry—high-pitched • cyanosis • decerebrate posture • decorticate posture • de
hyperactive • deep tendon reflexes—hypoactive • depression • diaphoresis • d
dizziness • doll's eye sign—absent • drooling • dysarthria • dysmenorrhea •
dyspepsia • dysphagia • dyspnea • dystonia • dysuria • earache • edema—ge
arms • edema of the face • edema of the legs • enophthalmos • enuresis • ep
erythema • exophthalmos • eye discharge • eye pain • facial pain • fascicula
incontinence • fetor hepaticus • fever • flank pain • flatulence • fontanelle bu
depression • footdrop • gag reflex abnormalities • gait—bizarre • gait—prop
gait—spastic • gait—steppage • gait—waddling • gallop—atrial • gallop—ve
in the male • grunting respirations • gum bleeding • gum swelling • gynecor
vision • headache • hearing loss • heat intolerance • Heberden's nodes • hem
hematochezia • hematuria • hemianopia • hemoptysis • hepatomegaly • hicc
hoarseness • Homans' sign • hyperpigmentation • hyperpnea • hypopigmenta
insomnia • intermittent claudication • Janeway's spots • jaundice • jaw pain
distention • Kehr's sign • Kernig's sign • leg pain • level of consciousness—d
flashes • low birth weight • lymphadenopathy • masklike facies • McBurney'
sign • melena • menorrhagia • metrorrhagia • miosis • moon face • mouth le
muscle atrophy • muscle flaccidity • muscle spasms • muscle spasticity • mu
mydriasis • myoclonus • nasal flaring • nausea • neck pain • night blindness
nipple retraction • nocturia • nuchal rigidity • nystagmus • ocular deviation
oliguria • opisthotonos • orofacial dyskinesia • orthopnea • orthostatic hypot
Osler's nodes • otorrhea • pallor • palpitations • papular rash • paralysis • p
nocturnal dyspnea • peau d'orange • pericardial friction rub • peristaltic wa
photophobia • pica • pleural friction rub • polydipsia • polyphagia • polyuri
priapism • pruritus • psoas sign • psychotic behavior • ptosis • pulse—abser
bounding • pulse pressure—narrowed • pulse pressure—widened • pulse rh
pulsus alternans • pulsus bisferiens • pulsus paradoxus • pupils—nonreactiv
purple striae • purpura • pustular rash • pyrosis • raccoon's eyes • rebound
retractions—costal and sternal • rhinorrhea • rhonchi • Romberg's sign • sal
salivation—increased • salt craving • scotoma • scrotal swelling • seizure—a
seizure—generalized tonic-clonic • seizure—psychomotor • setting-sun sign
skin—bronze • skin—clammy • skin—mottled • skin—scaly • skin turgor—
angioma • splenomegaly • stertorous respirations • stool—clay-colored • stri

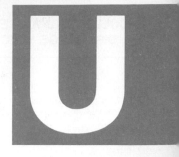

Uremic Frost

Uremic frost—a fine white powder, believed to be urate crystals, that covers the skin—is a characteristic sign of end-stage renal failure, or uremia. Urea compounds and other waste substances that can't be excreted by the kidneys in urine are excreted in sweat, and remain as powdery deposits on the skin when the sweat evaporates. The frost typically appears on the face, neck, axillae, groin, and genitalia.

Because of advances in managing renal failure, uremic frost is now relatively rare. However, it does occur in patients with chronic renal failure who, because of their advanced age or the severity of their accompanying illnesses (such as extensive neurologic deterioration), do not undergo dialysis.

Assessment
Uremic frost usually appears well after a diagnosis of chronic renal failure has been established. As a result, your assessment will be limited to inspecting the skin to determine the extent of uremic frost.

Medical cause
• *End-stage chronic renal failure.* Uremic frost heralds the preterminal stage of chronic renal failure. The patient may also have pruritus, hypertension, lassitude, fatigue, irritability, and decreased level of consciousness. Additional findings may include muscle cramps, gross myoclonus, peripheral neuropathies, and convulsions. Anorexia, nausea and vomiting, constipation or diarrhea, and oliguria or anuria may occur, along with GI bleeding, petechiae, and ecchymoses. Integumentary effects may include mouth and gum ulceration, skin pigment changes and excoriation, and brown arcs under nail margins. Acidosis results in Kussmaul's respirations; the patient may also have ammonia breath odor (uremic fetor).

Special considerations
Because this patient is prone to seizures from uremic encephalopathy, take seizure precautions. Monitor his vital signs frequently, pad the bed's side rails, and keep an artificial airway and suction equipment at hand.

Because the patient is also prone to respiratory or cardiac arrest from metabolic acidosis or hyperkalemia, constantly monitor his respiratory and cardiac status. As necessary, administer supplemental oxygen and be prepared to assist with intubation and mechanical ventilation. Establish an I.V. line to administer fluids and medication. Also begin cardiac monitoring, and be prepared to initiate cardiopulmonary

COLLECTING A URETHRAL DISCHARGE SPECIMEN

To obtain a urethral specimen from a male patient, follow these steps:

Instruct the patient not to void for 1 hour before specimen collection to prevent flushing secretions from the urethra.

Provide privacy for the patient. Position him supine on an examination table, and expose his penis. Have him grasp and raise his penis to allow visualization of the urethra.

Wash your hands and put on sterile gloves. Then insert a thin, sterile urogenital alginate swab no more than 2 cm (⅘″) into the urethra. Rotate the swab, and leave it in place for 10 to 30 seconds to absorb organisms.

Remove the swab, allow it to dry, and then send it to the laboratory. Assist the patient from the examination table and tell him to dress.

resuscitation, if indicated.

Enhance patient comfort by providing regular position changes to prevent skin breakdown and by bathing the patient often with tepid water and minimal soap to remove the frost. Trim his fingernails to prevent scratching.

Since the appearance of uremic frost invariably signals impending death, prepare the patient and his family for this eventuality, and provide emotional support. Death from uremia is generally peaceful, following a deep coma.

Pediatric pointers

Uremic frost is very rare in children, since most undergo dialysis or transplantation before the disease reaches the end stage.

Urethral Discharge

This excretion from the urinary meatus may be purulent, mucoid, or thin; sanguineous or clear; and scant or profuse. It usually develops suddenly, most commonly in men with a prostate infection. In children, urethral discharge indicates sexual abuse.

Assessment

Ask the patient when he first noticed the discharge, and have him describe its color, consistency, and quantity. Does he have any pain on urination? Any difficulty initiating a urinary stream? Ask about other associated symptoms, such as fever, chills, and perineal fullness. Explore his history for any incidence of prostate problems, sexually transmitted disease, or urinary tract infection. Ask if he's had recent sexual contacts or a new sexual partner.

Inspect the patient's urethral meatus for inflammation and swelling. Using proper technique, obtain a culture specimen. Then obtain a urine sample for urinalysis and possibly a three-glass urine sample (see *How to Perform the*

Three-Glass Urine Test, page 744). In a male patient, the doctor may palpate the prostate gland.

Medical causes

● *Prostatitis. Acute prostatitis* is characterized by purulent urethral discharge. Initial signs and symptoms include sudden fever, chills, low back pain, myalgia, perineal fullness, and arthralgia. Urination becomes increasingly frequent and urgent, and the urine may appear cloudy. Dysuria, nocturia, and some degree of urinary obstruction may also occur. When palpated rectally, the prostate is markedly tender, indurated, swollen, firm, and warm.

Chronic prostatitis, although often asymptomatic, may produce a persistent urethral discharge that's thin, milky or clear, and sometimes sticky. The discharge appears at the meatus after a long interval between voidings, as in the morning. Associated effects include a dull aching in the prostate or rectum, sexual dysfunction, and urinary disturbances, such as frequency, urgency, and dysuria.

● *Reiter's syndrome.* In this self-limiting syndrome that most commonly affects males, urethral discharge and other signs of acute urethritis occur 1 to 2 weeks after sexual contact. Arthritic and ocular symptoms and skin lesions usually develop within several weeks.

● *Urethral neoplasm.* This rare cancer is sometimes heralded by painless urethral discharge that's initially opaque and gray. Later, the discharge becomes yellowish and blood-tinged.

● *Urethritis.* This inflammatory disorder, which is often sexually transmitted (as in gonorrhea), commonly produces scant or profuse urethral discharge that's either thin and clear, mucoid, or thick and purulent. Other effects: urinary hesitancy, urgency, and frequency; dysuria; and itching and burning around the meatus.

Special considerations

Advise the patient with acute prostatitis to discontinue sexual activity until acute symptoms subside. However, encourage the patient with chronic prostatitis to regularly engage in sexual activity. To help this patient relieve symptoms, suggest that he take hot sitz baths several times daily, increase his fluid intake, void frequently, and avoid caffeine, tea, and alcohol. Monitor him for urinary retention.

Pediatric pointers

Carefully evaluate a child with urethral discharge for evidence of sexual and physical abuse.

Urinary Frequency

Urinary frequency refers to increased incidence of the urge to void. Usually resulting from decreased bladder capacity, frequency is a cardinal sign of urinary tract infection. However, it can also stem from other urologic disorders, neurologic dysfunction, and pressure on the bladder from a nearby tumor or from organ enlargement (as with pregnancy).

Urinary frequency may be reported by the patient with polyuria—an increase in total daily urine output. (See "Polyuria.")

Assessment

Ask the patient how many times a day he voids. How does this compare to his previous pattern of voiding? Ask about the onset and duration of the abnormal frequency and about any associated urinary symptoms, such as dysuria, urgency, incontinence, hematuria, or bladder cramps. Also ask about any neurologic symptoms, such as muscle weakness, numbness, or tingling. Explore the patient's medical history for urinary tract infection, other urologic problems or recent urologic procedures, and neurologic disorders. If the patient's a male, ask about a history of prostatic enlargement. If the patient's a female of childbearing age, ask whether she is or could be pregnant.

Obtain a clean-catch midstream sample for urinalysis and culture and sensitivity tests. Then palpate the patient's suprapubic area, abdomen, and flanks, noting any tenderness. Examine his urethral meatus for redness, discharge, or swelling. In a male patient, the doctor may palpate the prostate gland.

If the patient's medical history reveals symptoms or a history of neurologic disorders, perform a neurologic examination.

Medical causes

• *Anxiety neurosis.* Morbid anxiety produces urinary frequency and other types of genitourinary dysfunction, such as dysuria, impotence, and frigidity. Other findings include headache, diaphoresis, hyperventilation, palpitations, muscle spasm, polyphagia, constipation, and other GI complaints. Chest pain, tachycardia, and transient hypertension may also occur.

• *Benign prostatic hypertrophy.* Prostatic enlargement causes urinary frequency, along with nocturia and possibly incontinence and hematuria. Initial effects are those of prostatism: reduced caliber and force of the urinary stream, urinary hesitancy and tenesmus, a feeling of incomplete voiding, and occasionally urinary retention. Assessment reveals bladder distention.

• *Bladder calculus.* Bladder irritation may lead to urinary frequency and urgency, dysuria, hematuria, and suprapubic pain from bladder spasms. The patient may have overflow incontinence if the calculus lodges in the bladder neck.

• *Bladder cancer.* Urinary frequency, dribbling, and nocturia may develop from bladder irritation. The first sign of bladder cancer commonly is gross, painless, intermittent hematuria (often with clots). Patients with invasive lesions often have suprapubic pain from bladder spasms.

• *Multiple sclerosis (MS).* Urinary frequency, urgency, and incontinence are common urologic findings in MS. Signs and symptoms are highly variable, however, and tend to wax and wane. In most patients, visual problems (such as diplopia and blurred vision) and sensory impairment (such as paresthesias) are the earliest symptoms. Other signs and symptoms may include constipation, muscle weakness, paralysis, spasticity, hyperreflexia, intention tremor, ataxic gait, dysarthria, impotence, and emotional lability.

• *Prostatic cancer.* In advanced stages, urinary frequency may occur, along with hesitancy, dribbling, nocturia, dysuria, bladder distention, perineal pain, constipation, and a hard, irregularly shaped prostate. Pallor, weakness, and weight loss may also occur.

• *Prostatitis. Acute prostatitis* commonly produces urinary frequency, along with urgency, dysuria, nocturia, and purulent urethral discharge. Other findings include fever, chills, low back pain, myalgia, arthralgia, and perineal fullness. Rectal palpation reveals a markedly tender, indurated, swollen prostate. Clinical features of *chronic prostatitis* are usually the same as those of the acute form, but to a lesser degree. Other effects may include painful ejaculation, persistent urethral discharge, and sexual dysfunction.

• *Rectal tumor.* The pressure exerted by this tumor on the bladder may cause urinary frequency. Early findings include a change in bowel habits, often beginning with an urgent need to defecate on arising, or obstipation alternating with diarrhea; blood or mucus in the stool; and a sense of incomplete evacuation. Later, the patient may feel a dull ache in the rectum or sacral region.

• *Reiter's syndrome.* In this self-limiting syndrome, urinary frequency occurs with other symptoms of acute urethritis 1 to 2 weeks after sexual contact. Arthritic and ocular symptoms and skin lesions usually develop within several weeks.

• *Reproductive tract tumor.* A tumor in the female reproductive tract may compress the bladder, causing urinary frequency. Other findings vary but may include abdominal distention, menstrual disturbances, vaginal bleeding, weight loss, pelvic pain, and fatigue.

● *Spinal cord lesion.* Incomplete cord transection results in urinary frequency and urgency when voluntary control of sphincter function weakens. Added urologic effects may include hesitancy and bladder distention. Other effects occur below the level of the lesion and may include weakness, paralysis, sensory disturbances, hyperreflexia, and impotence.

● *Urethral stricture.* Bladder decompensation produces urinary frequency, along with urgency and nocturia. Early signs include hesitancy, tenesmus, and reduced caliber and force of the urinary stream. Eventually, overflow incontinence may occur.

● *Urinary tract infection.* Affecting the urethra (urethritis), the bladder (cystitis), or the kidneys (pyelonephritis), this common cause of urinary frequency also may produce urgency, dysuria, hematuria, cloudy urine and, in males, urethral discharge. The patient may report bladder spasms or a feeling of warmth during urination. He may also have fever, chills, malaise, nausea, vomiting, costovertebral angle tenderness, and suprapubic, lower back, or flank pain.

Other causes
● *Treatments.* Radiation therapy may cause bladder inflammation, leading to urinary frequency.

Special considerations
Prepare the patient for diagnostic tests, such as urinalysis, culture and sensitivity tests, imaging tests, ultrasonography, cystoscopy, cystometry, and a complete neurologic workup. If the patient's mobility is impaired, keep a bedpan or commode near his bed.

Pediatric pointers
Urinary tract infection is a common cause of urinary frequency in children, especially girls. Congenital anomalies that can cause urinary frequency include a duplicated ureter, congenital bladder diverticulum, and an ectopic ureteral orifice.

Urinary Hesitancy

Hesitancy—difficulty starting a urinary stream—can result from a urinary tract infection, a partial lower urinary tract obstruction, a neuromuscular disorder, or use of certain drugs. Occurring at all ages and in both sexes, it's most common in older men with prostatic enlargement. Hesitancy usually arises gradually, often going unnoticed until urinary ` retention causes bladder distention and discomfort.

Assessment
Ask the patient when he first noticed hesitancy and if he's ever had the problem before. Ask about other urinary problems, especially reduced force or interruption of the urinary stream. Ask the patient if he's ever been treated for a prostate problem or urinary tract infection or obstruction. Obtain a drug history.

Inspect the patient's urethral meatus for inflammation, discharge, and any other abnormalities. Test sensation in the perineum. Obtain a clean-catch sample for urinalysis. In a male patient, the doctor may palpate the prostate gland.

Medical causes
● *Benign prostatic hypertrophy.* Clinical features of this disorder depend on the extent of prostatic enlargement and the lobes affected. Characteristic early findings include urinary hesitancy, reduced caliber and force of urinary stream, a feeling of incomplete voiding and, occasionally, urinary retention. As obstruction increases, urination becomes more frequent, with nocturia,

HOW TO PERFORM CREDÉ'S MANEUVER

Dear Patient:

Credé's maneuver is a simple exercise that can help you start a stream of urine. Here's how to perform this maneuver:
• While sitting on the toilet, place your hands flat on your abdomen, just below the navel. Then, firmly stroke downward about six times. This puts pressure on the bladder and stimulates your urge to void. (Women can increase pressure further by bending forward at the hips.)
• Now, place one hand on top of the other above your pubic area, as shown. Then, press firmly inward and downward. This compresses the bladder and expels urine.

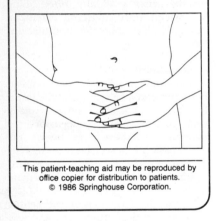

incontinence, bladder distention, and possibly hematuria.
• **Prostatic cancer.** In advanced stages of this disorder, urinary hesitancy may occur, accompanied by frequency, dribbling, nocturia, dysuria, bladder distention, perineal pain, and constipation. Palpation reveals a hard, irregularly shaped prostate. Pallor, weakness, and weight loss may also occur.
• **Spinal cord lesion.** A lesion below the micturition center that has destroyed the sacral nerve roots causes urinary hesitancy, tenesmus, and constant dribbling from retention and overflow incontinence. Associated findings are urinary frequency and urgency, dysuria, and nocturia. Other effects may include motor weakness or paralysis below the level of the lesion, paresthesias, fecal incontinence, and sexual dysfunction.
• **Urethral stricture.** Partial obstruction of the lower urinary tract secondary to trauma or infection produces urinary hesitancy, tenesmus, and decreased force and caliber of the urinary stream. Urinary frequency and urgency, nocturia, and eventually overflow incontinence may develop. Pyuria indicates accompanying infection.
• **Urinary tract infection.** Urinary hesitancy may be associated with this infection. Characteristic urinary changes include frequency, possible hematuria, dysuria, nocturia, and cloudy urine. Associated findings may include bladder spasms; costovertebral angle tenderness; suprapubic, low back, or flank pain; urethral discharge in males; and constitutional effects, such as fever, chills, malaise, nausea, and vomiting.

Other causes
• **Drugs.** Anticholinergics and drugs with anticholinergic properties (such as tricyclic antidepressants and some nasal decongestant preparations and cold remedies) may cause urinary hesitancy.

Special considerations
Monitor the patient's voiding pattern, and frequently palpate for bladder distention. Apply local heat to the perineum or the abdomen to enhance muscle relaxation and aid urination. Also teach the patient to perform Valsalva's maneuver or Credé's maneuver. As ordered, prepare the patient for appropriate diagnostic tests, such as cystometrography or observation cystourethroscopy.

Pediatric pointers
The most common cause of urinary hesitancy in male infants is obstruction caused by posterior urethral valves, thought to be vestigial embryonic

structures in the prostatic urethra. Besides other congenital causes of urethral obstruction, hesitancy in pediatric patients may result from hypospadias, epispadias, and neural tube defects. Teach Credé's maneuver to children with neural tube defects.

Urinary Incontinence

Incontinence, the uncontrollable passage of urine, results from bladder abnormalities or neurologic disorders. A common urologic sign, incontinence may be transient or permanent, and may involve large volumes of urine or scant dribbling. It can be classified as stress, overflow, urge, or total incontinence. *Stress incontinence* refers to intermittent leakage resulting from a sudden physical strain, such as a cough, sneeze, or quick movement. *Overflow incontinence* is a dribble resulting from urinary retention, which fills the bladder and prevents it from contracting with sufficient force to expel a urinary stream. *Urge incontinence* refers to the inability to suppress a sudden urge to urinate. *Total incontinence* is continuous leakage resulting from the bladder's inability to retain any urine.

Assessment

Ask the patient when he first noticed the incontinence and whether it began suddenly or gradually. Have him describe his typical urinary pattern: does incontinence usually occur during the day or at night? Does he have any urinary control, or is he totally incontinent? If he sometimes urinates with control, ask him the usual times and amounts voided. Determine his normal fluid intake. Ask about other urinary problems, such as hesitancy, frequency, urgency, nocturia, and decreased force or interruption of the urinary stream. Also ask if he's ever sought treatment for incontinence or found a way to deal with it himself.

Obtain a medical history, especially noting urinary tract infection, prostate conditions, spinal injury or tumor, cerebrovascular accident, or surgery involving the bladder, prostate, or pelvic floor.

After completing the history, have the patient empty his bladder. Inspect the urethral meatus for obvious inflammation or anatomic defect. Have female patients bear down; note any urine leakage. Gently palpate the abdomen for bladder distention, which signals urinary retention. Perform a complete neurologic assessment, noting motor and sensory function and obvious muscle atrophy.

Medical causes

• **Benign prostatic hypertrophy (BPH).** Overflow incontinence is common in this disorder as a result of urethral obstruction and urinary retention. BPH begins with a group of symptoms known as prostatism: reduced caliber and force of urinary stream, urinary hesitancy, and a feeling of incomplete voiding. As obstruction increases, urination becomes more frequent, with nocturia and, possibly, hematuria. Examination reveals bladder distention and an enlarged prostate.

• **Bladder calculus.** Overflow incontinence may occur if the stone lodges in the bladder neck. Associated findings depend on calculus size but may include those of an irritable bladder: urinary frequency and urgency, dysuria, hematuria, and suprapubic pain from bladder spasms.

• **Bladder cancer.** Obstruction by a tumor may produce overflow incontinence. The early stages are commonly asymptomatic, and the initial sign is usually gross, painless hematuria. Other urinary complaints may include frequency, dysuria, nocturia, dribbling, and suprapubic pain from bladder spasms after voiding.

• **Cerebrovascular accident.** Urinary incontinence may be transient or permanent. Associated findings reflect the site and extent of the lesion and may

CORRECTING INCONTINENCE WITH BLADDER RETRAINING

The incontinent patient typically feels frustrated, embarrassed, and sometimes hopeless. Fortunately, though, his problem can often be corrected by bladder retraining—a program that aims to establish a regular voiding pattern. Here are some guidelines for establishing such a program:

Before you start the program, assess the patient's intake pattern, voiding pattern, and behavior (for example, restlessness or talkativeness) before each voiding episode.

Encourage the patient to use the toilet 30 minutes before he's usually incontinent. If this isn't successful, readjust the schedule. Once he's able to stay dry for 2 hours, increase the time between voidings by 30 minutes each day until he achieves a 3- to 4-hour voiding schedule.

When your patient voids, make sure that the sequence of conditioning stimuli is always the same.

Ensure that the patient has privacy while voiding—any inhibiting stimuli should be avoided.

Keep a record of continence and incontinence for 5 days—this may reinforce your patient's efforts to remain continent.

Remember, both your positive attitude and your patient's are crucial to his successful bladder retraining. Here are some additional tips that may help your patient succeed:

Make sure the patient is close to a bathroom or portable toilet. Leave a light on at night.

If your patient needs assistance getting out of his bed or chair, promptly answer his call for help.

Encourage him to wear his accustomed clothing, as an indication that you're confident he can remain continent. Acceptable alternatives to diapers include condoms for the male patient and incontinence pads or panties for the female patient.

Encourage him to drink 2,000 to 2,500 ml of fluid each day. Less fluid doesn't prevent incontinence but does promote bladder infection. Limiting his intake after 5 p.m., however, will help him remain continent during the night.

Reassure your patient that any episodes of incontinence don't signal a failure of the program. Encourage him to maintain a persistent, tolerant attitude.

include impaired mentation, emotional lability, behavioral changes, altered level of consciousness, and seizures. Headache, vomiting, visual deficits, and decreased visual acuity are possible. Sensorimotor effects may include contralateral hemiplegia, dysarthria, dysphagia, ataxia, apraxia, agnosia, aphasia, and unilateral sensory loss.

● *Diabetic neuropathy.* Autonomic neuropathy may cause painless bladder distention with overflow incontinence. Related findings may include episodic constipation or diarrhea, impotence and retrograde ejaculation, orthostatic hypotension, syncope, and dysphagia.

● *Guillain-Barré syndrome.* Urinary incontinence may occur early in this disorder as a result of peripheral and autonomic nerve dysfunction. The most prominent sign is progressive, profound muscle weakness, which typically starts in the legs and extends to the arms and facial nerves within 24 to 72 hours. Associated findings may include paresthesias, dysarthria, nasal speech, dysphagia, orthostatic hypotension, fecal incontinence, diaphoresis, tachycardia, and possibly respiratory muscle paralysis and respiratory insufficiency.

● *Multiple sclerosis (MS).* Urinary incontinence, urgency, and frequency are common urologic findings in MS. In most patients, visual problems (such as diplopia and blurred vision) and sensory impairment (such as paresthesias) occur early. Other findings may include constipation, muscle weakness, paralysis, spasticity, hyperreflexia, intention tremor, ataxic gait, dysarthria, impotence, and emotional lability.

● *Prostatic cancer.* Urinary incontinence usually appears only in the advanced stages of this cancer. Urinary frequency and hesitancy, nocturia, dysuria, bladder distention, perineal pain, constipation, and a hard, irregularly shaped prostate are other common late findings, along with weight loss, pallor, and weakness.

● *Prostatitis (chronic).* Urinary incontinence may occur as a result of urethral obstruction from an enlarged prostate. Other findings may include urinary frequency and urgency, dysuria, hematuria, bladder distention, persistent urethral discharge, dull perineal pain that may radiate, decreased libido, and possibly impotence.

● *Spinal cord injury.* Complete cord transection above the sacral level causes flaccid paralysis of the bladder. Overflow incontinence follows rapid bladder distention. Other findings: paraplegia, sexual dysfunction, sensory loss, muscle atrophy, anhidrosis, and loss of reflexes distal to the injury.

● *Urethral stricture.* Eventually, overflow incontinence may occur here.

Other cause
● *Surgery.* Urinary incontinence may occur after prostatectomy as a result of urethral sphincter damage.

Special considerations
Prepare the patient for diagnostic tests, such as cystoscopy, cystometry, and a complete neurologic workup.

Begin management of incontinence by implementing a bladder retraining program (see *Correcting Incontinence with Bladder Retraining*). To prevent stress incontinence, teach exercises to help strengthen the pelvic floor muscles (see *Strengthening the Pelvic Floor Muscles,* page 742).

If the patient's incontinence has a neurologic basis, monitor for urinary retention, which may require periodic catheterizations. If appropriate, teach the patient self-catheterization techniques. A patient with permanent urinary incontinence may require surgical creation of a urinary diversion.

Pediatric pointers
Causes of incontinence in children include small-capacity hypertonic bladder, sphincter dyssynergia, epispadias, and ectopic ureteral orifice. Although children sometimes draw attention to themselves by feigning incontinence, a complete diagnostic evaluation usually is necessary to rule out organic disease.

Urinary Urgency

A sudden compelling urge to urinate, accompanied by bladder pain, is a classic symptom of urinary tract infection. As inflammation decreases bladder capacity, discomfort results from the accumulation of even small amounts of urine. Repeated, frequent voiding in an effort to alleviate this discomfort produces urine output of only a few milliliters at each voiding.

Urgency without bladder pain may point to an upper motor neuron lesion that has disrupted bladder control.

Assessment

Ask the patient about the onset of urinary urgency and whether he's ever experienced it before. Ask about other urologic symptoms, such as dysuria and cloudy urine. Also ask about neurologic symptoms, such as paresthesias. Examine his medical history for recurrent or chronic urinary tract infections or for surgery or procedures involving the urinary tract.

Obtain a clean-catch sample for urinalysis. Note urine character, color, and odor, and use a reagent strip to test for pH, glucose, and blood. Then palpate the suprapubic area and both flanks for tenderness. If the patient's history or symptoms suggest neurologic dysfunction, perform a neurologic examination.

Medical causes

• *Amyotrophic lateral sclerosis (ALS).* ALS occasionally produces urinary urgency. More common findings include muscle weakness, cramping, atrophy, and coarse fasciculations in the forearms and hands. Brain stem involvement produces speech, chewing, swallowing, and breathing difficulty.

• *Bladder calculus.* Bladder irritation can lead to urinary urgency and frequency, dysuria, hematuria, and suprapubic pain from bladder spasms.

• *Multiple sclerosis (MS).* Urinary urgency can occur with or without the frequent urinary tract infections that often accompany MS. Like MS's other variable effects, urinary urgency may wax and wane. Commonly, visual and sensory impairments are the earliest findings. Others include urinary frequency, incontinence, constipation, muscle weakness, paralysis, spasticity, intention tremor, hyperreflexia, ataxic gait, dysphagia, dysarthria, impotence, and emotional lability.

• *Reiter's syndrome.* In this self-limiting syndrome that primarily affects males, urgency occurs with other symptoms of acute urethritis 1 to 2 weeks after sexual contact. Arthritic and ocular symptoms and skin lesions usually develop within several weeks.

• *Spinal cord lesion.* Urinary urgency can result from incomplete cord transection when voluntary control of sphincter function weakens. Urinary frequency, difficulty initiating and inhibiting a urinary stream, and bladder distention and discomfort may also occur. Neuromuscular effects distal to the lesion may include weakness, paralysis, hyperreflexia, sensory disturbances, and impotence.

• *Urethral stricture.* Bladder decompensation produces urinary urgency, frequency, and nocturia. Early signs include hesitancy, tenesmus, and reduced caliber and force of the urinary stream. Eventually, overflow incontinence may occur.

• *Urinary tract infection.* Urinary urgency is commonly associated with this infection. Other characteristic urinary changes include frequency, hematuria, dysuria, nocturia, and cloudy urine. Urinary hesitancy may also occur. Associated findings may include bladder spasms; costovertebral angle tenderness; suprapubic, low back, or flank pain; urethral discharge in males; and constitutional effects, such as fever, chills, malaise, nausea, and vomiting.

Other causes

• *Treatments.* Radiation therapy may irritate and inflame the bladder, causing urinary urgency.

Special considerations

Prepare the patient for the diagnostic workup, including a complete urinalysis, culture and sensitivity studies, and possibly neurologic tests.

Increase the patient's fluid intake, if not contraindicated, to dilute the urine and diminish the feeling of urgency. As ordered, administer antibiotics and urinary anesthetics (such as phenazopyridine).

Pediatric pointers

In young children, urinary urgency may appear as a change in toilet habits, such as a sudden onset of bed-wetting or daytime accidents in a toilet-trained child. Urgency may also result from urethral irritation by bubble bath salts.

Urine Cloudiness

Cloudy, murky, or turbid urine reflects the presence of bacteria, mucus, leukocytes or erythrocytes, epithelial cells, fat, or phosphates (in alkaline urine). It's characteristic of urinary tract infection but can also result from prolonged storage of a urine specimen at room temperature.

Assessment

Ask about symptoms of urinary tract infection, such as dysuria, urinary urgency or frequency, or pain in the flank, lower back, or suprapubic area. Also ask about recurrent urinary tract infections, or recent surgery or treatment involving the urinary tract.

Obtain a urine sample to check for pus or mucus (see *How to Perform the Three-Glass Urine Test*, page 744). Using a reagent strip, test for blood, glucose, and pH. Palpate the suprapubic area and flanks for tenderness.

If you note cloudy urine in a patient with an indwelling (Foley) catheter, especially with concurrent fever, remove the catheter immediately (or change it if the patient must have one in place).

Medical cause

• *Urinary tract infection.* Cloudy urine is common here. Other urinary changes include urgency, frequency, hematuria, dysuria, nocturia, and, in males, urethral discharge. Urinary hesitancy, bladder spasms, costovertebral angle tenderness, and suprapubic, lower back, or flank pain may occur. Other effects: fever, chills, malaise, nausea, and vomiting.

Special considerations

Collect urine samples, as ordered, for urinalysis and culture and sensitivity tests. Increase the patient's fluid intake and administer antibiotics and urinary anesthetics (such as phenazopyridine), as ordered. Continue checking the ap-

HOW TO PERFORM THE THREE-GLASS URINE TEST

If your male patient complains of urinary frequency and urgency, dysuria, flank or lower back pain, or other signs of urethritis, and if his urine specimen is cloudy, perform the three-glass urine test.

First ask him to void into three conical glasses labeled with numbers 1, 2, and 3. First-voided urine goes into glass #1; midstream urine goes into #2; and the remainder goes into glass #3. Tell the patient to avoid interrupting the stream of urine when shifting glasses, if possible.

Now observe each glass for pus and mucus shreds. Also note urine color and odor. Glass #1 will contain matter from the anterior urethra; glass #2 will contain bladder contents; and glass #3 will contain sediment from the prostate and seminal vesicles.

Some common findings are shown here. However, confirming diagnosis requires microscopic examination and a bacteriology report.

	SPECIMEN I	SPECIMEN II	SPECIMEN III
Acute or subacute urethritis	Cloudy	Clear	Clear
Acute posterior urethritis	Cloudy	Clear or cloudy	Cloudy
Chronic anterior urethritis	Small comma shreds	Clear	Clear
Chronic posterior urethritis	Large shreds	Clear	Clear
Chronic urethritis (anterior and posterior)	Small and large shreds	Clear	Clear
Prostatitis	Clear or large shreds	Clear	Cloudy or large shreds
Cystitis and pyelonephritis	Cloudy	Cloudy	Cloudy

pearance of the patient's urine to monitor the effectiveness of therapy.

Pediatric pointers
Cloudy urine in children also points to urinary tract infection.

Urticaria
[Hives]

Urticaria is a vascular skin reaction characterized by the eruption of pruritic wheals—smooth, slightly elevated patches with well-defined erythematous margins and pale centers. It's produced by the local release of histamine or other vasoactive substances as part of a hypersensitivity reaction. (See *Recognizing Common Skin Lesions,* pages 558 and 559.)

Acute urticaria evolves rapidly and usually has a detectable cause, commonly hypersensitivity to certain drugs, foods, insect bites, inhalants, or contactants, or emotional stress. Although individual lesions usually subside within 12 to 24 hours, new crops of lesions may erupt continuously, thus prolonging the attack.

Urticaria lasting longer than 6 weeks is classified as chronic. The lesions may recur for months or years, and the underlying cause is usually unknown. Occasionally, a diagnosis of psychogenic urticaria is made.

Angioedema, or giant urticaria, is characterized by the acute eruption of wheals involving the mucous membranes and, occasionally, the arms, legs, or genitals.

Assessment

If the patient's urticaria is acute, quickly assess his respiratory status and take his vital signs. If you note any respiratory difficulty (such as air hunger, dyspnea, wheezing, or stridor) or signs of impending anaphylactic shock (apprehension and uneasiness; warm, moist skin; or edema, especially facial), have another nurse call the doctor immediately. Start an I.V. infusion of dextrose 5% in water and, as appropriate, administer local epinephrine or apply ice to the affected site to decrease absorption through vasoconstriction. Clear and maintain the airway, administer oxygen as needed, and institute cardiac monitoring. Have resuscitation equipment at hand, and be prepared to begin cardiopulmonary resuscitation or to assist with emergency intubation or tracheostomy if necessary.

If the patient's not in distress, obtain a complete history. Does the urticaria follow any seasonal pattern? Do certain foods or drugs seem to aggravate it? Is there any relationship to physical exertion? Is the patient routinely exposed to any chemicals on the job or at home? Obtain a detailed drug history, including prescription and over-the-counter drugs. Note any history of chronic or parasitic infections, skin disease, or gastrointestinal (GI) disorders.

Medical causes

● *Anaphylaxis.* This acute reaction is marked by the rapid eruption of diffuse urticaria and angioedema, with wheals ranging from pinpoint to palm-sized or larger. Lesions are usually pruritic and stinging; paresthesias

---

COMMON DRUGS THAT CAUSE URTICARIA

Many drugs can produce urticaria. Among the most common are:

aspirin	immune serums	penicillin
atropine		quinine
codeine	insulin	sulfonamides
dextrans	morphine	vaccines

In addition, radiographic contrast medium commonly produces urticaria, especially when administered intravenously.

---

commonly precede their eruption. Other acute findings include profound anxiety, weakness, diaphoresis, sneezing, shortness of breath, profuse rhinorrhea, nasal congestion, dysphagia, and warm, moist skin. Severe reactions may be life-threatening and are marked by signs of respiratory distress (due to upper airway edema), cardiac dysrhythmias, hypotension, and shock.

● *Hereditary angioedema.* In this autosomal-dominant disorder, cutaneous involvement is manifested by nonpitting, nonpruritic edema of an extremity or the face. Respiratory mucosal involvement can produce life-threatening acute laryngeal edema.

Special considerations

To help relieve the patient's discomfort, apply a bland skin emollient or one containing menthol and phenol, as ordered. Expect to give antihistamines, systemic corticosteroids, or, if stress is a suspected contributing factor, tranquilizers. Tepid baths and cool compresses may also enhance vasoconstriction and decrease pruritus.

Teach the patient to avoid the causative stimulus, if identified.

Pediatric pointers

Pediatric causes of urticaria include acute papular urticaria (usually after insect bites), hereditary angioedema, and urticaria pigmentosa (rare).

vaginal bleeding—postmenopausal • vaginal discharge • venous hum • vertigo • violent behavior • vision loss • visual blurring • visual floaters • vomiting • vu gain—excessive • weight loss—excessive • wheezing • wristdrop• abdominal mass • abdominal pain • abdominal rigidity • accessory muscle use • agitatio amenorrhea • amnesia • analgesia • anhidrosis • anorexia • anosmia • anuria apnea • apneustic respirations • apraxia • arm pain • asterixis • ataxia • athe reflex • back pain • barrel chest • Battle's sign • Biot's respirations • bladder o pressure decrease • blood pressure increase • bowel sounds—absent • bowel s bowel sounds—hypoactive • bradycardia • bradypnea • breast dimpling • bre pain • breast ulcer • breath with ammonia odor • breath with fecal odor • br Brudzinski's sign • bruits • buffalo hump • butterfly rash • café-au-lait spots • prolonged • carpopedal spasm • cat cry • chest expansion—asymmetrical • ch respirations • chills • chorea • Chvostek's sign • clubbing • cogwheel rigidity confusion • conjunctival injection • constipation • corneal reflex—absent • cos tenderness • cough—barking • cough—nonproductive • cough—productive • bony • crepitation—subcutaneous • cry—high-pitched • cyanosis • decerebrat posture • deep tendon reflexes—hyperactive • deep tendon reflexes—hypoacti diaphoresis • diarrhea • diplopia • dizziness • doll's eye sign—absent • drooli dysmenorrhea • dyspareunia • dyspepsia • dysphagia • dyspnea • dystonia • e edema—generalized • edema of the arms • edema of the face • edema of the enuresis • epistaxis • eructation • erythema • exophthalmos • eye discharge • fasciculations • fatigue • fecal incontinence • fetor hepaticus • fever • flank pa fontanelle bulging • fontanelle depression • footdrop • gag reflex abnormalitie propulsive • gait—scissors • gait—spastic • gait—steppage • gait—waddling • gallop—ventricular • genital lesions in the male • grunting respirations • gun swelling • gynecomastia • halitosis • halo vision • headache • hearing loss • h Heberden's nodes • hematemesis • hematochezia • hematuria • hemianopia • hepatomegaly • hiccups • hirsutism • hoarseness • Homans' sign • hyperpign hypopigmentation • impotence • insomnia • intermittent claudication • Janew jaw pain • jugular vein distention • Kehr's sign • Kernig's sign • leg pain • le decreased • lid lag • light flashes • low birth weight • lymphadenopathy • ma McBurney's sign • McMurray's sign • melena • menorrhagia • metrorrhagia • mouth lesions • murmurs • muscle atrophy • muscle flaccidity • muscle spasr muscle weakness • mydriasis • myoclonus • nasal flaring • nausea • neck pai nipple discharge • nipple retraction • nocturia • nuchal rigidity • nystagmus oligomenorrhea • oliguria • opisthotonos • orofacial dyskinesia • orthopnea • Ortolani's sign • Osler's nodes • otorrhea • pallor • palpitations • papular ras paresthesias • paroxysmal nocturnal dyspnea • peau d'orange • pericardial fr waves—visible • photophobia • pica • pleural friction rub • polydipsia • poly postnasal drip • priapism • pruritus • psoas sign • psychotic behavior • ptosi weak • pulse—bounding • pulse pressure—narrowed • pulse pressure—wide abnormality • pulsus alternans • pulsus bisferiens • pulsus paradoxus • pupil pupils—sluggish • purple striae • purpura • pustular rash • pyrosis • raccoo tenderness • rectal pain • retractions—costal and sternal • rhinorrhea • rhon salivation—decreased • salivation—increased • salt craving • scotoma • scrot absence • seizure—focal • seizure—generalized tonic-clonic • seizure—psych sign • shallow respirations • skin—bronze • skin—clammy • skin—mottled • turgor—decreased • spider angioma • splenomegaly • stertorous respirations stridor • syncope • tachycardia • tachypnea • taste abnormalities • tearing—i tic • tinnitus • tracheal deviation • tracheal tugging • tremors • trismus • tu

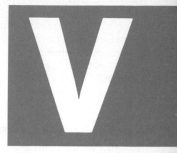

Vaginal Bleeding—Postmenopausal

Postmenopausal vaginal bleeding—bleeding that occurs 6 or more months after menopause—is an important indicator of gynecologic cancer. However, it can also result from infection, local pelvic disorders, estrogenic stimulation, and physiologic thinning and drying of the vaginal mucous membranes. It usually occurs as slight, brown or red spotting either spontaneously or following coitus or douching, but it may also occur as oozing of fresh blood or as bright red hemorrhage. Many patients—especially those with a history of heavy menstrual flow—minimize the importance of this bleeding, seriously delaying diagnosis.

Assessment

Determine the patient's current age and her age at menopause. Ask when she first noticed the abnormal bleeding. Then obtain a thorough obstetric and gynecologic history. When did she begin menstruating? Were her periods regular? If not, ask her to describe any menstrual irregularities. How old was she when she first had intercourse? How many sexual partners has she had? Has she had any children? Has she had fertility problems? If possible, obtain an obstetric and gynecologic history of the patient's mother, and ask about a family history of gynecologic cancer. Determine if the patient has any associated symptoms and if she's currently taking estrogen.

Observe the external genitalia, noting the character of any vaginal discharge and the appearance of the labia, vaginal rugae, and clitoris. Carefully palpate the patient's breasts and lymph nodes for nodules or enlargement. As ordered, assist the doctor with pelvic and rectal examinations.

Medical causes

• *Atrophic vaginitis.* When bloody staining occurs, it usually follows coitus or douching. Characteristic white vaginal discharge may be accompanied by pruritus, dyspareunia, and a burning sensation in the vagina and labia. Sparse pubic hair, a pale vagina with decreased rugae and small hemorrhagic spots, clitoral atrophy, and shrinking of the labia minora may also occur.

• *Cervical cancer.* Early invasive cervical cancer causes vaginal spotting or heavier bleeding, usually after coitus or douching but occasionally spontaneously. Related findings include persistent vaginal discharge and postcoital pain. As the cancer spreads, back and sciatic pain, leg swelling, anorexia, weight loss, and weakness may occur.

• *Cervical or endometrial polyps.* These small, pedunculated growths may cause spotting (possibly as a muco-purulent, pink discharge) after coitus, douching, or straining at stool. Endometrial polyps are often asymptomatic, however.

• *Endometrial cancer.* Bleeding occurs early and can be brownish and scant or bright red and profuse. It often follows coitus or douching. Bleeding later becomes heavier, more frequent, and of longer duration, and may be accompanied by pelvic, rectal, lower back, and leg pain.

• *Ovarian tumors (feminizing).* Estrogen-producing ovarian tumors can stimulate endometrial shedding and cause heavy bleeding unassociated with coitus or douching. A palpable pelvic mass, increased cervical mucus, breast enlargement, and spider angiomas may be present.

• *Vaginal cancer.* Characteristic spotting or bleeding may be preceded by a thin, watery vaginal discharge. Bleeding may be spontaneous but usually follows coitus or douching. A firm, ulcerated vaginal lesion may be present; dyspareunia, urinary frequency, bladder and pelvic pain, rectal bleeding, and vulvar lesions may develop later.

Other causes

• *Drugs.* Excessive or prolonged estrogen administration is the most common drug cause of postmenopausal vaginal bleeding.

Special considerations

Prepare the patient for diagnostic tests, such as ultrasonography to outline a cervical or uterine tumor; endometrial biopsy and dilation and fractional curettage to obtain tissue for histologic examination; testing for occult blood in the stool; and vaginal and cervical cultures to detect infection. Discontinue estrogens, as ordered, until a diagnosis is made.

Pediatric pointers

None.

Vaginal Discharge

Common in women of childbearing age, physiologic vaginal discharge is mucoid, clear or white, nonbloody, and odorless. Produced by the cervical mucosa and, to a lesser degree, by the vulvar glands, this discharge may occasionally be scant or profuse without pathologic significance. However, a marked increase in discharge or a change in discharge color, odor, or consistency can signal disease. Often, the abnormal discharge stems from altered estrogen production. However, it may also result from infection, sexually transmitted disease, reproductive tract disease, fistulas, and certain drugs. In addition, the prolonged presence of a foreign body, such as a tampon or diaphragm, in the vagina can cause excessive mucus production, as can irritation from frequent douching, feminine hygiene products, contraceptive products, bubble baths, and colored or perfumed toilet papers.

Assessment

Ask the patient to describe the onset, color, consistency, odor, and texture of her vaginal discharge. How does the discharge differ from her usual vaginal secretions? Is the onset related to her menstrual cycle? Also ask about associated symptoms, such as dysuria and perineal pruritus and burning. Does she have spotting after coitus or douching? Ask about recent changes in her sexual habits and hygiene practices. Is she or could she be pregnant? Next, ask if she has had vaginal discharge before or has ever been treated for a vaginal infection. What treatment did she receive? Did she complete the course of medication? Ask about her current use of medications, especially antibiotics, oral estrogens, and contraceptives.

Examine the external genitalia and note the character of the discharge (see *Identifying Causes of Vaginal Dis-*

IDENTIFYING CAUSES OF VAGINAL DISCHARGE

The color, consistency, amount, and odor of your patient's vaginal discharge provide important clues about the underlying disorder. For quick reference, use this chart to match common characteristics of vaginal discharge and their possible causes.

CHARACTERISTICS	POSSIBLE CAUSES
Thin, scant, white discharge	Atrophic vaginitis
White, curdlike, profuse discharge with yeasty, sweet odor	Candidiasis
Mucopurulent, foul-smelling discharge	Chancroid
Yellow, mucopurulent, odorless or acrid discharge	*Chlamydia* infection
Scant, serosanguineous discharge with foul odor	Endometritis
Thin, green or grayish white, foul-smelling discharge	*Gardnerella* vaginitis
Copious, mucoid discharge	Genital herpes
Profuse, mucopurulent discharge, possibly foul-smelling	Genital warts
Yellow or green, foul-smelling discharge, expressed from Bartholin's or Skene's ducts	Gonorrhea
Chronic, watery, bloody or purulent discharge, possibly foul-smelling	Gynecologic cancer
Frothy, greenish yellow, and profuse (or thin, white, and scant) foul-smelling discharge	Trichomoniasis

charge). Observe vulvar and vaginal tissues for redness, edema, and excoriation. Palpate the inguinal lymph nodes to detect tenderness or enlargement, and palpate the abdomen for tenderness. As ordered, assist with a pelvic examination and obtain vaginal discharge specimens for testing.

Medical causes

• *Atrophic vaginitis.* In this disorder, a thin, scant, white vaginal discharge may be accompanied by pruritus, burning, tenderness, and bloody spotting after coitus or douching. Sparse pubic hair, a pale vagina with decreased rugae and small hemorrhagic spots, clitoral atrophy, and shrinking of the labia minora may also occur.

• *Candidiasis.* Infection with *Candida albicans* causes a profuse, white, curdlike discharge with a yeasty, sweet odor. Onset is abrupt, usually just before menses. Exudate may be lightly attached to the labia and vaginal walls and is often accompanied by vulvar redness and edema. The inner thighs may be covered with a fine, red dermatitis. Intense labial itching and burning may also occur.

• *Chancroid.* This rare, sexually transmitted disease produces a mucopurulent, foul-smelling discharge and vulvar lesions that are initially erythematous and later ulcerated. Within 2 to 3 weeks, inguinal lymph nodes may become tender and enlarged, with pruritus, suppuration, and spontaneous drainage of nodes. Headache, malaise, and fever to 102.2° F. (39° C.) are common.

• Chlamydia *infection.* This infection causes a yellow, mucopurulent, odorless or acrid vaginal discharge. Other findings may include dysuria, dyspareunia, and vaginal bleeding after douching or coitus, especially following menses.

• *Endometritis.* A scant, serosanguineous discharge with a foul odor can result from bacterial invasion of the endometrium. Associated findings may include fever, lower back and abdominal pain, abdominal muscle spasm, malaise, and dysmenorrhea.

• **Gardnerella** *vaginitis.* This infection (by *Gardnerella vaginalis,* formerly called *Hemophilus vaginalis*) causes a thin, foul-smelling, green or grayish white discharge. It adheres to the vaginal walls and can be easily wiped away, leaving healthy-looking tissue. Pruritus, redness, and other signs of vaginal irritation may occur.

• *Genital warts.* Characteristic vulvar lesions can cause a profuse, mucopurulent vaginal discharge, which may be foul-smelling if the warts are infected. Pruritus and erythema are common.

• *Gonorrhea.* Although 80% of women with gonorrhea are asymptomatic, others have a yellow or green, foul-smelling discharge that can be expressed from Bartholin's or Skene's ducts. Other findings: dysuria, urinary frequency and incontinence, and vaginal redness and swelling. Severe pelvic and lower abdominal pain may develop.

• *Gynecologic cancer.* Endometrial or cervical cancer produces a chronic, watery, bloody or purulent vaginal discharge that may be foul-smelling. Other findings: abnormal vaginal bleeding and, later, weight loss; pelvic, back, and leg pain; fatigue; and abdominal distention.

• *Herpes simplex (genital).* A copious, mucoid discharge results from this disorder, but the initial complaint is painful, indurated vesicles and ulcerations on the labia, vagina, cervix, anus, thighs, or mouth. Erythema, marked edema, and tender inguinal lymph nodes may occur with fever, malaise, and dysuria.

• *Trichomoniasis.* This infection can cause a foul-smelling discharge, which may be frothy, greenish yellow, and profuse or thin, white, and scant. Other findings may include pruritus; a red, inflamed vagina with tiny petechiae; dysuria and urinary frequency; and dyspareunia, postcoital spotting, menorrhagia, or dysmenorrhea. However, about 70% of patients are asymptomatic.

Other causes

• *Contraceptive cream and jellies.* These products can increase vaginal secretions.

• *Drugs.* Estrogen-containing drugs, including oral contraceptives, can cause increased mucoid vaginal discharge. Antibiotics, such as tetracycline, can predispose the patient to vaginal infection and discharge.

• *Radiation therapy.* Irradiation of the reproductive tract can cause a watery, odorless vaginal discharge.

Special considerations

Teach the patient to keep her perineum clean and dry. Also tell her to avoid wearing tight-fitting clothing and nylon underwear, and instead to wear cotton-crotched underwear and pantyhose. If appropriate, suggest that the patient douche with a solution of 5 tablespoons of white vinegar to 2 quarts of warm water to help relieve her discomfort.

If the patient has a vaginal infection, tell her to continue taking the prescribed medication even if her symptoms clear or she menstruates. Also advise her to avoid intercourse until her symptoms clear, and then to have her partner use condoms until she completes her course of medication.

Pediatric pointers

Female newborns who have been exposed to maternal estrogens in utero may have a white mucous vaginal discharge for the first month after birth; a yellow mucous discharge indicates a pathologic condition. In the older child, a purulent, foul-smelling, and possibly bloody vaginal discharge commonly results from a foreign object placed in the vagina.

Venous Hum

A venous hum is a functional or in-nocent murmur heard above the clav-icles throughout the cardiac cycle. Loudest during diastole, it's low-pitched, rough, or noisy. The hum often accompanies a thrill or, possibly, a high-pitched whine. It's best heard by applying the bell of the stethoscope to the medial aspect of the right supra-clavicular area, with the patient seated upright (see *Detecting a Venous Hum*).

A venous hum is a common and nor-mal finding in children and pregnant women. However, it also occurs in hy-perdynamic states, such as anemia and thyrotoxicosis. The hum results from increased blood flow through the in-ternal jugular veins, especially on the right side, which causes audible vibra-tions in the tissues.

Occasionally, a venous hum may be mistaken for an intracardiac murmur or a thyroid bruit. However, a venous hum disappears with jugular vein compression and waxes and wanes with head-turning. In contrast, both an intracardiac murmur and a thyroid bruit persist despite jugular compres-sion and head-turning.

Assessment

Determine if the patient has a history of anemia or thyroid disorders. If he does, ask what medication or other treatments he has received. If he doesn't have a history of these disorders, ask if he has experienced any associated symptoms, such as palpitations, dys-pnea, nervousness, tremors, heat in-tolerance, weight loss, fatigue, weak-ness, or malaise.

Take the patient's vital signs, noting especially tachycardia, hypertension, a bounding pulse, and widened pulse pressure. Auscultate the patient's heart for gallops or murmurs. Examine his skin and mucous membranes for pal-lor.

DETECTING A VENOUS HUM

To detect a venous hum, have your patient sit upright and then place the bell of the stethoscope over his right supraclavicular area. Gently lift his chin and turn his head toward the left, which increases the loudness of the hum (top). If you still can't hear the hum, press his jugular vein with your thumb (bottom). The hum will disappear with pressure but will suddenly return, temporarily louder than before, when you release your thumb—a result of the turbulence created by pressure changes.

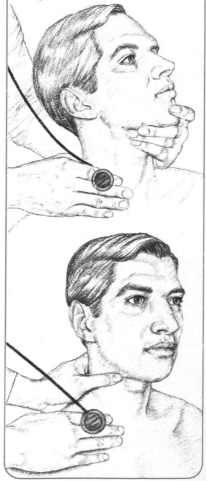

Medical causes

• *Anemia.* A venous hum is common with severe anemia (hemoglobin level below 7 g/dl). Additional findings may include pale skin and mucous membranes, dyspnea, crackles, tachycardia, bounding pulse, atrial gallop, systolic bruits over both carotid arteries, bleeding tendencies, weakness, fatigue, and malaise.

• *Thyrotoxicosis.* This disorder may cause a loud venous hum, audible whether the patient's sitting or supine. Auscultation may also reveal an atrial or ventricular gallop. Additional findings commonly include tachycardia, palpitations, weight loss despite increased appetite, an enlarged thyroid, dyspnea, nervousness and tremors, diaphoresis, and heat intolerance. Exophthalmos may be present.

Special considerations

Prepare the patient for diagnostic tests, which may include an EKG, complete blood count, and thyroid hormone (T_3 and T_4) assays.

Pediatric pointers

A cervical venous hum occurs normally in more than two thirds of children between the ages of 5 and 15.

Vertigo

Vertigo is an illusion of movement in which the patient feels that he's revolving in space (subjective vertigo) or that his surroundings are revolving around him (objective vertigo). He may complain of feeling pulled sideways, as though drawn by a magnet.

A common symptom, vertigo usually begins abruptly and may be temporary or permanent, mild or severe. It worsens when the patient moves and often subsides when he lies down. Frequently, it's confused with dizziness— a sensation of imbalance and lightheadedness that does not include a whirling sensation. However, unlike dizziness, vertigo is often accompanied by nausea, vomiting, nystagmus, and tinnitus or hearing loss. Although limb coordination is unaffected, vertiginous gait may occur.

Vertigo may result from neurologic or otologic disorders that affect the equilibratory apparatus (the vestibule, semicircular canals, eighth cranial nerve, vestibular nuclei in the brain stem and their temporal lobe connections, and eyes). However, this symptom may also result from alcohol intoxication, hyperventilation, postural changes (benign postural vertigo), and the effects of certain drugs, tests, and procedures.

Assessment

Ask your patient to describe the onset and duration of his vertigo, being careful to distinguish this symptom from dizziness. Does he feel that he's moving or that his surroundings are moving around him? How often do the attacks occur? Do they follow position changes, or are they unpredictable? Find out if the patient can walk during an attack, if he leans to one side, and if he's ever fallen. Ask if he experiences motion sickness and if he prefers one position during an attack. Obtain a recent drug history and note any evidence of alcohol abuse.

Perform a neurologic assessment, focusing particularly on eighth cranial nerve function. Observe the patient's gait and posture for abnormalities.

Medical causes

• *Acoustic neuroma.* This tumor of the eighth cranial nerve causes mild, intermittent vertigo several months after onset of unilateral sensorineural hearing loss. Other findings: tinnitus, postauricular or suboccipital pain, and— with cranial nerve compression—facial paralysis.

• *Brain stem ischemia.* This condition produces sudden, severe vertigo that becomes episodic and later persistent. Associated findings include ataxia, nausea, vomiting, increased blood pressure, tachycardia, nystagmus, and lateral deviation of the eyes toward the side of the lesion. Hemiparesis and paresthesias may also occur.

• **Head trauma.** Persistent vertigo, occurring soon after injury, accompanies spontaneous or positional nystagmus and, if the temporal bone is fractured, hearing loss. Associated findings include headache, nausea, vomiting, and decreased level of consciousness. Behavioral changes, diplopia or visual blurring, seizures, motor or sensory deficits, and signs of increased intracranial pressure may also occur.

• **Herpes zoster.** Infection of the eighth cranial nerve produces sudden onset of vertigo accompanied by facial paralysis, hearing loss in the affected ear, and herpetic vesicular lesions in the auditory canal.

• **Labyrinthitis.** Severe vertigo begins abruptly with this inner ear infection. Vertigo may occur in a single episode or may recur over months or years. Associated findings may include nausea, vomiting, progressive sensorineural hearing loss, and nystagmus.

• **Ménière's disease.** In this disease, labyrinthine dysfunction causes abrupt onset of vertigo, lasting minutes, hours, or days. Unpredictable episodes of severe vertigo and unsteady gait may cause the patient to fall. During an attack, any sudden motion of the head or eyes can precipitate nausea and vomiting. Other findings include hearing loss that can progress to deafness, worsening tinnitus and a sensation of fullness in the affected ear, diaphoresis, and nystagmus.

• **Multiple sclerosis (MS).** Episodic vertigo may occur early and become persistent. Other early findings include diplopia, visual blurring, and paresthesias. MS may also produce nystagmus, constipation, muscle weakness, paralysis, spasticity, hyperreflexia, intention tremor, and ataxia. Other effects include dysphagia, dysarthria, urinary dysfunction, impotence, and emotional lability.

• **Posterior fossa tumor.** In this disorder, positional vertigo lasts for a few seconds. The patient may have papilledema, headache, memory loss, nausea, vomiting, nystagmus, apneustic or ataxic respirations, and increased blood pressure. He may also fall sideways.

• **Vestibular neuritis.** In this disorder, severe vertigo usually begins abruptly and lasts several days, without tinnitus or hearing loss. Other findings include nausea, vomiting, and nystagmus.

Other causes

• **Diagnostic tests.** Caloric testing (irrigating the ears with warm or cold water) can induce vertigo.

• **Drugs and alcohol.** High doses and toxic levels of certain drugs may produce vertigo. These include salicylates, aminoglycosides (such as streptomycin and gentamicin), antibiotics (such as minocycline, capreomycin, and polymyxin), quinine, and oral contraceptives. Alcohol intoxication may also produce vertigo.

• **Surgery and other procedures.** Middle ear surgery may cause vertigo that lasts for several days. In addition, administration of overly warm or cold ear drops or irrigating solutions may cause vertigo.

Special considerations

Place the patient in a comfortable position, and monitor his vital signs and level of consciousness. Keep the side rails up if he's in bed, or help him to a chair if he's standing when vertigo occurs. Darken the room and keep him calm. If ordered, administer drugs to control nausea and vomiting, and meclizine or dimenhydrinate to decrease labyrinthine irritability.

Prepare the patient for diagnostic tests, such as electronystagmography, and X-rays of the middle and inner ears.

Pediatric pointers

Ear infection is a common cause of vertigo in children. Vestibular neuritis may also cause this symptom.

Vesicular Rash

A vesicular rash is a scattered or linear distribution of vesicles—sharply circumscribed lesions filled with clear, cloudy, or bloody fluid. The lesions, which are usually less than 0.5 cm in diameter, may occur singly or in groups. (See *Recognizing Common Skin Lesions,* pages 558 and 559.) They sometimes occur with bullae—fluid-filled lesions larger than 0.5 cm in diameter.

A vesicular rash may be mild or severe and temporary or permanent. It can result from infection, inflammation, or allergic reactions.

Assessment

Ask your patient when the rash began, how it spread, and whether it has appeared before. Did other skin lesions precede eruption of the vesicles? Obtain a thorough drug history. If the patient has used any topical medication, what type did he use and when was it last applied? Also ask about associated signs and symptoms. Find out if he has a family history of skin disorders, and ask about allergies, recent infections, insect bites, and exposure to allergens.

Examine the patient's skin, noting if it's dry, oily, or moist. Observe the general distribution of the lesions and record their exact location. Note the color, shape, and size of the lesions, and check for crusts, scales, scars, macules, papules, or wheals. Palpate the vesicles or bullae to determine if they're flaccid or tense. Slide your finger across the skin to see if the outer layer of epidermis separates easily from the basal layer (Nikolsky's sign).

Medical causes

- **Burns.** Thermal burns that affect the epidermis and part of the dermis often cause vesicles and bullae, with erythema, swelling, pain, and moistness.
- **Dermatitis.** In *contact dermatitis,* a severe hypersensitivity reaction produces an eruption of small vesicles surrounded by redness and marked edema. The vesicles may ooze, scale, and cause severe pruritus.

Dermatitis herpetiformis, occurring most often in men between the ages of 20 and 50, produces a chronic inflammatory eruption marked by vesicular, papular, bullous, pustular, or erythematous lesions. Usually, the rash is symmetrically distributed on the buttocks, shoulders, extensor surfaces of the elbows and knees, and sometimes the face, scalp, and neck. Other symptoms include severe pruritus, burning, and stinging.

In *nummular dermatitis,* groups of pinpoint vesicles and papules appear on erythematous or pustular lesions that are nummular (coinlike) or annular (ringlike). Often, the pustular lesions ooze a purulent exudate, itch severely, and rapidly become crusted and scaly. Two or three lesions may develop on the hands, but the lesions most commonly develop on the extensor surfaces of the limbs and on the buttocks and posterior trunk.

- **Dermatophytid.** This allergic reaction to fungal infection produces vesicular lesions on the hands, usually in response to tinea pedis. The lesions are extremely pruritic and tender and may be accompanied by fever, anorexia, generalized adenopathy, and splenomegaly.
- **Erythema multiforme.** This acute inflammatory skin disease is heralded by a sudden eruption of erythematous macules, papules, and, occasionally, vesicles and bullae. The characteristic rash appears symmetrically over the hands, arms, feet, legs, face, and neck and tends to reappear. Vesicles and bullae may also erupt on the eyes and genitalia. Most often, though, vesiculobullous lesions appear on the mucous membranes—especially the lips and buccal mucosa—where they rupture and ulcerate, producing a thick, yellow or white exudate. Bloody, painful crusts, a foul-smelling oral dis-

charge, and difficulty chewing may develop. Lymphadenopathy may also occur.

● **Herpes simplex.** This common viral infection produces vesicles on an erythematous base, and usually affects the lips. About 25% of patients develop lesions on the genitalia. Vesicles are preceded by itching, tingling, burning, or pain; develop singly or in groups; are 2 to 3 mm in size; and do not coalesce. Eventually, they rupture, forming a painful ulcer followed by a yellowish crust.

● **Herpes zoster.** A vesicular rash is preceded by erythema and, occasionally, by a nodular skin eruption and unilateral, sharp, shooting chest pain that mimics a myocardial infarction. About 5 days later, the lesions erupt and commonly spread unilaterally over the thorax or vertically over the arms and legs. The pain becomes burning. Vesicles dry and scab about 10 days after eruption. Associated findings include fever, malaise, pruritus, and paresthesia or hyperesthesia of the involved area. Occasionally, herpes zoster involves the cranial nerves, producing facial palsy, hearing loss, dizziness, loss of taste, eye pain, and impaired vision.

● **Insect bites.** Vesicles appear on red hivelike papules and may become hemorrhagic.

● **Pemphigoid (bullous).** Generalized pruritus or an urticarial or eczematous eruption may precede the classic bullous rash. Bullae are large, tense, and irregular, and most often form on an erythematous base. They usually appear on the lower abdomen, groin, inner thighs, and forearms.

● **Pemphigus.** In *chronic familial pemphigus*, groups of tiny vesicles erupt on erythematous or normal skin. The vesicles are flaccid and easily broken, producing small denuded areas that become covered with crust; itching and burning are common. The eruption remits spontaneously but recurs.

Pemphigus foliaceus usually develops slowly and may begin with bullous lesions, commonly on the head and trunk. As these lesions spread to other areas, they become moist, scaly, and foul-smelling. Nikolsky's sign is present, and denudation of lesions results in extensive erythema, with large, loose scales and crusts. Pruritus and burning are common.

Pemphigus vulgaris may be acute and rapidly progressive, or chronic. The bullae may be tender or painful and large or small, and are usually flaccid. When they rupture, denuded skin exudes a clear, bloody, or purulent discharge. Commonly, the bullae first erupt in a specific location, such as the mouth or scalp, and eventually become widespread. Nikolsky's sign and pruritus may be present.

● **Pompholyx.** This common, recurrent disorder produces symmetrical vesicular lesions that can become pustular. The pruritic lesions appear on the palms more frequently than on the soles and may be accompanied by minimal erythema.

● **Porphyria cutanea tarda.** Bullae—especially on areas exposed to sun, fric-

---

DRUGS CAUSING TOXIC EPIDERMAL NECROLYSIS

A variety of drugs can trigger toxic epidermal necrolysis (TEN)—a rare but potentially fatal immune reaction characterized by a vesicular rash. TEN produces large, flaccid bullae that rupture easily, exposing extensive areas of denuded skin. The resulting loss of fluid and electrolytes—along with widespread systemic involvement—can lead to such life-threatening complications as pulmonary edema, shock, renal failure, sepsis, and disseminated intravascular coagulation. Here's a list of some drugs that can cause TEN:

- allopurinol
- aspirin
- barbiturates
- chloramphenicol
- chlorpropamide
- gold salts
- nitrofurantoin

- penicillin
- phenolphthalein
- phenylbutazone
- phenytoin
- primidone
- sulfonamides
- tetracycline

tion, trauma, or heat—result from the characteristic photosensitivity that develops between the ages of 20 and 40. Papulovesicular lesions evolving to erosions or ulcers and scars may appear. Chronic skin changes include hyperpigmentation or hypopigmentation, hypertrichosis, and sclerodermoid lesions. Urine is pink to brown.

• *Scabies.* Small vesicles erupt on an erythematous base and may be located at the end of a curved, threadlike burrow. The lesions are 1 to 10 cm long, with a swollen nodule or red papule that contains the itch mite. Pustules and excoriations may also occur. Men may develop lesions on the glans, shaft, and scrotum; women may develop lesions on the nipples. Both sexes may develop lesions on the wrists, elbows, axilla, and waistline. Associated pruritus worsens with inactivity and warmth.

• *Tinea pedis.* This fungal infection causes vesicles and scaling between the toes and, possibly, dry scaling over the entire sole. Severe infection causes inflammation, pruritus, and difficulty walking.

• *Toxic epidermal necrolysis.* In this immune reaction to drugs or other toxins, vesicles and bullae are preceded by a diffuse, erythematous rash and followed by large-scale epidermal necrolysis and desquamation. Large, flaccid bullae develop after mucous membrane inflammation, a burning sensation in the conjunctivae, malaise, fever, and generalized skin tenderness. The bullae rupture easily, exposing extensive areas of denuded skin.

Special considerations

Any skin eruption that covers a large area may cause substantial fluid loss through the vesicles, bullae, or other weeping lesions. If necessary, start an I.V. to replace fluids and electrolytes. Keep the patient's environment warm and free from drafts, cover him with sheets or blankets as necessary, and take his rectal temperature every 4 hours, since increased fluid loss and increased blood flow to inflamed skin

may lead to hyperthermia.

Obtain cultures, as ordered, to determine the causative organism. Use sterile technique and observe isolation procedures until infection is ruled out. Tell the patient to wash his hands often and not to touch the lesions. Report any signs of secondary infection, such as swelling and purulent drainage. Give antibiotics and apply corticosteroid or antimicrobial ointment to the lesions.

Pediatric pointers

Vesicular rashes in children are usually caused by varicella, hand-foot-and-mouth disease, and miliaria rubra.

Violent Behavior

Marked by sudden loss of self-control, violent behavior refers to the use of physical force to violate, injure, or abuse an object or person. This behavior may also be self-directed. It may result from organic and psychiatric disorders and the effects of drugs.

Assessment

During your assessment, determine if the patient has a history of violent behavior. Is he intoxicated or suffering symptoms of alcohol or drug withdrawal? Does he have a history of family violence, including corporal punishment and child or spouse abuse?

Watch for clues indicating that the patient is losing control and may become violent. Has he exhibited abrupt behavioral changes? Is he unable to sit still? Increased activity may indicate an attempt to discharge aggression. Does he suddenly cease activity (suggesting the calm before the storm)? Does he make verbal threats or angry gestures? Is he jumpy, extremely tense, or laughing? Such intensifing of emotion may herald loss of control.

If your patient's violent behavior is a new development, he may have an organic disorder. Obtain a medical his-

UNDERSTANDING FAMILY VIOLENCE

Effectively managing the violent patient requires an understanding of the roots of his behavior. For example, his behavior may be spawned by a family history of corporal punishment or child or spouse abuse. His violent behavior may also be associated with drug or alcohol abuse and fixed family roles that stifle growth and individuality.

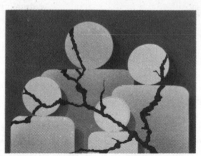

What causes family violence? Social scientists suggest that it stems from cultural attitudes fostering violence and from the frustration and stress associated with overcrowded living conditions and poverty. Albert Bandura, a social learning theorist, believes that individuals learn violent behavior by observing and imitating other family members who vent their aggressive feelings through verbal abuse and physical force. (They also learn from television and the movies, especially when the violent hero gains power and recognition.) Members of families with these characteristics may have an increased potential for violent behavior, initiating a cycle of violence that passes from generation to generation.

tory and perform a physical examination. Watch for a sudden change in his level of consciousness. Disorientation, failure to recall recent events, or display of tics, jerks, tremors, or asterixis all suggest an organic disorder.

Medical causes

• *Organic disorders.* Many disorders may cause violent behavior due to metabolic and neurologic dysfunction. Common causes include epilepsy, brain tumor, encephalitis, head injury, endocrine disorders, metabolic disorders (such as uremia and calcium imbalance), and severe physical trauma.

• *Psychiatric disorders.* Violent behavior occurs as a protective mechanism in response to a perceived threat in psychotic disorders, such as schizophrenia. A similar response may occur in personality disorders, such as antisocial or borderline personality.

Other causes

• *Drugs and alcohol.* Various drugs, such as lidocaine and procaine penicillin, may cause violent behavior as an adverse effect. Alcohol abuse or withdrawal, hallucinogens, amphetamines, and barbiturate withdrawal may also cause violent behavior.

Special considerations

Violent behavior is most prevalent in certain hospital areas—emergency rooms, critical care units, and crisis and acute psychiatric units. Natural disasters and accidents also increase the potential for violent behavior, so be on guard in these situations.

If your patient becomes violent or potentially violent, your goal is to remain composed and to establish environmental control. First, protect yourself. Remain at a distance from the patient, call for assistance, and don't overreact. Remain calm, and make sure you have enough personnel for a show of force or, if necessary, for subduing him. Encourage the patient to move to a quiet location—free of noise, activity, and people—to avoid frightening or stimulating him further. Reassure him, explain what's happening, and tell him that he's safe. If he makes violent threats, take them seriously, and inform those at whom the threats are directed. If ordered, give drugs to combat his psychotic symptoms.

Remember, your own attitudes can affect your ability to care for a violent patient. If you feel fearful or judgmental, ask another staff member for help.

Pediatric pointers

Adolescents and younger children often make threats resulting from violent dreams or fantasies or unmet needs. Adolescents who exhibit extreme violence can be from families with a history of physical or psychological abuse. These children may display violent behavior toward their peers, siblings, and pets.

Vision Loss

Vision loss—the inability to perceive visual stimuli—can be sudden or gradual and temporary or permanent. The deficit can range from a slight impairment of vision to total blindness. It results from ocular, neurologic, and systemic disorders, as well as from trauma and reactions to certain drugs.

Assessment

If the patient reports sudden vision loss, inform the doctor immediately since such loss can signal an ocular emergency. (See *Managing Sudden Vision Loss.*) Don't touch the eye if the patient has perforating or penetrating ocular trauma.

If the patient's vision loss occurred gradually, ask him if it affects one eye or both, and all or only part of the visual field. Ask if he's experienced photosensitivity, and about the location, intensity, and duration of any eye pain. Obtain an ocular history and a family history of eye problems or systemic diseases that may lead to eye problems, such as hypertension; diabetes mellitus; thyroid, rheumatic, or vascular disease; infections; and cancer.

Carefully inspect both eyes, noting edema, foreign bodies, drainage, or conjunctival or scleral redness. Observe whether lid closure is complete or incomplete, and check for ptosis. Using a flashlight, examine the cornea and iris for scars, irregularities, and foreign bodies. Observe the size, shape, and color of the pupils, and test the direct and consensual light reflex (see "Pupils—Nonreactive") and the effect of accommodation. Evaluate extraocular muscle function by testing the six cardinal fields of gaze (see *Testing Extraocular Muscles,* page 235). Evaluate the extent of vision loss by testing visual acuity in each eye (see *Testing Visual Acuity,* page 762).

Medical causes

● *Amaurosis fugax.* In this disorder, recurrent attacks of unilateral vision loss may last from a few seconds to a few minutes. Vision is normal at other times. Transient unilateral weakness, hypertension, and elevated intraocular pressure in the affected eye may also occur.

● *Cataract.* Typically, painless and gradual visual blurring precedes vision loss. As the cataract progresses, the pupil turns milky white.

● *Concussion.* Immediately or shortly after blunt head trauma, vision may be blurred, double, or lost. Generally, vision loss is temporary. Other findings may include headache, anterograde and retrograde amnesia, transient loss of consciousness, nausea, vomiting, dizziness, irritability, confusion, lethargy, and aphasia.

● *Diabetic retinopathy.* Retinal edema and hemorrhage lead to visual blurring, which may progress to blindness.

● *Endophthalmitis.* Typically, this intraocular infection follows penetrating trauma, intravenous drug use, or intraocular surgery, causing possibly permanent unilateral vision loss; a sympathetic inflammation may affect the other eye.

● *Glaucoma.* This disorder produces gradual visual blurring that may progress to total blindness. *Acute closed-angle glaucoma* is an ocular emergency that may produce blindness within 3

MANAGING SUDDEN VISION LOSS

Sudden vision loss can signal central retinal artery occlusion or acute closed-angle glaucoma—ocular emergencies that require immediate intervention. If your patient reports sudden vision loss, immediately notify an ophthalmologist for an emergency examination, and perform these interventions as ordered:

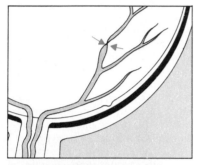

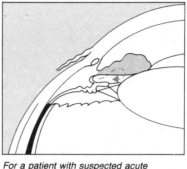

For a patient with suspected central retinal artery occlusion, perform light massage over his closed eyelid. Increase his carbon dioxide level, as ordered, by administering a set flow of oxygen and carbon dioxide through a Venturi mask. Or have the patient rebreathe in a paper bag to retain exhaled carbon dioxide. These steps will dilate the artery and, possibly, restore blood flow to the retina.

For a patient with suspected acute closed-angle glaucoma, help the doctor measure intraocular pressure with a tonometer, as ordered. (You can also estimate intraocular pressure without a tonometer by placing your fingers over the patient's closed eyelid. A rock-hard eyeball usually indicates increased intraocular pressure.) Expect to administer timolol drops and I.V. acetazolamide to help decrease intraocular pressure.

---

to 5 days. Findings are rapid onset of unilateral inflammation and pain, pressure over the eye, moderate pupil dilation, nonreactive pupillary response, a cloudy cornea, reduced visual acuity, photophobia, and perception of blue or red halos around lights. Nausea and vomiting may also occur.

Chronic closed-angle glaucoma has a gradual onset and usually produces no symptoms, although blurred or halo vision may occur. If untreated, it progresses to blindness and extreme pain.

Chronic open-angle glaucoma is usually bilateral, with an insidious onset and a slowly progressive course. It causes peripheral vision loss, aching eyes, halo vision, and reduced visual acuity (especially at night).

● *Hereditary corneal dystrophies.* Some dystrophies cause vision loss with associated pain, photophobia, tearing, and corneal opacities.

● *Herpes zoster.* When this disorder affects the nasociliary nerve, bilateral vision loss is accompanied by eyelid lesions, conjunctivitis, skin lesions that usually appear on the nose, and ocular muscle palsies.

● *Keratitis.* This inflammation of the cornea may lead to complete unilateral vision loss. Other findings include an opaque cornea, increased tearing, irritation, and photophobia.

● *Ocular trauma.* Following eye injury, sudden unilateral or bilateral vision loss may occur. Vision loss may be total or partial, and permanent or temporary. The eyelids may be reddened, edematous, and lacerated; and intraocular contents may be extruded.

● *Optic neuritis.* An umbrella term for inflammation, degeneration, or demyelinization of the optic nerve, optic neuritis usually produces temporary but severe unilateral vision loss. Pain around the eye occurs, especially with movement of the globe. This may be accompanied by visual field defects and a sluggish pupillary response to light. Ophthalmoscopic examination commonly reveals hyperemia of the optic disk, blurred disk margins, and filling of the physiologic cup.

● *Paget's disease.* Bilateral vision loss may develop as a result of bony impingements on the cranial nerves. This is accompanied by hearing loss, tinnitus, vertigo, and severe, persistent bone pain. Cranial enlargement may be noticeable frontally and occipitally, and headaches may occur. Kyphosis, barrel chest, and asymmetrical bowing of the legs may also occur. Sites of bone involvement are warm and tender, and impaired mobility and pathologic fractures are common.

● *Pituitary tumor.* As a pituitary adenoma grows, blurred vision progresses to hemianopia and, possibly, unilateral blindness. Double vision, nystagmus, ptosis, limited eye movement, and headaches may also occur. Other findings are rare but may include seizures, hypothermia, and somnolence. If the tumor secretes prolactin or excessive growth hormone, extensive changes may occur in all body systems.

● *Retinal artery occlusion (central).* This painless ocular emergency causes sudden, unilateral vision loss, which may be partial or complete. Pupil examination reveals a sluggish direct pupillary response and a normal consensual response. Permanent blindness may occur within hours.

● *Retinal detachment.* Depending on the degree and location of detachment, painless vision loss may be gradual or sudden and total or partial. Macular involvement will cause total blindness.

With partial vision loss, the patient may describe visual field defects or a shadow or curtain over the visual field, as well as visual floaters.

● *Retinal vein occlusion (central).* Most common in geriatric patients, this painless disorder causes a unilateral decrease in visual acuity with variable vision loss. Intraocular pressure may be elevated in both eyes.

● *Senile macular degeneration.* Occurring in elderly patients, this disorder causes painless blurring or loss of central vision. Vision loss may proceed slowly or rapidly, eventually affecting both eyes. Visual acuity may be worse at night.

● *Stevens-Johnson syndrome.* Corneal scarring from associated conjunctival lesions produces marked vision loss. Purulent conjunctivitis, eye pain, and difficulty opening the eyes occur. Additional findings may include widespread bullae, fever, malaise, cough, drooling, inability to eat, sore throat, chest pain, vomiting, diarrhea, myalgias, arthralgias, hematuria, and possibly signs of renal failure.

● *Temporal arteritis.* Vision loss and visual blurring with a throbbing, unilateral headache characterize this disorder. Other findings include malaise, anorexia, weight loss, weakness, low-grade fever, generalized muscle aches, and confusion.

● *Trachoma.* This rare disorder may initially produce varying vision loss and a mild infection resembling bacterial conjunctivitis. Conjunctival follicles, red and edematous eyelids, pain, photophobia, tearing, and exudation also occur. After about 1 month, conjunctival follicles enlarge into inflamed yellow or gray papillae.

● *Uveitis.* Inflammation of the uveal tract may result in unilateral vision loss. *Anterior uveitis* produces moderate to severe eye pain, severe conjunctival injection, photophobia, and a small, nonreactive pupil. *Posterior uveitis* may produce insidious onset of blurred vision, conjunctival injection, visual floaters, pain, and photophobia.

Associated posterior scar formation distorts the shape of the pupil.

● *Vitreous hemorrhage.* In this condition, sudden unilateral vision loss may result from intraocular trauma, ocular tumors, or systemic disease (especially diabetes, hypertension, sickle cell anemia, or leukemia). Visual floaters and partial vision with a reddish haze may occur. The patient's vision loss may be permanent.

Other causes
● *Drugs.* Chloroquine therapy may cause gradual vision loss that's not arrested by discontinuing the drug; prolonged use causes irreversible vision loss. Phenylbutazone may cause vision loss and increased susceptibility to retinal detachment. Digitalis derivatives, indomethacin, ethambutol, quinine sulfate, and methanol toxicity may also cause vision loss.

Special considerations
Any degree of vision loss is extremely frightening to your patient. To ease his fears, orient him to his environment, and announce your presence each time you approach him. If the patient reports photophobia, darken the room and suggest that he wear sunglasses during the day. Obtain cultures of any drainage, and instruct him not to touch the unaffected eye with anything that has come in contact with the affected eye. Instruct him to wash his hands often and to avoid rubbing his eyes. If necessary, prepare him for surgery.

Pediatric pointers
Children who complain of slowly progressive vision loss may have an optic nerve glioma (a slow-growing, usually benign tumor) or retinoblastoma (a malignant tumor of the retina). Congenital rubella and syphilis may cause vision loss in infants. Retrolental fibroplasia may cause vision loss in premature infants. Other congenital causes of vision loss include Marfan's syndrome, retinitis pigmentosa, and amblyopia.

Visual Blurring

This common symptom refers to the loss of visual acuity with indistinct visual details. It may result from eye injury, neurologic and eye disorders, or disorders with vascular complications, such as diabetes mellitus. Visual blurring may also result from mucus passing over the cornea, refractive errors, improperly fitted contact lenses, or the effects of drugs.

Assessment
If your patient has visual blurring accompanied by sudden, severe eye pain, a history of trauma, or sudden vision loss, call the doctor immediately (see *Managing Sudden Vision Loss,* page 759). If the patient has a penetrating or perforating eye injury, don't touch the eye.

If the patient isn't in distress, ask him how long he has had the visual blurring. Does it occur only at certain times? Ask about associated symptoms, such as pain or discharge. If visual blurring followed injury, obtain details of the accident, and ask if vision was impaired immediately after the injury. Obtain a medical and drug history.

Inspect the patient's eye, noting lid edema, drainage, or conjunctival or scleral redness. Also note an irregularly shaped iris, which may indicate previous trauma, and excessive blinking, which may indicate corneal damage. Assess for pupillary changes, and test visual acuity in both eyes. (See *Testing Visual Acuity,* page 762.)

Medical causes
● *Brain tumor.* Visual blurring may occur with a brain tumor. Associated findings may include decreased level of consciousness, headache, apathy, behavioral changes, memory loss, decreased attention span, dizziness, and confusion. A tumor can also cause aphasia, seizures, ataxia, and signs of

hormonal imbalance. Its later effects are papilledema, vomiting, increased systolic blood pressure, widened pulse pressure, and decorticate posture.

• *Cataract.* This painless disorder causes gradual visual blurring. Other effects include halo vision (an early sign), visual glare in bright light, progressive vision loss, and a gray pupil that later turns milky white.

• *Cerebrovascular accident (CVA).* Brief attacks of bilateral visual blurring may precede or accompany a CVA. Associated findings may include a decreased level of consciousness, contralateral hemiplegia, dysarthria, dysphagia, ataxia, unilateral sensory loss, and apraxia. CVA may also cause agnosia, aphasia, homonymous hemianopia, diplopia, disorientation, memory loss, and poor judgment. Other features include urinary retention or inconti-

---

TESTING VISUAL ACUITY

Use a Snellen letter chart to test visual acuity in the literate patient over age 6. Have the patient sit or stand 20′ (6 m) from the chart. Then, tell him to cover his left eye and read aloud the smallest line of letters that he can see. Record the fraction assigned to that line (the numerator indicates distance from the chart; the denominator indicates the distance at which a normal eye can read the chart). Normal vision is 20/20. Repeat the test with the patient's right eye covered.

If your patient can't read the largest letter from a distance of 20 feet, have him approach the chart until he can read it. Then, record the distance between him and the chart as the numerator of the fraction. For example, if he can see the top line of the chart at a distance of 3′ (1 m), record the test result as 3/200.

Use a Snellen symbol chart to test children aged 3 to 6 and illiterate patients. Follow the same procedure as for the Snellen letter chart, but ask the patient to indicate the direction of the E's fingers as you point to each symbol.

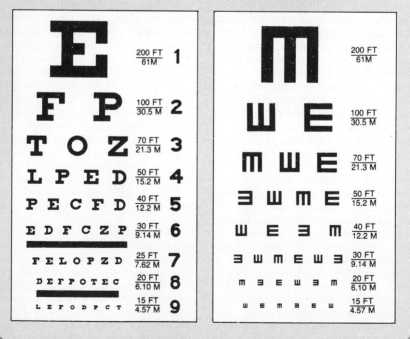

SNELLEN LETTER CHART

SNELLEN SYMBOL CHART

nence, constipation, personality changes, emotional lability, headache, vomiting, and seizures.

● *Concussion.* Immediately or shortly after blunt head trauma, vision may be blurred, double, or temporarily lost. Other findings include changes in level of consciousness and behavior.

● *Conjunctivitis.* Visual blurring may be accompanied by photophobia, pain, burning, tearing, itching, and a feeling of fullness around the eyes. Other findings: redness near the fornices (brilliant red suggests a bacterial cause; milky red, an allergic cause) and drainage (copious, mucopurulent, and flaky in bacterial conjunctivitis; stringy in allergic conjunctivitis). Copious tearing, minimal exudate, and an enlarged preauricular lymph node occur with viral conjunctivitis.

● *Corneal abrasions.* Visual blurring may occur with severe eye pain, photophobia, redness, and excessive tearing.

● *Corneal foreign bodies.* Visual blurring may accompany a foreign body sensation, excessive tearing, photophobia, intense eye pain, miosis, conjunctival injection, and a dark corneal speck.

● *Diabetic retinopathy.* Retinal edema and hemorrhage produce gradual blurring, which may progress to blindness.

● *Dislocated lens.* Dislocation of the lens, especially beyond the line of vision, causes visual blurring and (with trauma) redness.

● *Eye tumor.* If the tumor involves the macula, visual blurring may be the presenting symptom. Related findings include varying visual field losses.

● *Glaucoma.* In *acute closed-angle glaucoma,* an ocular emergency, unilateral visual blurring and severe pain begin suddenly. Other findings: halo vision; a moderately dilated, nonreactive pupil; conjunctival injection; a cloudy cornea; and decreased visual acuity. Severely elevated intraocular pressure may cause nausea and vomiting.

In *chronic closed-angle glaucoma,* transient visual blurring and halo vision may precede pain and blindness.

● *Hereditary corneal dystrophies.* Visual blurring may remain stable or may progressively worsen throughout life. Some dystrophies cause associated pain, vision loss, photophobia, tearing, and corneal opacities.

● *Hypertension.* This disorder may cause visual blurring and a constant morning headache that decreases in severity during the day. If diastolic blood pressure exceeds 120 mm Hg, the patient may report a severe, throbbing headache. Associated findings may include restlessness, confusion, nausea, vomiting, seizures, and decreased level of consciousness.

● *Hyphema.* Blunt eye trauma with hemorrhage into the anterior chamber causes visual blurring. Other effects include moderate pain, diffuse conjunctival injection, visible blood in the anterior chamber, ecchymoses, eyelid edema, and a hard eye.

● *Iritis.* Acute iritis causes sudden visual blurring, moderate to severe eye pain, photophobia, conjunctival injection, and a constricted pupil.

● *Migraine headache.* This disorder may cause visual blurring and paroxysmal attacks of severe, throbbing, unilateral or bilateral headache. Other effects: nausea, vomiting, sensitivity to light and noise, and sensory or visual auras.

● *Multiple sclerosis.* Blurred vision, diplopia, and paresthesias may occur early in this disorder. Later effects vary and may include nystagmus, muscle weakness, paralysis, spasticity, hyperreflexia, intention tremor, and ataxic gait. Urinary frequency, urgency, and incontinence may also occur.

● *Optic neuritis.* Inflammation, degeneration, or demyelinization of the optic nerve usually causes an acute attack of visual blurring and vision loss. Related findings include scotomas and eye pain. Ophthalmoscopic examination reveals hyperemia of the optic disk, large vein distention, blurred disk margins, and filling of the physiologic cup.

● *Retinal detachment.* Sudden visual blurring may be the initial symptom of this disorder. Blurring worsens, accompanied by visual floaters and recurring flashes of light. Progressive detachment increases vision loss.

• *Retinal vein occlusion (central).* This disorder causes gradual unilateral visual blurring and varying degrees of vision loss.

• *Senile macular degeneration.* This retinal disorder may cause visual blurring (initially worse at night) and slowly or rapidly progressive vision loss.

• *Serous retinopathy (central).* Visual blurring may accompany darkened vision in the affected eye.

• *Temporal arteritis.* Most common in women over age 60, this disorder causes sudden blurred vision accompanied by vision loss and a throbbing unilateral headache in the temporal or frontotemporal region. Prodromal symptoms include malaise, anorexia, weight loss, weakness, low-grade fever, and generalized muscle aches. Other findings include confusion; disorientation; swollen, nodular, tender temporal arteries; and erythema of overlying skin.

• *Uveitis (posterior).* This disorder may produce insidious onset of blurred vision, conjunctival injection, visual floaters, pain, and photophobia.

• *Vitreous hemorrhage.* Sudden unilateral visual blurring and varying vision loss occur with this condition. Visual floaters or dark streaks may also occur.

Other causes
• *Drugs.* Visual blurring may stem from the effects of cycloplegics, guanethidine, reserpine, clomiphene, phenylbutazone, thiazide diuretics, antihistamines, anticholinergics, and phenothiazines.

Special considerations
Prepare the patient for diagnostic tests, such as tonometry, slit-lamp examination, X-rays of the skull and orbit, and, if a neurologic lesion is suspected, a computed tomography scan. As necessary, teach him how to instill ophthalmic medication. If visual blurring leads to permanent vision loss, provide emotional support, orient him to his surroundings, and provide for his safety. If necessary, prepare him for surgery.

Pediatric pointers
Visual blurring in children may stem from congenital syphilis, congenital cataracts, refractive errors, eye injuries or infections, and increased intracranial pressure. Refer the child to an ophthalmologist if appropriate.

Test vision in school-age children as you would in adults; test children aged 3 to 6 with the Snellen symbol chart (see *Testing Visual Acuity,* page 762). Test toddlers with Allen cards, each illustrated with a familiar object, such as an animal. Ask the child to cover one eye and identify the objects as you flash them. Then, ask him to identify them as you gradually back away. Record the maximum distance at which he can identify at least three pictures.

Visual Floaters

Visual floaters are particles of blood or cellular debris that move about in the vitreous. As these enter the visual field, they appear as spots or dots. Chronic floaters may occur normally in elderly or myopic patients. However, the sudden onset of visual floaters often signals retinal detachment, an ocular emergency.

Assessment
If your patient reports sudden onset of visual floaters, suspect retinal detachment. Ask if he also sees flashing lights or spots in the affected eye, and if he's experiencing a curtainlike loss of vision. If so, notify an ophthalmologist immediately. Restrict the patient's eye movements until the diagnosis is made.

If the patient's condition permits, obtain a drug and allergy history. Ask about any nearsightedness (a predisposing factor), use of corrective lenses, eye trauma, or other eye disorders. Also ask about a history of granulomatous disease, diabetes mellitus, or hypertension, which may have predisposed him to retinal detachment, vitreous hemorrhage, or uveitis. If appropriate, inspect his eyes for signs of injury, such as bruising or edema, and assess his visual acuity. (See *Testing Visual Acuity*, page 762.)

Medical causes

• *Retinal detachment.* Floaters and light flashes appear suddenly in the portion of the visual field where the retina is detached. As the retina detaches further (a painless process), gradual vision loss occurs, likened to a cloud or curtain falling in front of the eyes. Ophthalmoscopic examination reveals a gray, opaque, detached retina with an indefinite margin. Retinal vessels appear almost black.

• *Uveitis (posterior).* This disorder may cause visual floaters accompanied by gradual eye pain, photophobia, blurred vision, and conjunctival injection.

• *Vitreous hemorrhage.* Rupture of retinal vessels produces a shower of red or black dots or a red haze across the visual field. Vision is suddenly blurred in the affected eye, and visual acuity may be greatly reduced.

Special considerations

Encourage bed rest and provide a calm environment. Depending on the cause, the patient may require eye patches, surgery, and corticosteroids or other drug therapy. If bilateral eye patches are necessary—as with retinal detachment—ensure the patient's safety. Identify yourself when you approach him, and orient him to time frequently. Provide sensory stimulation, such as a radio or tape player. Check the doctor's orders to determine the appropriate patient position, and place pillows or towels behind the patient's head to maintain it. Warn him not to touch or rub his eyes and to avoid straining or sudden movements.

Pediatric pointers

Visual floaters in children usually follow trauma that causes retinal detachment or vitreous hemorrhage. However, they may also result from vitreous debris, a benign congenital condition with no other signs or symptoms.

Vomiting

Vomiting is the forceful expulsion of gastric contents through the mouth. Characteristically preceded by nausea, vomiting results from a coordinated sequence of abdominal muscle contractions and reverse esophageal peristalsis.

A common sign of GI disorders, vomiting also occurs with fluid and electrolyte imbalances; infections; and metabolic, endocrine, labyrinthine, central nervous system (CNS), and cardiac disorders. It can also result from drug therapy, surgery, and radiation.

Vomiting occurs normally during the first trimester of pregnancy, but its subsequent development may signal complications. It can also result from stress, anxiety, pain, alcohol intoxication, overeating, or ingestion of distasteful foods or liquids.

Assessment

Ask your patient to characterize the onset, duration, and intensity of his vomiting. What precipitated the vomiting? What makes it subside? If possible, collect and measure the patient's vomitus (see *Vomitus: Characteristics and Causes,* page 767). Explore any associated complaints, particularly nausea, abdominal pain, anorexia and weight loss, changes in bowel habits or stool character, excessive belching or flatus, and bloating or fullness.

Obtain a medical history, noting GI, endocrine, and metabolic disorders; recent infections; and cancer, including chemotherapy or radiation therapy. Ask about current medication use and alcohol consumption. If the patient's female of childbearing age, ask if she is or could be pregnant.

Inspect the abdomen for distention, and auscultate for bowel sounds and bruits. Palpate for rigidity and tenderness, and test for rebound tenderness. Next, palpate and percuss the liver for enlargement. Assess other body systems as appropriate.

During the assessment, keep in mind that projectile vomiting *unaccompanied* by nausea may indicate increased intracranial pressure, a life-threatening emergency. If this occurs in a patient with CNS injury, quickly check his vital signs. Notify the doctor immediately if you detect widened pulse pressure or bradycardia.

Medical causes

● *Adrenal insufficiency.* Common GI findings in the disorder include vomiting, nausea, anorexia, and diarrhea. Other findings include weakness, fatigue, weight loss, bronze skin, hypotension, and weak, irregular pulse.

● *Appendicitis.* Vomiting and nausea may follow or accompany abdominal pain. Pain typically begins as vague epigastric or periumbilical discomfort and rapidly progresses to severe, stabbing pain in the right lower quadrant (McBurney's sign). Associated findings usually include abdominal rigidity and tenderness, anorexia, constipation or diarrhea, cutaneous hyperalgesia, fever, tachycardia, and malaise.

● *Cholecystitis (acute).* In this disorder, nausea and mild vomiting often follow severe upper quadrant pain that may radiate to the back or shoulders. Associated findings include abdominal tenderness and, possibly, rigidity and distention, fever, and diaphoresis.

● *Cholelithiasis.* Nausea and vomiting accompany severe right upper quadrant or epigastric pain following ingestion of fatty foods. Other findings include abdominal tenderness and guarding, flatulence, belching, epigastric burning, pyrosis, tachycardia, and restlessness. Common bile duct occlu-

sion may cause jaundice, clay-colored stools, fever, and chills.

● *Cirrhosis.* Insidious early symptoms of cirrhosis typically include nausea and vomiting, anorexia, aching abdominal pain, and constipation or diarrhea. Later findings include jaundice, hepatomegaly, and abdominal distention. Hematologic, endocrine, and mental changes occur as well.

● *Congestive heart failure.* Nausea and vomiting may occur, especially in right-heart failure. Associated findings include tachycardia, ventricular gallop, fatigue, dyspnea, crackles, peripheral edema, and jugular vein distention.

● *Ectopic pregnancy.* Vomiting, nausea, vaginal bleeding, and lower abdominal pain occur in this potentially life-threatening disorder.

● *Electrolyte imbalances.* Such disturbances as hyponatremia, hypernatremia, hypokalemia, and hypercalcemia frequently cause nausea and vomiting. Other effects may include dysrhythmias, tremors, seizures, anorexia, malaise, and weakness.

● *Food poisoning.* Certain toxins, such as *Salmonella*, cause vomiting, nausea, and diarrhea.

● *Gastric cancer.* This rare cancer may produce mild nausea, vomiting (possibly of mucus or blood), anorexia, upper abdominal discomfort, and chronic dyspepsia. Fatigue, weight loss, weakness, melena, and altered bowel habits are also common.

● *Gastritis.* Nausea and vomiting of mucus or blood are common here, especially after ingestion of alcohol, aspirin, spicy foods, or caffeine. Epigastric pain, belching, fever, and malaise may also occur.

● *Gastroenteritis.* This disorder causes nausea, vomiting (often of undigested food), diarrhea, and abdominal cramping. Fever, malaise, hyperactive bowel sounds, and abdominal pain and tenderness may also occur.

● *Hepatitis.* Vomiting often follows nausea as an early sign of viral hepatitis. Fatigue, myalgia, arthralgia, headache, photophobia, anorexia, pharyngitis, cough, and fever also occur early.

• *Hyperemesis gravidarum.* Unremitting nausea and vomiting that last beyond the first trimester characterize this disorder of pregnancy. Vomitus contains undigested food, mucus, and small amounts of bile early in the disorder; later, it has a "coffee-ground" appearance. Associated findings include weight loss, headache, and delirium.

• *Increased intracranial pressure.* Projectile vomiting that *isn't* preceded by nausea is a sign of increased intracranial pressure. The patient may exhibit a decreased level of consciousness and Cushing's triad (bradycardia, hypertension, and respiratory pattern changes). He may also have headache, widened pulse pressure, impaired motor movement, visual disturbances, and pupillary changes.

• *Infection.* Acute localized or systemic infection may cause vomiting and nausea. Other findings commonly include fever, headache, malaise, and fatigue.

• *Intestinal obstruction.* Nausea and vomiting (bilious or fecal) frequently occur with obstruction, especially of the upper small intestine. Abdominal pain is usually episodic and colicky but can become severe and steady. Constipation occurs early in large intestinal obstruction and late in small intestinal obstruction. Obstipation, however, may signal complete obstruction. Bowel sounds are typically high-pitched and hyperactive in partial obstruction; hypoactive or absent in complete obstruction. Abdominal distention and tenderness also occur, possibly with visible peristaltic waves and a palpable abdominal mass.

• *Labyrinthitis.* Nausea and vomiting commonly occur with this acute inner ear inflammation. Other findings: severe vertigo, dizziness, progressive hearing loss, nystagmus, and possibly otorrhea.

• *Ménière's disease.* This disorder causes sudden, brief, recurrent attacks of nausea and vomiting, dizziness, vertigo, hearing loss, tinnitus, diaphoresis, and nystagmus.

VOMITUS: CHARACTERISTICS AND CAUSES

When you collect a sample of the patient's vomitus, observe it carefully for clues to the underlying disorder. Here's what this vomitus may indicate:

Bile-stained (greenish) vomitus
Obstruction below the pylorus, as from a duodenal lesion

Bloody vomitus
Upper GI bleeding, as from gastritis or peptic ulcer if bright red; if dark red, as from esophageal or gastric varices

Brown vomitus with a fecal odor
Intestinal obstruction or infarction

Burning, bitter-tasting vomitus
Excessive hydrochloric acid in gastric contents

Coffee-ground vomitus
Digested blood from slowly bleeding gastric or duodenal lesion

Undigested food
Gastric outlet obstruction, as from gastric tumor or ulcer

• *Mesenteric artery ischemia.* This life-threatening disorder may cause nausea and vomiting and severe, cramping abdominal pain, especially after meals. Other findings: diarrhea or constipation, abdominal tenderness and bloating, anorexia, weight loss, and abdominal bruits.

• *Mesenteric venous thrombosis.* Insidious or acute onset of nausea, vomiting, and abdominal pain occur here, with diarrhea or constipation, abdominal distention, hematemesis, and melena.

• *Metabolic acidosis.* This imbalance may produce nausea, vomiting, anorexia, diarrhea, Kussmaul's respirations, and decreased level of consciousness.

• *Migraine headache.* Nausea and vomiting are prodromal symptoms, with fatigue, photophobia, light flashes, increased noise sensitivity, and possibly partial vision loss and paresthesias.

● *Motion sickness.* Nausea and vomiting may be accompanied by headache, dizziness, fatigue, diaphoresis, and dyspnea.

● *Myocardial infarction.* Nausea and vomiting may occur here, but the cardinal symptom is severe substernal chest pain that may radiate to the left arm, jaw, or neck. Dyspnea, pallor, clammy skin, diaphoresis, and restlessness also occur.

● *Pancreatitis (acute).* Vomiting, usually preceded by nausea, is an early symptom of pancreatitis. Associated findings include steady, severe epigastric or left upper quadrant pain that may radiate to the back, abdominal tenderness and rigidity, hypoactive bowel sounds, and fever. Tachycardia, restlessness, hypotension, skin mottling, and cold, sweaty extremities may occur in severe cases.

● *Peptic ulcer.* Nausea and vomiting may follow sharp or burning epigastric pain, especially when the stomach is empty or after ingestion of alcohol, caffeine, or aspirin. Attacks are relieved by eating or antacids. Hematemesis or melena may also occur.

● *Peritonitis.* Nausea and vomiting usually accompany acute abdominal pain in the area of inflammation. Other findings may include high fever with chills; tachycardia; hypoactive or absent bowel sounds; abdominal distention and tenderness; weakness; pale, cold skin; diaphoresis; hypotension; signs of dehydration; and shallow respirations.

● *Preeclampsia.* Nausea and vomiting are common in this disorder of pregnancy. Rapid weight gain, epigastric pain, generalized edema, elevated blood pressure, oliguria, severe frontal headache, and blurred or double vision also occur.

● *Renal and urologic disorders.* Cystitis, pyelonephritis, calculi, and other disorders of this system can cause vomiting. Accompanying findings reflect the specific disorder.

● *Thyrotoxicosis.* Nausea and vomiting may accompany the classic findings of severe anxiety, heat intolerance, weight loss despite increased appetite, diaphoresis, diarrhea, tremors, tachycardia, and palpitations. Other findings may include exophthalmos, ventricular or atrial gallop, and an enlarged thyroid gland.

● *Ulcerative colitis.* Vomiting, nausea, and anorexia may occur here, but the most common sign is recurrent diarrhea with blood, pus, and mucus.

Other causes

● *Drugs.* Drugs that commonly cause vomiting include antineoplastic agents, opiates, ferrous sulfate, levodopa, oral potassium, chloride replacements, estrogens, sulfasalazine, antibiotics, quinidine, anesthetic agents, and overdoses of digitalis and theophylline.

● *Radiation and surgery.* Radiation therapy may cause nausea and vomiting if it disrupts the gastric mucosa. Postoperative nausea and vomiting are common, especially after abdominal surgery.

Special considerations

As ordered, draw blood to determine fluid, electrolyte, and acid-base balance. (Prolonged vomiting can cause dehydration, electrolyte imbalances, and metabolic alkalosis.) Have the patient breathe deeply to ease his nausea and help prevent further vomiting. Keep his room fresh and clean-smelling by removing bedpans and emesis basins promptly after use. Elevate his head or position him on his side to prevent aspiration of vomitus. Continuously monitor vital signs and intake and output (including vomitus and liquid stools). If necessary, administer I.V. fluids or have the patient sip clear liquids to maintain hydration.

Because pain can precipitate or intensify nausea and vomiting, administer ordered pain medications promptly. If possible, give these by injection or suppository to prevent exacerbating associated nausea. If you administer antiemetics, be alert for abdominal distention and hypoactive bowel sounds, which may indicate gastric retention. If this occurs, insert a nasogastric tube, as ordered.

Pediatric pointers
In a newborn, pyloric obstruction may cause projectile vomiting, whereas Hirschsprung's disease may cause fecal vomiting. Intussusception may lead to vomiting of bile and fecal matter in an infant or toddler. Because an infant may aspirate vomitus as a result of his immature cough and gag reflexes, position him on his side or abdomen and clear any vomitus immediately.

Vulvar Lesions

These cutaneous lumps, nodules, papules, vesicles, or ulcers result from benign or malignant tumors, dystrophies, dermatoses, or infection. They can appear anywhere on the vulva and may go undetected until a gynecologic examination. Usually, however, the patient notices lesions because of associated symptoms, such as pruritus, dysuria, or dyspareunia.

Assessment
Ask the patient when she first noticed a vulvar lesion, and find out about associated features, such as swelling, pain, tenderness, itching, or discharge. Does she have lesions elsewhere on her body? Ask about signs of systemic illness, such as malaise, fever, or rash on other body areas. Is the patient sexually active? Could she have been exposed to a sexually transmitted disease?

Examine the lesion, and be prepared to assist the doctor with a pelvic examination and to obtain cultures.

Medical causes
● *Basal cell carcinoma.* Occurring most often in postmenopausal women, this nodular tumor has a central ulcer and a raised, rolled border. Typically asymptomatic, the tumor may occa-

sionally cause pruritus, bleeding, discharge, and a burning sensation.
● *Benign cysts. Epidermal inclusion cysts,* the most common vulvar cysts, appear primarily on the labia majora and are usually round and asymptomatic. *Bartholin's duct cysts* are usually tense, nontender, and palpable. They appear on the posterior labia minora and may cause minor discomfort during intercourse or, when large, difficulty with intercourse or even walking. *Bartholin's abscess,* infection of a Bartholin's duct cyst, causes gradual pain and tenderness and possibly vulvar swelling, redness, and deformity.
● *Benign vulvar tumors.* Cystic or solid benign vulvar tumors are usually asymptomatic.
● *Chancroid.* This rare, sexually transmitted disease causes painful vulvar lesions. Headache, malaise, and fever to 102.2° F. (39° C.) may occur, with enlarged, tender inguinal lymph nodes.
● *Dermatoses (systemic).* Psoriasis, seborrheic dermatitis, and other skin conditions may produce vulvar lesions.
● *Genital warts.* This sexually transmitted disease produces painless warts on the vulva, vagina, and cervix. Warts start as tiny red or pink swellings that grow (sometimes to 4″, or 10 cm) and become pedunculated. Multiple swellings with a cauliflower appearance are common. Other findings: pruritus, erythema, and a profuse, mucopurulent vaginal discharge.
● *Gonorrhea.* Vulvar lesions may develop along with pruritus, a burning sensation, pain, and a greenish yellow vaginal discharge, but most patients are asymptomatic. Other findings, if any, may include dysuria and urinary incontinence; vaginal redness, swelling, and engorgement; and severe pelvic and lower abdominal pain.
● *Granuloma inguinale.* Initially, a single painless macule or papule appears on the vulva, ulcerating into a raised, beefy-red lesion with a granulated, friable border. Other painless and possibly foul-smelling lesions may occur on the labia, vagina, or cervix. These

RECOGNIZING COMMON VULVAR LESIONS

Various disorders can cause vulvar lesions. For example, sexually transmitted diseases account for most vulvar lesions in premenopausal women, whereas vulvar tumors and cysts account for most lesions in women aged 50 to 70. The illustrations below will help you recognize some of the most common lesions.

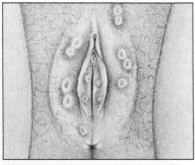

Primary genital herpes produces multiple ulcerated lesions surrounded by red halos.

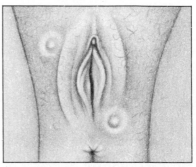

Primary syphilis produces chancres, which appear as ulcerated lesions with raised borders.

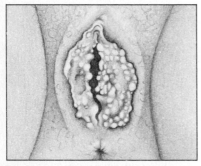

Squamous cell carcinoma can produce a large, granulomatous-appearing ulcer.

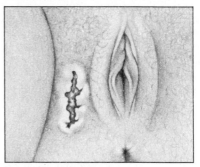

Basal cell carcinoma can produce an ulcerated lesion with raised, rolled edges.

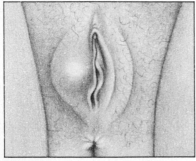

Epidermal inclusion cysts produce a round lump that usually appears on the labia majora.

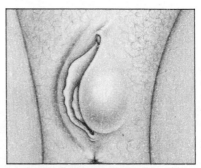

Bartholin's duct cysts produce a tense, nontender, palpable lump that usually appears on the labia minora.

become infected and painful, and regional lymph nodes enlarge and may become tender. Systemic effects include fever, weight loss, and malaise.

● *Herpes simplex (genital).* In this disorder, fluid-filled vesicles appear on the cervix and, possibly, on the vulva, labia, perianal skin, vagina, or mouth. The vesicles, initially painless, may rupture and develop into extensive, shallow, painful ulcers, with redness, marked edema, and tender inguinal lymph nodes. Other findings may include fever, malaise, and dysuria.

● *Herpes zoster.* This viral infection may produce vulvar lesions, although other areas are more commonly affected. Small, red nodular lesions erupt on painful erythematous areas. The lesions quickly evolve into vesicles or pustules, which dry and form scabs about 10 days later. Other findings: fever, malaise, paresthesia or hyperesthesia, and pain.

● *Hyperplastic dystrophy.* Vulvar lesions may be well delineated or poorly defined; localized or extensive; and red, brown, white, or both red and white. However, intense pruritus, possibly with vulvar pain and dyspareunia, is the cardinal symptom. In *lichen sclerosus,* a type of vulvar dystrophy, vulvar skin has a parchment-like appearance. Fissures may develop between the clitoris and urethra or other vulvar areas.

● *Lymphogranuloma venereum.* This bacterial infection commonly presents with a single, painless papule or ulcer on the posterior vulva that heals in a few days. Inguinal lymphadenopathy develops about 2 weeks later. Other findings may include fever, chills, headache, anorexia, myalgias, arthralgias, weight loss, and perineal edema.

● *Malignant melanoma.* This disorder causes irregular, pigmented vulvar lesions that enlarge rapidly. Lesions may ulcerate and bleed.

● *Molluscum contagiosum.* This viral infection produces raised vulvar papules that are 1 to 2 mm in diameter and have a white core. Pruritic lesions may also appear on the face, eyelids, breasts, and inner thighs.

● *Pediculosis pubis.* This parasitic infection produces erythematous vulvar papules with pruritus and skin irritation. Pubic lice nits are visible on pubic hair with magnification.

● *Squamous cell carcinoma. Invasive carcinoma* occurs primarily in postmenopausal women and may produce vulvar pruritus and a vulvar lump. As the tumor enlarges, it may encroach on the vagina, anus, and urethra. *Carcinoma in situ* occurs most often in premenopausal women, producing a vulvar lesion that may be white or red, raised, well defined, moist, crusted, and isolated.

● *Syphilis.* Chancres, the primary vulvar lesions of this sexually transmitted disease, may appear on the vulva, vagina, or cervix 10 to 90 days after initial contact. Usually painless, they start as papules that then erode, with indurated, raised edges and clear bases. Condylomata lata, highly contagious secondary vulvar lesions, are raised, gray, flat-topped, and frequently ulcerated. Other findings: a maculopapular, pustular, or nodular rash; headache; malaise; anorexia; weight loss; fever; nausea; vomiting; generalized lymphadenopathy; and a sore throat.

● *Viral disease (systemic).* Varicella, measles, and other systemic viral diseases may produce vulvar lesions.

Special considerations

Expect to administer systemic antibiotics, antiviral agents, topical corticosteroids, topical testosterone, or an antipruritic agent. If ordered, show the patient how to give herself a sitz bath to promote healing and comfort. If she has a sexually transmitted disease, encourage her to inform her sexual partners and persuade them to be treated. Advise her to avoid sexual contact until the lesions are no longer contagious.

Pediatric pointers

Vulvar lesions in children may result from congenital syphilis or gonorrhea.

weight gain—excessive • weight loss—excessive • wheezing • wristdrop• abd
abdominal mass • abdominal pain • abdominal rigidity • accessory muscle us
alopecia • amenorrhea • amnesia • analgesia • anhidrosis • anorexia • anosm
aphasia • apnea • apneustic respirations • apraxia • arm pain • asterixis • at
Babinski's reflex • back pain • barrel chest • Battle's sign • Biot's respirations
blood pressure decrease • blood pressure increase • bowel sounds—absent • l
hyperactive • bowel sounds—hypoactive • bradycardia • bradypnea • breast c
nodule • breast pain • breast ulcer • breath with ammonia odor • breath with
with fruity odor • Brudzinski's sign • bruits • buffalo hump • butterfly rash •
capillary refill time—prolonged • carpopedal spasm • cat cry • chest expansic
pain • Cheyne-Stokes respirations • chills • chorea • Chvostek's sign • clubbin
cold intolerance • confusion • conjunctival injection • constipation • corneal r
costovertebral angle tenderness • cough—barking • cough—nonproductive • c
crackles • crepitation—bony • crepitation—subcutaneous • cry—high-pitched
posture • decorticate posture • deep tendon reflexes—hyperactive • deep tend
depression • diaphoresis • diarrhea • diplopia • dizziness • doll's eye sign—a
dysarthria • dysmenorrhea • dyspareunia • dyspepsia • dysphagia • dyspnea •
earache • edema—generalized • edema of the arms • edema of the face • ede
enophthalmos • enuresis • epistaxis • eructation • erythema • exophthalmos •
pain • facial pain • fasciculations • fatigue • fecal incontinence • fetor hepatic
flatulence • fontanelle bulging • fontanelle depression • footdrop • gag reflex a
bizarre • gait—propulsive • gait—scissors • gait—spastic • gait—steppage • g
gallop—atrial • gallop—ventricular • genital lesions in the male • grunting re
bleeding • gum swelling • gynecomastia • halitosis • halo vision • headache •
intolerance • Heberden's nodes • hematemesis • hematochezia • hematuria • l
hemoptysis • hepatomegaly • hiccups • hirsutism • hoarseness • Homans' sig
hyperpnea • hypopigmentation • impotence • insomnia • intermittent claudica
jaundice • jaw pain • jugular vein distention • Kehr's sign • Kernig's sign • le
consciousness—decreased • lid lag • light flashes • low birth weight • lympha
facies • McBurney's sign • McMurray's sign • melena • menorrhagia • metror
face • mouth lesions • murmurs • muscle atrophy • muscle flaccidity • muscle
spasticity • muscle weakness • mydriasis • myoclonus • nasal flaring • nause
blindness • nipple discharge • nipple retraction • nocturia • nuchal rigidity •
deviation • oligomenorrhea • oliguria • opisthotonos • orofacial dyskinesia • c
hypotension • Ortolani's sign • Osler's nodes • otorrhea • pallor • palpitations
paralysis • paresthesias • paroxysmal nocturnal dyspnea • peau d'orange • p
peristaltic waves—visible • photophobia • pica • pleural friction rub • polydi
polyuria • postnasal drip • priapism • pruritus • psoas sign • psychotic beha
absent or weak • pulse—bounding • pulse pressure—narrowed • pulse press
rhythm abnormality • pulsus alternans • pulsus bisferiens • pulsus paradoxu
pupils—sluggish • purple striae • purpura • pustular rash • pyrosis • raccoo
tenderness • rectal pain • retractions—costal and sternal • rhinorrhea • rhon
salivation—decreased • salivation—increased • salt craving • scotoma • scrot
absence • seizure—focal • seizure—generalized tonic-clonic • seizure—psych
sign • shallow respirations • skin—bronze • skin—clammy • skin—mottled •
turgor—decreased • spider angioma • splenomegaly • stertorous respirations
stridor • syncope • tachycardia • tachypnea • taste abnormalities • tearing—i
tic • tinnitus • tracheal deviation • tracheal tugging • tremors • trismus • tur
frost • urethral discharge • urinary frequency • urinary hesitancy • urinary i
urgency • urine cloudiness • urticaria • vaginal bleeding—postmenopausal •

Weight Gain—Excessive

Weight gain occurs when ingested calories exceed body requirements for energy, causing increased adipose tissue storage. It can also occur when fluid retention causes edema. When weight gain results from overeating, emotional factors—most commonly anxiety, guilt, and depression—and social factors may be the primary causes.

Among the elderly, weight gain often reflects a sustained food intake in the presence of the normal, progressive fall in basal metabolic rate. Among women, a progressive weight gain occurs with pregnancy, whereas a periodic weight gain usually occurs with menstruation.

Weight gain, a primary symptom of many endocrine disorders, also occurs with conditions that limit activity, especially cardiovascular and pulmonary disorders. It can also result from drug therapy that increases appetite or causes fluid retention and from cardiovascular, hepatic, and renal disorders that cause edema.

Assessment

Determine your patient's previous patterns of weight gain and loss. Does he have a family history of obesity, thyroid disease, or diabetes mellitus? Assess his eating and activity patterns. Has his appetite increased? Does he exer-

cise regularly or at all? Next, ask about associated symptoms. Has he experienced visual disturbances, hoarseness, paresthesias, or increased urination and thirst? Has he become impotent? If the patient's a female, has she had menstrual irregularities or experienced weight gain during menstruation?

Form an impression of the patient's mental status. Is he anxious or depressed? Does he respond slowly? Is his memory poor? What medications is he currently using?

During your physical examination, measure skinfold thickness to estimate fat reserves (see *Assessing Nutritional Status,* pages 774 and 775). Note fat distribution and the presence of localized or generalized edema. Inspect for other abnormalities, such as abnormal body hair distribution or hair loss and dry skin. Take and record the patient's vital signs.

Medical causes

● *Acromegaly.* This disorder causes moderate weight gain. Other findings include coarsened facial features, prognathism, enlarged hands and feet, increased sweating, oily skin, deep voice, back and joint pain, lethargy, sleepiness, and heat intolerance. Occasionally, hirsutism may occur.

● *Congestive heart failure.* Despite anorexia, weight gain may result from edema. Other typical findings include paroxysmal nocturnal dyspnea, orthopnea, and fatigue.

• **Diabetes mellitus.** The increased appetite associated with this disorder may lead to weight gain, although weight loss sometimes occurs instead. Other findings may include fatigue, polydipsia, polyuria, nocturia, weakness, polyphagia, and somnolence.

• **Hypercortisolism.** Excessive weight gain, usually over the trunk and the back of the neck (buffalo hump), characteristically occurs in this disorder. Other cushingoid features include slender extremities, moon face, weakness, purple striae, emotional lability, and increased susceptibility to infection. Gynecomastia may occur in men; hirsutism, acne, and menstrual irregularities may occur in women.

• **Hyperinsulinism.** This disorder increases appetite, leading to weight gain. Emotional lability, indigestion, weakness, diaphoresis, tachycardia, visual disturbances, and syncope also occur.

• **Hypogonadism.** Weight gain is common in this disorder. *Prepubertal hypogonadism* causes eunuchoid body proportions with relatively sparse facial and body hair and a high-pitched voice. *Postpubertal hypogonadism* causes loss of libido, impotence, and infertility.

• **Hypothalamic dysfunction.** Such conditions as Laurence-Moon-Biedl and Morgagni-Stewart-Morel syndromes cause a voracious appetite with subsequent weight gain, along with altered body temperature and sleep rhythms.

• **Hypothyroidism.** In this disorder, weight gain occurs despite anorexia. Related signs and symptoms include fatigue; cold intolerance; constipation; menorrhagia; slowed intellectual and motor activity; dry, pale, cool skin; dry, sparse hair; and thick, brittle nails. Myalgia, hoarseness, hypoactive deep tendon reflexes, bradycardia, and abdominal distention may occur. Eventually, the face assumes a dull expres-

ASSESSING NUTRITIONAL STATUS

If your patient has excessive weight loss or gain, you can help assess his nutritional status by measuring his skinfold thickness and midarm circumference and by calculating his midarm muscle circumference. Skinfold measurements reflect adipose tissue mass (subcutaneous fat accounts for about 50% of the body's adipose tissue). Midarm measurements reflect both skeletal muscle and adipose tissue mass.

Use the steps described on the next page to gather these measurements. Then express them as a percentage of standard by using this formula:

$$\frac{\text{actual measurement}}{\text{standard measurement}} \times 100 = \underline{\hspace{1cm}}\%$$

Standard anthropometric measurements vary according to the patient's age and sex, and can be found in a chart of normal anthropometric values. The abridged chart below lists standard arm measurements for adult men and women.

TEST	STANDARD	
Triceps skinfold	Men	12.5 mm
	Women	16.5 mm
Midarm circumference	Men	29.3 cm
	Women	28.5 cm
Midarm muscle circumference	Men	25.3 cm
	Women	23.2 cm

A triceps or subscapular skinfold measurement below 60% of the standard value indicates severe depletion of fat reserves; a measurement between 60% and 90% indicates moderate to mild depletion; and above 90% indicates significant fat reserves. A midarm circumference of less than 90% of the standard value indicates caloric deprivation; greater than 90% indicates adequate or ample muscle and fat. A midarm muscle circumference of less than 90% indicates protein depletion; over 90% indicates adequate or ample protein reserves.

To measure the triceps skinfold, locate the midpoint of the patient's upper arm, using a nonstretch tape measure. Mark the midpoint with a felt-tip pen. Then grasp the skin with your thumb and forefinger about 1 cm above the midpoint. Place the calipers at the midpoint and squeeze them for about 3 seconds. Record the measurement registered on the handle gauge to the nearest 0.5 mm. Take two more readings and average all three to compensate for any measurement error.

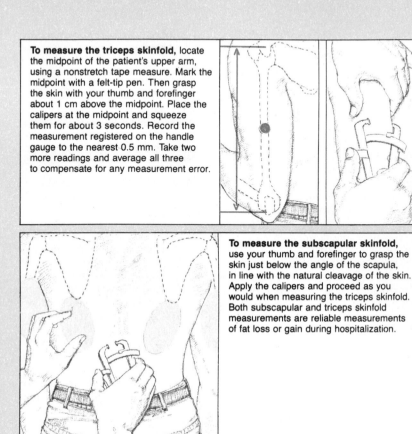

To measure the subscapular skinfold, use your thumb and forefinger to grasp the skin just below the angle of the scapula, in line with the natural cleavage of the skin. Apply the calipers and proceed as you would when measuring the triceps skinfold. Both subscapular and triceps skinfold measurements are reliable measurements of fat loss or gain during hospitalization.

To measure midarm circumference, return to the midpoint you marked on the patient's upper arm. Then use a tape measure to determine the arm circumference at this point. This measurement reflects both skeletal muscle and adipose tissue mass and helps evaluate protein and calorie reserves. *To calculate midarm muscle circumference,* multiply the triceps skinfold thickness (in centimeters) by 3.143, and subtract this figure from the midarm circumference. Midarm muscle circumference reflects muscle mass alone, providing a more sensitive index of protein reserves.

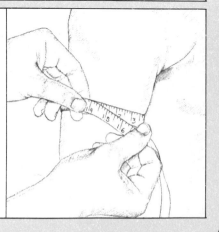

sion with periorbital edema.

• *Nephrotic syndrome.* In this syndrome, weight gain results from edema. In severe cases, anasarca develops—increasing body weight up to 50%. Related effects include abdominal distention, orthostatic hypotension, and lethargy.

• *Pancreatic islet cell tumor.* This disorder causes excessive hunger, which leads to weight gain. Other findings include emotional lability, weakness, malaise, fatigue, restlessness, diaphoresis, palpitations, tachycardia, visual disturbances, and syncope.

• *Preeclampsia.* In this disorder, rapid weight gain (exceeding the normal weight gain of pregnancy) may accompany nausea and vomiting, epigastric pain, elevated blood pressure, and blurred or double vision.

• *Sheehan's syndrome.* Most common in women who experience severe obstetric hemorrhage, this syndrome may cause weight gain.

Other causes

• *Drugs.* Corticosteroids, phenothiazines, and tricyclic antidepressants cause weight gain from fluid retention and increased appetite. Other drugs that can lead to weight gain include oral contraceptives, which cause fluid retention; cyproheptadine, which increases appetite; and lithium, which can induce hypothyroidism.

Special considerations

Psychological counseling may be necessary for patients with weight gain, particularly when it results from emotional problems or when uneven weight distribution alters body image. If the patient is obese or has a cardiopulmonary disorder, seek a doctor's advice before recommending exercise.

Pediatric pointers

Weight gain in children can result from endocrine disorders, such as hypercortisolism. Other causes include inactivity caused by prolonged bed rest, Werdnig-Hoffmann disease, Down's syndrome, late stages of muscular dystrophy, and severe cerebral palsy.

Nonpathologic causes include poor eating habits, sedentary recreations, and emotional problems, especially among adolescents. Regardless of the cause, discourage fad diets and provide a balanced weight loss program.

Weight Loss—Excessive

Weight loss can reflect decreased food intake, increased metabolic requirements, or a combination of the two. Its causes include endocrine, neoplastic, GI, and psychiatric disorders; nutritional deficiencies; infections; and neurologic lesions that cause paralysis and dysphagia. However, weight loss may accompany conditions that prevent sufficient food intake, such as painful oral lesions, ill-fitting dentures, and loss of teeth. It may be the metabolic sequela of poverty, fad diets, excessive exercise, and certain drugs.

Weight loss may occur as a late sign in such chronic diseases as congestive heart failure and renal disease. In these diseases, however, it's the result of anorexia (see "Anorexia").

Assessment

Begin your assessment with a thorough diet history since weight loss may be caused by inadequate caloric intake. If your patient hasn't been eating properly, try to determine why. Ask about his previous weight and if the recent loss was intentional. Be alert to lifestyle or occupational changes that may be a source of anxiety or depression. For example, has the patient gotten separated or divorced? Has he recently changed jobs?

Inquire about recent changes in bowel habits, such as diarrhea or bulky, floating stools. Has the patient had nausea, vomiting, or abdominal pain, which may indicate a GI disorder? Has he had excessive thirst, excessive urination, or heat intolerance, which may signal an endocrine disorder? Take a careful drug history, noting especially any use of diet pills and laxatives.

Carefully check the patient's height and weight, and ask about his previous weight. Take his vital signs and note his general appearance: is he well nourished? Do his clothes fit? Is muscle wasting evident?

Now, examine the patient's skin for turgor and abnormal pigmentation, especially around the joints. Does he have pallor or jaundice? Examine his mouth, including the condition of his teeth or dentures. Look for signs of infection or irritation on the roof of the mouth, and note any hyperpigmentation of the buccal mucosa. Also check the patient's eyes for exophthalmos and his neck for swelling, and evaluate his lungs for adventitious sounds. Inspect his abdomen for signs of wasting, and palpate for masses, tenderness, and an enlarged liver.

Medical causes

● *Adrenal insufficency.* Weight loss occurs in this disorder, along with anorexia, weakness, fatigue, irritability, syncope, nausea, vomiting, abdominal pain, and diarrhea or constipation. Hyperpigmentation over the joints, belt line, palmar creases, lips, gums, tongue, and buccal mucosa ranges from tan, brown, or bronze to black. Other possible findings include postural hypotension; weak, irregular pulse; a craving for salty food; decreased libido; and amenorrhea.

● *Anorexia nervosa.* This psychogenic disorder, most common in young women, is characterized by a severe, self-imposed weight loss ranging from 10% to 50% of premorbid weight, which typically was normal or not more than 5 lb (2.3 kg) over ideal weight. Related findings include skeletal muscle atrophy, loss of fatty tissue, hypotension, constipation, dental caries, susceptibility to infection, blotchy or

sallow skin, cold intolerance, hairiness on the face and body, dryness or loss of scalp hair, and amenorrhea. The patient usually demonstrates restless activity and vigor and may also have a morbid fear of becoming fat. Self-induced vomiting or self-administration of laxatives or diuretics may lead to dehydration or to metabolic alkalosis or acidosis.

● *Cancer.* Weight loss is frequently a sign of cancer. Associated signs and symptoms reflect the type, location, and stage of the tumor, and often include fatigue, pain, nausea, vomiting, anorexia, abnormal bleeding, and a palpable mass.

● *Crohn's disease.* Weight loss occurs with chronic cramping abdominal pain and anorexia. Other signs and symptoms may include diarrhea (possibly bloody) or constipation, nausea, fever, tachycardia, abdominal tenderness and guarding, hyperactive bowel sounds, abdominal distention, and pain. Perianal lesions and a palpable mass in the right or left lower quadrant may also be present.

● *Depression.* Weight loss may occur with severe depression, along with insomnia or hypersomnia, anorexia, apathy, fatigue, and feelings of worthlessness. Indecisiveness, incoherence, and suicidal thoughts or behavior may also occur.

● *Diabetes mellitus.* Weight loss may occur with this disorder, despite increased appetite (polyphagia). Other characteristics include polydipsia, weakness, fatigue, and polyuria with nocturia.

● *Esophagitis.* Painful inflammation of the esophagus leads to temporary avoidance of eating and subsequent weight loss. Intense pain in the mouth and anterior chest occurs, along with hypersalivation, dysphagia, tachypnea, and hematemesis. If a stricture develops, dysphagia and weight loss will recur.

● *Gastroenteritis.* Malabsorption and dehydration cause weight loss in this disorder. The loss may be sudden in acute viral infections or reactions, or gradual in parasitic infection. Other findings include poor skin turgor, dry mucous membranes, tachycardia, hypotension, diarrhea, abdominal pain and tenderness, hyperactive bowel sounds, nausea, vomiting, fever, and malaise.

• *Leukemia. Acute leukemia* causes progressive weight loss accompanied by severe prostration; high fever; swollen, bleeding gums; and bleeding tendencies. Dyspnea, tachycardia, palpitations, and abdominal or bone pain may occur. As the disease progresses, neurologic symptoms may eventually develop.

Chronic leukemia, which occurs insidiously in adults, causes progressive weight loss with malaise, fatigue, pallor, enlarged spleen, bleeding tendencies, anemia, skin eruptions, anorexia, and fever.

• *Lymphoma. Hodgkin's disease* and *non-Hodgkin's lymphoma* cause gradual weight loss. Associated findings include fever, fatigue, night sweats, malaise, hepatosplenomegaly, and lymphadenopathy. Scaly rashes and pruritus may develop.

• *Pulmonary tuberculosis.* This disorder causes gradual weight loss, along with fatigue, weakness, anorexia, night sweats, and low-grade fever. Other clinical effects include a cough with bloody or mucopurulent sputum, dyspnea, and pleuritic chest pain. Examination may reveal dullness upon percussion, crackles after coughing, increased tactile fremitus, and amphoric breath sounds.

• *Stomatitis.* Inflammation of the oral mucosa (usually red, swollen, and ulcerated) in this disorder causes weight loss due to decreased eating. Associated findings may include fever, increased salivation, malaise, mouth pain, anorexia, and swollen, bleeding gums.

• *Thyrotoxicosis.* In this disorder, increased metabolism causes weight loss. Other characteristic signs and symptoms include nervousness, heat intolerance, diarrhea, increased appetite, palpitations, tachycardia, diaphoresis, fine tremor, and possibly an enlarged thyroid and exophthalmos. A ventricular or atrial gallop may be heard.

• *Ulcerative colitis.* Weight loss is a late sign of this disorder, which is initially characterized by bloody diarrhea with pus or mucus. Weakness, crampy lower abdominal pain, tenesmus, anorexia, low-grade fever, and occasional nausea and vomiting may also occur. Bowel sounds are hyperactive, and constipation may occur late. With fulminant colitis, severe and steady abdominal pain and diarrhea, high fever, and tachycardia occur.

• *Whipple's disease.* This rare disease causes progressive weight loss along with abdominal pain, diarrhea, steatorrhea, arthralgia, fever, hyperpigmentation, lymphadenopathy, and splenomegaly.

Other causes

• *Drugs.* Amphetamines and inappropriate dosage of thyroid preparations commonly lead to weight loss. Laxative abuse may cause a malabsorptive state that leads to weight loss. Chemotherapeutic agents cause stomatitis, which, when severe, causes weight loss.

Special considerations

Refer your patient for psychological counseling if weight loss negatively affects his body image. If he has a chronic disease, administer hyperalimentation or tube feedings, as ordered, to maintain nutrition and to prevent edema, poor healing, and muscle wasting. Take daily calorie counts and weigh him weekly. Consult a dietitian, if necessary.

Pediatric pointers

In infants, weight loss may be caused by failure-to-thrive syndrome. In children, severe weight loss may be the first indication of diabetes mellitus. Chronic, gradual weight loss occurs in children with marasmus—nonedematous protein-calorie malnutrition.

Weight loss may also occur as a result of child abuse or neglect, infections causing high fevers, GI disorders causing vomiting and diarrhea, or celiac disease.

Wheezing

[Sibilant rhonchi]

Wheezes are adventitious breath sounds with a high-pitched, musical, squealing, creaking, or groaning quality. When they originate in the large airways, they can be heard by placing an unaided ear over the chest wall or at the mouth. When they originate in smaller airways, they can be heard by placing a stethoscope over the anterior or posterior chest. Unlike crackles and rhonchi, wheezes can't be cleared by coughing.

Usually, prolonged wheezing occurs during expiration when bronchi are shortened and narrowed. Causes of airway narrowing include bronchospasm; mucosal thickening or edema; partial obstruction from a tumor, a foreign body, or secretions; and extrinsic pressure, as in tension pneumothorax or goiter. With airway obstruction, wheezing occurs during inspiration.

Assessment

If you detect wheezing, determine the degree of the patient's respiratory distress. Is he responsive? Is he restless, confused, anxious, or afraid? Are his respirations abnormally fast, slow, shallow, or deep? Are they irregular? Can you hear wheezing through his mouth? Does he have increased use of accessory muscles; increased chest wall motion; intercostal, suprasternal, or supraclavicular retractions; stridor; or nasal flaring? Take the patient's other vital signs, noting hypotension or hypertension and an irregular, weak, rapid, or slow pulse. Help him relax, and administer humidified oxygen by face mask. Suction him, and encourage coughing and slow, deep breathing. Be sure to have intubation and emergency resuscitation equipment readily available. As ordered, call the respiratory therapy department to supply intermittent positive pressure breathing (IPPB) and nebulization treatments with bronchodilators. Insert an I.V. line to allow for administration of fluids and drugs, such as diuretics, bronchodilators, and sedatives.

If the patient's not in respiratory distress, obtain a history. What provokes his wheezing? Does he have asthma or allergies? Does he smoke or have a history of pulmonary, cardiac, or circulatory disorders? Does he have cancer? Ask about recent surgery, illness, or trauma, and obtain a drug history. Ask about changes in appetite, weight, exercise tolerance, or sleep patterns. If he has a cough, ask how it sounds, when it starts, and how often it occurs. Does he have paroxysms of coughing? Is his cough dry, sputum-producing, or bloody?

Ask the patient about chest pain. If he reports pain, determine its quality, onset, duration, intensity, and radiation. Does it increase with breathing, coughing, or certain positions?

Examine the patient's nose and mouth for congestion, drainage, or signs of infection, such as halitosis. If he produces sputum, obtain a sample for examination. Check for cyanosis, pallor, clamminess, masses, tenderness, swelling, distended neck veins, and enlarged lymph nodes. Inspect his chest for abnormal configuration and asymmetrical motion, and determine if the trachea is midline (see *Detecting Slight Tracheal Deviation,* page 723). Percuss for dullness or hyperresonance, and auscultate for crackles, rhonchi, or pleural friction rubs. Note absent or hypoactive breath sounds, abnormal heart sounds, gallops, or murmurs. Also note dysrhythmias, bradycardia, or tachycardia.

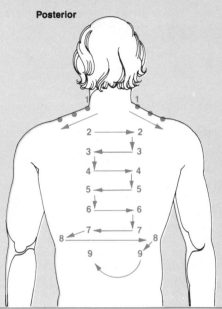

ASSESSING ABNORMAL BREATH SOUNDS

Follow the auscultation sequences shown here to assess airflow through the patient's respiratory system and to detect abnormal breath sounds. Have the patient take full, deep breaths, and compare sound variations from one side to the other. Note the location and timing of any abnormal breath sounds, and characterize them as follows:

• *Wheezes* sound like high-pitched, musical squeaks. They may be detected anywhere in the chest and are usually more prominent on expiration.

• *Rhonchi* are loud, low, coarse, rattling sounds that may be sonorous, bubbling, and rumbling. They're generally detected in larger airways during expiration.

• *Crackles* are popping, nonmusical sounds that may be high- or low-pitched. They may be detected anywhere in the chest and are usually heard best during inspiration.

Posterior

Medical causes

• *Anaphylaxis.* This allergic reaction can cause tracheal edema or bronchospasm, resulting in severe wheezing and stridor. Initial symptoms include fright, weakness, sneezing, dyspnea, nasal pruritus, urticaria, erythema, and angioedema. Respiratory distress occurs with nasal flaring, accessory muscle use, and intercostal retractions. Other findings include nasal edema and congestion; profuse, watery rhinorrhea; chest or throat tightness; and dysphagia. Cardiac effects include dysrhythmias and hypotension.

• *Aspiration of a foreign body.* Partial obstruction by a foreign body produces sudden onset of wheezing and possibly stridor; a dry, paroxysmal cough; gagging; and hoarseness. Other findings include tachycardia, dyspnea, decreased breath sounds, and possibly cyanosis. A retained foreign body may cause inflammation leading to fever, pain, and swelling.

• *Aspiration pneumonitis.* In this disorder, wheezing may accompany tachypnea, marked dyspnea, cyanosis, tachycardia, fever, productive (eventually purulent) cough, and pink, frothy sputum.

• *Asthma.* Wheezing is an initial and cardinal sign of asthma. It's heard at the mouth during expiration. An initially dry cough later becomes productive with thick mucus. Other findings include apprehension, prolonged expiration, intercostal and supraclavicular retractions, rhonchi, accessory muscle use, nasal flaring, and tachypnea. Asthma also produces tachycardia, diaphoresis, and flushing or cyanosis.

• *Bronchial adenoma.* This insidious disorder produces unilateral, possibly severe wheezing. Common features are chronic cough and recurring hemoptysis. Symptoms of airway obstruction may occur later.

• *Bronchiectasis.* Excessive mucous commonly causes intermittent and localized or diffuse wheezing. A copious,

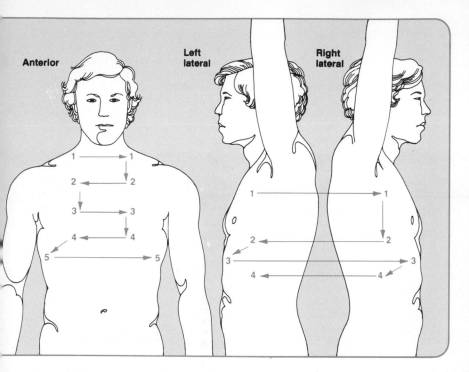

foul-smelling, mucopurulent cough is classic. It's accompanied by hemoptysis, rhonchi, and coarse crackles. Weight loss, fatigue, weakness, dyspnea on exertion, fever, malaise, halitosis, and late-stage clubbing may also occur.

• *Bronchitis (chronic).* This disorder causes wheezing that varies in severity, location, and intensity. Associated findings include prolonged expiration, coarse crackles, scattered rhonchi, and a hacking cough that later becomes productive. Other effects include dyspnea, accessory muscle use, barrel chest, tachypnea, clubbing, edema, weight gain, and cyanosis.

• *Bronchogenic carcinoma.* Obstruction may cause localized wheezing. Typical findings include a productive cough, dyspnea, hemoptysis (initially blood-tinged sputum, possibly leading to massive hemorrhage), anorexia, and weight loss. Upper extremity edema and chest pain may also occur.

• *Chemical pneumonitis (acute).* Mucosal injury causes increased secretions and edema, leading to wheezing, dyspnea, orthopnea, crackles, malaise, fever, and a productive cough with purulent sputum. The patient may also have signs of conjunctivitis, pharyngitis, laryngitis, and rhinitis.

• *Emphysema.* Mild to moderate wheezing may occur in this form of COPD. Related findings include dyspnea, malaise, tachypnea, diminished breath sounds, peripheral cyanosis, pursed-lip breathing, anorexia, and malaise. Accessory muscle use, barrel chest, a chronic productive cough, and clubbing may also occur.

• *Inhalation injury.* Wheezing can eventually occur here. Early findings include hoarseness and coughing, singed nasal hairs, orofacial burns, and soot-stained sputum. Later effects are crackles, rhonchi, and respiratory distress.

• *Pneumothorax (tension).* This life-threatening disorder causes respiratory distress with possible wheezing, dyspnea, tachycardia, tachypnea, and sudden, severe, sharp chest pain (often unilateral). Other findings include a dry cough, cyanosis, accessory muscle use, asymmetrical chest wall movement, anxiety, and restlessness. Examination reveals hyperresonance or tympany and diminished or absent breath sounds on the affected side, subcutaneous crepitation, decreased vocal fremitus, and tracheal deviation.

• *Pulmonary coccidioidomycosis.* This disorder may cause wheezing and rhonchi along with cough, fever, chills, pleuritic chest pain, headache, weakness, malaise, anorexia, and macular rash.

• *Pulmonary edema.* Wheezing may occur with this life-threatening disorder. Other symptoms include coughing, exertional and paroxysmal nocturnal dyspnea and, later, orthopnea. Examination reveals tachycardia, tachypnea, dependent crackles, and a diastolic gallop. Severe pulmonary edema produces rapid, labored respirations; diffuse crackles; a productive cough with frothy, bloody sputum; dysrhythmias; cold, clammy, cyanotic skin; hypotension; and thready pulse.

• *Pulmonary embolus.* Rarely, diffuse, mild wheezing occurs in this disorder.

• *Pulmonary tuberculosis.* In late stages, fibrosis causes wheezing. Common findings include a mild to severe productive cough with pleuritic chest pain and fine crackles, night sweats, anorexia, weight loss, fever, malaise, dyspnea, and fatigue. Other features are dullness to percussion, increased tactile fremitus, and amphoric breath sounds.

• *Thyroid goiter.* This disorder may be asymptomatic, or it may cause wheezing, dysphagia, and respiratory difficulty related to a compressed airway.

• *Tracheobronchitis.* Auscultation may detect wheezing, rhonchi, and crackles. The patient also has a cough, slight fever, sudden chills, muscle and back pain, and substernal tightness.

• *Wegener's granulomatosis.* This disorder may cause mild to moderate wheezing if it compresses major airways.

Other findings include a cough (possibly bloody), dyspnea, pleuritic chest pain, hemorrhagic skin lesions, and progressive renal failure. Epistaxis and severe sinusitis are common.

Special considerations

Prepare the patient for diagnostic tests, such as chest X-rays, arterial blood gas analysis, and sputum culture.

Ease the patient's breathing by placing him in a semi-Fowler's position and repositioning him frequently. If appropriate, encourage increased activity to promote drainage and prevent pooling of secretions. Encourage regular deep breathing and coughing. Perform pulmonary physiotherapy as necessary.

As ordered, administer antibiotics to treat infection, bronchodilators to relieve bronchospasm and open airways, and mucolytics and expectorants to increase the flow of secretions. Provide humidification to relieve mucous membrane inflammation and to thin secretions. Encourage the patient to drink plenty of fluids to liquefy secretions and prevent dehydration.

Pediatric pointers

Children are especially susceptible to wheezing because their small airways allow rapid obstruction. Primary causes of wheezing include bronchospasm, mucosal edema, and accumulation of secretions. These may occur with such disorders as cystic fibrosis, aspiration of a foreign body, acute bronchiolitis, and pulmonary hemosiderosis.

Wristdrop

In wristdrop, the hand remains flexed due to paresis of the extensor muscles of the hand and fingers. This weakness may be slight or severe and temporary or permanent. Wristdrop may occur unilaterally and suddenly with a radial nerve injury, or bilaterally and gradually with neurologic disorders, such as myasthenia gravis, Guillain-Barré syndrome, and multiple sclerosis.

Assessment

If the patient complains of wristdrop, ask when it began and if he can extend his hand at all. Also ask about associated symptoms, such as visual disturbances, difficulty swallowing or chewing, and urinary incontinence. Has he recently injured his arm or axilla? Test the extent of his wristdrop by asking the patient to make a fist. Then, grasp his fist and attempt to pull it down—if he can't resist your pull, his extensor muscles are weak. Test complete range of motion in the arm to detect radial nerve injury.

If the patient reports leg or arm weakness or visual disturbances, proceed with a complete neurologic examination. Assess his level of consciousness; cranial nerve, motor, and sensory functions; and reflexes. Are other areas weak? If so, does the weakness increase with fatigue and decrease with rest, as in myasthenia gravis? Does the patient have exacerbations and remissions of signs and symptoms, suggesting multiple sclerosis, or rapidly ascending weakness, indicating Guillain-Barré syndrome?

Medical causes

● *Guillain-Barré syndrome.* Wristdrop may occur in this syndrome, but the primary neurologic sign is muscle weakness that typically begins in the legs and ascends to the arms and facial nerves within 24 to 72 hours. Associated findings include paresthesias, diminished or absent corneal reflexes, dysarthria, hypernasality, dysphagia, respiratory insufficiency, and possibly respiratory paralysis. Sympathetic nerve dysfunction, such as postural hypotension, loss of bladder and bowel control, sweating, and tachycardia, may also occur.

● *Multiple sclerosis.* This disorder may cause wristdrop, but the earliest symptoms are usually diplopia, blurred vi-

sion, and paresthesias. Other findings include nystagmus, constipation, muscle weakness, paralysis, spasticity, hyperreflexia, intention tremor, gait ataxia, dysphagia, and dysarthria. Multiple sclerosis also causes urinary dysfunction, impotence, and emotional lability.

● *Myasthenia gravis.* In this disorder, weakness causes wristdrop. Associated findings vary with the muscle group affected and may include weak eye closure, ptosis, diplopia, masklike facies, difficulty chewing and swallowing, nasal regurgitation of fluids, and hypernasality. Weakened neck muscles may lead to head bobbing. Respiratory muscle weakness produces myasthenic crisis marked by dyspnea, shallow respirations, and cyanosis, and perhaps leading to respiratory failure.

● *Radial nerve injury.* Compression, severance, or inflammation of the radial nerve causes a loss of motor and sensory function in the involved area. Wristdrop may occur; it may be temporary if injury is incomplete. Other findings in radial nerve injury include loss of finger and elbow extension, forearm supination, and thumb abduction; paresthesias; and hand muscle atrophy.

Special considerations

Help the patient with wristdrop perform routine tasks of eating and personal hygiene. If his wristdrop is permanent, contact a physical therapist to teach him range-of-motion exercises to strengthen weakened muscles. Contact an occupational therapist to provide assistive devices, such as a swivel spoon with a cuff that enables the patient to feed himself. Apply splints, as ordered, to help prevent contractures. Remind the patient to avoid holding hot objects in the affected hand. Also teach the family to help the patient with routine activities.

Pediatric pointers

Radial nerve injury is the most common cause of wristdrop in children.

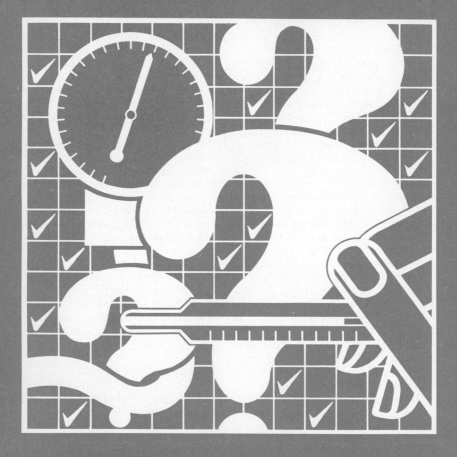

Appendices and Index

Selected Signs and Symptoms

This appendix supplements the main text of *Signs & Symptoms,* which provides detailed coverage of 300 signs and symptoms that are familiar, diagnostically significant, or indicative of an emergency. The appendix, in contrast, provides the definition and common causes of about 250 less familiar, accessory, or nonspecific signs and symptoms. For an elicited sign, such as Chaddock's sign, it also includes the technique for evoking the patient's response.

The appendix also covers selected pediatric signs, such as low-set ears and Allis' sign; psychiatric symptoms, such as delusions and hallucinations; and nail and tongue signs, such as nail plate hypertrophy and tongue discoloration.

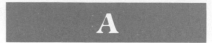

Aaron's sign • Pain in the chest or abdominal area that's elicited by applying gentle but steadily increasing pressure over McBurney's point. A positive sign indicates appendicitis.

Abadie's sign • Spasm of the levator muscle of the upper eyelid. This sign may be slight or pronounced and may affect one eye or both. It reflects an exophthalmic goiter in Graves' disease.

adipsia • Abnormal absence of thirst. This sign commonly occurs in hypothalamic injury or tumor, head injury, bronchial tumor, and cirrhosis.

agnosia • Inability to recognize and interpret sensory stimuli. *Auditory agnosia* refers to the inability to recognize familiar sounds. *Astereognosis*, or *tactile agnosia*, is the inability to recognize objects by touch or feel. *Anosmia* is the inability to recognize familiar smells; *gustatory agnosia,* the inability to recognize familiar tastes. *Visual agnosia* refers to the inability to recognize familiar objects by sight. *Autotopagnosia* is the inability to recognize body parts. *Anosognosia* refers to the denial or lack of awareness of a disease or defect (especially paralysis).

Agnosias stem from lesions that affect the association areas of the parietal sensory cortex. They're common sequelae of cerebrovascular accident.

agraphia • Inability to express thoughts in writing. *Aphasic agraphia* is associated with spelling and grammatical errors, whereas *constructional agraphia* refers to the reversal or incorrect ordering of correctly spelled words. *Apraxic agraphia* refers to the inability to form letters in the absence of significant motor impairment.

Agraphia commonly results from cerebrovascular accident.

Allis' sign • In an adult: relaxation of the fascia lata between the iliac crest and greater trochanter due to fracture of the neck of the femur. To detect this sign, place a finger over the area between the iliac crest and greater trochanter and press firmly. If your finger sinks deeply into this area, you've detected Allis' sign.

In an infant: unequal leg lengths due to hip dislocation. To detect this sign, place the infant on his back with his pelvis flat. Then flex both legs at the knee and hip with the feet even. Next compare the height of the knees. If they differ, suspect hip dislocation in the shorter leg.

ambivalence • Simultaneous existence of conflicting feelings about a person, idea, or object. It causes uncertainty or indecisiveness about which course to follow. Severe, debilitating ambivalence can occur in schizophrenia.

Amoss' sign • A sparing maneuver to avoid pain upon flexion of the spine. To detect this sign, ask the patient to rise from a supine to a sitting position. If he supports himself by placing his hands far behind him on the examining table, you've observed this sign.

anesthesia • Absence of cutaneous sensation of touch, temperature, and pain. This sensory loss may be partial or total, unilateral or bilateral. To detect anesthesia, ask the patient to close his eyes. Then touch him and ask him to specify the location. If the patient's verbal skills are immature or poor, watch for movement or changes in facial expression in response to your touch.

anisocoria • A difference of 0.5 to 2 mm in pupil size. Anisocoria occurs normally in about 2% of people, in whom the pupillary inequality remains constant over time and despite changes in light. However, if anisocoria results from fixed dilation or constriction of one pupil or slowed or impaired constriction of one pupil in response to light, it may indicate neurologic disease.

apathy • Absence or suppression of emotion or interest in the external envi-

ALLIS' SIGN

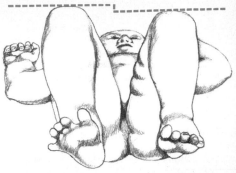

ronment and personal affairs. This indifference can result from many disorders—chiefly neurologic, psychological, respiratory, and renal—as well as from alcohol and drug use and abuse. It's associated with many chronic disorders that cause personality changes and depression. In fact, apathy may be an early indicator of a severe disorder, such as a brain tumor.

aphonia • Inability to produce speech sounds. This sign may result from overuse of the vocal cords, disorders of the larynx or laryngeal nerves, psychological disorders, or muscle spasm.

Argyll Robertson pupil • A small, irregular pupil that constricts normally in accommodation for near vision, but poorly or not at all in response to light. Response to mydriatic drugs also is poor or absent. This condition may be unilateral or bilateral and most commonly results from chronic syphilitic meningitis or other forms of late syphilis.

arthralgia • Joint pain. This symptom may have no pathologic importance or may indicate such disorders as arthritis or systemic lupus erythematosus.

ANISOCORIA

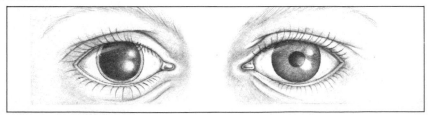

asthenocoria • Slow dilation or constriction of the pupils in response to light changes. Photophobia may be present if constriction occurs slowly. Asthenocoria occurs in adrenal insufficiency.

asynergy • Impaired coordination of muscles or organs that normally function harmoniously. This extrapyramidal symptom stems from disorders of the basal ganglia and cerebellum.

attention span decrease • Inability to focus selectively on a task while ignoring extraneous stimuli. Anxiety, emotional upset, and any dysfunction of the central nervous system may decrease the attention span.

autistic behavior • Exaggerated self-centered behavior marked by a lack of responsiveness to other people. It's characterized by highly personalized speech and actions that are not meaningful to an observer. For example, the patient may rock his body or repeatedly bang his head against the floor or wall. Autistic behavior may occur in schizophrenic children and adults.

B

Ballance's sign • A fixed mass or area of dullness found by palpation and percussion of the left upper quadrant of the abdomen. It may indicate subcapsular or extracapsular hematoma following splenic rupture.

BEAU'S LINES

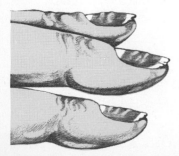

Ballet's sign • Ophthalmoplegia, or paralysis of the external ocular muscles. The patient displays no control of voluntary eye movement but has normal reflexive movement and pupillary light reflexes. This sign is an indicator of thyrotoxicosis.

Bárány's symptom • With warm water irrigation of the ear, rotary nystagmus toward the irrigated side; with cold water irrigation, rotary nystagmus away from the irrigated side. Absence of this symptom indicates labyrinthine dysfunction.

Barlow's sign • An indicator of congenital dislocation of the hip, detected in the first 6 weeks of life. To elicit this sign, place the infant supine with the hips flexed 90° and the knees fully flexed. Then place your palm over the infant's knee, your thumb in the femoral triangle opposite the lesser trochanter, and your index finger over the greater trochanter. Bring the hip into midabduction while gently exerting posterior and lateral pressure with your thumb and posterior and medial pressure with your palm. If you detect a click of the femoral head as it dislocates across the posterior lip of the acetabular socket, you've elicited this sign.

Barré's pyramidal sign • Inability to hold the lower legs still with the knees flexed. To detect this sign, place the patient prone and flex his knees 90°. Then ask him to hold his lower legs still. If he can't maintain this position, you've observed this sign of pyramidal tract disease.

Barré's sign • Delayed contraction of the iris, seen in mental deterioration.

Beau's lines • Transverse linear depressions on the fingernails. These lines may develop after any severe illness or toxic reaction. Other common causes include malnutrition, nail bed trauma, and coronary artery occlusion.

Beevor's sign • Upward movement of the umbilicus upon contraction of the abdominal muscles. To detect this sign, position the patient supine and ask him to sit up. If the umbilicus moves upward, you've observed this sign—an indicator of paralysis of the lower recti abdominis muscles associated with lesions at T10.

Bell's sign • Reflexive upward and outward deviation of the eyes that occurs when the patient attempts to close his eyes. It occurs on the affected side in Bell's palsy and indicates that the defect is supranuclear.

Bezold's sign • Swelling and tenderness of the mastoid area. Resulting from formation of an abscess beneath the sternocleidomastoid muscle, Bezold's sign indicates mastoiditis.

Bitot's spots • White or foamy gray superficial spots, varying from a few bubbles to a frothy white coating. Appearing on the conjunctiva at the lateral margin of the cornea, they're associated with vitamin A deficiency.

blepharoclonus • Excessive blinking of the eyes. This extrapyramidal sign occurs with disorders of the basal ganglia and cerebellum.

blocking • A cognitive disturbance resulting in interruption of a stream of speech or thought. It usually occurs in midsentence or before completion of a thought. Generally, the patient is unable to explain the interruption. Blocking may occur in normal individuals but most commonly occurs in schizophrenics.

Bonnet's sign • Pain on adduction of the thigh, seen in sciatica.

Bozzolo's sign • Pulsation of arteries in the nasal mucous membrane, seen occasionally with thoracic aortic aneurysms. To detect this sign, examine both nostrils, using a speculum and light.

Braunwald sign • Occurrence of a weak pulse rather than a strong pulse immediately after a premature ventricular contraction (PVC). To detect this sign, watch for a PVC during cardiac monitoring and check the quality of the pulse after it. Braunwald sign may indicate idiopathic hypertrophic subaortic stenosis.

breath sounds—absent or decreased • Diminished loudness of breath sounds—or their absence—detected by auscultation. This sign may reflect reduced airflow to a lung segment caused by a tumor, foreign body, mucous plug, or mucosal edema. It may also re-

flect hyperinflation of the lungs in emphysema or an asthmatic attack. Or it may reflect the presence of air or fluid in the pleural cavity from a pneumothorax, hemothorax, pleural effusion, atelectasis, or empyema. In an obese or extremely muscular patient, breath sounds may be diminished or inaudible because of increased thickness of the chest wall.

Broadbent's inverted sign • Pulsations on the left posterolateral chest wall during ventricular systole. To detect this sign, palpate the patient's chest with your fingers and palm over areas of visible pulsation while auscultating for ventricular systole. When you feel pulsations, note their rate, rhythm, and intensity. This sign may indicate gross dilatation of the left atrium.

Broadbent's sign • Visible retraction of the left posterior chest wall near the 11th and 12th ribs, occurring during systole. To detect this sign, inspect the chest wall while standing at the patient's right side. Position a strong light so that it casts rays tangential to the skin. While auscultating the heart, watch for retraction of the skin and muscles and determine its timing in the cardiac cycle. Broadbent's sign may occur in extensive adhesive pericarditis.

BEZOLD'S SIGN

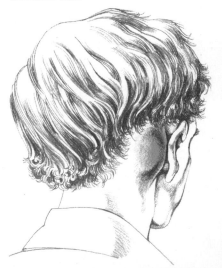

C

catatonia • Marked inhibition or excitation in motor behavior, occurring in psychotic disorders. *Catatonic stupor* refers to extreme inhibition of spontaneous activity or movement. *Catatonic excitement* refers to extreme psychomotor agitation.

Chaddock's sign • Chaddock's toe sign: extension of the great toe and fanning of the other toes. To elicit this sign, firmly stroke the side of the patient's foot just distal to the lateral malleolus. A positive sign indicates pyramidal tract disorders.

Chaddock's wrist sign: flexion of the wrist and extension of the fingers. To elicit this sign, stroke the ulnar surface of the patient's forearm near the wrist. A positive sign occurs on the affected side in hemiplegia.

Although Chaddock's sign signals pathology in children and adults, it's a normal finding in infants up to 7 months of age.

cherry red spot • The choroid appearing as a red circular area surrounded by an abnormal gray-white retina. It's viewed through the fovea centralis of the eye with an ophthalmoscope. A cherry red spot appears in infantile cerebral sphingolipidosis; for example, this spot appears in over 90% of patients with Tay-Sachs disease.

circumstantiality • Speech in which the main point is obscured by minute detail. Although the speaker may recognize his main point and return to it after many digressions, the listener may fail to recognize it. Circumstantiality commonly occurs in compulsive disorders, organic brain disorders, and schizophrenia.

Claude's hyperkinesis sign • Increased reflex activity of paretic muscles, elicited by painful stimuli.

clavicular sign • Swelling, puffiness, or edema at the medial third of the right clavicle, most often seen in congenital syphilis.

Cleeman's sign • Slight linear depression or wrinkling of the skin superior to the patella. It usually indicates a femoral fracture with overriding bone fragments.

clenched fist sign • The patient's placement of a clenched fist against his chest. This gesture may be performed by patients with angina pectoris when they're asked to indicate the location of their pain. The patient's gesture conveys the constricting, oppressive quality of substernal pain.

clicks • Brief, high-frequency heart sounds auscultated during systole or diastole. *Ejection clicks* occur soon after the first heart sound. Presumably, they result from sudden distention of a dilated pulmonary artery or the aorta or from forceful opening of the pulmonic or aortic valves. Associated with increased pulmonary resistance and hypertension, they occur most commonly with septal defects or patent ductus arteriosus. To detect ejection clicks best, have the patient sit upright or lie down, then auscultate the heart with the diaphragm of the stethoscope.

Systolic clicks occur most often in mid- to late systole. They're characteristic of mitral valve prolapse. To detect systolic clicks, auscultate over the mitral valve with the diaphragm of the stethoscope.

CHADDOCK'S TOE SIGN

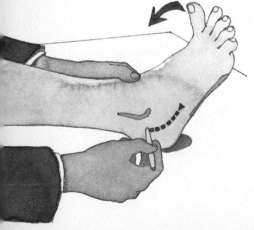

Codman's sign • Pain resulting from rupture of the supraspinatus tendon. To elicit this sign, have the patient relax the arm on the affected side while you abduct it. If the patient reports no pain until you remove your support and the deltoid muscle contracts, you've detected Codman's sign.

Comolli's sign • Triangular swelling over the scapula that matches its shape. This sign indicates scapular fracture.

complementary opposition sign • Increased effort in lifting a paretic leg, demonstrated in the opposite leg. To elicit this sign, position the patient supine and place your hand under the heel of the unaffected leg. Then ask the patient to lift the paretic leg. If his effort produces marked downward pressure on your hand, you've detected this sign.

compulsion • Stereotyped, repetitive behavior in which the individual recognizes the irrationality of his actions but is unable to stop them. An example is constant handwashing. Compulsion occurs in obsessive-compulsive disorders and occasionally in schizophrenia.

confabulation • Fabrication to cover gaps in memory. Confabulation is most often seen in alcoholism and Korsakoff's syndrome.

conjunctival paleness • Lack of color in the tissues inside the eyelid. Although the conjunctiva is a transparent mucous membrane, the portion lining the eyelids normally appears pink or red because it overlies the vasculature of the inner lid. Pale conjunctiva indicates anemia. To detect this sign, separate the eyelids widely by applying gentle pressure against the orbit of the eye. Ask the patient to look up, down, and to each side.

conversion • An alteration in physical activity or function that resembles an organic disorder but lacks an organic cause. Occurring without voluntary control, conversion is generally considered symbolic of psychological conflict and most commonly occurs in conversion disorders.

Coopernail sign • Ecchymoses on the perineum, scrotum, or labia. This sign indicates pelvic fracture.

Corrigan's pulse • A jerky pulse in which a strong surge precedes an abrupt collapse. To detect this sign, hold the patient's hand above his head and palpate the carotid artery. Corrigan's pulse occurs in aortic insufficiency. It may also occur in severe anemia, patent ductus arteriosus, coarctation of the aorta, and systemic arteriosclerosis.

Cowen's sign • A jerky consensual pupillary light reflex. To detect this sign, observe for constriction and dilation of one pupil while the other is stimulated by increased and decreased light.

crossed extensor reflex • Extension of one leg in response to stimulation of the opposite leg; a normal reflex in newborn infants. It's mediated at the spinal cord level and should disappear after 6 months of age. To elicit this sign, place the infant supine with his legs extended. Tap the medial aspect of the thigh just above the patella. The infant should respond by extending and adducting the opposite leg and fanning the toes of that foot. Persistence of this reflex beyond 6 months of age indicates anoxic brain damage. Its appearance in a child signals a central nervous system lesion or injury.

COMOLLI'S SIGN

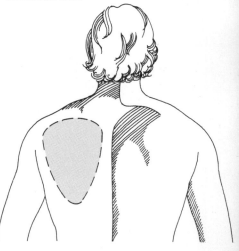

crowing respirations • Slow, deep inspirations accompanied by a high-pitched crowing sound—the characteristic whoop of the paroxysmal stage of pertussis.

Cruveilhier's sign • Swelling in the groin associated with inguinal hernia. To detect this sign, ask the patient to flex one knee slightly while you insert your index finger in the inguinal canal on the same side. When your finger is inserted as deeply as possible, ask the patient to cough. If a hernia is present, you'll feel a mass of tissue that meets your finger and then withdraws.

Cullen's sign • Irregular, bluish hemorrhagic patches on the skin around the umbilicus and occasionally around abdominal scars. Cullen's sign indicates massive hemorrhage after trauma or rupture in such disorders as duodenal ulcer, ectopic pregnancy, abdominal aneurysm, gallbladder or common bile duct obstruction, or acute hemorrhagic pancreatitis. Usually, Cullen's sign appears gradually; blood travels from a retroperitoneal organ or structure to the periumbilical area, where it diffuses through subcutaneous tissues. It may be difficult to detect in a dark-skinned patient. The extent of discoloration depends on the extent of bleeding. In time, the bluish discoloration fades to greenish yellow and then yellow before disappearing.

CULLEN'S SIGN

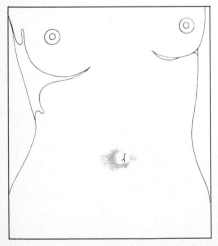

D

Dalrymple's sign • Abnormally wide palpebral fissures associated with retraction of the upper eyelids. To detect this sign of thyrotoxicosis, observe the eyes while the patient focuses on a fixed point or ask him to close his eyes. There may be infrequent blinking and noticeable restriction of lid movement. The patient may not be able to close his eyes completely.

Darier's sign • Whealing and itching of the skin upon rubbing the macular lesions of urticaria pigmentosa (mastocytosis). To elicit this sign, vigorously rub the pigmented macules with the blunt end of a pen or a similar blunt object. The appearance of pruritic, red, palpable wheals around the macules—a positive Darier's sign—follows the release of histamine when mast cells are irritated.

Dawbarn's sign • Pain on palpation of the acromial process in acute subacromial bursitis. To elicit this sign, palpate the patient's shoulder while his arm hangs at his side and as he abducts it. If palpation causes pain that disappears on abduction, you've detected Dawbarn's sign.

Delbet's sign • Adequate collateral circulation to the distal portion of a limb associated with aneurysmal occlusion of the main artery. To detect this sign, check pulses, color, and temperature in the affected limb. If you find absent pulses but normal color and temperature, you've detected Delbet's sign.

delirium • Acute confusion characterized by restlessness, agitation, incoherence, and often hallucinations. Typically, delirium develops suddenly and lasts for a short period. It's a common effect of drug and alcohol abuse, metabolic disorders, and high fever. Delirium may also follow head trauma or seizure.

delusion • A persistent false belief held despite invalidating evidence. A *delusion of grandeur*, which may occur in schizophrenia and bipolar disorders, refers to an exaggerated belief in one's importance, wealth, or talent. The patient may take a powerful figure, such as Napoleon, as his persona. In a *paranoid delusion*, which may occur in schizophrenia and paranoid disorders, the patient believes that he or someone close to him is the victim of an attack, harrassment, or conspiracy. In a *somatic delusion*, which may occur in psychotic disorders, the patient believes that his body is diseased or distorted.

Demianoff's sign • Lumbar pain caused by stretching the sacrolumbalis muscle. To elicit this sign, place the patient supine on the examining table and raise his extended leg. Lumbar pain that prevents lifting the leg high enough to form a 10° angle to the table—a positive Demianoff's sign—occurs in lumbago.

denial • An unconscious defense mechanism used to ward off distressing feelings, thoughts, wishes, or needs. Denial occurs in normal and pathologic mental states. In terminal illness, it represents the first stage of the response to dying.

depersonalization • Perception of the self as strange or unreal. For example, a person may report feeling as if he's observing himself from a distance. This symptom occurs in patients with schizophrenia and depersonalization disorders and in normal individuals during periods of great stress or anxiety.

Desault's sign • Alteration of the arc made by the greater trochanter upon rotation of the femur; seen in fracture of the intracapsular region of the femur. In this fracture, the greater trochanter rotates only on the axis of the femur, making a much smaller arc than it does upon normal rotation of the femur in the capsule of the hip joint.

disorientation • Inaccurate perception of time, place, or identity. Disorientation may occur in organic brain disorders, cerebral anoxia, and drug and alcohol intoxication. It occurs occasionally after prolonged, severe stress.

Dorendorf's sign • Fullness at the supraclavicular groove. This sign may occur in an aneurysm of the aortic arch.

Duchenne's sign • Inward movement of the epigastrium during inspiration. This may indicate diaphragmatic paralysis or accumulation of fluid in the pericardium.

Dugas' sign • An indicator of a dislocated shoulder. To detect this sign, ask the patient to place the hand of the affected side on his opposite shoulder and to move his elbow toward his chest. The inability to perform this maneuver—a positive Dugas' sign—indicates dislocation.

Duroziez's sign • A double murmur heard over a large peripheral artery. To detect this sign, auscultate over the femoral artery, alternately compressing the vessel proximally and then distally. If you hear a systolic murmur with proximal compression and a diastolic murmur with distal compression, you've detected Duroziez's sign—an indicator of aortic insufficiency.

dysdiadochokinesia • Difficulty in stopping one movement and starting another. This extrapyramidal sign occurs with disorders of the basal ganglia and cerebellum.

dysphonia • Hoarseness or difficulty in producing voice sounds. This sign may reflect disorders of the larynx or laryngeal nerves, overuse or spasm of the vocal cords, or central nervous system disorders, such as Parkinson's disease. It may also occur at puberty.

DORENDORF'S SIGN

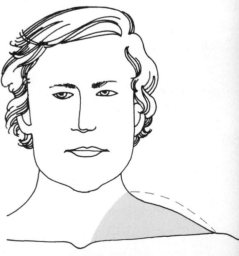

E

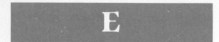

echolalia • In an adult: repetition of another's words or phrases with no comprehension of their meaning. This sign occurs in schizophrenia and frontal lobe disorders.

In a child: an imitation of sounds or words produced by others.

echopraxia • Repetition of another's movements with no comprehension of their meaning. This sign may occur in catatonic schizophrenia and certain neurologic disorders.

ectropion • Eversion of the eyelid. It may affect the lower eyelid or both lids, exposing the palpebral conjunctiva. If the lacrimal puncta are everted, the eye cannot drain properly, and tearing occurs. Ectropion may occur gradually as part of aging

ECTROPION

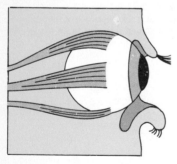

ENTROPION

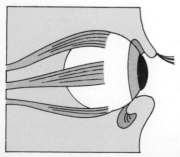

but may also occur with injury or paralysis of the facial nerve.

entropion • Inversion of the eyelid. It typically affects the lower lid but may also affect the upper lid. The eyelashes may touch and irritate the cornea. Most commonly associated with aging, entropion may also stem from chemical burns, mechanical injuries, spasm of the orbicularis muscle, pemphigoid, Stevens-Johnson syndrome, and trachoma.

epicanthal folds • Vertical skin folds that partially or fully obscure the inner canthus of the eye. These folds may make the eyes appear crossed, since the pupil lies closer to the inner canthus than to the outer canthus. Epicanthal folds are a normal characteristic in many young children and Orientals. They also occur as a familial trait in other ethnic groups, and as an acquired trait in aging. However, the presence of epicanthal folds along with oblique palpebral fissures in non-Oriental children indicates Down's syndrome.

Erben's reflex • Slowing of the pulse when the head and trunk are forcibly bent forward. It may indicate vagal excitability.

Erb's sign. • In tetany, increased irritability of motor nerves, detected by electromyography. Erb's sign also refers to dullness on percussion over the sternum's manubrium in acromegaly.

Escherich's sign • Contraction of the lips, tongue, and masseters, occurring in tetany. To elicit Escherich's sign, percuss the inner surface of the lips or the tongue.

euphoria • A feeling of great happiness or well-being. When euphoria doesn't accompany enlightening experiences or superb achievements, it may reflect bipolar disorders, organic brain disease, or use of such drugs as heroin, cocaine, and amphetamines.

Ewart's sign • Bronchial breathing heard on auscultation of the lungs and dullness heard on percussion below the angle of the left scapula. These compression signs commonly occur in pericardial effusion.

extensor thrust reflex • Extension of the leg upon stimulation of the sole of the foot; a normal reflex in newborn infants. This reflex is mediated at the spinal cord level and should disappear after 6 months of age.

To elicit the extensor thrust reflex, place the infant supine with the leg flexed; then stimulate the sole of the foot. If the extensor thrust reflex is present, the leg will slowly extend. In premature infants, this reflex may be weak. Its persistence beyond 6 months of age indicates anoxic brain damage. Its recurrence in a child signals a central nervous system lesion or injury.

extinction • In neurology: inability to perceive one of two stimuli presented simultaneously. To detect this sign, simultaneously stimulate two corresponding areas on opposite sides of the body. Extinction is present if the patient fails to perceive one sensation.

In neurophysiology: loss of excitability of a nerve, synapse, or nervous tissue in response to stimuli that were previously adequate.

In psychology: disappearance of a conditioned reflex resulting from lack of reinforcement.

extrapyramidal signs and symptoms • Movement and posture disturbances characteristically resulting from disorders of the basal ganglia and cerebellum. These disturbances include asynergy, ataxia, athetosis, blepharoclonus, chorea, dysarthria, dysdiadochokinesia, dystonia, muscle rigidity and spasticity, myoclonus, spasmodic torticollis, and tremors.

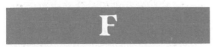

F

fabere sign • Pain produced by maneuvers used in Patrick's test. It indicates an arthritic hip. The name is an acronym for maneuvers used to elicit the sign: flexion, abduction, external rotation, and extension. Begin by placing the patient supine and asking him to flex the thigh and knee of the leg being examined. Then have him externally rotate the leg and place the lateral malleolus on the patella of the opposite leg. Depress the knee. If he experiences pain, you've detected the fabere sign.

Fajersztajn's crossed sciatic sign • In sciatica, pain on the affected side caused by lifting the extended opposite leg. To elicit this sign, place the patient supine and have him flex his unaffected hip, keeping his knee extended. Flexion at the hip will cause pain on the affected side by stretching the irritated sciatic nerve.

fan sign • A component of Babinski's reflex. This sign refers to the spreading apart of the patient's toes after firmly stroking his foot.

flexor withdrawal reflex • Flexion of the knee upon stimulation of the sole of the foot; a normal reflex in newborn infants. This reflex is mediated at the spinal cord level and should disappear after 6 months of age.

To elicit this reflex, place the infant supine, extend his legs, and pinch the sole of his foot. Normally, an infant younger than 6 months of age will respond with slow, uncontrolled flexion of the knee. This reflex may be weak in premature infants. Its persistence beyond 6 months of age may indicate anoxic brain damage. Its recurrence signals a central nervous system lesion or injury.

flight of ideas • Continuous, often seemingly pressured speech with abrupt changes of topic. In contrast with *looseness of association*, a listener can discern the connection between topics based on word similarities or sounds. This sign characteristically occurs in the manic phase of a bipolar disorder.

foot malposition—congenital • Anomalous positioning of the foot, present at birth in roughly 0.4 % of infants. It may reflect the fetal position of comfort, neuromuscular disease, or malformation of a joint or connective tissue. To assess this sign, observe the resting infant's foot to determine the position of comfort. Then observe the foot during spontaneous activity. Using gentle passive maneuvers, determine the full range of motion of the foot and ankle.

Fränkel's sign • In tabes dorsalis, the excessive range of passive motion at the hip joint. This excessive motion stems from decreased tone in the surrounding muscles.

G

Galant's reflex • Movement of the pelvis toward the stimulated side when the back is stroked laterally to the spinal column. Normally present at birth, this reflex disappears by 2 months of age. To elicit this reflex, place the infant prone on the examining table or on your hand. Then, using a pin or your finger, stroke the back laterally to the midline. Normally, the infant responds by moving the pelvis toward the stimulated side, indicating integrity of the spinal cord from T1 to S1. The absence, irregularity, or asymmetry of this reflex may indicate a spinal cord lesion.

Galeazzi's sign • Unequal leg lengths in an infant, seen in congenital dislocation of the hip. To detect this sign, place the infant supine on a flat, hard surface. Flex the knees and hips 90° and compare the heights of the knees. With dislocation of the hip, the knee will be lower and the femur will appear shortened on the affected side.

Gifford's sign • Resistance to everting the upper eyelid, seen in thyrotoxicosis. To detect this sign, attempt to raise the eyelid and evert it over a blunt object.

glabella reflex • Persistent blinking in response to repeated light tapping on the forehead between the eyebrows. This reflex occurs in Parkinson's disease, presenile dementia, and diffuse tumors of the frontal lobes.

Goldthwait's sign • Pain elicited by maneuvers of the leg, pelvis, and lower back to differentiate irritation of the sacroiliac joint from irritation of the lumbosacral or sacroiliac articulation. To elicit this sign, position the patient supine and place one hand under the small of his back. With your other hand, raise the patient's leg. If the patient reports pain, suspect sacroiliac joint irritation. If he reports no pain, place your hand under his lower back and apply pressure. If the patient reports pain, suspect irritation of the lumbosacral or sacroiliac articulation.

Gowers' sign • In an adult: irregular contraction of the iris, occurring when the eye is illuminated. This sign can be detected in certain stages of tabes dorsalis.

In a child: the characteristic maneuver used to rise from the floor or a low sitting position to compensate for proximal muscle weakness in Duchenne's or Becker's muscular dystrophy. See "Gait—Waddling," page 340.

grasp reflex • Flexion of the fingers when the palmar surface is touched, and of the toes when the plantar surface is touched; a normal reflex in infants.

In an infant: this reflex develops at approximately 26 to 28 weeks gestational age but may be weak until term. The absence, weakness, or asymmetry of this reflex during the neonatal period may indicate paralysis, central nervous system depression, or injury. To elicit this reflex, place a finger in each of the infant's palms. His reflexive grasping should be symmetrical and strong enough at term to allow him to be lifted. Elicit flexion of the toes by gently touching the ball of the foot.

In an adult: the grasp reflex is an *abnormal* finding, indicating a disorder of the premotor cortex.

Grasset's phenomenon • Inability to raise both legs simultaneously, even though each can be raised separately. In an adult: this phenomenon occurs in incomplete organic hemiplegia. To elicit it, place the patient supine and lift and support the affected leg; then attempt to lift the opposite leg. In Grasset's phenome-

GALANT'S REFLEX

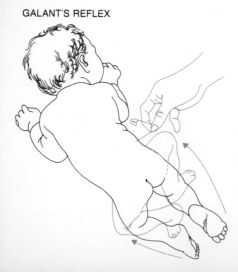

non, the unaffected leg will drop—the result of an upper motor neuron lesion.

In an infant: this sign is normally present until 5 to 7 months of age.

Grey Turner's sign • A bruiselike discoloration of the skin of the flanks. This sign appears 6 to 24 hours after onset of retroperitoneal hemorrhage in acute pancreatitis.

grief • Deep anguish or sorrow typically felt upon the loss of a loved one, a job, a goal, or an ideal. In patients with terminal illness, grief may precede acceptance of dying. Unlike depression, grief proceeds in stages and often resolves with the passage of time.

Griffith's sign • Lagging motion of the lower eyelids during upward rotation of the eyes, seen in thyrotoxicosis. To detect this sign, ask the patient to focus on a steadily rising point, such as your moving finger. If the lower lid doesn't follow eye motion smoothly, you've observed this sign.

Guilland's sign • Quick, energetic flexion of the hip and knee in response to pinching the contralateral quadriceps muscle. This sign indicates meningeal irritation.

H

hallucination • A sensory perception without corresponding external stimuli. Hallucinations may occur in depression, schizophrenia, bipolar disorder, organic brain disorders, and drug-induced and toxic conditions.

An *auditory hallucination* refers to the perception of nonexistent sounds—typically voices but occasionally music or other sounds. Occurring in schizophrenia, this is the most common type of hallucination.

An *olfactory hallucination*—a perception of nonexistent odors from the patient's own body or from some other person or object—is typically associated with somatic delusions. It occurs most often in temporal lobe lesions and may also occur in schizophrenia.

A *tactile hallucination* refers to the perception of nonexistent tactile stimuli, generally described as something crawling on or under the skin. It occurs mainly in toxic conditions and addiction to certain drugs. Formication—the sensation of insects crawling on the skin—most often occurs in alcohol withdrawal syndrome and cocaine abuse.

A *visual hallucination* is a perception of nonexistent images of people, flashes of light, or other scenes. It occurs most often in acute, reversible organic brain disorders but may also occur in drug and alcohol intoxication, schizophrenia, febrile illness, and encephalopathy.

A *gustatory hallucination* refers to the perception of nonexistent, usually unpleasant tastes.

Hamman's sign • A loud, crushing, crunching sound synchronous with the heart beat. Auscultated over the precordium, it reflects mediastinal emphysema, which occurs in such life-threatening conditions as pneumothorax or rupture of the trachea or bronchi. To detect this sign, place the patient in a left lateral recumbent position and gently auscultate over the precordium.

harlequin sign • A benign, erythematous color change occurring especially in low-birth-weight infants. This reddening of one longitudinal half of the body appears when the infant is placed on either side for a few minutes. When he's placed on his back, the sign usually disappears immediately but may persist up to 20 minutes.

hemorrhage—subungual • Bleeding under the nail plate. Hemorrhagic lines,

SUBUNGUAL HEMORRHAGE

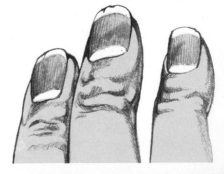

called splinter hemorrhages, run proximally from the distal edge and serve as an indicator of subacute bacterial endocarditis and trichinosis. Large hemorrhagic areas generally reflect nail bed injury.

high birth weight • Neonatal weight that exceeds the 90th percentile for the gestational age of the infant. The high-birth-weight neonate is at increased risk for birth trauma, respiratory distress, hypocalcemia, hypoglycemia, and polycythemia.

Hill's sign • A femoral systolic pulse pressure 60 to 100 mm Hg higher in the right leg than in the right arm. Hill's sign may indicate severe aortic insufficiency. To detect this sign, place the patient in a supine position and take blood pressure readings, first in the right arm and then in the right leg, noting the difference.

Hoehne's sign • Absence of uterine contractions during delivery, despite repeated doses of oxytocic drugs. This sign indicates a ruptured uterus.

Hoffmann's sign • Flexion of the terminal phalanx of the thumb and the second and third phalanx of another finger when the nail of the index, middle, or ring finger is snapped. A bilateral or strongly

unilateral response suggests a pyramidal tract disorder, such as spastic hemiparesis. To elicit this sign, dorsiflex the patient's wrist, have him flex his fingers, and then snap the nail of his index, middle, or ring finger.

Hoffmann's sign also refers to increased sensitivity of sensory nerves to electrical stimulation, as in tetany.

Hoover's sign • Inward movement of one or both costal margins with inspiration. Bilateral movement occurs in emphysema with acute respiratory distress. Unilateral movement occurs in intrathoracic disorders that cause flattening of one half of the diaphragm.

hyperacusis • Abnormally acute hearing resulting from increased irritability of the auditory neural mechanism.

hyperesthesia • Increased cutaneous sensitivity to touch, temperature, or pain.

hypernasality • A voice quality reflecting excessive expiration of air through the nose during speech. It's often associated with symptoms of dysarthria and possibly with swallowing defects. The sudden onset of hypernasality may indicate a neuromuscular disorder. This sign may also accompany cleft palate, a short soft and hard palate, abnormal nasopharyngeal size, and partial or complete velar paralysis. To detect this sign, ask the patient to extend vowel sounds first with the nostrils open, then closed (pinched). A significant shift in tone may indicate hypernasality.

hypoesthesia • Decreased cutaneous sensitivity to touch, temperature, or pain.

I

idea of reference • A delusion that other people, statements, actions, or events have a meaning specific to oneself. This delusion occurs in schizophrenia and paranoid states.

illusion • A misperception of external stimuli—usually visual or auditory. An example: the sound of the wind being perceived as a voice. Illusions occur normally as well as in schizophrenia and toxic states.

KOPLIK'S SPOTS

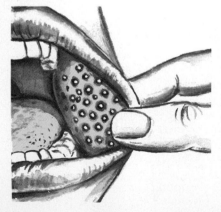

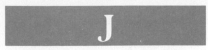

Jellinek's sign • Brownish pigmentation on the eyelids, usually more prominent on the upper lid than on the lower one. This sign appears in Graves' disease.

Joffroy's sign • Immobility of the facial muscles with upward rotation of the eyes, associated with exophthalmos in Graves' disease. To detect this sign, observe the patient's forehead as he quickly rotates his eyes upward.

Joffroy's sign also refers to the inability to perform simple mathematics—a possible early sign of organic brain disorders.

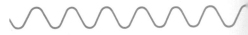

KUSSMAUL'S RESPIRATIONS

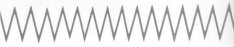

NORMAL RESPIRATIONS

Kussmaul's sign • Distention of the jugular veins on inspiration, occurring in constrictive pericarditis and mediastinal tumor.

Kussmaul's sign also refers to a paradoxical pulse and to seizures and coma that result from absorption of toxins.

K

Kanavel's sign • An area of tenderness in the palm, caused by inflammation of the tendon sheath of the little finger. To detect this sign, apply pressure to the palm proximal to the metacarpophalangeal joint of the little finger.

Kashida's sign • Hyperesthesia and muscle spasms produced by application of heat or cold. This sign occurs in tetany.

Keen's sign • Increased ankle circumference in Pott's fracture of the fibula. To detect this sign, measure the ankles at the malleoli and compare their circumferences.

Kleist's sign • Flexion, or hooking, of the fingers when passively raised, associated with frontal lobe and thalamic lesions. To elicit this sign, have the patient turn his palms down, then gently raise his fingers. If his fingers hook onto yours, you've detected this sign.

Koplik's spots • Small red spots with bluish white centers on the lingual and buccal mucosa characteristic of measles. After this sign appears, the measles rash usually erupts in 1 to 2 days.

Kussmaul's respirations • An abnormal breathing pattern characterized by deep, rapid sighing respirations, generally associated with metabolic acidosis.

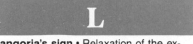

Langoria's sign • Relaxation of the extensor muscles of the thigh and hip joint, resulting from intracapsular fracture of the femur. To elicit this sign, place the patient in a prone position, then press firmly on the gluteus maximus and hamstring muscles on both sides, noting greater muscle relaxation on the affected side. (The muscles are soft and spongy.)

Lasègue's sign • Pain upon passive movement of the leg that distinguishes hip joint disease from sciatica. To elicit this sign, place the patient supine, raise one of his legs, and bend the knee to flex the hip joint. Pain with this movement indicates hip joint disease. With the hip still flexed, slowly extend the knee. Pain with this movement results from stretching an irritated sciatic nerve, indicating sciatica.

Laugier's sign • An abnormal spatial relationship of the radial and ulnar styloid processes, resulting from fracture of the distal radius. To detect this sign, compare the patient's wrists. Normally more distal than the ulnar process, the radial process may migrate proximally in fracture of the distal radius, so that it's level with the ulnar process.

lead-pipe rigidity • Diffuse muscle stiffness occurring, for example, in Parkinson's disease.

Leichtenstern's sign • Pain upon gentle tapping of the bones of an extremity. This sign occurs in cerebrospinal meningitis. The patient may wince, draw back suddenly, or cry out loudly.

Lhermitte's sign • Sensations of sudden, transient, electriclike shocks spreading down the back and into the extremities, precipitated by forward flexion of the head. This sign occurs in multiple sclerosis, spinal cord degeneration, and cervical spinal cord injury.

Lichtheim's sign • An inability to speak associated with subcortical aphasia. However, the patient can indicate with his fingers the number of syllables in the word he wants to say.

Linder's sign • Pain upon neck flexion, indicating sciatica. To elicit this sign, place the patient in a supine or sitting position with his legs fully extended. Then passively flex his neck, noting if he experiences pain in the lower back or the affected leg, resulting from stretching the irritated sciatic nerve.

Lloyd's sign • Referred loin pain elicited by deep percussion over the kidney. This sign is associated with renal calculi.

looseness of association • A cognitive disturbance marked by absence of a logical link between spoken statements. It occurs in schizophrenia, bipolar disorders, or other psychotic disorders.

low-set ears • A position of the ears in which the superior helix lies lower than the eyes. This sign appears in several genetic syndromes, including Down's, Apert's, Turner's, Noonan's, and Potter's, and may also appear in other congenital abnormalities.

Ludloff's sign • Inability to raise the thigh while sitting, along with edema and ecchymosis at the base of Scarpa's triangle (the depressed area just below the fold of the groin). Occurring in children, this sign indicates traumatic separation of the epiphyseal growth plate of the greater trochanter.

lumbosacral hair tuft • Abnormal growth of hair over the lower spine, possibly accompanied by skin depression or discoloration. This may mark the site of spina bifida occulta or spina bifida cystica.

M

Macewen's sign • A "cracked pot" sound heard on light percussion with one finger over an infant's or young child's anterior fontanelle. An early indicator of hydrocephalus, this sign may also occur in cerebral abscess.

Maisonneuve's sign • Hyperextension of the wrist in Colles' fracture. Hyperextension results when a fracture of the lower radius causes posterior displacement of the distal fragment.

malaise • Listlessness, weariness, or absence of the sense of well-being. This nonspecific symptom may begin suddenly or gradually and may precede characteristic signs of an illness by several days or weeks. Malaise may reflect the metabolic alterations that precede or accompany infectious, endocrine, or neurologic disorders.

LUMBOSACRAL HAIR TUFT

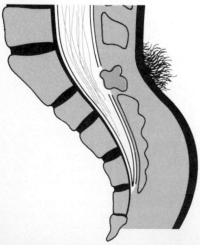

malingering • Exaggeration or simulation of symptoms to avoid an unpleasant situation or to gain attention or some other goal.

mania • An alteration in mood characterized by increased psychomotor activity, euphoria, flight of ideas, and pressured speech. It occurs most often in the manic phase of a bipolar disorder.

Mannkopf's sign • Elevated pulse rate upon application of pressure over a painful area. It can help distinguish real pain from simulated pain.

Marcus Gunn phenomenon • Unilateral reflexive elevation of an upper ptotic eyelid, associated with movement of the lower jaw. This occurs in misdirectional syndrome, involving the oculomotor and trigeminal nerves (cranial nerves III and V). To elicit this sign, ask the patient to open his mouth and move his lower jaw from side to side.

Marcus Gunn's pupillary sign • Paradoxical dilatation of a pupil in response to afferent visual stimuli. This sign results from an optic nerve lesion or severe retinal dysfunction. However, visual loss in the affected eye is minimal. To detect this pupillary sign, darken the room and instruct the patient to focus on a distant object. Shine a bright beam of light into the unaffected eye, and observe for bilateral pupillary constriction. Then shine the light into the affected eye; you'll observe brief bilateral dilatation. Next, return the light beam to the unaffected eye; you'll observe prompt and persistent bilateral pupillary constriction.

Mayo's sign • In deep anesthesia, relaxation of the muscles controlling the lower jaw.

Means' sign • Lagging eye motion when the patient looks upward. In this sign of Graves' disease, the globe of the eye moves more slowly than the upper lid.

meconium staining of amniotic fluid • The presence of greenish brown or yellow meconium in the amniotic fluid during labor. Although not necessarily indicative of distress, this sign signals the need for close fetal monitoring to detect decreased variability or deceleration of

heart rate. It may also signal the need for infant intubation and resuscitation at delivery to prevent meconium aspiration into the lungs.

menometrorrhagia • An abnormal menstrual cycle marked by a prolonged flow (menorrhagia) with irregular, intermittent spotting between menses (metrorrhagia). Its causes include adenoacanthoma, endometriosis, follicular ovarian cysts, ovarian tumors, polycystic ovary disease, and submucosal leiomyoma.

Möbius' sign • Inability to maintain convergence of the eyes. To detect this sign of Graves' disease, observe the patient's attempt to focus on any small object, such as a pencil, as you move it toward him in line with his nose.

Moro's reflex • An infant's generalized response to a loud noise or sudden movement. Usually, this reflex disappears by about age 3 months. Its persistence after 6 months of age may indicate brain damage. To elicit this reflex, make a sudden loud noise near the infant, or carefully hold his body with one hand, while allowing his head to drop a few centimeters with the other hand. In a complete response, the infant's arms extend and abduct, and his fingers open; then his arms adduct and flex over his chest in a grasping motion. The infant may also extend his hips and legs and cry briefly. A bilaterally equal response is normal; an asymmetrical response may indicate a fractured clavicle or brachial nerve damage. The absence of a response may indicate hearing loss or severe central nervous system depression.

MORO'S REFLEX

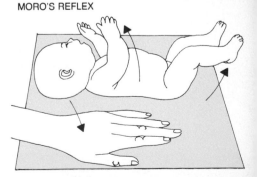

Murphy's sign • The arrest of inspiratory effort when gentle finger pressure beneath the right subcostal arch and below the margin of the liver causes pain during deep inspiration. This classic (but not always present) sign of acute cholecystitis may also occur in hepatitis.

muscle rigidity • Muscle tension, stiffness, and resistance to passive movement. This extrapyramidal symptom occurs in disorders affecting the basal ganglia and cerebellum, such as Parkinson's disease, Wilson's disease, Hallervorden-Spatz disease in adults, and kernicterus in infants.

N

nail dystrophy • Changes in the nail plate, such as pitting, furrowing, splitting, or fraying. It most often results from injury, chronic nail infections, neurovascular disorders affecting the extremities, or collagen disorders.

nail plate discoloration • A change in the color of the nail plate, resulting from infection or drugs. Blue-green discoloration may occur with *Pseudomonas* infection; brown or black, with fungal infection or fluorosis; and bluish gray, with excessive use of silver salts.

nail plate hypertrophy • Thickening of the nail plate resulting from the accumulation of irregular keratin layers. This condition is often associated with fungal infections of the nails, although it can be hereditary.

NAIL SEPARATION

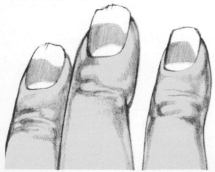

nail separation • The separation of the nail plate from the nail bed. This occurs primarily in injury or infection of the nail, and thyrotoxicosis.

neologism • A new word or condensation of several words with special meaning for the patient but not readily understood by others. This coining occurs in schizophrenia and organic brain disorders.

neuralgia • Severe, paroxysmal pain over an area innervated by specific nerve fibers. The cause is often unknown, but it may be precipitated by pressure, cold, movement, or stimulation of a trigger zone. Usually brief, neuralgia may be accompanied by vasomotor symptoms, such as sweating or tearing.

Nicoladoni's sign • Bradycardia resulting from finger pressure on an artery proximal to an arteriovenous fistula.

nodules • Small, solid, circumscribed masses of differentiated tissue, detected on palpation.

O

obsession • A persistent, usually disturbing thought or image that can't be eliminated by reason or logic. It's associated with an obsessive-compulsive disorder and occasionally schizophrenia.

obturator sign • Pain in the right hypogastric region, occurring with flexion of the right leg at the hip with the knee bent and internally rotated. It indicates irritation of the obturator muscle.
  In children, this sign may signal acute appendicitis since the appendix lies rectocecally over the obturator muscle.

oculocardiac reflex • Bradycardia in response to vagal stimulation, caused by application of pressure to the eyeball or carotid sinus. This reflex can help diagnose angina or relieve anginal pain. *Caution:* Repeated application of pressure to the eye to elicit this response may precipitate retinal detachment.

orbicularis sign • Inability to close one eye at a time, occurring in hemiplegia.

orgasmic dysfunction • Transient or persistent inhibition of the orgasmic phase of sexual excitement. In the female: delayed or absent orgasm following a phase of sexual excitement. This results most commonly from psychological or interpersonal problems. It may also result from chronic disorders, congenital anomalies, and chronic vaginal or pelvic infections.

In the male: delayed or absent ejaculation following a phase of sexual excitement. Its causes include psychological problems, neurologic disorders, and the effects of antihypertensive drugs. See "Impotence," page 423.

orthotonos • A form of tetanic spasm producing a rigid, straight line of the neck, limbs, and body.

ostealgia • Bone pain associated with such disorders as osteomyelitis.

otorrhagia • Bleeding from the ear occurring with a tumor, severe infection, or injury affecting the auricle, external canal, tympanic membrane, or temporal bone.

P

palmar crease abnormalities • An abnormal line pattern on the palms, resulting from faulty embryonic development during the second and fourth months of gestation. This pattern may occur normally but most commonly appears in Down's syndrome (called the *simian crease*) as a single transverse crease formed by fusion of the proximal and distal palmar creases. It also appears in Turner's syndrome and congenital rubella syndrome.

paradoxical respirations • An abnormal breathing pattern marked by paradoxical movement of an injured portion of the chest wall—it contracts on inspiration and bulges on expiration. This ominous sign is characteristic of flail chest—a thoracic injury involving multiple free-floating, fractured ribs.

paranoia • Extreme suspiciousness related to delusions of persecution by another person, group, or institution. This may occur in schizophrenia, drug-induced or toxic states, or paranoid disorders.

Pastia's sign • Petechiae appearing along skin creases in such areas as the antecubital fossa, the groin, and the wrists. They accompany the rash of scarlet fever as a response to the erythrogenic toxin produced by scarlatinal strains of group A streptococci.

Pel-Ebstein fever • A recurrent pattern characterized by several days of high fever alternating with afebrile periods that last for days or weeks. Typically, the fever becomes progressively higher and continuous. Pel-Ebstein fever occasionally occurs in Hodgkin's disease.

Perez's sign • Crackles auscultated over the lungs when a seated patient raises and lowers his arms. This sign commonly occurs in fibrous mediastinitis and may also occur in aortic arch aneurysm.

peroneal sign • Dorsiflexion and abduction of the foot upon tapping over the common peroneal nerve. To elicit this sign of latent tetany, tap over the lateral neck of the fibula with the patient's knee relaxed and slightly flexed.

phobia • An irrational and persistent fear of an object, situation, or activity. Occurring in phobic disorders, it may interfere with normal functioning. Typical manifestations include faintness, fatigue, palpitations, diaphoresis, nausea, tremor, and panic.

Piotrowski's sign • Dorsiflexion and supination of the foot on percussion of the anterior tibial muscle. Excessive flexion may indicate a central nervous system disorder.

Pitres' sign • In tabes dorsalis, hyperesthesia of the scrotum. This sign also refers to the anterior deviation of the sternum in pleural effusion.

Plummer's sign • Inability to ascend stairs or step up onto a chair. This sign can be demonstrated in Graves' disease.

pneumaturia • The passage of gas in the urine while voiding. Causes include a fistula between the bowel and bladder, sigmoid diverticulitis, rectosigmoid cancer, and gas-forming urinary tract infections.

Pool-Schlesinger sign • In tetany, muscle spasm of the forearm, hand, and fingers or of the leg and foot. To detect this sign, forcefully abduct and elevate the patient's arm with his forearm extended. Or forcefully flex the patient's extended leg at the hip. Spasm results from tension on the brachial plexus or the sciatic nerve.

Potain's sign • Dullness on percussion over the aortic arch, extending from the manubrium to the third costal cartilage on the right. This occurs in aortic dilatation.

Prehn's sign • Relief of pain with elevation and support of the scrotum, occurring in epididymitis. This sign differentiates epididymitis from testicular torsion. Both disorders produce severe pain, tenderness, and scrotal swelling.

pressured speech • Verbal expression that is accelerated, difficult to interrupt, and at times unintelligible. This may accompany flight of ideas in the manic phase of a bipolar disorder.

Prévost's sign • Conjugate deviation of the head and eyes in hemiplegia. Typically, the eyes gaze toward the affected hemisphere.

prognathism • An enlarged, protuberant jaw associated with normal mandible condyles and temporomandibular joints. This sign most commonly appears in acromegaly.

Q

Quinquaud's sign • Trembling of the fingers, in alcoholism. To detect this sign, have the patient spread his hand, flex his fingers at the metacarpophalangeal joints, and touch your palm with his fingers at a 90° angle to your hand.

R

rectal tenesmus • Spasmodic contraction of the anal sphincter with a persistent urge to defecate and involuntary, ineffective straining. This occurs in inflammatory bowel disorders, such as ulcerative colitis and Crohn's disease, and in rectal tumors. Often painful, rectal tenesmus usually accompanies passage of small amounts of blood, pus, or mucus.

regression • Return to a behavioral level appropriate to an earlier developmental age. This defense mechanism may occur in various psychiatric and organic disorders.

repression • The unconscious retreat from awareness of unacceptable ideas or impulses. This defense mechanism may occur normally or may accompany psychiatric disorders.

Rockley's sign • In a depressed fracture of the zygomatic arch, the difference in the angle created by two straight edges placed vertically against the orbits and zygomatic bones. To detect this sign, rest two rulers or other straight-edged objects on the outer edge of the ocular orbits and zygomatic arches. In a positive Rockley's sign, the angle on the affected side is smaller—the straight edge is more nearly parallel to the basic plane of the patient's face.

PROGNATHISM

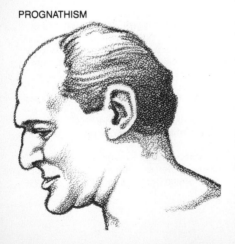

RUMPEL-LEEDE SIGN

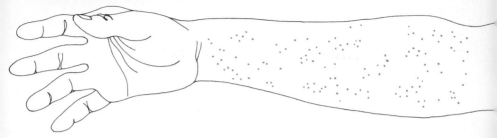

Rosenbach's sign • Absence of the abdominal skin reflex, associated with intestinal inflammation and hemiplegia. This sign also refers to the fine, rapid tremor of gently closed eyelids in Graves' disease.

Rotch's sign • Dullness on percussion over the right lung at the fifth intercostal space. This sign occurs in pericardial effusion.

Rovsing's sign • Pain in the right lower quadrant upon palpation and quick withdrawal of the fingers in the left lower quadrant. This referred rebound tenderness suggests appendicitis.

Rumpel-Leede sign • Extensive petechiae distal to a tourniquet placed around the upper arm, indicating capillary fragility in scarlet fever and in severe thrombocytopenia. To elicit this sign, place a tourniquet around the upper arm for 5 to 10 minutes and observe for distal petechiae.

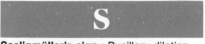

S

Seeligmüller's sign • Pupillary dilation on the affected side, in facial neuralgia.

Siegert's sign • Short, inwardly curved little fingers, typically appearing in Down's syndrome.

Signorelli's sign • Extreme tenderness on palpation of the area anterior to the mastoid; associated with meningitis.

Simon's sign • Incoordination of the

movements of the diaphragm and thorax, occurring early in meningitis.

Soto-Hall sign • Pain in the area of a lesion, occurring on passive flexion of the spine. To elicit this sign, place the patient supine and progressively flex his spine from the neck downward. The patient will complain of pain at the area of the lesion.

spasmodic torticollis • Intermittent or continuous spasms of the shoulder and neck muscles that turn the head to one side. Often transient and idiopathic, this sign can occur in extrapyramidal disorders. It can also occur in patients with shortened neck muscles. See "Dystonia," page 264.

SIEGERT'S SIGN

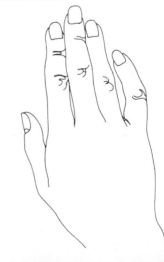

spine sign • Resistance to anterior flexion of the spine, resulting from pain in poliomyelitis.

spoon nails • Malformation of the nails characterized by a concave instead of the normal convex outer surface. This commonly occurs in severe hypochromic anemia but occasionally may be hereditary.

Stellwag's sign • Incomplete and infrequent blinking, usually related to exophthalmos in Graves' disease.

stepping reflex • In the neonate, spontaneous stepping movements that simulate walking. This reciprocal flexion and extension of the legs disappears after about age 4 weeks. To elicit this sign, hold the infant erect with the soles of his feet touching a hard surface. However, scissoring movements with persistent extension and crossing of the legs or asymmetrical stepping is abnormal, possibly indicating central nervous system damage.

Strunsky's sign • Pain on plantar flexion of the toes and forefoot, caused by inflammatory disorders of the anterior arch. To detect this sign, have the patient assume a relaxed position with his foot exposed, then grasp his toes and quickly plantar-flex his toes and forefoot.

STEPPING REFLEX

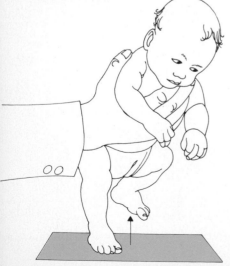

succussion splash • A splashing sound heard over a hollow organ or body cavity, such as the stomach or thorax, after rocking or shaking the patient's body. Indicating the presence of fluid or air and gas, this sound may be auscultated in pyloric or intestinal obstruction, a large hiatal hernia, or hydropneumothorax. However, it may also be auscultated over a normal, empty stomach.

sucking reflex • Involuntary circumoral sucking movements in response to stimulation. Present at about 26 weeks gestational age, this reflex is initially weak and not synchronized with swallowing. It persists through infancy, becoming more discriminating during the first few months and disappearing by age 1. To elicit this response, place your finger in the infant's mouth. Rhythmic sucking movements are normal. Weakness or absence of these movements may indicate elevated intracranial pressure.

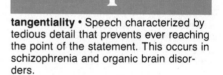

T

tangentiality • Speech characterized by tedious detail that prevents ever reaching the point of the statement. This occurs in schizophrenia and organic brain disorders.

Terry's nails • A white, opaque surface over more than 80% of the nail and a normal pink distal edge. This sign is often associated with cirrhosis.

testicular pain • Unilateral or bilateral pain localized in or around the testicle and possibly radiating along the spermatic cord and into the lower abdomen. It usually results from trauma, infection, or torsion. Typically, its onset is sudden and severe; however, its intensity can vary from sharp pain accompanied by nausea and vomiting to a chronic, dull ache. In a child, sudden onset of severe testicular pain is a urologic emergency. Assume torsion is the cause until disproven. If a young male complains of abdominal pain, always carefully examine the scrotum because abdominal pain often precedes testicular pain in testicular torsion.

Thornton's sign • Severe flank pain resulting from nephrolithiasis.

thrill • A palpable sensation resulting from the vibration of a loud murmur or from turbulent blood flow in an aneurysm. Thrills are associated with heart murmurs of grades IV to VI and may be palpable over major arteries. See "Bruits," page 136, and "Murmurs," page 484.

tibialis sign • Involuntary dorsiflexion and inversion of the foot upon brisk, voluntary flexion of the patient's knee and hip, occurring in spastic paralysis of the lower limb.

To detect this sign, place the patient supine and have him flex his leg at the hip and knee so that the thigh touches the abdomen. Or you can place the patient prone, and have him flex his leg at the knee so that the calf touches the thigh. If this sign is present, you may observe dorsiflexion of the great toe or of all toes as the foot dorsiflexes and inverts. Normally, plantar flexion of the foot occurs with this action.

Tinel's sign • Distal paresthesias on percussion over an injured nerve in an extremity, as in carpal tunnel syndrome. To elicit this sign in the patient's wrist, tap over the median nerve on the wrist's flexor surface. This sign indicates a partial lesion or the early regeneration of the nerve.

Tommasi's sign • Absence of hair on the posterolateral calf, occurring in males with gout.

tongue enlargement • An increase in the tongue's size, causing it to protrude from the mouth. Its causes include Down's syndrome, acromegaly, lymphangioma, Beckwith's syndrome, and congenital micrognathia. An enlarged tongue can also stem from cancer of the tongue, amyloidosis, and neurofibromatosis.

tongue fissures • Shallow or deep grooving of the dorsum of the tongue. Usually a congenital defect, tongue fissures occur normally in about 10% of the population. However, deep fissures may promote collection of food particles, leading to chronic inflammation and tenderness.

tongue—hairy • Hypertrophy and elongation of the tongue's filiform papillae. Normally white, the papillae may turn yel-

low, brown, or black from bacteria, food, tobacco, coffee, or dyes in drugs and food. Hairy tongue may also result from antibiotic therapy, irradiation of the head and neck, chronic debilitating disorders, and habitual use of mouthwashes containing oxidizing or astringent agents.

tongue—magenta cobblestone • Swelling and hyperemia of the tongue, forming rows of elevated fungiform and filiform papillae that give the tongue a magenta-colored, cobblestone appearance. It's most often a sign of vitamin B_2 (riboflavin) deficiency.

TONGUE FISSURES

HAIRY TONGUE

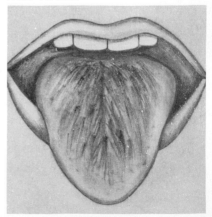

tongue—red • Patchy or uniform redness (ranging from pink to magenta) of the tongue, which may be swollen and smooth, rough, or fissured. It usually indicates glossitis, resulting from emotional stress or nutritional disorders, such as pernicious anemia, Plummer-Vinson syndrome, pellagra, sprue, and folic acid and vitamin B deficiency.

tongue—smooth • Absence or atrophy of the filiform papillae, causing a smooth (patchy or uniform), glossy, red tongue. This primary sign of undernutrition results from anemia and vitamin B deficiency.

tongue swelling • Edema of the tongue, most commonly associated with pernicious anemia, pellagra, hypothyroidism, and allergic angioneurotic edema.

tongue ulcers • Circumscribed necrotic lesions of the dorsum, margin, tip, and inferior surface of the tongue. Ulcers most commonly result from biting, chewing, or burning of the tongue. They may also stem from Type I herpes simplex virus, tuberculosis, histoplasmosis, and cancer of the tongue.

TONIC NECK REFLEX

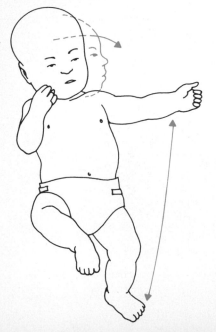

tongue—white • A uniform white coating or plaques on the tongue. Lesions associated with a white tongue may be premalignant or malignant and may require a biopsy. *Necrotic white lesions*—collections of cells, bacteria, and debris—are painful and can be scraped from the tongue. They often appear in children, commonly resulting from candidiasis and thermal burns. *Keratotic white lesions*—thickened, keratinized patches—are usually asymptomatic and can't be scraped from the tongue. These lesions commonly result from alcohol use and local irritation from tobacco smoke or other substances.

tonic neck reflex • Extension of the limbs on the side to which the head is turned and flexion of the opposite limbs. In the neonate, this normal reflex appears between 28 and 32 weeks gestational age, diminishes as voluntary muscle control increases, and disappears by 3 or 4 months of age. The absence or persistence of this reflex may indicate central nervous system damage. To elicit this response, place the infant supine, then turn his head to one side.

tooth discoloration • Bluish yellow or gray teeth may result from hypoplasia of the dentin and pulp, nerve damage, or caries. Yellow teeth may indicate caries. Mottling and staining suggest fluorine excess and may also be associated with the effects of certain drugs, such as tetracycline. Tooth discoloration (and small tooth size) may occur in osteogenesis imperfecta.

tophi • Deposits of sodium urate crystals in cartilage, soft tissue, synovial membranes, and tendon sheaths, producing painless nodular swellings, a classic symptom of gout. Tophi appear commonly on the ears, hands, and feet. They may erode the skin, producing open lesions, and cause gross deformity, limiting joint mobility. Inflammatory flare-ups may occur.

transference • Unconscious process of transferring feelings and attitudes originally associated with important figures, such as parents, to another. Used therapeutically in psychoanalysis, transference can also occur in other settings and relationships.

Trendelenburg's test • A demonstration of valvular incompetence of the saphenous vein and inefficiency of the communicating veins at different levels. To perform this test, raise the patient's legs above the heart level until the veins empty; then rapidly lower his legs. If the valves are incompetent, the veins immediately distend.

Troisier's sign • Enlargement of a single lymph node, usually in the left supraclavicular group. It indicates metastasis from a primary carcinoma in the upper abdomen, often the stomach. To detect this sign, have the patient sit erect facing you. Palpate the region behind the sternocleidomastoid muscle as the patient performs Valsalva's maneuver. Although the enlarged node often lies so deep that it escapes detection, it may rise and become palpable with this maneuver.

Trousseau's sign • In tetany, carpopedal spasm upon ischemic compression of the upper arm. To elicit this sign, apply a blood pressure cuff to the patient's arm; then inflate the cuff to a pressure between the patient's diastolic and systolic readings, maintaining it for 4 minutes. The patient's hand and fingers assume the "obstetrical hand" position, with wrist and metacarpophalangeal joints flexed, interphalangeal joints extended, and fingers and thumb adducted. See also "Carpopedal Spasm," page 147.

twitching • Nonspecific intermittent contraction of muscles or muscle bundles. See "Fasciculations," page 307, and "Tics," page 718.

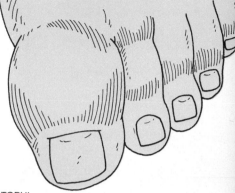

TOPHI

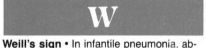

U

urinary tenesmus • Persistent, ineffective, painful straining to empty the bladder. This results from irritation of nerve endings in the bladder mucosa, caused by infection or an indwelling catheter.

V

vaginal bleeding abnormalities • Passage of blood from the vagina at times other than menses. It may indicate abnormalities of the uterus, cervix, ovaries, fallopian tubes, or vagina. It may also indicate an abnormal pregnancy. See also "Menorrhagia," page 475, "Metrorrhagia," page 476, and "Vaginal Bleeding—Postmenopausal," page 747.

vein sign • A palpable, bluish cordlike swelling along the line formed in the axilla by the junction of the thoracic and superficial epigastric veins. This sign appears in tuberculosis and obstruction of the superior vena cava.

W

Weill's sign • In infantile pneumonia, absence of expansion in the subclavicular area of the affected side on inspiration.

Westphal's sign • Absence of the knee jerk reflex, occurring in tabes dorsalis.

Wilder's sign • Subtle twitching of the eyeball on medial or lateral gaze. This early sign of Graves' disease is discernible as a slight jerk of the eyeball when the patient changes the direction of his gaze.

Y

yawning—excessive • Persistent involuntary opening of the mouth, accompanied by attempted deep inspiration. In the absence of sleepiness, excessive yawning may indicate cerebral hypoxia.

References and Acknowledgments

References

Adams, Raymond, and Victor, Maurice. *Principles of Neurology,* 2nd ed. New York: McGraw-Hill Book Co., 1981.

American Hospital Formulary Service: Drug Information '85. Bethesda, Md.: American Society of Hospital Pharmacists.

Assessment. Nurse's Reference Library. Springhouse, Pa.: Springhouse Corp., 1982.

Avery, Mary E., and Taeusch, H. William, Jr. *Shaffer's Diseases of the Newborn,* 5th ed. Philadelphia: W.B. Saunders Co., 1984.

Bates, Barbara. *A Guide to Physical Examination,* 3rd ed. Philadelphia: J.B. Lippincott Co., 1983.

Baum, Gerald L., ed. *Textbook of Pulmonary Diseases,* 3rd ed. Boston: Little, Brown & Co., 1983.

Behrman, Richard E., and Vaughan, Victor C., III. *Nelson Textbook of Pediatrics,* 12th ed. Philadelphia: W.B. Saunders Co., 1983.

Blacklow, Robert S., ed. *MacBryde's Signs and Symptoms: Applied Pathologic Physiology and Clinical Interpretation,* 6th ed. Philadelphia: J.B. Lippincott Co., 1983.

Braunwald, Eugene, ed. *Heart Disease: A Textbook of Cardiovascular Medicine,* 2 vols. Philadelphia: W.B. Saunders Co., 1984.

Bricker, Neal S., and Kirschenbaum, Michael A. *The Kidney: Diagnosis and Management.* New York: John Wiley & Sons, 1984.

Brunner, Lillian, and Suddarth, Doris. *Textbook of Medical-Surgical Nursing,* 5th ed. Philadelphia: J.B. Lippincott Co., 1984.

Bullock, Barbara, et al., eds. *Pathophysiology: Adaptations and Alterations in Function.* Boston: Little, Brown & Co., 1984.

Cardiovascular Disorders. Nurse's Clinical Library. Springhouse, Pa.: Springhouse Corp., 1984.

Cavenar, Jesse O., Jr., and Brodie, Keith H., eds. *Signs and Symptoms in Psychiatry.* Philadelphia: J.B. Lippincott Co., 1983.

Danforth, David N., ed. *Obstetrics and Gynecology,* 4th ed. Philadelphia: J.B. Lippincott Co., 1982.

Diseases, 2nd ed. Nurse's Reference Library. Springhouse, Pa.: Springhouse Corp., 1986.

Duane, Thomas D., and Jaeger, Edward A., eds. *Clinical Ophthalmology.* Philadelphia: Harper & Row Publishers, 1983.

Endocrine Disorders. Nurse's Clinical Library. Springhouse, Pa.: Springhouse Corp., 1984.

Glauser, Frederick L., ed. *Signs and Symptoms in Pulmonary Medicine.* Philadelphia: J.B. Lippincott Co., 1983.

Grant, A., and Skyring, A., eds. *Clinical Diagnosis of Gastrointestinal Disease.* Boston: Blackwell Scientific Publications, 1981.

Greenspan, Francis, S., and Forsham, Peter H., eds. *Basic and Clinical Endocrinology.* Los Altos, Calif.: Lange Medical Pubns., 1983.

Herten, R.J. "Nonscarring Hair Loss Disorders: The Basis for Recognition and Treatment," *Postgraduate Medicine* 72(4):231-36, 243-46, October 1982.

Hickey, Joanne V.X. *The Clinical Practice of Neurological and Neurosurgical Nursing.* Philadelphia: J.B. Lippincott Co., 1981.

Horwitz, L., and Groves, B. *Signs and Symptoms in Cardiology.* Philadelphia: J.B. Lippincott Co., 1985.

Hurst, J.W., et al. *The Heart,* 5th ed. New York: McGraw-Hill Book Co., 1982.

Jacobs, Margaret, and Geels, Wilma. *Signs and Symptoms in Nursing Interpretation and Management.* Philadelphia: J.B. Lippincott Co., 1985.

Kempe, C. Henry, et al., eds. *Current Pediatric Diagnosis and Treatment,* 8th ed. Los Altos, Calif.: Lange Medical Pubns., 1984.

Krause, Marie V., and Mahan, Kathleen. *Food, Nutrition and Diet Therapy: A Textbook of Nutritional Care,* 7th ed. Philadelphia: W.B. Saunders Co., 1984.

Krupp, Marcus A., et al., eds. *Current Medical Diagnosis and Treatment.* Los Altos, Calif.: Lange Medical Pubns., 1985.

Leitman, Mark, et al. *Manual for Eye Examination and Diagnosis.* Oradell, N.J.: Medical Economics Books, 1983.

Lerner, Judith, and Khan, Zafar. *Mosby's Manual of Urologic Nursing.* St. Louis: C.V. Mosby Co., 1982.

Loustau, A., and Lee, K. "Dealing With the Dangers of Dysphagia," *Nursing85* 15(2):47-50, February 1985.

Lucente, Frank E., and Sobol, Stephen M. *Essentials of Otolaryngology.* New York: Raven Press Pubs., 1983.

Luckmann, Joan, and Sorensen, Karen. *Medical-Surgical Nursing: A Psychophysiologic Approach,* 2nd ed. Philadelphia: W.B. Saunders Co., 1980.

Malasanos, Lois, et al. *Health Assessment,* 2nd ed. St. Louis: C.V. Mosby Co., 1981.

Metz, Robert, and Larson, Eric B. *Blue Book of Endocrinology.* Philadelphia: W.B. Saunders Co., 1984.

Moschella, Samuel L., and Hurley, Harry J. *Dermatology,* 2nd ed. Philadelphia: W.B. Saunders Co., 1985.

Moser, Kenneth M., and Spragg, Roger G. *Respiratory Emergencies,* 2nd ed. St. Louis: C.V. Mosby Co., 1982.

Norman, S. "The Pupil Check," *American Journal of Nursing* 82(4):588-91, April 1982.

Nursing86 Drug Handbook. Springhouse, Pa.: Springhouse Corp., 1986.

Peckham, Ben M., and Shapiro, Sander S. *Signs and Symptoms in Gynecology.* Philadelphia: J.B. Lippincott Co., 1983.

Petersdorf, Robert G., and Adams, Raymond D., eds. *Harrison's Principles of Internal Medicine,* 10th ed. New York: McGraw-Hill Book Co., 1983.

Phipps, Wilma J., et al. *Medical-Surgical Nursing: Concepts and Clinical Practice,* 2nd ed. St. Louis: C.V. Mosby Co., 1983.

Respiratory Disorders. Nurse's Clinical Library. Springhouse, Pa.: Springhouse Corp., 1984.

Rudy, Ellen B. *Advanced Neurological and Neurosurgical Nursing.* St. Louis: C.V. Mosby Co., 1984.

Shafer, William G., et al. *Textbook of Oral Pathology,* 4th ed. Philadelphia: W.B. Saunders Co., 1983.

Sleisenger, Marvin H., and Fordtran, John S. *Gastrointestinal Disease: Pathophysiology, Diagnosis, Management,* 3rd ed. Philadelphia: W.B. Saunders Co., 1983.

Smith, Donald R. *General Urology,* 11th ed. Los Altos, Calif.: Lange Medical Pubns., 1984.

Spiro, Howard M. *Clinical Gastroenterology,* 3rd ed. New York: Macmillan Publishing Co., 1983.

Spodick, D.H. "Answers to Questions on Acute Pericarditis and Pericardial Effusion," *Hospital Medicine* 19(4):219, 223-26, 228, April 1983.

Suitor, Carol J., and Crowley, Merrily F. *Nutrition: Principles and Application in Health Promotion,* 2nd ed. Philadelphia: J.B. Lippincott Co., 1984.

Swanson, Phillip D. *Signs and Symptoms in Neurology.* Philadelphia: J.B. Lippincott Co., 1984.

Thomas, D.O., "Are You Sure It's Only Croup?" *RN* 47(12):40-43, December 1984.

Vararinsh, P. *Clinical Dermatology: Diagnosis and Therapy of Common Skin Diseases.* Woburn, Mass.: Butterworth Pubs., 1982.

Vaughan, Daniel, and Asbury, Taylor. *General Ophthalmology,* 10th ed. Los Altos, Calif.: Lange Medical Pubns., 1983.

Whaley, Lucille F., and Wong, Donna L. *Nursing Care of Infants and Children,* 2nd ed. St. Louis: C.V. Mosby Co., 1983.

Wilson, William B., and Nadol, Joseph B., Jr. *Quick Reference to Ear, Nose and Throat Disorders.* Philadelphia: J.B. Lippincott Co., 1982.

Wyngaarden, James B., and Smith, Lloyd H. *Cecil Textbook of Medicine,* 16th ed. Philadelphia: W.B. Saunders Co., 1982.

Acknowledgments

p. 437: Illustration adapted from an original drawing by David E. Cook.

pp. 462-63: Scale adapted from M.H. Klaus and A.A. Fanaroff, *Care of the High Risk Neonate,* 2nd ed. (Philadelphia: W.B. Saunders Co., 1979, p. 79). Used with permission of the publisher and Dr. J.L. Ballard.

p. 731: Photo courtesy of H. Armstrong Roberts, Inc.

Index

A

Aaron's sign, 786
Abadie's sign, 786
Abasia, 333
Abdominal aortic aneurysm,
   abdominal mass in, 8
Abdominal aortic
   atherosclerosis, bruits in,
   138
Abdominal cancer
   abdominal distention in, 3
   abdominal pain in, 14
Abdominal distention, **1-7**
   associated findings, 4-5t
   causes, 3, 4-5t, 6-7
   hiccups in, 405
Abdominal guarding. *See*
   Abdominal rigidity.
Abdominal mass, **8-12**
   causes, 8-9, 10i, 11
   locations, 10i
Abdominal muscle spasm.
   See Abdominal rigidity.
Abdominal pain, **12-22**. *See*
   also Psoas sign.
   associated findings, 16-19t
   causes, 13-15, 16-19t, 20-
   22
   types and locations, 12, 13t
Abdominal rigidity, **22-24**
   causes, 23-24
   voluntary vs. involuntary, 23
   in child, 24
Absence seizure. *See*
   Seizure—absence.
Accessory muscles, 25i
   use of, **24-28**
Acetone breath. *See* Breath
   with fruity odor.
Achalasia
   drooling in, 241
   dysphagia in, 255
   hematemesis in, 381
Achilles tendon reflex,
   innervation of, 219i
Acne vulgaris
   papular rash in, 558
   pustular rash in, 633
Acoustic neuroma
   absent corneal reflex in,
   184
   drooling in, 241
   hearing loss in, 375
   tinnitus in, 719
   vertigo in, 752
Acquired immunodeficiency
   syndrome, 226

Acrocyanosis, 680. *See also*
   Cyanosis.
Acromegaly
   diaphoresis in, 226
   excessive weight gain in,
   773
   hirsutism in, 407
   hyperpigmentation in, 414
Actinomycosis, productive
   cough in, 194
Acute adrenal insufficiency
   blood pressure decrease in,
   99
   mouth lesions in, 482
Acute closed-angle glaucoma,
   eye pain in, 301
Acute tubular necrosis
   anuria in, 56
   oliguria in, 534-535
   polyuria in, 585
Adenofibroma, 120
Adenoid hypertrophy, 375
Adenomyosis, 247
Adie's syndrome
   nonreactive pupils in, 623
   sluggish pupils in, 625
Adipsia, 786
Adrenal carcinoma
   gynecomastia in, 362
   hirsutism in, 407
Adrenal crisis
   abdominal pain in, 14
   decreased level of
   consciousness in, 452
Adrenal hyperplasia
   bronze skin in, 677
   oligomenorrhea in, 533
Adrenal insufficiency
   amenorrhea in, 37
   anorexia in, 50
   bronze skin in, 677
   excessive weight loss in,
   777
   fatigue in, 309
   hyperpigmentation in, 414
   nausea in, 509
   orthostatic hypotension in,
   543
   salt craving in, 656
   tachycardia in, 699
   vomiting in, 766
Adrenal tumor, amenorrhea
   in, 37
Adrenergics, 57
Adrenocortical hypofunction.
   See Adrenal insufficiency.

Adult respiratory distress
   syndrome
   accessory muscle use in,
   26
   anxiety in, 58
   crackles in, 201
   dyspnea in, 260
   nasal flaring in, 507
   rhonchi in, 649
   tachycardia in, 699
   tachypnea in, 704
Aerophagia, 1, 290
   cause, 324
   prevention, 291
   signs, 323
Affective disorders
   anxiety in, 58
   insomnia in, 426
Ageusia, 52, 708
Agitation, **28-30**
   causes, 29-30
Agnogenic myeloid
   metaplasia, jaundice in,
   434-435
Agnosia, 786
Agranulocytosis
   gum bleeding in, 356
   throat pain in, 714
Agraphia, 786
Airway obstruction
   accessory muscle use in,
   26
   apnea in, 64
   cough in, 189
   dysphagia in, 255
   nasal flaring in, 507
   stertorous respirations in,
   691
Albright's syndrome, 145
Alcoholic cerebellar
   degeneration, dysarthria
   in, 245
Alcoholism
   anorexia in, 50
   bounding pulse in, 606
   ptosis in, 600
Alcohol withdrawal syndrome
   agitation in, 29
   generalized tonic-clonic
   seizure in, 666
   insomnia in, 426
   tachypnea in, 704
   tremors in, 726
Aldosteronism, blood pressure
   increase in, 105
Alkalosis, tremors in, 726
Allen cards, 764
Allergic reaction
   erythema in, 292
   facial edema in, 279

Bronchitis—cont'd.
  hemoptysis in, 399
  nonproductive cough in,
    189
  productive cough in, 195
  rhonchi in, 649
  shallow respirations in, 675
  tachypnea in, 705
  throat pain in, 716
  wheezing in, 781
Bronchogenic carcinoma
  nonproductive cough in,
    189
  wheezing in, 781
Bronchoscopy, 650, 696
Bronze skin. See
    Hyperpigmentation and
    Skin—bronze.
Brown-Séquard syndrome,
    pathophysiology of, 565i
Brucellosis
  lymphadenopathy in, 464
  splenomegaly in, 687-688
Brudzinski's sign, **134-136**
  causes, 136
  test for, 135i
Bruits, **136-139**
  auscultation of, 137i
  causes, 138-139
  false, prevention of, 137i
Buerger's disease
  cyanosis in, 210
  intermittent claudication in,
    430
  mottled skin in, 681
  paresthesias in, 567
  prolonged capillary refill
    time in, 146
Buffalo hump, **139-141**
  causes, 141
  in hypercortisolism, 140i
Bulbar palsy
  fasciculations in, 308
  gag reflex abnormalities in,
    332
Bulimia, 584
Bulging fontanelle. See
    Fontanelle bulging.
Bulla, 558i
Burns
  alopecia in, 32
  anhidrosis in, 48
  edema in, 276, 278, 282
  erythema in, 292
  eye pain in, 301
  hypopigmentation in, 420-
    421
  muscle atrophy in, 490
  photophobia in, 575
  vesicular rash in, 754
Busulfan, 39
Butterfly rash, **141-143**, 142i
  associated findings, 143t
  causes, 141-143, 143t

C

Cacogeusia, 708
Café-au-lait spots, **145-146**
  causes, 145-146
Calcium channel blockers,
    102
Calculi. See also Bladder
    calculi and Renal calculi.
  costovertebral angle
    tenderness in, 185-186
  flank pain in, 322
  hematuria in, 388
  oliguria in, 535
Caloric response, See
    Bárány's symptom.
Calorie reserves
  assessment of, 774-775i
Cancer. See also specific
    types of cancer.
  anorexia in, 50
  excessive weight loss in,
    777
  fatigue in, 310
Candida albicans infection,
    breast ulcer in, 129
Candidiasis
  erythema in, 292
  genital lesions in male with,
    348
  mouth lesions in, 482
  vaginal discharge in, 749
Cantelli's sign. See Doll's eye
    sign—absent.
Capillary refill time—
    prolonged, **146-147**
  causes, 146-147
Carbamazepine, 35
Carbon monoxide poisoning
  chorea in, 168
  masklike facies in, 469
  propulsive gait in, 334
Carcinoid syndrome, diarrhea
    in, 231
Carcinoma, jaundice in, 435
Cardarelli's sign. See Tracheal
    tugging.
Cardiac contusion
  blood pressure decrease in,
    101
  tachycardia in, 701
Cardiac tamponade
  absent or weak pulse in,
    601
  blood pressure decrease in,
    101
  jugular vein distention in,
    443
  narrowed pulse pressure in,
    608
  prolonged capillary refill
    time in, 146-147
  pulsus paradoxus in, 621
  tachycardia in, 701
  tachypnea in, 705
Cardinal fields of gaze, 235i

Cardiogenic shock
  anxiety in, 58
  blood pressure decrease in,
    101
  clammy skin in, 678
  narrowed pulse pressure in,
    609
  tachycardia in, 701
  tachypnea in, 705
Cardiomyopathy
  atrial gallop in, 343
  bradycardia in, 114
  chest pain in, 157
  murmur in, 486
  pulsus bisferiens in, 620
  ventricular gallop in, 347
Carotid artery aneurysm
  hemianopia in, 396
  mydriasis in, 503
Carotid artery stenosis, bruits
    in, 138
Carotid sinus hypersensitivity
  dizziness in, 237
  syncope in, 697
Carpopedal spasm, **147-149**,
    148i
  causes 148-149
Carvallo's sign, 487
Castellino's sign. See Tracheal
    tugging.
Cataract
  halo vision in, 368
  night blindness in, 517
  vision loss in, 758
  visual blurring in, 762
Catatonia, 790
Cat cry, **149**
  cause, 149
Catheterization, bladder
    distention in, 98
Causalgia, 439
Cavernous sinus thrombosis
  diplopia in, 234
  edema of the face in, 279
  exophthalmos in, 296
  ocular deviation in, 530
Celiac disease, hematochezia
    in, 385
Cellulitis, 70
Central cord syndrome
  analgesia in, 43
  pathophysiology of, 565i
Central nervous system
    depressants, 65
Central nervous system
    stimulants, 60, 107
Cerebellar abscess, ataxia in,
    75
Cerebellar disease, 239, 493,
    726
Cerebral aneurysm
  decreased level of
    consciousness in, 453
  generalized tonic-clonic
    seizure in, 668

Esophageal spasm
  chest pain in, 157
  dysphagia in, 256
Esophageal trauma, 513
Esophageal tubes, 383i
Esophageal varices
  hematemesis in, 382
  hematochezia in, 386
  melena in, 473
Esophagitis
  cough in, 191
  dysphagia in, 256
  weight loss in, 777
Estrogens, 363, 748, 750
Ethmoiditis, rhinorrhea in, 647
Euphoria, 794
Eustachian tube patency,
  tinnitus in, 720
Ewald tube, 382i
Ewart's sign, 794
Excessive eating. See
  Polyphagia.
Exfoliative dermatitis, alopecia
  in, 32
Exhaustion. See Fatigue.
Exophthalmometer, 248i
Exophthalmos, **295-297**
  causes, 296-297
  unilateral, assessment for,
    296i
Expectoration of blood. See
  Hemoptysis.
Expiration
  accessory muscle use in,
    25i
  asymmetrical chest
    expansion and, 151i
Expressive aphasia, 62t
Extension, abnormal. See
  Decerebrate posture.
Extensor plantor reflex. See
  Babinski's reflex.
Extensor reflex, abnormal.
  See Decerebrate posture.
Extensor thrust reflex, 794-
  795
Extinction, 795
Extraocular movements, test
  of, 235i
Extrapyramidal signs and
  symptoms, 795
Eye
  examination of, 301i
  redness. See Conjunctival
    injection.
Eyeache. See Eye pain.
Eyeballs
  involuntary oscillations of.
    See Nystagmus.
  protrusion of. See
    Exophthalmos.
Eye discharge, **298-300**
  causes, 298-300
  sources, 299i

Eyelid, drooping. See Ptosis.
Eye movement, abnormal.
  See Ocular deviation.
Eye pain, **300-303**
  causes, 301-301
Eye tumor, 763

F

Fabere sign, 795
Facial adiposity. See Moon
  face.
Facial burns, 280
Facial edema. See Edema of
  the face.
Facial expression, loss of.
  See Masklike facies.
Facial nerve, pathways of,
  306i
Facial pain, **305-307**
  causes, 305-307
Facial tic. See Orofacial
  dyskinesia and Tics.
Facial trauma, 280
Faint. See Syncope.
Fajersztajn's crossed sciatic
  sign, 795
Familial spastic paralysis,
  Babinski's reflex in, 84
Family violence, 757
Fan sign, 795
Fasciculations, **307-309**
  causes, 308-309
Fatigue, **309-312**
  causes, 309-311
Fat necrosis
  breast dimpling in, 119
  breast nodule in, 124
  breast pain in, 126
  nipple retraction in, 521
Fat reserves, assessment of,
  774-775i
Febrile disorders
  bounding pulse in, 606
  pulse pressure changes in,
    610
  tachycardia in, 701
  tachypnea in, 705
Fecal breath odor. See Breath
  with fecal odor.
Fecal incontinence, **312-315**
  bowel retraining in, 314
  causes, 312, 314
Felty's syndrome, 689
Festinating gait. See Gait—
  propulsive.
Festination, 333
Fetor hepaticus, **315-316**
  cause, 315
Fever, **316-319**
  causes, 316-317
  chills and, 164i
  pathogenesis, 318-319
Finger(s)
  clubbed. See Clubbing.

Finger(s)—cont'd.
  joints, bony enlargement of.
    See Heberden's nodes.
Fixed pupils. See Pupils—
  nonreactive.
Flaccid muscles. See Muscle
  flaccidity.
Flail chest
  asymmetrical chest
    expansion in, 152
  dyspnea in, 261
  shallow respirations in, 675
  tachypnea in, 705
Flank pain, **319-323**
  associated findings, 320-
    321t
  causes, 320-321t, 322-323
Flapping tremor. See
  Asterixis.
Flatulence, **323-325**
  causes, 324-325
  diet to reduce, 324
Flexor withdrawal reflex, 795
Flight of idea, 795
Floaters. See Light flashes
  and Visual floaters.
Fluid balance, regulation of,
  275i
Fluorouracil, 35
Focal seizure. See Seizure—
  focal.
Follicular mucinosis, 559
Folliculitis
  decalvans, alopecia in, 32
  genital lesions in male with,
    349
  pustular rash in, 633
Fontanelle bulging, **325-326**
  cause, 326
Fontanelle depression, **326-
  327**
  cause, 327
Fontanelles, location of, 326i
Food poisoning
  hematochezia in, 386
  vomiting in, 766
Footdrop, **327-329**
  associated findings, 329t
  causes, 328-329, 329t
  steppage gait and, 338
Foot eversion. See Foot
  malposition—congenital.
Foot inversion. See Foot
  malposition—congenital.
Foot malposition—congenital,
  795
Foot pain, causes of, 450.
  See also Leg pain.
Formication sign. See Tinel's
  sign.
Forschheimer's spots, 295
Fox-Fordyce disease, 560
Fractures
  arm pain in, 71-72

Boldface page numbers indicate major entries; i refers to an illustration, t to a table.

Ovarian tumor
dyspareunia in, 250
hirsutism in, 409
postmenopausal vaginal
bleeding in, 748

P

Pain
abdominal, **12-22.** *See also*
Psoas sign.
absense of sensitivity to.
See Analgesia.
arm, **69-72**
back, **86-91**
breast, **125-128**
chest, **153-162**
eye, **300-303**
facial, **305-307**
flank, **319-323**
insomnia and, 427t
jaw, **438-441**
leg, **449-451**
limb. *See* Intermittent
claudication.
neck, **512-517**
rectal, **642-643**
throat, **714-718**
Pallor, **553-555**
causes, 554-555
pathophysiology, 554i
Palmar crease abnormalities,
803
Palpitations, **555-557**
causes, 556-557
Pancreatic abscess,
abdominal mass in, 11
Pancreatic cancer
clay-colored stool in, 693
hepatomegaly in, 404
splenomegaly in, 690
Pancreatic pseudocysts,
abdominal mass in, 11
Pancreatitis
abdominal pain in, 20
back pain in, 88
chest pain in, 160
clay-colored stool in, 692
dyspepsia in, 254
flank pain in, 322
hiccups in, 405
jaundice in, 436
nausea in, 511
vomiting in, 768
Papillary muscle rupture,
murmur in, 487
Papillary necrosis
anuria in, 56
flank pain in, 322
Papular rash, **557-562**
causes, 558-562

Papule, 559i
Paradoxical pulse. *See* Pulsus
paradoxus.
Paradoxical respirations, 803
Paralysis, **562-566**
causes, 563-566
Paralytic ileus
abdominal distention in, 6-7
absent bowel sounds in,
109
hypoactive bowel sounds in,
113
Paralytic poliomyelitis,
drooling in, 242
Paranasal sinus pain. *See*
Facial pain.
Paranoia, 803
Paraplegia, 562
Parapsoriasis
papular rash in, 561
scaly skin in, 683
Parasympatholytics, bladder
distention in, 98
Paresis, 562
Paresthesias, **567-569**
causes, 567-569
Parietal lobe lesion,
hemianopia in, 396
Parkinson's disease
cogwheel rigidity in, 172
drooling in, 242
dysarthria in, 246
dysphagia in, 258
dystonia in, 265
masklike facies in, 469
muscle atrophy in, 491
muscle weakness in, 499
paralysis in, 564
propulsive gait in, 334
shallow respirations in, 675
tremors in, 727
Parotitis, jaw pain in, 440
Paroxysmal atrial tachycardia,
612-613i
Paroxysmal nocturnal
dyspnea, **570**
causes, 570
Parry-Romberg syndrome
enophthalmos in, 284
miosis in, 479
ptosis in, 601
Pastia's sign, 803
Patellar reflexes, 219i
Patent ductus arteriosus,
murmur in, 489t
Patient-teaching aid
antiflatulence diet, 324
bedwetting, preventive
measures for, 285
bleeding gums, prevention
of, 358
breast self-examination,
122-123i
circulation in legs, exercises
to improve, 431i
Credé's maneuver, 738i

Patient-teaching aid—*cont'd.*
itching, preventive and relief
measures for, 593
Kegel exercises, 250
low back pain, chronic,
exercises for, 89i
orthostatic hypotension,
preambulation
exercises to minimize
effects of, 544i
stress incontinence,
exercises to minimize,
742
testicular self-examination,
660i
urinary tract infections,
prevention of, 267
Peau d'orange, **570-571,** 571i
causes, 571
Pediatric vital signs, 706-707t
Pediculosis
genital lesions in male with,
351
pruritus in, 593
vulvar lesions in, 771
Pel-Ebstein fever, 803
Pellagra, ataxia in, 77
Pelvic inflammatory disease
abdominal pain in, 20
amenorrhea in, 38
chills in, 166
dysmenorrhea in, 248
dyspareunia in, 250
Pemphigus
eye discharge in, 300
eye pain in, 303
mouth lesions in, 483
vesicular rash in, 755
Penicillin, 294, 317, 684
Penile cancer, 350i
genital lesions in male with,
351
priapism in, 590
Penile discharge. *See*
Urethral discharge.
Penile trauma, 590
Peptic ulcer
chest pain in, 160
eructation in, 291
hematemesis in, 383
hematochezia in, 386
melena in, 474
nausea in, 511
pyrosis in, 635
vomiting in, 768
Percussion, of liver, 403i
Perez's sign, 803
Perforated ulcer
abdominal pain in, 20
back pain in, 88-89
Periarteritis nodosa, mottled
skin in, 681

Boldface page numbers indicate major entries; i refers to an illustration, t to a table.

838

S

S$_1$, interpretation of, 344-345t
S$_2$, interpretation of, 344-345t
S$_3$. See Gallop—ventricular.
S$_4$. See Gallop—atrial.
Sacroiliac strain, back pain in, 90
Salem-Sump tube, 382i
Salicylates, 22
Salivary duct obstruction, 653
Salivary glands, assessment of, 654i
Salivation—decreased, **653-654**
  causes, 653-654
Salivation, excessive. See Drooling.
Salivation—increased, **654-655**
  causes, 655
Salt craving, **656-657**
  cause, 656
Sarcoidosis
  alopecia in, 34
  cough in, 192
  crackles in, 204
  epistaxis in, 288
  lymphadenopathy in, 465
  rash in, 561
  seizures in, 664, 669
  splenomegaly in, 690
Scabies
  genital lesions in, 351
  pruritus in, 594
  rash in, 634, 756
Scaly skin. See Skin—scaly.
Schistosomiasis, 395
Schlesinger's sign. See Pool-Schlesinger sign.
Sciatica, 450
Scissors gait. See Gait—scissors.
Scleritis
  conjunctival injection in, 179
  exophthalmos in, 297
  eye pain in, 303
  photophobia in, 577
Scleroderma, 415, 469-470, 636
Sclerokeratitis, 303, 577
Scleroma, 288, 648
Scotoma, **657-658**
  causes, 657-658
  classification, 658i
Scrotal trauma, 661
Scrotal swelling, **659-661**
  causes, 659, 661
Scurvy, 288
Seizure—absence, **661-662**
  cause, 662
Seizure—focal, **662-665**
  body functions affected by, 664i
  causes, 663-664

Seizure—generalized tonic-clonic, **665-670**
  causes, 666-669
  phases of, 668i
Seizure—psychomotor, **670-671**
  causes, 670-671
Seizure, unilateral. See Seizure—focal.
Seizure disorders
  confusion in, 176
  decreased level of consciousness in, 456
  muscle changes in, 493, 502
  paralysis in, 565
  paresthesias in, 569
  trismus in, 729
Self-examination
  of breast, 122-123i
  of testicles, 660i
Sengstaken-Blakemore tube, 383i
Sentinel node. See Troisier's sign.
Sepsis
  dyspnea in, 264
  hyperpnea in, 420
  oliguria in, 538
Septicemia, 631
Septic shock
  blood pressure decrease in, 102
  chills in, 166
  clammy skin in, 679-680
  edema in, 276
  pulse pressure changes in, 609
  tachycardia in, 702-703
Sertoli-Leydig cell tumor, 39
Setting-sun sign, **671-672**, 672i
  cause, 672
Shallow respirations, **672-677**
  causes, 673-676
Sheehan's syndrome
  oligomenorrhea in, 533
  polydipsia in, 583
  polyuria in, 587
  weight gain in, 776
Shifting dullness. See Abdominal distention.
Shock
  cyanosis in, 211
  decreased level of consciousness in, 456
  dyspnea in, 264
  hyperpnea in, 420
  pallor in, 555
  pulse changes in, 603, 608-609
Shortness of breath. See Dyspnea.
Shoulder pain, causes of, 70. See also Arm pain.

Sibilant rhonchi. See Wheezing.
Sickle cell anemia
  hematuria in, 395
  jaundice in, 436, 438
  polydipsia in, 583
  polyuria in, 587
  priapism in, 590-591
Sickle cell crisis
  abdominal pain in, 21
  chest pain in, 161
Siegert's sign, 805
Signorelli's sign, 805
Silent abdomen. See Bowel sounds—absent.
Silicosis
  cough in, 198
  crackles in, 204
  hemoptysis in, 401
Simon's sign, 805
Simple partial seizure. See Seizure—focal.
Singultus. See Hiccups.
Sinus arrhythmia, 612-613i
Sinus carcinoma, 306
Sinus discharge. See Postnasal drip.
Sinuses, palpation of, 589i
Sinusitis
  anosmia in, 54-55
  chills in, 167
  cough in, 192
  epistaxis in, 288-289
  facial pain in, 306-307
  halitosis, 367
  headache in, 371-372
  postnasal drip in, 589
  rhinorrhea in, 648
  sore throat in, 717
Sjögren's syndrome
  decreased salivation in, 653
  hoarseness in, 410
  lymphadenopathy in, 465
  taste abnormalities in, 711
Skin—bronze, **677-678.** See also Hyperpigmentation.
  causes, 677-678
Skin—clammy, **678-680**
  causes, 678-680
Skin—mottled, **680-682**
  causes, 680-682
Skin—scaly, **682-684**
  causes, 682-684
Skin, moist. See Diaphoresis and Skin—clammy.
Skin color
  decreased. See Hypopigmentation.
  excessive. See Hyperpigmentation.
  loss of. See Pallor.
Skinfold thickness measurement, 774-775i
Skin inflammation. See Erythema.

Boldface page numbers indicate major entries; i refers to an illustration, t to a table.